MOVEMENT DISORDERS 4

MOVEMENT DISORDERS 4

Edited by

ANTHONY H. V. SCHAPIRA, DSc, MD, FRCP, FMedSci

Professor of Neurology and Chair
University Department of Clinical Neurosciences
Institute of Neurology
University College London
London, United Kingdom

ANTHONY E. T. LANG, MD, FRCPC

Professor, Department of Medicine
Director, Division of Neurology
Jack Clark Chair for Parkinson's Disease Research
University of Toronto
Director, Morton and Gloria Shulman Movement Disorders Centre
Toronto Western Hospital
Toronto, Ontario, Canada

STANLEY FAHN, MD

Movement Disorder Division Chief
H. Houston Merritt Professor of Neurology
The Neurological Institute
Columbia University
New York, New York

SAUNDERS

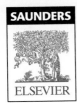

ELSEVIER

SAUNDERS
ELSEVIER

1600 John F. Kennedy Blvd.
Ste 1800
Philadelphia, PA 19103-2899

MOVEMENT DISORDERS 4   ISBN: 978-1-4160-6641-5
Copyright © 2010 by Saunders, an imprint of Elsevier Inc.

Notice

Knowledge and best practice in this field are constantly changing. As new research and experience broaden our knowledge, changes in practice, treatment, and drug therapy may become necessary or appropriate. Readers are advised to check the most current information provided (i) on procedures featured or (ii) by the manufacturer of each product to be administered to verify the recommended dose or formula, the method and duration of administration, and contraindications. It is the responsibility of the practitioners, relying on their own experience and knowledge of the patient, to make diagnoses, to determine dosages and the best treatment for each individual patient, and to take all appropriate safety precautions. To the fullest extent of the law, neither the Publisher nor the Editors assume any liability for any injury and/or damage to persons or property arising out of or related to any use of the material contained in this book.

The Publisher

Library of Congress Cataloging-in-Publication Data
Movement disorders 4 / [edited by] Stanley Fahn, Anthony E. T. Lang, Anthony H. V. Schapira.—1st ed.
    p. cm.—(Blue books of neurology series; 34)
  ISBN 978-1-4160-6641-5
1. Movement disorders. I. Fahn, Stanley. II. Lang, Anthony E. III. Schapira, Anthony H. V.
  (Anthony Henry Vernon) IV. Title: Movement disorders four. V. Series: Blue books of
  neurology; 34.
  [DNLM: 1. Movement Disorders. W1 BU9749 v.34 2009 / WL 390 M935723 2009]
  RC376.5.M684 2009
  616.8'3—dc22
  2009005736

Acquisitions Editor: Adrianne Brigido
Developmental Editor: Joan Ryan
Publishing Services Manager: Hemamalini Rajendrababu
Project Manager: Anitha Rajarathnam
Design Direction: Steve Stave

**Working together to grow
libraries in developing countries**

www.elsevier.com | www.bookaid.org | www.sabre.org

ELSEVIER   BOOK AID International   Sabre Foundation

Printed in the USA
Last digit is the print number: 9 8 7 6 5 4 3 2 1

BLUE BOOKS OF NEUROLOGY

CONTENTS

CONTRIBUTING AUTHORS

KAILASH BHATIA, MD
Institute of Neurology
University College London
London, United Kingdom

VINCENZO BONIFATI, MD, PhD
Associate Professor
Department of Clinical Genetics
Erasmus Medical Centre
Rotterdam, The Netherlands

DAVID JAMES BROOKS, MD, DSc, FRCP, FM
Hartnett Professor of Neurology
MRC Clinical Science Centre
Division of Neuroscience
Faculty of Medicine
Imperial College London
London, United Kingdom

JONATHAN M. BROTCHIE, PhD
Senior Scientist
University Health Network
Toronto Western Research Institute
Toronto, Ontario, Canada

DAVID JOHN BURN, FRCP, MD
Professor of Movement Disorders
Clinical Ageing Research Unit
Campus for Ageing and Health
Newcastle University
Newcastle upon Tyne, United Kingdom

YAROSLAU COMPTA, MD
Department of Neurology
Neurology Service
Institute Clinic of Neurosciences
Hospital Clinic Universitari
Centro de Investigación
Biomédica En Red Sobre Enfermedades Neurodegenrativas (Ciberned)
University of Barcelona
Barcelona, Spain

TED M. DAWSON, MD, PhD
Leonard and Madlyn Abramson Professor in Neurodegenerative Diseases
Neuroregeneration and Stem Cell Programs
Institute for Cell Engineering
Johns Hopkins University School of Medicine
Baltimore, Maryland

GUNTHER DEUSCHL, MD
Professor of Neurology
Universitätsklinikum Schleswig-Holstein and Christian-Albrechts University
Kiel, Germany

DENNIS W. DICKSON, MD
Professor of Pathology and Neuroscience
Mayo Clinic
Jacksonville, Florida

STANLEY FAHN, MD
Movement Disorder Division Chief and H. Houston Merritt Professor of
  Neurology
The Neurological Institute
Columbia University
New York, New York

MATTHEW JAMES FARRER, PhD
Professor of Molecular Neuroscience
Department of Neuroscience
Mayo Clinic
Jacksonville, Florida

ALFONSO FASANO, MD
Consultant Neurologist
Department of Neurology
Universite Cattolica del Sacro Cuore
Rome, Italy

ALESSANDRO FERRARIS, MD, PhD
Researcher
Neurogenetics Unit
CSS-Mendel Institute
Rome, Italy

SUSAN FOX, MRCP(UK), PhD
Assistant Professor of Neurology
Movement Disorder Clinic
Toronto Western Hospital
Toronto, Ontario, Canada

CARLES GAIG, MD
Department of Neurology
Neurology Service
Institute Clinic of Neurosciences
Hospital Clinic Universitari
Centro de Investigación
Biomédica En Red Sobre Enfermedades Neurodegenrativas (Ciberned)
University of Barcelona
Barcelona, Spain

THOMAS GASSER, MD
Head of the Department
Professor of Medicine
Neurologische University of Tubingen Klinik
Tübingen, Germany

FELIX GESER, MD
Department of Neurology
Parkinson and Movement Disorders Centre
Medical University Innsbruck
Innsbruck, Austria

AMITABH GUPTA, MD, PhD
Clinical Fellow in Movement Disorders
Toronto Western Hospital
Morton and Gloria Shulman Movement Disorders Centre
University of Toronto
Toronto, Ontario, Canada

GLENDA HALLIDAY, PhD
Principal Research Fellow
Director, Human Tissue Resource Centre
Prince of Wales Medical Research Institute;
Professor of Neuroscience
Faculty of Medicine
School of Medical Sciences
University of New South Wales
Sydney, Australia

CLEMENT HAMANI, MD

Division of Neurosurgery
Toronto Western Hospital
University of Toronto
Toronto, Ontario, Canada

TAKU HATANO, MD

Department of Neurology
Juntendo University School of Medicine
Tokyo, Japan

NOBUTAKA HATTORI, MD

Professor and Chairman
Department of Neurology
Juntendo University School of Medicine
Tokyo, Japan

†WAYNE HENING, MD

Robert Wood Johnson School of Medicine
University of Medicine and Dentistry of New Jersey
New Brunswick, New Jersey

JOSEPH JANKOVIC, MD

Professor of Neurology
Distinguished Chair in Movement Disorders
Department of Neurology
Director
Parkinson's Disease Center and Movement Disorders Clinic
Baylor College of Medicine
Houston, Texas

KURT JELLINGER, MD

Parkinson and Movement Disorders Centre
Department of Neurology
Medical University Innsbruck
Innsbruck, Austria

KEITH A. JOSEPHS Jr, MST, MD, MS

Associate Professor and Consultant of Neurology
Department of Behavioral Neurology and Movement Disorders
Mayo Clinic
Rochester, Minnesota

---

†Deceased

CHRISTINE KLEIN, MD
Schilling Professor of Clinical and Molecular Neurogenetics
Section of Neurogenetics
Department of Neurology
University of Lübeck
Lübeck, Germany

MARTIN KÖLLENSPERGER, MD
Parkinson and Movement Disorders Centre
Department of Neurology
Medical University Innsbruck
Innsbruck, Austria

SHIN-ICHIRO KUBO, MD
Department of Neurology
Juntendo University School of Medicine
Tokyo, Japan

G. B. LANDWEHRMEYER, MD
Medical Director
University Clinic Ulm
Neurological University Ambulance in the RKU
Ulm, Germany

ANTHONY E. T. LANG, MD, FRCPC
Professor
Department of Medicine
Director
Division of Neurology
Jack Clark Chair for Parkinson's Disease Research
University of Toronto;
Director
Morton and Gloria Shulman Movement Disorders Centre
Toronto Western Hospital
Toronto, Ontario, Canada

ADRIAN W. LAXTON, MD
Neurosurgery Resident
Division of Neurosurgery
Toronto Western Hospital
University Health Network
University of Toronto
Toronto, Ontario, Canada

ANDRES M. LOZANO, MD, PhD
Division of Neurosurgery
Toronto Western Hospital
University of Toronto
Toronto, Ontario, Canada

ALBERT C. LUDOLPH, MD
Medical Director
University Clinic Ulm
Neurological University Ambulance in the RKU
Ulm, Germany

YUTAKA MACHIDA, MD
Department of Neurology
Juntendo University School of Medicine
Tokyo, Japan

ELENA MORO, MD, PhD
Toronto Western Hospital
Toronto, Ontario, Canada

HUW R. MORRIS, PhD, FRCP
Senior Lecturer in Neurology and Neurogenetics
Department of Neurology and Neurogenetics Neurology
University Hospital of Wales
Cardiff, United Kingdom

KAREN MURPHY, BSc (Hons)
Research Assistant
Prince of Wales Medical Research Institute
Sydney, Australia

JOSÉ A. OBESO, MD, PhD
Consultant and Professor of Neurology and Senior Researcher
Clinica Universitaria and Medical School
CIMA and CIBERNED
University of Navarra
Pamplona, Spain

C. WARREN OLANOW, MD, FRCPC
Department of Neurology
Mount Sinai School of Medicine
New York, New York

WERNER POEWE, MD
Professor of Neurology
Director
Department of Neurology
Medical University Innsbruck
Innsbruck, Austria

ROSA RADEMAKERS, PhD
Assistant Professor of Neuroscience
Department of Neuroscience
Mayo Clinic
Jacksonville, Florida

JOAN SANTAMARIA, MD
Department of Neurology
Neurology Service
Institute Clinic of Neurosciences
Hospital Clinic Universitari
Centro de Investigación
Biomédica En Red Sobre Enfermedades Neurodegenrativas (Ciberned)
University of Barcelona
Barcelona, Spain

SHIGETO SATO, MD
Department of Neurology
Juntendo University School of Medicine
Tokyo, Japan

ANTHONY H. V. SCHAPIRA, DSc, MD, FRCP, FMedSci
Professor of Neurology and Chair
University Department of Clinical Neurosciences
Institute of Neurology
University College London
London, United Kingdom

SUSANNE A. SCHNEIDER, MD, PhD
Sobell Department of Motor Neuroscience and Movement Disorders
Institute of Neurology
University College London
London, United Kingdom;
Department of Neurogenetics
University of Lübeck
Lübeck, Germany

KLAUS SEPPI, MD

Professor of Neurology
Department of Neurology
Medical University Innsbruck
Innsbruck, Austria

IRA SHOULSON, MD

Louis C. Lasagna Professor in Experimental Therapeutics and Professor
Departments of Neurology and Pharmacology and Physiology
University of Rochester
Rochester, New York

HARVEY S. SINGER, MD

Haller Professor of Pediatric Neurology
Director
Division of Pediatric Neurology
Child Neurology
Johns Hopkins Hospital
Baltimore, Maryland

NADIA STEFANOVA, MD

Parkinson and Movement Disorders Centre
Department of Neurology
Medical University Innsbruck
Innsbruck, Austria

CAROLINE M. TANNER, MD, PhD

Director of Clinical Research
Parkinson's Institute
Sunnyvale, California

MADHAVI THOMAS, MD

Associate Attending Neurologist
Baylor University Medical Center
Dallas, Texas

PHILIP THOMPSON, MB, PhD, FRACP

Professor of Neurology
University Department of Medicine
University of Adelaide;
Department of Neurology
Royal Adelaide Hospital
Adelaide, South Australia

EDUARDO TOLOSA, MD

Neurology Service
Department of Neurology
Institute Clinic of Neurosciences
Hospital Clinic Universitari
Centro de Investigación
Biomédica En Red Sobre Enfermedades Neurodegenrativas (Ciberned)
University of Barcelona
Barcelona, Spain

CLAUDIA TRENKWALDER, MD

Professor of Clinical Neurophysiology
University of Goettingen
Goettingen;
Medical Director
Center of Parkinsonism and Movement Disorders
Paracelsus-Elena Klinik
Kassel, Germany

ENZA MARIA VALENTE, MD, PhD

Associate Professor of Medical Genetics
University of Messina and CSS-Mendel Institute
Rome, Italy

MARIE VIDAILHET, MD

Head of the Movement Disorders Group
Federation of Neurology
Salpêtrière Hospital
Paris, France

RUTH H. WALKER, MB, CHB, PhD

Associate Professor
Department of Neurology
Mount Sinai School of Medicine;
James J. Peters Veterans Affairs Medical Center
New York, New York

THOMAS T. WARNER, BA, BM, BCh, PhD, FRCP

Reader in Clinical Neurosciences
Department of Clinical Neurosciences
Institute of Neurology
University College London
London, United Kingdom

DANIEL WEINTRAUB, MD

Assistant Professor of Psychiatry
University of Pennsylvania
Philadelphia, Pennsylvania

GREGOR K. WENNING, MD, MSc, PhD

Head
Section of Clinical Neurobiology
Parkinson and Movement Disorder Centre
Department of Neurology
Medical University Innsbruck
Innsbruck, Austria

PATRICK WEYDT, MD

Resident Physician
Department of Neurology
University of Ulm
Ulm, Germany

CHRISTIAN W. WIDER, MD

Visiting Scientist
Department of Neurology
Mayo Clinic
Jacksonville, Florida

ZBIGNIEW K. WSZOLEK, MD

Professor of Neurology
Department of Neurology
Mayo Clinic
Jacksonville, Florida

SERIES PREFACE

The *Blue Books of Neurology* have a long and distinguished lineage. The life of these books began as the *Modern Trends in Neurology* series and continued with the monographs forming *BIMR Neurology*. The present series was first edited by David Marsden and Arthur Asbury and saw the publication of 25 volumes over 18 years.

The guiding principle of each volume, the topic of which is selected by the Series Editors, was that each should cover an area in which there had been significant advances in research, and that such progress had been translated to new or improved patient management. This has been the guiding spirit behind each volume, and we expect it to continue. In effect, we emphasize basic, translational, and clinical research, but principally to the extent that this research changes our collective attitudes and practices in caring for those who are neurologically afflicted.

Tony Schapira took over as joint editor in 1999 following David's death, and together with Art oversaw the publication and preparation of a further 8 volumes. In 2005, Art Asbury ended his exceptional co-editorship after 25 years of distinguished contribution, and Martin Samuels was asked to continue the co-editorship with Tony.

The current volumes represent the beginning of the next stage in the development of the Blue Books. The editors intend to build on the excellent reputation established by the Series with a new and attractive visual style incorporating the same level of high-quality review. The ethos of the Series remains the same: up-to-date reviews of topic areas in which there have been important and exciting advances of relevance to the diagnosis and treatment of patients with neurological diseases. The intended audience remains neurologists in training and practicing clinicians in search of a contemporary, valuable, and interesting source of information.

ANTHONY H. V. SCHAPIRA
MARTIN A. SAMUELS
Series Editors

PREFACE

The Blue Books of Neurology series has proven to be an enduring and popular series. David Marsden and Art Asbury were the first editors, beginning in 1982. In 1999 Tony Schapira joined the editorship following David's death, and Marty Samuels took over in 2005 when Art retired from the series. Three of the most popular editions of the series were *Movement Disorders 1, 2,* and *3,* edited by Drs. Marsden and Fahn. It is 15 years since the last was published in 1994.

We felt that *Movement Disorders 4* was long overdue! The science and practice of neurology have been transformed by advances in our understanding, particularly of the etiology and pathogenesis of neurological diseases. The field of movement disorders is at the forefront of this progress. Several disciplines have contributed to this effort, including molecular biology, genetics, imaging, physiology, epidemiology, and phenomenology. These advances have enabled us not only to better define the different diseases that encompass movement disorders, but also to appreciate the common areas that exist among them.

Progress has led to improvements in clinical practice and patient management. New therapies have become available, including new drugs and novel surgical techniques. Exciting areas for future development are cell-based therapies and gene therapies, which may find application in several movement disorders.

We have been fortunate to be able to recruit an extraordinary group of authors to contribute to this edition. In truth, this was not a difficult task and reflects the high esteem in which the series and particularly *Movement Disorders 1* through *3* are held. The leading authorities in the various fields represented within this book were approached and, despite extremely busy schedules and over-commitment that has become the norm, gave generously of their time to produce truly outstanding chapters.

During the writing of this book and his chapter, Wayne Hening tragically died prematurely. He was a master of his field of movement disorders and of his selected area of restless legs research. He will be sadly missed by all who were privileged to know him. We thank Claudia Trenkwalder for working with Wayne on their chapter and producing such an excellent contribution in difficult circumstances.

We have sought to focus on those areas of the field where most advances have been made and where there is the real prospect of translation into new treatments or management strategies now or in the near future. This edition is comprehensive, but it is not intended to be all inclusive. Any omissions are our responsibility and not those of the authors. We thank them for their enthusiasm, diligence, and forbearance!

We must also thank Adrianne Brigido for her support and encouragement; Susan Pioli, who sponsored and championed both the series and this edition; Joan Ryan, who once again proved how indispensable she is as the organizer who finally delivers the finished product; and Anitha Raj, who proved indispensable as the organizer who delivered the finished product.

ANTHONY SCHAPIRA
ANTHONY LANG
STANLEY FAHN

CURRENT CONCEPTS IN THE ANATOMY AND PHYSIOLOGY OF THE BASAL GANGLIA

1 Functional Anatomy and Pathophysiology of the Basal Ganglia

JONATHAN M. BROTCHIE • JOSÉ A. OBESO

Introduction

The basal ganglia are a collection of functionally related nuclei that work in concert and with many other areas spread across the neuraxis to provide crucial functions, not only in movement control, but also in learning, planning, working memory, and emotions. Most, if not all, of these domains frequently become abnormal in patients with movement disorders such as Parkinson's disease (PD), Huntington's disease, progressive supranuclear palsy, and Gilles de la Tourette syndrome. This chapter provides an overview of the functional organization of the basal ganglia and briefly reviews the current status of understanding regarding how these circuits function abnormally in movement disorders.

Functional Anatomy

The basal ganglia are classically described as comprising the striatum, globus pallidus, substantia nigra, and subthalamic nucleus (STN). These component nuclei can be divided as follows:

1. The striatum, comprising the caudate nucleus, putamen, and nucleus accumbens
2. The globus pallidus, divided into an external segment (GPe), located laterally adjacent to the striatum, and an internal segment (GPi), located more medially
3. The substantia nigra, composed of a cell-dense, pigmented region, the substantia nigra pars compacta (SNc), and an unpigmented region, the substantia nigra pars reticulata (SNr)

Although described as three separate structures, the caudate, putamen, and nucleus accumbens have a similar functional organization. In contrast, the components of the globus pallidus and substantia nigra, the GPe/GPi and SNr/SNc, have distinct functional roles. The functions of the GPi and SNr are, as described subsequently, very similar. The STN is typically considered to function as a single unit, although there is clear topography in its connections.

The basal ganglia act to integrate and process information, provided by diverse inputs from the cerebral cortex and thalamus, and provide output to a range of brain structures, particularly the ventral thalamus, and the cerebral cortex, superior colliculus nucleus, and lateral habenula nucleus. The principal region receiving inputs from outside the basal ganglia is the striatum. The output regions, projecting beyond the basal ganglia, are the GPi and SNr.

The functional organization of the basal ganglia can be described in simple terms as a series of connections by which information flows from the striatum to the GPi and SNr (Fig. 1–1). The input and output regions of the basal ganglia are connected via either a direct pathway or an indirect pathway or network.[1,2] The direct pathway arises from medium-sized spiny neurons (MSNs) in the striatum and projects, as its name implies, directly to the output regions of the basal ganglia. The indirect network, also arising from striatal MSNs, takes a more circuitous route to the GPi and SNr, involving the GPe. MSNs of the indirect network project from the striatum to the GPe. The GPe influences basal ganglia output via a GPe to GPi/SNr connection, and via the intermediary of the STN, via a GPe to STN connection, and then a projection from the STN to the GPi and SNr (see Fig. 1–1). Neurons of the GPi and SNr that receive inputs from the direct and indirect pathways form the outputs of the basal ganglia and project to the ventral thalamus, superior colliculus, pedunculopontine nucleus, and reticular formation.[3,4]

Alongside this indirect/direct pathway organization lies a loop involving the striatum and SNc. The striatum projects to the SNc (using γ-aminobutyric acid [GABA] as the neurotransmitter), and the SNc projects back onto the striatum. The latter is the well-known dopaminergic pathway. Most neurons within the basal ganglia use the inhibitory neurotransmitter GABA. In rats, it has been estimated that 98.9% of basal ganglia neurons are GABAergic.[5] For the purpose of the simple description of basal ganglia anatomy, presented earlier and in Figure 1–1, the MSNs of the striatum contribute to the "direct" striato-GPi/SNr pathway, and the "indirect" striato-GPe projections are GABAergic. Likewise, the neurons

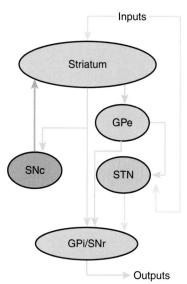

Figure 1–1 Circuitry of the basal ganglia. This figure represents schematically the core components of the basal ganglia and the connections between them. Although it is an oversimplification of a complex neural network, this circuit provides a powerful framework for discussing the pathophysiology of movement disorders. The striatum represents the major input region of the basal ganglia. The internal segment of the globus pallidus (GPi) and substantia nigra pars reticulata (SNr) are the output regions of the basal ganglia. The striatum projects to the GPi/SNr, the direct pathway. The striatum also projects to the external globus pallidus (GPe), which projects to the subthalamic nucleus (STN), which then innervates the GPi/SNr. This link between striatum and GPi/SNr is known as the indirect pathway or network. The substantia nigra pars compacta (SNc) is dopaminergic. Regions and connections that are inhibitory, using GABA as a principal neurotransmitter, are colored blue. Excitatory regions and connections, using glutamate, are colored pink. The substantia nigra pars corpacta (SNc), uses dopamine, and is colored green.

of the GPe, from which GPe-GPi/SNr and GPe-STN projections arise, are also GABAergic, as are the basal ganglia outputs from the GPi and SNr. The principal exceptions to the GABAergic nature of basal ganglia neurons are the neurons of the STN, which are excitatory, using glutamate as transmitter, and the pigmented dopaminergic neurons of the SNc.

The major inputs to the basal ganglia target the striatum and come from almost all regions of the cerebral cortex and the intralaminar (i.e., centromedian/parafascicular) nuclei of the thalamus. Both of these projections are excitatory and use glutamate as a neurotransmitter. Glutamate provides excitation by activation of a combination of all major classes of glutamate receptor, including the N-methyl-D-aspartate (NMDA), alpha-amino-3-hydroxy-5-methyl-4-isoxazolepropionate (AMPA), kainic acid, and metabotropic glutamate receptors (mGluR). These projections are extensive, accounting for 85% of all synapses in the striatum.[6]

Within the striatum, the distribution of projections from specific cortical regions is diffuse, being spread in bands along the rostrocaudal plane. Each corticostriatal neuron typically provides only one or two synapses to each MSN and can influence on average 1000 MSNs; an individual MSN may receive 15,000 cortical inputs overall.[6-8] There is significant convergence of cortical inputs onto individual MSNs. Dopaminergic nigrostriatal inputs act to modulate corticostriatal excitation. While corticostriatal inputs impinge on the heads of the spines of MSNs, the dopaminergic inputs are focused on the bases of the spines or on dendrites, being localized in a manner by which they can gate the spread of excitation from the spines, down dendrites to the soma.[6]

This basic circuitry, although an oversimplification of detailed anatomical connectivity, has proved extremely valuable in providing a simple heuristic model of basal ganglia function in health and disease. This model is considered in more detail subsequently. In oversimplifying the circuitry, however, much of the richness of basal ganglia anatomy is lost. In particular, the following additional information should be appreciated:

1. Although MSNs may form 75% to 95% of neurons in the striatum (depending on the species examined), there is a significant population of striatal interneurons.[9] Most of these are GABAergic, of which there are three clearly distinct classes. A fourth class, the large aspiny interneurons, use acetylcholine.[10] Interneurons act to regulate the activity of MSNs. A major role of the GABAergic interneurons is to provide strong inhibition of MSNs and influence the timing of firing of MSNs individually and in groups. This activity is crucial to the patterning of information flow through basal ganglia. The cholinergic interneurons act more to control the threshold for cortical or thalamic derived excitation of MSNs. These interneurons are tonically active; they are often termed *tonically active neurons*. Suppression of their firing contributes to motivation and reward-related functions.[11-13]

2. The striatum is organized into two subcompartments, termed striosome and matrix.[14] In cross-section, the striosomes can be seen as small "islands" of cells floating in a "sea" of matrix. In three dimensions, this organization is more complex. The striosome-matrix compartmentalization has functional significance. MSNs of the direct and indirect pathways arise almost exclusively from the matrix, whereas the striato-SNc projection arises from striosomes. The dopaminergic SNc-striatum connection does not complete a closed striato-SNc-striatum loop because it innervates striosomes and matrix.

3. Although MSNs of the direct and indirect pathways look identical on a morphological level and are all GABAergic, there are significant differences with respect to the details of their chemical neuroanatomy. Although both pathways use peptides as cotransmitters with GABA, MSNs of the direct pathways employ the tachykinin substance P and opioids derived from the precursor pre–proenkephalin B (PPE-B), including dynorphins, leu-enkephalin, and α-neoendorphin. In contrast, MSNs of the indirect network use peptides produced from pre–proenkephalin A (PPE-A), predominantly met-enkephalin, and neurotensin as cotransmitters with GABA.[15]

4. Subtypes of dopamine receptors are distributed differentially within the striatum. D2 dopamine receptors are found predominantly on MSNs of the indirect pathway, whereas D_1 receptors are located on the direct pathway.[16] In the normal state, D3 dopamine receptors are located on MSNs of the direct pathway and concentrated ventrally within the striatum, being found primarily in the nucleus accumbens.[17] This distribution may change in pathologic states, and as described in this text, may be important in the response to dopaminergic antiparkinsonian therapy.

5. Nondopaminergic receptors also are distributed differentially across neurons of the striatum. One of the clearest examples of this is the A_{2A} adenosine receptor, which is almost exclusively expressed by MSNs of the indirect, rather than direct, pathway.[18,19] Similarly, although the M_1 class of muscarinic acetylcholine receptor is expressed on MSNs of the direct and the indirect pathway, the M_4 muscarinic acetylcholine receptor is expressed more robustly on neurons of the direct pathway.[20,21]

6. The STN receives significant inputs from outside the basal ganglia. The glutamatergic corticosubthalamic pathway may have great functional impact. This pathway has been referred to as the "hyperdirect" pathway because it allows the cerebral cortex to influence the GPi and SNr more rapidly than via the striatum and direct/indirect pathway circuits. The centromedian/parafascicular thalamus also projects to the STN.

7. Although the dopaminergic projections from the SNc to the striatum are undoubtedly crucial to basal ganglia function, increasingly additional dopaminergic projections from the SNc to the STN, GPe, and GPi and SNr need to be considered in defining the pathophysiology of movement disorders.

Pathophysiology of the Parkinsonian State

The principal characteristic of the parkinsonian state from a pathophysiological point of view is striatal dopamine depletion; this leads to increased neuronal activity in the output nuclei of the basal ganglia, the GPi and SNr (Fig. 1–2A). Overactivity of the GPi and SNr produces excessive inhibition of the thalamocortical and brainstem motor systems, interfering with normal speed of movement onset and execution.[1,2,22] The classic model of the basal ganglia function in parkinsonism was based on the idea that striatal dopamine deficiency reduces inhibition of indirect pathway neurons and decreases excitation of direct pathway neurons.[2,23] Increased activity of MSNs in the indirect pathway leads to overinhibition of the GPe, disinhibition of the STN, and increased excitation of the GPi and SNr, whereas decreased activation of MSNs in the direct pathway reduces their inhibitory influence on the GPi and SNr, and contributes to excessive neuronal activity in basal ganglia output neurons. A large body of evidence supports key features of the model in the parkinsonian state, although over the years numerous unexplained observations and questions have arisen. These data are reviewed and summarized.

DATA SUPPORTING THE MODEL

A lesion of the nigrostriatal projection in animal models of PD (i.e., the rat with a 6-hydroxydopamine [6-OHDA] lesion and the monkey intoxicated with 1-methyl-4-phenyl-1,2,3,6-tetrahydropyridine [MPTP]) is associated with increased expression of D2 receptor and PPE-A mRNA in striatal neurons constituting the indirect pathway, whereas expression of D_1 receptor, substance P, and PPE-B mRNA is decreased in neurons of the direct pathway.[24-27] Several markers of cellular activity have been shown to be increased in the STN or GPi and SNr in these models. In direct support of the models, 2-deoxyglucose uptake as a marker of synaptic afferent activity,[28] in situ hybridization of cytochrome oxidase I mRNA

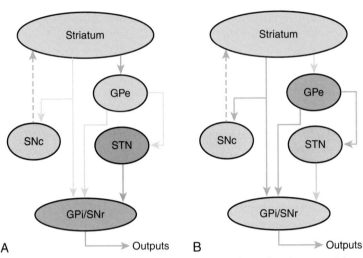

Figure 1–2 A and **B,** Pathophysiology of movement disorders—the classic model. In disease states, the balance of activity in the circuit outlined in Figure 1–1 changes such that in hypokinetic movement disorders, such as Parkinson's disease (**A**), the outputs of the basal ganglia are overactive, a result of overactivity of the indirect pathway and underactivity of the direct pathway. In contrast, in hyperkinetic movement disorders, such as levodopa-induced dyskinesia (**B**), the outputs of the basal ganglia are underactive, a result of overactivity of the direct pathway and underactivity of the indirect pathway. Underactive pathways and regions are signified by thinner lines and pale shading; overactive pathways and regions are signified by thicker lines and darker shading. See legend for Figure 1–1 for abbreviations.

as a measure of cellular mitochondrial activity,[29] and glutamic acid decarboxylase (GAD) mRNA as a measure of GABA activity[30] have been found abnormal.

Mean neuronal firing rate evaluated by single cell recordings also has been reported as increased in the STN and GPi in the parkinsonian state, although there is some inconsistency among publications.[31] This inconsistency could be related to differences in the experimental paradigm. The firing rate ratio between GPe/GPi is clearly shifted toward a reduction (i.e., relative hypoactivity of GPe and hyperactivity of GPi) in MPTP-treated monkeys and patients with PD.[32] Lesions of the STN and GPi induce marked motor improvement in MPTP-treated monkeys in association with reduced neuronal activity in GPi and SNr neurons.[33-35]

OBSERVATIONS AT ODDS WITH THE CLASSIC MODEL

According to the model, in parkinsonism, the GPi and SNr are pushed into overdrive by increased excitatory activity in the STN; these features represent the pathophysiologic hallmark of the parkinsonian state. How such STN overactivity arises is unclear. GPe hypoactivity resulting from the loss of the inhibitory influence of dopamine on striatal neurons in the indirect pathway is the classic presumed mechanism (see Fig. 1–2A). Studies in MPTP-treated monkeys and PD patients indicate that the neuronal firing rate in GPe is reduced, particularly compared with GPi, but metabolic markers such as cytochrome oxidase I or GAD mRNA expression are increased, not decreased, in the GPe of MPTP-treated parkinsonian monkeys[30] and the rodent GPe homologue, termed simply "globus pallidus," of 6-OHDA–lesioned rodents.[36]

A study in 6-OHDA–lesioned rats[37] showed that increased STN firing preceded significant striatal dopamine depletion and was without a concomitant reduction in GPe discharge rate in MPTP-treated monkeys.[38] These findings suggest that the origin of STN hyperactivity in the parkinsonian state is not as clear as what is portrayed in the model, and may not depend solely on a reduction in inhibitory tone from the GPe. STN hyperactivity in the parkinsonian state could depend not only on a reduction in inhibitory tone from the GPe, but also on reduction of the "direct" SNc-STN dopaminergic projection and increased excitatory input from the centromedian/parafascicular complex of the thalamus and the pendunculopontine nucleus.[39]

Two more recent studies in monkeys have provided support for the key role of the GPe in modulating STN activity as originally proposed by the model. First, Soares and colleagues[40] found that neuronal discharge rate in the GPe is reduced in the parkinsonian state and showed (by microdialysis) that GABA release is reduced in the STN, whereas GAD (measured by immunoradiography) was elevated in the GPe. This latter finding corroborates previous studies assessing GAD expression in the GPe, but casts some doubts about the validity of this assay to assess the output of a given nucleus. A study by Zhang and coworkers[41] showed that a unilateral lesion of the GPe led to further increase of GPi firing activity in MPTP-treated monkeys and significant deterioration in spontaneous movement and timed tests.[41] These results, albeit in a small number of animals, established a clear-cut relationship between reduced inhibition from the GPe and increased GPi firing rate and severity of parkinsonism.

Another major area where pathophysiology needs further advances is in the model's ability to provide an adequate explanation of basic clinical manifestations. Akinesia/bradykinesia is perhaps the best understood problem in terms of basic mechanism. In the parkinsonian state, the basal ganglia function is shifted toward inhibiting cortically aided movements by an increased influence of the STN-GPi microcircuitry and by reduced excitability in the "direct" corticostriato-GPi projection. In addition, reduction in automatic movements, such as reduced blinking rate, decreased arm swing, and short stepping on walking are probably mediated by brainstem mechanisms, which are also functionally impaired by excessive basal ganglia inhibitory outputs, perhaps via the pendunculopontine nucleus. Other features of akinesia/bradykinesia, such as the movement deterioration associated with the performance of simultaneous and sequential movements, the reduction in amplitude when undertaking a repetitive movement, and the striking improvement in gait freezing induced by visual cues, are not explained by the current model.

The understanding of tremor or rigidity with respect to the model is even more difficult when using the simple scheme of excessive output basal ganglia activity as the fundamental explanation. Recording neuronal activity in the MPTP-intoxicated monkeys[42] and in patients with PD[43] has revealed a definite correlation between tremor in the limbs and rhythmical 4- to 6-Hz firing in the basal ganglia (GPe, GPi, STN) and in the ventralis intermedius nucleus of the thalamus.[44] In addition, lesion or deep brain stimulation of the STN, GPi, and ventralis intermedius nucleus may stop tremor in PD patients. It may be that the multiple circuits and feedback loops that characterize the organization of the basal ganglia have a tendency to generate oscillatory activity that produces tremor in PD.

In this regard, in organotypic cultures (from mice brains), the GPe and STN have an enhanced tendency to rhythmical and reciprocal firing, giving rise to 4- to 5-Hz bursting activity.[45]

It remains to be elucidated if mechanisms engaging tremor are primarily mediated and depend on striatal dopamine deficiency or the consequence of impairment of direct dopaminergic projection to the STN, GPe, and GPi or the thalamus.[46] How the ventralis intermedius nucleus, which is not directly connected with the basal ganglia, becomes engaged in parkinsonian tremor requires elucidation.

Pathophysiology of the Dyskinetic State

The model proposes that dyskinesia (i.e., chorea or ballism) results from reduced activity in the STN-GPi projection leading to decreased firing in GPi output.[1,2,22] In essence, the pathophysiology of dyskinesias can be seen as the opposite of parkinsonism. Dyskinesias secondary to focal lesion of the basal ganglia or induced by levodopa in patients with PD share a similar common pathophysiological mechanism[47,48]—reduced GPi/SNr activity. The original model conceives that levodopa-induced dyskinesia (LID) in dopamine-deficient animals or PD patients arises by excessive inhibition of MSNs giving rise to the indirect striato-GPe projections, which leads to disinhibition of GPe, overinhibition of STN, reduced STN excitatory drive, and consequent hypoactivity in GPi/SNr output neurons (see Fig. 1–2B). In addition, abnormal striatal dopaminergic stimulation enhances activity of D_1 receptor–bearing MSNs of the direct pathway augmenting inhibition onto the GPi. This "double whammy" provides reduction in GPi and SNr activity, and leads to reduced inhibitory basal ganglia output, disinhibiting release of the thalamocortical projection. Dyskinesias are seen as the parallel facilitation of movement fragments owing to inefficient basal ganglia filtering action.

DATA SUPPORTING THE MODEL

The initial evidence supported a major role of the indirect pathway in the induction of dyskinesias. Choreic dyskinesias were induced in normal monkeys by disinhibition of the GPe (by local administration of bicuculline) and blockade or lesioning of the STN.[49,50] The model explained these results as blockade of the striato-GPe inhibitory projection increasing GPe efferent activity, resulting in overinhibition of the STN and, as a consequence, decreased glutamatergic excitatory activity onto the GPi.[50,51] Electrophysiological and metabolic studies showed increased neuronal activity in the GPe, decreased STN activation, and reduced neuronal firing in the GPi recorded during surgery in dyskinetic MPTP-treated monkeys[52] and PD patients.[53]

Metabolic markers are not in keeping with the suggested role of the indirect pathway. Expression of mRNA for striatal met-enkephalin remains increased, and expression of GAD mRNA (an index of GABA activity) and cytochrome oxidase mRNA (an index of cellular activation) were not above normal in the GPe of dyskinetic monkeys.[27,29,54] Lesion of the GPe did not block LID in MPTP-treated monkeys.[55] The prediction of the model whereby levodopa induces hyperactivity of the GPe leading to overinhibition of the STN is not fully supported by experimental data.

In recent years, interest has been centered on the direct pathway as a mediator of LID. Hypoactivity of the GPi also may occur by increased GABAergic input in the "direct" striatopallidal pathway, and evidence has accumulated for abnormal D_1 receptor activation in the striatum of dyskinetic animals. Expression of D_1 striatal receptors is unchanged in relation to LID in MPTP-treated monkeys, confirming previous data from PD patients, but there was increased binding of [^{35}S]GTP gamma-S, indicating increased efficiency of receptor signaling.[56] Levels of Cdk5 (cyclin-dependent protein kinase 5) and DARP-32, two pivotal players in D_1 signal transduction pathway, are increased in the striatum of dyskinetic monkeys.[56] Such abnormalities were not seen in other equally parkinsonian but nondyskinetic monkeys despite receiving the same regimen of levodopa treatment. In addition, LID in MPTP-treated monkeys correlated linearly with D3 receptor binding levels.[57] Markers of MSN activity in the direct pathway such as D_1 and D3 receptors seem to be directly related to LID.[58]

OBSERVATIONS AT ODDS WITH THE CLASSIC MODEL

According to the firing rate–based model, lesioning or blockade of basal ganglia output should lead to dyskinesias. Direct administration of the GABA agonist muscimol into the GPi has been associated mainly, however, with cocontraction of antagonist muscles, provoking dystonic postures, and secondary slowness of movement initiation.[59,60] The strongest argument against the notion that GPi hypoactivity is the primary mechanism responsible for the development of LID is the finding that pallidotomy, which by definition reduces GPi neuronal output, consistently ameliorates or actually abolishes chorea or ballism secondary to lesioning of the STN and LID.[47,61] This consistent observation obliges one to reconsider the pathophysiologic model of the basal ganglia in general and the mechanisms of LID in particular.

❙ Therapeutic Applications

Perhaps the greatest impact, to date, on therapy resulting from the classic pathophysiologic model is the surgical targeting of STN in parkinsonism. The convincing evidence that neuronal activity is increased in the STN and GPi, as predicted by the model, has served as the basis for surgical treatments in PD designed to reduce excess neuronal activity in these structures.[62] It is now well established that lesioning or high-frequency deep brain stimulation of these brain targets provides dramatic benefit to PD patients and restores thalamocortical activity.[63,64] The understanding of the role of overactivity of the indirect pathway in parkinsonism has supported the use of D2 dopamine receptor selective agonists, and the development of A_{2A} adenosine receptor antagonists as antiparkinsonian symptomatic therapy.[19]

With respect to LID, the appreciation of the role of overactivity of the direct pathway has led to attempts to define pharmacology to reduce that drive. The use of amantadine to reduce LID is thought to result from its ability to antagonize NMDA receptors on MSNs of the direct pathway and reduce the activity of that pathway.[65,66] Other means to achieve this goal, including AMPA and mGluR antagonists, also are in development.[67,68] Although the model led to the targeting of the GPi in an attempt to reduce parkinsonian symptoms, as described previously, the finding that LID can also be reduced by lesioning of the GPi suggests that simple underactivity of the GPi and SNr cannot completely explain the mechanisms underlying LID generation. Beyond firing rate, we need to move toward theoretical models incorporating descriptions of firing pattern and rate.[45] The anticonvulsant levetiracetam has been suggested as an antidyskinetic agent because it can alter neuronal synchronization rather than rate.[69]

Conclusions

The last 2 decades have seen significant advances in understanding the functional anatomy and pathophysiology of movement disorders. This increased understanding has led to a greater appreciation of neural mechanisms of disease and encouraged the development of novel therapies.[19,70] Increasingly, the basal ganglia are seen as a more dynamic system, however, with new, evolving models incorporating concepts beyond rate of firing, particularly involving the importance of pattern of firing, synchronization, or coincidence.[45,71] To date, these new models have not had a great impact on treatment, although they will undoubtedly be important in explaining the benefits of deep brain stimulation and have potential to identify novel drug therapies. These models also may, in time, help explain the enigma of why, in certain situations, hyperkinetic and hypokinetic symptoms can coexist, and, perhaps the greatest paradox of all,[72] why it is possible to disrupt the basal ganglia surgically with little or no apparent deficits.[73]

REFERENCES

1. Albin RL, Young AB, Penney JB: The functional anatomy of basal ganglia disorders. Trends Neurosci 1989;12:366-375.
2. DeLong MR: Primate models of movement disorders of basal ganglia origin. Trends Neurosci 1990;13:281-285.
3. Parent M, Parent A: The pallidofugal motor fiber system in primates. Parkinsonism Relat Disord 2004;10:203-211.
4. Mena-Segovia J, Bolam JP, Magill PJ: Pedunculopontine nucleus and basal ganglia: distant relatives or part of the same family? Trends Neurosci 2004;27:585-588.
5. Oorschot DE: Total number of neurons in the neostriatal, pallidal, subthalamic, and substantia nigral nuclei of the rat basal ganglia: a stereological study using the cavalieri and optical dissector methods. J Comp Neurol 1996;366:580-599.
6. Tepper JM, Abercrombie ED, Bolam JP: Basal ganglia macrocircuits. Prog Brain Res 2007;160:3-7.
7. Kincaid AE, Zheng T, Wilson CJ: Connectivity and convergence of single corticostriatal axons. J Neurosci 1998;18:4722-4731.
8. Zheng T, Wilson CJ: Corticostriatal combinatorics: the implications of corticostriatal axonal arborizations. J Neurophysiol 2002;87:1007-1017.
9. Tepper JM, Bolam JP: Functional diversity and specificity of neostriatal interneurons. Curr Opin Neurobiol 2004;14:685-692.
10. Pisani A, Bernardi G, Ding J, Surmeier DJ: Re-emergence of striatal cholinergic interneurons in movement disorders. Trends Neurosci 2007;30:545-553.
11. Morris G, Nevet A, Arkadir D, et al: Midbrain dopamine neurons encode decisions for future action. Nat Neurosci 2006;9:1057-1063.
12. Apicella P: Tonically active neurons in the primate striatum and their role in the processing of information about motivationally relevant events. Eur J Neurosci 2002;16:2017-2026.
13. Apicella P: Leading tonically active neurons of the striatum from reward detection to context recognition. Trends Neurosci 2007;30:299-306.

14. Gerfen CR: The neostriatal mosaic: multiple levels of compartmental organization. Trends Neurosci 1992;15:133-139.
15. Steiner H, Gerfen CR: Role of dynorphin and enkephalin in the regulation of striatal output pathways and behavior. Exp Brain Res 1998;123:60-76.
16. Surmeier DJ, Song WJ, Yan Z: Coordinated expression of dopamine receptors in neostriatal medium spiny neurons. J Neurosci 1996;16:6579-6591.
17. Le Moine C, Bloch B: Expression of the D3 dopamine receptor in peptidergic neurons of the nucleus accumbens: comparison with the D1 and D2 dopamine receptors. Neuroscience 1996;73:131-143.
18. Fredholm BB, Svenningsson P: Striatal adenosine A2A receptors—where are they? What do they do? Trends Pharmacol Sci 1998;19:46-48.
19. Schapira AH, Bezard E, Brotchie J, et al: Novel pharmacological targets for the treatment of Parkinson's disease. Nat Rev Drug Discov 2006;5:845-854.
20. Yan Z, Flores-Hernandez J, Surmeier DJ: Coordinated expression of muscarinic receptor messenger RNAs in striatal medium spiny neurons. Neuroscience 2001;103:1017-1024.
21. Harrison MB, Tissot M, Wiley RG: Expression of m1 and m4 muscarinic receptor mRNA in the striatum following a selective lesion of striatonigral neurons. Brain Res 1996;734:323-326.
22. Crossman AR: Primate models of dyskinesia: the experimental approach to the study of basal ganglia-related involuntary movement disorders. Neuroscience 1987;21:1-40.
23. Gerfen CR, Engber TM, Mahan LC, et al: D1 and D2 dopamine receptor-regulated gene expression of striatonigral and striatopallidal neurons. Science 1990;250:1429-1432.
24. Betarbet R, Greenamyre JT: Regulation of dopamine receptor and neuropeptide expression in the basal ganglia of monkeys treated with MPTP. Exp Neurol 2004;189:393-403.
25. Herrero MT, Augood SJ, Asensi H, et al: Effects of L-DOPA-therapy on dopamine D2 receptor mRNA expression in the striatum of MPTP-intoxicated parkinsonian monkeys. Brain Res Mol Brain Res 1996;42:149-155.
26. Soghomonian JJ, Chesselet MF: Effects of nigrostriatal lesions on the levels of messenger RNAs encoding two isoforms of glutamate decarboxylase in the globus pallidus and entopeduncular nucleus of the rat. Synapse 1992;11:124-133.
27. Herrero MT, Augood SJ, Hirsch EC, et al: Effects of L-DOPA on preproenkephalin and preprotachykinin gene expression in the MPTP-treated monkey striatum. Neuroscience 1995;68:1189-1198.
28. Brotchie JM: The neural mechanisms underlying levodopa-induced dyskinesia in Parkinson's disease. Ann Neurol 2000;47:S105-S112.
29. Vila M, Levy R, Herrero MT, et al: Consequences of nigrostriatal denervation on the functioning of the basal ganglia in human and nonhuman primates: an in situ hybridization study of cytochrome oxidase subunit I mRNA. J Neurosci 1997;17:765-773.
30. Herrero MT, Levy R, Ruberg M, et al: Consequence of nigrostriatal denervation and L-dopa therapy on the expression of glutamic acid decarboxylase messenger RNA in the pallidum. Neurology 1996;47:219-224.
31. Filion, M., Tremblay, L: Abnormal spontaneous activity of globus pallidus neurons in monkeys with MPTP-induced parkinsonism. Brain Res 1991;547:142-151.
32. Obeso JA, Rodriguez-Oroz MC, Rodriguez M, et al: Pathophysiology of the basal ganglia in Parkinson's disease. Trends Neurosci 2000;23:S8-S19.
33. Bergman H, Wichmann T, DeLong MR: Reversal of experimental parkinsonism by lesions of the subthalamic nucleus. Science 1990;249:1436-1438.
34. Aziz TZ, Peggs D, Sambrook MA, Crossman AR: Lesion of the subthalamic nucleus for the alleviation of 1-methyl-4-phenyl-1,2,3,6-tetrahydropyridine (MPTP)-induced parkinsonism in the primate. Mov Disord 1991;6:288-292.
35. Guridi J, Herrero MT, Luquin MR, et al: Subthalamotomy in parkinsonian monkeys: behavioural and biochemical analysis. Brain 1996;119(Pt 5):1717-1727.
36. Delfs JM, Anegawa NJ, Chesselet MF: Glutamate decarboxylase messenger RNA in rat pallidum: comparison of the effects of haloperidol, clozapine and combined haloperidol-scopolamine treatments. Neuroscience 1995;66:67-80.
37. Hassani OK, Mouroux M, Feger J: Increased subthalamic neuronal activity after nigral dopaminergic lesion independent of disinhibition via the globus pallidus. Neuroscience 1996;72:105-115.
38. Bezard E, Boraud T, Bioulac B, Gross CE: Involvement of the subthalamic nucleus in glutamatergic compensatory mechanisms. Eur J Neurosci 1999;11:2167-2170.
39. Blandini F, Levandis G, Bazzini E, et al: Time-course of nigrostriatal damage, basal ganglia metabolic changes and behavioural alterations following intrastriatal injection of 6-hydroxydopamine in the rat: new clues from an old model. Eur J Neurosci 2007;25:397-405.

40. Soares J, Kliem MA, Betarbet R, et al: Role of external pallidal segment in primate parkinsonism: comparison of the effects of 1-methyl-4-phenyl-1,2,3,6-tetrahydropyridine-induced parkinsonism and lesions of the external pallidal segment. J Neurosci 2004;24:6417-6426.
41. Zhang J, Russo GS, Mewes K, et al: Lesions in monkey globus pallidus externus exacerbate parkinsonian symptoms. Exp Neurol 2006;199:446-453.
42. Bergman H, Wichmann T, Karmon B, DeLong MR: The primate subthalamic nucleus, II: neuronal activity in the MPTP model of parkinsonism. J Neurophysiol 1994;72:507-520.
43. Rodriguez MC, Guridi OJ, Alvarez L, et al: The subthalamic nucleus and tremor in Parkinson's disease. Mov Disord 1998;13(Suppl 3):111-118.
44. Ohye C, Shibazaki T, Hirai T, et al: Tremor-mediating thalamic zone studied in humans and in monkeys. Stereotact Funct Neurosurg 1993;60:136-145.
45. Bevan MD, Magill PJ, Terman D, et al: Move to the rhythm: oscillations in the subthalamic nucleus-external globus pallidus network. Trends Neurosci 2002;25:525-531.
46. Garcia-Cabezas MA, Rico B, Sanchez-Gonzalez MA, Cavada C: Distribution of the dopamine innervation in the macaque and human thalamus. Neuroimage 2007;34:965-984.
47. Suarez JI, Metman LV, Reich SG, et al: Pallidotomy for hemiballismus: efficacy and characteristics of neuronal activity. Ann Neurol 1997;42:807-811.
48. Obeso JA, Rodriguez-Oroz MC, Rodriguez M, et al: Pathophysiology of levodopa-induced dyskinesias in Parkinson's disease: problems with the current model. Ann Neurol 2000;47: S22-S32.
49. Carpenter MB, Whittier JR, Mettler FA: Analysis of choreoid hyperkinesia in the Rhesus monkey: surgical and pharmacological analysis of hyperkinesia resulting from lesions in the subthalamic nucleus of Luys. J Comp Neurol 1950;92:293-331.
50. Crossman AR, Sambrook MA, Jackson A: Experimental hemichorea/hemiballismus in the monkey: studies on the intracerebral site of action in a drug-induced dyskinesia. Brain 1984;107(Pt 2):579-596.
51. Mitchell IJ, Jackson A, Sambrook MA, Crossman AR: The role of the subthalamic nucleus in experimental chorea: evidence from 2-deoxyglucose metabolic mapping and horseradish peroxidase tracing studies. Brain 1989;112(Pt 6):1533-1548.
52. Papa SM, Desimone R, Fiorani M, Oldfield EH: Internal globus pallidus discharge is nearly suppressed during levodopa-induced dyskinesias. Ann Neurol 1999;46:732-738.
53. Merello M, Balej J, Delfino M, et al: Apomorphine induces changes in GPi spontaneous outflow in patients with Parkinson's disease. Mov Disord 1999;14:45-49.
54. Levy R, Herrero MT, Ruberg M, et al: Effects of nigrostriatal denervation and L-dopa therapy on the GABAergic neurons in the striatum in MPTP-treated monkeys and Parkinson's disease: an in situ hybridization study of GAD67 mRNA. Eur J Neurosci 1995;7:1199-1209.
55. Blanchet PJ, Boucher R, Bedard PJ: Excitotoxic lateral pallidotomy does not relieve L-dopa-induced dyskinesia in MPTP parkinsonian monkeys. Brain Res 1994;650:32-39.
56. Aubert I, Guigoni C, Hakansson K, et al: Increased D1 dopamine receptor signaling in levodopa-induced dyskinesia. Ann Neurol 2005;57:17-26.
57. Bezard E, Ferry S, Mach U, et al: Attenuation of levodopa-induced dyskinesia by normalizing dopamine D3 receptor function. Nat Med 2003;9:762-767.
58. Bezard E, Brotchie JM, Gross CE: Pathophysiology of levodopa-induced dyskinesia: potential for new therapies. Nat Rev Neurosci 2001;2:577-588.
59. Inase M, Buford JA, Anderson ME: Changes in the control of arm position, movement, and thalamic discharge during local inactivation in the globus pallidus of the monkey. J Neurophysiol 1996;75:1087-1104.
60. Mink JW, Thach WT: Basal ganglia motor control, I: nonexclusive relation of pallidal discharge to five movement modes. J Neurophysiol 1991;65:273-300.
61. Alkhani A, Lozano AM: Pallidotomy for parkinson disease: a review of contemporary literature. J Neurosurg 2001;94:43-49.
62. Obeso JA, Guridi J, Obeso JA, DeLong M: Surgery for Parkinson's disease. J Neurol Neurosurg Psychiatry 1997;62:2-8.
63. Jahanshahi M, Ardouin CM, Brown RG, et al: The impact of deep brain stimulation on executive function in Parkinson's disease. Brain 2000;123(Pt 6):1142-1154.
64. Rodriguez-Oroz MC, Obeso JA, Lang AE, et al: Bilateral deep brain stimulation in Parkinson's disease: a multicentre study with 4 years follow-up. Brain 2005;128:2240-2249.
65. Blanchet PJ, Konitsiotis S, Chase TN: Amantadine reduces levodopa-induced dyskinesias in parkinsonian monkeys. Mov Disord 1998;13:798-802.

66. Verhagen Metman L, Del Dotto P, van den Munckhof P, et al: Amantadine as treatment for dyskinesias and motor fluctuations in Parkinson's disease. Neurology 1998;50:1323-1326.
67. Fabbrini G, Brotchie JM, Grandas F, et al: Levodopa-induced dyskinesias. Mov Disord 2007;22: 1379-1389.
68. Bibbiani F, Oh JD, Kielaite A, et al: Combined blockade of AMPA and NMDA glutamate receptors reduces levodopa-induced motor complications in animal models of PD. Exp Neurol 2005;196: 422-429.
69. Bezard E, Hill MP, Crossman AR, et al: Levetiracetam improves choreic levodopa-induced dyskinesia in the MPTP-treated macaque. Eur J Pharmacol 2004;485:159-164.
70. Johnston TH, Brotchie JM: Drugs in development for Parkinson's disease. Curr Opin Invest Drugs 2004;5:720-726.
71. Montgomery EB Jr: Basal ganglia physiology and pathophysiology: a reappraisal. Parkinsonism Relat Disord 2007;13:455-465.
72. Brown P, Eusebio A: Paradoxes of functional neurosurgery: clues from basal ganglia recordings. Mov Disord 2008;23:12-20.
73. Marsden CD, Obeso JA: The functions of the basal ganglia and the paradox of stereotaxic surgery in Parkinson's disease. Brain 1994;117(Pt 4):877-897.

2 Genetics of Parkinson's Disease—An Overview

CHRISTINE KLEIN

Introduction

The etiology of Parkinson's disease (PD) currently remains a complex puzzle of genes, the environment, and an aging brain. Over the past decade, however, the identification of single genes for familial forms of parkinsonism has dismantled the previously held dogma of a largely nongenetic etiology for this progressive movement disorder, and has greatly advanced our understanding of the preclinical and clinical, morphological, and pathological changes seen in parkinsonism.[1]

Studying the effect of mutations in PD genes has provided unique opportunities to pursue the mechanisms of neuronal degeneration in parkinsonism, highlighting the significance of oxidative stress, mitochondrial dysfunction, and impaired protein turnover. Variants in the aforementioned genes seem to play a role in the development of the much more common, sporadic form of parkinsonism (i.e., idiopathic PD). Figure 2-1 presents a model of common pathways underlying genetic parkinsonism and idiopathic PD.

PD is clinically characterized by classic parkinsonism, which has been defined phenomenologically as the triad of bradykinesia, rigidity, and rest tremor (not all features mandatory) with a therapeutic response to levodopa, and the frequent development of motor complications.[2] The term *Parkinson's disease* historically also implies the identification of Lewy-type synucleinopathy,[3] a diagnostic feature found on autopsy that is not available in the clinical setting. Regardless of the etiology and autopsy data, in this chapter, the term *classic parkinsonism* refers to patients with the aforementioned classic clinical characteristics.

The identification of several monogenic forms of classic parkinsonism that are frequently clinically indistinguishable from idiopathic PD has shown that there are multiple known causes of parkinsonism. Although a genetic contribution to the patient's disease remains mostly untested in the clinical setting and thus unknown, the degree of genetic contributors may be significant, as convincingly shown in multigenerational population studies.[4] When estimating the percentage of all known forms of familial parkinsonism, about 2% to 3% of "idiopathic" cases can currently be identified as PD caused by a single genetic factor. This proportion may be significantly higher, however, in select populations; about 40% of PD patients of North African Arab descent and about 20% of the patients of Ashkenazi Jewish descent have been identified to carry the G2019S founder mutation in the *LRRK2* gene.[5,6]

The genes and chromosomal loci linked to familial forms of parkinsonism have been designated as PARK1 through PARK13 (Table 2–1). These loci include five autosomal dominant forms (PARK1/4, PARK3, PARK5, PARK8, and PARK13), four recessive forms (PARK2, PARK6, PARK7, and PARK9), one X-linked form (PARK12), and two forms with an as yet unknown mode of transmission (PARK10, PARK11). Mutations in two other genes have been linked to classic parkinsonism in a few families or in individual cases, but have not (yet) been assigned a PARK locus number (see Table 2–1). Also, a heterogeneous group of other monogenic conditions may include prominent parkinsonian features (Table 2–2). Finally, classic parkinsonism has been associated with numerous genetic polymorphisms in various genes that are neither sufficient nor necessary to cause disease, but may act as susceptibility factors (Table 2–3). These four different scenarios of a genetic

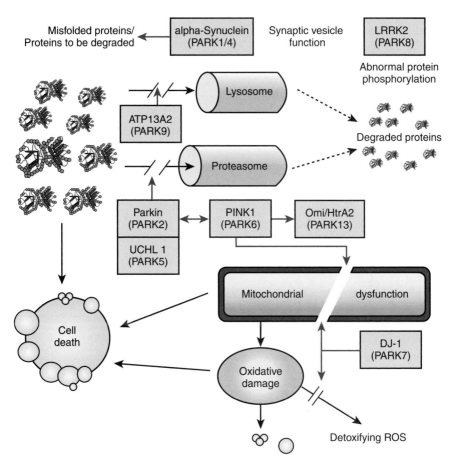

Figure 2–1 Model of common pathways underlying genetic parkinsonism (and idiopathic Parkinson's disease) with impaired protein degradation, mitochondrial dysfunction, and oxidative damage as key elements. ROS, reactive oxygen species.

contribution to the etiology of parkinsonism are reviewed, followed by a brief discussion of genetic testing of PD genes and of novel therapeutic strategies.

Monogenic Parkinsonism with a PARK Acronym

In this section, monogenic forms of parkinsonism with a PARK acronym are grouped according to their mode of inheritance. This is in agreement with functional findings that suggest a gain-of-function mechanism for dominant and a loss-of-function mechanism for recessive forms. In reality, the situation may be more complex, and this classification has been challenged by a remarkably reduced penetrance (percentage of mutation carriers that develop the disease) in dominant forms and by a putative role of single heterozygous mutations in recessive forms.[7]

TABLE 2–1	Monogenic Forms of Parkinsonism with Known Gene/Protein with or without PARK Acronym				
Acronym	Mode of Inheritance	Locus	Gene/Protein	Main Clinical Features	OMIM #
PARK1/PARK4	Autosomal dominant	4q21-q23	SNCA (α-synuclein)	Early-onset parkinsonism (~40 yr), dementia, reduced life span	168601
PARK5	Autosomal dominant	4p14	UCHL1 (ubiquitin carboxy-terminal hydrolase 1)	Classic parkinsonism	191342
PARK8	Autosomal dominant	12q12	LRRK2 (leucine-rich repeat kinase 2)	Classic parkinsonism	607060
PARK13	Probably autosomal dominant	2p12	Omi/HtrA2	Classic parkinsonism	610297
PARK2	Autosomal recessive	6q25.2-q27	Parkin	Early onset (~30-40 yr), rarely juvenile, slow disease progression, exquisite response to levodopa	600116
PARK6	Autosomal recessive	1p35-p36	PINK1 (PTEN-induced putative kinase 1)	Early onset (~30-40 yr), rarely juvenile, onset slow disease progression, exquisite response to levodopa, frequently psychiatric features	605909
PARK7	Autosomal recessive	1p36	DJ-1	Early onset (~30-40 yr), rarely juvenile onset	606324
PARK9	Autosomal recessive	1p36	ATP13A2	Juvenile or early onset, dementia, spasticity, supranuclear gaze palsy; classic early-onset parkinsonism in carriers of heterozygous mutations	606693
Not assigned	Probably autosomal dominant	5q23.1-q23.3	Synphilin-1	Classic parkinsonism	603779
Not assigned	Probably autosomal dominant	2q22-q23	NR4A2/Nurr1	Classic parkinsonism	601828

TABLE 2–2	Parkinsonism Associated with Mutations in Non-PARK Genes			
Condition	Gene	Predominant Clinical Features Other than Parkinsonism	Additional Investigations	OMIM #
Gaucher's disease	Glucocerebrosidase (GBA)	Hepatosplenomegaly, anemia	Gaucher cells on bone marrow biopsy sample; reduction in β-glucosidase activity	230800
Mitochondrial gene mutations	Polymerase gamma	Progressive external ophthalmoplegia	Ragged red fibers and Cox-negative fibers on muscle biopsy sample	174763
X-linked dystonia-parkinsonism (lubag; DYT3)	DYT3/TATA-box binding protein-associated factor 1 (TAF1)	Dystonia-parkinsonism with poor response to levodopa in male patients from the Filipino Island of Panay	Neuronal loss and astrocytosis in caudate nucleus and lateral putamen on postmortem analysis	314250
Dopa-responsive dystonia (Segawa's disease; DYT5)	GTP-cyclohydrolase I (GCHI)	Dystonia with onset in the legs and diurnal fluctuation of symptoms and worsening after exercise	Decreased levels of neopterin and biopterin in CSF	128230
Rapid-onset dystonia-parkinsonism (DYT12)	Na⁺,K⁺-ATPase alpha 3 gene (ATP1A3)	Rapid development of severe dystonia-parkinsonism with prominent bulbar features	Decreased levels of homovanillic acid in CSF in some mutation carriers	128235
Spinocerebellar ataxia 2	ATXN2	Ataxia, extremely slow saccades, dementia, facial myokymia, areflexia	Olivopontocerebellar atrophy on MRI	183090
Spinocerebellar ataxia 3	MJD/ATXN3	Ataxia, progressive supranuclear palsy, dysarthria, dysphagia, dysphonia, facial fasciculations, peripheral neuropathy	Simple enlargement of fourth ventricle to severe spinopontine atrophy sparing the olives	109150

Table continued on following page

TABLE 2–2	Parkinsonism Associated with Mutations in Non-PARK Genes (Continued)			
Condition	Gene	Predominant Clinical Features Other than Parkinsonism	Additional Investigations	OMIM #
Spinocerebellar ataxia 6	CACNA1A	Ataxia, noncerebellar signs less frequent, milder disease course than in other SCAs	Cerebellar atrophy	183086
Spinocerebellar ataxia 8	ATXN8	Ataxia, eye movement abnormalities, dysphagia, dysarthria	Cerebellar atrophy	603680
Spinocerebellar ataxia 17	TATA-binding protein (TBP)	Ataxia, dystonia, dementia, behavioral changes	Cerebellar atrophy	607136
Fragile X–associated tremor-ataxia syndrome	Premutations in the FMR1 gene	Tremor	T2 signal intensity of middle cerebellar peduncle	300623
Familial dementias	Microtubule-associated protein tau (MAPT); PROGRANULIN (GRN)	Dementia	Tau-positive neuronal and glial inclusions (MAPT); neuronal intranuclear ubiquitin-positive and TDP43-positive inclusions (PROGRANULIN)	157140
Prion disease	Prion protein	Dementia, myoclonus, ataxia	14-3-3 and other proteins in CSF; hyperintensities in putamen and caudate on MRI; periodic biphasic and triphasic sharp wave complexes on EEG	138945
Wilson's disease	ATP7B	"Flapping" tremor, dystonia, psychiatric symptoms, liver damage	Kayser-Fleischer rings; elevated copper and low ceruloplasmin levels	277990

Iron overload conditions	HFE; ferritin light chain (FTL1)	Chorea, dystonia	Granular nuclear inclusion bodies in muscle or nerve biopsy samples in neuroferritinopathy	235200
Chorea-acanthocytosis	CHAC	Facial hyperkinesias, dysarthria, dysphagia, chorea and less often dystonia, psychopathology and cognitive changes, muscle wasting and weakness	Acanthocytosis; caudate atrophy on MRI	134790
Panthothenate kinase-associated neurodegeneration	PANK2	Dysarthria, dystonia, corticospinal tract signs, neurobehavioral and cognitive problems	"Eye-of-the-tiger" sign on MRI; acanthocytosis in a subset of patients	606157
Huntington's disease–like 2	Junctophilin-3 (JPH3)	Cognitive deficits, chorea, dystonia in patients of African descent	Severe atrophy of caudate and putamen and cortical atrophy on MRI; acanthocytosis in a subset of patients	605267
Juvenile Huntington's disease	Huntington	Chorea, but juvenile parkinsonism may be the only disease manifestation; seizures in ~30%	Caudate atrophy on MRI	143100

CSF, cerebrospinal fluid; EEG, electroencephalogram; MRI, magnetic resonance imaging; SCAs, spinocerebellar ataxias.

TABLE 2–3	Genes Implicated as Susceptibility Factors Based on Association Studies*	
Chromosome	**Genes**	**OMIM #**
1	*PINK1*	605909
	ELAVL4	168360
	GSTM1	138350
2	GWA_2q.36.3	N/A
3	None	N/A
4	*UCHL1*	191342
	SNCA	168601
5	*SEMA5A*	609297
6	None	N/A
7	GWA_7p.14.2	N/A
8	None	N/A
9	None	N/A
10	None	N/A
11	None	N/A
12	*LRRK2*	607060
13	None	N/A
14	None	N/A
15	None	N/A
16	None	N/A
17	*MAPT*	157140
18	None	N/A
19	*ApoE*	107741
20	None	N/A
21	None	N/A
22	*CYP2D6*	124030
X/Y	None	N/A

*As published under "top results" at www.pdgene.org. "Top results" are derived from a continuously updated list displaying the most strongly associated genes with classic parkinsonism. The list is ranked by effect size, and includes only genes that contain at least one variant showing a nominally significant summary odds ratio in the analysis of all ethnic groups ("All"), or those limited to samples of white ancestry ("Caucasian only"). This list represents an up-to-date summary of particularly promising Parkinson's disease candidate genes that warrant follow-up with high priority; however, many may represent false-positive findings, in particular, those based on small (<10) sample sizes.

GWA, genome-wide association; N/A, not applicable.

From PDGene Website. Available at www.pdgene.org. Accessed December 18, 2007.

PARK1/4 (DOMINANT): α-SYNUCLEIN, A MAJOR COMPONENT OF LEWY BODIES

In 1997, the α-synuclein (*SNCA*) gene was the first one to be unequivocally associated with familial parkinsonism.[8] In addition to the three point mutations known to cause disease, a handful of families with parkinsonism have been identified that carry single allele triplications (initially assigned as PARK4[9]) or duplications of the wild-type *SNCA* gene.[10-13] Penetrance has been described to be 33%.[11]

The results of single photon emission computed tomography scanning were normal in unaffected mutation carriers and not different from nonmutation carriers from the same family.[14] This excludes any preclinical nigrostriatal dopaminergic deficit in these asymptomatic carriers of *SNCA* mutations that is observed (e.g., in asymptomatic carriers of heterozygous mutations in recessive PD genes). Although reduced penetrance of *SNCA* mutations may result in "pseudosporadic" occurrence of parkinsonism,[15] an *SNCA* de novo mutation has been described as a rare cause of early-onset disease without a positive family history of parkinsonism.[16] For many of the *SNCA*-linked cases, the severity of the phenotype seems to depend on gene dosage, and patients with *SNCA* duplications clinically resemble idiopathic PD patients more than patients with triplications, although the phenotypic spectrum can be remarkably broad.[12] Although missense mutations and multiplication events are extremely rare,[17] an elevated expression rate of the two wild-type *SNCA* gene copies—as a result of increased transcriptional activity—may play a role in some cases of idiopathic PD.[18]

SNCA is abundantly expressed as a 140-residue cytosolic and lipid-binding protein in the vertebrate nervous system, where it is believed to participate in the maturation of presynaptic vesicles and to function as a negative coregulator of neurotransmitter release.[19] The SNCA protein also localizes to the cytosol and the nucleus, with mutants exhibiting increased nuclear targeting in cell culture.[20] SNCA has a propensity to aggregate owing to its hydrophobic non–amyloid-beta domain. Oligomer-forming species of SNCA, along with truncated, oxidized, and phosphorylated variants, have been found in insoluble inclusions (Lewy bodies and Lewy neurites) of the human brain including *SNCA*-linked cases.[21,22]

Implications and Perspectives

Misprocessing of SNCA—at the level of its amino acid sequence, its expression rate, its post-translational modifications, or its efficient degradation—plays a key role in the development of very rare familial *and* common sporadic parkinsonism. Regarding the latter, it is crucial to elucidate the mechanism underlying *SNCA* overexpression that is represented by different, ethnically dependent patterns of association to various *SNCA* polymorphisms.

PARK5 (DOMINANT): UBIQUITIN CARBOXY-TERMINAL HYDROLASE 1, A COMPONENT OF PROTEIN DEGRADATION

A single mutation was found in the *UCHL1* (ubiquitin carboxyterminal hydrolase 1; PARK5) gene in one family with parkinsonism and caused partial loss of the hydrolytic activity of the gene product in vitro (I93M).[23] Expression of *UCHL1* is highly specific to neurons, and UCHL1 composes 2% of total soluble brain protein. UCHL1 is involved in ubiquitin-related post-translational modifications in in vitro and cell culture models; the bifunctional enzyme weakly hydrolyzes small covalent adducts of ubiquitin to release ubiquitin monomers. In addition, UCHL1 exhibits a dimerization-dependent ubiquitin ligase activity on substrates that include exogenously expressed SNCA to promote di-ubiquitylated protein modification.[24] The possible role of *UCHL1* as a susceptibility gene for PD is highly debated (see next).

Implications and Perspectives

UCHL1 as one of the key players in protein degradation is a plausible candidate to be involved in the pathogenesis of parkinsonism. Its potential role is not unequivocal, however, because a mutation has been found in a single family only, and the results of association studies are inconclusive.

PARK8 (DOMINANT): LRRK2, A MULTIDOMAIN PROTEIN WITH KINASE ACTIVITY

The *LRRK2* (leucine-rich repeat kinase 2) gene has been identified by two independent groups,[25,26] and is now recognized as the most common known cause of familial and sporadic parkinsonism. Mutations in the *LRRK2* gene are often, but not exclusively,[27-29] associated with late-onset, classic parkinsonism. *LRRK2* is a large gene that consists of 51 exons encoding a 2527-amino acid protein named LRRK2 featuring several functional domains.[25,26] To date, more than 50 variants have been reported in this gene.[30-38] Because of often markedly reduced penetrance and a possible gender effect,[39] the role of some of these variants currently remains uncertain, and it is possible that certain genotypes represent a susceptibility factor. The most frequent and best studied mutation is the c.6055G>A (p.G2019S) substitution, which accounts for approximately 1.5% of all index cases with late-onset, classic parkinsonism.[36,40] At least 29 patients have been described to carry the frequent p.G2019S mutation in the homozygous state. There were no observable differences, however, between the homozygous and the heterozygous carriers, arguing against a gene dosage effect.[41] There is a high degree of neuropathological heterogeneity even in members of the same family carrying an identical mutation, ranging from Lewy body–positive parkinsonism, to diffuse Lewy body disease, to nigral degeneration without distinctive histopathology, to progressive supranuclear palsy–like pathology.[42]

The multidomain LRRK2 functions as a protein kinase in ex vivo studies, mutations of which alter its phosphorylation activity through a proposed gain-of-function mechanism.[43-48] Unexpectedly, the expression rate of the *LRRK2* gene (e.g., compared with the *parkin* or *DJ-1* gene) in mammalian brain is low in the predominantly affected dopamine neurons of the human substantia nigra,[49] whereas high expression rates of *LRRK2* were found in striatal neurons that receive dopaminergic input.[49]

Implications and Perspectives

LRRK2 is the only gene that plays a considerable, albeit mostly small, role in late-onset sporadic parkinsonism, with mutation frequencies ranging from 2% to 40% in different populations. Important research questions include the exact function of the LRRK2 protein, the range of physiological (and possibly pathological) substrates for the kinase activity, and factors influencing (reduced) penetrance of *LRRK2* mutations.

PARK13 (DOMINANT): OMI/HTRA2, A SERINE PROTEASE

In contrast to the other known PD genes, the *Omi/HtrA2* gene was not discovered by linkage analysis in families with multiple affected members, but was selected as an attractive PD candidate gene based on the observation that loss of Omi/HtrA2 causes neurodegeneration with parkinsonian features in mice.[50] This observation led to the detection of a novel heterozygous missense mutation (G399S) in four unrelated patients with classic parkinsonism.[51] Further supporting a possible role of this gene in the etiology of parkinsonism, a polymorphism (A141S) was significantly more common among patients and controls.

In vitro studies showed that both sequence variants induced mitochondrial dysfunction and were associated with altered mitochondrial morphology. In addition, cells overexpressing the G399S mutation were more susceptible to stress-induced cell death than wild-type cells.[51] Omi/HtrA2 was identified as a component of about a third of the stained Lewy bodies, predominantly in the halo (i.e., in a similar distribution as SNCA).[51] More recently, Omi/HtrA2 has been shown to be regulated by PINK1, another known PD protein.[52] Both proteins apparently are components of the same stress-sensing pathway. Omi/HtrA2 is phosphorylated on activation of the p38 pathway, in a PINK1-dependent manner, at an amino acid adjacent to G399. Omi/HtrA2 phosphorylation was decreased in brains of patients with PINK1-associated parkinsonism.[52]

Implications and Perspectives

The mutation frequency of *Omi/HtrA2* (in classic parkinsonism) remains to be determined, as does its putative role as a susceptibility factor in idiopathic PD. The discovery of Omi/HtrA2 as an important interactor of *PINK1* (and *parkin*) stresses its importance and adds crucial momentum to the concept that mitochondrial dysfunction is a key element in the pathogenesis of parkinsonism.

PARK2 (RECESSIVE): PARKIN, AN E3-UBIQUITIN LIGASE

Overall, *parkin* mutation carriers tend to have an earlier age at disease onset, tend to have a slower disease progression, and often show a better response to levodopa than patients without *parkin* mutations.[53] Only two of the six *parkin* mutant PD brains that have been autopsied showed typical Lewy bodies, whereas the other four did not.[54] Today, mutations in the *parkin* gene[55] represent the most common known factor responsible for early-onset parkinsonism (10% to 20%), and have been found across all tested ethnic groups.[56] The large number and wide spectrum of *parkin* mutations include small mutations and exon rearrangements in each of its 12 exons.[57]

The gene product, called parkin, is an E3-type ubiquitin ligase that is involved in the proteasomal degradation of target proteins.[58] The available E3 activity of many (but not all) PD-linked mutants is disrupted in ex vivo experiments; others affect the solubility, localization, and binding properties of parkin.[59,60] Parkin has been shown to mediate proteasome-independent mono-ubiquitylation[61] and proteasome-linked poly-ubiquitylation of target proteins, which—when taken together with the neuropathological evidence—led several authors to postulate that the parkin protein is essential in Lewy body formation.[62-63] Reduced ubiquitin ligase activity may only be one of several pathogenetic mechanisms,[64] however, because in vivo studies have delineated an essential role for fly and mouse parkin in mitochondrial integrity.[65-67]

Implications and Perspectives

parkin mutations are the most common known cause of early-onset classic parkinsonism, and modifications of wild-type parkin activity may be involved in sporadic disease. Important future research aims include further elucidation of the different mechanisms of action of *parkin* mutants and the validation of suggested and identification of novel, relevant parkin substrates.

PARK6 (RECESSIVE): PINK1, A MITOCHONDRIAL PROTEIN KINASE

Two homozygous mutations in the *PINK1* (PTEN-induced kinase 1) gene were initially described in three consanguineous families with autosomal recessive (and "*parkin*-negative"), early-onset parkinsonism.[68] The frequency of *PINK1* mutations ranges from 1% to 8% in patients of different ethnicities (often selected for their young age of onset and positive family history).[69-74] Most of the currently described mutations are located near or within the functional serine/threonine kinase domain of PINK1. Wild-type PINK1 protein is mainly located inside mitochondria.[75-80]

A pro-mitochondrial function has been shown for endogenous pink1 in elegant fly models,[81-84] in human cells,[85] and in conjunction with Omi/HtrA2 as described previously. The first identified cellular substrate for PINK1 was TNF receptor–associated protein 1 (TRAP1), a mitochondrial molecular chaperone, also known as heat shock protein 75. PINK1 binds and colocalizes with TRAP1 in mitochondria and phosphorylates TRAP1 in vitro and in vivo. The ability of PINK1 to promote TRAP1 phosphorylation and cell survival is impaired by known pathogenic PINK1 mutations.[86] In human brain, PINK1 occurs as a full-length preprotein (66 kD) and as an N-terminally truncated mature form (55 kD). More recently, PINK1 has been identified as a client kinase of the Cdc37/Hsp90 chaperone system and was shown not to localize exclusively to mitochondria.[87]

The Cdc37/Hsp90 chaperone system influences the 66 kD-to-55 kD protein ratio and the subcellular localization of PINK1. Cells show an increased mitochondrial pool of PINK1 in the presence of overexpressed parkin, providing further evidence for a common pathogenic pathway involving PINK1 and parkin.[87] Evoked dopamine release in striatal slices from a PINK1 mouse model with a germline deletion of exons 4 through 7 was reduced, and intracellular recordings of striatal medium spiny neurons, the major dopaminergic target, showed specific impairments of corticostriatal long-term potentiation and depression that could be rescued by levodopa and dopamine agonists.[88] Loss of PINK1 function in mouse brain did not cause severe mitochondrial morphological defects, however, further highlighting the lack of genetic mouse models that replicate the clinical and pathological findings in humans.[89]

Implications and Perspectives

PINK1 mutations are rarer than *parkin* mutations, but still explain numerous early-onset cases. Future research is expected to establish and clarify further the role of PINK1 in (impaired) mitochondrial function in *PINK1*-associated and non-genetic classic parkinsonism, and its interplay with other PD proteins, such as parkin, TRAP1, and Omi/HtrA2.

PARK7 (RECESSIVE): DJ-1, A PROTEIN WITH ANTIOXIDATIVE FUNCTION

The *DJ-1* gene[90] is associated with early-onset parkinsonism in about 1% to 2% of cases.[91] The *DJ-1* gene is ubiquitously expressed, and was initially described in association with oncogenesis and male rat infertility. DJ-1 has been shown in mice to coregulate D2 dopamine receptor signaling.[92] The protein has also been found to confer chaperone-like activity, and several more recent reports convincingly showed that DJ-1 functions as an intracellular sensor of oxidative stress.[93] Within the conserved sequence of DJ-1, the oxidation of Cys106 seems to play a crucial role in the response to oxidative stress in vivo.[93-95] Although DJ-1 knockout mice lacking exons 2 and 3 do not display any observable degeneration of central dopaminergic pathways, and are anatomically and behaviorally similar to wild-type mice, there is upregulation of mitochondrial manganese superoxide dismutase and glutathione peroxidase in older mice.[96] Knockout mice have a deficit in scavenging mitochondrial hydrogen peroxide owing to the impaired function of DJ-1 as an atypical peroxiredoxin-like peroxidase.[96]

Implications and Perspectives

Clinically, *DJ-1* mutations play only a minor role even among patients with early-onset disease. DJ-1 function seems to be at an important juncture, however, of maintaining mitochondrial function and redox equilibrium with possible implications in sporadic disease, which need to be elucidated further.

PARK9 (RECESSIVE): ATP13A2, A LYSOSOMAL ATPASE

In 2006, mutations in the *ATP13A2* gene were detected in patients from two families with recessively inherited Kufor-Rakeb syndrome.[97] These patients have early-onset, atypical parkinsonism that features rapid progression, a transient response to levodopa treatment, and additional neurological findings including pyramidal signs and dementia.[98] Single heterozygous *ATP13A2* mutations have been associated more recently with juvenile or early-onset but otherwise classic parkinsonism in three patients.[99]

The *ATP13A2* gene encodes a previously uncharacterized, predominantly neuronal ATPase. The ATP13A2 protein has 10 transmembrane domains that are affected by known mutations. In transiently transfected cells, the wild-type protein is localized to the lysosomes, whereas truncated mutants were retained in the endoplasmic reticulum and degraded by the proteasome.[97] The *ATP13A2* gene product joins a growing list of proteins linking central nervous system diseases with abnormal function of lysosomes and related macroautophagy.[100,101]

ATP13A2 is predominantly expressed in brain tissues. About 10-fold higher *ATP13A2* mRNA levels were detected in substantia nigra dopaminergic neurons from patients with sporadic disease compared with control brains.[97]

Implications and Perspectives

Kufor-Rakeb syndrome is not a form of classic parkinsonism and is probably a rare condition. Mutational analysis of this gene and association studies in larger patient samples with atypical and classic parkinsonism should elucidate further the role of this gene (and the role of heterozygous mutations) in different forms of parkinsonism. Future research also is expected to explore further the suggested link of parkinsonism pathogenesis to lysosomal pathways of protein degradation.

DIGENIC PARKINSONISM

Numerous patients have been reported with mutations in more than one of the known PD genes, including one patient with heterozygous missense mutations in *DJ-1* and *PINK1*. Coexpression of both mutants in a cell culture model significantly potentiated susceptibility to 1-methyl-4-phenylpyridinium (MPP) (+)-induced cell death, suggesting a neuroprotective collaboration of DJ-1 and PINK1.[102]

Several patients carried combined mutations in *LRRK2* and *parkin*.[5,33,103,104] These patients did not present with an earlier age at onset or a faster disease progression compared with patients with a single *LRRK2* or *parkin* mutation, not supporting a synergistic effect of *LRRK2* and *parkin*. In cultured cells, a direct interaction of both proteins has been shown, however, by coimmunoprecipitation with overexpressed *LRRK2*.[46]

Implications and Perspectives

These findings of digenic inheritance further support the notion that there may be interactions of different (mutated) proteins in individual patients with genetic parkinsonism. Similarly, variants of different proteins that are not pathogenic by themselves but increase disease susceptibility may act together to increase the risk for the much more frequent idiopathic PD.

Monogenic Parkinsonism without a PARK Acronym

ADDITIONAL CANDIDATE GENES FOR PARKINSONISM: *NURR1* AND SYNPHILIN-1

Two different mutations in the 5′-untranslated region of *Nurr1* (*NR4A2*), a member of a nuclear receptor family, were found in 10 European families with parkinsonism. They resulted in a marked decrease in *Nurr1* mRNA levels in transfected cell lines and in lymphocytes of affected individuals.[105] A third, novel mutation has been identified in a sporadic patient and has been predicted to affect phosphorylation.[106] *Nurr1* is highly expressed in brain and is crucial to the development and survival of dopaminergic cells. All other studies searching for *Nurr1* mutations in European patients with parkinsonism failed, however, to detect either of the two known or any other mutations in this gene,[107-109] suggesting that *Nurr1* mutations are a very rare cause of parkinsonism.

A mutation in synphilin-1, a gene encoding an α-synuclein–interacting protein and a substrate of *parkin* in cellular coexpression studies,[110,111] has been found in two individuals.[112] Synphilin-1 is expressed in the heart, placenta, and many regions of the brain, including the substantia nigra pars compacta, and is present in Lewy bodies. In cell culture models, it is capable of producing cytoplasmic inclusions.

Implications and Perspectives

Although a role of the candidate genes *Nurr1* and synphilin-1 in the etiology of parkinsonism is conceivable, confirmation in larger patient series is awaited.

Parkinsonism Associated with Mutations in Non-PARK Genes

HETEROZYGOUS MUTATIONS IN THE GLUCOCEREBROSIDASE GENE: ASSOCIATION WITH CLASSIC PARKINSONISM

Gaucher's disease is the most common of the lipidoses and among the most frequently inherited recessive disorders in Ashkenazi Jews. An association between Gaucher's disease and PD has been suggested by the co-occurrence of parkinsonism in rare cases on the one hand, and by the identification of glucocerebrosidase (*GBA*) mutations in probands with PD on the other.[113,114] Further supporting this link, obligate or confirmed carriers of *GBA* mutations from 10 families developed parkinsonism.[115] While *GBA* mutations have been found, mostly in the heterozygous state, in 31% of patients with classic parkinsonism from Israel,[113] these mutations accounted for 12% in a Venezuelan cohort with very early onset,[116] 6% in a sample of white patients from Canada,[117] 4.3% in ethnic Chinese patients,[118] and only 2.3% in Norwegian patients with PD.[119]

MITOCHONDRIAL GENE MUTATIONS: A VERY RARE CAUSE OF CLASSIC PARKINSONISM

Autosomal dominant mutations in the DNA polymerase gamma (*POLG*) and the twinkle genes are found in patients who present with predominant progressive external ophthalmoplegia and in some of the mutation carriers with concomitant features of parkinsonism.[120,121] Although compound heterozygous *POLG* mutations have been identified in two sisters with early-onset parkinsonism in the absence of progressive external ophthalmoplegia,[122] *POLG* mutations seem to be an exceedingly rare cause of classic parkinsonism. In single families, several different point mutations of mitochondrial genes have been identified in patients with maternally inherited parkinsonism, including the cytochrome b gene, the *12sRNA* gene, and *tRNA* genes.[123,124] Patients from such families usually present with additional signs, however, such as deafness and neuropathy.

DYSTONIA-PARKINSONISM: DYSTONIA-PLUS SYNDROMES THAT MAY MANIFEST WITH PARKINSONISM (DYT3, DYT5, DYT12)

DYT3 dystonia is inherited in an X-linked recessive fashion with complete penetrance by the end of the fifth decade. Specific sequence changes in a multiple transcript system "DYT3" are associated with X-linked dystonia-parkinsonism.[125] This multiple transcript system has been shown to contain several of the *TAF1* (TATA-box binding protein-associated factor 1) exons.[126,127] X-linked dystonia-parkinsonism is clinically characterized by dystonia-parkinsonism and occurs almost exclusively in men from the Island of Panay in the Philippines.[128] Parkinsonism commonly is an early sign and may precede the onset of dystonia.

The dominantly inherited form of levodopa-responsive dystonia (DYT5; Segawa's disease) is associated with mutations in the GTP cyclohydrolase I (*GCHI*) gene (DYT5a). *GCHI* encodes the enzyme GTPCH, which catalyzes the first step in the biosynthesis of tetrahydrobiopterin (cofactor for TH) as a homodecamer.[129] In patients, there is a decrease in GTPCH activity as a result of a dominant negative effect of the mutated allele, leading to dopamine depletion and explaining the remarkable therapeutic effect of levodopa substitution. Levodopa-responsive dystonia is usually characterized by childhood onset of dystonia, diurnal fluctuation of symptoms, and a dramatic response to levodopa therapy. Later in the course of the disease, parkinsonian features frequently occur,[130] or may even be the sole clinical manifestation.[131]

Rapid-onset dystonia-parkinsonism (DYT12) is a rare, autosomal dominant movement disorder associated with different mutations in the Na+, K+-ATPase alpha 3 gene (*ATP1A3*).[132] Symptoms usually manifest over hours to weeks and may be followed by moderate or no progression, and are sometimes preceded by mild (focal) dystonia.[133] Parkinsonian features of rapid-onset dystonia-parkinsonism primarily include bradykinesia and postural instability[133] with or without rigidity[134] but rarely tremor.

SPINOCEREBELLAR ATAXIAS: CLASSIC PARKINSONISM CAUSED BY SPINOCEREBELLAR ATAXIA MUTATIONS

Patients with mutations in some of the dominant ataxia genes that are associated with ataxia and degeneration of other neuronal systems (*ADCAI*) may present with parkinsonian features and, rarely, with isolated, classic parkinsonism.[135] Parkinsonism has been described as a prominent sign in some patients and families with SCA2, SCA3, SCA8, and SCA17, and may occur as a mild, additional feature in some of the other spinocerebellar ataxia gene (*SCA*) mutations, such as SCA6.[136]

A detailed review of other hereditary conditions sometimes associated with (atypical) parkinsonism is beyond the scope of this chapter. These conditions include an assortment of different diseases, such as the fragile X–associated tremor/ataxia syndrome, familial dementias, prion disease, Wilson's disease, iron overload conditions, neuroacanthocytosis, panthothenate kinase–associated neurodegeneration, juvenile Huntington's disease, and Huntington's disease–like 2.

Implications and Perspectives

Although none of the diseases discussed in this section are usually characterized by isolated classic parkinsonism, some cases with mutations in non-PARK genes may clinically mimic idiopathic PD: Patients in this mixed category harbor mutations in genes associated with metabolic or mitochondrial disorders or in one of the dystonia (*DYT*) or spinocerebellar ataxia (*SCA*) genes, and should be considered in the differential diagnosis of genetic parkinsonism.

Genetic Susceptibility Factors for Parkinson Disease

As outlined previously, monogenic forms of parkinsonism and their potential additive and interacting effects account only for rare cases. There are different ways to identify genetic susceptibility factors for parkinsonism: case-control studies of candidate genes that are selected based on their known involvement in parkinsonism or their function, genome-wide association studies, or large-scale expression studies. A growing body of conflicting data has accumulated in the literature, however, raising important questions regarding the exact role of susceptibility genes in parkinsonism.

Several common variants in genes implicated in hereditary forms of parkinsonism have been investigated as predisposing factors for sporadic, classic parkinsonism (see Table 2–3). A detailed list of published association studies and meta-analyses is available at the following website: www.pdgene.org.

Single heterozygous mutations in some of the "recessive" parkinsonism-linked genes (e.g., *parkin* and *PINK1*) are frequently found in patients with parkinsonism and seem to act as susceptibility factors.[7] This has been widely noticed for *PINK1* mutations.[73,137-141] Further supporting a role of heterozygous *PINK1* mutations, 6 of 11 heterozygous offspring of affected homozygous carriers presented with mild signs of parkinsonism.[141] For *parkin,* the role of single heterozygous mutations is less well defined. Two of three case-control studies found similar frequencies of heterozygous mutations in patients and healthy controls.[142,143] In contrast, one study could not detect *parkin* alterations in more than 100 comprehensively tested controls.[144] A correlation of the age at onset and the number of mutated alleles had been suggested[145] and was confirmed more recently: Individuals with only one mutated allele had disease onset about 10 years later than individuals with two mutated alleles.[146]

As previously mentioned, genetic polymorphisms in PD genes (i.e., nucleotide variations that are found within a given species at a frequency of >1%) may be associated with disease, such as the p.G2385 LRRK2 polymorphism that seems to confer an increased risk to develop parkinsonism in ethnic Chinese patients.[147] In contrast, the widely cited role of the p.S18Y polymorphism in UCHL-1 as a protective factor for parkinsonism has been questioned by a new large case-control study comprising more than 3000 individuals that did not find such an association.[148] One more recent paper reported a screen of 121 functional candidate genes known to be involved in mitochondrial functions, oxidative stress, and proteasome function, and revealed a single nucleotide polymorphism in the *SNCA* gene as a susceptibility factor,[149] stressing the proposed role of *SNCA* in the etiology of sporadic PD.[18]

A second way to identify susceptibility genes is genome-wide genotyping. One study identified 26 single nucleotide polymorphisms with notably different allele frequencies between patients and controls.[150] Replication studies could not confirm the suggested associations, however,[151,152,153] or even showed an opposite effect.[154] Publicly available genome-wide single nucleotide polymorphism genotype data have been provided on 267 patients and 270 neurologically normal control subjects.[155]

Third, a microarray-based gene expression study on different brain regions from patients compared with controls showed an altered expression pattern for 11 genes in most studied regions. Their function was related to apoptosis, cell signaling, and cell cycle control.[156] It is unclear, however, whether these changes are a cause or a consequence of the cell loss. Similarly, a quantitative approach on protein levels identified 119 of 842 tested nigral mitochondrial proteins to display significant differences in their relative abundance between patients and age-matched controls.[157]

Implications and Perspectives

Only a few polymorphisms in candidate genes have clearly stood the test of replication. Even for those, their exact contribution to sporadic PD remains largely elusive, especially in the individual patient, and depends on ethnicity. Although it seems likely that several polymorphisms, in the same or in different genes, act together to confer susceptibility, it is highly difficult to disentangle these interactions and to take into account the probable additional roles of epigenetics (reversible, heritable changes in gene expression without a change in DNA sequence) or of the environment.

Genetic Testing for Parkinsonism

Mutation screening has become available on a commercial basis for most of the monogenic forms of parkinsonism. Genetic testing is complicated, however, by the fact that there are few clinically recognizable features that might aid in prioritizing patients for screening of specific genes. In addition, the analysis of all parkinsonism genes is laborious and expensive because of the large size of many genes and the variability of gene mutations. Further adding to the complexity of genetic testing in classic parkinsonism, the interpretation of the results is often difficult because of the issues of reduced penetrance of mutations in dominant genes, variable disease expressivity, and the uncertain role of heterozygous mutations in recessive genes and of susceptibility genes. Finally, the diagnosis of a positively identified, genetic form of parkinsonism does not yet lead to any different therapeutic intervention.[158-160]

Although guidelines for genetic parkinsonism have yet to be established, progress has been made regarding improved screening of large patient and control cohorts for common mutations in a single experiment: First, for gene dosage alterations that are frequent in several genes associated with parkinsonism, multiplex ligation-dependent probe amplification has been shown to be a reliable method for cost-effective identification of this type of mutations.[161] Second, a microarray detects 65 known *parkin* mutations (single base pair substitutions and small deletions/insertions) using arrayed primer extension technology.[162]

Implications and Perspectives

Although molecular genetic testing has become available for most known forms of hereditary parkinsonism, genetic testing guidelines are still lacking. A particular challenge in genetic counseling of patients is posed by the markedly reduced penetrance of mutations in dominant PD genes, and by the likely role of heterozygous mutations in recessive genes as a susceptibility factor.

Novel Therapeutic Strategies

Based on the proposed loss-of-function or gain-of-function mechanisms of mutated proteins, an increase of parkin, PINK1, and DJ-1 and a decrease of SNCA and LRRK2 levels and function might be considered beneficial. Toxicity conferred by increased nuclear targeting of SNCA mutants can be reduced by cytoplasmic sequestration. Because of direct binding of SNCA to histones and involvement in histone acetylation, toxicity can be rescued by histone deacetylase inhibitors, offering a potential therapeutic mechanism.[20] Similarly, blocking self-association of LRRK2 may be a novel therapeutic strategy.[89] Many other potential future therapeutic strategies are based on genetics, including modulation of calcium currents,[163,164] modification of the effects of noncoding microRNAs,[165] or induction of pluripotent stem cells from adult human fibroblasts through genetic reprogramming followed by differentiation into dopaminergic neurons.[166]

Implications and Perspectives

The past decade has witnessed the molecular genetic revolution of parkinsonism. It is hoped that the anticipated next phase will see the successful translation of genetic clues into therapies for patients that specifically and causally treat the different forms of parkinsonism.

Acknowledgment

Christine Klein is supported by a Lichtenberg Grant from the Volkswagen Foundation and a career development award from the Hermann and Lilly Schilling foundation.

REFERENCES

1. Thomas B, Beal MF: Parkinson's disease. Hum Mol Genet 2007;16(Spec No. 2):R183-R194.
2. Galpern WR, Lang AE: Interface between tauopathies and synucleinopathies: a tale of two proteins. Ann Neurol 2006;59:449-458.
3. Gibb WR, Lees AJ: The relevance of the Lewy body to the pathogenesis of idiopathic Parkinson's disease. J Neurol Neurosurg Psychiatry 1988;51:745-752.
4. Sveinbjornsdottir S, Hicks AA, Jonsson T, et al: Familial aggregation of Parkinson's disease in Iceland. N Engl J Med 2000;343:1765-1770.
5. Lesage S, Durr A, Tazir M, et al: LRRK2 G2019S as a cause of Parkinson's disease in North African Arabs. N Engl J Med 2006;354:422-423.
6. Ozelius LJ, Senthil G, Saunders-Pullman R, et al: LRRK2 G2019S as a cause of Parkinson's disease in Ashkenazi Jews. N Engl J Med 2006;354:424-425.
7. Klein C, Lohmann-Hedrich K, Rogaeva E, et al: Deciphering the role of heterozygous mutations in genes associated with parkinsonism. Lancet Neurol 2007;6:652-662.
8. Polymeropoulos MH, Lavedan C, Leroy E, et al: Mutation in the alpha-synuclein gene identified in families with Parkinson's disease. Science 1997;276:2045-2047.
9. Singleton AB, Farrer M, Johnson J, et al: alpha-Synuclein locus triplication causes Parkinson's disease. Science 2003;302:841.
10. Singleton A, Gwinn-Hardy K: Parkinson's disease and dementia with Lewy bodies: a difference in dose? Lancet 2004;364:1105-1107.
11. Nishioka K, Hayashi S, Farrer MJ, et al: Clinical heterogeneity of alpha-synuclein gene duplication in Parkinson's disease. Ann Neurol 2006;59:298-309.
12. Fuchs J, Nilsson C, Kachergus J, et al: Phenotypic variation in a large Swedish pedigree due to SNCA duplication and triplication. Neurology 2007;68:916-922.
13. Farrer MJ: Genetics of Parkinson disease: paradigm shifts and future prospects. Nat Rev Genet 2006;7:306-318.
14. Ahn TB, Kim SY, Kim JY, et al: Alpha-synuclein gene duplication is present in sporadic Parkinson disease. Neurology 2008;1;70(1):43-9:E7.
15. Troiano AR, Cazeneuve C, Le Ber I, et al: Alpha-synuclein gene duplication is present in sporadic Parkinson disease. Neurology 2008;71(16):1295.

16. Brueggemann N, Per O, Grünewald A, et al: Alpha-synuclein gene duplication is present sporadic Parkinson disease. Neurology.
17. Berg D, Niwar M, Maass S, et al: Alpha-synuclein and Parkinson's disease: implications from the screening of more than 1,900 patients. Mov Disord 2005;20:1191-1194.
18. Maraganore DM, de Andrade M, Elbaz A, et al: Collaborative analysis of alpha-synuclein gene promoter variability and Parkinson disease. JAMA 2006;296:661-670.
19. Vekrellis K, Rideout HJ, Stefanis L: Neurobiology of alpha-synuclein. Mol Neurobiol 2004;30: 1-22.
20. Kontopoulos E, Parvin JD, Feany MB: Alpha-synuclein acts in the nucleus to inhibit histone acetylation and promote neurotoxicity. Hum Mol Genet 2006;15:3012-3023.
21. Anderson JP, Walker DE, Goldstein JM, et al: Phosphorylation of Ser-129 is the dominant pathological modification of alpha-synuclein in familial and sporadic Lewy body disease. J Biol Chem 2006;281:29739-29752.
22. Spillantini MG, Schmidt ML, Lee VM, et al: Alpha-synuclein in Lewy bodies. Nature 1997;388: 839-840.
23. Leroy E, Boyer R, Auburger G, et al: The ubiquitin pathway in Parkinson's disease. Nature 1998;395:451-452.
24. Liu Y, Fallon L, Lashuel HA, et al: The UCH-L1 gene encodes two opposing enzymatic activities that affect alpha-synuclein degradation and Parkinson's disease susceptibility. Cell 2002;111: 209-218.
25. Zimprich A, Biskup S, Leitner P, et al: Mutations in LRRK2 cause autosomal-dominant parkinsonism with pleomorphic pathology. Neuron 2004;44:601-607.
26. Paisan-Ruiz C, Jain S, Evans EW, et al: Cloning of the gene containing mutations that cause PARK8-linked Parkinson's disease. Neuron 2004;44:595-600.
27. Kay DM, Zabetian CP, Factor SA, et al: Parkinson's disease and LRRK2: frequency of a common mutation in U.S. movement disorder clinics. Mov Disord 2006;21:519-523.
28. Goldwurm S, Di Fonzo A, Simons EJ, et al: The G6055A (G2019S) mutation in LRRK2 is frequent in both early and late onset Parkinson's disease and originates from a common ancestor. J Med Genet 2005;42:e65.
29. Hedrich K, Winkler S, Hagenah J, et al: Recurrent LRRK2 (Park8) mutations in early-onset Parkinson's disease. Mov Disord 2006;21:1506-1510.
30. Funayama M, Hasegawa K, Ohta E, et al: An LRRK2 mutation as a cause for the parkinsonism in the original PARK8 family. Ann Neurol 2005;57:918-921.
31. Zabetian CP, Samii A, Mosley AD, et al: A clinic-based study of the LRRK2 gene in Parkinson disease yields new mutations. Neurology 2005;65:741-744.
32. Farrer M, Stone J, Mata IF, et al: LRRK2 mutations in Parkinson disease. Neurology 2005;65:738-740.
33. Paisan-Ruiz C, Lang AE, Kawarai T, et al: LRRK2 gene in Parkinson disease: mutation analysis and case control association study. Neurology 2005;65:696-700.
34. Mata IF, Kachergus JM, Taylor JP, et al: Lrrk2 pathogenic substitutions in Parkinson's disease. Neurogenetics 2005;6:171-177.
35. Kachergus J, Mata IF, Hulihan M, et al: Identification of a novel LRRK2 mutation linked to autosomal dominant parkinsonism: evidence of a common founder across European populations. Am J Hum Genet 2005;76:672-680.
36. Lesage S, Ibanez P, Lohmann E, et al: G2019S LRRK2 mutation in French and North African families with Parkinson's disease. Ann Neurol 2005;58:784-787.
37. Berg D, Schweitzer K, Leitner P, et al: Type and frequency of mutations in the LRRK2 gene in familial and sporadic Parkinson's disease. Brain 2005;128:3000-3011.
38. Di Fonzo A, Tassorelli C, De Mari M, et al: Comprehensive analysis of the LRRK2 gene in sixty families with Parkinson's disease. Eur J Hum Genet 2006;14:322-331.
39. Orr-Urtreger A, Shifrin C, Rozovski U, et al: The LRRK2 G2019S mutation in Ashkenazi Jews with Parkinson disease: is there a gender effect? Neurology 2007;69:1595-1602.
40. Kay DM, Kramer P, Higgins D, et al: Escaping Parkinson's disease: a neurologically healthy octogenarian with the LRRK2 G2019S mutation. Mov Disord 2005;20:1077-1078.
41. Ishihara L, Warren L, Gibson R, et al: Clinical features of Parkinson disease patients with homozygous leucine-rich repeat kinase 2 G2019S mutations. Arch Neurol 2006;63:1250-1254.
42. Wszolek ZK, Pfeiffer RF, Tsuboi Y, et al: Autosomal dominant parkinsonism associated with variable synuclein and tau pathology. Neurology 2004;62(9):1619-1622.
43. Gloeckner CJ, Kinkl N, Schumacher A, et al: The Parkinson disease causing LRRK2 mutation I2020T is associated with increased kinase activity. Hum Mol Genet 2006;15:223-232.

44. Smith WW, Pei Z, Jiang H, et al: Kinase activity of mutant LRRK2 mediates neuronal toxicity. Nat Neurosci 2006;9:1231-1233.
45. West AB, Moore DJ, Biskup S, et al: Parkinson's disease-associated mutations in leucine-rich repeat kinase 2 augment kinase activity. Proc Natl Acad Sci U S A 2005;102:16842-16847.
46. Smith WW, Pei Z, Jiang H, et al: Leucine-rich repeat kinase 2 (LRRK2) interacts with parkin, and mutant LRRK2 induces neuronal degeneration. Proc Natl Acad Sci U S A 2005;102:18676-18681.
47. Greggio E, Jain S, Kingsbury A, et al: Kinase activity is required for the toxic effects of mutant LRRK2/dardarin. Neurobiol Dis 2006;23:329-341.
48. Mata IF, Wedemeyer WJ, Farrer MJ, et al: LRRK2 in Parkinson's disease: protein domains and functional insights. Trends Neurosci 2006;29:286-293.
49. Galter D, Westerlund M, Carmine A, et al: LRRK2 expression linked to dopamine-innervated areas. Ann Neurol 2006;59:714-719.
50. Martins LM, Morrison A, Klupsch K, et al: Neuroprotective role of the Reaper-related serine protease HtrA2/Omi revealed by targeted deletion in mice. Mol Cell Biol 2004;24:9848-9862.
51. Strauss KM, Martins LM, Plun-Favreau H, et al: Loss of function mutations in the gene encoding Omi/HtrA2 in Parkinson's disease. Hum Mol Genet 2005;14:2099-2111.
52. Plun-Favreau H, Klupsch K, Moisoi N, et al: The mitochondrial protease HtrA2 is regulated by Parkinson's disease-associated kinase PINK1. Nat Cell Biol 2007;9:1243-1252.
53. Lohmann E, Periquet M, Bonifati V, et al: How much phenotypic variation can be attributed to parkin genotype? Ann Neurol 2003;54:176-185.
54. Pramstaller PP, Schlossmacher MG, Jacques TS, et al: Lewy body Parkinson's disease in a large pedigree with. 77 Parkin mutation carriers. Ann Neurol 2005;58:411-422.
55. Kitada T, Asakawa S, Hattori N, et al: Mutations in the parkin gene cause autosomal recessive juvenile parkinsonism. Nature 1998;392:605-608.
56. Hedrich K, Eskelson C, Wilmot B, et al: Distribution, type, and origin of Parkin mutations: review and case studies. Mov Disord 2004;19:1146-1157.
57. Hedrich K, Kann M, Lanthaler AJ, et al: The importance of gene dosage studies: mutational analysis of the parkin gene in early-onset parkinsonism. Hum Mol Genet 2001;10:1649-1656.
58. Shimura H, Hattori N, Kubo S, et al: Familial Parkinson disease gene product, parkin, is a ubiquitin-protein ligase. Nat Genet 2000;25:302-305.
59. Sriram SR, Li X, Ko HS, et al: Familial-associated mutations differentially disrupt the solubility, localization, binding and ubiquitination properties of parkin. Hum Mol Genet 2005;14:2571-2586.
60. Matsuda N, Kitami T, Suzuki T, et al: Diverse effects of pathogenic mutations of Parkin that catalyze multiple monoubiquitylation in vitro. J Biol Chem 2006;281:3204-3209.
61. Hampe C, Ardila-Osorio H, Fournier M, et al: Biochemical analysis of Parkinson's disease-causing variants of Parkin, an E3 ubiquitin-protein ligase with monoubiquitylation capacity. Hum Mol Genet 2006;15:2059-2075.
62. Shimura H, Schlossmacher MG, Hattori N, et al: Ubiquitination of a new form of alpha-synuclein by parkin from human brain: implications for Parkinson's disease. Science 2001;293:263-269.
63. Schlossmacher MG, Frosch MP, Gai WP, et al: Parkin localizes to the Lewy bodies of Parkinson disease and dementia with Lewy bodies. Am J Pathol 2002;160:1655-1667.
64. Feany MB, Pallanck LJ: Parkin: a multipurpose neuroprotective agent? Neuron 2003;38:13-16.
65. Greene JC, Whitworth AJ, Kuo I, et al: Mitochondrial pathology and apoptotic muscle degeneration in Drosophila parkin mutants. Proc Natl Acad Sci U S A 2003;100:4078-4083.
66. Palacino JJ, Sagi D, Goldberg MS, et al: Mitochondrial dysfunction and oxidative damage in parkin-deficient mice. J Biol Chem 2004;279:18614-18622.
67. Rosen KM, Veereshwarayya V, Moussa CE, et al: Parkin protects against mitochondrial toxins and beta-amyloid accumulation in skeletal muscle cells. J Biol Chem 2006;281:12809-12816.
68. Valente EM, Abou-Sleiman PM, Caputo V, et al: Hereditary early-onset Parkinson's disease caused by mutations in PINK1. Science 2004;304:1158-1160.
69. Healy DG, Abou-Sleiman PM, Gibson JM, et al: PINK1 (PARK6) associated Parkinson disease in Ireland. Neurology 2004;63:1486-1488.
70. Rogaeva E, Johnson J, Lang AE, et al: Analysis of the PINK1 gene in a large cohort of cases with Parkinson disease. Arch Neurol 2004;61:1898-1904.
71. Li Y, Tomiyama H, Sato K, et al: Clinicogenetic study of PINK1 mutations in autosomal recessive early-onset parkinsonism. Neurology 2005;64:1955-1957.
72. Klein C, Djarmati A, Hedrich K, et al: PINK1, Parkin, and DJ-1 mutations in Italian patients with early-onset parkinsonism. Eur J Hum Genet 2005;13:1086-1093.

73. Bonifati V, Rohe CF, Breedveld GJ, et al: Early-onset parkinsonism associated with PINK1 mutations: frequency, genotypes, and phenotypes. Neurology 2005;65:87-95.
74. Tan EK, Yew K, Chua E, et al: PINK1 mutations in sporadic early-onset Parkinson's disease. Mov Disord 2006;21:789-793.
75. Gandhi S, Muqit MM, Stanyer L, et al: PINK1 protein in normal human brain and Parkinson's disease. Brain 2006;129:1720-1731.
76. Silvestri L, Caputo V, Bellacchio E, et al: Mitochondrial import and enzymatic activity of PINK1 mutants associated to recessive parkinsonism. Hum Mol Genet 2005;14:3477-3492.
77. Petit A, Kawarai T, Paitel E, et al: Wild-type PINK1 prevents basal and induced neuronal apoptosis, a protective effect abrogated by Parkinson disease-related mutations. J Biol Chem 2005;280:34025-34032.
78. Beilina A, Van Der Brug M, Ahmad R, et al: Mutations in PTEN-induced putative kinase 1 associated with recessive parkinsonism have differential effects on protein stability. Proc Natl Acad Sci U S A 2005;102:5703-5708.
79. Sim CH, Lio DS, Mok SS, et al: C-terminal truncation and Parkinson's disease-associated mutations down-regulate the protein serine/threonine kinase activity of PTEN-induced kinase-1. Hum Mol Genet 2006;15:3251-3262.
80. Muqit MM, Abou-Sleiman PM, Saurin AT, et al: Altered cleavage and localization of PINK1 to aggresomes in the presence of proteasomal stress. J Neurochem 2006;98:156-169.
81. Greenamyre JT, Hastings TG: Biomedicine: Parkinson's—divergent causes, convergent mechanisms. Science 2004;304:1120-1122.
82. Clark IE, Dodson MW, Jiang C, et al: Drosophila pink1 is required for mitochondrial function and interacts genetically with parkin. Nature 2006;441:1162-1166.
83. Park J, Lee SB, Lee S, et al: Mitochondrial dysfunction in Drosophila PINK1 mutants is complemented by parkin. Nature 2006;441:1157-1161.
84. Yang Y, Gehrke S, Imai Y, et al: Mitochondrial pathology and muscle and dopaminergic neuron degeneration caused by inactivation of Drosophila Pink1 is rescued by Parkin. Proc Natl Acad Sci U S A 2006;103:10793-10798.
85. Exner N, Treske B, Paquet D, et al: Loss-of-function of human PINK1 results in mitochondrial pathology and can be rescued by parkin. J Neurosci 2007;27:12413-12418.
86. Pridgeon JW, Olzmann JA, Chin LS, Li L: PINK1 protects against oxidative stress by phosphorylating mitochondrial chaperone TRAP1. PLoS Biol 2007;5:e172.
87. Weihofen A, Ostaszewski B, Minami Y, Selkoe DJ: Pink1 Parkinson mutations, the Cdc37/Hsp90 chaperones and Parkin all influence the maturation or subcellular distribution of Pink1. Hum Mol Genet 2007;17:602-616.
88. Kitada T, Pisani A, Porter DR, et al: Impaired dopamine release and synaptic plasticity in the striatum of PINK1-deficient mice. Proc Natl Acad Sci U S A 2007;104:11441-11446.
89. Cookson MR, Dauer W, Dawson T, et al: The roles of kinases in familial Parkinson's disease. J Neurosci 2007;27:11865-11868.
90. Bonifati V, Rizzu P, van Baren MJ, et al: Mutations in the DJ-1 gene associated with autosomal recessive early-onset parkinsonism. Science 2003;299:256-259.
91. Hedrich K, Djarmati A, Schafer N, et al: DJ-1 (PARK7) mutations are less frequent than Parkin (PARK2) mutations in early-onset Parkinson disease. Neurology 2004;62:389-394.
92. Goldberg MS, Pisani A, Haburcak M, et al: Nigrostriatal dopaminergic deficits and hypokinesia caused by inactivation of the familial Parkinsonism-linked gene DJ-1. Neuron 2005;45:489-496.
93. Canet-Aviles RM, Wilson MA, Miller DW, et al: The Parkinson's disease protein DJ-1 is neuroprotective due to cysteine-sulfinic acid-driven mitochondrial localization. Proc Natl Acad Sci U S A 2004;101:9103-9108.
94. Kim RH, Smith PD, Aleyasin H, et al: Hypersensitivity of DJ-1-deficient mice to 1-methyl-4-phenyl-1,2,3,6-tetrahydropyridine (MPTP) and oxidative stress. Proc Natl Acad Sci U S A 2005;102:5215-5220.
95. Meulener MC, Xu K, Thomson L, et al: Mutational analysis of DJ-1 in Drosophila implicates functional inactivation by oxidative damage and aging. Proc Natl Acad Sci U S A 2006;103:12517-12522.
96. Andres-Mateos E, Perier C, Zhang L, et al: DJ-1 gene deletion reveals that DJ-1 is an atypical peroxiredoxin-like peroxidase. Proc Natl Acad Sci U S A 2007;104:14807-14812.
97. Ramirez A, Heimbach A, Grundemann J, et al: Hereditary parkinsonism with dementia is caused by mutations in ATP13A2, encoding a lysosomal type 5 P-type ATPase. Nat Genet 2006;38:1184-1191.

98. Williams DR, Hadeed A, al-Din AS, et al: Kufor Rakeb disease: autosomal recessive, levodopa-responsive parkinsonism with pyramidal degeneration, supranuclear gaze palsy, and dementia. Mov Disord 2005;20:1264-1271.

99. Di Fonzo A, Chien HF, Socal M, et al: ATP13A2 missense mutations in juvenile parkinsonism and young onset Parkinson disease. Neurology 2007;68:1557-1562.

100. Massey AC, Zhang C, Cuervo AM: Chaperone-mediated autophagy in aging and disease. Curr Top Dev Biol 2006;73:205-235.

101. Rubinsztein DC: The roles of intracellular protein-degradation pathways in neurodegeneration. Nature 2006;443:780-786.

102. Tang B, Xiong H, Sun P, et al: Association of PINK1 and DJ-1 confers digenic inheritance of early-onset Parkinson's disease. Hum Mol Genet 2006;15:1816-1825.

103. Dachsel JC, Mata IF, Ross OA, et al: Digenic parkinsonism: investigation of the synergistic effects of PRKN and LRRK2. Neurosci Lett 2006;410:80-84.

104. Ferreira JJ, Guedes LC, Rosa MM, et al: High prevalence of LRRK2 mutations in familial and sporadic Parkinson's disease in Portugal. Mov Disord 2007;22:1194-1201.

105. Le WD, Xu P, Jankovic J, et al: Mutations in NR4A2 associated with familial Parkinson disease. Nat Genet 2003;33:85-89.

106. Grimes DA, Han F, Panisset M, et al: Translated mutation in the Nurr1 gene as a cause for Parkinson's disease. Mov Disord 2006;21:906-909.

107. Wellenbrock C, Hedrich K, Schafer N, et al: NR4A2 mutations are rare among European patients with familial Parkinson's disease. Ann Neurol 2003;54:415.

108. Zimprich A, Asmus F, Leitner P, et al: Point mutations in exon 1 of the NR4A2 gene are not a major cause of familial Parkinson's disease. Neurogenetics 2003;4:219-220.

109. Hering R, Petrovic S, Mietz EM, et al: Extended mutation analysis and association studies of Nurr1 (NR4A2) in Parkinson disease. Neurology 2004;62:1231-1232.

110. Engelender S, Kaminsky Z, Guo X, et al: Synphilin-1 associates with alpha-synuclein and promotes the formation of cytosolic inclusions. Nat Genet 1999;22:110-114.

111. Chung KK, Zhang Y, Lim KL, et al: Parkin ubiquitinates the alpha-synuclein-interacting protein, synphilin-1: implications for Lewy-body formation in Parkinson disease. Nat Med 2001;7:1144-1150.

112. Marx FP, Holzmann C, Strauss KM, et al: Identification and functional characterization of a novel R621C mutation in the synphilin-1 gene in Parkinson's disease. Hum Mol Genet 2003;12:1223-1231.

113. Aharon-Peretz J, Rosenbaum H, Gershoni-Baruch R: Mutations in the glucocerebrosidase gene and Parkinson's disease in Ashkenazi Jews. N Engl J Med 2004;351:1972-1977.

114. Goker-Alpan O, Giasson BI, Eblan MJ, et al: Glucocerebrosidase mutations are an important risk factor for Lewy body disorders. Neurology 2006;67:908-910.

115. Goker-Alpan O, Schiffmann R, LaMarca ME, et al: Parkinsonism among Gaucher disease carriers. J Med Genet 2004;41:937-940.

116. Eblan MJ, Scholz S, Stubblefield B, et al: Glucocerebrosidase mutations are not found in association with LRRK2 G2019S in subjects with parkinsonism. Neurosci Lett 2006;404:163-165.

117. Sato C, Morgan A, Lang AE, et al: Analysis of the glucocerebrosidase gene in Parkinson's disease. Mov Disord 2005;20:367-370.

118. Ziegler SG, Eblan MJ, Gutti U, et al: Glucocerebrosidase mutations in Chinese subjects from Taiwan with sporadic Parkinson disease. Mol Genet Metab 2007;91:195-200.

119. Toft M, Pielsticker L, Ross OA, et al: Glucocerebrosidase gene mutations and Parkinson disease in the Norwegian population. Neurology 2006;66:415-417.

120. Mancuso M, Filosto M, Bellan M, et al: POLG mutations causing ophthalmoplegia, sensorimotor polyneuropathy, ataxia, and deafness. Neurology 2004;62:316-318.

121. Luoma P, Melberg A, Rinne JO, et al: Parkinsonism, premature menopause, and mitochondrial DNA polymerase gamma mutations: clinical and molecular genetic study. Lancet 2004;364:875-882.

122. Davidzon G, Greene P, Mancuso M, et al: Early-onset familial parkinsonism due to POLG mutations. Ann Neurol 2006;59:859-862.

123. Thyagarajan D, Bressman S, Bruno C, et al: A novel mitochondrial 12SrRNA point mutation in parkinsonism, deafness, and neuropathy. Ann Neurol 2000;48:730-736.

124. Grasbon-Frodl EM, Kosel S, Sprinzl M, et al: Two novel point mutations of mitochondrial tRNA genes in histologically confirmed Parkinson disease. Neurogenetics 1999;2:121-127.

125. Nolte D, Niemann S, Muller U: Specific sequence changes in multiple transcript system DYT3 are associated with X-linked dystonia parkinsonism. Proc Natl Acad Sci U S A 2003;100:10347-10352.

126. Makino S, Kaji R, Ando S, et al: Reduced neuron-specific expression of the TAF1 gene is associated with X-linked dystonia-parkinsonism. Am J Hum Genet 2007;80:393-406.
127. Muller U, Herzfeld T, Nolte D: The TAF1/DYT3 multiple transcript system in X-linked dystonia-parkinsonism. Am J Hum Genet 2007;81:415-417.
128. Lee LV, Pascasio FM, Fuentes FD, Viterbo GH: Torsion dystonia in Panay, Philippines. Adv Neurol 1976;14:137-151.
129. Nar H, Huber R, Auerbach G, et al: Active site topology and reaction mechanism of GTP cyclohydrolase I. Proc Natl Acad Sci U S A 1995;92:12120-12125.
130. Segawa M, Hosaka A, Miyagawa F, et al: Hereditary progressive dystonia with marked diurnal fluctuation. Adv Neurol 1976;14:215-233.
131. Grimes DA, Barclay CL, Duff J, et al: Phenocopies in a large GCH1 mutation positive family with dopa responsive dystonia: confusing the picture? J Neurol Neurosurg Psychiatry 2002;72:801-804.
132. de Carvalho Aguiar P, Aguiar P, Sweadner K, et al: Mutations in the Na+/K+-ATPase alpha3 gene ATP1A3 are associated with rapid-onset dystonia parkinsonism. Neuron 2004;43:169-175.
133. Brashear A, Dobyns WB, de Carvalho Aguiar P, et al: The phenotypic spectrum of rapid-onset dystonia-parkinsonism (RDP) and mutations in the ATP1A3 gene. Brain 2007;130:828-835.
134. Lee JY, Gollamudi S, Ozelius LJ, et al: ATP1A3 mutation in the first Asian case of rapid-onset dystonia-parkinsonism. Mov Disord 2007;22:1808-1809.
135. Schols L, Peters S, Szymanski S, et al: Extrapyramidal motor signs in degenerative ataxias. Arch Neurol 2000;57:1495-1500.
136. Schols L, Kruger R, Amoiridis G, et al: Spinocerebellar ataxia type 6: genotype and phenotype in German kindreds. J Neurol Neurosurg Psychiatry 1998;64:67-73.
137. Abou-Sleiman PM, Muqit MM, McDonald NQ, et al: A heterozygous effect for PINK1 mutations in Parkinson's disease? Ann Neurol 2006;60:414-419.
138. Criscuolo C, Volpe G, De Rosa A, et al: PINK1 homozygous W437X mutation in a patient with apparent dominant transmission of parkinsonism. Mov Disord 2006;21:1265-1267.
139. Toft M, Myhre R, Pielsticker L, et al: PINK1 mutation heterozygosity and the risk of Parkinson's disease. J Neurol Neurosurg Psychiatry 2007;78:82-84.
140. Djarmati A, Hedrich K, Svetel M, et al: Heterozygous PINK1 mutations: a susceptibility factor for Parkinson disease? Mov Disord 2006;21:1526-1530.
141. Hedrich K, Hagenah J, Djarmati A, et al: Clinical spectrum of homozygous and heterozygous PINK1 mutations in a large German family with Parkinson disease: role of a single hit? Arch Neurol 2006;63:833-838.
142. Lincoln SJ, Maraganore DM, Lesnick TG, et al: Parkin variants in North American Parkinson's disease: cases and controls. Mov Disord 2003;18:1306-1311.
143. Kay DM, Moran D, Moses L, et al: Heterozygous parkin point mutations are as common in control subjects as in Parkinson's patients. Ann Neurol 2007;61:47-54.
144. Clark LN, Afridi S, Karlins E, et al: Case-control study of the parkin gene in early-onset Parkinson disease. Arch Neurol 2006;63:548-552.
145. Hedrich K, Marder K, Harris J, et al: Evaluation of. 50 probands with early-onset Parkinson's disease for Parkin mutations. Neurology 2002;58:1239-1246.
146. Sun M, Latourelle JC, Wooten GF, et al: Influence of heterozygosity for parkin mutation on onset age in familial Parkinson disease: the GenePD study. Arch Neurol 2006;63:826-832.
147. Tan EK, Zhao Y, Skipper L, et al: The LRRK2 Gly2385Arg variant is associated with Parkinson's disease: genetic and functional evidence. Hum Genet 2006;120:857-863.
148. Healy DG, Abou-Sleiman PM, Casas JP, et al: UCHL-1 is not a Parkinson's disease susceptibility gene. Ann Neurol 2006;59:627-633.
149. Mizuta I, Satake W, Nakabayashi Y, et al: Multiple candidate gene analysis identifies alpha-synuclein as a susceptibility gene for sporadic Parkinson's disease. Hum Mol Genet 2006;15:1151-1158.
150. Maraganore DM, de Andrade M, Lesnick TG, et al: High-resolution whole-genome association study of Parkinson disease. Am J Hum Genet 2005;77:685-693.
151. Elbaz A, Nelson LM, Payami H, et al: Lack of replication of thirteen single-nucleotide polymorphisms implicated in Parkinson's disease: a large-scale international study. Lancet Neurol 2006;5:917-923.
152. Farrer MJ, Haugarvoll K, Ross OA, et al: Genomewide association, Parkinson disease, and PARK10. Am J Hum Genet 2006;78:1084-1088.
153. Bialecka M, Kurzawski M, Klodowska-Duda G, et al: Polymorphism in semaphorin 5A (Sema5A) gene is not a marker of Parkinson's disease risk. Neurosci Lett 2006;399:121-123.

154. Clarimon J, Scholz S, Fung HC, et al: Conflicting results regarding the semaphorin gene (SEMA5A) and the risk for Parkinson disease. Am J Hum Genet 2006;78:1082-1084.
155. Fung HC, Scholz S, Matarin M, et al: Genome-wide genotyping in Parkinson's disease and neurologically normal controls: first stage analysis and public release of data. Lancet Neurol 2006;5:911-916.
156. Papapetropoulos S, Ffrench-Mullen J, McCorquodale D, et al: Multiregional gene expression profiling identifies MRPS6 as a possible candidate gene for Parkinson's disease. Gene Expr 2006;13:205-215.
157. Jin J, Hulette C, Wang Y, et al: Proteomic identification of a stress protein, mortalin/mthsp70/GRP75: relevance to Parkinson disease. Mol Cell Proteomics 2006;5:1193-1204.
158. Klein C: Implications of genetics on the diagnosis and care of patients with Parkinson disease. Arch Neurol 2006;63:328-334.
159. Klein C, Schlossmacher M: The genetics of Parkinson disease. Nat Clin Pract Neurol 2006;2:136-146.
160. McInerney-Leo A, Hadley DW, Gwinn-Hardy K, Hardy J: Genetic testing in Parkinson's disease. Mov Disord 2005;20:1-10.
161. Djarmati A, Guzvic M, Grunewald A, et al: Rapid and reliable detection of exon rearrangements in various movement disorders genes by multiplex ligation-dependent probe amplification. Mov Disord 2007;22:1708-1714.
162. Clark LN, Haamer E, Mejia-Santana H, et al: Construction and validation of a Parkinson's disease mutation genotyping array for the Parkin gene. Mov Disord 2007;22:932-937.
163. Chan CS, Guzman JN, Ilijic E, et al: 'Rejuvenation' protects neurons in mouse models of Parkinson's disease. Nature 2007;447:1081-1086.
164. Sulzer D, Schmitz Y: Parkinson's disease: return of an old prime suspect. Neuron 2007;55:8-10.
165. Hebert SS, De Strooper B: Molecular biology: miRNAs in neurodegeneration. Science 2007;317:1179-1180.
166. Takahashi K, Tanabe K, Ohnuki M, et al: Induction of pluripotent stem cells from adult human fibroblasts by defined factors. Cell 2007;131:861-872.

3 α-Synuclein and Parkinson's Disease

THOMAS GASSER

Introduction

Parkinson's disease (PD) is traditionally defined as a clinicopathological entity with variable combinations of akinesia, rigidity, tremor, and postural instability, and a characteristic pattern of neurodegeneration, affecting dopaminergic neurons of the substantia nigra, but also many other brain areas. Characteristic eosinophilic inclusions, the Lewy bodies, are found in surviving dopaminergic neurons and, although less abundantly, in other parts of the brain, and have been considered to be essential for the pathological diagnosis of PD.

Genetic research, in particular the mapping and cloning of numerous genes that cause, when mutated, monogenically inherited forms of PD, has shown that this disorder is actually not a single disease entity, but rather a heterogeneous group of diseases associated with an overlapping spectrum of clinical and pathological changes. Although the mutations and genes identified so far seem to be directly causative in only a few families each, there is accumulating evidence that the molecular pathways identified, and in some cases also "normal" genetic variability in "PD genes," may predispose to the common sporadic disease. This evidence holds the promise that the study of monogenic disease variants in model systems and in patients will provide a better understanding of the disease processes in a wider sense and eventually will be relevant for the discovery of new drug targets for the treatment of PD in general.

A major breakthrough on the way to a better understanding of the molecular pathogenesis of PD was the discovery that point mutations,[1-3] and duplications and triplications,[4,5] of the SNCA gene, the gene encoding the α-synuclein protein (αSYN), cause an autosomal dominantly inherited form of PD, which is clinically and pathologically well within the spectrum of Lewy body diseases as they are defined today: a group of disorders that comprises classic PD, PD with dementia, and diffuse Lewy body disease (this term is used interchangeably with *dementia with Lewy bodies* [DLB]). These disorders are considered by many researchers today to be a continuum of conditions, characterized and possibly caused by the abnormal processing and aggregation of a key protein—αSYN.

The pathogenic relevance of this protein may extend beyond the group of Lewy body disorders proper because αSYN aggregates are also an indispensable pathological feature of other diverse neurodegenerative diseases, such as multiple systems atrophy (where they take the form of flame-shaped "glial fibrillary inclusions" and are found in oligodendrocytes[6]), and neurodegeneration with brain iron accumulation (formerly known as Hallervorden-Spatz disease, and now recognized to be most commonly caused by mutations in the pantothenate kinase 2 gene [*PANK2*] and also referred to as pantothenate kinase–associated neurodegeneration, PKAN). Because much less is known about the role of αSYN in these disorders, they are not discussed in this chapter.

❚ *SNCA* Mutations

The genetic locus bearing the *SNCA* gene (called the PARK1 locus) was mapped to the long arm of chromosome 4 in a large family of Italian ancestry with dominantly inherited PD and Lewy body pathology,[7] and the mutated gene was later identified by the same group as αSYN (*SNCA*).[1] Over the years, several families have been identified that carry the same mutation, the exchange of an alanine by a threonine at position 53 of the protein (A53T), in different regions of the world, but it could be shown by examining genetic markers closely surrounding the gene (a method called *haplotype analysis*) that affected members in all these families share the identical mutation "by descent"—they all are likely to originate from a single ancestor in whom this mutation occurred for the first time, probably a few thousand years ago ("founder effect"). It was only in 2006 that a truly independent A53T mutation was discovered in a Korean family with PD,[8] indicating, first, that this amino acid may be of particular relevance to the pathogenic process leading to PD because it is the only residue affected twice independently, and, second, that mutational events are exceedingly rare. Only two additional point mutations have been recognized,[2,3] each in dominant families with multiple affected family members, reflecting the high penetrance of these mutations. Both also lead to an amino acid exchange (A30P, E46K). SNCA point mutations are very rare and have not been found in sporadic PD.[9]

The clinical picture associated with these *SNCA* point mutations extends over the full spectrum of Lewy body disorders, as they are recognized today, from classic late-onset PD without prominent cognitive deterioration (particularly in the German family carrying the A30P mutation[2]) to PD of earlier onset with frequent and early dementia and rapid progression (a mean age of onset of 44 years and a mean survival time of <10 years were described for the original A53T mutation family). There is a high variability in age of onset and severity of symptoms even in families with a single mutation, as best shown in the extensive A53T kindred, but there also seem to be some mutation-specific features.

In several members of an A53T family,[10] and even more so in the E46K family,[3] clinical symptoms of early dementia and prominent autonomic disturbances suggested a diagnosis of DLB, rather than classic PD. In the A30P mutation family, onset is later, dementia less common, and the course generally more benign[2] (R. Krüger, personal communication). These observations support the notion that Lewy body diseases form a continuum, rather than representing distinct nosological entities, and that modifying factors (genetic or nongenetic) in addition to the causative mutation are also responsible for the variability in clinical presentation.

SNCA MULTIPLICATIONS

An even more direct causative link between αSYN and PD on the genetic level is provided by the more recent discovery that not only point mutations, but also multiplications of the entire wild-type sequence of the SNCA gene (duplications and triplications) cause autosomal dominant parkinsonism with or without dementia with extensive αSYN inclusions,[4,5] suggesting that a mere increase in αSYN protein levels can be directly toxic to neurons. The disease in these families recapitulates the anatomical pattern and pathological and clinical features of sporadic Lewy body diseases. The first family discovered with this type of mutation, the so-called Spellman-Muenter kindred (also known as the Iowa kindred), was initially described as a family with early-onset parkinsonism, dementia, and prominent autonomic disturbances by Muenter and colleagues.[11,12] Pathologically, αSYN staining showed widespread aggregates of different forms and shapes, which the authors called *pleomorphic Lewy bodies*; severe neuritic changes; vacuolar changes in the temporal cortex; and, notably, αSYN aggregates in oligodendroglial cells (which is the prominent pathological feature of multiple systems atrophy).[13]

In this family, Singleton and colleagues[4] discovered the first SNCA genomic triplication as a cause of disease. In these cases, a cellular overload of "healthy" (wild-type) αSYN is apparently sufficient to cause the disease. A triplication of the gene on one chromosome leads to the effective doubling of the gene dose on the protein level (four instead of two copies), which, as predicted, leads approximately to a doubling of the αSYN protein level in brain tissue from affected members of this kindred. Subsequently, it was found that not only triplications, but also duplications of the SNCA locus (theoretically corresponding to a 50% increase in protein load) can lead to dominantly inherited PD.[14]

Multiplications seem to be considerably more common than point mutations. In particular, duplications sometimes can be found in patients with seemingly sporadic disease, owing to the late onset of the disease.[15] Later age at onset and milder disease in the duplication families compared with the triplication families point to a dosage effect, which was confirmed in a family in which a duplication and a triplication of the identical SNCA-bearing genomic fragment segregated in two family branches.[5]

Based on these findings, there is general consensus today that SNCA mutations are a direct cause of PD, at least in these dominant families. Because αSYN has been found to be the principal fibrillar component of Lewy bodies[16] also in sporadic PD, it is likely that the protein plays a more general role in the pathogenic process. The precise nature of this process is unclear. It also is unclear whether the pathogenic role of αSYN has anything to do with its physiological function, and how exactly it relates to cellular dysfunction and cell death. These issues are discussed next.

α-Synuclein Normal Localization, Regulation, and Function

SNCA is located on the long arm of chromosome 4, consists of six exons, and spans a genomic region of about 120 kb. It encodes a small 14-kD protein of 140 amino acids. Alternative splicing has been described resulting in two less prevalent, smaller isoforms, αSYN126 (lacking exon 3[17]) and αSYN112 (lacking exon 5[18]). Although it is possible that alternative splicing may contribute to the normal, cell-specific function and the pathological aggregation of αSYN,[19] its role has not yet been studied in detail.

αSYN is ubiquitously expressed, but expression levels are particularly high in the brain, where it is estimated to account for about 1% of the total protein. Under normal conditions, its expression is highest in neurons, whereas only very low expression is observed in glia; in multiple systems atrophy, one of the atypical parkinsonian syndromes, and in patients with SNCA triplications, αSYN forms characteristic cytoplasmic inclusions in oligodendroglial cells (cytoplasmic glial inclusions). αSYN is particularly abundant in dopaminergic and noradrenergic neurons, and in cortical neurons and neurons in the amygdalae.

Under physiological conditions, αSYN is an unfolded protein with little or no ordered structure when it is in solution in the cytosol. With its N-terminal domain, it can bind to lipid membranes (e.g., to vesicles containing neurotransmitters), which are enriched in presynaptic terminals. This localization suggests that physiologically αSYN may be involved in synaptic vesicle recycling, storage, and compartmentalization of neurotransmitters, and the regulation of neurotransmitter release. One of the earliest indications in this direction was that its ortholog in birds, called synelfin, has been found to be upregulated developmentally during song learning, a period of particularly high synaptic activity.[20] αSYN knockout mice behave grossly normally and display no obvious pathological phenotype, but they show subtle alterations of neurotransmitter release in the basal ganglia under certain experimental conditions in vitro.[21] Electrophysiological studies in mouse primary cortical neurons have also provided more direct evidence for the role of αSYN in synaptic transmission. Application of glutamate increased αSYN immunoreactivity and functional bouton number in the presynaptic terminals, whereas presynaptic injection of αSYN increased neurotransmitter release, an effect that was mediated by the production of nitric oxide.[22,23]

α-SYNUCLEIN REGULATION

Numerous pathological conditions seem to alter the abundance and distribution of αSYN in the brain. It has been shown that αSYN immunoreactivity rapidly accumulates after brain trauma in mice[24] and in humans.[25] This observation has been attributed to a disturbance of the axonal transport of the protein, but it recapitulates some features of synucleinopathies, and may contribute to the increased vulnerability of the brain after trauma to neurodegeneration.

αSYN is also strongly upregulated after 1-methyl-4-phenyl-1,2,3,6-tetrahydropyridine (MPTP) administration in nonhuman primates.[26] αSYN knockout mice are resistant to MPTP toxicity,[27] and overexpression of mutated αSYN potentiates the deleterious action of this mitochondrial toxin.[28] It is conceivable that upregulation of αSYN and mitochondrial toxins act synergistically.

α-SYNUCLEIN CATABOLISM

Proteins can be degraded in several different ways. Given the involvement of the ubiquitin-dependent proteasomal protein degradation system in PD, which is suggested by the discovery of mutations in the ubiquitin-ligase parkin as a cause for autosomal recessive early-onset parkinsonism,[29] it was tempting to speculate that impaired αSYN degradation through this pathway might contribute to the pathogenesis of PD. No direct link between parkin-mediated proteasomal protein degradation and αSYN has been shown convincingly; however, αSYN itself has not been shown to be one of the confirmed parkin substrates, and the relevance of the observation that an O-glycosylated form of αSYN may be a substrate of parkin[30] is still unclear.

More recently, the lysosomal pathway of chaperone-mediated autophagy was implicated in αSYN degradation; it was shown that wild-type αSYN is selectively translocated into lysosomes for degradation by the pathway. The pathogenic A53T and A30P αSYN mutants seemed to act as uptake blockers, inhibiting their own degradation and that of other substrates.[31] It is likely that αSYN can be degraded by both systems, depending on the conditions,[32] so both could play a role in the pathogenesis of PD, when the reduced ability to clear excess αSYN may become a problem.

Aggregate Formation

Shortly after the discovery of the *SNCA* A53T mutation as a cause for familial PD, Spillantini and coworkers[16] identified the αSYN protein as the major component of the Lewy body, the characteristic cytoplasmic inclusion body of sporadic and most familial forms of PD and DLB. Lewy bodies contain many other proteins as well, but it is generally believed that the aggregation of the highly ordered αSYN fibrils[33] are crucial to the process, although its precise relationship to neuronal damage is still controversial.

The central core region of the αSYN protein (residues 61 through 95), containing a high proportion of hydrophobic amino acids (also referred to as the non–β-amyloid component precursor [NACP] region), is indispensable for fibril formation, owing to its propensity to adopt a β-sheet conformation in a concentration-dependent and nucleation-dependent manner.[34] It has been shown that overexpression of a construct lacking amino acids of the NACP domain (amino acids 71 through 82) in *Drosophila*, which has been one of the better models to study the pathological consequences of αSYN toxicity,[35] did not lead to aggregation and dopaminergic degeneration, whereas a truncated species (amino acids 1 through 120) containing the amyloidogenic NACP domain induced increased aggregation and dopaminergic neurotoxicity.[36]

Nevertheless, amino acid alterations outside this region (e.g., the pathogenic mutations A53T and A30P) and the pathologically relevant phosphorylation of the protein at residue ser129 are able to modify this process. N-terminal and

C-terminal domains of wild-type αSYN may "shield" the amyloidogenic core region of the protein through long-range interactions. Using nuclear magnetic resonance spectroscopy, Bertoncini and coworkers[37] showed a loss of native conformations and the disruption of autoinhibitory long-range interactions in A53T and A30P mutant αSYN. These findings suggest a potential mechanism for the toxic gain of functions conveyed by pathogenic αSYN mutations.

At least in vitro, the A53T mutation seems to accelerate fibril formation, whereas the A30P mutation retards it.[38] This is one of the reasons why it is often assumed that smaller oligomers or protofibrils, containing only one to three dozen αSYN molecules and taking many geometric shapes, rather than the mature fibrils themselves, are the true toxic species, and that formation of fibrils and sequestration into Lewy bodies is an attempt of the cell to protect itself.

In addition to the influence of the protein concentration and the role of pathogenic point mutations, post-translational modifications of αSYN may influence its propensity to form aggregates. Using antibodies to specific nitrated tyrosine residues in αSYN, it has been shown that a high proportion of the protein that accumulates within Lewy bodies and Lewy neurites is nitrated, providing evidence for a role of oxidative and nitrative damage in the onset and progression of the disease.[39]

Many groups have shown with different methods that the Ser129 residue of αSYN is selectively and extensively (hyper-) phosphorylated in synucleinopathy lesions. This is true in transgenic mouse models[40] and in Lewy bodies isolated from brains of patients with PD, DLB, and multiple systems atrophy, and in families with *SNCA* mutations, suggesting that phosphorylation enhances inclusion formation. In vitro, phosphorylation at Ser129 also promoted insoluble fibril formation, and more recently it has been shown that G protein–coupled receptor kinase 5 is responsible for catalyzing this phosphorylation step, enhancing the formation of soluble oligomers and aggregates.[41]

Animal Models

Numerous animal models for αSYN-related neurodegeneration have been generated in a whole array of organisms, from yeast and worms to vertebrates and even nonhuman primates: each organism allows the study of specific features of the molecular pathogenesis of the disease, but none recapitulates all aspects of the human disorder.

Many aspects of the maturation, processing, and degradation of proteins and their cell toxicity can best be studied in simple organisms, such as baker's yeast, *Saccharomyces cerevisiae*. Many mammalian disease genes have orthologs in yeast, and disease-associated molecular pathways are conserved across species; this also proved to be the case for αSYN. αSYN, when expressed in yeast, associated with the plasma membrane in a highly selective manner, before forming cytoplasmic inclusions through a concentration-dependent, nucleated process.[42] Yeast models have the advantages of being readily manipulatable and of lending themselves to high-throughput screening procedures, whether genetic or pharmacological. More recently, these studies led to the discovery that inhibitors of SIRT2 (a histone deacetylase implicated in aging) protect against αSYN-mediated toxicity.[43] This may be one of many starting points to develop disease-modifying treatment strategies.

The worm *Caenorhabditis elegans* is another simple model system that is well suited to study the molecular mechanisms of human diseases. With respect to the analysis of the pathological basis of PD, *C. elegans* possesses exactly eight dopaminergic neurons, and its transparency provides the exceptional advantage to visualize directly protein inclusions in a living animal. Springer and associates[44] proposed a two-hit model for αSYN neurotoxicity and *parkin* mutations, providing a functional link. Synthetic combination of human αSYN A53T and a neomorphic worm *parkin* mutant results in exacerbating phenotypes expressed by a dose-dependent and temperature-dependent lethality of the double mutant. More recently, systematic and genome-wide screening approaches for modifiers of αSYN inclusion formation[45,46] have identified, besides factors involved in protein quality control and vesicle-mediated trafficking, aging-associated proteins such as SIRT1 and LAG1/LASS2,[45] underscoring the results obtained from other model systems.

Drosophila models have proven to be extremely useful in the study of αSYN neurotoxicity. Overexpression of human wild-type and mutated αSYN resulted in an age-dependent specific degeneration of dopaminergic neurons, a motor phenotype, and αSYN-positive intracytoplasmic inclusions.[35] In this model, the suspected crucial role of Ser129 phosphorylation could be experimentally corroborated. Mutation of Ser129 to alanine to prevent phosphorylation completely suppressed dopaminergic neuronal loss produced by expression of human αSYN. In contrast, altering Ser129 to the negatively charged residue aspartate, to mimic phosphorylation, significantly enhances αSYN toxicity. Ser129 phosphorylation status is crucial in mediating αSYN neurotoxicity and inclusion formation. Because increased number of inclusion bodies correlates with reduced toxicity, these experiments have been interpreted to support the hypothesis that inclusion bodies may protect neurons from αSYN toxicity.[47]

Despite these insights provided by invertebrate models for synucleinopathies, a caveat is the fact that the invertebrate genome does not encode αSYN, and may not have evolved the cellular antiaggregation systems against the formation of αSYN fibrils that may be found in mammals. This difference poses limits to the validity of these models for the human disease.

Mouse and other mammalian models are still an important tool to study the pathological processes of αSYN aggregation and its relationship to neurodegeneration. Numerous transgenic mouse models have been generated, using wild-type and mutated, full-length and truncated forms of the *SNCA* gene. As stated earlier, none of the models is able to recapitulate all pathological features of the human disease, but each of them allows one to study specific aspects. Transgenic mice expressing mutational and wild-type αSYN under the control of the tyrosine hydroxylase promoter express the transgene selectively in catecholaminergic neurons. These mice did not show an obvious phenotype[48,49] and no increased sensitivity to MPTP, possibly because of powerful defense mechanisms present in the mouse dopaminergic system. If the propensity of the transgene for aggregation is increased by cutting off 20 or 10 amino acids of the C-terminus (truncated αSYN120 or αSYN130), transgenic animals showed significantly reduced spontaneous locomotion, which could be treated with levodopa, corresponding to an impressive loss of nigrostriatal dopaminergic neurons.[50,51] In contrast to human disease, the neuronal loss was not progressive, but seemed to occur during embryogenesis, and no fibrillar inclusions resembling Lewy bodies were observed.

The use of the pan-neuronal promoter Thy1 allows the expression of wild-type and mutational αSYN widely throughout the brain. In these mice, prominent somatodendritic accumulation of granular and detergent-insoluble αSYN throughout the brain and the spinal cord could be shown, accompanied by a progressive age-related motor phenotype.[52] This deficit is not predominantly caused by damage to the nigrostriatal dopaminergic system, however, because this region is remarkably spared in transgenic αSYN mice even in late stages, but rather by pathology (neuronal loss and astrogliosis) in the lower brainstem and the spinal cord.[53,54]

Nevertheless, transgenic mouse models using the Thy1 promoter showed a remarkable consistency of αSYN fibrillation (Fig. 3–1) and neurodegeneration in affected brain areas, which parallels the human disease, even if it does not reflect its topographical distribution.[40] These models are particularly useful to study the relationship between aggregation, neuronal dysfunction, and cell death, and possibly to identify ways to ameliorate this deleterious process.

To overcome the remaining limitations of existing animal models, innovative approaches are being used. The long-term expression of wild-type and mutational αSYN using recombinant adeno-associated viral vectors applied to the ventral midbrain of marmosets has been shown to induce a parkinsonian-like state with motor incoordination. This motor phenotype was accompanied by the accumulation of pathologically phosphorylated αSYN, the formation of ubiquitinated aggregates, and dopaminergic neurodegeneration, suggesting that this model may reflect important aspects of the human disease and be of potential value to test novel therapeutic targets for neuroprotective strategies.[55]

Although many questions remain to be answered, astonishing progress has been made since the discovery of pathogenic αSYN mutations in familial PD in the elucidation of the sequence of events that lead to dopaminergic cell death. To apply this new knowledge and emerging therapies to all PD patients, it is crucial to show that in sporadic PD as well, αSYN is not just an innocent bystander, but a primary cause of the neurodegenerative process.

Association Studies: SNCA Genetics in Sporadic Disease

Alterations of the SNCA gene (point mutations and multiplications) that lead to autosomal dominantly inherited parkinsonism are not found in the common sporadic form of the disease (clinically diagnosed as idiopathic PD and DLB). This has been shown by searching for these alterations in very large patient cohorts.[9,56]

The fact that an increase of the *normal* cellular αSYN protein load by 50% to 100% (as found in gene duplication and triplication patients) causes familial PD with high penetrance suggests that alterations in regulatory regions of the gene that could cause increased gene expression may be associated with a higher disease risk. There is now increasing evidence that this is the case from multiple studies, many of which had been performed long before the discovery of SNCA multiplications.

Several case-control studies found a complex polymorphic dinucleotide repeat polymorphism (NACP-Rep1) located close to the promoter region to be associated with sporadic PD,[57,58] whereas other studies have been unable to reproduce these initial findings.[59,60] Nevertheless, a large collaborative study using pooled

Brainstem

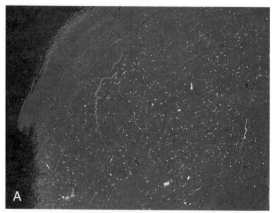

A

Cerebellum

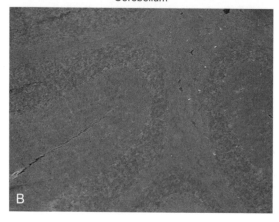

B

Figure 3–1 A and **B,** Thioflavin S stains amyloid protein (fibrils featuring β-pleated structure) derived from α-synuclein in an aged (Thy1)-h[A30P] αSYN mouse. The brainstem **(A)** shows numerous Lewy bodies (*dots*) and Lewy neurites composed of aggregated α-synuclein, whereas the cerebellum **(B)** shows only background staining.

populations confirmed the positive findings,[61] and an appealing mechanism explaining this association—the allele-specific binding of the transcriptional regulator poly-(ADP-ribose) transferase/polymerase-1 (PARP-1)—has been suggested.[62] In cell culture experiments, specific binding of PARP-1 to NACP-Rep1 could be shown. Inhibition of the catalytic domain of PARP-1 increased the endogenous *SNCA* mRNA levels in cultured cells, whereas PARP-1 binding to NACP-Rep1 specifically reduced the transcriptional activity of the *SNCA* promoter/enhancer in luciferase reporter assays. The association of different NACP-Rep1 alleles with PD may be mediated partly by the effect on PARP-1.

The reality of SNCA regulation may be more complex. In a more comprehensive approach, Mueller and colleagues[63] first analyzed the entire *SNCA* gene using more than 50 single nucleotide polymorphisms, and found a strong association of the disease with a haplotype block comprising exons 5 and 6 and the 3'-UTR of the gene. This finding has been confirmed in a Japanese study,[64] suggesting that despite different haplotype structures, the effect can be detected in different populations, and in another more recent study analyzing patients from northern

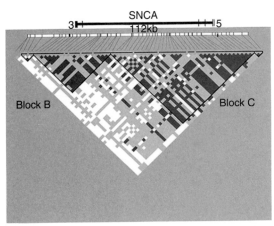

Figure 3–2 The genomic and haplotype structure of the *SNCA* gene (encoding α-synuclein, drawn to scale). Exons are the *small vertical lines* crossing the black bar on the top; the gene is transcribed from 5′ to 3′. Fifty-three analyzed single nucleotide polymorphisms (SNPs) are symbolized by the *thin vertical lines* in the second horizontal bar from the top. The haplotype structure is depicted in the *triangle*. The higher the intercorrelation between SNPs (also called "linkage disequilibrium"), the darker the color of the intersecting lines symbolizing SNP position. Two darkly colored "sub-triangles" denote two blocks of highly intercorrelated SNPs (i.e., two "haplotype blocks"). Reproduced with permission from [63].

Germany and Serbia.[65] Figure 3–2 shows the genomic and haplotype structure of the *SNCA* gene.

In a follow-up first study, Fuchs and associates[66] showed that specific alleles found in the risk haplotype also influenced reporter gene expression in a luciferase assay and that there was a correlation with measurable αSYN levels in human peripheral blood mononuclear cells and brain tissue. It is conceivable that more than one genetic mechanism contributes in a relevant way to *SNCA* expression, influencing the risk of developing PD. If confirmed, pharmacological manipulation of *SNCA* expression may be a possible therapeutic or preventive strategy in susceptible individuals.

Although the extent of *SNCA* expression regulation is not understood, it may still be simplistic to assume that expression levels, as determined by multiple genetic variations, are the only, or even the dominant, contributor to the susceptibility to sporadic PD and DLB. Odds ratios for risk alleles discovered so far in most studies were on the order of 1.5 to 2.2, indicating that many other genetic or nongenetic factors are likely to be involved to determine an individual's fate.

Further Considerations

As shown in cellular and animal models described previously, post-translational modifications, such as phosphorylation at Ser129, or oxidation and nitrosylation as a result of oxidative stress, may have a profound influence on the propensity of αSYN to form oligomers, protofibrils, and fibrils. Post-translational modification may be crucial to determine whether αSYN aggregation leads to the predominant formation of small oligomers, which are regarded by many as the true toxic species, or rather to the rapid formation of fibrils, which ideally can be degraded or, at least, sequestered into less harmful inclusions. Dopamine itself may be the cause of one particularly important modification of αSYN,[67] possibly explaining the high vulnerability of these neurons.

A possible link between an important class of cellular regulating proteins, the sirtuins, and αSYN aggregation and PD has emerged more recently. The sirtuins (there are seven forms in mammals, SIRT1 through SIRT7) are a group of NAD+-dependent histone deacetylases that participate in numerous age-related phenomena, including life span extension, glucose homeostasis, and neurodegeneration.[68] Outeiro and colleagues identified a potent inhibitor of one of the sirtuins (SIRT2) and found that inhibition of SIRT2 rescued αSYN toxicity in a cellular model of PD, possibly by favoring the formation of large aggregates over the presence of small toxic oligomers.[69] A suggested mechanism for this effect is the inhibition of the deacetylation of tubulin, one of the known physiological actions of SIRT2. SIRT2 inhibition also protected against dopaminergic cell death in a *Drosophila* model of PD.

Alternative splicing is another process that is still poorly understood with respect to its potential influence on the pathogenic potential of αSYN. There is initial evidence that splice variants may influence aggregability, with the αSYN126 variant, which lacks exon 3, exerting an antiaggregation effect, whereas αSYN112, lacking much of the C-terminal domain owing to skipping of exon 5, may favor or seed aggregation.[70] It is still largely unclear, however, if those splice variants are expressed to any relevant degree at the protein level in affected brain regions.

Also, the crosstalk between αSYN and other PD genes is still not understood. As far as we know today, there seems to be no direct interaction between αSYN and other PD genes, such as *parkin* (with the possible exception of *parkin* mediating the proteasomal degradation of a rare *O*-glycosylated species of αSYN[30]) or *LRRK2*. At least in the case of *LRRK2*, an indirect interaction is highly likely because the major pathological phenotype of patients with *LRRK2* mutations is indistinguishable from typical αSYN-positive Lewy body PD. *LRRK2* mutations may be located upstream of αSYN, leading, via still unknown signaling pathways, to an increase in αSYN aggregability.

Finally, upregulation of *SNCA* expression in response to external influences, such as trauma[25] or toxins,[26] may help to bridge the gap between "genetic" and "environmental" models of the causation of PD. It is becoming increasingly clear that αSYN protein levels are regulated in response to numerous stimuli or conditions, such as in cocaine[71,72] and alcohol[73] addiction. A better understanding of these mechanisms and their interactions may provide new approaches to the treatment or even prevention of synucleinopathies.

Conclusions

Although genes that are linked to monogenic forms of PD and other closely related neurodegenerative diseases are, at first glance, not related to a common causative pathway, genetic, pathological, and molecular studies have strengthened the evidence that there is probably more crosstalk between the different pathways, on several levels, than previously appreciated. These findings support the existence of common pathogenic mechanisms, including protein aggregation, mitochondrial dysfunction, and oxidative stress, which had been suspected as major culprits of neurodegeneration for many years.

The pathogenic link between *SNCA* point mutations and multiplications in large dominant families with a range of clinical phenotypes from classic PD to DLB is well established and positions αSYN at the center of the pathogenetic network leading to these disorders. The fact that Lewy bodies and Lewy neurites composed of fibrillar αSYN are the most consistent feature and the pathological hallmark of the common sporadic synucleinopathies, including PD and DLB, supports a crucial role of this protein for this group of neurodegenerative diseases. Just exactly what leads to αSYN oligomerization and fibrillation, and eventually to neuronal dysfunction and cell loss, remains largely unknown. Based on many more recent genetic studies and on the insight gained from the cellular and the animal models described in this chapter, a complex picture of interactions is beginning to emerge that is expected eventually to lead to clearly testable hypotheses and potential targets for intervention.

REFERENCES

1. Polymeropoulos MH, Lavedan C, Leroy E, et al: Mutation in the α-synuclein gene identified in families with Parkinson's disease. Science 1997;276:2045-2047.
2. Krüger R, Kuhn W, Müller T, et al: Ala39Pro mutation in the gene encoding a-synuclein in Parkinson's disease. Nat Genet 1998;18:106-108.
3. Zarranz JJ, Alegre J, Gomez-Esteban JC, et al: The new mutation, E46K, of alpha-synuclein causes Parkinson and Lewy body dementia. Ann Neurol 2004;55:164-173.
4. Singleton AB, Farrer M, Johnson J, et al: α-Synuclein locus triplication causes Parkinson's disease. Science 2003;302:841.
5. Fuchs J, Nilsson C, Kachergus J, et al: Phenotypic variation in a large Swedish pedigree due to SNCA duplication and triplication. Neurology 2007;68:916-922.
6. Dickson DW, Lin W, Liu WK, Yen SH: Multiple system atrophy: a sporadic synucleinopathy. Brain Pathol 1999;9:721-732.
7. Polymeropoulos MH, Higgins JJ, Golbe LI, et al: Mapping of a gene for Parkinson's disease to chromosome 4q21-q23. Science 1996;274:1197-1199.
8. Ki CS, Stavrou E, Davanos N, et al: The Ala53Thr mutation in the alpha-synuclein gene in a Korean family with Parkinson disease. Clin Genet 2007;71:471-473.
9. Berg D, Niwar M, Maass S, et al: Alpha-synuclein and Parkinson's disease: implications from the screening of more than 1,900 patients. Mov Disord 2005;20:1191-1194.
10. Spira PJ, Sharpe DM, Halliday G, et al: Clinical and pathological features of a parkinsonian syndrome in a family with an Ala53Thr alpha-synuclein mutation. Ann Neurol 2001;49:313-319.
11. Muenter M, Howard FM Jr, Okazaki H: A familial Parkinson-dementia syndrome. Neurology 1986;36(Suppl 1):115.
12. Muenter MD, Forno LS, Hornykiewicz O, et al: Hereditary form of parkinsonism—dementia. Ann Neurol 1998;43:768-781.
13. Gwinn-Hardy K, Mehta ND, Farrer M, et al: Distinctive neuropathology revealed by alpha-synuclein antibodies in hereditary parkinsonism and dementia linked to chromosome 4p. Acta Neuropathol (Berl) 2000;99:663-672.
14. Ibanez P, Bonnet AM, Debarges B, et al: Causal relation between alpha-synuclein gene duplication and familial Parkinson's disease. Lancet 2004;364:1169-1171.
15. Ahn TB, Kim SY, Kim JY, et al: alpha-Synuclein gene duplication is present in sporadic Parkinson disease. Neurology 2008;70:43-49.
16. Spillantini MG, Schmidt ML, Lee VM, et al: Alpha-synuclein in Lewy bodies. Nature 1997;388:839-840.
17. Campion D, Martin C, Heilig R, et al: The NACP/synuclein gene: chromosomal assignment and screening for alterations in Alzheimer disease. Genomics 1995;26:254-257.
18. Ueda K, Saitoh T, Mori H: Tissue-dependent alternative splicing of mRNA for NACP, the precursor of non-A beta component of Alzheimer's disease amyloid. Biochem Biophys Res Commun 1994;205:1366-1372.

19. Beyer K, Humbert J, Ferrer A, et al: A variable poly-T sequence modulates alpha-synuclein isoform expression and is associated with aging. J Neurosci Res 2007;85:1538-1546.
20. Jin H, Clayton DF: Synelfin regulation during the critical period for song learning in normal and isolated juvenile zebra finches. Neurobiol Learn Mem 1997;68:271-284.
21. Abeliovich A, Schmitz Y, Farinas I, et al: Mice lacking alpha-synuclein display functional deficits in the nigrostriatal dopamine system. Neuron 2000;25:239-252.
22. Liu S, Fa M, Ninan I, et al: Alpha-synuclein involvement in hippocampal synaptic plasticity: role of NO, cGMP, cGK and CaMKII. Eur J Neurosci 2007;25:3583-3596.
23. Liu S, Ninan I, Antonova I, et al: alpha-Synuclein produces a long-lasting increase in neurotransmitter release. EMBO J 2004;23:4506-4516.
24. Uryu K, Giasson BI, Longhi L, et al: Age-dependent synuclein pathology following traumatic brain injury in mice. Exp Neurol 2003;184:214-224.
25. Uryu K, Chen XH, Martinez D, et al: Multiple proteins implicated in neurodegenerative diseases accumulate in axons after brain trauma in humans. Exp Neurol 2007;208:185-192.
26. Purisai MG, McCormack AL, Langston WJ, et al: Alpha-synuclein expression in the substantia nigra of MPTP-lesioned nonhuman primates. Neurobiol Dis 2005;20:898-906.
27. Dauer W, Kholodilov N, Vila M, et al: Resistance of alpha-synuclein null mice to the parkinsonian neurotoxin MPTP. Proc Natl Acad Sci U S A 2002;99:14524-14529.
28. Yu WH, Matsuoka Y, Sziraki I, et al: Increased dopaminergic neuron sensitivity to 1-methyl-4-phenyl-1,2,3,6-tetrahydropyridine (MPTP) in transgenic mice expressing mutant A53T alpha-synuclein. Neurochem Res 2008;33(5):902-911.
29. Shimura H, Hattori N, Kubo S, et al: Familial parkinson disease gene product, parkin, is a ubiquitin-protein ligase. Nat Genet 2000;25:302-305.
30. Shimura H, Schlossmacher MG, Hattori N, et al: Ubiquitination of a new form of alpha-synuclein by parkin from human brain: implications for Parkinson's disease. Science 2001;293:263-269.
31. Cuervo AM, Stefanis L, Fredenburg R, et al: Impaired degradation of mutant alpha-synuclein by chaperone-mediated autophagy. Science 2004;305:1292-1295.
32. Shin Y, Klucken J, Patterson C, et al: The co-chaperone carboxyl terminus of Hsp70-interacting protein (CHIP) mediates alpha-synuclein degradation decisions between proteasomal and lysosomal pathways. J Biol Chem 2005;280:23727-23734.
33. Spillantini MG, Crowther RA, Jakes R, et al: alpha-Synuclein in filamentous inclusions of Lewy bodies from Parkinson's disease and dementia with Lewy bodies. Proc Natl Acad Sci U S A 1998;95:6469-6473.
34. Wood SJ, Wypych J, Steavenson S, et al: alpha-Synuclein fibrillogenesis is nucleation-dependent: implications for the pathogenesis of Parkinson's disease. J Biol Chem 1999;274:19509-19512.
35. Feany MB, Bender WW: A Drosophila model of Parkinson's disease. Nature 2000;404:394-398.
36. Periquet M, Fulga T, Myllykangas L, et al: Aggregated alpha-synuclein mediates dopaminergic neurotoxicity in vivo. J Neurosci 2007;27:3338-3346.
37. Bertoncini CW, Jung YS, Fernandez CO, et al: Release of long-range tertiary interactions potentiates aggregation of natively unstructured alpha-synuclein. Proc Natl Acad Sci U S A 2005;102:1430-1435.
38. Conway KA, Lee SJ, Rochet JC, et al: Acceleration of oligomerization, not fibrillization, is a shared property of both alpha-synuclein mutations linked to early-onset Parkinson's disease: implications for pathogenesis and therapy. Proc Natl Acad Sci U S A 2000;97:571-576.
39. Giasson BI, Duda JE, Murray IV, et al: Oxidative damage linked to neurodegeneration by selective alpha-synuclein nitration in synucleinopathy lesions. Science 2000;290:985-989.
40. Neumann M, Kahle PJ, Giasson BI, et al: Misfolded proteinase K-resistant hyperphosphorylated alpha-synuclein in aged transgenic mice with locomotor deterioration and in human alpha-synucleinopathies. J Clin Invest 2002;110:1429-1439.
41. Arawaka S, Wada M, Goto S, et al: The role of G-protein-coupled receptor kinase 5 in pathogenesis of sporadic Parkinson's disease. J Neurosci 2006;26:9227-9238.
42. Outeiro TF, Lindquist S: Yeast cells provide insight into alpha-synuclein biology and pathobiology. Science 2003;302:1772-1775.
43. Outeiro TF, Kontopoulos E, Altmann SM, et al: Sirtuin 2 inhibitors rescue alpha-synuclein-mediated toxicity in models of Parkinson's disease. Science 2007;317:516-519.
44. Springer W, Hoppe T, Schmidt E, Baumeister R: A Caenorhabditis elegans Parkin mutant with altered solubility couples alpha-synuclein aggregation to proteotoxic stress. Hum Mol Genet 2005;14:3407-3423.
45. van Ham TJ, Thijssen KL, Breitling R, et al: C. elegans model identifies genetic modifiers of alpha-synuclein inclusion formation during aging. PLoS Genet 2008;4:e1000027.

46. Hamamichi S, Rivas RN, Knight AL, et al: Hypothesis-based RNAi screening identifies neuroprotective genes in a Parkinson's disease model. Proc Natl Acad Sci U S A 2008;105:728-733.
47. Chen L, Feany MB: Alpha-synuclein phosphorylation controls neurotoxicity and inclusion formation in a *Drosophila* model of Parkinson disease. Nat Neurosci 2005;8:657-663.
48. Matsuoka Y, Vila M, Lincoln S, et al: Lack of nigral pathology in transgenic mice expressing human alpha-synuclein driven by the tyrosine hydroxylase promoter. Neurobiol Dis 2001;8:535-539.
49. Rathke-Hartlieb S, Kahle PJ, Neumann M, et al: Sensitivity to MPTP is not increased in Parkinson's disease-associated mutant alpha-synuclein transgenic mice. J Neurochem 2001;77:1181-1184.
50. Wakamatsu M, Ishii A, Iwata S, et al: Selective loss of nigral dopamine neurons induced by overexpression of truncated human alpha-synuclein in mice. Neurobiol Aging 2008;29(4):574-585.
51. Wakamatsu M, Ishii A, Ukai Y, et al: Accumulation of phosphorylated alpha-synuclein in dopaminergic neurons of transgenic mice that express human alpha-synuclein. J Neurosci Res 2007;85:1819-1825.
52. Fleming SM, Salcedo J, Fernagut PO, et al: Early and progressive sensorimotor anomalies in mice overexpressing wild-type human alpha-synuclein. J Neurosci 2004;24:9434-9440.
53. Lee MK, Stirling W, Xu Y, et al: Human alpha-synuclein-harboring familial Parkinson's disease-linked Ala-53-Thr mutation causes neurodegenerative disease with alpha-synuclein aggregation in transgenic mice. Proc Natl Acad Sci U S A 2002;99:8968-8973.
54. Martin LJ, Pan Y, Price AC, et al: Parkinson's disease alpha-synuclein transgenic mice develop neuronal mitochondrial degeneration and cell death. J Neurosci 2006;26:41-50.
55. Eslamboli A, Romero-Ramos M, Burger C, et al: Long-term consequences of human alpha-synuclein overexpression in the primate ventral midbrain. Brain 2007;130;(Pt 3):799-815.
56. Hofer A, Berg D, Asmus F, et al: The role of alpha-synuclein gene multiplications in early-onset Parkinson's disease and dementia with Lewy bodies. J Neural Transm 2005;112:1249-1254.
57. Chiba-Falek O, Nussbaum RL: Effect of allelic variation at the NACP-Rep1 repeat upstream of the alpha-synuclein gene (SNCA) on transcription in a cell culture luciferase reporter system. Hum Mol Genet 2001;10:3101-3109.
58. Kruger R, Vieira-Saecker AM, Kuhn W, et al: Increased susceptibility to sporadic Parkinson's disease by a certain combined alpha-synuclein/apolipoprotein E genotype. Ann Neurol 1999;45:611-617.
59. Khan N, Graham E, Dixon P, et al: Parkinson's disease is not associated with the combined alpha-synuclein/apolipoprotein E susceptibility genotype. Ann Neurol 2001;49:665-668.
60. Spadafora P, Annesi G, Pasqua AA, et al: NACP-REP1 polymorphism is not involved in Parkinson's disease: a case-control study in a population sample from southern Italy. Neurosci Lett 2003;351:75-78.
61. Maraganore DM, de Andrade M, Elbaz A, et al: Collaborative analysis of alpha-synuclein gene promoter variability and Parkinson disease. JAMA 2006;296:661-670.
62. Chiba-Falek O, Kowalak JA, Smulson ME, Nussbaum RL: Regulation of alpha-synuclein expression by poly (ADP ribose) polymerase-1 (PARP-1) binding to the NACP-Rep1 polymorphic site upstream of the SNCA gene. Am J Hum Genet 2005;76:478-492.
63. Mueller JC, Fuchs J, Hofer A, et al: Multiple regions of alpha-synuclein are associated with Parkinson's disease. Ann Neurol 2005;57:535-541.
64. Mizuta I, Satake W, Nakabayashi Y, et al: Multiple candidate gene analysis identifies α-synuclein as a susceptibility gene for sporadic Parkinson's disease. Hum Mol Genet 2006;15:1151-1158.
65. Winkler S, Hagenah J, Lincoln S, et al: alpha-Synuclein and Parkinson disease susceptibility. Neurology 2007;69:1745-1750.
66. Fuchs J, Tichopad A, Golub Y, et al: Genetic variability in the SNCA gene influences α-synuclein levels in the blood and brain. FASEB J 2008;22:1327-1334.
67. Martinez-Vicente M, Talloczy Z, Kaushik S, et al: Dopamine-modified alpha-synuclein blocks chaperone-mediated autophagy. J Clin Invest 2008;118(2):777-788.
68. Michan S, Sinclair D: Sirtuins in mammals: insights into their biological function. Biochem J 2007;404:1-13.
69. Outeiro TF, Kontopoulos E, Altmann SM, et al: Sirtuin 2 inhibitors rescue alpha-synuclein-mediated toxicity in models of Parkinson's disease. Science 2007;317:516-519.
70. Beyer K: Mechanistic aspects of Parkinson's disease: alpha-synuclein and the biomembrane. Cell Biochem Biophys 2007;47:285-299.
71. Mash DC, Adi N, Duque L, et al: Alpha synuclein protein levels are increased in serum from recently abstinent cocaine abusers. Drug Alcohol Depend 2008;94(1-3):246-250.
72. Mash DC, Ouyang Q, Pablo J, et al: Cocaine abusers have an overexpression of alpha-synuclein in dopamine neurons. J Neurosci 2003;23:2564-2571.
73. Liang T, Carr LG: Regulation of alpha-synuclein expression in alcohol-preferring and -non preferring rats. J Neurochem 2006;99:470-482.

4 PARK2: *Parkin* Mutations Responsible for Familial Parkinson's Disease

NOBUTAKA HATTORI • TAKU HATANO •
YUTAKA MACHIDA • SHIGETO SATO •
SHIN-ICHIRO KUBO

Introduction

Clinical Features

Function of Parkin Protein

Parkin Gene Therapies for Synucleinopathies

Conclusions

Introduction

Parkinson's disease (PD) is the second most common neurodegenerative disease after Alzheimer's disease, affecting approximately 0.3% of the general population and 3% of people older than 65 years.[1] PD should be considered as not only a movement disorder, but also a neuropsychiatric disorder. Depression and dementia are major symptoms that affect the level of daily activities of PD patients. PD could be recognized as multicentric neurodegeneration including dopamine, serotonin, norepinephrine, and acetylcholine.

Mitochondrial dysfunction and oxidative stress are crucial components of most current theories of nigral degeneration in PD[2-5]; however, the mechanisms responsible for the cell death are largely unknown. More recently, there has been increasing evidence that genetic factors play an important role in PD. Although most PD is sporadic, a few cases show a mendelian inheritance. The identification of responsible genes for rare familial forms of PD has provided vital clues to understanding the molecular pathogenesis of the more common sporadic forms of this disease. To date, at least nine distinct genetic loci have been recognized to be linked to PD (PARK1, PARK2, PARK3, PARK5, PARK6, PARK7, PARK8, PARK10, and PARK11).[6-14] The family that was originally mapped to PARK4 has been assigned to PARK1.[15] PARK9 has been found not to be a genetic locus for PD because of the atypical associated phenotypes, such as spasticity resulting from corticospinal tract degeneration, a supranuclear upward-gaze paresis, and the development of dementia in all affected subjects.[16] Most patients linked to PARK9 have been shown to respond to levodopa therapies for a long time, however.

More recently, *ATP13A2* has been identified as the causative gene for PARK9. *ATP13A2* is associated with the autophagy-lysosomal system. In addition to parkin, protein degradation systems such as ubiquitin-proteasome and autophagy-lysosomal systems could be involved in dopaminergic neuronal cell loss.[17] Among the PD-associated loci, mutations have been identified in six genes (α-synuclein,[18] *parkin*,[19] *PINK1*,[20] *DJ-1*,[21] *LRRK2*,[22,23] *ATP13A2*[17]) that definitely cause familial forms of PD. The most common genetic causes of PD are *parkin* mutations, responsible for PARK2, and *LRRK2* mutations. *parkin* mutations can be directly linked to the neuronal cell loss by loss-of-function effects because of the recessive mode of inheritance. It is suggested that *parkin* is essential for the survival of dopaminergic neurons. This chapter reviews the clinical findings linked to *parkin* mutations, the molecular biology of *parkin*, and the potential therapeutic roles for *parkin*.

Clinical Features

Clinical manifestations of PARK2 were originally characterized by parkinsonism associated with early onset before age 40, wearing-off phenomenon, foot dystonia, hyperreflexia, diurnal fluctuations, sleep benefit, and early susceptibility to levodopa-induced dyskinesias.[24-27] In addition, most patients with *parkin* mutations had slow disease progression.[24] More recent studies have suggested a broader phenotypic spectrum of PARK2 that includes later age at onset and tremor-dominant manifestations without typical features as mentioned earlier. Many PARK2 patients seem to be clinically indistinguishable from patients with sporadic PD. A wide variation of age at onset has been reported, even within single families with mutations in the *parkin* gene,[26] suggesting that additional genetic or environmental factors contribute to the phenotype. Lohmann and colleagues[28] reported, however, that PARK2 patients tend to have earlier and more symmetrical onset, slow progression of the disease, and greater response to levodopa despite low doses compared with patients with early-onset PD without *parkin* mutations. Clinical features including atypical phenotypes are summarized in Table 4–1.[28-31] Although the pathology associated with *parkin*-positive PD is based on only a few cases, Lewy bodies are absent[32-36] except in two reported cases with compound heterozygous mutations.[37,38] Atypical pathological findings have been reported in PARK2, such as tau pathology in the cerebral cortex and brainstem nuclei,[39] degeneration of the spinocerebellar system, and α-synuclein–positive inclusions in the neuropils of the pedunculopontine nucleus.[34] The presence of α-synuclein–positive inclusions, including Lewy bodies, although detected in only a few patients, suggests a possible relationship between PARK2 and idiopathic PD.

The gene responsible for PARK2, *parkin*,[18] contains 12 exons spanning over 1.4 Mb and encodes a 465-amino acid protein with moderate homology to ubiquitin at the amino-terminus (ubiquitin-like domain) and two RING finger motifs at the carboxy-terminus. Various *parkin* mutations have been reported worldwide, including exonic deletions, exonic duplications, insertions, and many different point mutations.[27,31,40,41] Mutations in the *parkin* gene are a frequent cause of early-onset PD, especially in cases with a positive family history and an autosomal recessive mode of transmission. To date, more than 95 different mutations in approximately 400 patients have been reported worldwide. Frequency

TABLE 4–1	Clinical Features of PARK2

Age of onset usually <40 yr
Typical presenting phenotype: young-onset PD
Normal cognition
Frequent foot dystonia
Early instability, freezing, festination, or retropulsion in some cases
Dramatic response to levodopa, and dose-sensitive motor and psychiatric
   complications of medication
Excellent response to anticholinergics in some cases
Usually benign and slow disease course
Atypical presenting phenotypes
   Later onset, mimicking idiopathic PD
   Psychosis, panic attacks, depression, obsessive-compulsive behavior
   Exercise-induced dystonia
   Atremulous bilateral akinetic rigid syndrome
   Focal dystonia (writer's cramp, cervical)
   Autonomic or peripheral neuropathy
   Cerebellar and pyramidal tract dysfunction

PD, Parkinson disease.

of the mutations in early-onset PD has been estimated at 40% to 50% in familial cases[42] and at 10% to 20% in idiopathic cases.[42] Numerous patients carry a single heterozygous mutation. Clinical features of the carriers of heterozygous *parkin* mutations are more similar to the clinical features of idiopathic PD, including a significantly later age at onset and more asymmetrical disease presentation, than those of carriers of two mutations.[28,43-45]

Because PARK2 is considered to be an autosomal recessively transmitted disease, the role of mutations in the single heterozygous state is difficult to interpret. There are two possibilities: haploinsufficiency effect and dominant negative. Another possible explanation is that still unknown factors, such as mutations located elsewhere in the genome[46] and environmental factors, act in combination to cause the disease. In a North American study of more than 300 PD patients unselected for age at onset or family history, the frequency of *parkin* mutations reported as pathogenic in homozygous or compound heterozygous individuals was essentially the same in PD patients (3.8%) and controls (3.1%).[47] Whether the single heterozygous state in *parkin* is a risk factor for developing PD remains to be elucidated.

Function of Parkin Protein

The gene product, *parkin*, is localized to the Golgi complex in addition to the cytoplasm in human brain, although parkin has no transmembrane domain.[48] In cultured cells and rat brain, parkin also associates with synaptic vesicles as a peripheral membrane protein.[49] More recently, parkin was implicated in the ubiquitin-proteasome system as an E3 ubiquitin ligase, and mutations in the *parkin* gene are reported to result in loss of ligase function.[50] The ubiquitin-proteasome system is involved in two tasks. One is the accurate timely regulation of the level of short-lived proteins that play a role in processes such as cell-cycle regulation, signal transduction, and metabolism. The other task is protein quality control. Polyubiquitination of the target proteins for degradation by proteasomes is catalyzed by three enzymes: E1 (ubiquitin-activating enzyme), E2 (ubiquitin-conjugating enzyme), and E3 ubiquitin ligase. Parkin has been shown to catalyze the proteasomal degradation of target proteins by interacting with E2 and target proteins through its RING domain[50-52] and by binding the Rpn10 subunit of 26S proteasomes through its ubiquitin-like domain.[53]

Parkin is also reported to exhibit E3 activity by interacting with components of SCF complexes (Skp1-Cullin-F-box protein).[54] In addition, parkin forms a complex with Hsp70 and CHIP, resulting in enhancement of its E3 enzymatic activity.[55] Because PARK2 is recessively inherited, that is, loss-of-function of parkin leads to development of PARK2, substrates for parkin (for its E3 function) would be expected to accumulate in the brain. Substrates identified to date include cell division control-related protein 1 (CDCrel-1),[51] parkin-associated endothelin receptor-like receptor (Pael-R),[52] the *O*-glycosylated form of α-synuclein (aSp22),[56] synphilin-1,[57] synaptotagmin XI,[58] SEPT5_v/CDCrel-2,[59] cyclin E,[54] the p38 subunit of the aminoacyl-tRNA synthetase complex,[60] and α/β-tubulin.[61] In addition to the substrates, several interactive molecules have been reported.[62]

One may postulate that the substrates that escape ubiquitination by parkin for degradation by the proteasome accumulate in PARK2 brains, leading to nigral degeneration. Three of the substrates (CDCrel-1,[51] Pael-R,[52] αSp22[56]) have been reported to accumulate in PARK2 brains. An important caveat is that the most substrates have been identified by in vitro experiments and remain to be validated.[63] Parkin has been shown more recently to catalyze Lys63 (K63)-linked ubiquitination, which is not recognized by the proteasome.[64,65] Assembly of polyubiquitination occurs through the sequential formation of an isopeptide bond between the carboxy-terminal glycine residue and specific lysine residues in ubiquitin. Substrates tagged with the polyubiquitin chain linked via K29 or K48 are recognized and degraded by the proteasome.[66] In contrast, K63-linked ubiquitination is involved in diverse cellular processes, such as endocytosis[67-70] and protein sorting and trafficking.[71-73] Although the relevance of K63-linked ubiquitination by parkin in the pathogenesis of PARK2 remains unclear, this insight might facilitate elucidation of the pathogenesis. In addition, it has been reported that parkin catalyzed multiple mono-ubiquitination, although the role of mono-ubiquitination remains to be elucidated.[74]

With regard to loss-of-function of parkin as a mechanism underlying PARK2, parkin-knockout animal models should help to elucidate the mechanisms of the disease. Although several lines of parkin-knockout mice have been reported,[75-77] none of these develops a PD-like phenotype or PD pathology. Two exon 3–disrupted knockouts show subtle motor and cognitive deficits, inhibition of amphetamine-induced dopamine release and glutamate neurotransmission, and abnormal dopamine metabolism, but no loss of substantia nigra (SN) or locus caeruleus catecholaminergic neurons. Meanwhile, an exon 7–disrupted knockout exhibits loss of noradrenergic locus caeruleus neurons, although the locus caeruleus in autopsied brains with *parkin* mutations has been generally damaged less than SN.

None of the previously reported substrates for parkin in the ubiquitin-proteasome system accumulated in the knockout brains,[76,77] suggesting that parkin might function as an E3 for K63-linked polyubiquitination. Proteomic analysis of ventral midbrain from the exon 3–disrupted mice revealed decreased abundance of numerous proteins involved in mitochondrial function or oxidative stress.[78] Consistent with reduction of these proteins, the mice exhibited decreased respiratory capacity of striatal mitochondria, and reduced serum antioxidant capacity and increased protein and lipid peroxidation. In addition, we reported a decline of endogenous dopamine release in parkin-null mice after methamphetamine challenge.[79] Parkin-null mice led to a considerable increase of binding potentials for D1 and D2 dopamine receptors in the striatum and dopamine levels in the midbrain.[79] These phenomena may be associated with the early appearance of drug-induced dyskinesias after induction of levodopa therapies. The level of dopamine was also increased in the midbrain of parkin-null mice, although it was unchanged in the striatum.[79] It is unclear why the dopamine levels are increased in association with impairment of parkin function. It is plausible, however, that the decrease of dopamine release is linked to this issue, and consequently dopamine D1 and D2 are increased as a compensatory response. An abnormality of the dopamine signaling pathway caused by impairment of parkin may be an important factor in the pathogenesis of Park2 PD (Fig. 4–1).

A study in *Drosophila* with an inactivated orthologue of human parkin also suggested mitochondrial dysfunction.[80] The parkin-null mutants exhibited reduced longevity, locomotor defects, and sterility.[80,81] Mitochondrial pathology has been the earliest manifestation of muscular degeneration and defective spermatogenesis in the parkin mutants. These observations suggest a new role for parkin in the

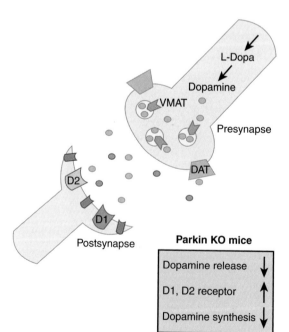

Figure 4–1 Summary of *Parkin* knockout (KO) mice. (1) Decreasing of dopamine release; (2) increasing of binding potential for D1 and D2. *Parkin* KO mice have no locomotion deficits. Dopamine releasing could be impaired as in *PINK1* or *DJ-1* KO mice. L-Dopa, levodopa. DAT, Dopamine transporter; VMAT, Vesicular monoamine transporter.

regulation of normal mitochondrial function. Parkin overexpression in cultured cells protects against mitochondria-dependent apoptosis and parkin associates with the outer mitochondrial membrane.[82] Parkin has been shown to have cytoprotective effects against diverse cellular insults, including dopamine-mediated toxicity,[83] kainate-induced excitotoxicity,[54] overexpression of Pael-R[55] or the p38 subunit,[60] and toxicity induced by proteasomal inhibition or overexpression of mutant α-synuclein.[84]

More recently, antisense knockdown of parkin was reported to cause apoptotic cell death of human dopaminergic cells associated with caspase activation, accompanied by accumulation of oxidative dopamine metabolites owing to auto-oxidation of DOPA and dopamine.[85] These results suggest that parkin may function as a multipurpose neuroprotectant.[86] Parkin has been shown to be S-nitrosylated in vitro and in brains of patients with idiopathic PD.[87,88] Chung and associates[87] reported that S-nitrosylation of parkin impaired its E3 activity and its protective function. Yao and colleagues[88] showed that S-nitrosylation increased, rather than decreased, the E3 activity of parkin. Several technical differences may explain the discrepancy between them. These findings may provide a molecular link between PARK2 and sporadic PD.

More recently, we identified 14-3-3η as a regulator molecule for ubiquitin ligase activities of parkin.[89] This binding of 14-3-3η to parkin suppressed the ubiquitin-ligase activity, suggesting that the complex formation between parkin and 14-3-3η acts as a negative regulator for ubiquitin ligase activities of parkin and might be essential to maintain the nigral neurons. Certain parkin bound to 14-3-3η is present in latent form in the brain. In addition, 14-3-3η is located within Lewy bodies. The latent parkin can be activated by α-synuclein, which has strong affinity to 14-3-3η over parkin, and can capture 14-3-3η from the latent parkin-14-3-3η complex (Fig. 4–2).[89]

Parkin and α-synuclein might share a protein degradation system. More recently, biochemical and morphological studies using *Drosophila* suggested that *parkin* and *PINK1* act in a common pathway to maintain mitochondrial function. *Parkin* functions downstream of *PINK1*.[90,91] *DJ-1* also may play a role to maintain the function of mitochondria, including antioxidative stress. *Parkin* interacts with *DJ-1*.[92] Dominant or recessive PD gene products share a common pathway, including mitochondrial functions. Considering the roles of parkin as a protein downstream of other proteins involved in PD pathogenesis, parkin has the

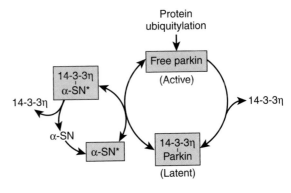

Figure 4–2 Schematic model for regulation of *Parkin* activity by 14-3-3η and modified α-synuclein (α-SN*). The enzymes catalyzing phosphorylation and dephosphorylation of α-SN are unknown. See text for details.

potential to rescue neurons in not only *parkin*-linked familial PD but also other forms of familial PD.

Parkin Gene Therapies for Synucleinopathies

α-Synuclein is a major component of Lewy bodies. It is crucial to elucidate the relationship between its functions and Lewy body formation. In contrast, several studies using human brain specimens have suggested the possibility of a direct interaction between parkin and α-synuclein, co-immunoprecipitation of both proteins,[93] the presence of ubiquitinated α-synuclein in synucleinopathy lesions,[94,95] and the presence of parkin in the Lewy body.[96] Parkin can mitigate the neuronal cell death induced by several cytotoxic insults, such as tunicamycin, ceramide, kainite excitotoxicity, manganese, dopamine, and overexpression of α-synuclein.[54,55,82-84,97,99,100]

Besides these studies, it has been reported that *parkin* can mitigate the dopaminergic neuronal cell death induced by α-synuclein overexpression in rat SN.[101] The amelioration of behavioral deficits is necessary, however, for further confirmation of the potential suitability of *parkin* gene therapy for synucleinopathy. We examined the effects of *parkin* on the synucleinopathy in rat SN, including aspects of motor function. To coexpress genes of interest in rat SN, we used the recombinant adeno-associated viral (rAAV) vector system. It has already reported that targeted overexpression of α-synuclein in SN via rAAV (rAAV-α-synuclein) induces dopaminergic neuronal cell death.[102-104] Based on the implication of α-synuclein in the pathogenesis of PD, the use of α-synuclein–based methods, such as transgenic animals or the viral vector delivery, is a more appropriate model of synucleinopathy. Synucleinopathy induced by rAAV-α-synuclein resembles the pathological changes in PD.[104]

The ameliorative effects of *parkin* on α-synuclein toxicity from the pathology and motor function perspectives have been reported.[105] This effect of *parkin* on synucleinopathy in rat SN may add further support to the applicability of *parkin* gene therapy for patients with PD. Because *parkin* is expressed throughout the brain,[106] epigenetic and additional expressions of *parkin* gene are probably less adverse. Human *parkin* expression in rat SN induced neither dopaminergic neuron loss nor motor dysfunction.[104] *Parkin* gene therapy also can be effective in PD caused by *parkin* gene mutations. In contrast to genes of an apoptosis inhibitor, such as *bcl-2*, *parkin* does not seem to be associated with oncogenesis. To assess the ameliorative effects of *parkin* on synucleinopathy, we used the rAAV-based method to deliver α-synuclein gene and induce the loss of dopaminergic neurons in SN. The rAAV-based method has already been confirmed to cause the loss of dopaminergic neurons in SN, in contrast to α-synuclein transgenic mice.[107]

Previous studies revealed the presence of *parkin* in Lewy bodies,[96] and mutations in the *parkin* gene have been linked to autosomal recessive juvenile parkinsonism, in which Lewy bodies are hardly detected in the brain.[36,48] These findings imply the involvement of *parkin* in Lewy body formation; however, we were unable to detect the large inclusions reminiscent of Lewy bodies even in SN coexpressed *parkin* and α-synuclein. It is possible that the presence of *parkin* and α-synuclein is necessary for the formation of Lewy bodies in the brain. In fact, a recent study suggested that other proteins such as synphilin-1 are probably involved in Lewy body formation, in addition to *parkin* and α-synuclein.[108] More recently, similar findings have been reported by Lo Bianco and coworkers[109]; these investigators documented the ameliorative effect of *parkin* on synucleinopathy using the lentiviral vector delivery. It has also been indicated that the inhibition of dopaminergic neuron death by *parkin* resulted in accumulation of phosphorylated α-synuclein inclusions. Viral vector–based methods are likely to be quite useful not only for the development of the *parkin* gene therapy, but also for the elucidation of mechanisms of α-synuclein and *parkin* that underlie Lewy body formation, dopaminergic neuron loss, and amelioration of synucleinopathy. In addition, the other major finding of our study is the ameliorative effect of *parkin* on the motor dysfunction induced by α-synuclein.

Conclusions

The discovery of *parkin* mutations as a cause of familial PD has provided valuable insights into the pathogenesis of sporadic disease. Importantly in terms of developing neuroprotective therapies, downstream effects of *parkin* mutations have converged with the effects induced by other mutations. The position of *parkin* as a component perhaps of the final common pathway to cell damage and death offers the opportunity to consider *parkin* expression as a potential therapy for dopaminergic cells in PD.

REFERENCES

1. Lang AE, Lozano AM: Parkinson's disease: first of two parts. N Engl J Med 1998;339:1044-1053.
2. Schapira AH, Cooper JM, Dexter D, et al: Mitochondrial complex I deficiency in Parkinson's disease. J Neurochem 1990;54:823-827.
3. Hattori N, Tanaka M, Ozawa T, Mizuno Y: Immunohistochemical studies on complexes I, II, III, and IV of mitochondria in Parkinson's disease. Ann Neurol 1991;30:563-571.
4. Ben-Shachar D, Riederer P, Youdim MB: Iron-melanin interaction and lipid peroxidation: implications for Parkinson's disease. J Neurochem 1991;57:1609-1614.
5. Jenner P: Oxidative stress in Parkinson's disease. Ann Neurol 2003;53;(Suppl 3):S26-S36.
6. Polymeropoulos MH, Higgins JJ, Golbe LI, et al: Mapping of a gene for Parkinson's disease to chromosome 4q21-q23. Science 1996;274:1197-1199.
7. Matsumine H, Saito M, Shimoda-Matsubayashi S, et al: Localization of a gene for an autosomal recessive form of juvenile parkinsonism to chromosome 6q25.2-27. Am J Hum Genet 1997;60:588-596.
8. Gasser T, Muller-Myhsok B, Wszolek ZK, et al: A susceptibility locus for Parkinson's disease maps to chromosome 2p13. Nat Genet 1998;18:262-265.
9. Leroy E, Boyer R, Auburger G, et al: The ubiquitin pathway in Parkinson's disease. Nature 1998;395:451-452.
10. Valente EM, Bentivoglio AR, Dixon PH, et al: Localization of a novel locus for autosomal recessive early-onset parkinsonism, PARK6, on human chromosome 1p35-p36. Am J Hum Genet 2001;68:895-900.
11. van Duijn CM, Dekker MC, Bonifati V, et al: Park7, a novel locus for autosomal recessive early-onset parkinsonism, on chromosome 1p36. Am J Hum Genet 2001;69:629-634.
12. Funayama M, Hasegawa K, Kowa H, et al: A new locus for Parkinson's disease (PARK8) maps to chromosome 12p11.2-q13.1. Ann Neurol 2002;51:296-301.
13. Hicks AA, Petursson H, Jonsson T, et al: A susceptibility gene for late-onset idiopathic Parkinson's disease. Ann Neurol 2002;52:549-555.
14. Pankratz N, Nichols WC, Uniacke SK, et al: Significant linkage of Parkinson disease to chromosome 2q36-37. Am J Hum Genet 2003;72:1053-1057.

15. Singleton AB, Farrer M, Johnson J, et al: alpha-Synuclein locus triplication causes Parkinson's disease. Science 2003;302:841.
16. Hampshire DJ, Roberts E, Crow Y, et al: Kufor-Rakeb syndrome, pallido-pyramidal degeneration with supranuclear upgaze paresis and dementia, maps to 1p36. J Med Genet 2001;38:680-682.
17. Ramirez A, Heimbach A, Gründemann J, et al: Hereditary parkinsonism with dementia is caused by mutations in ATP13A2, encoding a lysosomal type 5 P-type ATPase. Nat Genet 2006;38:1184-1191.
18. Polymeropoulos MH, Lavedan C, Leroy E, et al: Mutation in the alpha-synuclein gene identified in families with Parkinson's disease. Science 1997;276:2045-2047.
19. Kitada T, Asakawa S, Hattori N, et al: Mutations in the parkin gene cause autosomal recessive juvenile parkinsonism. Nature 1998;392:605-608.
20. Valente EM, Abou-Sleiman PM, Caputo V, et al: Hereditary early-onset Parkinson's disease caused by mutations in PINK1. Science 2004;304:1158-1160.
21. Bonifati V, Rizzu P, van Baren MJ, et al: Mutations in the DJ-1 gene associated with autosomal recessive early-onset parkinsonism. Science 2003;299:256-259.
22. Paisan-Ruiz C, Jain S, Evans EW, et al: Cloning of the gene containing mutations that cause PARK8-linked Parkinson's disease. Neuron 2004;44:595-600.
23. Zimprich A, Biskup S, Leitner P, et al: Mutations in LRRK2 cause autosomal-dominant parkinsonism with pleomorphic pathology. Neuron 2004;44:601-607.
24. Yamamura Y, Sobue I, Ando K, et al: Paralysis agitans of early onset with marked diurnal fluctuation of symptoms. Neurology 1973;23:239-244.
25. Abbas N, Lucking CB, Ricard S, et al: A wide variety of mutations in the parkin gene are responsible for autosomal recessive parkinsonism in Europe. French Parkinson's Disease Genetics Study Group and the European Consortium on Genetic Susceptibility in Parkinson's Disease. Hum Mol Genet 1999;8:567-574.
26. Klein C, Pramstaller PP, Kis B, et al: Parkin deletions in a family with adult-onset, tremor-dominant parkinsonism: expanding the phenotype. Ann Neurol 2000;48:65-71.
27. Lucking CB, Durr A, Bonifati V, et al: Association between early-onset Parkinson's disease and mutations in the parkin gene. French Parkinson's Disease Genetics Study Group. N Engl J Med 2000;342:1560-1567.
28. Lohmann E, Periquet M, Bonifati V, et al: How much phenotypic variation can be attributed to parkin genotype? Ann Neurol 2003;54:176-185.
29. Morales B, Martinez A, Gonzalo I, et al: Steele-Richardson-Olszewski syndrome in a patient with a single C212Y mutation in the parkin protein. Mov Disord 2002;17:1374-1380.
30. Khan NL, Graham E, Critchley P, et al: Parkin disease: a phenotypic study of a large case series. Brain 2003;126:1279-1292.
31. Periquet M, Latouche M, Lohmann E, et al: Parkin mutations are frequent in patients with isolated early-onset parkinsonism. Brain 2003;126:1271-1278.
32. Gouider-Khouja N, Larnaout A, Amouri R, et al: Autosomal recessive parkinsonism linked to parkin gene in a Tunisian family: clinical, genetic and pathological study. Parkinsonism Relat Disord 2003;9:247-251.
33. Hayashi S, Wakabayashi K, Ishikawa A, et al: An autopsy case of autosomal-recessive juvenile parkinsonism with a homozygous exon 4 deletion in the parkin gene. Mov Disord 2000;15:884-888.
34. Sasaki S, Shirata A, Yamane K, Iwata M: Parkin-positive autosomal recessive juvenile parkinsonism with alpha-synuclein-positive inclusions. Neurology 2004;63:678-682.
35. Mori H, Kondo T, Yokochi M, et al: Pathologic and biochemical studies of juvenile parkinsonism linked to chromosome 6q. Neurology 1998;51:890-892.
36. Takahashi H, Ohama E, Suzuki S, et al: Familial juvenile parkinsonism: clinical and pathologic study in a family. Neurology 1994;44:437-441.
37. Farrer M, Chan P, Chen R, et al: Lewy bodies and parkinsonism in families with parkin mutations. Ann Neurol 2001;50:293-300.
38. Pramstaller PP, Schlossmacher MG, Jacques TS, et al: Lewy body Parkinson's disease in a large pedigree with 77 Parkin mutation carriers. Ann Neurol 2005;58:411-422.
39. van de Warrenburg BP, Lammens M, Lucking CB, et al: Clinical and pathologic abnormalities in a family with parkinsonism and parkin gene mutations. Neurology 2001;56:555-557.
40. Hattori N, Kitada T, Matsumine H, et al: Molecular genetic analysis of a novel Parkin gene in Japanese families with autosomal recessive juvenile parkinsonism: evidence for variable homozygous deletions in the Parkin gene in affected individuals. Ann Neurol 1998;44:935-941.

41. Khan NL, Graham E, Critchley P, et al: Parkin disease: a phenotypic study of a large case series. Brain 2003;126:1279-1292.
42. Hedrich K, Eskelson C, Wilmot B, et al: Distribution, type, and origin of Parkin mutations: review and case studies. Mov Disord 2004;19:1146-1157.
43. Kann M, Jacobs H, Mohrmann K, et al: Role of parkin mutations in 111 community-based patients with early-onset parkinsonism. Ann Neurol 2002;51:621-625.
44. Hedrich K, Marder K, Harris J, et al: Evaluation of 50 probands with early-onset Parkinson's disease for Parkin mutations. Neurology 2002;58:1239-1246.
45. Foroud T, Uniacke SK, Liu L, et al: Heterozygosity for a mutation in the parkin gene leads to later onset Parkinson disease. Neurology 2003;60:796-801.
46. Pankratz N, Nichols WC, Uniacke SK, et al: Genome-wide linkage analysis and evidence of gene-by-gene interactions in a sample of 362 multiplex Parkinson disease families. Hum Mol Genet 2003;12:2599-2608.
47. Lincoln SJ, Maraganore DM, Lesnick TG, et al: Parkin variants in North American Parkinson's disease: cases and controls. Mov Disord 2003;18:1306-1311.
48. Shimura H, Hattori N, Kubo S, et al: Immunohistochemical and subcellular localization of Parkin protein: absence of protein in autosomal recessive juvenile parkinsonism patients. Ann Neurol 1999;45:668-672.
49. Kubo S, Kitami T, Noda S, et al: Parkin is associated with cellular vesicles. J Neurochem 2001;78:42-54.
50. Shimura H, Hattori N, Kubo S, et al: Familial Parkinson disease gene product, parkin, is a ubiquitin-protein ligase. Nat Genet 2000;25:302-305.
51. Zhang Y, Gao J, Chung KK, et al: Parkin functions as an E2-dependent ubiquitin-protein ligase and promotes the degradation of the synaptic vesicle-associated protein, CDCrel-1. Proc Natl Acad Sci U S A 2000;97:13354-13359.
52. Imai Y, Soda M, Inoue H, et al: An unfolded putative transmembrane polypeptide, which can lead to endoplasmic reticulum stress, is a substrate of Parkin. Cell 2001;105:891-902.
53. Sakata E, Yamaguchi Y, Kurimoto E, et al: Parkin binds the Rpn10 subunit of 26S proteasomes through its ubiquitin-like domain. EMBO Rep 2003;4:301-306.
54. Staropoli JF, McDermott C, Martinat C, et al: Parkin is a component of an SCF-like ubiquitin ligase complex and protects postmitotic neurons from kainate excitotoxicity. Neuron 2003;37:735-749.
55. Imai Y, Soda M, Hatakeyama S, et al: CHIP is associated with Parkin, a gene responsible for familial Parkinson's disease, and enhances its ubiquitin ligase activity. Mol Cell 2002;10:55-67.
56. Shimura H, Schlossmacher MG, Hattori N, et al: Ubiquitination of a new form of alpha-synuclein by parkin from human brain: implications for Parkinson's disease. Science 2001;293:263-269.
57. Chung KK, Zhang Y, Lim KL, et al: Parkin ubiquitinates the alpha-synuclein-interacting protein, synphilin-1: implications for Lewy-body formation in Parkinson disease. Nat Med 2001;7:1144-1150.
58. Huynh DP, Scoles DR, Nguyen D, Pulst SM: The autosomal recessive juvenile Parkinson disease gene product, parkin, interacts with and ubiquitinates synaptotagmin XI: Hum Mol Genet, 2003;12:2587-2597.
59. Choi P, Snyder H, Petrucelli L, et al: SEPT5_v2 is a parkin-binding protein. Brain Res Mol Brain Res 2003;117:179-189.
60. Corti O, Hampe C, Koutnikova H, et al: The p38 subunit of the aminoacyl-tRNA synthetase complex is a Parkin substrate: linking protein biosynthesis and neurodegeneration. Hum Mol Genet 2003;12:1427-1437.
61. Ren Y, Zhao J, Feng J: Parkin binds to alpha/beta tubulin and increases their ubiquitination and degradation. J Neurosci 2003;23:3316-3324.
62. Hattori N, Mizuno Y: Pathogenetic mechanisms of parkin in Parkinson's disease. Lancet 2004;364:722-724.
63. Mata IF, Lockhart PJ, Farrer MJ: Parkin genetics: one model for Parkinson's disease. Hum Mol Genet 2004;13;(Spec No 1):R127-R133.
64. Doss-Pepe EW, Chen L, Madura K: Alpha-synuclein and parkin contribute to the assembly of ubiquitin lysine63-linked multiubiquitin chains. J Biol Chem 2005;280:16619-16624.
65. Lim KL, Chew KC, Tan JM, et al: Parkin mediates nonclassical, proteasomal-independent ubiquitination of synphilin-1: implications for Lewy body formation. J Neurosci 2005;25:2002-2009.
66. Hershko A, Ciechanover A: The ubiquitin system for protein degradation. Annu Rev Biochem 1992;61:761-807.

67. Haglund K, Sigismund S, Polo S, et al: Multiple monoubiquitination of RTKs is sufficient for their endocytosis and degradation. Nat Cell Biol 2003;5:461-466.
68. Nakatsu F, Sakuma M, Matsuo Y, et al: A Di-leucine signal in the ubiquitin moiety; possible involvement in ubiquitination-mediated endocytosis. J Biol Chem 2000;275:26213-26219.
69. Roth AF, Davis NG: Ubiquitination of the PEST-like endocytosis signal of the yeast α-factor receptor. J Biol Chem 2000;275:8143-8153.
70. Shih SC, Sloper-Mould KE, Hicke L: Monoubiquitin carries a novel internalization signal that is appended to activated receptors. EMBO J 2000;19:187-198.
71. Hicke L: Ubiquitin-dependent internalization and down-regulation of plasma membrane proteins. FASEB J 1997;11:1215-1226.
72. Hicke L: Protein regulation by monoubiquitin. Nat Rev Mol Cell Biol 2001;2:195-201.
73. Katzmann DJ, Odorizzi G, Emr SD: Receptor downregulation and multivesicular-body sorting. Nat Rev Mol Cell Biol 2002;3:893-905.
74. Matsuda N, Kitami T, Suzuki T, et al: Diverse effects of pathogenic mutations of Parkin that catalyze multiple monoubiquitylation in vitro. J Biol Chem 2006;281:3204-3209.
75. Itier JM, Ibanez P, Mena MA, et al: Parkin gene inactivation alters behaviour and dopamine neurotransmission in the mouse. Hum Mol Genet 2003;12:2277-2291.
76. Goldberg MS, Fleming SM, Palacino JJ, et al: Parkin-deficient mice exhibit nigrostriatal deficits but not loss of dopaminergic neurons. J Biol Chem 2003;278:43628-43635.
77. Von Coelln R, Thomas B, Savitt JM, et al: Loss of locus coeruleus neurons and reduced startle in parkin null mice. Proc Natl Acad Sci U S A 2004;101:10744-10749.
78. Palacino JJ, Sagi D, Goldberg MS, et al: Mitochondrial dysfunction and oxidative damage in parkin-deficient mice. J Biol Chem 2004;279:18614-18622.
79. Sato S, Chiba T, Nishiyama S, et al: Decline of striatal dopamine release in parkin-deficient mice shown by ex vivo autoradiography. J Neurosci Res 2006;84:1350-1357.
80. Greene JC, Whitworth AJ, Kuo I, et al: Mitochondrial pathology and apoptotic muscle degeneration in Drosophila parkin mutants. Proc Natl Acad Sci U S A 2003;100:4078-4083.
81. Pesah Y, Pham T, Burgess H, et al: Drosophila parkin mutants have decreased mass and cell size and increased sensitivity to oxygen radical stress. Development 2004;131:2183-2194.
82. Darios F, Corti O, Lucking CB, et al: Parkin prevents mitochondrial swelling and cytochrome c release in mitochondria-dependent cell death. Hum Mol Genet 2003;12:517-526.
83. Jiang H, Ren Y, Zhao J, Feng J: Parkin protects human dopaminergic neuroblastoma cells against dopamine-induced apoptosis. Hum Mol Genet 2004;13:1745-1754.
84. Petrucelli L, O'Farrell C, Lockhart PJ, et al: Parkin protects against the toxicity associated with mutant alpha-synuclein: proteasome dysfunction selectively affects catecholaminergic neurons. Neuron 2002;36:1007-1019.
85. Machida Y, Chiba T, Takayanagi A, et al: Common anti-apoptotic roles of parkin and alpha-synuclein in human dopaminergic cells. Biochem Biophys Res Commun 2005;332:233-240.
86. Feany MB, Pallanck LJ: Parkin: a multipurpose neuroprotective agent? Neuron 2003;38:13-16.
87. Chung KK, Thomas B, Li X, et al: S-nitrosylation of parkin regulates ubiquitination and compromises parkin's protective function. Science 2004;304:1328-1331.
88. Yao D, Gu Z, Nakamura T, et al: Nitrosative stress linked to sporadic Parkinson's disease: S-nitrosylation of parkin regulates its E3 ubiquitin ligase activity. Proc Natl Acad Sci U S A 2004;101:10810-10814.
89. Sato S, Chiba T, Sakata E, et al: 14-3-3eta is a novel regulator of parkin ubiquitin ligase. EMBO J 2006;25:211-221.
90. Park J, Lee SB, Lee S, et al: Mitochondrial dysfunction in Drosophila PINK1 mutants is complemented by parkin. Nature 2006;441:1157-1161.
91. Clark IE, Dodson MW, Jiang C, et al: Drosophila pink1 is required for mitochondrial function and interacts genetically with parkin. Nature 2006;441:1162-1166.
92. Moore DJ, Zhang L, Troncoso J, et al: Association of DJ-1 and parkin mediated by pathogenic DJ-1 mutations and oxidative stress. Hum Mol Genet 2005;14:71-84.
93. Choi P, Golts N, Snyder H, et al: Co-association of parkin and alpha-synuclein. Neuroreport 2001;12:2839-2843.
94. Hasegawa M, Fujiwara H, Nonaka T: Phosphorylated alpha-synuclein is ubiquitinated in alpha-synucleinopathy lesions. J Biol Chem 2002;277:49071-49076.
95. Tofaris GK, RazzaqA Ghetti B, et al: Ubiquitination of alpha-synuclein in Lewy bodies is a pathological event not associated with impairment of proteasome function. J Biol Chem 2003;278:44405-44411.

96. Schlossmacher MG, Frosch MP, Gai WP, et al: Parkin localizes to the Lewy bodies of Parkinson disease and dementia with Lewy bodies. Am J Pathol 2002;160:1655-1667.
97. Kim SJ, Sung JY, Um JW, et al: Parkin cleaves intracellular alpha-synuclein inclusions via the activation of calpain. J Biol Chem 2003;278:41890-41899.
98. Oluwatosin-Chigbu Y, Robbins A, Scott CW, et al: Parkin suppresses wild-type alpha-synuclein-induced toxicity in SHSY-5Y cells. Biochem Biophys Res Commun 2003;309:679-684.
99. Yang Y, Nishimura I, Imai Y, et al: Parkin suppresses dopaminergic neuron-selective neurotoxicity induced by Pael-R in *Drosophila*. Neuron 2003;37:911-924.
100. Higashi Y, Asanuma M, Miyazaki I, et al: Parkin attenuates manganese-induced dopaminergic cell death. J Neurochem 2004;89:1490-1497.
101. Lo Bianco C, Ridet JL, Schneider BL, et al: Alpha-synucleinopathy and selective dopaminergic neuron loss in a rat lentiviral-based model of Parkinson's disease. Proc Natl Acad Sci U S A 2002;99:10813-10818.
102. Kirik D, Rosenblad C, Burger C, et al: Parkinson-like neurodegeneration induced by targeted overexpression of alpha-synuclein in the nigrostriatal system. J Neurosci 2002;22:2780-2791.
103. Klein RL, King MA, Hamby ME, Meyer EM: Dopaminergic cell loss induced by human A30P alpha-synuclein gene transfer to the rat substantia nigra. Hum Gene Ther 2002;13:605-612.
104. Yamada M, Iwatsubo T, Mizuno Y, Mochizuki H: Overexpression of α-synuclein in rat substantia nigra results in loss of dopaminergic neurons, phosphorylation of α-synuclein and activation of caspase-9: resemblance to pathogenetic changes in Parkinson's disease. J Neurochem 2004;91:451-461.
105. Yamada M, Mizuno Y, Mochizuki H: Parkin gene therapy for alpha-synucleinopathy: a rat model of Parkinson's disease. Hum Gene Ther 2005;16:262-270.
106. Zarate-Lagunes M, Gu WL, Blanchard V, et al: Parkin immunoreactivity in the brain of human and non-human primates: an immunohistochemical analysis in normal conditions and in parkinsonian syndromes. J Comp Neurol 2001;432:184-196.
107. Hashimoto M, Rockenstein E, Masliah E: Transgenic models of alpha-synuclein pathology: past, present, and future. Ann N Y Acad Sci 2003;991:171-188.
108. Chung KK, Zhang Y, Lim KL, et al: Parkin ubiquitinates the alpha-synuclein-interacting protein, synphilin-1: implications for Lewy-body formation in Parkinson disease. Nat Med 2001;7:1144-1150.
109. Lo Bianco C, Schneider BL, Bauer M, et al: Lentiviral vector delivery of parkin prevents dopaminergic degeneration in an alpha-synuclein rat model of Parkinson's disease. Proc Natl Acad Sci U S A 2004;101:17510-17515.

5 PINK1 (PARK6) and Parkinson's Disease

ENZA MARIA VALENTE • ALESSANDRO FERRARIS

Clinical and Molecular Genetic Studies
Identification of the PINK1 Gene
PINK1 Homozygous and Compound Heterozygous Mutations
PINK1 Heterozygous Rare Variants

Functional Studies
PINK1 Localization in Human Brain
PINK1 as a Serine-Threonine Kinase

Subcellular Localization of PINK1
PINK1 as Protective from Different Types of Cellular Stress
Regulatory Mechanisms of PINK1

PINK1 Animal Models
Mouse Models
Drosophila Models

Clinical and Molecular Genetic Studies

IDENTIFICATION OF THE PINK1 GENE

The PARK6 locus was mapped to chromosome 1p35-36 through a genome-wide scan in a large Sicilian family (the Marsala kindred) with autosomal recessive parkinsonism (ARP).[1] Four affected subjects (two siblings and two first cousins) presented a typical parkinsonian phenotype with onset between 32 and 48 years, slow progression, sustained response to levodopa, and occurrence of levodopa-associated dyskinesias of variable severity. Subsequent mapping of two additional consanguineous families from central Italy and Spain allowed refining the PARK6 locus to 2.8 Mb of genomic DNA, containing approximately 40 genes. Candidate sequence analysis led us to identify homozygous mutations in the PTEN-induced putative kinase 1 (PINK1) gene in the three families.[2] Both Italian families carried the nonsense mutation W437X, whereas the missense change G309D was detected in affected members from the Spanish family.

Since the gene identification in 2004, several groups have screened the PINK1 gene in large cohorts of parkinsonian patients, allowing the identification of several biallelic (homozygous and compound heterozygous) and single heterozygous mutations. While biallelic mutations are unequivocally causative of ARP with full penetrance, the significance of single heterozygous mutations is still debated, although they have been proposed to play a minor role in genetic susceptibility to idiopathic Parkinson's disease (PD). This chapter discusses the mutational spectrum, prevalence, and phenotypes of biallelic and single heterozygous mutations. Table 5–1 reports the frequencies of biallelic and single heterozygous mutations in all *PINK1* mutation screens including 50 or more patients, that have been published up to December 31, 2007.

PINK1 HOMOZYGOUS AND COMPOUND HETEROZYGOUS MUTATIONS

Mutational Spectrum

More than 30 different *PINK1* mutations have been described in homozygous or compound heterozygous state (Fig. 5–1). Mutations were distributed across the whole gene, but most of them clustered in exons encoding for the large kinase domain of the protein. Only a few mutations (R246X, L347P, W437X, Q456X, and R492X) recurred in more than two unrelated families, and for two of them (W437X found in Italian families and L347P found in Filipino families), a common ancestor has been suggested.[2-6]

TABLE 5–1	Frequencies of Biallelic and Single Heterozygous Mutations*					
Reference	No. of Probands	Two Mutations (%)†	One Mutation (%)‡	Country	Selection	Age at Onset (yr)
6, 7	90	8.9	0	Mainly Japan	ARP	NA
22	177	4	0.6	Mainly Europe	ARP	NA (<60)
9	116	3.4	3.4	Mainly Italy	EOP	36 (18-45)
11	80	2.5	1.3	Singapore	EOP	44 (<55)
3	58	1.7	0	Italy	EOP	NA (<50)
15	127	1.6	0.8	Taiwan	EOP	33 (5-40)
10	65	1.5	3.1	Italy	EOP	43 (25-51)
4	289	0.7	2.1	North America	Mix	51 (14-83)
2, 8, 16, 31,u.d.§	1130	0.5	1.8	Italy	Mix	50 (17-85)
12	92	0	3.3	South Tyrol, Serbia	EOP	39 (26-45)
19	131	0	2.3	Norway	Mix	50 (31-75)
13	73	0	1.4	Taiwan	EOP	48 (24-55)
33	768	0	1.2	England	Mix	NA
18	290	0	0.3	Ireland	Mix	70% >45
17	175	0	0	Norway, Germany	LOP	61 (45-79)
14	55	0	0	Korea	EOP	<50

*In all *PINK1* mutation screens including ≥50 patient, published by December 31, 2007.
†Homozygotes or compound heterozygotes.
‡Heterozygotes.
§u.d. = unpublished data.
ARP, autosomal recessive parkinsonism; EOP, early-onset parkinsonism; LOP, late-onset parkinsonism; Mix, cohorts including familial and sporadic cases, regardless of age at onset; NA, not available.

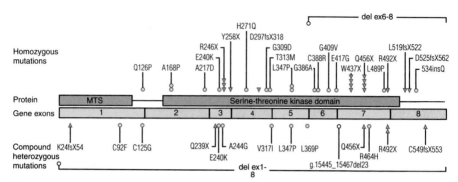

Figure 5–1 *PINK1* homozygous and compound heterozygous mutations, published by December 31, 2007.

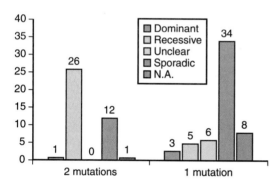

Figure 5–2 Distribution of family history for PD in probands with two *PINK1* mutations (*n* = 40)[2-11,15,16,20-22,30,32,36,71] and in single heterozygous carriers (*n* = 56).[4,9-13,15,18,19,22,31-36] N.A., not available.

Most mutations were missense or nonsense, whereas small insertions or deletions have been rarely identified. Exonic multiplications have never been reported; deletions have been detected in two probands only, one carrying a homozygous deletion of exons 6 to 8,[7] and one with a heterozygous deletion of the whole *PINK1* gene, who also carried a 23-bp deletion affecting exon 7 splicing.[8] Genomic rearrangements seem to be a rare mutational mechanism underlying *PINK1*-related parkinsonism.

Prevalence

Biallelic mutations in the *PINK1* gene represent the second cause of ARP after *parkin*, and have been reported in 40 probands so far. Their frequency varied from 0% to 8.9% in distinct studies, likely depending on the different inclusion criteria adopted by each molecular screening (i.e., early onset only, autosomal recessive only) (see Table 5–1). The highest mutation rate (8.9%) was found among a selected cohort of *parkin*-negative probands with autosomal recessive inheritance and mostly early onset of the disease.[6,7] Among the 40 probands carrying biallelic mutations, 26 (65%) had a family history compatible with recessive inheritance (multiple affected cases in the same generation or parental consanguinity or both), whereas 12 (30%) were sporadic (Fig. 5–2).

Considering early-onset cases (<40 to 50 years old) unselected for family history, mutation frequency ranged from 0% to 3.4%.[3,9-16] Conversely, mutation

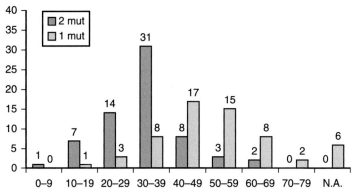

Figure 5–3 Distribution of PD ages at onset in patients (including probands and relatives for whom information was available) with two *PINK1* mutations (*n* = 66)[2-11,15,16,20-22,30,32,36,71,72] and with one heterozygous mutation (*n* = 60).[3,4,9-13,15,18,19,22,31-36] N.A., not available.

screens of patients with late-onset PD generally failed to identify *PINK1* biallelic mutations,[4,17-19] and in our large cohort of late-onset cases (602 probands with onset ≥50 years old), only one patient with sporadic PD was compound heterozygous for two *PINK1* missense mutations.

Phenotypes

Similar to other genes causative of ARP, *PINK1*-related phenotype differs from idiopathic PD in the earlier age at onset, slower progression, and better and sustained response to levodopa. The disease usually becomes clinically manifest in the third or fourth decade (45 out of 66 reported cases—68.2%), with a mean age at onset of 32.7 years (standard deviation 11.2; range 9 to 67 years). The range of ages at onset is wide, and patients have been reported with onset in the first and second decades and the seventh decade of life (Fig. 5–3).[15,20,21,73] Patients with onset after age 50 years are rare, however, and nearly invariably found among relatives of early-onset probands.[11,21,22] Progression is generally slow, and many patients maintain relatively low Unified Parkinson's Disease Rating Scale Part III (UPDRSIII) motor scores and preserved functional and working abilities after many years of disease. Response to treatment is good or excellent in most cases, and remains sustained for many years, although drug-related dyskinesias and fluctuations of symptoms often occur early.

Atypical features at onset, such as dystonia and diurnal fluctuations, seem to be rarer in *PINK1*-related than in *parkin*-related ARP, being reported in less than one third of *PINK1* biallelic mutation carriers, mostly with very early onset.[5,20,23] Leutenegger and colleagues[20] reported a large inbred family from Sudan with eight patients homozygous for the A217D mutation, presenting with juvenile-onset parkinsonism (range 9 to 17 years old) with diurnal fluctuations and sleep benefit, which in some cases resembled levodopa-responsive dystonia.[20] Other peculiar features that have been described in association with the *PINK1* phenotype include hyperreflexia,[22] hypo-osmia,[5] and restless legs syndrome.[11,21]

Psychiatric disturbances, in particular, depression and anxiety, have been reported in about one third of patients with *PINK1* mutations regardless of onset age, often appearing early in the course of the disease and even before the manifestation of motor symptoms.[3,7,9,22-25] In a few *PINK1* families, psychiatric symptoms were more severe and invalidating, and included major depression, dysphoria, obsessive-compulsive and psychotic traits, hallucinations, and other behavioral disturbances.[9,22,24,25] Two affected siblings from one of these families also presented with progressive cognitive decline with frontal-type dementia 20 years after onset,[25] and two other early-onset patients were reported with an association of dementia, depression, and visual hallucinations.[7,22] Other than these cases, cognitive impairment seems to be a rare feature in *PINK1*-related parkinsonism, even after a prolonged disease course.

Functional neuroimaging techniques (single photon emission computed tomography and positron emission tomography) have been employed in *PINK1* patients to investigate the nigrostriatal dopaminergic pathway at presynaptic and postsynaptic levels. Carriers of two mutations overall presented with a significant loss of presynaptic dopaminergic terminals in the putamen and caudate nucleus compared with normal controls, with normal postsynaptic function.[3,5,10,15,21,26-29] Possible differences compared with idiopathic PD, not observed in all patients, include a more symmetrical reduction of dopamine reuptake with less evident anteroposterior gradient and a slower progression of dopaminergic neuronal loss. These results suggest a more uniform loss of nigrostriatal projections and the possible presence of compensatory mechanisms in *PINK1*-related parkinsonism.[15,26]

To evaluate the integrity of sympathetic cardiac innervation, which is usually compromised in idiopathic PD, two different studies assessed the myocardial [123]metaiodobenzylguanidine (MIBG) uptake in three *PINK1* homozygous patients, obtaining variable results ranging from normal to markedly decreased values.[28,30] No neuropathological data are available on patients carrying two *PINK1* mutations.

PINK1 HETEROZYGOUS RARE VARIANTS

Carriers of single heterozygous variants have been identified in most *PINK1* studies (see Table 5–1). In this chapter, we discuss only heterozygous changes with allelic frequency in controls less than 1%, which are predicted to affect the protein primary structure (excluding synonymous changes and intronic variants not obviously affecting splicing). These are designated as "rare variants" to distinguish them from the more plainly pathogenic homozygous or compound heterozygous mutations.[31]

Mutational Spectrum

Up to December 31st, 2007, 47 variants have been reported (Fig. 5–4).[15,31,32] Of these variants, 43 (91.5%) were missense and have been identified only in the heterozygous state in patients, controls, or both, with the exception of the L347P variant. This variant was identified in homozygosity in three Filipino patients and in heterozygosity in three of 50 Filipino controls, likely secondary to a founder effect in this population.[4-6] All four nonmissense variants (two nonsense, one splice-site mutation, and one 3-bp insertion) also have been found in homozygosity or compound heterozygosity in autosomal recessive families. Bioinformatic anaylysis using the PolyPhen (polymorphism phenotyping) software (at http://coot.embl. de/PolyPhen) for the 43 *PINK1* missense variants predicted that only 24 (55.8%) were possibly or probably pathogenic, whereas 19 (44.2%) were likely benign, and often affected residues that were poorly conserved among orthologues.

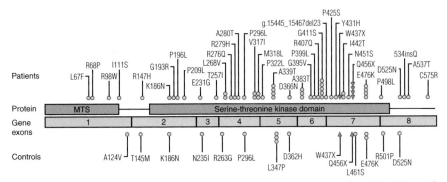

Figure 5–4   *PINK1* single heterozygous mutations reported in patients and unaffected controls, published by December 31st, 2007.

Taken together, these findings suggest that some variations would not substantially affect the protein's structure or function, although in some cases they are challenged by contradictory *in vitro* functional results. The E476K variant has been detected only in the heterozygous state in patients and controls, is predicted to be benign, and affects a poorly conserved residue,[9] but it has been shown to impair PINK1 protective activity severely in conditions of cellular stress.[33]

Prevalence and Phenotypes

The prevalence of heterozygous rare variants in mixed patients' cohorts, including sporadic and familial cases of all onset ages, ranged from 0.3% to 2.3% in different studies (see Table 5–1).[4,18,19,31,33] These variants were rarely detected in large screenings of ARP probands,[6,7,22,31] and only 5 of 56 (8.9%) heterozygous patients had a family history compatible with autosomal recessive inheritance, including the family also found to carry a heterozygous mutation in the *DJ-1* gene.[12,22,33-35] Conversely, most heterozygous carriers (34 of 56—60.7%) were sporadic (see Fig. 5–2).

In contrast to biallelic mutations, the phenotype associated with heterozygous rare variants was generally indistinguishable from that of idiopathic PD. The mean age at onset of *PINK1* heterozygotes was 48.6 years (standard deviation 12.4; range 13 to 73 years), about 15 years older than that of *PINK1* biallelic carriers, and half of the heterozygous patients (32 of 60—53.3%) had onset in the fifth or sixth decade (see Fig. 5–3).

Significance of *PINK1* Heterozygous Rare Variants

There is growing consensus on the hypothesis that single heterozygous variants in *PINK1* and other ARP genes could act as risk factors increasing the susceptibility to PD in a multifactorial model of disease pathogenesis. This hypothesis is mostly supported by functional neuroimaging studies, which showed significant 20% to 30% reduction of striatal dopamine reuptake in healthy *PINK1* heterozygotes, whereas affected carriers behaved similarly to patients with idiopathic PD.[15,26,36] Subclinical abnormalities in the nigrostriatal function of healthy heterozygous carriers also have been suggested in a study of voxel-based morphometry applied to high-resolution structural magnetic resonance imaging.[37] This hypothesis would justify the occurrence of heterozygous variants in unaffected controls and in individuals with very mild parkinsonian signs.[9,21]

Case-control studies also represent a valid research strategy to evaluate whether the risk of developing PD is increased in heterozygous carriers. We performed a meta-analysis of published screens that analyzed the whole *PINK1* gene in parkinsonian cases and healthy controls.[31] Overall, *PINK1* heterozygotes were more frequent among cases than controls (1.7% versus 1%), with an odds ratio of 1.62 (95% confidence interval 0.88 to 2.99), which did not reach statistical significance ($P = .121$). The contribution of *PINK1* heterozygous rare variants to PD genetic susceptibility seems to be minor. Heterozygotes would have a risk increased less than twofold compared with wild-type individuals, and most of them are likely to remain unaffected throughout their life span. Long-term follow-up studies of healthy carriers and functional assays are needed to decipher better the actual role of heterozygous rare variants, and at present genetic counseling should be performed with the utmost caution.

Functional Studies

PINK1 was first identified as a novel gene, the transcription of which was upregulated by the oncosuppressor gene *PTEN*.[38] The *PINK1* mRNA transcript is ubiquitously expressed, with the highest concentration in heart and skeletal muscle and testis, and encodes a 581-amino acid protein with a predicted molecular mass of 62.8 kD.

PINK1 LOCALIZATION IN HUMAN BRAIN

Only a few studies have explored the localization of wild-type PINK1 in human brains. Gandhi and coworkers[39] raised rabbit polyclonal antibodies and probed brains from two control subjects, two patients with idiopathic PD, and four patients single heterozygous for *PINK1* rare variants, and selected regions of brains from patients with other neurodegenerative conditions. The PINK1 protein was detected mostly in the gray matter, but also in the white matter in all regions studied (frontal cortex, hippocampus, putamen, caudate, thalamus, subthalamic nucleus, cerebellum, pons, medulla, and midbrain), within neurons and glial cells. No obvious differences in PINK1 localization were evident between normal and PD brains, and between brains with or without heterozygous *PINK1* mutations. In PD brains, including brains of *PINK1* heterozygotes, the protein was also detected in about 5% to 10% of α-synuclein–positive brainstem Lewy bodies, but not in glial inclusions from multiple systems atrophy brains. In another study, a different antibody detected PINK1 within most Lewy bodies from brains of patients with PD and with Lewy body dementia, and within multiple systems atrophy glial cytoplasmic inclusions.[40] These controversial results may depend on the variable sensitivity and specificity of the antibodies against native PINK1, and need further confirmation.

Two other studies have used a different approach based on in situ hybridization histochemistry using riboprobes to detect *PINK1* mRNA expression in different brain areas. *PINK1* mRNA was found to be broadly and uniformly expressed in most brain regions, including cortex, striatum, brainstem, thalamus, hippocampus, and cerebellum, whereas glial cells appeared negative for mRNA expression.[41,42] No significant differences were found in brains from five patients with PD versus five healthy controls.[42]

PINK1 AS A SERINE-THREONINE KINASE

On bioinformatic analysis, the PINK1 protein was shown to have a highly conserved protein kinase domain spanning amino acids 156 to 509-511, with homology to the serine/threonine kinases of the Ca^{2+} calmodulin family.[2] The kinase activity of PINK1 was explored in distinct studies that used *in vitro* kinase assays to measure [^{32}P] incorporation into PINK1 itself (autophosphorylation) or external substrates.[43-45] Different PINK1 constructs have been created for these purposes, expressing a protein either lacking the N-terminus (amino acids 112-581)[45] or the N-terminus and C-terminus (amino acids 112-496)[43,44] or expressing the kinase domain only (amino acids 148-515).[46] Various amino acid changes have been inserted in these constructs, representing either missense or truncating mutations previously reported in parkinsonian patients, or changes within key domains predicted to reduce or abolish the kinase activity of the protein.

Autophosphorylation Activity

PINK1(112-496) and PINK1(112-581) were capable of autophosphorylation.[43-45] This ability, which is common to many kinases, may represent a regulatory mechanism through which the protein is post-transductionally activated or deactivated in response to specific cellular signaling. Removal of the C-terminus, such as for the PINK1(112-437) construct, expressing the truncating mutation W437X, resulted in a marked increase of autophosphorylating activity, suggesting that the C-terminal portion of the protein could play a negative role in regulating autophosphorylation.[45] In the absence of the C-terminus, PINK1 protein expressing the missense mutations G309D, A168P, and L347P autophosphorylated less efficiently than the wild-type protein, implying an overall reduction of kinase activity in line with the expected loss-of-function model.[44,45] In particular, the striking reduction of kinase activity shown by PINK1(L347P) could be related to the reduced stability of the mutant protein, which would lead to premature degradation and reduced half-life.[44] The PINK1(148-515) and PINK1(148-581) proteins showed no autophosphorylating activity, suggesting that the autophosphorylation site is placed between amino acids 112 and 148,[46] a unique region with no homology with other known proteins.

Phosphorylation of External Substrates

Although the C-terminus region downregulates PINK1 autophosphorylation, the same region seems to enhance the kinase activity of the protein strongly toward some external substrates, such as histone H1, at the same time influencing substrate recognition and selectivity of phosphorylation sites. These effects seem to be restricted to selected substrates because they are not observed when using casein.[45,46] In a phosphorylation assay with the kinase domain of PINK1 (amino acids 148-515), expression of the PD-associated mutations G386A and G409V was shown to reduce markedly the ability to phosphorylate histone H1.[46]

Major progress came with the identification of the first specific PINK1 substrate, the mitochondrial chaperone TRAP1 (*T*NF *R*eceptor *A*ssociated *P*rotein 1), also known as heat shock protein 75 (Hsp75).[47] The role of TRAP1 is still poorly understood, but it has been proposed as a modulator of the apoptotic cascade. TRAP1 is specifically phosphorylated by wild-type PINK1, in a way that directly correlates with increased PINK1 expression and with levels of oxidative stress within cells. This mechanism has been proven to be highly protective against oxidative stress–induced mitochondrial cytochrome *c* release and apoptotic cell death (see later). PD-associated missense mutations G309D and L347P virtually abolished the ability of PINK1 to phosphorylate TRAP1 in vitro and in vivo, whereas the truncating mutation W437X caused a 30% to 45% reduction of TRAP1 phosphorylation in vivo.[47] Very recently, another relevant substrate of PINK1 has been identified: the PD-related protein Parkin. Both in *Drosophila* and mammalian cell systems, PINK1 was found to regulate the phosphorylation and to directly phosphorylate Parkin, promoting its translocation within mitochondria.[74]

SUBCELLULAR LOCALIZATION OF PINK1

Mitochondrial Localization

Bioinformatic analysis of PINK1 predicted a mitochondrial targeting sequence (MTS) at the N-terminus of the protein. PINK1 mitochondrial localization has been confirmed by many research groups using alternative strategies such as immunofluorescence (see an example in Fig. 5–5), immunogold analysis, and Western blotting on mitochondrial enriched subcellular fractions.[2,44,45,48,49] Two main PINK1 bands of about 66 kD and 55 kD are visualized on Western blotting that correspond to the full-length protein and to a shorter "mature" form obtained by cleavage of the MTS. Based on bioinformatic predictions, it has been long debated whether the MTS cleavage site would fall between amino acids 34 and 35, 77 and 78, or even farther down in the protein.

Another study has shown that a PINK1 fragment lacking the first 112 amino acids ran on Western blots as the same size of mature PINK1, suggesting that the cleavage site might occur between residues 111 and 112.[50] A PINK1 mutant lacking the first 108 amino acids was found to localize exclusively in the cytosol.[49] Despite this, it has been shown that the first 34 amino acids of PINK1 are sufficient for mitochondrial targeting,[48,49] suggesting that residues 34 through 112 may contain additional information other than that necessary for mitochondrial import. Within mitochondria, PINK1 seems to localize mainly to the inner and outer membranes, and is likely exposed to the intermembrane space.[39,45,48,51] Yet a recent study has proposed a further localization of PINK1, with the N-terminus region inserted in the outer mitochondrial membrane and the kinase domain facing the cytosol.[75] Moreover, PINK1 has been reported as part of a protein complex including the proteins Miro and Milton, that resides at the outer mitochondrial membrane and is implicated in trafficking of mitochondria along microtubules.[76] Studies of mitochondrial import in vitro have confirmed that maintenance of inner membrane potential ($\Delta\Psi$) is essential for correct PINK1 processing because no mature protein was formed in the presence of valinomycin, a mitochondrial uncoupler.[45]

Extramitochondrial Localization

Besides its obvious mitochondrial localization, several groups have reported that PINK1 is not exclusively found in the mitochondria. After transient PINK1 overexpression, PINK1 and mitochondrial markers showed only partial overlap in confocal microscopy images (see Fig. 5–5), and Western blotting after subcellular fractionation showed the presence of full-length and mature PINK1 in the

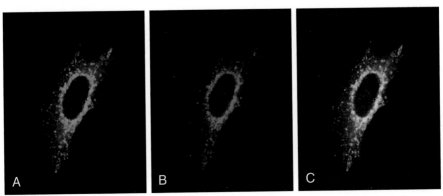

Figure 5–5 **A-C,** Immunofluorescence analysis showing partial overlap (yellow, **C**) between HA-tagged PINK1 (revealed with an anti-HA antibody, green **A**) and the mitochondrial marker TIM20 (red, **B**).

cytoplasmic and microsomal fractions.[2,44,45,49,52,53] Not only full-length, but also the mature form of PINK1 has been detected outside mitochondria, suggesting a retrograde transport of the protein from mitochondria to cytosol after MTS cleavage.[44,49] In some cells, PINK1 was shown to accumulate partly in multiple small cytosolic puncta or in single large perinuclear inclusions, a behavior reminiscent of insoluble aggregating proteins.[44]

In line with these findings, Muqit and coworkers[48] reported that, on proteasome inhibition with MG-132, PINK1 and other mitochondrial proteins were detected within aggresomes, perinuclear inclusions forming in the presence of an excess of misfolded or damaged proteins that could serve as cellular accessory protein degradation centers. It has been suggested that the mechanism of aggresome formation resembles that of Lewy bodies, which could also represent processing centers of misfolded proteins within neurons under stressing conditions.[54] The detection of PINK1 and of other mitochondrial proteins within aggresomes has been linked to the recruitment of whole mitochondria to the aggresome.[48] This finding, and the identification of autophagic bodies around aggresomes, could reflect the activation of the autophagy pathway, a key mechanism aimed at clearing misfolded proteins and damaged organelles to prevent neuronal death.[48,55] Proteasomal inhibition also increased the amount of cleaved PINK1, and this isoform was shown to be a constitutive target of proteasomal degradation, with a half-life (<30 minutes) much shorter than that of the full-length protein (12 hours).[48,49]

Elevated levels of cleaved PINK1 were found in the substantia nigra and cerebellum of PD patients, further suggesting that the ratio between full-length and cleaved protein ("66/55 ratio") might be relevant for PINK1 function within neuronal cells. It is known that some kinases have distinct and possibly divergent functions according to their subcellular localization. This has been explored by Weihofen and collaborators,[50] who characterized the relative amount of 66-kD and 55-kD isoforms of endogenous and exogenous PINK1 in different subcellular compartments and under different conditions. Both 66-kD and 55-kD isoforms were detected in variable proportions in all subcellular compartments (mitochondrial, cytoplasmic, and microsomal). In particular, the detection of both PINK1 isoforms in microsome-rich fractions that normally consist of fragments of plasma membrane and the endoplasmic reticulum is in line with previously reported findings of PINK1 within cytosolic inclusions reminiscent of aggregates or within aggresomes.[44,48] The 66/55 ratio was significantly reduced by PD-associated or kinase-dead PINK1 mutations, whereas overexpression of wild-type parkin, and of the Miro-Milton complex strongly increased the 66/55 ratio and the relative mitochondrial localization of PINK1. These findings suggest for the first time that not only the global level of PINK1 expression, but also the relative amounts of full-length versus cleaved PINK1 and their subcellular distribution may correlate with neuronal dysfunction leading to PD.[50,76]

PINK1 AS PROTECTIVE IN DIFFERENT TYPES OF CELLULAR STRESS

Several lines of evidence indicate that wild-type PINK1 protects cells from different types of stress, including proteasomal inhibition, oxidative stress, mitochondrial blockers, and apoptotic inducers. Conversely, this protective effect is abolished in the presence of PD-associated mutations, or when wild-type PINK1 is silenced through small interfering RNA (siRNA) approaches. The protective effect of wild-type PINK1 has been evaluated assessing different parameters, such as $\Delta\Psi$, cell viability, apoptotic rate, apoptotic markers (cytochrome c release, activation of caspases), and markers of oxidative stress. We first showed that wild-type PINK1 was able to maintain $\Delta\Psi$ and significantly reduce apoptosis in dopaminergic cells treated with the proteasomal inhibitor MG-132,[2] whereas several missense mutations abolished this protective effect.[2,33] Petit and coworkers[52] showed that over-expression of wild-type but not mutant PINK1 prevented staurosporine-induced apoptosis by blocking cytochrome c release from mitochondria and consequent caspase activation. Similarly, when treated with the mitochondrial stressor MPP+, SH-SY5Y cells stably expressing wild-type PINK1 showed significantly increased viability compared with cells expressing L399P mutant PINK1.[35]

The protective role of PINK1 against mitochondrial respiratory chain complex I blockers also was assessed by Deng and collaborators,[56] who studied the effects of siRNA-based PINK1 silencing in cells exposed to MPP+ or rotenone. PINK1 suppression was sufficient per se to cause a decrease in cell viability, and dramatically enhanced apoptotic cell death induced by mitochondrial stressors. PINK1 silencing also was shown to reduce $\Delta\Psi$ and induce severe morphological abnormalities of mitochondria, which appeared truncated and fragmented and showed reduced or absent cristae. This phenotype could be rescued by expression of wild-type, but not mutant, PINK1.[51] Finally, the pro-survival effect of PINK1 was also confirmed in different models by its ability to counteract toxicity induced by alpha-synuclein, a PD-related protein playing a well known role in neurodegeneration.[77,78] The identification of the first specific PINK1 substrate, TRAP1, also confirmed the protective properties of PINK1. Pridgeon and coworkers[47] showed that wild-type PINK1 protected dopaminergic cells from oxidative stress by suppressing mitochondrial cytochrome c release, and that this effect was mediated by phosphorylation of TRAP1. Conversely, several missense and truncating mutations were shown to impair TRAP1 phosphorylation *in vitro* and *in vivo,* abolishing the cytoprotective effect of PINK1 and, in some cases, exacerbating oxidative stress–induced cellular damage.

Plun-Favreau and collaborators[53] have identified HtrA2 (also known as Omi), a mitochondrial serine protease, as a novel interactor of PINK1. Two point mutations deregulating the protease activity of HtrA2 have been implicated in PD,[57] and gene inactivation in mice induced a parkinsonian neurodegenerative phenotype and premature death,[58,59] suggesting that this protease may be protective from certain stress conditions. In particular, the phosphorylation of HtrA2 at Ser142 was shown to be necessary for its protease activity and stress protection. Although it is currently unknown whether PINK1 can directly phosphorylate HtrA2, it has been shown to regulate HtrA2 phosphorylation on activation of the p38 stress pathway in vitro, and brains with heterozygous *PINK1* mutations have shown nearly abolished levels of phosphorylated HtrA2, possibly resulting in increased vulnerability to stressful stimuli.[53] Besides these functions, PINK1 has been very recently implicated in other protective mechanisms, such as the regulation of intramitochondrial calcium levels,[77,79] the activation of the ubiquitin-proteasome pathway through a multiprotein complex with Parkin and DJ-1,[80] and the regulation of mitochondrial clearance through autophagy.[81] These preliminary evidences require further studies to be confirmed and fully characterized in distinct experimental settings.

Although several in vitro models have confirmed that overexpression of mutant PINK1 results in loss of its protective abilities, only a few studies have explored the deleterious effect of *PINK1* mutations in lymphoblastoid or fibroblastoid cell lines of PD patients. Petit and coworkers[52] compared levels of basal caspase 3 activity in primary cultures of human skin fibroblasts from a neurologically normal elderly man and from a 74-year-old PD patient compound heterozygous for *PINK1* E204K and L489P mutations. Levels of caspase 3 activity seemed to be much higher (+147%) in fibroblast lysates from the patient than in the lysates from the age-matched control. Similarly, Hoepken and colleagues[60] assessed the levels of oxidative stress and mitochondrial damage in primary fibroblasts and immortalized lymphoblasts from three affected siblings homozygous for the G309D mutation, three unaffected siblings heterozygous for the same mutation, and two healthy controls. Cells from homozygous patients showed reduction of complex I activity, increased lipid peroxidation, and overactivation of two main antioxidant pathways, the manganese superoxide dismutase and the glutathione pathway. The same G309D fibroblasts and cells from patients homozygous for the Q126P mutation also showed severe defects in mitochondrial morphology, especially under low-glucose conditions.[51] Overall, these findings are suggestive of oxidative stress and mitochondrial dysfunction in unaffected peripheral tissues that could well reflect higher levels of damage in the degenerating substantia nigra neurons of PINK1-mutated patients.[60]

REGULATORY MECHANISMS OF PINK1

The data presented so far suggest that PINK1 functions to maintain mitochondrial and cellular integrity in various conditions of cellular stress. This activity requires a tight regulation of PINK1 expression and functioning, acting at the transcriptional, transductional, or post-transductional level. A possible pathway of PINK1 regulation could run through the PTEN-AKT network because *PINK1* has been initially identified as a gene transcriptionally transactivated in the presence of the oncosuppressor gene *PTEN*.[38] Despite this early report, the cellular mechanisms underlying PINK1 regulation have remained largely obscure until more recently.

Using different complementary strategies, Weihofen and collaborators[50] identified PINK1 as a novel Cdc37/Hsp90 client kinase. Cdc37 is a molecular cochaperone that functions with Hsp90 to promote folding of many kinases. This chaperone system was shown to influence the subcellular distribution and the

66/55 protein ratio of PINK1. Relative mitochondrial levels of PINK1 66-kD and 55-kD isoforms were differently regulated in the presence of the Cdc37/Hsp90 complex or Cdc37 alone, suggesting that distinct mechanisms influence the mitochondrial localization of the two isoforms. Overexpression of parkin strongly increased the 66/55 ratio and the mitochondrial localization of PINK1, and could rescue the mitochondrial morphological abnormalities,[50,51] strengthening the PINK1-parkin connection already emerged from studies on *Drosophila* models.[61-63]

Scheele and collaborators[64] identified in human neuroblastoma cells and skeletal muscle tissue a novel splice variant of *PINK1* (svPINK1) homologous to the C-terminus regulatory region of the protein and a human-specific noncoding antisense RNA regulating the *PINK1* locus (naPINK1). In particular, naPINK1 was shown to stabilize and promote the expression of svPINK1, which could play a major role in regulating PINK1 physiological activity in vivo. This regulatory effect and the relative importance of these novel species in PD pathogenesis need to be clarified further. Recently FOXO3a, a member of the FOXO transcription factors family implicated in pro-survival responses to oxidative stress-induced cell death, was identified as a positive modulator of PINK1 expression in response to growth factor deprivation, both in mouse and human cells.[82]

PINK1 Animal Models

MOUSE MODELS

Three *PINK1* mouse models have been reported to date. In the first one, transgenic mice were created that could conditionally express siRNA against *PINK1*, resulting in tightly regulated temporal and spatial silencing of the target gene. The suppression of *PINK1* expression in embryonic mouse tissues (including central nervous system, heart, liver, kidney, muscle, spleen, and testis) did not produce gross abnormalities in 6-month-old animals, and did not result in dopaminergic neuronal loss from the substantia nigra pars compacta. In line with these findings, motor function and behavior of these mice were also normal.[65]

The second model is a knockout mouse homozygous for a large deletion (exons 4 through 7) of the *PINK1* gene (PINK1−/−). The deletion removed most of the kinase domain and created a nonsense mutation at the beginning of exon 8, generating a truncated mRNA likely to be degraded through nonsense-mediated decay. Similar to *PINK1* siRNA mice, PINK1−/− mice showed no obvious abnormalities in morphology and density of dopaminergic cells; unaltered numbers of dopaminergic neurons in the substantia nigra pars compacta; and normal striatal levels of tyrosine hydroxylase, dopamine, and its metabolites DOPAC and HVA at the ages of 2 to 3 months and 8 to 9 months, suggesting normal dopamine synthesis and turnover in the absence of PINK1. Nevertheless, sophisticated neurophysiological recordings from striatal medium spiny neurons revealed a reduction in evoked dopamine release and specific impairments of corticostriatal long-term potentiation and long-term depression that could be rescued by either dopamine receptor agonists or agents increasing dopamine release, such as amphetamine or levodopa.

These results reveal a crucial role for PINK1 in dopamine release and striatal synaptic plasticity in the nigrostriatal circuit, and suggest that altered dopaminergic physiology may precede degeneration.[66] These mice also showed a significant reduction in the mitochondrial respiratory capacity, involving not only complex I but also complex II and aconitase, a key enzyme in the Krebs cycle. These functional defects were detected in the striatum and, in older mice, in the cerebral cortex, and could be exacerbated by exposure to oxidative stress or mild heat-shock.[83] In a third study, measurements of enzymatic activity of respiratory chain complexes in brain mitochondria from PINK1 knock-out mice showed functional defects in complex I activity that could be rescued by over-expression of human wild type PINK1, indicating a direct role for PINK1 in modulating complex I function.[84] Although it cannot be excluded that PINK1[-/-] mice could develop nigral degeneration at an older age, this possibility is unlikely, given that *parkin* and *DJ-1* knockout mice failed to develop significant dopaminergic neurodegeneration at age 24 months.[66-68] Striatal dopamine release was reduced in all mouse models, however, suggesting a common pathogenetic mechanism.

DROSOPHILA MODELS

The generation of PINK1 loss-of-function mutant *Drosophila* represented a major step toward understanding the complex pathogenetic mechanisms that underlie PD neurodegeneration. PINK1 suppression in flies was shown to induce a peculiar severe phenotype characterized by sterility; shorter life span; and age-dependent movement abnormalities resulting from progressively altered, disorganized, and apoptotic muscle fibers. At a cellular level, this phenotype could be related directly to the massive mitochondrial abnormalities observed especially within muscle cells, with dramatically altered mitochondrial morphology, marked reduction in ATP levels, and increased sensitivity to multiple stresses including oxidative stress.[61-63] Some authors observed dopaminergic neuronal degeneration and reduction of brain dopamine levels.[62,63,69] This phenotype highly resembled that caused by parkin suppression, and it could be rescued by overexpression not only of PINK1, but also of parkin.

Double mutant flies lacking PINK1 and parkin showed phenotypes that were indistinguishable from those of each single mutant, whereas *PINK1* knockdown flies also showed significantly reduced levels of parkin protein. Taken together, these results strongly suggested that PINK1 and parkin could act in the same pathway implicated in the maintenance of mitochondrial integrity and function, with parkin downstream of PINK1.[61-63] Wang and colleagues[69] also showed that dopaminergic degeneration induced by *PINK1* silencing in *Drosophila* could be rescued by antioxidant strategies, such as overexpression of the human *SOD1* gene or vitamin E treatment, in line with in vitro studies showing a protective role of wild-type PINK1 against oxidative stress.[47]

Neither *PINK1*-defective mouse nor *Drosophila* models fully recapitulate the complex neuropathological and clinical phenotype of PD. Although the neurological phenotype is subtle or absent in both models, *Drosophila* display a dramatic muscle phenotype that has no counterpart in humans or mice with similar genetic depletions. Possibly, the short life span of these animals prevents them from developing a neurological phenotype that may require a longer time, and possibly prevents the co-occurrence of other genetic or environmental susceptibility factors from developing fully. For this reason, although PD genetic animal models have proven extremely useful in understanding some key processes, such as the connection between PINK1 and *parkin* within the same neuroprotective pathway, the leap to PD-related neurodegeneration should be made with caution.[70]

REFERENCES

1. Valente EM, Bentivoglio AR, Dixon PH, et al: Localization of a novel locus for autosomal recessive early-onset parkinsonism, PARK6, on human chromosome 1p35-p36. Am J Hum Genet 2001;68:895.
2. Valente EM, bou-Sleiman PM, Caputo V, et al: Hereditary early-onset Parkinson's disease caused by mutations in PINK1. Science 2004;304:1158.
3. Criscuolo C, Volpe G, De RA, et al: PINK1 homozygous W437X mutation in a patient with apparent dominant transmission of parkinsonism. Mov Disord 2006;21:1265.
4. Rogaeva E, Johnson J, Lang AE, et al: Analysis of the PINK1 gene in a large cohort of cases with Parkinson disease. Arch Neurol 2004;61:1898.
5. Doostzadeh J, Tetrud JW, len-Auerbach M, et al: Novel features in a patient homozygous for the L347P mutation in the PINK1 gene. Parkinsonism Relat Disord 2007;13:359.
6. Hatano Y, Li Y, Sato K, et al: Novel PINK1 mutations in early-onset parkinsonism. Ann Neurol 2004;56:424.
7. Li Y, Tomiyama H, Sato K, et al: Clinicogenetic study of PINK1 mutations in autosomal recessive early-onset parkinsonism. Neurology 2005;64:1955.
8. Marongiu R, Brancati F, Antonini A, et al: Whole gene deletion and splicing mutations expand the PINK1 genotypic spectrum. Hum Mutat 2007;28:98.
9. Bonifati V, Rohe CF, Breedveld GJ, et al: Early-onset parkinsonism associated with PINK1 mutations: frequency, genotypes, and phenotypes. Neurology 2005;65:87.
10. Klein C, Djarmati A, Hedrich K, et al: PINK1, Parkin, and DJ-1 mutations in Italian patients with early-onset parkinsonism. Eur J Hum Genet 2005;13:1086.
11. Tan EK, Yew K, Chua E, et al: PINK1 mutations in sporadic early-onset Parkinson's disease. Mov Disord 2006;21:789.
12. Djarmati A, Hedrich K, Svetel M, et al: Heterozygous PINK1 mutations: a susceptibility factor for Parkinson disease? Mov Disord 2006;21:1526.
13. Fung HC, Chen CM, Hardy J, et al: Analysis of the PINK1 gene in a cohort of patients with sporadic early-onset parkinsonism in Taiwan. Neurosci Lett 2006;394:33.
14. Chung EJ, Ki CS, Lee WY, et al: Clinical features and gene analysis in Korean patients with early-onset Parkinson disease. Arch Neurol 2006;63:1170.
15. Weng YH, Chou YH, Wu WS, et al: PINK1 mutation in Taiwanese early-onset parkinsonism: clinical, genetic, and dopamine transporter studies. J Neurol 2007;254:1347.
16. Valente EM, Salvi S, Ialongo T, et al: PINK1 mutations are associated with sporadic early-onset parkinsonism. Ann Neurol 2004;56:336.
17. Schlitter AM, Kurz M, Larsen JP, et al: Exclusion of PINK1 as candidate gene for the late-onset form of Parkinson's disease in two European populations. J Negat Results Biomed 2005;4:10.
18. Healy DG, bou-Sleiman PM, Gibson JM, et al: PINK1 (PARK6) associated Parkinson disease in Ireland. Neurology 2004;63:1486.
19. Toft M, Myhre R, Pielsticker L, et al: PINK1 mutation heterozygosity and the risk of Parkinson's disease. J Neurol Neurosurg Psychiatry 2007;78:82.
20. Leutenegger AL, Salih MA, Ibanez P, et al: Juvenile-onset Parkinsonism as a result of the first mutation in the adenosine triphosphate orientation domain of PINK1. Arch Neurol 2006;63:1257.
21. Hedrich K, Hagenah J, Djarmati A, et al: Clinical spectrum of homozygous and heterozygous PINK1 mutations in a large German family with Parkinson disease: role of a single hit? Arch Neurol 2006;63:833.
22. Ibanez P, Lesage S, Lohmann E, et al: Mutational analysis of the PINK1 gene in early-onset parkinsonism in Europe and North Africa. Brain 2006;129:686.
23. Rohe CF, Montagna P, Breedveld G, et al: Homozygous PINK1 C-terminus mutation causing early-onset parkinsonism. Ann Neurol 2004;56:427.
24. Steinlechner S, Stahlberg J, Volkel B, et al: Co-occurrence of affective and schizophrenia spectrum disorders with PINK1 mutations. J Neurol Neurosurg Psychiatry 2007;78:532.
25. Ephraty L, Porat O, Israeli D, et al: Neuropsychiatric and cognitive features in autosomal-recessive early parkinsonism due to PINK1 mutations. Mov Disord 2007;22:566.
26. Khan NL, Valente EM, Bentivoglio AR, et al: Clinical and subclinical dopaminergic dysfunction in PARK6-linked parkinsonism: an 18F-dopa PET study. Ann Neurol 2002;52:849.
27. Kessler KR, Hamscho N, Morales B, et al: Dopaminergic function in a family with the PARK6 form of autosomal recessive Parkinson's syndrome. J Neural Transm 2005;112:1345.
28. Albanese A, Valente EM, Romito LM, et al: The PINK1 phenotype can be indistinguishable from idiopathic Parkinson disease. Neurology 2005;64:1958.

29. Lu CS, Chou YH, Weng YH, et al: Genetic and DAT imaging studies of familial parkinsonism in a Taiwanese cohort. J Neural Transm Suppl 2006:235.
30. Quattrone A, Bagnato A, Annesi G, et al: Myocardial (123)metaiodobenzylguanidine uptake in genetic Parkinson's disease. Mov Disord 2008;23:21.
31. Marongiu R, Ferraris A, Ialongo T, et al: PINK1 heterozygous rare variants: prevalence, significance and phenotypic spectrum. Hum Mutat 2008;29:565.
32. Schweitzer KJ, Brussel T, Leitner P, et al: Transcranial ultrasound in different monogenetic subtypes of Parkinson's disease. J Neurol 2007;254:613.
33. Abou-Sleiman PM, Muqit MM, McDonald NQ, et al: A heterozygous effect for PINK1 mutations in Parkinson's disease? Ann Neurol 2006;60:414.
34. Tan EK, Yew K, Chua E, et al: Analysis of PINK1 in Asian patients with familial parkinsonism. Clin Genet 2005;68:468.
35. Tang B, Xiong H, Sun P, et al: Association of PINK1 and DJ-1 confers digenic inheritance of early-onset Parkinson's disease. Hum Mol Genet 2006;15:1816.
36. Zadikoff C, Rogaeva E, Djarmati A, et al: Homozygous and heterozygous PINK1 mutations: considerations for diagnosis and care of Parkinson's disease patients. Mov Disord 2006;21:875.
37. Binkofski F, Reetz K, Gaser C, et al: Morphometric fingerprint of asymptomatic Parkin and PINK1 mutation carriers in the basal ganglia. Neurology 2007;69:842.
38. Unoki M, Nakamura Y: Growth-suppressive effects of BPOZ and EGR2, two genes involved in the PTEN signaling pathway. Oncogene 2001;20:4457.
39. Gandhi S, Muqit MM, Stanyer L, et al: PINK1 protein in normal human brain and Parkinson's disease. Brain 2006;129:1720.
40. Murakami T, Moriwaki Y, Kawarabayashi T, et al: PINK1, a gene product of PARK6, accumulates in alpha-synucleinopathy brains. J Neurol Neurosurg Psychiatry 2007;78:653.
41. Taymans JM, Van den HC, Baekelandt V: Distribution of PINK1 and LRRK2 in rat and mouse brain. J Neurochem 2006;98:951.
42. Blackinton JG, Anvret A, Beilina A, et al: Expression of PINK1 mRNA in human and rodent brain and in Parkinson's disease. Brain Res 2007;1184:10.
43. Nakajima A, Kataoka K, Hong M, et al: BRPK, a novel protein kinase showing increased expression in mouse cancer cell lines with higher metastatic potential. Cancer Lett 2003;201:195.
44. Beilina A, van der BM, Ahmad R, et al: Mutations in PTEN-induced putative kinase 1 associated with recessive parkinsonism have differential effects on protein stability. Proc Natl Acad Sci U S A 2005;102:5703.
45. Silvestri L, Caputo V, Bellacchio E, et al: Mitochondrial import and enzymatic activity of PINK1 mutants associated to recessive parkinsonism. Hum Mol Genet 2005;14:3477.
46. Sim CH, Lio DS, Mok SS, et al: C-terminal truncation and Parkinson's disease-associated mutations down-regulate the protein serine/threonine kinase activity of PTEN-induced kinase-1. Hum Mol Genet 2006;15:3251.
47. Pridgeon JW, Olzmann JA, Chin LS, et al: PINK1 protects against oxidative stress by phosphorylating mitochondrial chaperone TRAP1. PLoS Biol 2007;5:e172.
48. Muqit MM, Abou-Sleiman PM, Saurin AT, et al: Altered cleavage and localization of PINK1 to aggresomes in the presence of proteasomal stress. J Neurochem 2006;98:156.
49. Takatori S, Ito G, Iwatsubo T: Cytoplasmic localization and proteasomal degradation of N-terminally cleaved form of PINK1. Neurosci Lett 2007;430:13.
50. Weihofen A, Ostaszewski B, Minami Y, et al: Pink1 Parkinson mutations, the Cdc37/Hsp90 chaperones and Parkin all influence the maturation or subcellular distribution of Pink1. Hum Mol Genet 2008;17:602.
51. Exner N, Treske B, Paquet D, et al: Loss-of-function of human PINK1 results in mitochondrial pathology and can be rescued by parkin. J Neurosci 2007;27:12413.
52. Petit A, Kawarai T, Paitel E, et al: Wild-type PINK1 prevents basal and induced neuronal apoptosis, a protective effect abrogated by Parkinson disease-related mutations. J Biol Chem 2005;280:34025.
53. Plun-Favreau H, Klupsch K, Moisoi N, et al: The mitochondrial protease HtrA2 is regulated by Parkinson's disease-associated kinase PINK1. Nat Cell Biol 2007;9:1243.
54. Olanow CW, Perl DP, DeMartino GN, et al: Lewy-body formation is an aggresome-related process: a hypothesis. Lancet Neurol 2004;3:496.
55. Martinez-Vicente M, Cuervo AM: Autophagy and neurodegeneration: when the cleaning crew goes on strike. Lancet Neurol 2007;6:352.
56. Deng H, Jankovic J, Guo Y, et al: Small interfering RNA targeting the PINK1 induces apoptosis in dopaminergic cells SH-SY5Y. Biochem Biophys Res Commun 2005;337:1133.

57. Strauss KM, Martins LM, Plun-Favreau H, et al: Loss of function mutations in the gene encoding Omi/HtrA2 in Parkinson's disease. Hum Mol Genet 2005;14:2099.

58. Jones JM, Datta P, Srinivasula SM, et al: Loss of Omi mitochondrial protease activity causes the neuromuscular disorder of mnd2 mutant mice. Nature 2003;425:721.

59. Martins LM, Morrison A, Klupsch K, et al: Neuroprotective role of the Reaper-related serine protease HtrA2/Omi revealed by targeted deletion in mice. Mol Cell Biol 2004;24:9848.

60. Hoepken HH, Gispert S, Morales B, et al: Mitochondrial dysfunction, peroxidation damage and changes in glutathione metabolism in PARK6. Neurobiol Dis 2007;25:401.

61. Clark IE, Dodson MW, Jiang C, et al: *Drosophila* pink1 is required for mitochondrial function and interacts genetically with parkin. Nature 2006;441:1162.

62. Park J, Lee SB, Lee S, et al: Mitochondrial dysfunction in Drosophila PINK1 mutants is complemented by parkin. Nature 2006;441:1157.

63. Yang Y, Gehrke S, Imai Y, et al: Mitochondrial pathology and muscle and dopaminergic neuron degeneration caused by inactivation of *Drosophila* Pink1 is rescued by Parkin. Proc Natl Acad Sci U S A 2006;103:10793.

64. Scheele C, Petrovic N, Faghihi MA, et al: The human PINK1 locus is regulated in vivo by a non-coding natural antisense RNA during modulation of mitochondrial function. BMC Genomics 2007;8:74.

65. Zhou H, Falkenburger BH, Schulz JB, et al: Silencing of the Pink1 gene expression by conditional RNAi does not induce dopaminergic neuron death in mice. Int J Biol Sci 2007;3:242.

66. Kitada T, Pisani A, Porter DR, et al: Impaired dopamine release and synaptic plasticity in the striatum of PINK1-deficient mice. Proc Natl Acad Sci U S A 2007;104:11441.

67. Goldberg MS, Pisani A, Haburcak M, et al: Nigrostriatal dopaminergic deficits and hypokinesia caused by inactivation of the familial Parkinsonism-linked gene DJ-1. Neuron 2005;45:489.

68. Goldberg MS, Fleming SM, Palacino JJ, et al: Parkin-deficient mice exhibit nigrostriatal deficits but not loss of dopaminergic neurons. J Biol Chem 2003;278:43628.

69. Wang D, Qian L, Xiong H, et al: Antioxidants protect PINK1-dependent dopaminergic neurons in Drosophila. Proc Natl Acad Sci U S A 2006;103:13520.

70. Tan JM, Dawson TM: Parkin blushed by PINK1. Neuron 2006;50:527.

71. Chishti MA, Bohlega S, Ahmed M, et al: T313M PINK1 mutation in an extended highly consanguineous Saudi family with early-onset Parkinson disease. Arch Neurol 2006;63:1483.

72. Bentivoglio AR, Cortelli P, Valente EM, et al: Phenotypic characterisation of autosomal recessive PARK6-linked parkinsonism in three unrelated Italian families. Mov Disord 2001;16:999.

73. Gelmetti V, Ferraris A, Brusa L, et al: Late onset sporadic Parkindon's disease caused by PINK1 mutations: clinical and functional study. Mov Disord 2008;23:881.

74. Kim Y, Park J, Kim S, et al: PINK1 controls mitochondrial localization of Parkin through direct phosphorylation. Biochem Biophys Res Commun 2008;377:975.

75. Zhou C, Huang Y, Shao Y, et al: The kinase domain of mitochondrial PINK1 faces the cytoplasm. Proc Natl Acad Sci U S A 2008;105:12022.

76. Weihofen A, Thomas KJ, Ostaszewski BL, Cookson MR, Selkoe DJ: Pink1 forms a multiprotein complex with Miro and Milton, Linking Pink1 function to mitochondrial trafficking (dagger). Biochemistry 2009;48:2045.

77. Marongiu R, Spencer B, Crews L, et al: Mutant Pink1 induces mitochondrial dysfunction in a neuronal cell model of Parkinson's disease by disturbing calcium flux. J Neurochem 2009;108:1561.

78. Todd AM, Staveley BE: Pink1 suppresses alpha-synuclein-induced phenotypes in a Drosophila model of Parkinson's disease. Genome 2008;51:1040.

79. Gandhi S, Wood-Kaczmar A, Yao Z, et al: PINK1-associated Parkinson's disease is caused by neuronal vulnerability to calcium-induced cell death. Mol Cell 2009;33:627.

80. Xiong H, Wang D, Chen L, et al: Parkin, PINK1, and DJ-1 form a ubiquitin E3 ligase complex promoting unfolded protein degradation. J clin Invest 2009;119:650.

81. Dagda RK, Cherra SJ, III, Kulich SM, et al: Loss of pink1 function promotes mitophagy through effects on oxidative stress and mitochondrial fission. J Biol Chem 2009;284:13843.

82. Mei Y, Zhang Y, Yamamoto K, et al: FOXO3a-dependent regulation of Pink1 (Park6) mediates survival signaling in response to cytokine deprivation. Proc Natl Acad Sci U S A 2009;106:5153.

83. Gautier CA, Kitada T, Shen J: Loss of PINK1 causes mitochondrial functional defects and increased sensitivity to oxidative stress. Proc Natl Acad Sci U S A 2008;105:11364.

84. Morais VA, Verstreken P, Roethig A, et al: Parkinson's disease mutations in PINK1 result in decreased Complex I activity and deficient synaptic function. Embo Mol Med 2009;doi/10.1002/emmm. 200900006.

6 DJ-1 (PARK7) and Parkinson's Disease

VINCENZO BONIFATI

Introduction

Mutations in the DJ-1 gene (approved gene symbol PARK7) cause a rare, autosomal recessive human neurodegenerative disease, which in most cases manifests clinically as levodopa-responsive parkinsonism of early onset (OMIM *602533).[1] The function of the protein encoded by the DJ-1 gene remains poorly understood, but the available evidence suggests an important role of DJ-1 in the protection of brain against oxidative stress, protein misfolding, or both. Whether the mechanisms of DJ-1–related neurodegeneration overlap with those of the disease caused by mutations in the other genes for autosomal recessive (parkin and PINK1) or autosomal dominant (SNCA and LRRK2) parkinsonism, and whether these mechanisms are also implicated in the pathogenesis of the common, late-onset forms of Parkinson's disease (PD) are important questions, which also remain currently unanswered. Despite its low frequency, DJ-1–related disease offers an exciting opportunity for understanding the mechanisms of brain maintenance and neurodegeneration. This chapter reviews more recent advances in the genetic and clinical aspects of PARK7. Also, the molecular biology of this form is discussed.

Genetics of PARK7—Nature and Frequency of DJ-1 Mutations

A third locus for autosomal recessive, early-onset parkinsonism (named PARK7, on chromosome 1p36) was mapped in 2001 by genome-wide linkage analysis in a large consanguineous family from a genetically isolated community in The Netherlands.[2] Linkage to the same genomic region was detected in a second family from Italy with early-onset parkinsonism.[3] A positional cloning effort led to the discovery of mutations in the *DJ-1* gene as the cause of disease in both families.[1] The four patients of the Dutch family carried a homozygous deletion that removes approximately 14,000 nucleotides, including the promoter and large part of the *DJ-1* gene. In the Italian family, the three patients were homozygous carriers of a point mutation, which replaces a highly conserved leucine by proline in the DJ-1 protein (p.L166P). The Dutch mutation represents a natural knockout of the *DJ-1* gene, confirmed by the absence of DJ-1 mRNA and protein in patient-derived cell lines.[1,4] The p.L166P mutation destabilizes dramatically the DJ-1 structure, leading to severely reduced steady-state protein levels.[4] Both mutations clearly lead to loss of the DJ-1 function, in keeping with a recessive mechanism of disease inheritance.

The identification of *DJ-1* as the causative gene at the PARK7 locus was rapidly followed by studies assessing frequency and spectrum of *DJ-1* mutations in PD.[5-17] The studies performed in large series of patients are shown in Table 6–1. Most of this work targeted early-onset PD.

Overall, the frequency of *DJ-1* mutations turned out to be low. About 1% to 2% of early-onset PD cases might be explained by pathogenic *DJ-1* mutations, present in the homozygous or compound heterozygous state. In other patients, a single heterozygous mutation has been detected, but whether these mutations are disease-causing remains unclear. The fact that the DJ-1 protein forms homodimers (discussed later) leaves open the possibility for some single heterozygous mutations to be disease-causing by dominant-negative mechanisms. This hypothesis remains to be shown experimentally, however; PARK7 was linked to parkinsonism under an autosomal recessive model of inheritance. The frequency of *DJ-1* mutations in patients with late-onset PD seems also very low, although fewer data are available in this regard.[6,17]

In many ways, the studies listed in Table 6–1 are not fully comparable. First, the mean onset age of the patients included differs (see Table 6–1), and it is known that the likelihood of finding mutations in a given gene might be a function of the disease onset age (e.g., consider the case of the *parkin* gene).[18] Second, the frequency of mutations might differ dramatically according to patient ethnicity[9,16,19]; most of the *DJ-1* studies have been performed in series from tertiary referral centers, representing collections of patients from disparate ethnic groups. Third, the mutation frequency depends on the sensitivity of the screening methods used. Different types of pathogenic mutations are known in the *DJ-1* gene, including point mutations and small deletions, but also large genomic rearrangements (leading to deletion of entire exons). A sensitive screening requires not only sequencing, but also exon copy number assay (gene dosage) to detect heterozygous genomic rearrangements. A similar situation is well known for the *parkin* gene.[18,20]

Gene dosage methods have been included in only a few *DJ-1* studies (see Table 6–1), and the sensitivity of other studies remained less than optimal. Some of the screening techniques used, such as Dematuring High-Performance Liquid Chromatography (DHPLC) might not detect all mutations, especially novel mutations. In some studies, only the coding exons of *DJ-1* were screened, excluding other exons (1A and 1B) where pathogenic mutations might also occur. Despite these methodological limitations, 18 different *DJ-1* mutations have been identified in patients with parkinsonism or PD (Table 6–2), including point mutations (missense, truncating, splice site mutations), and large genomic deletions removing one or more exons.

Most of the mutations have been detected in single families or patients. Of particular importance are the mutations found in the homozygous or compound heterozygous state because they are more likely disease-causing.

One patient of Hispanic ethnicity has been reported with a clinical diagnosis of sporadic, early-onset PD and two *DJ-1* heterozygous mutations (a frameshift mutation in exon 2, predicted to lead to protein truncation, and a splice site mutation in exon 7, also predicted to affect protein synthesis severely).[5] Both mutations are predicted to affect the DJ-1 protein markedly. The only caveat is that the phase of these mutations was not formally resolved, and the possibility (although very small) that these were both located on the same allele remains.

A different missense mutation predicted to lead to the missense change p.M26I in the DJ-1 protein was detected in the homozygous state in an Ashkenazi Jewish patient with sporadic, early-onset PD.[6] The p.M26I mutant affects an important helix for the DJ-1 dimerization, and shows evidence of impaired dimerization[21] and protein instability, although less than the p.L166P mutant.[22,23]

A third homozygous point mutation has been detected in a patient of Turkish ethnicity with sporadic, early-onset PD.[10] The mutation (c.192G→C) is predicted to lead to a missense p.E64D change in the DJ-1 protein. Because c.192G is the last nucleotide of exon 3, however, this mutation is also likely to affect mRNA splicing. In vitro data provide compelling evidence for c.192G→C being a severe splicing mutation, predicted to lead to marked abnormalities in DJ-1 protein expression.[24] Confirmation of this prediction by DJ-1 protein assays in patient-derived material would be of great value. The p.E64D mutation was absent from large series of controls, but, notably, was also present in the homozygous state in the proband's sister, who was asymptomatic at age 42, displaying only a mild hypomimia. By itself, this is not surprising because asymptomatic individuals or individuals with few symptoms have also been noted in the original Dutch PARK7-linked family,[25] and in some families with *parkin* and *PINK1* gene mutations.[26-28] Imaging the brain dopaminergic system using positron emission tomography (PET) in the sister homozygous for the DJ-1 p.E64D mutation revealed tracer uptake at the lower limits of the normal range, suggesting a subclinical impairment.

One of the mutations found in the single heterozygous state (p.A104T) has been detected in two studies, each time in only one patient (of Hispanic ethnicity in one study and Chinese ethnicity in the other) (see Table 6–2).[5,11] There is evidence that some of the mutations detected in patients in the single heterozygous state (p.A104T and p.D149A) impair DJ-1 homodimerization,[21] suggesting these variants might also be pathogenic through dominant-negative mechanisms.

Assessing the frequency of single heterozygous mutations in the whole coding region of a given gene in controls is an important issue, for a proper interpretation of the role of single heterozygous mutations detected in patients. Data (although limited) are available concerning *parkin*[29,30] and *PINK1*,[31] but not yet concerning *DJ-1*.

On the basis of the studies so far available, it is clear that *DJ-1* mutations are much less frequent than *parkin* mutations in early-onset PD. *DJ-1* mutations also seem less frequent than *PINK1* mutations, although mutations in both of these last two genes are rare. Because the frequency of mutations in each gene may be different in different populations, a rigorous comparison of the frequency of involvement of *parkin, PINK1,* and *DJ-1* requires testing all the above-mentioned genes in large series of ethnically homogeneous patients with early-onset PD. This strategy has been adopted in only one study so far.[16]

TABLE 6–1	Mutational Analyses of the *DJ-1* Gene in Large Series of Parkinson's Disease Patients		
Authors (yr)	Study Subjects	Screening Method	Main Results
Hague et al. (2003)	107 young-onset PD (median 38 yr)	Sequence all exons (1-7)	1 Hispanic case with heterozygous frameshift plus heterozygous splicing mutation (c.56delC;c.57G→A)+(IVS6-1G→C) (mutation phase not explored)
			1 Hispanic case with single heterozygous missense mutation (p.A104T) (cDNA analysis did not reveal a second mutation)
Abou-Sleiman et al. (2003)	185 young-onset PD (<40 yr)	Sequence coding exons (2-7)	1 Ashkenazi Jewish case with homozygous missense mutation (p.M26I)
			1 Afro-Caribbean case with single heterozygous missense mutation (p.D149A) (the same case also homozygous for p.G78G, likely a polymorphism in Afro-Caribbeans)
	190 pathologically proven PD (late-onset)	Sequence coding exons	1 case with single heterozygous silent mutation (p.A167A)
			1 case with single heterozygous mutation, noncoding region (3′-UTR+120insA)
			1 case with single heterozygous mutation, noncoding region (3′-UTR+203G→A)
Ibanez et al. (2003)	100 young-onset PD (mean 44 yr)	PARK7 allele sharing + sequence all exons	No mutations identified
Hedrich et al. (2004)	100 young-onset PD (mean 33 yr)	DHPLC and dosage—coding exons	1 Tyrolean case with single heterozygous large deletion (exon 5-7 del)
			1 Russian case with single heterozygous splicing mutation (IVS5+2-12 del)
Djarmati et al. (2004)	75 young-onset PD (mean 39 yr)	DHPLC and dosage—coding exons	1 Serbian case with single heterozygous large deletion (exon 5 del)

Reference	Cohort	Method	Findings
Hering et al. (2004)	104 young-onset PD (mean 44 yr)	DHPLC coding exons	1 Turkish case with homozygous missense mutation (p.E64D) (data from Sahashi et al. [2007] reveal p.E64D as a splicing mutation) 1 case with single heterozygous silent mutation (p.V186V) (gene dosage did not reveal other mutations)
Clark et al. (2004)	89 young-onset PD (mean 41 yr)	Sequence all exons	1 Chinese case with single heterozygous missense mutation (p.A104T) (cDNA or dosage analysis were not performed)
Lockhart et al. (2004a)	49 young-onset PD (mean 38 yr)	RT-PCR, cDNA sequence, exon dosage	No mutations identified (U.S. patients)
Lockhart et al. (2004b)	41 young-onset PD (mean 41 yr)	RT-PCR, cDNA sequence, exon dosage	No mutations identified (Taiwanese patients)
Healy et al. (2004)	39 autosomal recessive PD (onset age not reported)	Sequence coding exons	No mutations identified
Tan et al. (2004)	40 young-onset PD (mean 42 yr)	Sequence all exons	No mutations identified
	25 autosomal recessive PD (mean 57 yr)	Sequence all exons	No mutations identified
Klein et al. (2005)	65 young-onset PD (mean 43 yr)	DHPLC and dosage—coding exons	No mutations identified
Pankratz et al. (2006)	287 PD families (mean 61 yr)	PARK7 linkage support + sequence coding exons + dosage	1 case with single heterozygous silent mutation (p.T160T) 1 case with single heterozygous silent mutation (p.A167A)

Table continued on following page

TABLE 6–2   *DJ-1* Gene Mutations Reported in Patients with Neurodegenerative Disorders (Continued)

Mutation	Effect	Zygosity	Ethnicity	Author (yr)
exon 1-5 del	No mRNA expression	Homozygous	Dutch	Bonifati et al. (2003)
g.168_185dup	Unknown	Homozygous*	Italian	Annesi et al. (2005)
p.M26I	Missense	Homozygous	Jewish	Abou-Sleiman et al. (2003)
p.E64D	Splicing abnormality	Homozygous	Turkish	Hering et al. (2004)
p.E163K	Missense	Homozygous*	Italian	Annesi et al. (2005)
p.L166P	Protein instability	Homozygous	Italian	Bonifati et al. (2003)
c.56delC,c.57G→A	Protein truncation	Heterozygous†	Hispanic	Hague et al. (2003)
IVS6-1G→C	Splicing abnormality	Heterozygous†	Hispanic	Hague et al. (2003)
p.A39S	Missense	Heterozygous‡	Chinese	Tang et al. (2006)
exon 5 del	Protein truncation	Heterozygous	Serbian	Djarmati et al. (2004)
exon 5-7 del	Protein truncation	Heterozygous	Tyrolean	Hedrich et al. (2004)
IVS5+2-12 del	Splicing abnormality	Heterozygous	Russian	Hedrich et al. (2004)
p.A104T	Missense	Heterozygous	Hispanic	Hague et al. (2003)
			Chinese	Clark et al. (2004)
p.D149A	Missense	Heterozygous	Afro-Caribbean	Abou-Sleiman et al. (2003)
p.T160T	Unknown§	Heterozygous	Not reported	Pankratz et al. (2006)
p.A167A	Unknown§	Heterozygous	Not reported	Abou-Sleiman et al. (2003)
			Not reported	Pankratz et al. (2006)
p.V186V	Unknown§	Heterozygous	Not reported	Hering et al. (2004)
3′UTR+120insA	Unknown¶	Heterozygous	Not reported	Abou-Sleiman et al. (2003)
3′UTR+203G→A	Unknown¶	Heterozygous	Not reported	Abou-Sleiman et al. (2003)

*The promoter (g.168_185dup) mutation and the missense (p.E163K) mutation were detected in the homozygous state in patients with parkinsonism–dementia–amyotrophic lateral sclerosis complex.

†The c.56delC,c.57G→A and the IVS6-1G→C mutations were detected in the same patient with early-onset Parkinson's disease, and are likely compound heterozygous; however, phase was not formally resolved.

‡A second heterozygous mutation (p.P399L) was present in the *PINK1* gene in two Chinese sibs with early-onset Parkinson's disease, suggesting digenic disease inheritance.

§Silent mutation; effects on mRNA splicing, mRNA stability, and translation efficiency cannot be excluded.

¶Mutation in the 3′ untranslated region; effects on mRNA stability cannot be excluded.

In addition to the screening of large series (see Table 6–1), two reports have described families with neurodegenerative disorders and *DJ-1* mutations.[32,33] A combination of two novel homozygous mutations was detected in two patients from a consanguineous Italian family with a complex neurodegenerative disease including early-onset parkinsonism, motor neuron disease, behavioral disturbances, and severe cognitive decline.[32] A third deceased sibling was affected with a similar disease, but could not be genotyped. One of the mutations, a missense in exon 7, is predicted to replace the conserved, negatively charged glutamate163 by a positively charged lysine (p.E163K). The other mutation is a duplication of an imperfect repeat of 18 nucleotides located in intron 1, which is close to the *DJ-1* promoter and could affect gene expression. This study is especially relevant because it expands the genetic and the clinical spectrum of the *DJ-1*-related neurodegeneration. Whether *DJ-1* mutations are a cause of pure forms of motor neuron disease or dementia (particularly frontotemporal dementia) remains unknown.

More recently, a Chinese family with two siblings affected by early-onset PD was reported to carry single heterozygous mutations in the *DJ-1* and the *PINK1* gene.[33] Both mutations replace highly conserved amino acids and likely affect the function of the proteins. These single heterozygous mutations could represent disease-unrelated coincidental findings. Functional data presented in the same study suggest, however, that the DJ-1 and PINK1 protein interact in a common neuroprotective pathway, raising the question whether early-onset PD is explained by a digenic inheritance, at least in some cases.

DJ-1 POLYMORPHISMS

The coding sequence of *DJ-1* has been highly conserved in evolution, but several polymorphic variants are known in the noncoding regions of the gene. Of particular interest is an 18-nucleotide insertion/deletion polymorphism in intron 1, which, owing to its proximity to the *DJ-1* promoter, could influence gene expression (g.168_185del),[34,35] and a coding polymorphism in exon 5, leading to the missense change p.R98Q.[12,17,36] The allelic frequency of the g.168_185del variant ranges from 20% to 30% in European populations. The R98Q variant is uncommon, being present in about 1.5% to 2% of alleles, but it also was detected in the homozygous state in one control individual, strongly suggesting that, even in the homozygous state, it is not pathogenic.[36]

Association between the g.168_185del polymorphism and common, late-onset PD or dementia with Lewy bodies was not found in two small case-control series from Finland[34] and England.[35] The role of common variants in the *DJ-1* locus in PD has been studied using a comprehensive, haplotype-tagging approach in a large case-control sample from North America, with substantially negative results.[37] Similar studies should be performed in other populations because the role of a given gene in the disease etiology might differ markedly in different ethnic groups.

CLINICAL PHENOTYPE ASSOCIATED WITH *DJ-1* MUTATIONS

The most important clinical features of patients with *DJ-1* mutations are reported in Table 6–3. The limited number of patients identified so far makes genotype-phenotype correlations and comparisons with other genetic forms of PD difficult. Overall, the clinical phenotype in patients with *DJ-1* mutations seems very similar

TABLE 6–3	Clinical Features Reported in Patients with *DJ-1* Gene Mutations				

Mutation	Zygosity	Ethnicity	Sex	Onset (yr)	Asymmetry of Signs at Onset
exon 1-5 del	HOM	Dutch	F	31	+
exon 1-5 del	HOM	Dutch	M	40	+
exon 1-5 del	HOM	Dutch	M	<40	–
exon 1-5 del	HOM	Dutch	M	27	+
p.L166P	HOM	Italian	M	28	NA
p.L166P	HOM	Italian	F	35	NA
p.L166P	HOM	Italian	M	27	NA
c.56delC;c.57G→A; IVS6-1G→C	dl.het	Hispanic	F	24	+
p.M26I	HOM	Jewish	NA	39	+
p.E64D	HOM	Turkish	M	34	+
p.E64D	HOM	Turkish	F	NA	–
[g.168_185dup; p.E163K]	HOM	Italian	M	36	NA
g.168_185dup; p.E163K	HOM	Italian	M	35	NA
g.168_185dup; p.E163K	HOM	Italian	M	24	NA
p.A39S (+PINK1 p.P399L)	dl.het	Chinese	F	26	+
p.A39S (+PINK1 p.P399L)	dl.het	Chinese	F	27	+
exon 5 del	het	Serbian	M	45	+
exon 5-7 del	het	Tyrolean	M	42	+
IVS5+2-12 del	het	Russian	F	17	–
p.A104T	het	Hispanic	M	35	+
p.A104T	het	Chinese	M	47	+
p.D149A	het	Afro-Caribbean	NA	36	+

ago, dopamine agonists; ALS, amyotrophic lateral sclerosis; behav dist, behavioral disturbance; dl.het, double heterozygous; dysk, levodopa-induced dyskinesias; fluct, motor fluctuations; HOM, homozygous; NA, not available or not applicable; NT, untreated; park, parkinsonism; psy, levodopa-induced hallucinations, or psychosis; +, present; –, absent.

to the phenotype of the other recessive forms of early-onset parkinsonism (*parkin*-related and *PINK1*-related disease).[26,27] In most cases with *DJ-1* mutations, and in all cases with homozygous or compound-heterozygous mutations, parkinsonism symptoms appeared before 40 years of age. The earliest reported onset age in a patient with *DJ-1* mutation has been 24 years old.[5] Onset age in some cases

Neurological Phenotype	Psychiatric Phenotype	Response to Levodopa	Levodopa-related Complications	Author (yr) (Clinical Data)
park, blepharospasm	anxiety	+ (ago)	–	Dekker et al. (2003)
park	psychosis	NT	NA	Dekker et al. (2003)
park, asymptomatic (age 40)	anxiety	NT	NA	Dekker et al. (2003)
park	–	++	fluct, dysk	Dekker et al. (2003)
park, blepharospasm	–	++	NA	Bonifati et al. (2002)
park, dystonia	behav dist	++	NA	Bonifati et al. (2002)
park	–	++	psy	Bonifati et al. (2002)
park	–	++	–	Hague et al. (2003)
park, leg dystonia	anxiety	++	dysk	Abou-Sleiman et al. (2003)
park, sleep dist	depression	+ (ago)	–	Hering et al. (2004)
hypomimic, asymptomatic (age 42)	–	NT	NA	Hering et al. (2004)
ALS, dementia, park	–	NA	NA	Annesi et al. (2005)
park, ALS, dementia	behav dist	NA	NA	Annesi et al. (2005)
park, ALS, dementia	behav dist	++	dysk, psy	Annesi et al. (2005)
park, sleep benefit	–	++	NA	Tang et al. (2006)
park, sleep benefit	–	++	NA	Tang et al. (2006)
park, rapid progression	–	+/–	–	Djarmati et al. (2004)
park	–	++	fluct, dysk	Hedrich et al. (2004)
park, hand dystonia	–	+ (ago)	–	Hedrich et al. (2004)
park	–	++	fluct, dysk, psy	Hague et al. (2003)
park	–	++	NA	Clark et al. (2004)
park	anxiety	++	NA	Abou-Sleiman et al. (2003)

with a single heterozygous mutation was later (latest onset reported has been 47 years old).[11] These statements are based on very few cases and should be considered with caution. Other characteristic features are a good or excellent response to levodopa or dopamine agonists, with, in some patients, early development of levodopa-related motor fluctuations and dyskinesias.

The phenotype might show a wide variability even in different patients from the same family. In the Dutch family with homozygous deletion of *DJ-1* (exon 1-5del), one patient had severe parkinsonism with levodopa-induced motor fluctuations and dyskinesias, whereas another two had only mild parkinsonism; yet another relative was asymptomatic, but had clear signs of parkinsonism on neurological examination.[25] The patients from the Italian family with p.L166P mutation broadly showed a similar phenotype,[3] although a detailed description has not been reported. In the Dutch family with homozygous deletion of *DJ-1* (exon 1-5del), short stature and brachydactyly were noted, in addition to parkinsonism.[38] These somatic features showed no cosegregation with parkinsonism, however, and they might be due to another genetic abnormality in the PARK7 region or elsewhere in the genome. Somatic abnormalities have not been reported in other patients with *DJ-1* mutations.

Progression of parkinsonism is reported to be slow in most cases with *DJ-1* mutations. Only one Serbian patient with a single heterozygous mutation had rapid progression and atypical features (early falls and vanishing response to levodopa).[9] The *DJ-1* mutation detected in that patient might represent a coincidental, non–disease-related finding, however.

In different patients with *DJ-1* mutations, dystonic features have been noted in the early phases of disease development (e.g., leg dystonia or blepharospasm). Anxiety disorder, panic attacks, and psychotic episodes unrelated to dopaminergic therapy have been reported, suggesting that patients with *DJ-1* mutations are particularly prone to develop psychiatric disturbances early in the course of disease. Other cases developed psychiatric complications related to levodopa therapy (see Table 6–3). Dystonic features at disease onset are well known to occur in young-onset PD, however, regardless of the presence of a certain genetic etiology.[26] Psychiatric disturbances are very frequent in the population in general, and they are frequent in PD, especially in early-onset cases (with or without mutations in the genes for autosomal recessive PD).[26,27,39,40] From the clinical standpoint, no clinical features enable cases with *DJ-1* mutations to be distinguished from cases with mutations in *parkin* or *PINK1*, or from cases without mutations in these three genes. Genetic testing is essential for an accurate diagnosis and distinction between the different recessive forms of early-onset parkinsonism. It is possible that *DJ-1* mutations are associated with different neurodegenerative phenotypes, including parkinsonism, dementia, and motor neuron disease, and further genetic screening is warranted.

Neuroimaging of PARK7

Structural brain imaging with computed tomography or magnetic resonance imaging in patients with *DJ-1* mutations was unremarkable. PET or single photon emission computed tomography (SPECT) studies of the nigrostriatal dopaminergic system are available from the original Dutch family with pathogenic homozygous *DJ-1* deletion (exon 1-5del)[25,41] and from the Turkish family with the pathogenic homozygous mutation (p.E64D).[10] The patients from the Dutch family (exon 1-5del) showed normal postsynaptic dopaminergic D2 receptor binding ([123 I] iodobezamide (IBZM) SPECT) and a clear presynaptic deficit, evident in SPECT and PET studies, as in idiopathic PD.[25,41] The deficit was bilateral, but more marked in the striatum opposite to the body side, which was most severely affected by parkinsonism, and the posterior part (putamen) was more severely abnormal than the anterior (caudate). Despite a disease duration of more than 15 years, the severity of F-DOPA uptake deficit was in the range observed in patients with idiopathic PD with a disease duration of about 2 years (de novo PD).[41] This suggests a very slow rate of disease progression, in agreement with the results of clinical studies.

Two healthy relatives, who were heterozygous carriers of the Dutch *DJ-1* mutation (exon 1-5del) and age 49 and 61 at the time of scanning, showed normal F-DOPA uptake, suggesting that a single heterozygous mutation in *DJ-1* is compatible with normal nigrostriatal dopaminergic function.[41] In heterozygous carriers of a *parkin* or *PINK1* mutation, evidence of a mild nigrostriatal dysfunction have been detected using PET.[42,43] The number of *DJ-1* cases is too small to draw firm conclusions, but the impact of single *DJ-1* mutations on the integrity of the nigrostriatal system might differ from the impact of single mutations in *parkin* or *PINK1*.

In a patient with the homozygous p.E64D mutation, there was a substantial loss of striatal [[18]]FP-CIT tracer uptake bilaterally, and more markedly in the striatum opposite to the body side, which was most severely affected by parkinsonism; the striatal anteroposterior gradient in the tracer uptake loss, typically observed in idiopathic PD, was also evident. The proband's sister, also a homozygous carrier of the p.E64D mutation, asymptomatic but hypomimic at age 42, showed tracer uptake values at the lower limits of the normal range, compatible with the initial stage of a neurogenerative process. In a different patient carrying a single heterozygous *DJ-1* mutation (IVS5+2-12del), Dopamine Transporter (DAT) scan and IBZM SPECT yielded a pattern similar to that observed in idiopathic PD.[8] Last, the myocardial [123]metaiodobenzylguanidine (MIBG) uptake was reduced in one patient with homozygous pathogenic *DJ-1* mutations (p.E163K; promoter duplication), suggesting the presence of cardiac sympathetic denervation, as typically observed in idiopathic PD.[44]

Pathological Correlates of *DJ-1* Mutations

The pathology of *DJ-1*–related human neurodegeneration is unknown because no autopsy studies are available. Lewy bodies from brains of patients with idiopathic PD are substantially not stained by anti–DJ-1 antibodies; however, DJ-1 immunoreactivity is increased in the insoluble fraction of brain extracts from patients with classic Lewy body–positive PD, patients with diffuse Lewy body disease,[21] and patients with Alzheimer's disease and Pick's disease.[45,46] DJ-1 immunoreactivity is found in pathological tau inclusions in different tauopathies,[45-48] and in glial inclusions in multiple systems atrophy,[47,48] suggesting further links between these seemingly different diseases, and a role of DJ-1 in their pathogenesis.

Proteomic analysis revealed the existence of several DJ-1 isoforms, which differ on the basis of their oxidative and monomeric/dimeric status.[46,49,50] The levels of total DJ-1 protein and of the most oxidized (possibly damaged) isoforms were increased in the brains of patients with common forms of PD and Alzheimer's disease.[46,50,51] These data are still based on small series of brains. If confirmed on larger studies, they would point to an involvement of the DJ-1 protein in the pathogenesis of these diseases.

The DJ-1 protein is present in the human serum and cerebrospinal fluid, and serum and cerebrospinal fluid levels of DJ-1 have been proposed as markers of

PD status and disease progression.[52,53] Results obtained in serum have not been replicated,[54] however, whereas levels in CSF await independent study.

Molecular Biology of *DJ-1*

The *DJ-1* gene has been highly conserved in evolution,[55] and is abundantly and ubiquitously expressed in the brain (in neurons and glia) and other body tissues.[56,57] The protein encoded by the human *DJ-1* gene possesses 189 amino acids, and belongs to the ThiJ/PfpI superfamily of proteins, which contain a highly conserved domain and include members in all kingdoms of life. The endogenous DJ-1 protein shows cytosolic and mitochondrial localization.[58] The crystal structure of the human DJ-1 protein has been resolved, leading to the discovery that it exists as a homodimer.[59-62]

The function of the DJ-1 protein remains poorly understood. Early after the identification of *DJ-1* as the PARK7 gene, a conservative model was proposed, in which the DJ-1 protein could react to cell stresses (oxidation or protein misfolding) at multiple levels: by directly scavenging hydrogen peroxide and other reactive molecules, by acting as a molecular chaperone, and by orchestrating the cell reaction to stress at transcriptional (nuclear) and post-transcriptional levels (cytosol, regulating the transport or availability of mRNAs) (reviewed previously).[63]

Subsequently, a large amount of functional data have been generated, which provide evidence in support of each component of the model. It is currently difficult, however, to disentangle direct from indirect and compensatory effects, and some of the activities reported in overexpression studies might not represent physiological functions of the endogenous DJ-1 protein. Confirmation of these effects in transgenic model organisms and in patient-derived material remains crucial.

Before the identification of *DJ-1* as a Parkinson-causing gene, work from different laboratories had linked the activity of DJ-1 to disparate biological processes, including oncogenesis, sperm maturation and fertilization, control of gene transcription, regulation of mRNA stability, and response to cell stress (reviewed previously).[63] More recent studies also suggest an important role of the DJ-1 protein in the protection of neurons from ischemic damage.[64,65] Of particular interest for the mechanisms of neurodegeneration, it was reported that DJ-1 is converted into a more acidic variant in response to exogenous or endogenous oxidative stress, suggesting a role for DJ-1 as an antioxidant, or a sensor of oxidative stress.[49,66] DJ-1 was exquisitely reactive to stress induced by hydrogen peroxide, similarly to the so-called peroxiredoxin proteins.[49,66] Many subsequent biochemical and structural studies confirmed a role of DJ-1 in the protection of cells against oxidative stress, particularly stress from hydrogen peroxide.[67-70] The oxidation of the Cys106 residue of DJ-1 into sulfinic acid seems to underlie the antioxidative and neuroprotective activity.[61,62,68,71] The protection against oxidative stress might also be mediated through increased cellular levels of glutathione.[70] More recent studies in *DJ-1*-knockout mice provide further evidence that the DJ-1 protein acts as a peroxiredoxin-like peroxidase, which scavenges hydrogen peroxide through oxidation of Cys106 residue.[72]

Another body of evidence supports the view that DJ-1 is a molecular chaperone. DJ-1 is homologous to Hsp31, a stress-inducible molecular chaperone in

Escherichia coli.[73] Chaperone activity of DJ-1 in vitro has been detected in some studies,[62] but denied in others.[74] This discrepancy might be explained, at least in part, by the fact that the chaperone activity of DJ-1 seems redox-dependent, being activated in response to oxidative stress, and able to inhibit aggregation of α-synuclein.[75,76] DJ-1 also might prevent aggregation of α-synuclein by increasing the levels of heat shock protein 70, a different well-known α-synuclein chaperone.[70] Other studies support the contention that DJ-1 has protease activity.[74]

A different, important contribution of DJ-1 for the PD research field has been to focus on the possible role of nuclear and cytoplasmic control of gene expression in the disease pathogenesis. It has long been proposed that DJ-1 influences gene expression by interacting with transcription factors.[63] From this perspective, novel putative partners of DJ-1 have been identified, which might be potentially relevant for the role of this protein in neurodegeneration.

In dopaminergic neuronal cell lines, DJ-1 interacts with the nuclear proteins p54nrb and pyrimidine tract–binding protein–associated splicing factor (PSF), two multifunctional regulators of transcription and RNA metabolism.[77] In this model, DJ-1 acts in concert with p54nrb and PSF to regulate the expression of a neuroprotective genetic program, including protection from toxicity of mutant α-synuclein.[77] The tyrosine hydroxylase gene might also be among the DJ-1–regulated PSF transcriptional targets,[78] linking directly DJ-1 dysfunction to decreased tyrosine hydroxylase expression. In another study, DJ-1 was found to stabilize Nrf2 (nuclear factor erythroid 2–related factor), a master regulator of antioxidant transcriptional responses[79] (including glutathione synthesis). There also is evidence for a role of the DJ-1 protein within mitochondria,[58,68] and for DJ-1 interaction with key proteins linked to apoptosis, such as PTEN[80] and Daxx,[81] delineating a possible involvement of DJ-1 in other pathways, which might be important for the survival and death of dopaminergic neurons, and for the pathogenesis of PD in general.

Of primary importance for the ongoing research is the clarification of the relationships between *DJ-1*–related disease and the other forms of monogenic parkinsonism caused by mutations in *parkin, PINK1, α-synuclein,* and *LRRK2*; are the products of these genes all involved in the same molecular pathway, or are there many, independent pathways leading to nigral neuronal death? Perhaps more importantly, to what extent is DJ-1 implicated in the pathogenesis of the classic, late-onset forms of PD and of other common neurodegenerative disorders? The proposed roles of DJ-1 as antioxidative protein and as a molecular chaperone are intriguing in the light of the evidence of oxidative stress and protein misfolding documented in the brains of patients with idiopathic PD and other common neurodegenerative disorders.

There is some preliminary evidence of direct or indirect functional interaction between the DJ-1 protein and parkin,[21,82,83] PINK1,[33] and α-synuclein[48,77] pathways. Some of these proposed interactions seem validated by independent observations. As an example, the levels of DJ-1 protein were reduced in the brain of patients with early-onset PD caused by *parkin* mutations, supporting the idea that parkin activity promotes the stability of DJ-1.[21] If confirmed, these interactions would link the pathogenesis of different forms of monogenic parkinsonism. Evidence from biochemical and proteomic studies also suggests an involvement of DJ-1 in the pathogenesis of common forms of PD and Alzheimer's disease (see also the discussion of the pathological correlates of *DJ-1* mutations).

DJ-1–Related Neurodegeneration in Model Organisms

Because *DJ-1* mutations cause human disease by a loss of function, it is logical to try to replicate the *DJ-1*–related disease in model organisms by removing the *DJ-1* homologue gene. Several *DJ-1* gene knockout mice have been generated.[72,84-88] These mice are viable and fertile (which denies an essential role for DJ-1 in fertilization), they display a normal number of brain dopaminergic neurons, and they develop no α-synuclein–containing or ubiquitin-containing intraneuronal inclusions, even at advanced ages for mice.[88,89] These mice show marked neurophysiological abnormalities in the central dopaminergic neurotransmission (especially implicating the dopamine D2 receptors[84]), however, and they develop age-related motor hypoactivity. How these mice phenotypes relate to the neurodegeneration seen in patients with *DJ-1* mutations remains unclear, but the DJ-1 protein might play important roles in the physiology of the brain dopaminergic systems.

In mice, the inactivation of a single gene, such as *DJ-1, parkin,* or *PINK1,* is insufficient to replicate the age-dependent loss of nigral dopaminergic neurons, seen in the patients with mutations in these genes (nigral cell loss is documented histologically only in *parkin*-related patients so far, but functional imaging data suggest that nigral neuronal loss also occurs in patients with *PINK1* and *DJ-1* mutations). Species-specific differences might exist between humans and mice in the effects of these single-gene defects, or there could be additional, still unknown factors (genetic, nongenetic, or both), which lead to disease in patients, in combination with mutations in the above-mentioned genes. *DJ-1* knockout mice, or neuronal lines generated from them, display increased sensitivity to oxidative stress and to toxins, such as MPTP,[87] paraquat,[90] and rotenone,[91] which have been independently implicated in PD pathogenesis.

The *DJ-1*–related neurodegeneration also has been modeled in *Drosophila melanogaster* (the fruit fly),[92-97] *Danio rerio* (zebrafish),[98,99] and *Caenorhabditis elegans* (nematode).[100] *Drosophila* possess two *DJ-1* homologues termed *DJ-1a* (mainly expressed in testis) and *DJ-1b* (ubiquitously expressed). The phenotypes resulting by inactivation of the *Drosophila DJ-1* homologue differ markedly, owing to different strategies used for targeting *DJ-1a, DJ-1b,* or both; the possible compensatory induction of the remaining gene; the effect of other modifier loci in different fly strains; and other differences (e.g., the methods used to detect neuronal death). In most of these studies, however, transgenic flies are viable and fertile, they do not display loss of dopaminergic neurons, but they are much more sensitive to oxidative stress–inducing toxins, such as paraquat and rotenone, a scenario similar to that obtained in transgenic *DJ-1* mice and worms. Last, the inactivation of the *DJ-1* gene in zebrafish led to loss of dopaminergic neurons only in combination with oxidative stress or proteasomal inhibition.[99]

Conclusions

The discovery that loss of the DJ-1 function causes rare forms of early-onset parkinsonism links DJ-1 to the mechanisms of maintenance of brain dopamine neurons and the DJ-1 dysfunction to neurodegeneration. From the clinical standpoint,

DJ-1 mutations are very rare in early-onset PD, and screening of this gene might be indicated only after the exclusion of mutations in the more commonly involved genes, *parkin* and *PINK1*.

Knowledge of the *DJ-1* mutational spectrum and the associated clinical phenotype should be considered as still incomplete, and the pathological phenotype remains totally unknown. Much more work is ahead to understand the normal function of the DJ-1 protein in the brain, and the mechanisms by which *DJ-1* mutations lead to neurodegeneration. Available data are compatible with DJ-1 being a multifunctional neuroprotective protein, which might act as an antioxidant, a molecular chaperone, and a regulator of neuronal survival and death. Unraveling the mysteries of this fascinating protein might ultimately promote understanding of the pathogenesis of the common forms of PD and other, related neurodegenerative disorders.

Acknowledgments

This chapter was supported by research grants from the Internationaal Parkinson Fonds (The Netherlands).

REFERENCES

1. Bonifati V, Rizzu P, van Baren MJ, et al: Mutations in the DJ-1 gene associated with autosomal recessive early-onset parkinsonism. Science 2003;299:256-259.
2. van Duijn CM, Dekker MC, Bonifati V, et al: Park7, a novel locus for autosomal recessive early-onset parkinsonism, on chromosome 1p36. Am J Hum Genet 2001;69:629-634.
3. Bonifati V, Breedveld GJ, Squitieri F, et al: Localization of autosomal recessive early-onset parkinsonism to chromosome 1p36 (PARK7) in an independent dataset. Ann Neurol 2002;51:253-256.
4. Macedo MG, Anar B, Bronner IF, et al: The DJ-1L166P mutant protein associated with early onset Parkinson's disease is unstable and forms higher-order protein complexes. Hum Mol Genet 2003;12:2807-2816.
5. Hague S, Rogaeva E, Hernandez D, et al: Early-onset Parkinson's disease caused by a compound heterozygous DJ-1 mutation. Ann Neurol 2003;54:271-274.
6. Abou-Sleiman PM, Healy DG, Quinn N, et al: The role of pathogenic DJ-1 mutations in Parkinson's disease. Ann Neurol 2003;54:283-286.
7. Ibanez P, De Michele G, Bonifati V, et al: Screening for DJ-1 mutations in early onset autosomal recessive parkinsonism. Neurology 2003;61:1429-1431.
8. Hedrich K, Djarmati A, Schafer N, et al: DJ-1 (PARK7) mutations are less frequent than Parkin (PARK2) mutations in early-onset Parkinson disease. Neurology 2004;62:389-394.
9. Djarmati A, Hedrich K, Svetel M, et al: Detection of Parkin (PARK2) and DJ1 (PARK7) mutations in early-onset Parkinson disease: Parkin mutation frequency depends on ethnic origin of patients. Hum Mutat 2004;23:525.
10. Hering R, Strauss KM, Tao X, et al: Novel homozygous p.E64D mutation in DJ1 in early onset Parkinson disease (PARK7). Hum Mutat 2004;24:321-329.
11. Clark LN, Afridi S, Mejia-Santana H, et al: Analysis of an early-onset Parkinson's disease cohort for DJ-1 mutations. Mov Disord 2004;19:796-800.
12. Lockhart PJ, Lincoln S, Hulihan M, et al: DJ-1 mutations are a rare cause of recessively inherited early onset parkinsonism mediated by loss of protein function. J Med Genet 2004;41:e22.
13. Lockhart PJ, Bounds R, Hulihan M, et al: Lack of mutations in DJ-1 in a cohort of Taiwanese ethnic Chinese with early-onset parkinsonism. Mov Disord 2004;19:1065-1069.
14. Healy DG, Abou-Sleiman PM, Valente EM, et al: DJ-1 mutations in Parkinson's disease. J Neurol Neurosurg Psychiatry 2004;75:144-145.
15. Tan EK, Tan C, Zhao Y, et al: Genetic analysis of DJ-1 in a cohort Parkinson's disease patients of different ethnicity. Neurosci Lett 2004;367:109-112.

16. Klein C, Djarmati A, Hedrich K, et al: PINK1, Parkin, and DJ-1 mutations in Italian patients with early-onset parkinsonism. Eur J Hum Genet 2005;13:1086-1093.
17. Pankratz N, Pauciulo MW, Elsaesser VE, et al: Mutations in DJ-1 are rare in familial Parkinson disease. Neurosci Lett 2006;408:209-213.
18. Lucking CB, Durr A, Bonifati V, et al: Association between early-onset Parkinson's disease and mutations in the parkin gene. N Engl J Med 2000;342:1560-1567.
19. Bonifati V: LRRK2 Low-penetrance mutations (Gly2019Ser) and risk alleles (Gly2385Arg)-linking familial and sporadic Parkinson's disease. Neurochem Res 2007;32:1700-1708.
20. Hedrich K, Kann M, Lanthaler AJ, et al: The importance of gene dosage studies: mutational analysis of the parkin gene in early-onset parkinsonism. Hum Mol Genet 2001;10:1649-1656.
21. Moore DJ, Zhang L, Troncoso J, et al: Association of DJ-1 and parkin mediated by pathogenic DJ-1 mutations and oxidative stress. Hum Mol Genet 2005;14:71-84.
22. Hulleman JD, Mirzaei H, Guigard E, et al: Destabilization of DJ-1 by familial substitution and oxidative modifications: implications for Parkinson's disease. Biochemistry 2007;46:5776-5789.
23. Blackinton J, Ahmad R, Miller DW, et al: Effects of DJ-1 mutations and polymorphisms on protein stability and subcellular localization. Brain Res Mol Brain Res 2005;134:76-83.
24. Sahashi K, Masuda A, Matsuura T, et al: In vitro and in silico analysis reveals an efficient algorithm to predict the splicing consequences of mutations at the 5' splice sites. Nucleic Acids Res 2007;35:5995-6003.
25. Dekker M, Bonifati V, van Swieten J, et al: Clinical features and neuroimaging of PARK7-linked parkinsonism. Mov Disord 2003;18:751-757.
26. Lohmann E, Periquet M, Bonifati V, et al: How much phenotypic variation can be attributed to parkin genotype? Ann Neurol 2003;54:176-185.
27. Bonifati V, Rohe CF, Breedveld GJ, et al: Early-onset parkinsonism associated with PINK1 mutations: frequency, genotypes, and phenotypes. Neurology 2005;65:87-95.
28. Hedrich K, Hagenah J, Djarmati A, et al: Clinical spectrum of homozygous and heterozygous PINK1 mutations in a large German family with Parkinson disease: role of a single hit? Arch Neurol 2006;63:833-838.
29. Lincoln SJ, Maraganore DM, Lesnick TG, et al: Parkin variants in North American Parkinson's disease: cases and controls. Mov Disord 2003;18:1306-1311.
30. Kay DM, Moran D, Moses L, et al: Heterozygous parkin point mutations are as common in control subjects as in Parkinson's patients. Ann Neurol 2007;61:47-54.
31. Abou-Sleiman PM, Muqit MM, McDonald NQ, et al: A heterozygous effect for PINK1 mutations in Parkinson's disease? Ann Neurol 2006;60:414-419.
32. Annesi G, Savettieri G, Pugliese P, et al: DJ-1 mutations and parkinsonism-dementia-amyotrophic lateral sclerosis complex. Ann Neurol 2005;58:803-807.
33. Tang B, Xiong H, Sun P, et al: Association of PINK1 and DJ-1 confers digenic inheritance of early-onset Parkinson's disease. Hum Mol Genet 2006;15:1816-1825.
34. Eerola J, Hernandez D, Launes J, et al: Assessment of a DJ-1 (PARK7) polymorphism in Finnish PD. Neurology 2003;61:1000-1002.
35. Morris CM, O'Brien KK, Gibson AM, et al: Polymorphism in the human DJ-1 gene is not associated with sporadic dementia with Lewy bodies or Parkinson's disease. Neurosci Lett 2003;352:151-153.
36. Hedrich K, Schafer N, Hering R, et al: The R98Q variation in DJ-1 represents a rare polymorphism. Ann Neurol 2004;55:145.
37. Maraganore DM, Wilkes K, Lesnick TG, et al: A limited role for DJ1 in Parkinson disease susceptibility. Neurology 2004;63:550-553.
38. Dekker MC, Galjaard RJ, Snijders PJ, et al: Brachydactyly and short stature in a kindred with early-onset parkinsonism. Am J Med Genet A 2004;130:102-104.
39. Steinlechner S, Stahlberg J, Volkel B, et al: Co-occurrence of affective and schizophrenia spectrum disorders with PINK1 mutations. J Neurol Neurosurg Psychiatry 2007;78:532-535.
40. Khan NL, Graham E, Critchley P, et al: Parkin disease: a phenotypic study of a large case series. Brain 2003;126;(Pt 6):1279-1292.
41. Dekker MC, Eshuis SA, Maguire RP, et al: PET neuroimaging and mutations in the DJ-1 gene. J Neural Transm 2004;111:1575-1581.
42. Khan NL, Brooks DJ, Pavese N, et al: Progression of nigrostriatal dysfunction in a parkin kindred: an [18F]dopa PET and clinical study. Brain 2002;125;(Pt 10):2248-2256.
43. Khan NL, Valente EM, Bentivoglio AR, et al: Clinical and subclinical dopaminergic dysfunction in PARK6-linked parkinsonism: an 18F-dopa PET study. Ann Neurol 2002;52:849-853.

44. Quattrone A, Bagnato A, Annesi G, et al: Myocardial (123)metaiodobenzylguanidine uptake in genetic Parkinson's disease. Mov Disord 2008;23:21-27.
45. Rizzu P, Hinkle DA, Zhucareva V, et al: DJ-1 colocalizes with tau inclusions: a link between parkinsonism and dementia. Ann Neurol 2004;55:113-118.
46. Kumaran R, Kingsbury A, Coulter I, et al: DJ-1 (PARK7) is associated with 3R and 4R tau neuronal and glial inclusions in neurodegenerative disorders. Neurobiol Dis 2007;28: 122-132.
47. Neumann M, Muller V, Gorner K, et al: Pathological properties of the Parkinson's disease-associated protein DJ-1 in alpha-synucleinopathies and tauopathies: relevance for multiple system atrophy and Pick's disease. Acta Neuropathol (Berl) 2004;107:489-496.
48. Meulener MC, Graves CL, Sampathu DM, et al: DJ-1 is present in a large molecular complex in human brain tissue and interacts with alpha-synuclein. J Neurochem 2005;93:1524-1532.
49. Mitsumoto A, Nakagawa Y, Takeuchi A, et al: Oxidized forms of peroxiredoxins and DJ-1 on two-dimensional gels increased in response to sublethal levels of paraquat. Free Radic Res 2001;35:301-310.
50. Choi J, Sullards MC, Olzmann JA, et al: Oxidative damage of DJ-1 is linked to sporadic Parkinson and Alzheimer diseases. J Biol Chem 2006;281:10816-10824.
51. Bandopadhyay R, Kingsbury AE, Cookson MR, et al: The expression of DJ-1 (PARK7) in normal human CNS and idiopathic Parkinson's disease. Brain 2004;127;(Pt 2):420-430.
52. Waragai M, Nakai M, Wei J, et al: Plasma levels of DJ-1 as a possible marker for progression of sporadic Parkinson's disease. Neurosci Lett 2007;425:18-22.
53. Waragai M, Wei J, Fujita M, et al: Increased level of DJ-1 in the cerebrospinal fluids of sporadic Parkinson's disease. Biochem Biophys Res Commun 2006;345:967-972.
54. Maita C, Tsuji S, Yabe I, et al: Secretion of DJ-1 into the serum of patients with Parkinson's disease. Neurosci Lett 2008;431:86-89.
55. Lucas JI, Marin I: A new evolutionary paradigm for the Parkinson disease gene DJ-1. Mol Biol Evol 2007;24:551-561.
56. Bader V, Ran Zhu X, Lubbert H, Stichel CC: Expression of DJ-1 in the adult mouse CNS. Brain Res 2005;1041:102-111.
57. Galter D, Westerlund M, Belin AC, Olson L: DJ-1 and UCH-L1 gene activity patterns in the brains of controls, Parkinson and schizophrenia patients and in rodents. Physiol Behav 2007;92; (1-2):46-53.
58. Zhang L, Shimoji M, Thomas B, et al: Mitochondrial localization of the Parkinson's disease related protein DJ-1: implications for pathogenesis. Hum Mol Genet 2005;14:2063-2073.
59. Honbou K, Suzuki NN, Horiuchi M, et al: The crystal structure of DJ-1, a protein related to male fertility and Parkinson's disease. J Biol Chem 2003;278:31380-31384.
60. Tao X, Tong L: Crystal structure of human DJ-1, a protein associated with early-onset Parkinson's diseasec. J Biol Chem 2003;278:31372-31379.
61. Wilson MA, Collins JL, Hod Y, et al: The 1.1-A resolution crystal structure of DJ-1, the protein mutated in autosomal recessive early onset Parkinson's disease. Proc Natl Acad Sci U S A 2003;100:9256-9261.
62. Lee SJ, Kim SJ, Kim IK, et al: Crystal structures of human DJ-1 and *Escherichia coli* Hsp31, which share an evolutionarily conserved domain. J Biol Chem 2003;278:44552-44559.
63. Bonifati V, Oostra BA, Heutink P: Linking DJ-1 to neurodegeneration offers novel insights for understanding the pathogenesis of Parkinson's disease. J Mol Med 2004;82:163-174.
64. Yanagisawa D, Kitamura Y, Inden M, et al: DJ-1 protects against neurodegeneration caused by focal cerebral ischemia and reperfusion in rats. J Cereb Blood Flow Metab 2008;28:563-578.
65. Aleyasin H, Rousseaux MW, Phillips M, et al: The Parkinson's disease gene DJ-1 is also a key regulator of stroke-induced damage. Proc Natl Acad Sci U S A 2007;104:18748-18753.
66. Mitsumoto A, Nakagawa Y: DJ-1 is an indicator for endogenous reactive oxygen species elicited by endotoxin. Free Radic Res 2001;35:885-893.
67. Taira T, Saito Y, Niki T, et al: DJ-1 has a role in antioxidative stress to prevent cell death. EMBO Rep 2004;5:430.
68. Canet-Aviles RM, Wilson MA, Miller DW, et al: The Parkinson's disease protein DJ-1 is neuroprotective due to cysteine-sulfinic acid-driven mitochondrial localization. Proc Natl Acad Sci U S A 2004;101:9103-9108.
69. Martinat C, Shendelman S, Jonason A, et al: Sensitivity to oxidative stress in DJ-1-deficient dopamine neurons: an ES-derived cell model of primary parkinsonism. PLoS Biol 2004;2:e327.
70. Zhou W, Freed CR: DJ-1 up-regulates glutathione synthesis during oxidative stress and inhibits A53T alpha-synuclein toxicity. J Biol Chem 2005;280:43150-43158.

71. Kinumi T, Kimata J, Taira T, et al: Cysteine-106 of DJ-1 is the most sensitive cysteine residue to hydrogen peroxide-mediated oxidation in vivo in human umbilical vein endothelial cells. Biochem Biophys Res Commun 2004;317:722-728.

72. Andres-Mateos E, Perier C, Zhang L, et al: DJ-1 gene deletion reveals that DJ-1 is an atypical peroxiredoxin-like peroxidase. Proc Natl Acad Sci U S A 2007;104:14807-14812.

73. Quigley PM, Korotkov K, Baneyx F, Hol WG: The 1.6-A crystal structure of the class of chaperones represented by *Escherichia coli* Hsp31 reveals a putative catalytic triad. Proc Natl Acad Sci U S A 2003;100:3137-3142.

74. Olzmann JA, Brown K, Wilkinson KD, et al: Familial Parkinson's disease-associated L166P mutation disrupts DJ-1 protein folding and function. J Biol Chem 2004;279:8506-8515.

75. Shendelman S, Jonason A, Martinat C, et al: DJ-1 is a redox-dependent molecular chaperone that inhibits alpha-synuclein aggregate formation. PLoS Biol 2004;2:e362.

76. Zhou W, Zhu M, Wilson MA, et al: The oxidation state of DJ-1 regulates its chaperone activity toward alpha-synuclein. J Mol Biol 2006;356:1036-1048.

77. Xu J, Zhong N, Wang H, et al: The Parkinson's disease-associated DJ-1 protein is a transcriptional co-activator that protects against neuronal apoptosis. Hum Mol Genet 2005;14:1231-1241.

78. Zhong N, Kim CY, Rizzu P, et al: DJ-1 transcriptionally up-regulates the human tyrosine hydroxylase by inhibiting the sumoylation of pyrimidine tract-binding protein-associated splicing factor. J Biol Chem 2006;281:20940-20948.

79. Clements CM, McNally RS, Conti BJ, et al: DJ-1, a cancer- and Parkinson's disease-associated protein, stabilizes the antioxidant transcriptional master regulator Nrf2. Proc Natl Acad Sci U S A 2006;103:15091-15096.

80. Kim RH, Peters M, Jang Y, et al: DJ-1, a novel regulator of the tumor suppressor PTEN. Cancer Cell 2005;7:263-273.

81. Junn E, Taniguchi H, Jeong BS, et al: Interaction of DJ-1 with Daxx inhibits apoptosis signal-regulating kinase 1 activity and cell death. Proc Natl Acad Sci U S A 2005;102:9691-9696.

82. Baulac S, Lavoie MJ, Strahle J, et al: Dimerization of Parkinson's disease-causing DJ-1 and formation of high molecular weight complexes in human brain. Mol Cell Neurosci 2004;27:236-246.

83. Olzmann JA, Li L, Chudaev MV, et al: Parkin-mediated K63-linked polyubiquitination targets misfolded DJ-1 to aggresomes via binding to HDAC6. J Cell Biol 2007;178:1025-1038.

84. Goldberg MS, Pisani A, Haburcak M, et al: Nigrostriatal dopaminergic deficits and hypokinesia caused by inactivation of the familial Parkinsonism-linked gene DJ-1. Neuron 2005;45:489-496.

85. Kim RH, Smith PD, Aleyasin H, et al: Hypersensitivity of DJ-1-deficient mice to 1-methyl-4-phenyl-1,2,3,6-tetrahydropyrindine (MPTP) and oxidative stress. Proc Natl Acad Sci U S A 2005;102:5215-5220.

86. Chen L, Cagniard B, Mathews T, et al: Age-dependent motor deficits and dopaminergic dysfunction in DJ-1 null mice. J Biol Chem 2005;280:21418-21426.

87. Manning-Bog AB, Caudle WM, Perez XA, et al: Increased vulnerability of nigrostriatal terminals in DJ-1-deficient mice is mediated by the dopamine transporter. Neurobiol Dis 2007;27:141-150.

88. Chandran JS, Lin X, Zapata A, et al: Progressive behavioral deficits in DJ-1-deficient mice are associated with normal nigrostriatal function. Neurobiol Dis 2008;29:505-514.

89. Yamaguchi H, Shen J: Absence of dopaminergic neuronal degeneration and oxidative damage in aged DJ-1-deficient mice. Mol Neurodegener 2007;2:10.

90. Yang W, Chen L, Ding Y, et al: Paraquat induces dopaminergic dysfunction and proteasome impairment in DJ-1-deficient mice. Hum Mol Genet 2007;16:2900-2910.

91. Pisani A, Martella G, Tscherter A, et al: Enhanced sensitivity of DJ-1-deficient dopaminergic neurons to energy metabolism impairment: role of Na+/K+ ATPase. Neurobiol Dis 2006;23:54-60.

92. Meulener M, Whitworth AJ, Armstrong-Gold CE, et al: *Drosophila* DJ-1 mutants are selectively sensitive to environmental toxins associated with Parkinson's disease. Curr Biol 2005;15:1572-1577.

93. Menzies FM, Yenisetti SC, Min KT: Roles of *Drosophila* DJ-1 in survival of dopaminergic neurons and oxidative stress. Curr Biol 2005;15:1578-1582.

94. Yang Y, Gehrke S, Haque ME, et al: Inactivation of *Drosophila* DJ-1 leads to impairments of oxidative stress response and phosphatidylinositol 3-kinase/Akt signaling. Proc Natl Acad Sci U S A 2005;102:13670-13675.

95. Park J, Kim SY, Cha GH, et al: *Drosophila* DJ-1 mutants show oxidative stress-sensitive locomotive dysfunction. Gene 2005;361:133-139.

96. Meulener MC, Xu K, Thomson L, et al: Mutational analysis of DJ-1 in *Drosophila* implicates functional inactivation by oxidative damage and aging. Proc Natl Acad Sci U S A 2006;103: 12517-12522.

97. Lavara-Culebras E, Paricio N: *Drosophila* DJ-1 mutants are sensitive to oxidative stress and show reduced lifespan and motor deficits. Gene 2007;400;(1-2):158-165.

98. Bai Q, Mullett SJ, Garver JA, et al: Zebrafish DJ-1 is evolutionarily conserved and expressed in dopaminergic neurons. Brain Res 2006;1113:33-44.

99. Bretaud S, Allen C, Ingham PW, Bandmann O: p53-dependent neuronal cell death in a DJ-1-deficient zebrafish model of Parkinson's disease. J Neurochem 2007;100:1626-1635.

100. Ved R, Saha S, Westlund B, et al: Similar patterns of mitochondrial vulnerability and rescue induced by genetic modification of alpha-synuclein, parkin, and DJ-1 in *Caenorhabditis elegans*. J Biol Chem 2005;280:42655-42668.

7 *LRRK2* and Parkinson's Disease

MATTHEW JAMES FARRER

PARK8 and *LRRK2*	Lrrk2 Pleomorphic Pathology
Lrrk2 Protein Structure	Lrrk2 Functional Neuroscience
Lrrk2 Pathogenic Mutations and Polymorphic Risk Factors—Families and Founders	Parsimonious Molecular Model of Lrrk2 Activity
	Future Research

PARK8 and *LRRK2*

The PARK8 linkage assignment (locus) was originally mapped to chromosome 12q12 in a Japanese family with asymmetric levodopa-responsive late-onset parkinsonism, consistent with a diagnosis of sporadic Parkinson's disease (PD).[1] Confirmation of the PARK8 locus came from Families A and D, which also have autosomal dominant late-onset parkinsonism.[2] Sequence analysis subsequently discovered the leucine-rich repeat kinase 2 gene (*LRRK2*) and disease-segregating R1441C and Y1699C coding substitutions.[3] The discovery was confirmed by genetic linkage in other families in which *LRRK2* sequencing has revealed additional mutations.[4-7]

LRRK2 comprises 51 exons and is expressed in most brain regions, including the striatum and substantia nigra (dopamine-receptive areas),[8-10] cortex, hippocampus, and subventricular zone.[11] Expression is also high in the kidneys, lungs, and leukocytes.[3,8,12] *LRRK1* is the closest human homologue on chromosome 15q26, and given their expression profile, *LRRK1* and *LRRK2* may be functionally redundant in early development.[13,14]

Lrrk2 Protein Structure

The *LRRK2* transcript encodes a 2527-amino acid protein (denoted Lrrk2), which contains several conserved domains, including ankyrin (ANK), leucine-rich repeat (LRR), GTPase (Roc), C-terminal of Roc spacer (COR), mitogen-activated protein kinase (MAPK), and WD40 repeats.[15] Each domain is potentially involved in multiple functions, including substrate binding, protein phosphorylation, and protein-protein interactions.[16-18] The combination of Roc-COR-MAPK motifs, encoding two distinct but functionally linked enzymatic domains, is highly conserved among vertebrates and shares homology to the ROCO protein family of receptor interacting protein kinases.[19] The protein is 286 kD, but biochemical evidence suggests Lrrk2 exists as a dimer, if not as part of a higher molecular weight complex[20-22] (unpublished data). Immunoprecipitation studies have favored many interacting proteins, including parkin and heat shock protein 90.[18,20,21,23-27] To date, few Lrrk2 MAPK substrates have been elucidated, but these include phosphorylation of moesin at threonine 588.[28] Moesin is a member of the ERM/merlin family of protein tethers that serve to link plasma membrane receptor complexes to the microfilament cytoskeleton.[29]

Lrrk2 Pathogenic Mutations and Polymorphic Risk Factors—Families and Founders

More than 75 Lrrk2 missense or nonsense mutations have been described[30-32] (see www.genetests.org), but genetic evidence for pathogenicity is proven only for R1441C/G, Y1699C, G2019S, and I2020T substitutions (by linkage)[3,5-7] and for Lrrk2 R1628P and G2385R (by association).[33-38] Although other sequence variants may be pathogenic, they might also represent benign mutations or polymorphisms. This is an important distinction in interpreting Lrrk2 function and for diagnosis; further discussion is focused on known pathogenic variants.

Lrrk2 R1441C, G, and H substitutions affect the Roc domain, a "Ras-like" part of the protein that binds and hydrolyzes GTP, which seems to be a prerequisite for Lrrk2 kinase activity.[15,16,39] Lrrk2 R1441C and R1441H families are worldwide, but rare, from which haplotype analysis suggests multiple independent founders.[40] For Lrrk2 R1441C carriers, the mean age at onset for parkinsonism is 60 years (range 30 to 79 years); less than 20% have symptoms before age 50, whereas by 75 years greater than 90% of carriers are affected.[41] By contrast, R1441G seems to be of Basque origin, appearing in 16% of familial parkinsonism and 4% of sporadic PD in this population, and is a frequent cause of PD in Spain.[7,42,43]

Lrrk2 Y1699C within the COR domain has been identified within two well-characterized families, the Lincolnshire kindred and Family A.[3,44,45] The mean age of onset for the Lincolnshire kindred is 57 ± 13 years with a clinical course similar to sporadic PD and Lewy body disease on autopsy.[44] In Family A, the predominant phenotype is levodopa-responsive clinical parkinsonism with a mean onset at 55 ± 13 years, but some family members also present with amyotrophy, dementia, dystonia, or postural tremor. Despite differences in their clinical and pathological presentations, chromosome 12q12 haplotype analysis suggests both families originate from the same ancestral founder (unpublished data).

Lrrk2 G2019S is within exon 41 and the "activation hinge" of the MAPK domain (Fig. 7–1). In the United States and Europe, the mutation is found in 0.5% to 2% of "seemingly sporadic" patients with PD and 5% of patients with familial parkinsonism in which it clearly segregates with autosomal dominant disease.[5,46-50] In Ashkenazi Jews, Lrrk2 G2019S is found in 13% of PD cases.[51,52] Lrrk2 G2019S is most frequent in North African Berber-Arabs, including 30% of "seemingly sporadic" PD cases in Tunisia, where it must contribute to the excess incidence of disease.[53-55] Lrrk2 G2019S is seldom found in aged, unaffected control subjects,[56] and early family-based studies show disease penetrance in Lrrk2 G2019S carriers is age dependent, increasing from 17% at age 50 to 85% at age 70.[5] A slightly lower

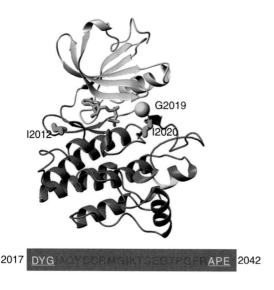

G2019

I2012

I2020

2017 DYG...APE 2042

Figure 7–1 Ribbon model of the MAPK domain of Lrrk2. The activation segment from 2017-2042 amino acids (*bottom*) is shown in the context of the MAPK domain hinged by DYG and APE "hinges" (in yellow) on either side (*top*). A central ATP molecule is shown in pale blue; the position of I2012T, G2019S, and I2020T mutations is highlighted. The activation segment typically blocks substrate access to the catalytic site. (Modified from Mata et al., 2006.)

but comparable family-based estimate has been derived through meta-analysis.[57] Although these figures are disputed, rigorous large-scale, population-based penetrance estimates are not yet available for genetic counseling.[58-60] In Tunisian Berbers, in whom Lrrk2 G2019S is most numerous, the odds ratio for disease is 22 (95% confidence interval 10 to 51, $P < 1E^{-6}$), and the lifetime penetrance for Lrrk2 G2019S carriers is 63%.[61]

The disease phenotype of Lrrk2 G2019S heterozygous carriers often varies within families and is comparable to patients with homozygous mutations.[62-65] The Lrrk2 G2019S mutation is primarily associated with one chromosome 12q12 haplotype inherited *identical-by-descent,* indicative of one ancestral founder.[5,55] The haplotype is shortest and most frequent in North African Berbers, consistent with its origin in this ethnic group.[5,66] Whether in the United States, Norway, Spain, Israel, or North Africa, almost all familial and "seemingly sporadic" patients with Lrrk2 G2019S and PD are genetically related; there are few exceptions.[67]

Lrrk2 I2012T and I2020T substitutions are also found within *LRRK2* exon 41 and the kinase domain, and similar to G2019S, each provides a potential site for phosphorylation.[6,50] Lrrk2 I2020T explains disease in the Japanese Sagamihara family in which the PARK8 locus was originally identified.[6] Clinically, patients have typical idiopathic PD and associated comorbidities, including cardiac denervation, and psychiatric and cognitive problems may develop.[50]

Lrrk2 G2385R is the most frequent polymorphic risk factor for PD. First described within a nuclear family of Taiwanese ethnic-Chinese descent,[31] the genetic association of Lrrk2 G2385R with PD has been reported in community-based studies in Taiwan, Singapore, and Japan.[33-37] Lrrk2 G2385R, inherited *identical-by-descent* from one ancient founder, is found in approximately 4% of the Southeast Asian population and represents a polymorphic "risk factor," rather than a pathogenic mutation.[34] Meta-analysis shows the variant increases disease risk by 2.5-fold (95% CI 1.9-3.3, p < 1.2 E-10) and may lower age at onset.[68] Pedigree studies suggest disease susceptibility is familial but otherwise affected carriers have clinical and imaging phenotypes consistent with idiopathic PD[69] Lrrk2 G2385R is located on the external surface of the C-terminal WD40 "barrel," a motif with multiple binding surfaces that typically enables protein-protein interactions.[15] Lrrk2 R1628P, within the COR domain, is the other common risk factor for PD in ethnic Chinese and contributes similar population and genotypic risk as Lrrk2 G2385R (OR 3.3, 95% CI 1.4-7.9, p < 0.007).[38-70]

Lrrk2 Pleomorphic Pathology

Lrrk2 has been dubbed the "Rosetta stone" of parkinsonism pathology. Most autopsy-examined cases of Lrrk2 parkinsonism (~80%) show typical Lewy body disease that is consistent with a postmortem diagnosis of "definite" PD.[47,64,71,72] Some brains have only tau-positive neurofibrillary tangles reminiscent of argyrophilic grains disease,[65,73] some have multiple ubiquitin-immunoreactive cytoplasmic or nuclear neuronal inclusions, and some show only nigral degeneration and gliosis without Lewy body pathology.[3,73,74] The latter have recently been reported to show TDP-43 immunopositive inclusions (D. Dickson personal communication).[75] The neuropathology may be pleomorphic even within members of a family with the same mutation.[3,75] The pathways that lead to clinical parkinsonism with α-synuclein–immunopositive Lewy body, ubiquitin, or neurofibrillary tangle pathology, often considered as distinct etiologies, may overlap.[76] Immunohistochemically, Lrrk2 does not seem to be a component of any neurodegenerative lesion,[11,77,78] although staining of inclusion bodies with less specific Lrrk2 antibodies has been reported.[11,14,79]

Lrrk2 Functional Neuroscience

In the slime mold *Dictyostelium discoideum*, *LRK-1*, the ancestral othologue of vertebrate *LRRK1/LRRK2*, encodes a homolog of GbpC, the main high-affinity cGMP-binding protein required for the normal phosphorylation and cytoskeletal assembly of myosin during chemotaxis.[13,80] In the nematode worm *C. elegans*, knockout of the orthologue *LRK-1* suggests the kinase determines the polarized sorting of synaptic vesicle proteins to axons by excluding them from dendrite-specific transport machinery in the Golgi.[81] *LRK-1 loss-of-function* worms also have a chemosensory deficit, but whether expression of human wild-type *LRRK2* rescues the phenotype has yet to be determined. Olfactory dysfunction (hyposmia) is a frequent and early abnormality in PD and Lrrk2 parkinsonism[82] suggesting a common biological pathway is affected.[83] In the fruit fly *D. melanogaster,* loss of the endogenous *LRRK* gene (CG5483) induces locomotive impairment and a reduction in tyrosine hydroxylase immunostaining within dopaminergic neurons and loss of fertility in females. In contrast, *LRRK* knockin of the Roc domain substitution R1069C (comparable to Lrrk2 R1441C in humans) produces no deleterious effects.[84] Neither observation is consistent with the genetic ethiology of Lrrk2 parkinsonisn in man.

In mammalian cells, Lrrk2 mutant transgenic overexpression induces a progressive reduction in neurite length and branching in primary neuronal cultures and in the intact rodent central nervous system.[85] In contrast, Lrrk2 deficiency induced by RNA interference leads to increased neurite length and branching.

In addition, neurons that express Lrrk2 mutations linked to PD may harbor prominent phospho-tau-immunopositive inclusions with lysosomal characteristics, and ultimately undergo apoptosis.[85] These phenotypes can be recapitulated in vertebrate models with more physiological patterns and levels of Lrrk2 expression. Indeed, mutant Lrrk2 R1441C BAC transgenic mice have been reported with dopaminergic and behavioral phenotypes, reminiscent of PD.[86]

Parsimonious Molecular Model of Lrrk2 Activity

Lrrk2 is postulated to be a member of the RIP kinase family of proteins, which are essential sensors of cellular stress.[19] These proteins integrate many different upstream signals to initiate a few specific responses, including cell survival and inflammatory-inducing or death-inducing programs that are mediated through the JNK, ERK, p38, and NF-κB signaling pathways. Changes in MAPK signaling are apparent in Lrrk2 parkinsonism and PD, and modulation of these pathways may have therapeutic potential.[12,87,88]

Fundamental to developing informative models and neuroprotective interventions is a physiological understanding of the function of Lrrk2. Based on homology to similar serine-threonine protein kinases, the G2019S substitution seems to be within the DY$\underline{G}$ hinge of the activation segment. This serves to anchor and close a ribbon of protein that protects the catalytic site. The G2019S mutation may keep "the door ajar," resulting in increased kinase activity consistent with a dominant gain-of-function (see Fig. 7–1).[5,89] Biochemical studies confirm Lrrk2 G2019S has twofold to threefold higher levels of intramolecular and intermolecular kinase activity.[17,28,85,90-92] Nevertheless, not all protein kinases identified by their primary sequence act as functional kinases[93]; and most mutations in recombinant Lrrk2 protein do not seem to increase kinase activity.[17,20,28,85,90,91,94] Lrrk2 may function as a MAPK scaffolding protein, given the protein-protein interaction domains at N-terminal and C-terminal ends. The complex may be involved but perhaps not directly responsible for substrate phosphorylation. It is even conceivable that Lrrk2 mutations cause loss-of-function, mutant protein acting in a dominant negative manner to impair signal transduction.

With this background, it remains unclear whether Lrrk2 kinase inhibition would be beneficial therapeutically. To add further to this complexity, empirical data suggest GTP binding to the Roc domain regulates Lrrk2 MAPK activity, intramolecular and intermolecular phosphorylation, and neuronal toxicity.[16,39,94-96] A parsimonious model of how mutations in Lrrk2 Roc, COR, MAPK, and WD40 domains lead to the same disease is required.

A simple solution is to consider the protein in its physiological context as a dimer or even higher molecular weight multimer (reminiscent of a "Chinese lantern") that requires GTP binding and intermolecular and intramolecular autophosphorylation to function (Fig. 7–2). Mutations in the Roc (R1441C/G/H), COR (Y1699C), MAPK (I2012T, G2019S, I2020T), and WD40 (G2385R susceptibility factor) domains all may increase intrinsic kinase activity (directly or indirectly); just one mutant Lrrk2 monomer would be sufficient to activate the protein complex; and patients with heterozygous or homozygous mutations may have comparable symptoms, age at onset, and progression.[17,63] The model may explain why in vitro GTPase and MAPK activity measurements using partial recombinant,

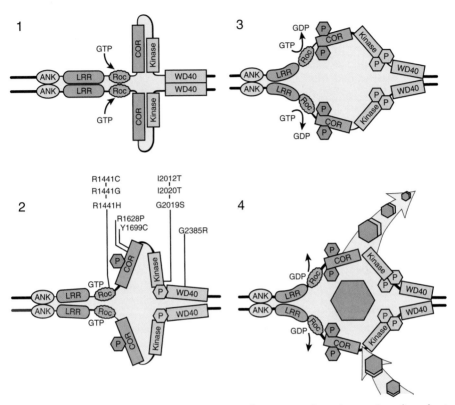

Figure 7–2 A parsimonious model of how genetically proven pathogenic mutations throughout Lrrk2 may affect its function. Dimeric Lrrk2 is postulated with intermolecular interactions between ANK or LRR and WD40 domains: (1) GTP binding to the Roc domain initially allows a "pore" to open between monomeric Lrrk2 subunits, attached via their N-terminal Ank/LRR and C-terminal WD40 domains; (2) this pore is progressively widened by autophosphorylation or extrinsic phosphorylation or both[16,17]; (3) the kinase domain has access to its appropriate substrate; and (4) ultimately the kinase domain has access to a GTPase/phosphatase that inactivates the dimeric Lrrk2 protein. Empirical data on Roc dimer structure, and intramolecular autophosphorylation, now support this hypothesis.

potentially monomeric Lrrk2 are low or suboptimal. The model also suggests there are several ways in which intrinsic kinase activity may be modulated. These include (1) inhibition of Lrrk2 dimerization and multimerization; (2) inhibition of the GTP and GDP binding and transition in the Roc domain; (3) inhibition of COR and MAPK phosphorylation (e.g., at T2031/S2032 and T2035[17]); and (4) direct inhibition of the active site of the MAPK domain.

Future Research

Pleomorphic pathology suggests that the normal function, and pathogenic mutations, of Lrrk2 must be more intimately associated with *successful aging* of the basal ganglia than a direct cause of disease. Most proteins genetically implicated in parkinsonism, whether involved in signaling, in synaptic connectivity, as chaperones, in redox sensing, or in protein degradation, may be considered in the same context.[76] PD is multifactorial disorder influenced by a combination of genetic, environmental, and stochastic factors for which age remains the greatest risk factor. Variable disease penetrance within genetically defined families, and the lack of late-onset disease concordance in monozygotic twins, should be expected.[97-99]

In humans, Lrrk2 mutations have accumulated within the locus, as they do not affect reproductive success; with aging, defective Lrrk2 protein provides a background of neuronal susceptibility on which subsequent triggers act. Lrrk2 mutations vary in frequency depending on ethnicity, and genetic screening in PD can inform a clinical diagnosis, but the results must be interpreted with caution because (1) most Lrrk2 coding substitutions have yet to be proven pathogenic, and (2) even pathogenic mutations have variable penetrance. Cross-sectional and longitudinal evaluation of Lrrk2 mutation carriers, including asymptomatic and affected subjects, is now warranted, and is likely to provide fundamental insight into the natural history of PD and other contributing environmental and genetic factors.

Future studies might define the earliest signs of the syndrome, such as rapid-eye-movement sleep behavior disorder, depression/apathy, constipation, or olfactory dysfunction. The natural progression of disability, the rate of decline, and frequency of associated comorbidities might also be followed. Special emphasis might be placed on "nonmotor" features to see which, if any, are an inevitable consequence of the disease process. Where possible, standardized methods should be used across centers to enable meta-analyses. Genetically diagnosed patients and asymptomatic "at-risk" subjects may provide a relatively uniform substrate to identify biomarkers of the disease process (trait, state, and rate) through imaging, RNA, and metabolomic and proteomic studies—and with which the efficacy of neuroprotection trials may be monitored.[12,45] From a clinical trials perspective, genetically diagnosed individuals may be most likely to participate and benefit from early intervention therapies.

The relationship between Lrrk2 pathogenesis, parkinsonism and end-stage pathology, and α-synuclein and tau remains enigmatic, and the biological switch between these different end states also has to be elucidated.[65] Perhaps a second hit is required.[100] Many common environmental risk factors have been nominated in PD, but none have been directly proven to have a causal role.[101,102] On a genetically defined background, however, more meaningful environmental exposures may yet be elucidated and tested. The role of normal endogenous Lrrk2 in normal aging and idiopathic PD also has to be defined.

Genetic models based on Lrrk2 transgenesis may be especially informative, and progress has already been rapid. In model organisms, it may be misleading, however, simply to overexpress the wild-type or mutant gene in inappropriate cell types at high concentrations with heterologous promoters. More physiological vertebrate models including LRRK2 knockouts, knockin mutations to the endogenous gene, BAC transgenics, and inducible systems may be insightful. In the creation of these models, it is important to consider the possibly redundant, compensatory function of LRRK1. Given the age-associated multifactorial etiology of PD, it is naive to expect that single transgenic models may recapitulate the phenotypic spectrum of disease.

It is important to consider the physiological, perhaps dimeric context in which Lrrk2 operates. Further evidence is required for the molecular dimer proposed and must be obtained through protein interaction and immunoprecipitation studies. In context, the search for interacting proteins may be especially worthwhile because these may be functional and phenotypic modifiers. In addition, directly identifying Lrrk2's biological substrates is likely to be of fundamental importance to developing novel therapeutics that modulate "Lrrk2 complex" activity.[18,21,23,28,96] Experimental concerns can be overcome; future prospects for a pharmaceutical approach that halts PD progression have never been more directed or more promising.

REFERENCES

1. Funayama M, et al: A new locus for Parkinson's disease (PARK8) maps to chromosome 12p11.2-q13.1. Ann Neurol 2002;51:296-301.
2. Zimprich A, et al: The PARK8 locus in autosomal dominant parkinsonism: confirmation of linkage and further delineation of the disease-containing interval. Am J Hum Genet 2004;74:11-19.
3. Zimprich A, et al: Mutations in LRRK2 cause autosomal-dominant parkinsonism with pleomorphic pathology. Neuron 2004;44:601-607.
4. Paisan-Ruiz C, et al: Cloning of the gene containing mutations that cause PARK8-linked Parkinson's disease. Neuron 2004;44:595-600.
5. Kachergus J, et al: Identification of a novel LRRK2 mutation linked to autosomal dominant parkinsonism: evidence of a common founder across European populations. Am J Hum Genet 2005;76:672-680.
6. Funayama M, et al: An LRRK2 mutation as a cause for the parkinsonism in the original PARK8 family. Ann Neurol 2005;57:918-921.
7. Paisan-Ruiz C, et al: Familial Parkinson's disease: clinical and genetic analysis of four Basque families. Ann Neurol 2005;57:365-372.
8. Biskup S, et al: Localization of LRRK2 to membranous and vesicular structures in mammalian brain. Ann Neurol 2006;60:557-569.
9. Melrose H, Lincoln S, Tyndall G, et al: Anatomical localization of leucine-rich repeat kinase 2 in mouse brain. Neuroscience 2006;139:791-794.
10. Higashi S, et al: Expression and localization of Parkinson's disease-associated leucine-rich repeat kinase 2 in the mouse brain. J Neurochem 2007;100:368-381.
11. Melrose HL, et al: A comparative analysis of leucine-rich repeat kinase 2 (Lrrk2) expression in mouse brain and Lewy body disease. Neuroscience 2007;147:1047-1058.
12. White LR, Toft M, Kvam SN, et al: MAPK-pathway activity, Lrrk2 G2019S, and Parkinson's disease. J Neurosci Res 2007;85:1288-1294.
13. Taylor JP, et al: Leucine-rich repeat kinase 1: a paralog of LRRK2 and a candidate gene for Parkinson's disease. Neurogenetics 2007;8:95-102.
14. Biskup S, et al: Dynamic and redundant regulation of LRRK2 and LRRK1 expression. BMC Neurosci 2007;8:102.
15. Mata IF, Wedemeyer WJ, Farrer MJ, et al: LRRK2 in Parkinson's disease: protein domains and functional insights. Trends Neurosci 2006;29:286-293.
16. Ito G, et al: GTP binding is essential to the protein kinase activity of LRRK2, a causative gene product for familial Parkinson's disease. Biochemistry 2007;46:1380-1388.
17. Luzon-Toro B, de la Torre ER, Delgado A, et al: Mechanistic insight into the dominant mode of the Parkinson's disease-associated G2019S LRRK2 mutation. Hum Mol Genet 2007;(16):2031-2039.
18. Dachsel JC, et al: Identification of potential protein interactors of Lrrk2. Parkinsonism Relat Disord 2007;13:382-385.
19. Meylan E, Tschopp J: The RIP kinases: crucial integrators of cellular stress. Trends Biochem Sci 2005;30:151-159.
20. Gloeckner CJ, et al: The Parkinson disease causing LRRK2 mutation I2020T is associated with increased kinase activity. Hum Mol Genet 2006;15:223-232.
21. Dachsel JC, et al: Digenic parkinsonism: investigation of the synergistic effects of PRKN and LRRK2. Neurosci Lett 2006;410:80-84.
22. Cookson MR, et al: The roles of kinases in familial Parkinson's disease. J Neurosci 2007;27:11865-11868.

23. Smith WW, et al: Leucine-rich repeat kinase 2 (LRRK2) interacts with parkin, and mutant LRRK2 induces neuronal degeneration. Proc Natl Acad Sci U S A 2005;102:18676-18681.
24. Imai Y, Gehrke S, Wang HQ, et al: Phosphorylation of 4E-BP by LRRK2 affects the maintenance of dopaminergic neurons in Drosophila. EMBO J 2008;27:2432-2443.
25. Gillardon F: Leucine-rich repeat kinase 2 phosphorylates brain tubulin-beta isoforms and modulates stability-a point of convergence in Parkinsonian neurodegeneration? J Neurochem 2009; [Epub ahead of print] PubMed PMID: 19545277.
26. Gillardon F: Interaction of elongation factor 1-alpha with leucine-rich repeat kinase 2 impairs kinase activity and microtubule bundling in vitro. Neuroscience 2009. [Epub ahead of print] PubMed PMID: 19559761.
27. Ko HS, Bailey R, Smith WW, et al: CHIP regulates leucine-rich repeat kinase-2 ubiquitination, degradation, and toxicity. Proc Natl Acad Sci U S A 2009;106:2897-2902.
28. Jaleel M, et al: LRRK2 phosphorylates moesin at threonine-558: characterization of how Parkinson's disease mutants affect kinase activity. Biochem J 2007;405:307-317.
29. Bretscher A, Edwards K, Fehon RG: ERM proteins and merlin: integrators at the cell cortex. Nat Rev Mol Cell Biol 2002;3:586-599.
30. Di Fonzo A, et al: Comprehensive analysis of the LRRK2 gene in sixty families with Parkinson's disease. Eur J Hum Genet 2006;14:322-331.
31. Mata IF, et al: Lrrk2 pathogenic substitutions in Parkinson's disease. Neurogenetics 2005;6: 171-177.
32. Nichols WC, et al: LRRK2 mutation analysis in Parkinson disease families with evidence of linkage to PARK8. Neurology 2007;69:1737-1744.
33. Di Fonzo A, et al: A common missense variant in the LRRK2 gene, Gly2385Arg, associated with Parkinson's disease risk in Taiwan. Neurogenetics 2006;7:133-138.
34. Farrer MJ, et al: Lrrk2 G2385R is an ancestral risk factor for Parkinson's disease in Asia. Parkinsonism Relat Disord 2007;13:89-92.
35. Fung HC, Chen CM, Hardy J, et al: A common genetic factor for Parkinson disease in ethnic Chinese population in Taiwan. BMC Neurol 2006;6:47.
36. Tan EK: Identification of a common genetic risk variant (LRRK2 Gly2385Arg) in Parkinson's disease. Ann Acad Med Singapore 2006;35:840-842.
37. Funayama M, et al: Leucine-rich repeat kinase 2 G2385R variant is a risk factor for Parkinson disease in Asian population. Neuroreport 2007;18:273-275.
38. Ross OA, Wu YR, Lee MC, et al: Analysis of Lrrk2 R1628P as a risk factor for Parkinson's disease. Ann Neurol 2008;64:88-92.
39. Lewis PA, et al: The R1441C mutation of LRRK2 disrupts GTP hydrolysis. Biochem Biophys Res Commun 2007;357:668-671.
40. Ross OA, Spanati C, Griffith A, et al: Haplotype analysis of Lrrk2 R1441H carriers with parkinsonism. Parkinsonism Relat Disord 2009;15:466-467.
41. Haugarvoll K, et al: Lrrk2 R1441C parkinsonism is clinically similar to sporadic Parkinson's disease. Neurology 2008;70:1456-1460.
42. Simon-Sanchez J, et al: Parkinson's disease due to the R1441G mutation in Dardarin: a founder effect in the Basques. Mov Disord 2006;21:1954-1959.
43. Gonzalez-Fernandez MC, et al: Lrrk2-associated parkinsonism is a major cause of disease in Northern Spain. Parkinsonism Relat Disord 2007;13:509-515.
44. Khan NL, et al: Mutations in the gene LRRK2 encoding dardarin (PARK8) cause familial Parkinson's disease: clinical, pathological, olfactory and functional imaging and genetic data. Brain 2005;128:2786-2796.
45. Adams JR, et al: PET in LRRK2 mutations: comparison to sporadic Parkinson's disease and evidence for presymptomatic compensation. Brain 2005;128:2777-2785.
46. Di Fonzo A, et al: A frequent LRRK2 gene mutation associated with autosomal dominant Parkinson's disease. Lancet 2005;365:412-415.
47. Gilks WP, et al: A common LRRK2 mutation in idiopathic Parkinson's disease. Lancet 2005;365:415-416.
48. Goldwurm S, et al: The G6055A (G2019S) mutation in LRRK2 is frequent in both early and late onset Parkinson's disease and originates from a common ancestor. J Med Genet 2005;42:e65.
49. Mata IF, et al: LRRK2 mutations are a common cause of Parkinson's disease in Spain. Eur J Neurol 2006;13:391-394.
50. Tomiyama H, et al: Clinicogenetic study of mutations in LRRK2 exon 41 in Parkinson's disease patients from 18 countries. Mov Disord 2006;21:1102-1108.

51. Orr-Urtreger A, et al: The LRRK2 G2019S mutation in Ashkenazi Jews with Parkinson disease: is there a gender effect? Neurology 2007;69:1595-1602.
52. Ozelius LJ, et al: LRRK2 G2019S as a cause of Parkinson's disease in Ashkenazi Jews. N Engl J Med 2006;354:424-425.
53. Gouider-Khouja N, Belal S, Hamida MB, Hentati F. Clinical and genetic study of familial Parkinson's disease in Tunisia. Neurology 2000;54:1603-1609.
54. Ishihara L, et al: Screening for Lrrk2 G2019S and clinical comparison of Tunisian and North American Caucasian Parkinson's disease families. Mov Disord 2007;22:55-61.
55. Lesage S, et al: LRRK2 G2019S as a cause of Parkinson's disease in North African Arabs. N Engl J Med 2006;354:422-423.
56. Kay DM, Kramer P, Higgins D, et al: Escaping Parkinson's disease: a neurologically healthy octogenarian with the LRRK2 G2019S mutation. Mov Disord 2005;20:1077-1078.
57. Healy DG, Falchi M, O'Sullivan SS, et al: International LRRK2 Consortium. Phenotype, genotype, and worldwide genetic penetrance of LRRK2-associated Parkinson's disease: a case-control study. Lancet Neurol 2008;7:583-590.
58. Kay DM, et al: Validity and utility of a LRRK2 G2019S mutation test for the diagnosis of Parkinson's disease. Genet Test 2006;10:221-227.
59. Goldwurm S, et al: Evaluation of LRRK2 G2019S penetrance: relevance for genetic counseling in Parkinson disease. Neurology 2007;68:1141-1143.
60. Clark LN, et al: Frequency of LRRK2 mutations in early- and late-onset Parkinson disease. Neurology 2006;67:1786-1791.
61. Hulihan MM, Ishihara-Paul L, Kachergus J, et al: LRRK2 Gly2019Ser penetrance in Arab-Berber patients from Tunisia: a case-control genetic study. Lancet Neurol 2008;7:591-594.
62. Aasly JO, et al: Clinical features of LRRK2-associated Parkinson's disease in central Norway. Ann Neurol 2005;57:762-765.
63. Ishihara L, et al: Clinical features of Parkinson disease patients with homozygous leucine-rich repeat kinase 2 G2019S mutations. Arch Neurol 2006;63:1250-1254.
64. Ross OA, et al: Lrrk2 and Lewy body disease. Ann Neurol 2006;59:388-393.
65. Rajput A, et al: Parkinsonism, Lrrk2 G2019S, and tau neuropathology. Neurology 2006;67:1506-1508.
66. Lesage S, et al: LRRK2 haplotype analyses in European and North African families with Parkinson disease: a common founder for the G2019S mutation dating from the 13th century. Am J Hum Genet 2005;77:330-332.
67. Zabetian CP, et al: LRRK2 G2019S in families with Parkinson disease who originated from Europe and the Middle East: evidence of two distinct founding events beginning two millennia ago. Am J Hum Genet 2006;79:752-758.
68. Tan EK, Peng R, Wu YR, et al: LRRK2 G2385R modulates age at onset in Parkinson's disease: a multi-center pooled analysis. Am J med Genet B Neuropsychiatr Genet 2009; [Epub ahead of print] PubMed PMID: 19152345.
69. Lin CH, Tzen KY, Yu CY, et al: LRRK2 mutation in familial Parkinson's disease in a Taiwanese population: clinical, PET, and functional studies. J Biomed Sci 2008;15:661-667.
70. Tan EK, Tan LC, Lim HQ, et al: LRRK2 R1628P increases risk of Parkinson's disease: replication evidence. Hum Genet 2008;124(3):287-288.
71. Hughes AJ, Ben-Shlomo Y, Daniel SE, Lees AJ: What features improve the accuracy of clinical diagnosis in Parkinson's disease: a clinicopathologic study. Neurology 1992;42:1142-1146.
72. Taylor JP, Mata IF, Farrer MJ: LRRK2: a common pathway for parkinsonism, pathogenesis and prevention? Trends Mol Med 2006;12:76-82.
73. Wszolek ZK, et al: Autosomal dominant parkinsonism associated with variable synuclein and tau pathology. Neurology 2004;62:1619-1622.
74. Gaig C, et al: G2019S LRRK2 mutation causing Parkinson's disease without Lewy bodies. J Neurol Neurosurg Psychiatry 2007;78:626-628.
75. Covy JP, Yuan W, Waxman EA, et al: Clinical and pathological characteristics of patients with leucine-rich repeat kinase-2 mutations. Mov Disord 2009;24:32-39.
76. Farrer MJ: Genetics of Parkinson disease: paradigm shifts and future prospects. Nat Rev Genet 2006;7:306-318.
77. Giasson BI, et al: Biochemical and pathological characterization of Lrrk2. Ann Neurol 2006;59:315-322.
78. Higashi S, et al: Localization of Parkinson's disease-associated LRRK2 in normal and pathological human brain. Brain Res 2007;1155:208-219.

79. Miklossy J, et al: LRRK2 expression in normal and pathologic human brain and in human cell lines. J Neuropathol Exp Neurol 2006;65:953-963.
80. Bosgraaf L, et al: A novel cGMP signalling pathway mediating myosin phosphorylation and chemotaxis in Dictyostelium. Embo J 2002;21:4560-4570.
81. Sakaguchi-Nakashima A, Meir JY, Jin Y, et al: LRK-1, a C: *elegans* PARK8-related kinase, regulates axonal-dendritic polarity of SV proteins. Curr Biol 2007;17:592-598.
82. Silveira-Moriyama L, Guedes LC, Kingsbury A, et al: Hyposmia in G20195 LRRK2-related Parkinsonism clinical and Pathologic data. Neurology 2008;71:1021-1026.
83. Katzenschlager R, Lees AJ: Olfaction and Parkinson's syndromes: its role in differential diagnosis. Curr Opin Neurol 2004;17:417-423.
84. Lee SB, Kim W, Lee S Chung J: Loss of LRRK2/PARK8 induces degeneration of dopaminergic neurons in Drosophila. Biochem Biophys Res Commun 2007;358:534-539.
85. MacLeod D, et al: The familial parkinsonism gene LRRK2 regulates neurite process morphology. Neuron 2006;52:587-593.
86. Li Y, Liu W, Oo TF, et al: Mutant LRRK2 (R1441G) BAC transgenic mice recapitulate cardinal features of Parkinson's disease. Nature Neuroscience 2009;12:826-828.
87. Burke RE: Inhibition of mitogen-activated protein kinase and stimulation of Akt kinase signaling pathways: two approaches with therapeutic potential in the treatment of neurodegenerative disease. Pharmacol Ther 2007;114:261-277.
88. Ho CC Rideout HJ, Ribe E, et al: The Parkinson disease Protein leucine-rich repeat kinase 2 transduces death signals via Fas-associated protein with death domain and capase-8 in a cellular model of neurodegeneration. J Neurosci 2009;29:1011-1016.
89. Toft M, Mata IF, Kachergus JM, et al: LRRK2 mutations and parkinsonism. Lancet 2005;365:1229-1230.
90. Smith WW, et al: Kinase activity of mutant LRRK2 mediates neuronal toxicity. Nat Neurosci 2006;9:1231-1233.
91. West AB, et al: Parkinson's disease-associated mutations in leucine-rich repeat kinase 2 augment kinase activity. Proc Natl Acad Sci U S A 2005;102:16842-16847.
92. Greggio E, et al: Kinase activity is required for the toxic effects of mutant LRRK2/dardarin. Neurobiol Dis 2006;23:329-341.
93. Claperon A, Therrien M: KSR and CNK: two scaffolds regulating RAS-mediated RAF activation. Oncogene 2007;26:3143-3158.
94. West AB, et al: Parkinson's disease-associated mutations in LRRK2 link enhanced GTP-binding and kinase activities to neuronal toxicity. Hum Mol Genet 2007;16:223-232.
95. Guo L, et al: The Parkinson's disease-associated protein, leucine-rich repeat kinase 2 (LRRK2), is an authentic GTPase that stimulates kinase activity. Exp Cell Res 2007;313:3658-3670.
96. Li X, et al: Leucine-rich repeat kinase 2 (LRRK2)/PARK8 possesses GTPase activity that is altered in familial Parkinson's disease R1441C/G mutants. J Neurochem 2007;103:238-247.
97. Dickson D, et al: Pathology of PD in monozygotic twins with a 20-year discordance interval. Neurology 2001;56:981-982.
98. Tanner CM: Is the cause of Parkinson's disease environmental or hereditary? Evidence from twin studies. Adv Neurol 2003;91:133-142.
99. Wirdefeldt K, Gatz M, Schalling M, Pedersen NL: No evidence for heritability of Parkinson disease in Swedish twins. Neurology 2004;63:305-311.
100. Hawkes CH, Del Tredici K, Braak H: Parkinson's disease: a dual-hit hypothesis. Neuropathol Appl Neurobiol 2007;33:599-614.
101. Di Monte DA: The environment and Parkinson's disease: is the nigrostriatal system preferentially targeted by neurotoxins? Lancet Neurol 2003;2:531-538.
102. Hardy J: No definitive evidence for a role for the environment in the etiology of Parkinson's disease. Mov Disord 2006;21:1790-1791.
103. Deng J, Lewis PA, Greggio E, et al: Structure of the ROC domain from the Parkinson's disease-associated leucine-rich repeat kinase 2 reveals a dimeric GTPase. Proc Natl Acad Sci U S A 2008;105:1499-1504.
104. Greggio E, Zambrano I, Kaganovich A, et al: The Parkinson disease-associated leucine-rich repeat kinase 2 (LRRK2) is a dimer that undergoes intramolecular autophosphorylation. J Biol Chem 2008;283:16906-16914.

8 | Environmental Factors and Parkinson's Disease

CAROLINE M. TANNER

Introduction

Exposure to the environmental factor 1-methyl-4-phenyl-1,2,3,6-tetrahydro-pyridine (MPTP) was one of the first single causes of parkinsonism identified.[1] Advances in molecular genetics have resulted in the identification of numerous genes causing parkinsonism, as detailed in the preceding chapters. Although the actual proportion of cases with parkinsonism resulting from any of these causes is unknown, most are rare. For most patients with Parkinson's disease (PD), a single cause cannot be identified. Failure to identify a single causative factor for most PD cases suggests that PD is a complex disorder, with genetic and environmental factors contributing to the underlying pathogenesis of disease. This chapter updates investigations of environmental determinants of PD, focusing on the last decade.

TABLE 8–1	Challenges in Studying Parkinson's Disease

No diagnostic test
    Examination by expert most reliable indicator
    No criterion always predicts
Long preclinical period
    Exposure may be years before signs
Late life disorder
    Risk factor identification retrospective
    Diagnostic accuracy in relatives poor
Relatively rare
    Large base population needed
No registries; not reported
    True distribution of disease uncertain

Patterns in Populations

Epidemiological investigations of PD must overcome several challenges (Table 8–1). Demographic patterns have been one source of hypotheses regarding environmental risks for PD. PD is associated with older age in all populations, suggesting an aging-related or time-dependent pathological process. Male preponderance, found in most countries, suggests either a biological predisposition or greater exposure of men to certain etiological agents. Unexpected frequency of parkinsonism (a disease cluster) has resulted in the identification of specific causes, including certain genes (familial clusters) and the toxicant MPTP. Whether the frequency of PD varies internationally or among racial or ethnic groups is controversial. Also unknown is whether the incidence of PD is changing with calendar time. Population-based methods with complete ascertainment of PD are needed to answer these questions.

Risk Factor Investigations

Ideally, risk factor investigations would focus on the time of life when the injury occurs, and the injurious environmental factors could most easily be identified. For PD, the time of this initial injury is unknown. Because nigrostriatal dopaminergic function is thought to be 50% depleted at the time motor symptoms manifest, most investigators believe that the pathogenesis of PD evolves over years. Suggestions that PD may have perinatal origins are intriguing, but populations appropriate for lifelong risk factor assessment have not been identified.[2] Instead, most studies of risk factors for PD have investigated adults. The correct time during adulthood for studying this late-life disorder is unknown.

Symptoms of dysfunction in other parts of the nervous system, such as constipation, impaired smell recognition, rapid-eye-movement sleep behavior disorder, and erectile dysfunction, have been observed years or decades before recognition of the motor symptoms of PD.[3-5] These features may represent an "at-risk" state, identifying individuals more likely to develop PD. Alternatively, these features may represent the earliest stages of PD. If these symptoms do reflect the earliest stages of PD, risk factor investigations involving individuals with one or more of these symptoms would be appropriate.

Risk factors for PD have been sought using two basic approaches. Patients with known PD have been compared with theoretically similar individuals without PD, and differences in putative risk factors have been sought. For most environmental risk factors, this investigation involves the ability of the individuals to remember experiences that occurred decades before the time of interview. Errors in recall are likely, and may differ between cases and controls, potentially biasing study results. A second approach takes advantage of existing prospective cohort studies. In this setting, risk factor information has been collected before disease is diagnosed, and participants are followed longitudinally, minimizing recall bias. Because existing cohorts have been established to investigate other medical conditions, such as cancer or heart disease, however, many putative risk factors for PD suggested by mechanistic laboratory studies cannot be assessed in these prospective cohorts.

Association between PD and an exposure suggests, but does not prove, a cause-and-effect relationship. Inverse association of an exposure and PD suggests that the factor protects against the development of PD. Direct association suggests that the exposure contributes to the development of PD. The likelihood that a risk factor causes or prevents PD can be judged by criteria of causality (Table 8–2).[6,7] Exposures fulfilling these criteria occur before PD onset, exhibit a dose-response association, are consistent over time, are replicated by other investigators, and have biological plausibility.

Tobacco Use

Cigarette smoking, use of smokeless tobacco, and passive exposure to cigarette smoke all have been associated with a lower risk of PD in populations worldwide, in reports spanning 4 decades.[8-10] Individuals ever smoking cigarettes had about 40% reduced risk of PD in one meta-analysis.[8] Lower risk is associated with a greater amount or longer duration of tobacco exposure. An analysis of more than 2000 cases from 11 U.S. studies replicated these findings overall, but not in subgroups of individuals with PD onset after age 75, African-Americans, or Hispanics; but whether these differences are due to biological differences is unknown.[11]

Animal studies suggest a neuroprotective effect for nicotine.[12] Some investigators have argued that the inverse association of smoking and PD reflects a "preparkinsonian personality" characterized by low sensation-seeking behavior and mediated by genetic factors also causing PD. Low sensation-seeking behavior was not associated with smoking, however, in one study of PD cases and controls.[13] In populations with similar genetic risk—two studies in twin pairs discordant for PD and one in nontwin sibling pairs—cigarette smoking was associated with a lower PD risk, most markedly in the genetically identical twins, supporting the hypothesis that a biological effect of nicotine may protect against PD.[14-16]

Cigarette smoking also may alter the course of PD, but results are contradictory. Smoking before PD onset is associated with increased risk of cognitive impairment,[17] but disease progression was not affected by cigarette smoking in PD

TABLE 8–2   Some Putative Protective Factors for Parkinson's Disease: Criteria for Causality

	Temporality	Strength of Association	Consistency	Replicability	Biological Plausibility
Tobacco use	Precedes PD in prospective and retrospective studies	Dose response: greater exposure → lower risk	Multiple populations over 40 years	Different populations worldwide; different forms of tobacco	Nicotine: acts in CNS; blocks injury in toxicant models of PD
Coffee, tea use	Precedes PD in prospective and retrospective studies	Dose-response: greater exposure → lower risk	Multiple populations over 15 years	Different populations worldwide; coffee and tea similar pattern	Caffeine: adenosine A2A receptor antagonist; blocks MPTP toxicity
Nonsteroidal anti-inflammatory drug use	Precedes PD in prospective and retrospective studies	Dose-response: greater exposure → lower risk	<10 studies over 10 years; specific drugs, gender effects vary	Found in ~50% of populations studied; most studies in U.S. and United Kingdom	Strong pathological and experimental evidence for inflammatory injury in PD

CNS, central nervous system; MPTP, 1-methyl-4-phenyl-1,2,3,6-tetrahydropyridine; PD, Parkinson's disease.
Adapted from references 6 and 7.

patients.[18] In one prospective study, men with PD who smoked cigarettes did not have the increased mortality expected.[19]

Caffeine Use

PD risk is reduced in habitual coffee or tea drinkers.[8,16] Higher intakes are associated with lower risk. The magnitude of risk reduction resembles that for tobacco use. The inverse association of caffeine and PD is less consistently found in women, although more recent prospective studies find women and men to be equally affected.[20,21] Caffeine is an adenosine A2A receptor antagonist, and can block MPTP toxicity in animal models, although the specific mechanism is uncertain.[22,23]

Nonsteroidal Anti-inflammatory Drugs

Pathological findings suggesting an active inflammatory process in PD prompted interest in a potential neuroprotective role for anti-inflammatory drugs.[24,25] Investigation of nonsteroidal anti-inflammatory drug (NSAID) use is limited by difficulties in measuring lifelong use because medications are available without a physician's prescription, and casual use is common. Nonetheless, many, although not all, studies have found PD risk to be decreased by 40% or more in habitual NSAID users.[26-30] Longer duration of use reduces risk further. Aspirin and non-aspirin NSAIDs are reported in different studies. Gender differences are observed in some studies, but these are inconsistent across populations. Plasma levels of the inflammatory biomarker interleukin-6 were elevated in blood collected on average 4 years before PD diagnosis.[31] If this observation is replicated, it may provide a biomarker of risk for PD.

Uric Acid

Uric acid is a potent antioxidant. In three prospective studies, high normal plasma urate levels are associated with reduced risk of PD.[32-34] Follow-up was for 30 years. Men with gout had a similar reduced risk of PD in a case-control study, but this was not observed in women.[35] Uric acid may serve as a biomarker of risk for PD. Elevation of uric acid has been proposed as a neuroprotective intervention, although this must be balanced against risks such as hypertension and gout.[36]

Physical Activity

Greater physical activity in adult life has been associated with lower risk of PD, but results are inconsistent. Strenuous physical activity during leisure hours was associated with 40% or greater reduction in PD risk in a prospective follow-up of several populations,[37,38] but not in men in another follow-up study.[39] In a case-control study, subjects with occupations presumed to involve high physical activity also had a decreased risk of PD.[40] In laboratory models, physical activity seems to counter oxidative stress and toxicant injury, and increase trophic factor release, all effects that could be expected to reduce risk of PD.[41]

Diet

Diets low in animal fats have long been suggested to reduce risk of PD, but this has not been seen in all studies.[42] A diet low in saturated fats but high in fruits and vegetables was associated with lower PD risk in a prospective study.[43] Dietary intake of dairy products has consistently been associated with higher PD risk in prospective cohort studies.[44-46] Whether this association implicates a specific effect of a constituent of dairy foods, such as calcium, or an effect of a toxicant carried in dairy foods (e.g., certain persistent organic pollutants or pesticides), or is simply a marker of a broader dietary or lifestyle pattern is uncertain.

Metabolic Conditions

Other factors associated with diet and physical activity have been linked with PD risk in some reports. Treatment with cholesterol-lowering agents has also been associated with lower PD risk in case-control studies,[47-49] but the significance of this association is unclear because higher serum cholesterol is associated with lower PD risk in prospective studies.[50,51] Measures of obesity in midlife are associated with higher PD risk.[52-54] Because similar determinants may influence all of these factors, future work to distinguish independent effects is important.

Estrogen Status

Because women are at lower risk of PD in most populations, female sex hormones have been proposed to protect against the development of PD. Results to date have been inconsistent. Younger age at menopause or surgical menopause has been associated with higher risk of PD in some,[55,56] but not all, studies.[57-59] Estrogen use after menopause also has been associated with lower PD risk,[56,60] but not in all studies.[58]

Head Injury

Head injury, particularly injury with loss of consciousness, is associated with increased risk of PD decades later.[61-63] More frequent injuries increase risk.[62-64] Head injury triggers an inflammatory cascade and causes mechanical stress, which can impair cellular repair mechanisms, such as the function of chaperones targeting misfolded proteins.[65] Head injury also can be associated with disruption of the blood-brain barrier, increasing risk of exposure to toxicants or infectious agents.

TABLE 8–3	Occupation as a Risk Factor for Parkinson's Disease: Selected Studies 2000-2007			
Location	Design	Occupation	OR/RR/RC (95% CI)	P
Scotland, Romania Sweden, Italy[95]	Clinic population; JEM	Processing occupations	0.7 (0.5-1.0)	.02
Illinois[96]	Case-control manufacturing plants	Welder	0.82 (0.36-1.86)	NS
Sweden[97]	National population-based registries	Welder	0.95 (0.7-1.28)	NS
South Korea[98]	Case-control: shipbuilding firms	Welding	0.7 (0.3-12.6)	NS
		White collar workers	1.29 (0.72-18.6)	NS
Denmark[99]	Metal manufacturing; hospital discharge database; focused questionnaire	Welding	SHR: 0.9 (0.4-1.5)	NS
		Metal manufacturing	SHR: 0.9 (0.4-1.8)	NS
Alabama[93]	Medicolegal litigant cases versus published prevalence	Welders, boiler makers	Prevalence ratio versus Copiah Co, MS: 10.19 (4.4-23.4)	NA
United States[68]	Clinic series versus expected derived Labor Bureau rates	Farming	3.0 (2.1-4.2)	.0001
		Physician/dentist	9.6 (6.9-13)	.0001
		Other medical	0.5 (0.3-0.6)	.0001
		Teacher	2.1 (1.8-2.4)	.0001
		Welder	0.91 (0.3-2.8)	NS
South Korea[100]	Case-control	*Industry*		
		Agriculture	2.0 (1.2-3.3)	NA
		Occupation		
		Farmer	1.6 (1.0-2.8)	NA
		Industrial machining	1.7 (0.3-10.4)	NA
		Health professionals	2.1 (0.2-19.7)	NA

Table continued on following page

TABLE 8–3	Occupation as a Risk Factor for Parkinson's Disease: Selected Studies 2000-2007(Continued)			
Location	Design	Occupation	OR/RR/RC (95% CI)	P
Michigan[101]	Health system –based; case-control	Farming	2.8 (1.0-7.5)	.04
		Copper work >20 yr	2.5 (1.1-5.9)	.04
		Manganese >20 yr	10.6 (1.1-106)	.04
		Lead/copper >20 yr	5.3 (1.6-17.3)	.006
		Lead/iron >20 yr	2.8 (1.1-7.5)	.04
		Copper/iron >20 yr	3.7 (1.4-9.7)	.008
Italy[102]	Case-control	Farming	7.7 (1.4-44.1)	0.02
India[103]	Case-control	Farming	2.4 (NA)	0.1

OR, odd ratio; RR, rate ratio; RC, regression coefficient; CI, confidence interval; JEM, job exposure matrix; NS, nonsignificant; SHR, standardized disease-specific hospitalization rate ratio; NA, not available

Occupation

Interest in occupation as a risk factor for PD derives from the idea that workers in certain occupations are more likely to be exposed to risk or protective factors for PD. Identification of such factors is difficult because the available information is often limited to job title. Some consistent associations of job title and PD have emerged (Table 8–3).[66] Agricultural work has been most consistently associated with PD risk. Certain industrial occupations have been associated with higher risk in some populations, but replication has been inconsistent. The unexpected finding of an increased risk of PD in teachers and health care workers has been proposed to be due to more frequent infections and a consequent chronic inflammatory process,[67,68] but proof of this hypothesis remains elusive. Occupations involving shift work and jobs with higher physical activity have been inversely associated with PD.[40,69]

Identification of specific occupational toxicant exposures is difficult. Ideally, direct monitoring of environmental exposures and exposure biomarkers of individual workers would be conducted throughout life, and monitored workers would be followed over years to document the development of parkinsonism. Direct exposure monitoring is rarely available, however. Toxicant exposure can also be inferred based on a lifelong occupational history detailing specific job tasks. Some studies have been able to identify classes of risk factors, or even specific compounds, that may cause or protect against PD. Some of these are addressed subsequently.

Specific Toxicants

PESTICIDES

Numerous case-control studies have implicated agricultural chemical exposures in the etiology of PD, and many others have found associations with rural living, farming, and gardening.[64,70-72] Pesticide exposure has been significantly associated

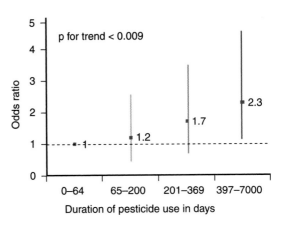

Figure 8–1 Longer duration of pesticide exposure was associated with higher risk of Parkinson's disease in a population of pesticide applicators and their spouses. Odds ratios were calculated by logistic regression with adjustment for age at enrollment, state, and type of participant (applicator or spouse). The test for trend was statistically significant.

with an increased PD risk in at least 16 studies, with odds ratios ranging from 1.6 to 7.0. Most of these studies were limited by broad measures of exposure, and in many, the proportion of exposed individuals was low, little was known about specific compounds, and validation of exposure was impossible.

Only a few studies have assessed classes of pesticides or individual chemicals, and even fewer have determined cumulative exposure. Specific pesticides associated with PD include paraquat, organochlorine pesticides, and carbamates.[72,73] In a study of pesticide applicators, longer duration of pesticide exposure was associated with increased risk of PD (Fig. 8–1).[72] Levels of the organochlorine insecticides dieldrin and lindane were elevated in brains of PD cases in postmortem analyses.[74] Many of the pathophysiological features of PD are replicated in laboratory studies of pesticides, including paraquat, rotenone, and dieldrin, providing biological plausibility for a causal effect of pesticides (Table 8–4).[75-80]

POLYCHLORINATED BIPHENYLS

Polychlorinated biphenyls (PCBs) were used extensively in industrial applications as coolants and lubricants, but their manufacture was stopped in the United States in 1977 because of evidence of environmental accumulation of these environmentally persistent compounds. PCB exposure in animal models causes a relatively selective, persistent reduction of dopamine, primarily affecting caudate, putamen, substantia nigra, and olfactory tract.[81-85] PCBs have been associated with PD in nigrostriatal regions in postmortem studies.[86,87] PCB-exposed female workers had greater mortality from PD in one study.[88] PCBs continue to cycle through soil, water, and air, and concentrate in animals higher on the food chain. Common sources of human exposure today are fish and marine mammals, meat, and dairy products. Dietary PCB intake has been proposed to explain an excess of PD in Greenland.[90]

METALS

Occupational exposure to metals, including manganese, iron, and lead, has been proposed to cause PD. A syndrome of atypical parkinsonism and behavioral changes resulting from high-dose exposure to manganese dust was described

TABLE 8–4	Biological Plausibility: Laboratory Studies of Toxicants Associated with Parkinson's Disease			
Biological Findings In Vitro and in Animal Models	MPTP/MPP+	Rotenone	Paraquat	Dieldrin
α-synuclein fibrillary aggregates	+		+	+
Mitochondrial dysfunction	+	+	+	+
Oxidative stress	+	+	+	+
Nigral injury	+	+	+	+
Behavioral changes	+	+	+	

MPTP/MPP+, 1-methyl-4-phenyl-1,2,3,6-tetrahydropyridine/1-methyl-4-phenylpyridinium

170 years ago.[91] Although high-dose exposure is now rare, the possibility that chronic low-dose exposure to manganese in welding fumes may cause PD has sparked debate in the clinic and in the courtroom.[92] In one clinical series and an occupational group referred for medicolegal evaluation, welding has been associated with earlier age at PD onset or higher than expected PD prevalence.[93,94] Welding or manganese exposure has not been associated with greater PD risk in other clinic-based studies, in industry-based case-control studies, or in studies linking national occupational databases and disease registries (see Table 8–3).[40,68,94-103]

Iron is increased in PD substantia nigra and has numerous effects in laboratory tests, suggesting iron may be a risk factor for PD. Iron can cause aggregation of α-synuclein, and may contribute to oxidative injury.[104] Chronic occupational exposure to lead has been suggested to be a risk factor for PD,[105] and iron in combination with copper or lead was associated with a modest increased risk in one study.[106] Studies of nonoccupational sources of iron have been unremarkable, and in one study of blood donors, more frequent donors, presumably with lower iron stores, had lower risk of PD.[107]

ENDOTOXINS (LIPOPOLYSACCHARIDES)

Endotoxins (lipopolysaccharides) are a component of gram-negative bacterial cell membranes and have inflammatory and toxic properties.[108,109] Lipopolysaccharide-stimulated microglia may express proinflammatory cytokines, chemokines, and reactive oxygen species to promote inflammation. Endotoxins are found in many agricultural, factory, and biotechnology settings. They have been proposed as risk factors for PD, although, to date, an association of lipopolysaccharides and PD has not been documented.[110] Nevertheless, animal studies indicate injection of endotoxin into the brain can result in PD-like effects.[108]

OTHER OCCUPATIONAL EXPOSURES

Exposure to the degreaser trichloroethylene has been reported in association with a cluster of PD cases working in one factory, and in related animal studies, trichloroethylene blocked mitochondrial complex I activity and caused the loss of substantia nigra dopaminergic neurons.[111] Dental technicians were found to have parkinsonism-like movement abnormalities, possibly resulting from exposure to solvents or metals.[112] Further investigation of trichloroethylene and other solvent exposure in PD is warranted.

Complex Interactions

The preceding sections provide evidence suggesting that many individual exposures may alter risk of PD. Although exposure to many of these putative risk factors is common, few individuals develop PD. The actual situation is undoubtedly more complex. Dose and duration of exposure likely play an important role, with larger doses and longer duration of exposure likely to be associated with greater risk. Several key factors are likely important.

First, the genetic and physiological state of the individual likely determines the response to toxicant exposure. A classic example of this is gene-environment interaction. Individuals with a particular susceptibility genotype may be more or less vulnerable to toxicant exposure (Table 8–5).[113-125] Variability in pesticide-metabolizing enzymes, such as cytochrome P450 2D6 (CYP2D6)[113] or GSTP1,[125] or in susceptible variants of *MnSOD* and *NQO1* genes[118] may influence the toxicity of pesticide exposures. Similarly, individuals with the GSTM1 null genotype exposed to solvents are at greater risk for PD.[116] Cigarette smoking may be inversely associated in PD only in individuals with certain variants of the *NOS2A* gene.[119] Physiological state, too, may be a determinant of the effect of toxicant exposure.[126]

Finally, most toxicant exposures involve combinations of chemicals. The toxicity of one pesticide may be enhanced by concomitant exposure to other pesticides[127-29] or proinflammatory agents such as lipopolysaccharides.[130,131] Exposure to putative protective agents may also modify the effect of toxicant exposure. Pesticide exposure was associated with a greater risk of PD in nonsmokers.[26] Different individuals are likely to have unique combinations of risk and protective factors. Understanding the common determinants of these would likely provide the key to understanding the pathophysiology of PD, and, it is hoped, lead to more effective treatment and even prevention.

Shared Risks for Neurodegenerative Disorders

Common mechanisms for neurodegeneration have been proposed for more than a century, yet underlying shared mechanisms remain elusive.[132,133] In human and experimental studies, multiple pesticides, including paraquat, rotenone, organochlorines, and dithiocarbamates, have been associated with increased PD risk (Table 8–6). Pesticides have less often been associated with increased risk of multiple system atrophy, Alzheimer's disease, or dementia in PD, but little work has been done on these outcomes, and specific agents have not been identified.

Family studies have documented the co-occurrence of PD and Alzheimer's disease in pedigrees, and epidemiological studies have implicated several common risk and protective factors.[134,135] Clinical disease features also overlap,

TABLE 8–5	Proposed Gene/Toxicant Interactions in Parkinson's Disease		
Polymorphism/ Allele/Marker	Gene + Pesticide	Gene + Solvent	Gene + Smoking
MDR1 e21/2677[113]	↑		
DAT[114]	↑		
ACHE/PON1[115]	↑		
Null GSTM1[116]		↑	
2 CYP2D6*4 (poor metabolizers)[117]	↑		
MnSOD[118]	↑		
NQO1[118]	↑		
NOS2A[119]			Δ
GSTP1[120]			Δ
MAOB (G allele)[121]			↓
MAOB (A allele)[121]			↑
COMT[122]			↓
GST[123]			↓
iNOS[124]			↓
Lower age at onset / GSTP1 (125)	+		

↑ = increased Parkinson's disease risk; ↓ = decreased Parkinson's disease risk; Δ = modifies inverse association; + = positive association.

TABLE 8–6	Examples of Shared Risk Factors for Neurodegenerative Disorders				
	MSA	Parkinsonism	Dementia	α-Synuclein Aggregation	Tau Aggregation
Pesticide exposure	↑	↑	↑	↑	↑
Head injury	↑	↑	↑		
NSAIDs		↓	↓		
Cigarette smoking	↓	↓	↑		
		PDD ↑			

↑ = direct association of exposure and disease; ↓ = inverse association of exposure and disease.
MSA, multiple system atrophy; NSAIDs, nonsteroidal anti-inflammatory drugs; PDD, parkinson's disease dementia, Alzheimer's disease or dementia in Parkinson's disease.

with dementia occurring in 20% to 50% of patients with PD,[136,137] and parkinsonism present in a similar proportion of patients with Alzheimer's disease.[138] In geographical isolates of atypical parkinsonism, such as the amyotrophic lateral sclerosis/parkinsonism-dementia complex (ALS/PDC) clusters on Guam and the Kii peninsula of Japan, features of multiple neurodegenerative diseases occur together.[139]

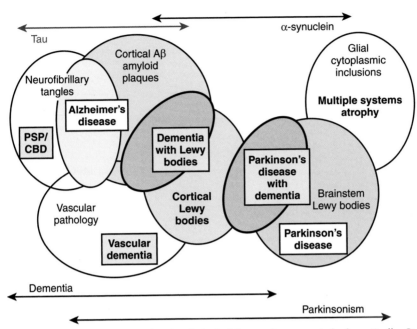

Figure 8–2 The overlap of clinical and pathological features is represented schematically. Overlap of clinical and pathological features among disorders is common, and more complex than shown here. A little-investigated factor is the contribution of cerebrovascular disease. PSP/CBD-progressive supranuclear palsy/corticobasilar degeneration.

The most convincing evidence of shared mechanisms of neurodegeneration comes from more recent histopathological studies, however, which show striking overlap of pathological features in human brain (Fig. 8–2). Specifically, aggregation of formerly soluble protein species occurs in virtually all sporadic or familial neurodegenerative diseases, and aggregates considered pathognomonic for one disorder are commonly seen in patients with another neurodegenerative disorder.[140] There is increasing evidence that aggregation of one protein species may synergistically enhance the aggregation of other species.[141,142] Investigations of etiological factors that may be shared among late-life neurodegenerative disorders are needed.

Conclusions

The pathophysiological mechanism of the rare forms of parkinsonism with a single genetic or toxicant cause have been assumed to apply to the more common cases of PD with unknown etiology. Although it is unknown whether this assumption is correct, many of the risk factors associated with common idiopathic PD have mechanisms in common with the rare forms. This situation supports the idea that the rare forms with single genetic or environmental causes can provide insights into the more common forms of PD with unknown cause. In most cases, PD is likely to be understood to be multifactorial, and genetic and environmental determinants are likely to be found important. Sophisticated methods of investigation are needed to arrive at an answer. These include investigations of large populations well characterized for genetic and for environmental factors. Close collaboration of epidemiologists, clinicians, and basic scientists involved in laboratory investigations of disease mechanisms is crucial.

Acknowledgments

The author acknowledges Jennifer Wright for editorial assistance. This chapter was supported by NIEHS RO1 ES10803, U54 ES012077; NINDS RO1 NS40467, PO1 NS44233; Parkinson's Disease Foundation; Michael J. Fox Foundation; Department of Defense NETRP; Former and Current Welding Products Manufacturers Group; James and Sharron Clark.

REFERENCES

1. Langston JW, Ballard P, Tetrud JW, Irwin I: Chronic Parkinsonism in humans due to a product of meperidine-analog synthesis. Science 1983;219:979-980.
2. Logroscino G: The role of early life environmental risk factors in Parkinson disease: what is the evidence? Environ Health Perspect 2005;113:1234-1238.
3. Abbott RD, Petrovitch H, White LR, et al: Frequency of bowel movements and the future risk of Parkinson's disease. Neurology 2001;57:456-462.
4. Ross GW, Petrovitch H, Abbott RD, et al: Association of olfactory dysfunction with risk for future Parkinson's disease. Ann Neurol 2008;63:167-173.
5. Gao X, Chen H, Schwarzschild MA, et al: Erectile function and risk of Parkinson's disease. Am J Epidemiol 2007;166:1446-1450.
6. Koch R: Die Aetiologie der Tuberkulose. Berliner Klin Wochenschr 1882;19:221-230.
7. Hill AB: The environment and disease: association or causation? Proc Roy Soc Med (Lond) 1965;58:295-300.
8. Hernán MA, Takkouche B, Caamaño-Isorna F, Gestal-Otero JJ: A meta-analysis of coffee drinking, cigarette smoking, and the risk of Parkinson's disease. Ann Neurol 2002;52:276-284.
9. Chade AR, Kasten M, Tanner CM: Nongenetic causes of Parkinson's disease. J Neural Transm Suppl 2006;70:147-151.
10. Mellick GD, Gartner CE, Silburn PA, Battistutta D: Passive smoking and Parkinson disease. Neurology 2006;67:179-180.
11. Ritz B, Ascherio A, Checkoway H, et al: Pooled analysis of tobacco use and risk of Parkinson disease. Arch Neurol 2007;64:990-997.
12. Quik M, O'Neill M, Perez XA: Nicotine neuroprotection against nigrostriatal damage: importance of the animal model. Trends Pharmacol Sci 2007;28:229-235.
13. Evans AH, Lawrence AD, Potts J, et al: Relationship between impulsive sensation seeking traits, smoking, alcohol and caffeine intake, and Parkinson's disease. J Neurol Neurosurg Psychiatry 2006;77:317-321.
14. Tanner CM, Ottman R, Goldman SM, et al: Parkinson disease in twins: an etiologic study. JAMA 1999;281:341-346.
15. Wirdefeldt K, Gatz M, Schalling M, Pedersen NL: No evidence for heritability of Parkinson disease in Swedish twins. Neurology 2004;63:305-311.
16. Hancock DB, Martin ER, Stajich JM, et al: Smoking, caffeine, and nonsteroidal anti-inflammatory drugs in families with Parkinson disease. Arch Neurol 2007;64:576-580.
17. Weisskopf MG, Grodstein F, Ascherio A: Smoking and cognitive function in Parkinson's disease. Mov Disord 2007;22:660-665.
18. Kandinov B, Giladi N, Korczyn AD: The effect of cigarette smoking, tea, and coffee consumption on the progression of Parkinson's disease. Parkinsonism Relat Disord 2007;13:243-245.
19. Chen H, Zhang SM, Schwarzschild MA, et al: Survival of Parkinson's disease patients in a large prospective cohort of male health professionals. Mov Disord 2006;21:1002-1007.
20. Hu G, Bidel S, Jousilahti P, et al: Coffee and tea consumption and the risk of Parkinson's disease. Mov Disord 2007;22:2242-2248.
21. Sääksjärvi K, Knekt P, Rissanen H, et al: Prospective study of coffee consumption and risk of Parkinson's disease. Eur J Clin Nutr 2008;62:908-915.

22. Chen JF, Moratalla R, Impagnatiello F, et al: The role of the D(2) dopamine receptor (D(2)R) in A(2A) adenosine receptor (A(2A)R)-mediated behavioral and cellular responses as revealed by A(2A) and D(2) receptor knockout mice. Proc Natl Acad Sci U S A 2001;98:1970-1975.
23. Ulanowska K, Piosik J, Gwizdek-Wiśniewska A, We Grzyn G: Formation of stacking complexes between caffeine (1,2,3-trimethylxanthine) and 1-methyl-4-phenyl-1,2,3,6-tetrahydropyridine may attenuate biological effects of this neurotoxin. Bioorg Chem 2005;33:402-413.
24. McGeer PL, Itagaki S, Boyes BE, McGeer EG: Reactive microglia are positive for HLA-DR in the substantia nigra of Parkinson's and Alzheimer's disease brains. Neurology 1988;38: 1285-1291.
25. Tansey MG, Frank-Cannon TC, McCoy MK, et al: Neuroinflammation in Parkinson's disease: is there sufficient evidence for mechanism-based interventional therapy? Front Biosci 2008;13: 709-717.
26. Abbott RD, Ross GW, White LR, et al: Environmental, life-style, and physical precursors of clinical Parkinson's disease: Recent findings from the Honolulu-Asia Aging Study. J Neurol 2003;250(Suppl 3):30-39.
27. Chen H, Zhang SM, Hernan MA, et al: Nonsteroidal anti-inflammatory drugs and the risk of Parkinson disease. Arch Neurol 2003;60:1059-1064.
28. Hernan MA, Logroscino G, Garcia Rodriguez LA: Nonsteroidal anti-inflammatory drugs and the incidence of Parkinson disease. Neurology 2006;66:1097-1099.
29. Esposito E, Di Matteo V, Benigno A, et al: Non-steroidal anti-inflammatory drugs in Parkinson's disease. Exp Neurol 2007;205:295-312.
30. Wahner AD, Bronstein JM, Bordelon YM, Ritz B: Nonsteroidal anti inflammatory drugs may protect against Parkinson disease. Neurology 2007;69:1836-1842.
31. Chen H, O'Reilly EJ, Schwarzschild MA, Ascherio A: Peripheral inflammatory biomarkers and risk of Parkinson's disease. Am J Epidemiol 2008;167:90-95.
32. Davis JW, Grandinetti A, Waslien CI, et al: Observations on serum uric acid levels and the risk of idiopathic Parkinson's disease. Am J Epidemiol 1996;144:480-484.
33. de Lau LM, Koudstaal PJ, Hofman A, Breteler MM: Serum uric acid levels and the risk of Parkinson disease. Ann Neurol 2005;58:797-800.
34. Weisskopf MG, O'Reilly E, Chen H, et al: Plasma urate and risk of Parkinson's disease. Am J Epidemiol 2007;166:561-567.
35. Alonso A, Rodríguez LA, Logroscino G, Hernán MA: Gout and risk of Parkinson disease: a prospective study. Neurology 2007;69:1696-1700.
36. Kutzing MK, Firestein BL: Altered uric acid levels and disease states. J Pharmacol Exp Ther 2008;324:1-7.
37. Chen H, Zhang SM, Schwarzschild MA, et al: Physical activity and the risk of Parkinson disease. Neurology 2005;64;(4):664-669.
38. Thacker EL, Chen H, Patel AV, et al: Recreational physical activity and risk of Parkinson's disease. Mov Disord 2008;23:69-74.
39. Logroscino G, Sesso HD, Paffenbarger RS Jr, Lee IM: Physical activity and risk of Parkinson's disease: a prospective cohort study. J Neurol Neurosurg Psychiatry 2006;77:1318-1322.
40. Frigerio R, Elbaz A, Sanft KR, et al: Education and occupations preceding Parkinson disease: a population-based case-control study. Neurology 2005;65:1575-1583.
41. Dishman RK, Berthoud HR, Booth FW, et al: Neurobiology of exercise. Obesity (Silver Spring) 2006;14:345-356.
42. Gaenslen A, Gasser T, Berg D: Nutrition and the risk for Parkinson's disease: review of the literature. J Neur Trans 2008;115:703-713.
43. Gao X, Chen H, Fung TT, et al: Prospective study of dietary pattern and risk of Parkinson disease. Am J Clin Nutr 2007;86:1486-1494.
44. Chen H, Zhang SM, Hernan MA, et al: Diet and Parkinson's disease: a potential role of dairy products in men. Ann Neurol 2002;52:793-801.
45. Park M, Ross GW, Petrovitch H, et al: Consumption of milk and calcium in midlife and the future risk of Parkinson disease. Neurology 2005;64:1047-1051.
46. Chen H, O'Reilly E, McCullough ML, et al: Consumption of dairy products and risk of Parkinson's disease. Am J Epidemiol 2007;165:998-1006.
47. Wolozin B, Wang SW, Li NC, et al: Simvastatin is associated with a reduced incidence of dementia and Parkinson's disease. BMC Med 2007;5:20.
48. Huang X, Chen H, Miller WC, et al: Lower low-density lipoprotein cholesterol levels are associated with Parkinson's disease. Mov Disord 2007;22:377-381.

49. Wahner AD, Bronstein JM, Bordelon YM, Ritz B: Statin use and the risk of Parkinson disease. Neurology 2008;70:1418-1422.
50. de Lau LM, Koudstaal PJ, Hofman A, Breteler MM: Serum cholesterol levels and the risk of Parkinson's disease. Am J Epidemiol 2006;164:998-1002.
51. Simon KC, Chen H, Schwarzschild M, Ascherio A: Hypertension, hypercholesterolemia, diabetes, and risk of Parkinson disease. Neurology 2007;69:1688-1695.
52. Abbott RD, Ross GW, White LR, et al: Midlife adiposity and the future risk of Parkinson's disease. Neurology 2002;59:1051-1057.
53. Hu G, Jousilahti P, Nissinen A, et al: Body mass index and the risk of Parkinson disease. Neurology 2006;67:1955-1959.
54. Chen H, Zhang SM, Schwarzschild MA, et al: Obesity and the risk of Parkinson's disease. Am J Epidemiol 2004;159:547-555.
55. Rocca WA, Bower JH, Maraganore DM, et al: Increased risk of parkinsonism in women who underwent oophorectomy before menopause. Neurology 2008;70:200-209.
56. Benedetti MD, Maraganore DM, Bower JH, et al: Hysterectomy, menopause, and estrogen use preceding Parkinson's disease: an exploratory case-control study. Mov Disord 2001;16:830-837.
57. Ragonese P, D'Amelio M, Callari G, et al: Age at menopause predicts age at onset of Parkinson's disease. Mov Disord 2006;21:2211-2214.
58. Popat RA, Van Den Eeden SK, Tanner CM, et al: Effect of reproductive factors and postmenopausal hormone use on the risk of Parkinson disease. Neurology 2005;65:383-390.
59. Ascherio A, Chen H, Schwarzschild MA, et al: Caffeine, postmenopausal estrogen, and risk of Parkinson's disease. Neurology 2003;60:790-795.
60. Currie LJ, Harrison MB, Trugman JM, et al: Postmenopausal estrogen use affects risk for Parkinson disease. Arch Neurol 2004;61:886-888.
61. Maher NE, Golbe LI, Lazzarini AM, et al: Epidemiologic study of 203 sibling pairs with Parkinson's disease: the GenePD study. Neurology 2002;58:79-84.
62. Goldman SM, Tanner CM, Oakes D, et al: Head injury and Parkinson's disease risk in twins. Ann Neurol 2006;60:65-72.
63. Bower JH, Maraganore DM, Peterson BJ, et al: Head trauma preceding PD: a case control study. Neurology 2003;60:1610-1615.
64. Dick FD, De Palma G, Ahmadi A, et al; Geoparkinson study group. Environmental risk factors for Parkinson's disease and parkinsonism: the Geoparkinson study. Occup Environ Med 2007;64:666-672.
65. Povlishock JT, Katz DI: Update of neuropathology and neurological recovery after traumatic brain injury. J Head Trauma Rehabil 2005;20:76-94.
66. Priyadarshi A, Khuder SA, Schaub EA, Priyadarshi SS: Environmental risk factors and Parkinson's disease: a metaanalysis. Environ Res 2001;86:122-127.
67. Tsui JK, Calne DB, Wang Y, et al: Occupational risk factors in Parkinson's disease. Can J Public Health 1999;90:334-337.
68. Goldman SM, Tanner CM, Olanow CW, et al: Occupation and parkinsonism in three movement disorders clinics. Neurology 2005;65:1430-1435.
69. Chen H, Schernhammer E, Schwarzschild MA, Ascherio A: A prospective study of night shift work, sleep duration, and risk of Parkinson's disease. Am J Epidemiol 2006;163:726-730.
70. Priyadarshi A, Khuder SA, Schaub EA, Shrivastava S: A meta-analysis of Parkinson's disease and exposure to pesticides. Neurotoxicology 2000;21:435-440.
71. Brown TP, Rumsby PC, Capleton AC, et al: Pesticides and Parkinson's disease—is there a link? Environ Health Perspect 2006;114:156-164.
72. Kamel F, Tanner C, Umbach D, et al: Pesticide exposure and self-reported Parkinson's disease in the agricultural health study. Am J Epidemiol 2007;165:364-374.
73. Firestone JA, Smith-Weller T, Franklin G, et al: Pesticides and risk of Parkinson disease: a population-based case-control study. Arch Neurol 2005;62:91-95.
74. Fleming L, Mann JB, Bean J, et al: Parkinson's disease and brain levels of organochlorine pesticides. Ann Neurol 1994;36:100-103.
75. Greenamyre JT, MacKenzie G, Peng TI, Stephans SE: Mitochondrial dysfunction in Parkinson's disease. Biochem Soc Symp 1999;66:85-97.
76. Manning-Bog AB, McCormack AL, Li J, et al: The herbicide paraquat causes up-regulation and aggregation of alpha-synuclein in mice: paraquat and alpha-synuclein. J Biol Chem 2002;277:1641-1644.
77. Fernagut PO, Hutson CB, Fleming SM, et al: Behavioral and histopathological consequences of paraquat intoxication in mice: Effects of alpha-synuclein over-expression. Synapse 2007;61:991-1001.

78. Watabe M, Nakaki T: Mitochondrial complex I inhibitor rotenone-elicited dopamine redistribution from vesicles to cytosol in human dopaminergic SH-SY5Y cells. J Pharmacol Exp Ther 2007;323:499-507.
79. Castello PR, Drechsel DA, Patel M: Mitochondria are a major source of paraquat-induced reactive oxygen species production in the brain. J Biol Chem 2007;282:14186-14193.
80. Hatcher JM, Richardson JR, Guillot TS, et al: Dieldrin exposure induces oxidative damage in the mouse nigrostriatal dopamine system. Exp Neurol 2007;204:619-630.
81. Seegal RF, Bush B, Brosch KO: Comparison of effects of Aroclors 1016 and 1260 on non-human primate catecholamine function. Toxicology 1991;66:145-163.
82. Seegal RF, Bush B, Brosch KO: Sub-chronic exposure of the adult rat to Aroclor 1254 yields regionally-specific changes in central dopaminergic function. Neurotoxicology 1991;12:55-65.
83. Seegal RF, Bush B, Brosch KO: Decreases in dopamine concentrations in adult non-human primate brain persist following removal from polychlorinated biphenyls. Toxicology 1994;86: 71-87.
84. Chu I, Villeneuve DC, Yagminas A, et al: Subchronic toxicity of 3,3′,4,4′,5-pentachlorobiphenyl in the rat, I: clinical, biochemical, hematological, and histopathological changes. Fundam Appl Toxicol 1994;22:457-468.
85. Chu I, Poon R, Yagminas A, et al: Subchronic toxicity of PCB 105 (2,3,3′,4,4′-pentachlorobiphenyl) in rats. J Appl Toxicol 1998;18:285-292.
86. Corrigan FM, Wienburg CL, Shore RF, et al: Organochlorine insecticides in substantia nigra in Parkinson's disease. J Toxicol Environ Health 2000;59:229-234.
87. Corrigan FM, Murray L, Wyatt CL, Shore RF: Diorthosubstituted polychlorinated biphenyls in caudate nucleus in Parkinson's disease. Exp Neurol 1998;150:339-342.
88. Steenland K, Hein MJ, Cassinelli RT 2nd, et al: Polychlorinated biphenyls and neurodegenerative disease mortality in an occupational cohort. Epidemiology 2006;17:8-13.
89. Caudle WM, Richardson JR, Delea KC, et al: Polychlorinated biphenyl-induced reduction of dopamine transporter expression as a precursor to Parkinson's disease-associated dopamine toxicity. Toxicol Sci 2006;92:490-499.
90. Wermuth L, Pakkenberg H, Jeune B: High age-adjusted prevalence of Parkinson's disease among Inuits in Greenland. Neurology 2002;58:1422-1425.
91. Jankovic J: Searching for a relationship between manganese and welding and Parkinson's disease. Neurology 2005;64:2021-2028.
92. Kaiser J: Manganese: a high-octane dispute. Science 2003;300:926-928.
93. Racette BA, McGee-Minnich L, Moerlein SM, et al: Welding-related parkinsonism: clinical features, treatment, and pathophysiology. Neurology 2001;56:8-13.
94. Racette BA, Tabbal SD, Jennings D, et al: Prevalence of parkinsonism and relationship to exposure in a large sample of Alabama welders. Neurology 2005;64:230-235.
95. Dick S, Semple S, Dick F, Seaton A: Occupational titles as risk factors for Parkinson's disease. Occup Med (Lond) 2007;57:50-56.
96. Marsh GM, Gula MJ: Employment as a welder and Parkinson disease among heavy equipment manufacturing workers. J Occup Environ Med 2006;48:1031-1046.
97. Fored CM, Fryzek JP, Brandt L, et al: Parkinson's disease and other basal ganglia or movement disorders in a large nationwide cohort of Swedish welders. Occup Environ Med 2006;63:135-140.
98. Park J, Yoo CI, Sim CS, et al: A retrospective cohort study of Parkinson's disease in Korean shipbuilders. Neurotoxicology 2006;27:445-449.
99. Fryzek JP, Hansen J, Cohen S, et al: A cohort study of Parkinson's disease and other neurodegenerative disorders in Danish welders. J Occup Environ Med 2005;47:466-472.
100. Park J, Yoo CI, Sim CS, et al: Occupations and Parkinson's disease: a multi-center case-control study in South Korea. Neurotoxicology 2005;26:99-105.
101. Gorell JM, Peterson EL, Rybicki BA, Johnson CC: Multiple risk factors for Parkinson's disease. J Neurol Sci 2004;217:169-174.
102. Zorzon M, Capus L, Pellegrino A, et al: Familial and environmental risk factors in Parkinson's disease: a case-control study in north-east Italy. Acta Neurol Scand 2002;105:77-82.
103. Behari M, Srivastava AK, Das RR, Pandey RM: Risk factors of Parkinson's disease in Indian patients. J Neurol Sci 2001;190;(1-2):49-55.
104. Uversky VN: Neuropathology, biochemistry, and biophysics of alpha synuclein aggregation. J Neurochem 2007;103:17-37.
105. Coon S, Stark A, Peterson E, et al: Whole-body lifetime occupational lead exposure and risk of Parkinson's disease. Environ Health Perspect 2006;114:1872-1876.

106. Gorell JM, Rybicki BA, Cole Johnson C, Peterson EL: Occupational metal exposures and the risk of Parkinson's disease. Neuroepidemiology 1999;18:303-308.

107. Logroscino G, Chen H, Wing A, Ascherio A: Blood donations, iron stores, and risk of Parkinson's disease. Mov Disord 2006;21:835-838.

108. Castaño A, Herrera AJ, Cano J, Machado A: The degenerative effect of a single intranigral injection of LPS on the dopaminergic system is prevented by dexamethasone, and not mimicked by rh-TNF-alpha, IL-1beta and IFN-gamma. J Neurochem 2002;81:150-157.

109. Hirsch EC, Hunot S: Nitric oxide, glial cells and neuronal degeneration in parkinsonism. Trends Pharmacol Sci 2000;21:163-165.

110. Niehaus I, Lange JH: Endotoxin: is it an environmental factor in the cause of Parkinson's disease? Occup Environ Med 2003;60:378.

111. Gash DM, Rutland K, Hudson NL, et al: Trichloroethylene: parkinsonism and complex 1 mitochondrial neurotoxicity. Ann Neurol 2008;63:184-192.

112. Fabrizio E, Vanacore N, Valente M, et al: High prevalence of extrapyramidal signs and symptoms in a group of Italian dental technicians. BMC Neurol 2007;7:24.

113. Elbaz A, Dutheil F, Alpérovitch A: Case-control study of the MDR1 gene in Parkinson disease. Mov Disord 2006;21(Suppl 15):S405.

114. Kelada SN, Checkoway H, Kardia SL, et al: 5′ and 3′ region variability in the dopamine transporter gene (SLC6A3), pesticide exposure and Parkinson's disease risk: a hypothesis-generating study. Hum Mol Genet 2006;15:3055-3062.

115. Benmoyal-Segal L, Vander T, Shifman S, et al: Acetylcholinesterase/paraoxonase interactions increase the risk of insecticide-induced Parkinson's disease. Faseb J 2005;19:452-454.

116. Dick FD, De Palma G, Ahmadi A, et al; Geoparkinson Study Group. Gene-environment interactions in parkinsonism and Parkinson's disease: the Geoparkinson study. Occup Environ Med 2007;64:673-680.

117. Elbaz A, Levecque C, Clavel J, et al: CYP2D6 polymorphism, pesticide exposure, and Parkinson's disease. Ann Neurol 2004;55:430-434.

118. Fong CS, Wu RM, Shieh JC, et al: Pesticide exposure on southwestern Taiwanese with MnSOD and NQO1 polymorphisms is associated with increased risk of Parkinson's disease. Clin Chim Acta 2007;378(1-2):136-141.

119. Hancock DB, Martin ER, Fujiwara K, et al: NOS2A and the modulating effect of cigarette smoking in Parkinson's disease. Ann Neurol 2006;60:366-373.

120. Deng Y, Newman B, Dunne MP, et al: Case-only study of interactions between genetic polymorphisms of GSTM1, P1, T1 and Z1 and smoking in Parkinson's disease. Neurosci Lett 2004;366:326-331.

121. Checkoway H, Franklin GM, Costa-Mallen P, et al: A genetic polymorphism of MAO-B modifies the association of cigarette smoking and Parkinson's disease. Neurology 1998;50:1458-1461.

122. Hernán MA, Checkoway H, O'Brien R, et al: MAOB intron 13 and COMT codon 158 polymorphisms, cigarette smoking, and the risk of PD. Neurology 2002;58:1381-1387.

123. Wahner AD, Glatt CE, Bronstein JM, Ritz B: Glutathione S-transferase mu, omega, pi, and theta class variants and smoking in Parkinson's disease. Neurosci Lett 2007;413:274-278.

124. Elbaz A, Dufouil C, Alpérovitch A: Interaction between genes and environment in neurodegenerative diseases. C R Biol 2007;330:318-328.

125. Wilk JB, Tobin JE, Suchowersky O, et al: Herbicide exposure modifies GSTP1 haplotype association to Parkinson onset age: the GenePD Study. Neurology 2006;67:2206-2210.

126. Aschner M, Erikson KM, Dorman DC: Manganese dosimetry: species differences and implications for neurotoxicity. Crit Rev Toxicol 2005;35:1-32.

127. Thiruchelvam M, Brockel BJ, Richfield EK, et al: Potentiated and preferential effects of combined paraquat and maneb on nigrostriatal dopamine systems: environmental risk factors for Parkinson's disease? Brain Res 2000;873:225-234.

128. Thiruchelvam M, Richfield EK, Baggs RB, et al: The nigrostriatal dopaminergic system as a preferential target of repeated exposures to combined paraquat and maneb: implications for Parkinson's disease. J Neurosci 2000;20:9207-9214.

129. Norris EH, Uryu K, Leight S, et al: Pesticide exposure exacerbates alpha-synucleinopathy in an A53T transgenic mouse model. Am J Pathol 2007;170:658-666.

130. Gao HM, Liu B, Zhang W, Hong JS: Synergistic dopaminergic neurotoxicity of MPTP and inflammogen lipopolysaccharide: relevance to the etiology of Parkinson's disease. Faseb J 2003;17:1957-1959.

131. Purisai MG, McCormack AL, Cumine S, et al: Microglial activation as a priming event leading to paraquat-induced dopaminergic cell degeneration. Neurobiol Dis 2007;25:392-400.
132. Gowers WR: A lecture on abiotrophy. Lancet 1902:1003-1007.
133. Calne DB, Langston JW: Aetiology of Parkinson's disease. Lancet 1983;2:1457-1459.
134. Marder K, Tang MX, Alfaro B, et al: Risk of Alzheimer's disease in relatives of Parkinson's disease patients with and without dementia. Neurology 1999;52:719-724.
135. Rosen AR, Steenland NK, Hanfelt J, et al: Evidence of shared risk for Alzheimer's disease and Parkinson's disease using family history. Neurogenetics 2007;8:263-270.
136. Aarsland D, Andersen K, Larsen JP, Lolk A: Prevalence and characteristics of dementia in Parkinson disease: an 8-year prospective study. Arch Neurol 2003;60:387-392.
137. Mayeux R, Denaro J, Hemenegildo N, et al: A population-based investigation of Parkinson's disease with and without dementia: relationship to age and gender. Arch Neurol 1992;49:492-497.
138. Ellis RJ, Caligiuri M, Galasko D, Thal LJ: Extrapyramidal motor signs in clinically diagnosed Alzheimer disease. Alzheimer Dis Assoc Disord 1996;10:103-114.
139. Forman MS, Schmidt ML, Kasturi S, et al: Tau and alpha-synuclein pathology in amygdala of Parkinsonism-dementia complex patients of Guam. Am J Pathol 2002;160:1725-1731.
140. Galpern WR, Lang AE: Interface between tauopathies and synucleinopathies: a tale of two proteins. Ann Neurol 2006;59:449-458.
141. Vieira MN, Forny-Germano L, Saraiva LM, et al: Soluble oligomers from a non-disease related protein mimic Abeta-induced tau hyperphosphorylation and neurodegeneration. J Neurochem 2007;103:736-748.
142. Giasson BI, Forman MS, Higuchi M, et al: Initiation and synergistic fibrillization of tau and alpha-synuclein. Science 2003;300:636-640.

9 Pathology of Parkinson's Disease

GLENDA HALLIDAY • KAREN MURPHY

Major Advances in Pathological Understanding of Parkinson's Disease

Numerous significant pathological findings in patients with Parkinson's disease (PD) were made around the turn of the 20th century. The pathological anatomy was first detailed by Lewy in 1912, who described the characteristic inclusions seen in postmortem specimens (Fig. 9–1), and the significant depigmentation and loss of neurons in the substantia nigra (Fig. 9–2) were brought to world attention in 1919 by Tretiakoff. Tretiakoff named the inclusions "*corps de Lewy.*" Lewy body inclusions, depigmentation, and cell loss in the substantia nigra are used today to arrive at definitive diagnosis of PD.

Some time after these advances, symptomatic treatment paradigms for PD were considered broadly successful. The surge in stereotaxic surgery in the latter half of the 20th century targeted the internal globus pallidus and the ventrolateral thalamus in patients with PD, providing relief for the symptoms of rigidity and tremor. In 1957, dopamine was identified by Carlsson as a neurotransmitter concentrating in the basal ganglia, and Hornykiewicz showed an absence of dopamine in the basal ganglia of postmortem brains from PD patients (see Fig. 9–2). The subsequent trial of injections of levodopa, the precursor of dopamine, into PD patients by Hornykiewicz was dramatically successful at relieving most of the movement disorder for these patients. Both of these different types of symptomatic treatments

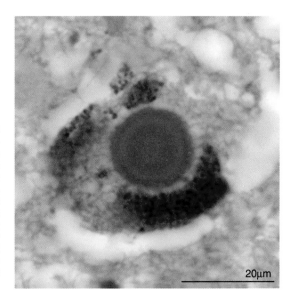

Figure 9–1 Photomicrograph of a Lewy body inclusion in a pigmented neuron of the substantia nigra from the brain of a patient with a diagnosis of levodopa-responsive idiopathic Parkinson's disease. Ultrastructural examination reveals the composition of Lewy bodies as radially arranged 7- to 20-nm filaments associated with a granular electron-dense coating material and vesicular structures with a core containing densely packed filaments and dense granular material.[165]

20μm

(stereotaxic surgery and dopamine replacement therapy) firmly identified the basal ganglia regions as important in the underlying pathogenesis of the major motor symptoms in PD. These treatments still remain the current gold standards for the treatment of PD.

Advances have occurred in the past decade through the identification of causal gene mutations for common and rare genetic forms of parkinsonism. The first mutations causing autosomal dominantly inherited PD were identified in the α-synuclein gene (*SNCA*),[1] which was subsequently discovered to be the major protein product in Lewy bodies.[2] Although many additional monogenic forms of PD with various mutations have since been identified, their pathogenic mechanisms remain unclear. Two main concepts currently prevail. Some mutations cause a toxic gain-of-function; these include the most common mutations causing autosomal dominant familial and sporadic forms of PD that occur in the *LRRK2*[3,4] and *SNCA* genes. The *LRRK2* gene codes for a large cytosolic protein with multiple functional domains, including kinase and GTPase domains. Increased enzymatic activity is thought to occur in PD. Other mutations cause a loss-of-function; these include the most common mutations causing autosomal recessive PD, which occur in the *parkin*[5] and *PINK1*[6] genes, and other rarer forms of PD with mutations in *DJ-1*,[7] *ATP132A*,[8] *UCH-L1*, synphilin-1, *Nurr1*, and *HtrA2*.[9]

The *parkin* gene codes for a neuroprotective E3 ligase, the *PINK1* gene codes for a neuroprotective mitochondrial kinase, the *ATP132A* gene codes for a lysosomal ATPase, and many of the other genes identified code for various proteins with neuroprotective functions, putting enzymatic dysfunction and loss of neuroprotection firmly in the limelight for causative abnormalities for PD. More proteins are likely to be involved in the pathogenesis of PD because there are several loci linked to different forms of familial PD in which the genes involved remain to be determined.[10,11] These genetic discoveries are providing new avenues to investigate the molecular pathogenesis of the more common sporadic form of PD (detailed later).

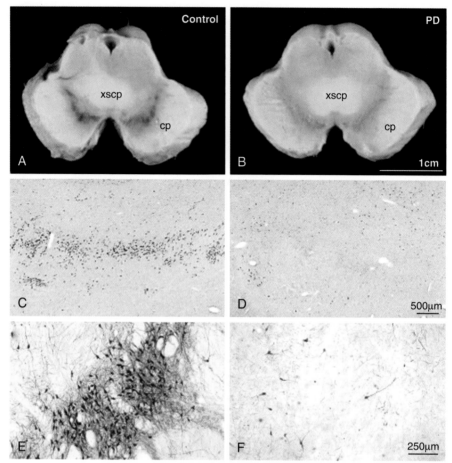

Figure 9–2 **A** and **B,** Photographs of transverse sections of human midbrain show the dark pigmentation of the substantia nigra between the decussation of the superior cerebellar peduncle (xscp) and the cerebral peduncle (cp) in a neurological control **(A)** and its reduction in Parkinson's disease **(B).** Depigmentation is one of the macroscopic features of the disease. **C** and **D,** Photomicrographs of Nissl-stained midbrain sections showing the severe loss of the naturally darkly pigmented neurons in the substantia nigra of Parkinson's disease patients **(D)** compared with neurological controls **(C).** **E** and **F,** Photomicrographs of dopaminergic neurons in the substantia nigra immunoreactive for the rate-limiting enzyme, tyrosine hydroxylase. There is a selective loss of these neurons in Parkinson's disease patients **(F)** but not in controls **(E).**

Clinicopathological Types of Parkinson's Disease

As stated previously, the pathological diagnosis of PD requires Lewy bodies (see Fig. 9–1), depigmentation, and cell loss in the substantia nigra (see Fig. 9–2). These features define the most common form, or idiopathic PD. The clinical course for idiopathic PD is long and slow, and most often there is very lengthy disease duration. The cardinal clinical features are bradykinesia, muscular rigidity, resting tremor, and postural instability, with greater certainty for this diagnosis when symptom onset is asymmetrical and there is a good response to levodopa therapy.[12] In addition to the predominant motor symptoms, PD patients can have a range of nonmotor symptoms, including autonomic dysfunction, olfactory dysfunction, depression, sleep disturbances, hallucinations, cognitive impairment and dementia.[12,13] Broader neuropathology in brainstem and cortical regions is associated with these nonmotor features.[14] The prevalence of this common form of PD is estimated at 0.3% of the entire population in industrialized countries, increasing to 1% in individuals older than 60 years, and 4% in individuals older than 85 years.[15]

Depigmentation and cell loss of the substantia nigra can occur without Lewy bodies, and the motor symptoms in such cases are extremely similar to the symptoms observed in idiopathic PD, including clinical benefit from dopaminergic replacement therapies. Rarely, circumscribed cerebrovascular disease can be responsible for a loss of dopamine neurons in the substantia nigra.[16] Also rare is the exposure to environmental toxins that seem to target substantia nigra neurons, such as 1-methyl-4-phenyl-1,2,3,6-tetrahydropyridine (MPTP), manganese, and pesticides. Accidental MPTP poisoning has induced acute clinical PD that does not recover over time, and with long survival can have Lewy bodies at postmortem.[17] Nigral cell loss and parkinsonism can also result from manganese toxicity, although additional basal ganglia neurons also degenerate.[18] The herbicide paraquat and the pesticide rotenone are used in animal studies to deplete dopaminergic neurons,[19] and although exposure to pesticides is considered a risk factor for developing PD,[20] these acute animal models do not form Lewy bodies. These forms of PD show that environmental toxins and focal vascular disease can have a profound impact on the substantia nigra, but usually do not produce Lewy bodies, unless the effect is sufficiently mild to set up a self-sustaining slow and protracted clinical course.

As discussed earlier, several genetic forms of PD have been identified. Ten percent of all PD cases are considered to have a strong genetic basis, although each of the genetic forms is very rare overall. On average, genetic forms of PD have a younger age of disease onset. Some mutations are most prevalent in certain ethnic groups suggesting more recent founder effects. Mutations in the *LRRK2* and glucocerebrosidase genes have a higher prevalence in Jewish populations.[21,22] Mutations in the *LRRK2* and *parkin* genes are high in North African Arab populations.[23,24] Mutations in the glucocerebrosidase gene are higher in Asians than general white populations,[25,26] whereas mutations in the *parkin* gene are comparatively higher in Indian PD patients.[27] Generally, the autosomal dominant *SNCA* and *LRRK2* mutant forms of PD mostly have Lewy bodies postmortem, aligning these forms with the common idiopathic form of the disease. In contrast, the autosomal recessive forms of PD generally do not have Lewy bodies at postmortem. Many risk genes are associated with the Lewy body form of PD, including mutations in the glucocerebrosidase gene.[28]

Widespread Pathology in the Common Form of Parkinson's Disease

ABNORMAL α-SYNUCLEIN DEPOSITION

As indicated earlier, the diagnostic pathology of idiopathic PD is characterized by the abnormal deposition of α-synuclein in intracytoplasmic Lewy body inclusions and dystrophic Lewy neurites.[2] The neuroanatomical regions accumulating α-synuclein pathology in idiopathic PD follow a consistent pattern as the disease progresses.[14,29] Pathology is initially confined to the olfactory bulbs and lower brainstem concentrating in the dorsal motor nucleus of the vagal nerve (stage 1) (Fig. 9–3A). In the second stage, the pathology spreads upward to include neuritic changes in the locus caeruleus (Fig. 9–3B).

Clinical symptoms of PD usually first manifest when stage 3 is reached, showing the appearance of Lewy neurites, granular α-synuclein aggregates, pale bodies, and then Lewy bodies in the substantia nigra in the absence of neuron loss; nigral cell loss is observed in stage 4 (Fig. 9–3C) when the basal forebrain and hippocampus become involved (Fig. 9–3D and E). In stage 5, neocortical α-synuclein Lewy body pathology first occurs concentrating in temporal regions (Fig. 9–3F), with α-synuclein deposition continuing its cortical spread in stage 6 of the disease. The common feature of the cell types developing α-synuclein inclusion pathology is proposed to be their long, thin, poorly myelinated or unmyelinated axons.[29]

α-Synuclein is normally concentrated at synaptic sites in mature neurons and is closely associated with synaptic vesicles in presynaptic terminals.[30,31] In healthy neurons, α-synuclein forms soluble monomers or oligomers, but it undergoes conformational change to precipitate into the stable fibrils that form Lewy pathologies.[32] The mechanisms that cause the conformational change of the protein include phosphorylation, C-terminal truncation, and ubiquitination. Lewy bodies in the substantia nigra of patients with PD are labeled with an antibody specifically recognizing the phosphorylated Ser129 residue of α-synuclein, and phosphorylation of α-synuclein at Ser129 promotes fibril formation in vitro.[33]

α-Synuclein is also deposited in glial cells in PD. Argyrophilic, α-synuclein–positive astrocytes have been reported in PD cases,[34] where they preferentially occur in the basal forebrain and limbic (see Fig. 9–3F) regions at pathological stages 4 through 6. Their topographical distribution pattern closely parallels the pattern for cortical Lewy pathology.[35] Astrocytes can react to damage by walling off a pathological target and stimulating surrounding microglia for damage control, while secreting protective agents into the surrounding area.[36] Pathology in this cell type may influence this neuroprotective capacity and participate in the further propagation of the disease process.

ATROPHY AND CELL LOSS

Despite widespread α-synuclein deposition, the macroscopic examination of PD brains shows no significant atrophy, consistent with magnetic resonance imaging findings.[37] A quantitative study comparing neocortical neuron number in PD cases with age-matched controls confirmed no global loss of neocortical neurons and no difference in neocortical volume.[38]

All patients with symptomatic PD have cell loss at least in the substantia nigra. This pigmented region typically has an obvious pallor (see Fig. 9–2A and B) owing to the severe loss of neuromelanin-pigmented dopaminergic neurons (see Fig. 9–2C and D), with an average 80% of pigmented nigral neurons lost in patients surviving 7 to 32 years after PD onset compared with controls without PD.[39] There is particular degeneration of the ventrolateral region of the substantia nigra, with greater than 90% neuron loss observed.[40] The cell loss begins before symptom onset with a logarithmic loss over time that correlates with increasing motor

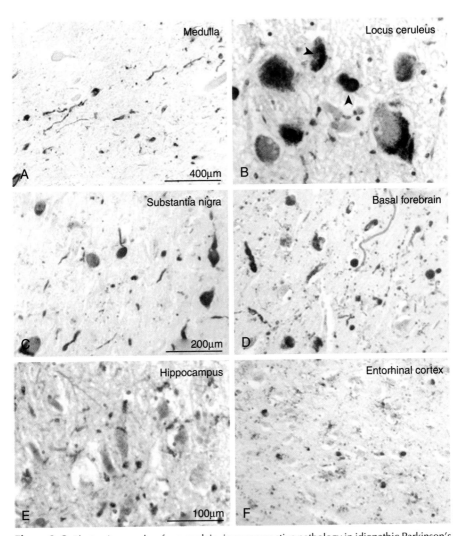

Figure 9–3 Photomicrographs of α-synuclein–immunoreactive pathology in idiopathic Parkinson's disease. Scale in **A** is equivalent for **B**, scale in **C** is equivalent for **D**, and scale in **E** is equivalent for **F. A,** Low magnification of abnormal α-synuclein pathology in dystrophic neurites and axonal Lewy bodies in and around the dorsal motor nucleus of the vagus nerve. Pathology in this area first appears in stage 1 disease, and remains present at all stages in virtually all cases of idiopathic Parkinsons disease. **B,** High magnification of abnormal α-synuclein deposition in neurons of the locus ceruleus. Note the round Lewy body inclusions (*arrowheads*), immunopositive Lewy neurites, and α-synuclein deposition on the pigment granules in some of the locus caeruleus neurons. Pathology in this area appears in stage 2 disease, and remains present at all later stages in virtually all cases of idiopathic Parkinson's disease. **C,** α-Synuclein deposition in Lewy bodies and Lewy neurites (stage 3) and cell loss (stage 4) in the substantia nigra are required for a definitive diagnosis of idiopathic Parkinson's disease. Patients progress to clinical disease only when pathology and degeneration have spread to include this region. **D** and **E,** At stage 4, α-synuclein deposition also occurs in the basal forebrain **(D)** and restricted regions of the hippocampus (CA2/3 region, **E**). **F,** By stage 5, neocortical regions have become involved, beginning in limbic and temporal cortices with increasing neocortical infiltration to stage 6 disease. Note the α-synuclein–positive Lewy bodies, Lewy neurites, and astrocytes in this case.

dysfunction.[41] The dopaminergic neurons targeted by PD project to the caudate nucleus and putamen, so the progressive degeneration of the nigrostriatal dopaminergic system results in dopaminergic denervation of the striatum.

The other dopaminergic cell groups in the midbrain, A8 and A10, show substantially less severe cell loss than the substantia nigra (30% and 50% loss). This less severe loss is most notable in the preservation of the adjacent dopaminergic neurons in the medial reticular formation.[42] These extranigral dopaminergic cell groups form the mesocortical dopaminergic system, innervating the thalamus, striatum, and prefrontal, motor, and premotor areas, and affecting the function of the basal ganglia and cerebral cortex.[43]

Degeneration of nondopaminergic neurons also occurs in patients with PD, but many of these regions are usually affected later in the disease course. Despite marked deposition of α-synuclein pathology, there is mild cell loss in the amygdala, even at end-stage disease.[44] The cholinergic nucleus basalis of Meynert experiences neuron loss and shrinkage with more severe disease.[45] Hypothalamic neurons containing the neurotransmitter hypocretin degenerate at later disease stages.[46] These neurons regulate sleep, appetite, and energy consumption. The noradrenergic locus caeruleus undergoes a change in cell phenotype without a substantial loss of neurons overall.[47] The nearby serotoninergic neurons of the raphe system are also lost at late stages.[48] The noradrenergic dorsal vagal nucleus shows comparatively mild neuron loss (5% to 17%)[48] despite frequent Lewy pathology (see Fig. 9–3A) from the earliest stages (see earlier).

In contrast, significant cell loss has been shown in previously unsuspecting regions that show limited Lewy body pathology. These include the striatal projection neurons from the caudal intralaminar nuclei of the thalamus and the corticocortical projection neurons in the presupplementary motor cortex.[49] The cortical changes are observed at the earliest onset of motor symptoms. The pattern and severity of cell loss is not the same as the pattern and severity of abnormal α-synuclein deposition in PD, possibly suggesting more separate degenerative processes (see later).

INFLAMMATION

Reactive microglia are found in abundance in the substantia nigra of PD cases agglomerated around the pigmented neurons (Fig. 9–4A) and extracellular neuromelanin,[50] indicating the presence of substantial inflammation. Microglia have also been identified in the putamen, hippocampus, and cerebral cortex of PD cases, in close proximity to Lewy bodies and independent of them.[51] Dopaminergic neurons seem particularly susceptible to degeneration through chronic microglial activation.[52] The release of neuromelanin from damaged dopaminergic neurons in the substantia nigra has been shown to activate microglia to cause further damage,[53] and the extent of extracellular neuromelanin deposits in normal aged human nigra correlates with the degree of increased microglial activation.[54]

The extent of microglial activation in the substantia nigra also correlates with the degree of α-synuclein deposition, although neither characteristic shows a relationship with indicators of the clinical progression of PD.[55] In vitro models have shown that α-synuclein can activate microglial cells, which generate oxygen free radicals that are toxic to dopaminergic neurons.[56] In many regions depositing α-synuclein, the upregulation of microglia may be a reaction to this

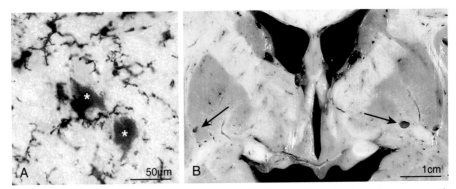

Figure 9–4 A, Photomicrograph of reactive microglia in the substantia nigra of a patient with idiopathic Parkinson's disease using a ligand for major histocompatibility complex II. Note the very enlarged phagocytic microglial cell (black peroxidase stain) directly engulfing a pigmented neuron (*asterisks*). Many of the surrounding microglia are also reactive and have some cell body enlargement. **B,** Photograph of a coronal 3-mm slice through the level of the basal ganglia in a patient with levodopa-responsive Parkinson's disease showing obvious small lacunes in the left putamen and right globus pallidus (*arrows*).

pathological change, although it seems to contribute to neuronal death in the substantia nigra. This finding is consistent with epidemiological studies of anti-inflammatory use in PD patients that show a slight protective effect, suggesting that microglia are involved in the disease attack, rather than just combating the ongoing damage owing to the pathological deposition of α-synuclein.[57] Further evidence for a self-sustaining inflammatory attack occurring in PD nigra is the observation of phagocytic microglia in postmortem specimens of this region from humans and monkeys with MPTP-induced parkinsonism many years after the acute insult.[58,59]

PREVALENCE OF OTHER COEXISTING PATHOLOGIES

Many retrospective postmortem studies have evaluated the prevalence of other co-existing pathologies in PD patients, with cerebrovascular lesions and Alzheimer's disease (AD) pathology the most prominent types encountered.[60] In a study of 617 autopsy-confirmed idiopathic PD cases, the frequency of all cerebrovascular lesions (lacunae, amyloid angiopathy, white matter lesions, old and recent ischemic infarcts, and hemorrhages) was 44%, which was higher than in an age-matched control cohort of 535 cases (33% frequency).[61] These lesions were mainly mild to moderate in severity. A smaller postmortem PD cohort study found similar frequencies of cerebrovascular lesions in PD patients and age-matched controls, with old subcortical lacunar infarcts (Fig. 9–4B) slightly more common than cortical infarcts in the PD group.[62] These results suggest that cerebrovascular pathology is common in PD patients, but its prevalence does not differ much from that seen in individuals without neurological abnormalities of the same age.

Investigation of a series of autopsy-confirmed PD cases for coexisting AD pathology showed 97% of nondemented PD patients had no morphological changes indicating probable or definite AD, with the remaining 3% reaching Consortium to Establish a Registry for Alzheimer Disease (CERAD) criteria for possible AD.[63]

There are considerable differences in the overlap of PD and AD pathologies in cases with dementia, and this is discussed further in the section on clinicopathological correlations.

Clinicopathological Correlations in Parkinson's Disease

The classic view of the pathological substrates of PD is that motor symptoms result from loss of substantia nigra neurons causing disruption of the dopaminergic nigrostriatal pathway,[64] with nondopaminergic cell dysfunction leading to the development of nonmotor features,[65,66] although evidence for this view was lacking until more recently.

CORE MOTOR SYMPTOMS

The severe neurodegeneration within the substantia nigra in PD disrupts transmission in the dopaminergic nigrostriatal pathway, causing significant dopaminergic striatal denervation. This dramatic insult to the nigrostriatal dopaminergic pathway induces a cascade of functional modifications to the motor circuitry of the basal ganglia and leads to the expression of motor dysfunction in PD. The clinical manifestation of motor symptoms occurs only after a critical threshold of dopamine depletion is reached—the loss of 30% to 50% of nigral dopaminergic neurons and a 50% to 80% reduction in striatal dopamine uptake.[67] This level of nigral degeneration becomes apparent when Lewy pathology has already reached stages 3 and 4, and other brainstem and forebrain nuclei are affected.[29]

The initial loss of nigral neurons before symptom onset is estimated to take approximately 5 years.[41] The degree of pigmented cell loss in the substantia nigra relates directly to the severity of bradykinesia and rigidity, but not tremor, and to disease duration.[41] Neuronal loss is more rapid over the initial 5 years of symptomatic disease and then tails off exponentially. The severity of bradykinesia and rigidity, but not tremor, also correlates with the loss of striatal fluorodopa F 18 (^{18}F-dopa) uptake (as seen in positron emission tomography scans), implying that the severity of tremor has a different mechanism from that of bradykinesia and rigidity.[68] This correlation is consistent with the frequent improvement in bradykinesia and rigidity shown by PD patients using dopaminergic agents, whereas tremor can be less responsive to this treatment.

Mounting evidence suggests that substantial compensatory remodeling occurs in the basal ganglia after the loss of substantia nigra neurons and ongoing denervation of dopaminergic axons in extrastriatal regions (nigra, pallidum, and subthalamic nucleus).[69,70] This remodeling causes further changes in regulation over time,[71,72] with the most prominent changes occurring in the subthalamic and pedunculopontine regions, which become hyperactive.[73] It has been suggested that overactivity of these nuclei also contributes to the neurodegenerative process in the substantia nigra as they provide excitatory input to this region.[74,75] There is an overall change in the pattern of basal ganglia discharge (e.g., the development of oscillatory phenomena and abnormal synchronization of neuron firing[76]) that is thought to contribute most to the expression of the clinical motor features of PD.[77] These changes over time may have a particular impact on the response to any therapeutic treatments.

The resting tremor in PD, but not bradykinesia, is successfully suppressed by lesions or chronic stimulation of the thalamus.[67,78-80] Tremor is associated with rhythmical synchronous neuronal discharges in various thalamic nuclei.[81] In particular, the cerebellothalamocortical loop plays a role in the frequency of PD tremor and is probably active during the suppression of resting tremor with voluntary movement.[82] A more recent study in PD patients found that stimulation of only two regions, the ventrolateral thalamus and the caudal zona incerta, can induce resting tremor in PD patients.[83] The caudal zona incerta inhibits the ventrolateral thalamus and the interpositus nucleus of the cerebellum, which also projects to the ventrolateral thalamus, and hyperactivity of this region occurs in concert with hyperactivity of the subthalamic nucleus in PD.[84,85] It is hypothesized that changes in dopaminergic and serotoninergic innervation are required to influence the firing pattern of the caudal zona incerta sufficiently to cause the tremor bursts at rest.[83]

There is no consensus on the pathological substrate for the postural instability and gait difficulties seen in patients with late onset of PD. The pedunculopontine nucleus is involved in the initiation and modulation of gait and other stereotyped movements,[86] but this region seems to be retrogradely affected in all types of PD as the disease progresses (see earlier). The caudal intralaminar thalamic projections regulating the striatum are more affected in older PD patients,[87] and in patients with progressive supranuclear palsy, a parkinsonian syndrome with early postural instability and gait problems.[88] Disruption of the striatum also underlies the postural instability and gait disorders observed in other parkinsonian syndromes, including multiple systems atrophy[89] and vascular parkinsonism.[16]

PAIN

Patients with PD commonly experience various types of pain, which can stem from neuropathic or nociceptive origin, or both. The basal ganglia have been implicated in the perception of pain, with dysfunction of dopaminergic and serotoninergic systems playing a significant role in pain perception.[90]

The medial and lateral pain systems are the two predominant pain systems involved in processing various aspects of pain.[91,92] Although the lateral pain system is important for processing sensory-discriminative aspects of pain, the medial pain system is involved in the motivational-affective aspects of pain, cognitive-evaluative aspects of pain, memory for pain, and autonomic responses to pain.[93] Regions of the medial pain system show evidence of Lewy pathology in the periaqueductal gray, parabrachial nucleus, and caeruleus-subcaeruleus area before the onset of cognitive dysfunction,[29,94] with neuronal loss in the caudal intralaminar thalamic nuclei disturbing glutamatergic regulation in the striatum.[88] There is little neuropathological impairment of the lateral pain system in PD.[95]

Differences in pain experience are observed between PD patients with and without dementia. Cognitively intact PD patients usually show an increase in all aspects of pain except for sensory-discriminative aspects, which are generally reduced.[92] A decline in the motivational-affective, cognitive-evaluative, and autonomic responses to pain may be the result of Lewy pathology in the caeruleus-subcaeruleus regions and intralaminar and medial thalamic nuclei, causing an increase in pain experience. Inhibition of the lateral thalamus may reduce the localization aspect of sensory-discrimination of pain, exemplified by the finding of a decreased threshold for heat pain in PD patients.[96] PD patients with cognitive impairment tend to show a reduction in the capacity to feel all aspects of pain, owing to a reduction in the motivational-affective, cognitive-evaluative, autonomic, and memory aspects of pain. This reduction results from the presence of Lewy pathology, but also occurs with AD pathology in subcortical and cortical areas, such as the anterior cingulate cortex, hippocampus, amygdala, and prefrontal cortex—regions that play a major role in the medial pain system, but are correlated with cognitive impairment in PD.[91,97]

AUTONOMIC DYSFUNCTION

Symptoms of autonomic dysfunction are common in PD patients and can occur at all stages of the disease. They are due primarily to the neurodegenerative processes at work in the autonomic nervous system, but also can be induced or exacerbated by drugs used in the treatment of motor symptoms. Autonomic dysfunction in PD patients can include cardiovascular, gastrointestinal, and urogenital systems, with central and peripheral degeneration and dysfunction of cholinergic, monoaminergic, and serotoninergic nuclei that mediate autonomic functions implicated in the development of symptoms.[98]

Cardiovascular autonomic dysfunction includes cardiac sympathetic denervation and orthostatic hypotension owing to peripheral sympathetic failure. Lewy pathology has been observed in neurons that affect cardiovascular function in the central and peripheral nervous systems. Lewy bodies are found in the cardiac plexus[99] and the heart of PD patients,[100] implicating postganglionic and intrinsic neurons of the heart in the PD disease process. More recent studies suggest that cardiac sympathetic denervation precedes neuronal cell loss and dysfunction in the dorsal vagal nucleus and sympathetic ganglia during the early disease process.[101,102] PD patients with orthostatic hypotension often exhibit reduced sympathetic noradrenergic innervation of left ventricular myocardium.[13]

Autonomic dysfunction of the gastrointestinal system includes constipation, bladder disturbances, excess saliva, and dysphagia, with disordered autonomic regulation caused by central and peripheral degeneration implicated in the underlying pathophysiology. Lewy pathology is present in the parasympathetic ganglia (enteric nervous system of the alimentary tract, pelvic plexus, submandibular ganglion, adrenal medulla, and dorsal vagus) and sympathetic ganglia (intermediolateral nucleus of the thoracic cord) of the gastrointestinal system.[99,103] Severe loss of central and peripheral dopaminergic neurons in PD is also observed, but symptoms of autonomic dysfunction do not respond well to dopaminergic treatment, indicating that nondopaminergic mechanisms play a larger role.[65]

OLFACTORY DYSFUNCTION

Olfactory dysfunction is a common feature of PD, especially early in the disease course, with evidence suggesting olfactory loss may be one of the first clinical signs of PD. A more recent clinical study showed that 4 years after baseline testing, 7% of individuals with idiopathic olfactory loss had newly developed clinical PD motor symptoms.[104] An association between olfactory dysfunction and incidental Lewy pathology in brains of men without clinical PD or dementia has been identified, suggesting that the cause of the olfactory deficits may be linked to the processes leading to Lewy body formation.[105] Neuropathological studies support the idea of early olfactory dysfunction in PD because the olfactory bulb, olfactory tract, and anterior olfactory nucleus together are some of the first sites of Lewy pathology in stages 1 and 2 of PD, before significant nigral degeneration.[29,106] In addition to early α-synuclein deposition in the olfactory structures, severe neuronal loss has been observed in the anterior olfactory nucleus of PD patients, with the degree of neuronal loss increasing with disease duration.[107]

Dopaminergic deficits also are implicated in the development of olfactory dysfunction in PD. Impairment in olfactory discrimination shows a strong correlation with nigrostriatal denervation, shown by positron emission tomography imaging of dopamine transporter activity.[108] Olfactory dysfunction may not be directly related to nigrostriatal abnormalities in PD, however, because patients with MPTP-induced toxic parkinsonism who have nigrostriatal dopaminergic denervation exhibit olfactory test scores similar to control subjects.[109] More likely, the number of dopaminergic cells in the olfactory bulb of PD patients may be relevant because these are found to increase in PD relative to age-matched and gender-matched controls.[110] This increase would lead to increased dopaminergic activity, which has an inhibitory role on olfactory transmission.[110]

PD-related neuropathology in certain subcortical regions may also contribute to olfactory dysfunction. The involvement of the cortical nucleus of the amygdala in olfactory function is well established.[111] In PD, this region of the amygdala shows significant Lewy body pathology.[44] Olfactory impairment could also be affected further in late-stage PD as limbic regions that provide higher level processing of olfactory discrimination become involved.

SLEEP DISORDERS

Nocturnal sleep disturbances and excessive daytime sleepiness are frequent clinical symptoms in PD, and although the causes are multifactorial, the pathological degeneration of central sleep regulation centers in brainstem, hypothalamus, and thalamocortical pathways are involved. Sleep disorders may manifest through abnormalities in the sleep-wake cycle–related pathway that mediates thalamocortical arousal (the "flip-flop switch" described by Lu and colleagues[112]), and includes the serotoninergic raphe nucleus, the noradrenergic locus caeruleus, the cholinergic pedunculopontine nucleus, and hypocretin neurons in the hypothalamus. Neuropathological examination of PD brains shows early Lewy body formation and later neuron loss in the these regions[46,48,113] that correlate with the early dysregulation and later degeneration of brainstem and hypothalamic neurotransmitter systems involved in arousal and sleep mechanisms.

Rapid-eye-movement (REM) sleep behavior disorder (RBD) is the most frequent of the nocturnal sleep disturbances exhibited by PD patients. RBD is frequently associated with neurodegenerative disorders with Lewy pathology and less often with nonsynucleinopathies, and RBD typically precedes the motor and cognitive symptoms of PD.[114] The degeneration of lower brainstem nuclei in the early PD stages (1 and 2) is thought to play a significant role in the pathogenesis of RBD. The human analogue of the rat sublaterodorsal nucleus and cat subcaerulus region has been proposed as the region crucial to RBD pathophysiology.[114] An imaging study of PD patients with and without RBD did not detect marked metabolic deficits in this pontine region, suggesting either insensitive methodology or that the primary site for RBD pathogenesis exists beyond the pons in other REM sleep–related regions.[115]

Excessive daytime sleepiness is also a frequent sleep disorder observed in PD. It has been associated with disease severity and duration of levodopa therapy,[116] with dopamine agonists significantly contributing to its presence.[117] A functional imaging study of excessive daytime sleepiness in PD patients showed that parietal and associated cortical hypofunction, relative to brainstem hyperfunction, is involved in excessive daytime sleepiness.[118]

DEPRESSION

Depression affects many PD patients, although the nature of the depression experienced remains unresolved. Depression may be a reaction to the disease diagnosis itself, but neuropathological mechanisms have also been implicated in the etiology of depression in PD.[119]

The two regions of the brain primarily implicated in the pathology of depression in PD are the noradrenergic locus caeruleus and the serotoninergic raphe nucleus. Depressed patients can have reduced noradrenergic innervation of the forebrain and neocortex, and there is a greater loss of locus caeruleus neurons in PD patients with depression.[120] An in vivo marker of catecholamine transporter binding showed that depression in PD patients is associated with a reduction of catecholaminergic innervation in the locus caeruleus and in several limbic regions, including the anterior cingulate cortex, amygdala, ventral striatum, and thalamus.[121] Depressed PD patients also have greater neuronal loss in the dorsal raphe and lower serotonin measures in the median raphe than PD patients without depression.[122] It has been suggested that PD patients with greater mesocortical dopaminergic disruption are more likely to exhibit depression than patients without this disruption[123] because the mesocortical dopaminergic pathway has an indirect impact on the serotoninergic system, and projects to the orbitofrontal cortex.

Neurosurgical stimulation of the rostral cingulate gyrus has been postulated as a target for treatment-refractory depression, based on its catalytic role in the integration of limbic-cortical pathways affected in depression.[124] There is significant Lewy body formation in the cingulate cortex in PD,[125] but it is currently unknown if there is any association with this pathology and depression. Reduced metabolism and perfusion have been observed in cingulate and frontal cortex in depressed PD patients.[126]

VISUAL HALLUCINATIONS

Visual hallucinations are present in more than 50% of PD patients, with occurrence often later in the disease course. Visual hallucinations are commonly viewed as side effects of dopaminergic therapy, but degeneration of the cholinergic pedunculopontine nucleus, noradrenergic locus caeruleus, and serotoninergic raphe nuclei has been implicated as related to the origin of visual hallucinations in PD.[127] The presence of visual hallucinations in PD has been significantly associated with the occurrence of RBD,[128] and PD patients with hallucinations but without dementia have deficits in executive function on par with demented PD patients.[129]

The most prominent pathological correlate for the presence visual hallucinations in PD is selective cortical Lewy body formation. The occurrence of visual hallucinations in life can predict postmortem Lewy pathology with 93% accuracy, indicating their high specificity for Lewy body parkinsonism.[130] High densities of Lewy bodies in the amygdala and parahippocampal cortex have been associated with the presence of visual hallucinations in PD,[44] with increasing numbers of Lewy bodies in the temporal lobe associated with an earlier onset of this nonmotor symptom.[131] In addition to selective Lewy body formation in the amygdala and temporal lobe, visual hallucinations have been associated with high Lewy body densities in frontal and parietal cortex.[132] The cortical areas associated with visual hallucinations show increased glucose metabolism, suggesting that cortical Lewy bodies may assist in increasing cortical neuronal activity.

A new model has been proposed for the origin of chronic visual hallucinations in PD that suggests their occurrence might reflect disturbed internal/external perception, depending on visual impairment and on dysfunction of the control system for REM sleep.[127] The inclusion of the retinal dopaminergic circuitry and REM sleep regulatory system into the putative neuroanatomical pathways underlying visual hallucinations is supported by significant correlations between hallucinations in PD, RBD, and dopaminergic therapy.[128]

COGNITIVE IMPAIRMENT

There is evidence of at least subtle cognitive impairment in the early stages of PD, with a very slow but continual cognitive decline over the disease course that often eventually culminates in dementia (see later). Cognitive impairment in PD is predominantly caused by disturbances of executive functions, leading to dysfunction of the mental processes involved in the elaboration and control of cognitive and behavioral responses to challenging situations.[133]

Dopaminergic deficiency has been implicated in cognitive impairment in PD because the severe loss of substantia nigra neurons in PD reduces the dopaminergic projection to the striatum. Although the depletion of the dopaminergic innervation to the putamen has an impact on motor function, the dopaminergic denervation of the projection to the caudate affects cognitive ability, particularly executive function.[134,135] An association between cognitive ability and decreased caudate activity has been shown in imaging studies in PD patients.[136,137] Caudate hypofunctioning from dopaminergic denervation affects frontal lobe circuits innervating the frontal lobe, leading to cognitive impairment.[138,139] Dopamine depletion in the frontal cortex can also occur from later stage disruption of the mesocortical dopaminergic system.[138-140]

Despite the evidence for the role of dopamine deficiency in the development of cognitive impairment in PD, the effects of dopaminergic therapy on these symptoms is heterogeneous, suggesting that nondopaminergic pathways are also involved.[141] The extent of neuronal loss in the noradrenergic locus caeruleus has been shown to be proportional to the severity of cognitive dysfunction in PD.[120] Adequate cholinergic tone is important for cognition,[142] and the degeneration of cholinergic neurons in the basal forebrain and other brainstem regions[143] is likely to affect cognition. The reduction of various cholinergic modulators correlates with the extent of cognitive impairment in PD patients.[143-145]

The presence and distribution of α-synuclein pathology have also been implicated in the underlying cognitive deficits in PD. Cognitive impairment in PD seems to occur when the spread of Lewy pathology goes from the brainstem (and is associated with motor symptoms) to higher cortical areas that are involved in cognitive function.[29,146,147] There is also some evidence that subcortical pathology alone might be sufficient to induce cognitive decline.[29,148]

DEMENTIA

The early cognitive impairment in PD often progresses to dementia, and various pathological substrates similar to the underlying cognitive deficits in other dementia syndromes can also exist in PD. In particular, the presence of concomitant AD pathology is commonly observed in association with early dementia in PD. The impact of neurotransmitter dysfunctions and Lewy pathology can independently influence dementia in PD patients, however.

The severity of dementia in PD has been correlated with the loss of dopaminergic neurons in the medial region of the substantia nigra, as these neurons project to the caudate nucleus.[135] The progression of cognitive deterioration has been correlated with the severity of damage to the locus caeruleus and raphe neurons, which causes noradrenergic and serotoninergic denervation of the forebrain and neocortex.[140] Reduction of cholinergic activity in the basal forebrain seems to be the most significant monoaminergic dysfunction associated with dementia in PD, however. There is a substantial and more severe depletion of cholinergic neurons in nucleus basalis of Meynert in PD patients with dementia compared with nondemented PD patients and patients with AD.[143,149] It is unclear whether the severity of cell loss in these neurotransmitter systems is predictive of PD.

Many neuropathological studies have found associations between dementia in PD with the progression of Lewy pathology from the brainstem to an extensive distribution within cortical regions. Cognitive status has been significantly correlated with the stage of PD Lewy pathology, with the risk of developing dementia increasing with disease progression from stage 3 to 6 as the Lewy pathology extends into the cortex.[150] The density of Lewy bodies in cortical limbic areas distinguishes PD cases with dementia from cases without dementia.[151] Compared with nondemented PD patients, patients with PD who develop dementia have a 10-fold increase of Lewy body inclusions in neocortex and limbic regions.[147,152-154] Lewy body load is not predictive of the onset or duration of dementia, however, and some studies have shown that some PD patients develop dementia with only mild Lewy pathology in cortical regions.[150,155,156] Overall cortical Lewy body load is not highly predictive of many dementia indices, but may predispose to dementia. This concept has been incorporated into a probability matrix for the neuropathological diagnosis of dementia in Lewy body disease.[157]

Although not present in all cases, concomitant AD pathology significantly contributes to the clinical phenotype when present. AD pathology has been shown to be more abundant in demented PD patients than in nondemented PD patients, particularly when patients are elderly, or when dementia occurs early in the disease course.[156,158] Numerous studies have shown differences in the severity and distribution of AD pathology in PD patients compared with patients with AD, suggesting that these neuropathological changes in the setting of PD may differ from the changes seen in cases with AD alone.[150,159,160] It is difficult to determine the true prevalence of AD pathology in cohorts of PD patients because most recent pathological screening studies have a broader cohort catchment that often includes dementia clinics as well. Large but typical neurological cohorts of PD patients, such as those seen at Queen Square, suggest that about one third of patients have dementia owing to AD.[161]

▍HYPOTHESES ON PATHOGENESIS

The cause of neuronal death in PD and its link to α-synuclein dysfunction are still unknown; however, investigations into the cellular mechanisms show evidence for apoptosis, excitotoxicity, and autophagy. In particular, the genes identified with causal mutations for PD are known to be involved in protein aggregation (α-synuclein), function of the ubiquitin-proteasome system (*parkin, UCHL-1*), and mitochondrial function (*PINK1, DJ-1, LRRK2*).[162] Dominant genetic findings implicate the ubiquitin-proteasome system, which facilitates the clearance of degraded proteins from neurons. Impairment of this system can result in the accumulation and aggregation of proteins and subsequent neuronal degeneration.

Mitochondrial dysfunction must also be considered because of the new genetic findings and the toxins used to model the disease. MPTP inhibits the mitochondrial respiratory complex I.[59] Oxidative stress can be linked to mitochondrial dysfunction and has long been considered a prominent pathogenic mechanism in PD because of some properties of substantia nigra neurons. These include the presence of neuromelanin pigment and high iron content, both of which would lead to a greater rate of reactive oxygen species formation. Last, a significant inflammatory response to neuronal death occurs in PD.

More recent work suggests that these potential pathogenic mechanisms do not work in isolation, but rather influence and exacerbate each other to affect neuronal function and survival. The complexity of such interactions gives this disorder its long and slow disease course. Deposition of α-synuclein in Lewy bodies and Lewy neurites is a consistent pathological feature of PD, with small prefibrillar oligomers of α-synuclein proposed as the toxic species. In vitro models have shown that dopamine-dependent oxidative modifications of α-synuclein can facilitate the accumulation of these toxic protofibrils in neurons.[163]

Impairment of the ubiquitin-proteasome system can result in the neuronal aggregation of toxic proteins, but can itself be inhibited by protein accumulation and be impaired through oxidative stress and mitochondrial dysfunction. Inflammation is initially a protective response to neuronal degeneration, but can drive oxidative stress through increased production of reactive oxygen species and can become a self-sustaining degenerative mechanism if the initial trigger for microglial activation is not rectified.[164] Mitochondrial dysfunction is also linked to oxidative stress because mitochondria themselves generate reactive oxygen species to facilitate oxidative mechanisms. The evidence suggests that the mechanisms leading to sporadic PD are linked and that PD is not the result of a single causative factor but is rather multifactorial, integrating many cellular systems to work in concert to induce progressive degeneration in vulnerable neuronal populations.

Implications for Clinical Practice

The current gold standards for symptomatic treatment of PD are neurosurgical intervention and dopamine replacement therapies. Dopamine replacement therapies have great benefit in noninvasively reducing the severity of motor symptoms in PD by redressing the dopamine deficiency in the nigrostriatal pathway. Long-term levodopa treatment can result in motor fluctuations and dyskinesia owing to remodeling in the basal ganglia, however, so the timing, initiation, and type of treatment are important considerations.

Nonmotor symptoms are now recognized as common features of PD and can occur at any stage during the course of the disease. Because the pathological basis for many of these nonmotor features is nondopaminergic, dopamine replacement therapies do not alleviate these symptoms. Alternative or additional measures may need to be considered when treating all aspects of PD. Many of these symptoms (i.e., constipation, olfactory dysfunction, RBD) are more prevalent early.

The increasing scope of genetic anomalies associated with PD provides the opportunity for genetic screening to identify definitively the pathological basis for the disease in life. Although known genetic mutations are rare, the identification of a pathogenic mutation could have significant ramifications for PD patients with family history of the disease.

Greater understanding of the pathological mechanisms of neuronal degeneration and death underlying PD has led to concepts for the development of potential neuroprotective strategies to avert or impede PD neurodegeneration. Examples include antioxidant trials to reduce oxidative stress, providing trophic factors to promote neuronal survival, and the use of anti-inflammatory medications to counteract any inflammatory attack. A significant limitation to the development of neuroprotective agents is the absence of robust biomarkers for the early diagnosis of PD, when such strategies may have the greatest effect, and for monitoring patient responses to such therapeutic interventions.

REFERENCES

1. Polymeropoulos MH, Lavedan C, Leroy E, et al: Mutation in the α-synuclein gene identified in families with Parkinson's disease. Science 1997;276:2045-2057.
2. Spillantini MG, Schmidt ML, Lee VM, et al: α-Synuclein in Lewy bodies. Nature 1997;388:839-840.
3. Zimprich A, Biskup S, Leitner P, et al: Mutations in LRRK2 cause autosomal-dominant parkinsonism with pleomorphic pathology. Neuron 2004;44:601-607.
4. Paisan-Ruiz C, Jain S, Evans EW, et al: Cloning of the gene containing mutations that cause PARK8-linked Parkinson's disease. Neuron 2004;44:595-600.
5. Kitada T, Asakawa S, Hattori N, et al: Mutations in the parkin gene cause autosomal recessive juvenile parkinsonism. Nature 1998;392:605-608.
6. Valente EM, Abou-Sleiman PM, Caputo V, et al: Hereditary early-onset Parkinson's disease caused by mutations in PINK1. Science 2004;304:1158-1160.
7. Bonifati V, Rizzu P, Squitieri F, et al: DJ-1(PARK7), a novel gene for autosomal recessive, early onset parkinsonism. Neurol Sci 2003;24:159-160.

8. Ramirez A, Heimbach A, Grundemann J, et al: Hereditary parkinsonism with dementia is caused by mutations in ATP13A2, encoding a lysosomal type 5 P-type ATPase. Nat Genet 2006;38: 1184-1191.

9. Klein C, Lohmann-Hedrich K: Impact of recent genetic findings in Parkinson's disease. Curr Opin Neurol 2007;20:453-464.

10. Sharma M, Mueller JC, Zimprich A, et al: The sepiapterin reductase gene region reveals association in the PARK3 locus: analysis of familial and sporadic Parkinson's disease in European populations. J Med Genet 2006;43:557-562.

11. Li YJ, Deng J, Mayhew GM, et al: Investigation of the PARK10 gene in Parkinson disease. Ann Hum Genet 2007;71:639-647.

12. Snyder CH, Adler CH: The patient with Parkinson's disease, part I: treating the motor symptoms; part II: treating the nonmotor symptoms. J Am Acad Nurse Pract 2007;19:179-197.

13. Ziemssen T, Reichmann H: Non-motor dysfunction in Parkinson's disease. Parkinsonism Rel Disord 2007;13:323-332.

14. Braak H, Bohl JR, Muller CM, et al: Stanley Fahn Lecture 2005: The staging procedure for the inclusion body pathology associated with sporadic Parkinson's disease reconsidered. Mov Disord 2006;21:2042-2051.

15. de Lau LM, Breteler MM: Epidemiology of Parkinson's disease. Lancet Neurol 2006;5:525-535.

16. Rektor I, Rektorova I, Kubova D: Vascular parkinsonism—an update. J Neurol Sci 2006;248: 185-191.

17. Langston JW, Ballard P, Tetrud JW, Irwin I: Chronic parkinsonism in humans due to a product of meperidine-analog synthesis. Science 1983;219:979-980.

18. Perl DP, Olanow CW: The neuropathology of manganese-induced parkinsonism. J Neuropathol Exp Neurol 2007;66:675-682.

19. Betarbet R, Sherer TB, MacKenzie G, et al: Chronic systemic pesticide exposure reproduces features of Parkinson's disease. Nat Neurosci 2000;3:1301-1306.

20. Lai BC, Marion SA, Teschke K, Tsui JK: Occupational and environmental risk factors for Parkinson's disease. Parkinsonism Rel Disord 2002;8:297-309.

21. Clark LN, Ross BM, Wang Y, et al: Mutations in the glucocerebrosidase gene are associated with early-onset Parkinson disease. Neurology 2007;69:1270-1277.

22. Clark LN, Wang Y, Karlins E, et al: Frequency of LRRK2 mutations in early- and late-onset Parkinson disease. Neurology 2006;67:1786-1791.

23. Lesage S, Durr A, Tazir M, et al: LRRK2 G2019S as a cause of Parkinson's disease in North African Arabs. N Engl J Med 2006;354:422-423.

24. Okubadejo NU: An analysis of genetic studies of Parkinson's disease in Africa. Parkinsonism Rel Disord 2008;14:177-182.

25. Tan EK, Tong J, Fook-Chong S, et al: Glucocerebrosidase mutations and risk of Parkinson disease in Chinese patients. Arch Neurol 2007;64:1056-1058.

26. Ziegler SG, Eblan MJ, Gutti U, et al: Glucocerebrosidase mutations in Chinese subjects from Taiwan with sporadic Parkinson disease. Mol Genet Metab 2007;91:195-200.

27. Biswas A, Maulik M, Das SK, et al: Parkin polymorphisms: risk for Parkinson's disease in Indian population. Clin Genet 2007;72:484-486.

28. Sidransky E: Gaucher disease: complexity in a "simple" disorder. Mol Genet Metab 2004;83:6-15.

29. Braak H, Del Tredici K, Rub U, et al: Staging of brain pathology related to sporadic Parkinson's disease. Neurobiol Aging 2003;24:197-211.

30. Iwai A, Masliah E, Yoshimoto M, et al: The precursor protein of non-Aβ component of Alzheimer's disease amyloid is a presynaptic protein of the central nervous system. Neuron 1995;14: 467-475.

31. Maroteaux L, Campanelli JT, Scheller RH: Synuclein: a neuron-specific protein localized to the nucleus and presynaptic nerve terminal. J Neurosci 1988;8:2804-2815.

32. Danzer KM, Haasen D, Karow AR, et al: Different species of α-synuclein oligomers induce calcium influx and seeding. J Neurosci 2007;27:9220-9232.

33. Fujiwara H, Hasegawa M, Dohmae N, et al: α-Synuclein is phosphorylated in synucleinopathy lesions. Nat Cell Biol 2002;4:160-164.

34. Wakabayashi K, Hayashi S, Yoshimoto M, et al: NACP/α-synuclein-positive filamentous inclusions in astrocytes and oligodendrocytes of Parkinson's disease brains. Acta Neuropathol 2000;99:14-20.

35. Braak H, Sastre M, Del Tredici K: Development of α-synuclein immunoreactive astrocytes in the forebrain parallels stages of intraneuronal pathology in sporadic Parkinson's disease. Acta Neuropathol 2007;114:231-241.

36. Teismann P, Schulz JB: Cellular pathology of Parkinson's disease: astrocytes, microglia and inflammation. Cell Tissue Res 2004;318:149-161.

37. Feldmann A, Illes Z, Kosztolanyi P, et al: Morphometric changes of gray matter in Parkinson's disease with depression: a voxel-based morphometry study. Mov Disord 2008;23:42-46

38. Pedersen KM, Marner L, Pakkenberg H, Pakkenberg B: No global loss of neocortical neurons in Parkinson's disease: a quantitative stereological study. Mov Disord 2005;20:164-171.

39. Damier P, Hirsch EC, Agid Y, Graybiel AM: The substantia nigra of the human brain, II: patterns of loss of dopamine-containing neurons in Parkinson's disease. Brain 1999;122:1437-1448.

40. Fearnley JM, Lees AJ: Ageing and Parkinson's disease: substantia nigra regional selectivity. Brain 1991;114:2283-2301.

41. Greffard S, Verny M, Bonnet AM, et al: Motor score of the Unified Parkinson Disease Rating Scale as a good predictor of Lewy body-associated neuronal loss in the substantia nigra. Arch Neurol 2006;63:584-588.

42. McRitchie DA, Cartwright HR, Halliday GM: Specific A10 dopaminergic nuclei in the midbrain degenerate in Parkinson's disease. Exp Neurol 1997;144:202-213.

43. Sanchez-Gonzalez MA, Garcia-Cabezas MA, Rico B, Cavada C: The primate thalamus is a key target for brain dopamine. J Neurosci 2005;25:6076-6083.

44. Harding AJ, Stimson E, Henderson JM, Halliday GM: Clinical correlates of selective pathology in the amygdala of patients with Parkinson's disease. Brain 2002;125:2431-2445.

45. Jellinger KA: Cell death mechanisms in Parkinson's disease. J Neural Transm 2000;107:1-29.

46. Thannickal TC, Lai YY, Siegel JM: Hypocretin (orexin) cell loss in Parkinson's disease. Brain 2007;130:1586-1595.

47. Hoogendijk WJ, Pool CW, Troost D, et al: Image analyser-assisted morphometry of the locus coeruleus in Alzheimer's disease, Parkinson's disease and amyotrophic lateral sclerosis. Brain 1995;118:131-143.

48. Halliday GM, Li YW, Blumbergs PC, et al: Neuropathology of immunohistochemically identified brainstem neurons in Parkinson's disease. Ann Neurol 1990;27:373-385.

49. Halliday GM, Macdonald V, Henderson JM: A comparison of degeneration in motor thalamus and cortex between progressive supranuclear palsy and Parkinson's disease. Brain 2005;128:2272-2280.

50. McGeer PL, McGeer EG: Glial reactions in Parkinson's disease. Mov Disord 2008;23:474-483.

51. Imamura K, Hishikawa N, Sawada M, et al: Distribution of major histocompatibility complex class II-positive microglia and cytokine profile of Parkinson's disease brains. Acta Neuropathol 2003;106:518-526.

52. Block ML, Hong JS: Chronic microglial activation and progressive dopaminergic neurotoxicity. Biochem Soc Trans 2007;35:1127-1132.

53. Zecca L, Zucca FA, Albertini A, et al: A proposed dual role of neuromelanin in the pathogenesis of Parkinson's disease. Neurology 2006;67(Suppl 2):S8-S11.

54. Beach TG, Sue LI, Walker DG, et al: Marked microglial reaction in normal aging human substantia nigra: correlation with extraneuronal neuromelanin pigment deposits. Acta Neuropathol 2007;114:419-424.

55. Croisier E, Moran LB, Dexter DT, et al: Microglial inflammation in the parkinsonian substantia nigra: relationship to α-synuclein deposition. J Neuroinflamm 2005;2:14.

56. Zhang W, Qin L, Wang T, et al: 3-Hydroxymorphinan is neurotrophic to dopaminergic neurons and is also neuroprotective against LPS-induced neurotoxicity. Faseb J 2005;19:395-397.

57. Chen H, Jacobs E, Schwarzschild MA, et al: Nonsteroidal antiinflammatory drug use and the risk for Parkinson's disease. Ann Neurol 2005;58:963-967.

58. McGeer PL, Schwab C, Parent A, Doudet D: Presence of reactive microglia in monkey substantia nigra years after 1-methyl-4-phenyl-1,2,3,6-tetrahydropyridine administration. Ann Neurol 2003;54:599-604.

59. Langston JW, Forno LS, Tetrud J, et al: Evidence of active nerve cell degeneration in the substantia nigra of humans years after 1-methyl-4-phenyl-1,2,3,6-tetrahydropyridine exposure. Ann Neurol 1999;46:598-605.

60. Jellinger KA: Morphological substrates of parkinsonism with and without dementia: a retrospective clinico-pathological study. J Neural Transm 2007;72:91-104.

61. Jellinger KA: Prevalence of cerebrovascular lesions in Parkinson's disease: a postmortem study. Acta Neuropathol 2003;105:415-419.

62. Mastaglia FL, Johnsen RD, Kakulas BA: Prevalence of stroke in Parkinson's disease: a postmortem study. Mov Disord 2002;17:772-774.

63. Jellinger KA: Prevalence of Alzheimer lesions in Parkinson's disease. Mov Disord 2003;18:1207-1208.
64. Albin RL, Young AB, Penney JB: The functional anatomy of basal ganglia disorders. Trends Neurosci 1989;12:366-375.
65. Chaudhuri KR, Healy DG, Schapira AH: Non-motor symptoms of Parkinson's disease: diagnosis and management. Lancet Neurol 2006;5:235-245.
66. Wolters EC: Variability in the clinical expression of Parkinson's disease. J Neurol Sci 2008;266:197-203.
67. Bernheimer H, Birkmayer W, Hornykiewicz O, et al: Brain dopamine and the syndromes of Parkinson and Huntington: clinical, morphological and neurochemical correlations. J Neurol Sci 1973;20:415-455.
68. Otsuka M, Ichiya Y, Kuwabara Y, et al: Differences in the reduced 18F-Dopa uptakes of the caudate and the putamen in Parkinson's disease: correlations with the three main symptoms. J Neurol Sci 1996;136:169-173.
69. Joel D, Weiner I: The connections of the dopaminergic system with the striatum in rats and primates: an analysis with respect to the functional and compartmental organization of the striatum. Neuroscience 2000;96:451-474.
70. Smith Y, Kieval JZ: Anatomy of the dopamine system in the basal ganglia. Trends Neurosci 2000;23(Suppl):S28-S33.
71. Obeso JA, Rodriguez-Oroz MC, Rodriguez M, et al: Pathophysiology of the basal ganglia in Parkinson's disease. Trends Neurosci 2000;23(Suppl):S8-S19.
72. Blandini F, Nappi G, Tassorelli C, Martignoni E: Functional changes of the basal ganglia circuitry in Parkinson's disease. Prog Neurobiol 2000;62:63-88.
73. Orieux G, Francois C, Feger J, et al: Metabolic activity of excitatory parafascicular and pedunculopontine inputs to the subthalamic nucleus in a rat model of Parkinson's disease. Neuroscience 2000;97:79-88.
74. Rodriguez MC, Obeso JA, Olanow CW: Subthalamic nucleus-mediated excitotoxicity in Parkinson's disease: a target for neuroprotection. Ann Neurol 1998;44;(Suppl 1):S175-S188.
75. Smith ID, Grace AA: Role of the subthalamic nucleus in the regulation of nigral dopamine neuron activity. Synapse 1992;12:287-303.
76. Brown P, Williams D: Basal ganglia local field potential activity: character and functional significance in the human. Clin Neurophysiol 2005;116:2510-2519.
77. DeLong MR, Wichmann T: Circuits and circuit disorders of the basal ganglia. Arch Neurol 2007;64:20-24.
78. Agid Y, Ahlskog E, Albanese A, et al: Levodopa in the treatment of Parkinson's disease: a consensus meeting. Mov Disord 1999;14:911-913.
79. Benabid AL, Pollak P, Gross C, et al: Acute and long-term effects of subthalamic nucleus stimulation in Parkinson's disease. Stereotact Funct Neurosurg 1994;62:76-84.
80. Hubble JP, Busenbark KL, Wilkinson S, et al: Effects of thalamic deep brain stimulation based on tremor type and diagnosis. Mov Disord 1997;12:337-341.
81. Bergman H, Feingold A, Nini A, et al: Physiological aspects of information processing in the basal ganglia of normal and parkinsonian primates. Trends Neurosci 1998;21:32-38.
82. Bergman H, Deuschl G: Pathophysiology of Parkinson's disease: from clinical neurology to basic neuroscience and back. Mov Disord 2002;17(Suppl 3):S28-S40.
83. Plaha P, Filipovic S, Gill SS: Induction of parkinsonian resting tremor by stimulation of the caudal zona incerta nucleus: a clinical study. J Neurol Neurosurg Psychiatry 2008;79:514-521
84. Merello M, Tenca E, Cerquetti D: Neuronal activity of the zona incerta in Parkinson's disease patients. Mov Disord 2006;21:937-943.
85. Perier C, Vila M, Feger J, et al: Functional activity of zona incerta neurons is altered after nigrostriatal denervation in hemiparkinsonian rats. Exp Neurol 2000;162:215-224.
86. Pahapill PA, Lozano AM: The pedunculopontine nucleus and Parkinson's disease. Brain 2000;123:1767-1783.
87. Henderson JM, Carpenter K, Cartwright H, Halliday GM: Degeneration of the centre median-parafascicular complex in Parkinson's disease. Ann Neurol 2000;47:345-352.
88. Henderson JM, Carpenter K, Cartwright H, Halliday GM: Loss of thalamic intralaminar nuclei in progressive supranuclear palsy and Parkinson's disease: clinical and therapeutic implications. Brain 2000;123:1410-1421.
89. Ozawa T, Paviour D, Quinn NP, et al: The spectrum of pathological involvement of the striato-nigral and olivopontocerebellar systems in multiple system atrophy: clinicopathological correlations. Brain 2004;127:2657-2671.

90. Drake DF, Harkins S, Qutubuddin A: Pain in Parkinson's disease: pathology to treatment, medication to deep brain stimulation. NeuroRehabilitation 2005;20:335-341.

91. Scherder EJ, Sergeant JA, Swaab DF: Pain processing in dementia and its relation to neuropathology. Lancet Neurol 2003;2:677-686.

92. Scherder E, Wolters E, Polman C, et al: Pain in Parkinson's disease and multiple sclerosis: its relation to the medial and lateral pain systems. Neurosci Biobehav Rev 2005;29:1047-1056.

93. Sewards TV, Sewards MA: The medial pain system: neural representations of the motivational aspect of pain. Brain Res Bull 2002;59:163-180.

94. Braak H, Rub U, Sandmann-Keil D, et al: Parkinson's disease: affection of brain stem nuclei controlling premotor and motor neurons of the somatomotor system. Acta Neuropathol 2000;99:489-495.

95. Rub U, Del Tredici K, Schultz C, et al: Parkinson's disease: the thalamic components of the limbic loop are severely impaired by α-synuclein immunopositive inclusion body pathology. Neurobiol Aging 2002;23:245-254.

96. Djaldetti R, Shifrin A, Rogowski Z, et al: Quantitative measurement of pain sensation in patients with Parkinson disease. Neurology 2004;62:2171-2175.

97. Jellinger KA: α-Synuclein lesions in normal aging, Parkinson disease, and Alzheimer disease: evidence from the Baltimore Longitudinal Study of Aging (BLSA). J Neuropathol Exp Neurol 2005;64:554.

98. Dubow JS: Autonomic dysfunction in Parkinson's disease. Dis Month 2007;53:265-274.

99. Wakabayashi K, Takahashi H: Neuropathology of autonomic nervous system in Parkinson's disease. Eur Neurol 1997;38(Suppl 2):2-7.

100. Iwanaga K, Wakabayashi K, Yoshimoto M, et al: Lewy body-type degeneration in cardiac plexus in Parkinson's and incidental Lewy body diseases. Neurology 1999;52:1269-1271.

101. Orimo S, Amino T, Itoh Y, et al: Cardiac sympathetic denervation precedes neuronal loss in the sympathetic ganglia in Lewy body disease. Acta Neuropathol 2005;109:583-588.

102. Orimo S, Takahashi A, Uchihara T, et al: Degeneration of cardiac sympathetic nerve begins in the early disease process of Parkinson's disease. Brain Pathol 2007;17:24-30.

103. Takeda S, Yamazaki K, Miyakawa T, Arai H: Parkinson's disease with involvement of the parasympathetic ganglia. Acta Neuropathol 1993;86:397-398.

104. Haehner A, Hummel T, Hummel C, et al: Olfactory loss may be a first sign of idiopathic Parkinson's disease. Mov Disord 2007;22:839-842.

105. Ross GW, Abbott RD, Petrovitch H, et al: Association of olfactory dysfunction with incidental Lewy bodies. Mov Disord 2006;21:2062-2067.

106. Del Tredici K, Rub U, De Vos RA, et al: Where does Parkinson disease pathology begin in the brain? J Neuropathol Exp Neurol 2002;61:413-426.

107. Pearce RK, Hawkes CH, Daniel SE: The anterior olfactory nucleus in Parkinson's disease. Mov Disord 1995;10:283-287.

108. Bohnen NI, Gedela S, Kuwabara H, et al: Selective hyposmia and nigrostriatal dopaminergic denervation in Parkinson's disease. J Neurol 2007;254:84-90.

109. Doty RL, Singh A, Tetrud J, Langston JW: Lack of major olfactory dysfunction in MPTP-induced parkinsonism. Ann Neurol 1992;32:97-100.

110. Huisman E, Uylings HB, Hoogland PV: A 100% increase of dopaminergic cells in the olfactory bulb may explain hyposmia in Parkinson's disease. Mov Disord 2004;19:687-692.

111. Swanson LW, Petrovich GD: What is the amygdala? Trends Neurosci 1998;21:323-331.

112. Lu J, Sherman D, Devor M, Saper CB: A putative flip-flop switch for control of REM sleep. Nature 2006;441:589-594.

113. Zweig RM, Jankel WR, Hedreen JC, et al: The pedunculopontine nucleus in Parkinson's disease. Ann Neurol 1989;26:41-46.

114. Boeve BF, Silber MH, Saper CB, et al: Pathophysiology of REM sleep behaviour disorder and relevance to neurodegenerative disease. Brain 2007;130:2770-2788.

115. Hanoglu L, Ozer F, Meral H, Dincer A: Brainstem 1H-MR spectroscopy in patients with Parkinson's disease with REM sleep behavior disorder and IPD patients without dream enactment behavior. Clin Neurol Neurosurg 2006;108:129-134.

116. Comella CL: Sleep disorders in Parkinson's disease: an overview. Mov Disord 2007;22;(S17): S367-S373.

117. Gjerstad MD, Alves G, Wentzel-Larsen T, et al: Excessive daytime sleepiness in Parkinson disease: is it the drugs or the disease? Neurology 2006;67:853-858.

118. Matsui H, Nishinaka K, Oda M, et al: Excessive daytime sleepiness in Parkinson disease: a SPECT study. Sleep 2006;29:917-920.

119. Mercury MG, Tschan W, Kehoe R, Kuechler A: The presence of depression and anxiety in Parkinson's disease. Dis Month 2007;53:296-301.
120. Zweig RM, Cardillo JE, Cohen M, et al: The locus ceruleus and dementia in Parkinson's disease. Neurology 1993;43:986-991.
121. Remy P, Doder M, Lees A, et al: Depression in Parkinson's disease: loss of dopamine and noradrenaline innervation in the limbic system. Brain 2005;128:1314-1322.
122. Mayberg HS, Solomon DH: Depression in Parkinson's disease: a biochemical and organic viewpoint. Adv Neurol 1995;65:49-60.
123. Torack RM, Morris JC: The association of ventral tegmental area histopathology with adult dementia. Arch Neurol 1988;45:497-501.
124. Sakas DE, Panourias IG: Rostral cingulate gyrus: a putative target for deep brain stimulation in treatment-refractory depression. Med Hypoth 2006;66:491-494.
125. Kovari E, Gold G, Herrmann FR, et al: Lewy body densities in the entorhinal and anterior cingulate cortex predict cognitive deficits in Parkinson's disease. Acta Neuropathol 2003;106:83-88.
126. Fregni F, Ono CR, Santos CM, et al: Effects of antidepressant treatment with rTMS and fluoxetine on brain perfusion in PD. Neurology 2006;66:1629-1637.
127. Diederich NJ, Goetz CG, Stebbins GT: Repeated visual hallucinations in Parkinson's disease as disturbed external/internal perceptions: focused review and a new integrative model. Mov Disord 2005;20:130-140.
128. Onofrj M, Bonanni L, Albani G, et al: Visual hallucinations in Parkinson's disease: clues to separate origins. J Neurol Sci 2006;248:143-150.
129. Imamura K, Wada-Isoe K, Kitayama M, Nakashima K: Executive dysfunction in non-demented Parkinson's disease patients with hallucinations. Acta Neurol Scand 2008;117:255-259.
130. Williams DR, Lees AJ: Visual hallucinations in the diagnosis of idiopathic Parkinson's disease: a retrospective autopsy study. Lancet Neurol 2005;4:605-610.
131. Harding AJ, Broe GA, Halliday GM: Visual hallucinations in Lewy body disease relate to Lewy bodies in the temporal lobe. Brain 2002;125:391-403.
132. Papapetropoulos S, McCorquodale DS, Gonzalez J, et al: Cortical and amygdalar Lewy body burden in Parkinson's disease patients with visual hallucinations. Parkinsonism Rel Disord 2006;12:253-256.
133. Caballol N, Marti MJ, Tolosa E: Cognitive dysfunction and dementia in Parkinson disease. Mov Disord 2007;22(Suppl 17):S358-S366.
134. Carbon M, Ma Y, Barnes A, et al: Caudate nucleus: influence of dopaminergic input on sequence learning and brain activation in parkinsonism. Neuroimage 2004;21:1497-1507.
135. Rinne JO, Rummukainen J, Paljarvi L, Rinne UK: Dementia in Parkinson's disease is related to neuronal loss in the medial substantia nigra. Ann Neurol 1989;26:47-50.
136. Lewis SJ, Dove A, Robbins TW, et al: Striatal contributions to working memory: a functional magnetic resonance imaging study in humans. Eur J Neurosci 2004;19:755-760.
137. Owen AM, Doyon J, Dagher A, et al: Abnormal basal ganglia outflow in Parkinson's disease identified with PET: implications for higher cortical functions. Brain 1998;121:949-965.
138. Dubois B, Pillon B: Cognitive deficits in Parkinson's disease. J Neurol 1997;244:2-8.
139. Pillon B, Czernecki V, Dubois B: Dopamine and cognitive function. Curr Opin Neurol 2003;16(Suppl 2):S17-S22.
140. Bosboom JL, Stoffers D, Wolters E: Cognitive dysfunction and dementia in Parkinson's disease. J Neural Transm 2004;111:1303-1315.
141. Levy G, Tang MX, Cote LJ, et al: Motor impairment in PD: relationship to incident dementia and age. Neurology 2000;55:539-544.
142. Everitt BJ, Robbins TW: Central cholinergic systems and cognition. Annu Rev Psychol 1997;48:649-684.
143. Perry EK, Curtis M, Dick DJ, et al: Cholinergic correlates of cognitive impairment in Parkinson's disease: comparisons with Alzheimer's disease. J Neurol Neurosurg Psychiatry 1985;48:413-421.
144. Dubois B, Ruberg M, Javoy-Agid F, et al: A subcortico-cortical cholinergic system is affected in Parkinson's disease. Brain Res 1983;288:213-218.
145. Rinne JO, Myllykyla T, Lonnberg P, Marjamaki P: A postmortem study of brain nicotinic receptors in Parkinson's and Alzheimer's disease. Brain Res 1991;547:167-170.
146. Haroutunian V, Serby M, Purohit DP, et al: Contribution of Lewy body inclusions to dementia in patients with and without Alzheimer disease neuropathological conditions. Arch Neurol 2000;57:1145-1150.
147. Hurtig HI, Trojanowski JQ, Galvin J, et al: α-Synuclein cortical Lewy bodies correlate with dementia in Parkinson's disease. Neurology 2000;54:1916-1921.

148. Galvin JE: Cognitive change in Parkinson disease. Alzheimer Dis Assoc Disord 2006;20:302-310.
149. Whitehouse PJ, Hedreen JC, White CL 3rd, Price DL: Basal forebrain neurons in the dementia of Parkinson disease. Ann Neurol 1983;13:243-248.
150. Braak H, Rub U, Del Tredici K: Cognitive decline correlates with neuropathological stage in Parkinson's disease. J Neurol Sci 2006;248:255-258.
151. Harding AJ, Halliday GM: Cortical Lewy body pathology in the diagnosis of dementia. Acta Neuropathol 2001;102:355-363.
152. Apaydin H, Ahlskog JE, Parisi JE, et al: Parkinson disease neuropathology: later-developing dementia and loss of the levodopa response. Arch Neurol 2002;59:102-112.
153. Mattila PM, Roytta M, Torikka H, et al: Cortical Lewy bodies and Alzheimer-type changes in patients with Parkinson's disease. Acta Neuropathol 1998;95:576-582.
154. Mattila PM, Rinne JO, Helenius H, et al: α-Synuclein-immunoreactive cortical Lewy bodies are associated with cognitive impairment in Parkinson's disease. Acta Neuropathol 2000;100: 285-290.
155. Colosimo C, Hughes AJ, Kilford L, Lees AJ: Lewy body cortical involvement may not always predict dementia in Parkinson's disease. J Neurol Neurosurg Psychiatry 2003;74:852-856.
156. de Vos RA, Jansen EN, Stam FC, et al: 'Lewy body disease': clinico-pathological correlations in 18 consecutive cases of Parkinson's disease with and without dementia. Clin Neurol Neurosurg 1995;97:13-22.
157. McKeith IG: Consensus guidelines for the clinical and pathologic diagnosis of dementia with Lewy bodies (DLB): report of the Consortium on DLB International Workshop. J Alzheimers Dis 2006;9(Suppl):417-423.
158. Jellinger KA, Seppi K, Wenning GK, Poewe W: Impact of coexistent Alzheimer pathology on the natural history of Parkinson's disease. J Neural Transm 2002;109:329-339.
159. Jendroska K: The relationship of Alzheimer-type pathology to dementia in Parkinson's disease. J Neural Transm 1997;49:23-31.
160. Vermersch P, Delacourte A, Javoy-Agid F, et al: Dementia in Parkinson's disease: biochemical evidence for cortical involvement using the immunodetection of abnormal Tau proteins. Ann Neurol 1993;33:445-450.
161. Hughes AJ, Daniel SE, Blankson S, Lees AJ: A clinicopathologic study of: 100 cases of Parkinson's disease. Arch Neurol 1993;50:140-148.
162. Thomas B, Beal MF: Parkinson's disease. Hum Mol Genet 2007;16;(Spec No: 2):R183-R194.
163. Ischiropoulos H: Oxidative modifications of α-synuclein. Ann N Y Acad Sci 2003;991:93-100.
164. Tansey MG, McCoy MK: Frank-Cannon TC: Neuroinflammatory mechanisms in Parkinson's disease: potential environmental triggers, pathways, and targets for early therapeutic intervention. Exp Neurol 2007;208:1-25.
165. Forno LS: Neuropathology of Parkinson's disease. J Neuropathol Exp Neurol 1996;55:259-272.

10 | Pathogenesis of Parkinson's Disease

AMITABH GUPTA • TED M. DAWSON

Introduction	**Observations beyond Known Parkinson's Disease Genes**
Insights from Genetics	Cellular Pacemaker Activity
α-Synuclein	and Parkinson's Disease
Parkin	Deacetylation and Parkinson's
LRRK2	Disease
DJ-1	
PINK1	**Conclusions**

Introduction

Since the clinical application of levodopa for the treatment of Parkinson's disease (PD), research into PD has yielded only incremental progress into understanding the mechanism of disease. The last decade has shown a revival of excitement and optimism, however, lending in great part to the tremendous progress made in the field of neurogenetics. Although familial cases make up only a small percentage of PD cases overall, the discovery of their underlying genetic defects has provided several novel proteins that—when mutated—are involved in the disease process. Essentially, the genetic approach has given the research community the future challenge to connect these proteins into a meaningful signaling cascade that may explain the pattern-selective neurodegeneration observed in PD.

Much of the drive to define signaling pathways is based on the assumption that PD is a single disease entity, implicating an expectation that pattern-selective cell death in PD can be explained in a uniform and all-encompassing fashion by disturbances at different points along a specific cell signaling network. This assumption may not hold true, however, in light of the clinical variability observed with idiopathic PD. This chapter primarily discusses more recent advances from neurogenetic research. At the end of this chapter, however, we will also highlight some observations from research that is not related to specific PD genes but appears to be converging with the insights obtained from neurogenetics.

Insights from Genetics

The currently known genes underlying familial PD cases are summarized in Table 10–1. They were discussed in detail in the context of genetics in the previous chapters. We focus here on the molecular research data available on the proteins

TABLE 10–1   Genetic Forms of Parkinson's Disease (PD)*

Form	Pattern of Inheritance	Chromosome Region	Name of Gene	Gene Identified	Name of Protein	Function of Protein
Familial PD	AD	4q21-q22	PARK1	Yes	α-Synuclein	Synaptic protein
Young-onset PD	AR/AD	6q25.2-q27	PARK2	Yes	Parkin	Ubiquitin-protein ligase
Susceptibility locus	AD	2p13	PARK3	No	N/I	N/I
Familial PD	AD	4q region	PARK4	Yes	Multiplication of α-synuclein chromosomal region	Excess α-synuclein protein
Familial PD	AR	4p15	PARK5	Yes	Ubiquitin carboxy-terminal hydrolase L1	Splits conjugated ubiquitin into monomers
Young-onset PD	AR	1p35-p36	PARK6	Yes	PINK1	Mitochondrial stress-induced degeneration
Young-onset PD	AR	1p36	PARK7	Yes	DJ-1	Sumoylation pathway, oxidative stress protection
Familial PD	AD	12p11.2-q13.1	PARK8	Yes	LRRK2 Dardarin	Protein Phosphorylation

Familial PD	AR	1p32	PARK10 (Iceland)	No	N/I	N/I
Familial PD	AD	2q36-q37	PARK11	Yes	N/I	N/I
Familial PD	X-linked recessive	Xq21-q25	PARK12	No	N/I	N/I
Familial PD	AD	2p12	PARK13	Yes	Serine protease HTRA2	Mitochondrial stress response
Familial PD	AD	1q21	Glucose cerebrosidase	Yes	Glucose cerebrosidase	Presumed membrane function
Familial PD	AD	2q22-q23	Nurr1	Yes	Nurr1	Transcriptional activator; dopaminergic neuronal development
Infantile/childhood PD	AR	11p11.5	Tyrosine hydroxylase	Yes	Tyrosine hydroxylase	Tyrosine to levodopa conversion
Familial PD	Mitochondrial	Mitochondria	N/I	No	N/I	Complex 1
Familial PD	Mitochondrial	Mitochondria	ND4	Yes	N/I	Complex 1
Familial PD	Susceptibility gene	17q21	Tau	Yes	Tau	Fibrils
Familial PD	AR	15q25	POLG	Yes	mtDNA polymerase gamma	Synthesis, replication, and repair of mtDNA

*Not included in table are Kufor-Rakeb syndrome (PARK9), dopa-responsive dystonia (DRD), and spinocerebellar ataxia 2 (SCA2) because PD symptoms are not the primary manifestation.

AD, autosomal dominant; AR, autosomal recessive; N/I, not identified.

Modified from Fahn S, Jankovic J: Principles and Practice of Movement Disorders. Churchill Livingston, NY 2007.

that these genes encode and the implications for future basic research and clinical investigation.

α-SYNUCLEIN

α-Synuclein was the first of the genes found to be mutated in a familial form of PD. Point mutations are located at three amino acids, A53T, A30P, and E46K, and act as gain-of-function mutations, consistent with the autosomal dominant pattern of inheritance.[1] Simple overexpression of wild-type α-synuclein also leads to PD.[1] Evidence for the toxic effect of α-synuclein in PD is solid, given that the requirement of α-synuclein for neurodegeneration is established in mouse models of PD.[2] In addition, α-synuclein is required for the degeneration of the nigrostriatal system induced by toxins such as 1-methyl-4-phenyl-1,2,3,6-tetrahydropyridine (MPTP) and 6-hydroxydopamine because mice lacking α-synuclein are resistant to these dopaminergic toxins.[3,4] Whether the toxic effect of α-synuclein is mediated through fibrils, protofibrils, small oligomers, or the large α-synuclein aggregates remains an open question. The toxicity of α-synuclein is related to its propensity to aggregate, and it is likely that toxicity of α-synuclein represents a continuum along the path to higher ordered aggregates.[5]

α-Synuclein comprises 140 amino acids. It is primarily localized to the cytoplasm and may be involved in a wide array of cellular functions, including vesicular dopamine release and synaptic plasticity. Results from mice that lack α-synuclein suggest that the protein acts as an activity-dependent presynaptic negative regulator of dopamine neurotransmission, although striatal dopamine levels are decreased in these mice.[6] Some investigators suggest that α-synuclein may regulate dopamine release through a complex protein scaffold, interacting with septin 4, the dopamine transporter, and other presynaptic proteins to maintain synaptic structural integrity.[7] Loss of septin 4 in mice that overexpress A53T human α-synuclein leads to increased neuropathology and locomotor disability, indicating that disruptions of the protein scaffold could affect α-synuclein function and induce neurodegeneration. Septin 4 may normally protect α-synuclein from phosphorylation at Ser129 and self-aggregation into toxic insoluble deposits.[7]

Other research suggests that α-synuclein aggregation perturbs the structural integrity of endosomes, lysosomes, and the plasma membrane at the synapse, and impedes the function of the endoplasmic reticulum and the Golgi apparatus. α-Synuclein aggregation can generally result in endoplasmic reticulum stress, but it also seems to inhibit specifically vesicular transport from the endoplasmic reticulum to the Golgi apparatus.[8] The guanosine triphosphatase Rab1 can rescue this inhibition of vesicular transfer, as it acts at the very same step, and protect against α-synuclein–induced dopaminergic neuron loss in animal models of PD.[8] α-Synuclein overexpression also rescues the neurodegenerative phenotype of cysteine-string protein knockout mice, suggesting that α-synuclein might function as a chaperone to maintain the integrity of the presynaptic terminal.[9]

Whatever the primary function of α-synuclein may be under healthy conditions, the accumulation of this protein in the disease state seems to be central to neurodegeneration.[10] An important aspect of understanding PD pathogenesis involves comprehension of how α-synuclein is cleared from the cell. Intervening with α-synuclein accumulation presents a tremendous opportunity for developing an effective treatment. α-Synuclein that accumulates in Lewy bodies may be degraded through the proteasome.[11,12] This observation led to the notion that abnormal function of the ubiquitin proteasome system (UPS) or proteasomal inability to degrade mutant α-synuclein may result in α-synuclein aggregation, inclusion body formation, and neurodegeneration in PD. In line with this possibility, proteasomal inhibition and overexpression of α-synuclein together with one of its targets, synphilin, resulted in increased cell death.[13,14]

The UPS usually degrades proteins with shorter half-life (<10 hours), and several investigators showed that the protein half-life of α-synuclein is often around 16 hours. Given that some investigators could not detect increased α-synuclein levels in the presence of proteasomal inhibition, and proteins with longer half-lives are degraded by autophagic pathways within lysosomes, it was subsequently found that α-synuclein can also be degraded by lysosomes. Such degradation can occur by the subtype of autophagy called chaperone-mediated autophagy (CMA) that involves the hsc70 chaperone and the lysosomal membrane receptor, lamp2a.[15]

Mutated α-synuclein is not properly degraded by CMA, although it still binds lamp2a. Mutant α-synuclein may act as an uptake blocker, inhibiting its own degradation and that of other autophagic substrates.[15] It seems that wild-type α-synuclein is degraded by CMA in addition to the UPS, whereas the mutant form of α-synuclein may be resistant to this pathway.[16] Other investigators have found that chaperone-independent autophagy, called macroautophagy, may play an important role in degrading aggregated α-synuclein.[17,18] Based on these findings, the notion has been entertained that wild-type α-synuclein is degraded by CMA, whereas mutant α-synuclein in aggregated form is cleared by the macroautophagy system.[17,18] The notion that perturbation of the autophagy system itself, as seen in settings of degenerative cellular stress, may facilitate α-synuclein toxicity also has been entertained.

As a result of the more recent advances in understanding the clearance mechanisms of α-synuclein aggregates, therapeutic strategies for facilitating α-synuclein clearance are actively pursued. Similar to the development of β-amyloid antibodies in Alzheimer's disease, one attractive approach is to develop immunoantibodies to oligomeric α-synuclein, using active immunization with corresponding α-synuclein material.[19] Active immunization reduced α-synuclein accumulation and pathology in PD mice models in preliminary tests. Based on data from these experiments, antibodies directed mostly against the C-terminus of α-synuclein were selected for passive immunization trials. Promising results were also obtained when the antibodies were injected intrathecally into PD mice models. The protective effect of the antibodies was reduced by lysosomal inhibitors, indicating that autophagy-mediated clearance may by involved in the degradation of α-synuclein aggregates.

Ongoing research in the related field of multiple systems atrophy has been therapeutically valuable as well. Multiple systems atrophy is a multisystem degenerative disease that can manifest with parkinsonism and shows α-synuclein aggregation mostly in glial cells. Because the consistent with the observation that the antibiotic rifampicin can inhibit α-Synuclein oligomerization,[20] application of rifampicin to the multiple systems atrophy mouse model reduces α-Synuclein aggregation and improves motor performance. In extension, rifampicin is being tested in PD mice models as well to assess its effectiveness. α-Synuclein is also cleaved by unknown α-synucleinases, which enhances its propensity to aggregate into toxic complexes.[21] Drugs that inhibit the cleavage of α-synuclein may provide great benefit to PD patients.

PARKIN

Parkin is an E3 ubiquitin ligase[22-24]; this supports the notion that UPS dysfunction may contribute to neurodegeneration in PD. Because mutant parkin is thought to be inherited in a recessive fashion, loss-of-function of parkin seems to lead to UPS dysfunction, the accumulation of parkin substrates, and subsequent neurodegeneration. Consistent with such a seemingly linear view of these events, overexpression of parkin improved UPS dysfunction and associated neurodegeneration,[25] whereas targeted reduction of parkin expression augmented neurodegeneration.[25] Importantly, however, it has not been clarified whether the accumulation of parkin substrates or UPS dysfunction directly causes cell death.

Because α-synuclein is a principal component of the Lewy body, a molecular interaction between parkin and α-synuclein would be an attractive unifying theory of PD pathogenesis. Because mutations in both proteins are also prominent genetic causes of familial PD, this would provide support for the notion that genetic interactions can indicate molecular interactions. In this sense, it could be envisioned that parkin loss-of-function results in defective degradation of α-synuclein in the UPS system, with subsequent aggregation and eventual accumulation of α-synuclein in Lewy bodies. It was observed that the phenotype of mice double mutant for parkin (loss-of-function) and human A53T α-synuclein (overexpression) was essentially identical to that of mice solely overexpressing A53T α-synuclein.[26] This observation indicates that parkin function does not have a significant impact on α-synuclein processing, implying that PD caused by parkin and α-synuclein mutations may have independent mechanisms.

In support of this idea, patients with PD caused by parkin—in contrast to patients with PD caused by α-synuclein—do not show Lewy body formation, which may indicate that proteins require further processing in the UPS before they eventually accumulate. The parkin substrate synphilin,[27] which also is an α-synuclein interacting protein,[28] forms Lewy body–like, ubiquitin-positive inclusions only when coexpressed with α-synuclein and wild-type parkin, but not with loss-of-function parkin.[27] These results suggest that loss of ubiquitination alone may not cause protein aggregation, and that a functional interaction between parkin and α-synuclein pathways in vivo may not be a logical consequence of (indirect) molecular interactions between these two proteins.

Aminoacyl-tRNA synthetase (ARS)–interacting multifunctional protein type 2 (AIMP2) (p38/JTV-1) and the Far Upstream Element-binding Protein-1 (FBP-1) seem to be authentic parkin substrates because they accumulate in parkin-deficient mice and in autosomal recessive PD caused by parkin mutations.[29,30] AIMP2 is selectively toxic to dopaminergic neurons.[30]

What are the ways in which parkin function is modulated? In line with abnormal protein degradation being important for the pathogenesis of PD, parkin has been shown to interact directly with Hsp70.[31] Because-Hsp70 is a heat shock protein that prevents protein misfolding when the cell is exposed to heat or other stressors, it is assumed that modulation of the parkin–Hsp70 interaction may result in proteins bypassing degradation, misfolding, and subsequently aggregating. Parkin E3 activity may be carefully regulated by Hsp70 protein complexes; this may explain partly how overexpression of the heat shock protein Hsp70 can reduce cell toxicity and enhance cell survival in PD models.[32] Alternatively, E4-like molecules, such as CHIP, may separate Hsp70 from parkin, allowing parkin to ubiquinate unfolded proteins, such as unfolded Parkin associated endothelin-receptor like (Pael) receptor, which would otherwise cause endoplasmic reticulum stress and cell death.[31] Finally, because neuroprotection by Hsp70 also occurs without affecting protein aggregation,[32,33] a direct inhibition of cell death mediators can be surmised.[34] Regardless of how heat shock proteins may prevent neurodegeneration, their overall importance in PD pathogenesis seems to be significant because drugs that activate the heat shock response, such as geldanamycin, prevent neurodegeneration in PD models.[35] Results such as these offer considerable hope for the development of new PD drugs.

Another way by which parkin function is modulated is through nitrosylation.[13,36] It has been shown in vitro and in vivo that parkin is S-nitrosylated in the disease state, including in PD mice models and brains of PD patients. S-nitrosylation of parkin inhibits its activity, leading to the notion that cellular stress can result in S-nitrosylation of parkin, decreased parkin activity, decreased ubiquitination of parkin substrates, accumulation of parkin substrates, protein aggregation, and neurodegeneration. Currently, the stress-signaling pathways that promote such S-nitrosylation are being investigated, which may offer an interesting angle on drug development in light of this unusual protein modification.

Parkin was shown to interact with BAG5.[37] In a differential display analysis, where changes in protein expression were detected in transected axons of rat substantia nigra neurons, BAG5 was identified and shown to interact with and inhibit Hsp70. Given that parkin and Hsp70 interact (see above), BAG5 was also shown to interact directly with parkin and inhibit its E3 ligase activity independent of Hsp70, as assessed by parkin autobiquitination and by synphilin ubiquitination. BAG5 also promotes parkin sequestration by inhibiting Hsp70, inhibits parkin-mediated suppression of UPS dysfunction and cell death in cell culture, and enhances the degeneration of substantia nigra neurons in vivo. Altogether, these results indicate that BAG5 may exert distinct molecular mechanisms to exert its antagonistic effects on parkin. Direct binding to parkin allows for reversal of the beneficial effects of parkin on UPS function and cell survival, whereas binding to Hsp70 and parkin may allow for parkin sequestration. Parkin sequestration and parkin-suppressed cell death may go hand in hand, supporting a potential role for cell toxicity mediated by protein aggregation or aberrant UPS function owing to loss-of-function of parkin. The precise mechanism by which BAG5 inhibits parkin is unknown. It can be hypothesized that BAG5 binding to parkin may block the RING finger domains at the C-terminus of parkin or, alternatively, change parkin's structural conformation. In either case, interaction with the E2s or parkin substrates may be compromised, explaining parkin loss-of-function and neurodegeneration.

LRRK2

Leucine-rich repeat kinase-2 (LRRK2) is another protein involved in PD pathogenesis.[38] It has an autosomal dominant inheritance pattern, indicating a gain-of-function mutation. Its particular appeal for research efforts is based on the fact that it is probably the most common mutation found in sporadic PD cases, with estimations of 4%. In familial PD cases of Ashkenazi Jews and North Africans, LRRK2 mutations can be found in 30% of Ashkenazi Jews and 40% of North

Africans. These numbers support the notion that defective signaling cascades in familial PD may likely contribute to disease pathogenesis in sporadic PD.

LRKK2 is a very large protein, with a molecular weight of 280 kD, and is organized into discrete protein modules. It is localized in the cytoplasm, associated with cellular membrane structures and the outer mitochondrial membrane.[39,40] LRRK2 is composed of several modules including the GTPase Roc and kinase domains. Based on these data, LRRK2 is considered to belong to the Roco family, a novel group of the Ras/GTPase superfamily. The type of kinase activity and the nature of substrates have not been clarified yet, but the kinase domain seems to have homology to the MAP kinase kinase kinases (MAP3K) of the mixed-lineage kinase class.[40]

It has been suggested that the kinase activity of LRRK2 actually is regulated by its GTPase Roc domain, with GTP binding being essential for kinase activity.[41,42] It was shown that alterations of LRRK2 protein that reduced kinase activity of mutant LRRK2 correspondingly reduced neuronal toxicity.[41,42] The latter result is significant because it strongly argues for the notion that increased kinase activity of mutant LRRK2 and potentially abnormal or excessive phosphorylation of LRRK2 substrates directly trigger neurodegeneration and PD pathogenesis. Increased autophosphorylation activity of LRRK2 seems to be important for the pathogenesis of PD caused by LRRK2 mutations because all mutations that segregate with disease have increased kinase activity.[42] In addition, it was found more recently that mutant LRRK2 can cause neuronal apoptosis, which was associated with prominent phospho-tau-positive inclusions with lysosomal characteristics and a reduction in neurite length and branching.[43]

Current LRRK2 research is focused on characterizing further the protein modules and defining their function. Part of this endeavor involves the search for LRRK2 interaction partners and kinase substrates, hoping that these proteins would aid in defining the molecular signaling pathways that LRRK2 modulates. LRRK2 has been shown to interact biochemically with parkin,[44] but the functional consequences of this interaction have remained elusive to date. Judging from the size of LRRK2 and the complexity of this protein, it would be a challenging undertaking to determine ultimately what interactions and what signaling pathways are primarily involved in the pathogenesis of PD with LRRK2 mutations. Nonetheless, the understanding that increased kinase activity is likely linked to PD pathogenesis invites a tremendous opportunity to develop new therapeutics that aim to inhibit LRRK2 kinase activity selectively.

DJ-1

DJ-1 is a protein found mutated in young-onset familial PD.[45] Because of the recessive character of inheritance, DJ-1–dependent pathogenesis is thought to result from a loss-of-function mutation. The nature of DJ-1 function is not well understood, however. DJ-1 knockout mice have shown deficits in the nigrostriatal system; this was reflected in decreased evoked dopaminergic transmission, in part owing to increased presynaptic transmitter reuptake, and in decreased D2 receptor–mediated functions, such as corticostriatal long-term depression.[46] The mechanism by which this DJ-1 function was mediated has remained elusive, however.

More recent data from DJ-1 knockout mice suggest that DJ-1 functions as an atypical peroxiredoxin-like peroxidase that scavenges mitochondrial peroxide through oxidation of its Cys106.[47] In mitochondria of aged DJ-1 knockout mice, levels of peroxide were found to be increased twofold. The phenotype of DJ-1 knockout mice was essentially identical to that of the wild-type counterparts. This finding may be explained by compensatory mechanisms that metabolize the added peroxide load, with a resulting twofold increase in peroxide insufficient to cause a phenotypic alteration. Consistent with that notion, increased levels of mitochondrial manganese superoxide dismutase and glutathione peroxidase were found in DJ-1 knockout mice. Altogether, these results suggest that DJ-1 may play a protective role against oxidative stress, participating in the mitochondrial response of scavenging toxic oxygen compounds.[48]

In support of a protective role for DJ-1 against oxidative stress, DJ-1 was shown to stabilize the antioxidant transcriptional master regulator, Nrf2, by preventing the association of Nrf2 with its inhibitor protein, Keap1, which would otherwise cause Nrf2 ubiquitination and degradation.[49] Loss of DJ-1 function results in loss of Nrf2, with subsequent loss of detoxification enzymes that are used for combating oxidative stress, including NAD(P)H quinone oxidoreductase-1 (NQO1). These effects were accomplished without physical interaction of DJ-1 with any of the involved proteins. DJ-1 plays a role in PD and cancer, emphasizing how oxidative stress can induce neuronal apoptosis (in PD) and genetic mutations leading to abnormal growth (in cancer). From the epidemiological standpoint, it would be interesting to see how prone DJ-1 patients are to developing cancer, given their specific DJ-1 mutations. This aspect underlines the need and the potential for the DJ-1–NRf2 interaction to be a therapeutic target.

In search of DJ-1 interaction partners that would aid in understanding DJ-1 function, several discoveries have been made. DJ-1 was shown to interact with the transcriptional corepressor pyrimidine tract-binding protein-associated splicing factor (PSF) to regulate the tyrosine hydroxylase promoter.[50] Specifically, DJ-1 acted as a transcriptional coactivator by inhibiting the sumoylation of PSF and preventing its sumoylation-dependent recruitment of histone deacetylase 1 to the promoter complex. This function of DJ-1 maintained the acetylation of tyrosine hydroxylase promoter–bound histones and facilitated expression of tyrosine hydroxylase, with the ultimate outcome of preserved dopamine synthesis. This mechanism may partly explain the observation that loss of DJ-1 is associated with decreased dopamine synthesis and nigrostriatal dopaminergic deficits.[46]

Another protein that interacts with DJ-1 is the proapoptotic protein Daxx. Specifically, it was shown that DJ-1 can sequester Daxx in the cell nucleus, preventing Daxx from reaching and activating the ASK1-mediated apoptotic pathway in the cytoplasm.[51] These findings reveal a cell-protective function for DJ-1 that has an impact on a signaling pathway independent of its peroxidase-scavenging activity. In this study, significant cell survival on oxidative stress was obtained only through both antiapoptotic functions of DJ-1.

PINK1

Phosphatase and tensin homologue (PTEN)–induced putative kinase 1 (PINK1) is a protein mutated in a subclass of familial young-onset PD.[38] Because of autosomal recessive inheritance, the PINK1 mutation is presumed to be a loss-of-function mutation. PINK1 encodes a putative serine/threonine kinase with a mitochondrial targeting sequence, indicating localization to the mitochondria that has been confirmed more recently.[52] Although not much is yet known about its molecular role in PD pathogenesis, expression of the PINK1 mutation in the *Drosophila* model has resulted in defects in mitochondrial morphology, reflected in fragmented mitochondrial cristae, and increased sensitivity to multiple stresses including oxidative stress.[53,54] This result indicates that the pathogenesis mechanism likely involves mitochondrial dysfunction.

More recently, inhibiting PINK1 with RNA interference in cell culture has also shown mitochondrial pathology,[55] extending the findings to the mammalian system. Mitochondrial pathology in PINK1 mutants could be alleviated with concomitant overexpression of wild-type parkin in the *Drosophila* model and in the mammalian cell culture system.[53-55] In the *Drosophila* model, flies double mutant for PINK1 and parkin had a phenotype identical to flies mutant in either protein alone.[53] These results suggest that PINK1 and parkin interact on a molecular level at least to some degree in the same signaling pathway, and that PINK1 is located upstream of parkin. This insight is genetically very appealing because both proteins cause young-onset forms of PD and are recessively inherited. Current research is exploring how PINK1 and parkin may intersect on a molecular level. Conceivably, the interaction is indirect, with the link between the proteosomal pathway and mitochondrial function obtained through mitochondrial proteins that require degradation by the UPS.[56]

Ongoing research has focused on PINK1 interaction partners, in the hope to elucidate the nature of the mitochondrial pathways in which PINK1 participates. One interacting partner of PINK1 is TRAP1, which is a heat shock protein that acts as a mitochondrial molecular chaperone.[57] PINK1 phosphorylates TRAP1, which seems to result in reduced cytochrome *c* release from mitochondria under conditions of oxidative stress, inhibiting cell death pathways and neurodegeneration. In contrast, the PD-linked G309D, L347P, and W437X mutations of PINK1 have an impaired ability to phosphorylate TRAP1 and rescue oxidative stress–induced cell death.[57] Taken together, these results begin to outline a signaling pathway that connects PINK1 to substrates that regulate mitochondria-dependent apoptotic pathways under conditions of oxidative stress.

Another interacting protein of PINK1 was identified more recently as HtrA2, which is a mitochondrial protein with serine protease activity that may regulate mitochondrial cell stress.[58] This interaction is particularly interesting from a genetic point of view because HtrA2 itself has been implicated in PD. Based on the observation that two HtrA2 mutations that affect the serine protease activity can be linked to PD, the HtrA2 gene was designated as the PD-13 locus.[59]

Knockout mice for HtrA2 and mice carrying a point mutation of HtrA2 that affects its serine protease activity showed a parkinsonian neurodegenerative phenotype.[60,61] Through this interaction, PINK1 directly phosphorylates HtrA2, which is consistent with the finding that phosphorylation of HtrA2 is reduced in brain tissue from patients with PD caused by PINK1. As PINK1 phosphorylates HtrA2 on activation of MEKK3-p38, PINK1 and HtrA2 constitute downstream components of the same stress-sending pathway. Although the phosphorylation occurs at a residue that is adjacent to the position that is mutated in PD patients, PINK1-dependent phosphorylation does seem to regulate the serine protease activity of HtrA2. Because mutations mimicking PINK1-phosphorylated HtrA2 were shown to enhance its proteolytic activity, PINK1 phosphorylation of HtrA2 is thought to allow for increased HtrA2 activity, which confers enhanced resistance to mitochondrial stress.[58,62]

Molecular approaches are being employed to define further components of the signaling pathways in which PINK1 is involved. Because PINK1 and HtrA2 are two proteins that produce a PD phenotype, directly affect mitochondrial function, and now are shown to interact physically in the cell, molecular identification of new components of PINK1 signaling pathways may reversely identify new genetic loci for inherited PD. Because PINK1 also phosphorylates TRAP, future molecular investigation also will aim to shed light on how the MEKKK3-p38 pathway may intersect with cytochrome *c* release–dependent apoptosis pathways through PINK1. Regardless of what future discoveries may reveal, what has already become obvious over a short time is how the PINK1-dependent signaling pathways are regulating the response of mitochondria to cell stress, emphasizing how mitochondrial dysfunction is central to PD pathogenesis.

Observations beyond Known Parkinson's Disease Genes

CELLULAR PACEMAKER ACTIVITY AND PARKINSON'S DISEASE

Aside from the advances in neurogenetics, various pathogenic insights have come from independent research avenues. A particularly exciting discovery was made more recently that connects the electrical discharge pattern of a subclass of substantia nigra neurons to PD.[63,64] Adult substantia nigra neurons are known to have intrinsic pacemaker activity that is thought to account for voluntary motor control.[65] This activity is based on calcium currents that are driven by L-type channels located in the somatodendritic compartment. These calcium currents are particularly strong because they occur during the relatively wide action potential and presumably when excitatory input triggers burst firing. In mice, inhibition of these L-type channels with the calcium antagonist isradipine resulted in protection of substantia nigra neurons in chemical PD models (MPTP, 6-hydroxydopamine, rotenone), indicating that high levels of intracellular calcium may play an important role in striatonigral degeneration, and that calcium antagonists may provide a new avenue of neuroprotective therapy for PD. On closer look, the study also showed that pacemaking is already present at the time of birth, when it is driven by sodium channels in coordination with hyperpolarization-activated and cyclic nucleotide–gated cation channels. Only in the second week after birth does a channel switch to the L-type calcium channels occur. Isradipine treatment resulted in a reversal to the birth-type pacemaking pattern within a few hours, as assessed in mouse midbrain slices.

What do we learn from these results? It is possible that calcium antagonists may provide neuroprotection in PD. A retrospective epidemiological analysis showed that patients taking dihydropyridines have substantially lower PD incidence rates. Prospective studies are needed to confirm this observation, but it seems to support the notion that L-type calcium channels operate similarly in human substantia nigra neurons. Treatment with dihydropyridine is not as straightforward as it might seem, however. Treatment in the mouse study was performed at high doses, which may prompt significant side effects in humans because PD patients are prone to orthostatic hypotension in the first place.

Dihydropyridines are most effective on the calcium 1.2 L-type channels, whereas the substantia nigra neurons express primarily calcium 1.3 channels. It is possible that drugs more specific to the 1.3 channel subtype may be developed to curb side effects and optimize treatment efficacy. Knockout mice for the 1.3 channel subunit show deafness,[66] consistent with the importance of L-type calcium channels in inner hair cell activity. This finding raises caution as to emerging unwanted severe side effects with the benefit of added channel specificity.

Another aspect that remains unresolved is how calcium currents cause neurodegeneration in PD. A genetic defect in an L-type calcium channel has not been linked to PD. A specific linkage of elevated intracellular calcium to the mutant proteins of familial PD has not been found. Because mitochondria are known to buffer calcium, however, and to be susceptible to oxidative stress that can be induced by high intracellular calcium,[67] a connection between the L-type calcium channel and the *PINK1, DJ-1,* and *LRRK2* genes may be invoked. Such investigation may provide important insight into the neuronal selectivity pattern in PD. In this regard, high levels of calbindin are found in dopaminergic neurons of the ventral tegmental area, which also express L-type calcium channels, but seem largely unaffected in PD. It may be speculated that mutated calcium binding proteins, including calbindin, may bridge a molecular connection between calcium channels and mitochondrial genes in substantia nigra neurons.

DEACETYLATION AND PARKINSON'S DISEASE

A separately emerging concept relates α-synuclein toxicity to histone deacetylases. In particular, the sirtuin family has received attention more recently. Originally recognized to play a role in aging, the sirtuins may be involved in neurodegeneration as well. In a screen to identify compounds that modulate α-synuclein aggregation,[68] AGK2 was identified as a compound that increased aggregate size by inhibiting sirtuin 2.[69] Inhibition of sirtuin2 (SIRT2) by AGK2 diminished α-synuclein–mediated toxicity in primary midbrain cultures and in a *Drosophila* model of PD, where tyrosine hydroxylase–positive neurons in the dorsomedial cluster were partly rescued. This finding indicates that aggregation may not simply induce neurotoxicity but may be neuroprotective. α-Synuclein oligomers may trigger neuronal cell death, and sequestration into large aggregates may promote cell survival.

The mechanism by which SIRT2 inhibition protects against cell death is not yet elucidated, but α-tubulin may be a potential target. Given that SIRT2 can deacetylate Lys40 of α-tubulin in vitro[69] and alpha-tubulin has been reported to interact with α-synuclein, modulation of tubulin by SIRT2 could potentially affect the aggregation behavior of α-synuclein. Alternatively, SIRT2 may affect autophagy, a cellular self-digestion process that has also been observed in PD.[70] Because histone deacetylases are required for this process, SIRT2 may be neuroprotective through deacetylation of histones important for autophagy. Because autophagy involves lysosomal recruitment to aggregated cellular proteins associated with the microtubule organizing center, a relationship between deacetylation of histones and tubulin can be envisioned as well. SIRT2 may promote the activity of apoptotic factors because antiapoptotic effects are observed in cells that have decreased SIRT2 expression. Finally, in a broader context, individual members of the sirtuin family seem to have opposing effects on α-synuclein–mediated neurodegeneration.[69,71] In contrast to SIRT2, increased SIRT1 activity was shown to delay α-synuclein toxicity.[72] Whether SIRT1 is involved in the dissemination of α-synuclein oligomers to monomers is currently an area of active investigation. It is possible that different sirtuins may work in opposing ways on the aggregation cascade of α-synuclein to mediate neurodegeneration.[71]

Conclusions

Since the identification of mutations in α-synuclein as a cause of autosomal dominant PD in 1997, there have been remarkable advances in the understanding of the molecular underpinnings of PD. One can expect that advances obtained from genetics will continue at a remarkable pace, and that new treatments that slow or reverse the process of neurodegeneration in PD will emerge from these studies.

Acknowledgments

This chapter was supported by the Morris K. Udall Parkinson's Disease Research Center and NIH/NINDS (NS38377) and NS04826. T.M.D. is the Leonard and Madlyn Abramson Professor in Neurodegenerative Diseases.

REFERENCES

1. Hardy J, Cai H, Cookson MR, et al: Genetics of Parkinson's disease and parkinsonism. Ann Neurol 2006;60:389-398.
2. Norris EH, Giasson BI, Lee VM: Alpha-synuclein: normal function and role in neurodegenerative diseases. Curr Top Dev Biol 2004;60:17-54.
3. Dauer W, Kholodilov N, Vila M, et al: Resistance of alpha-synuclein null mice to the parkinsonian neurotoxin MPTP. Proc Natl Acad Sci U S A 2002;99:14524-14529.
4. Drolet RE, Behrouz B, Lookingland KJ, Goudreau JL: Mice lacking alpha-synuclein have an attenuated loss of striatal dopamine following prolonged chronic MPTP administration. Neurotoxicology 2004;25:761-769.
5. Lee VM, Trojanowski JQ: Mechanisms of Parkinson's disease linked to pathological alpha-synuclein: new targets for drug discovery. Neuron 2006;52:33-38.
6. Abeliovich A, Schmitz Y, Farinas I, et al: Mice lacking alpha-synuclein display functional deficits in the nigrostriatal dopamine system. Neuron 2000;25:239-252.
7. Ihara M, Yamasaki N, Hagiwara A, et al: Sept4, a component of presynaptic scaffold and Lewy bodies, is required for the suppression of alpha-synuclein neurotoxicity. Neuron 2007;53:519-533.
8. Cooper AA, Gitler AD, Cashikar A, et al: Alpha-synuclein blocks ER-Golgi traffic and Rab1 rescues neuron loss in Parkinson's models. Science 2006;313:324-328.
9. Chandra S, Gallardo G, Fernandez-Chacon R, et al: Alpha-synuclein cooperates with CSPalpha in preventing neurodegeneration. Cell 2005;123:383-396.
10. Goedert M: Alpha-synuclein and neurodegenerative diseases. Nat Rev Neurosci 2001;2:492-501.
11. Bennett MC, Bishop JF, Leng Y, et al: Degradation of alpha-synuclein by proteasome. J Biol Chem 1999;274:33855-33858.
12. Tofaris GK, Layfield R, Spillantini MG: Alpha-synuclein metabolism and aggregation is linked to ubiquitin-independent degradation by the proteasome. Febs Lett 2001;509:22-26.
13. Chung KK, Thomas B, Li X, et al: S-nitrosylation of parkin regulates ubiquitination and compromises parkin's protective function. Science 2004;304:1328-1331.
14. Ihara M, Tomimoto H, Kitayama H, et al: Association of the cytoskeletal GTP-binding protein Sept4/H5 with cytoplasmic inclusions found in Parkinson's disease and other synucleinopathies. J Biol Chem 2003;278:24095-24102.
15. Cuervo AM, Stefanis L, Fredenburg R, et al: Impaired degradation of mutant alpha-synuclein by chaperone-mediated autophagy. Science 2004;305:1292-1295.
16. Martinez-Vicente M, Cuervo AM: Autophagy and neurodegeneration: when the cleaning crew goes on strike. Lancet Neurol 2007;6:352-361.
17. Rideout HJ, Lang-Rollin I, Stefanis L: Involvement of macroautophagy in the dissolution of neuronal inclusions. Int J Biochem Cell Biol 2004;36:2551-2562.
18. Williams A, Jahreiss L, Sarkar S, et al: Aggregate-prone proteins are cleared from the cytosol by autophagy: therapeutic implications. Curr Top Dev Biol 2006;76:89-101.

19. Masliah E, Rockenstein E, Adame A, et al: Effects of alpha-synuclein immunization in a mouse model of Parkinson's disease. Neuron 2005;46:857-868.

20. Li J, Zhu M, Rajamani S, et al: Rifampicin inhibits alpha-synuclein fibrillation and disaggregates fibrils. Chem Biol 2004;11:1513-1521.

21. Li W, West N, Colla E, et al: Aggregation promoting C-terminal truncation of alpha-synuclein is a normal cellular process and is enhanced by the familial Parkinson's disease-linked mutations. Proc Natl Acad Sci U S A 2005;102:2162-2167.

22. Imai Y, Soda M, Takahashi R: Parkin suppresses unfolded protein stress-induced cell death through its E3 ubiquitin-protein ligase activity. J Biol Chem 2000;275:35661-35664.

23. Shimura H, Hattori N, Kubo S, et al: Familial Parkinson disease gene product, parkin, is a ubiquitin-protein ligase. Nat Genet 2000;25:302-305.

24. Zhang Y, Gao J, Chung KK, et al: Parkin functions as an E2-dependent ubiquitin-protein ligase and promotes the degradation of the synaptic vesicle-associated protein, CDCrel-1. Proc Natl Acad Sci U S A 2000;97:13354-13359.

25. Petrucelli L, O'Farrell C, Lockhart PJ, et al: Parkin protects against the toxicity associated with mutant alpha-synuclein: proteasome dysfunction selectively affects catecholaminergic neurons. Neuron 2002;36:1007-1019.

26. von Coelln R, Thomas B, Andrabi SA, et al: Inclusion body formation and neurodegeneration are parkin independent in a mouse model of alpha-synucleinopathy. J Neurosci 2006;26:3685-3696.

27. Chung KK, Zhang Y, Lim KL, et al: Parkin ubiquitinates the alpha-synuclein-interacting protein, synphilin-1: implications for Lewy-body formation in Parkinson disease. Nat Med 2001;7:1144-1150.

28. Engelender S, Kaminsky Z, Guo X, et al: Synphilin-1 associates with alpha-synuclein and promotes the formation of cytosolic inclusions. Nat Genet 1999;22:110-114.

29. Ko HS, Kim SW, Sriram SR, et al: Identification of far upstream element-binding protein-1 as an authentic Parkin substrate. J Biol Chem 2006;281:16193-16196.

30. Ko HS, von Coelln R, Sriram SR, et al: Accumulation of the authentic parkin substrate aminoacyl-tRNA synthetase cofactor, p38/JTV-1, leads to catecholaminergic cell death. J Neurosci 2005;25:7968-7978.

31. Imai Y, Soda M, Hatakeyama S, et al: CHIP is associated with Parkin, a gene responsible for familial Parkinson's disease, and enhances its ubiquitin ligase activity. Mol Cell 2002;10:55-67.

32. Auluck PK, Chan HY, Trojanowski JQ, et al: Chaperone suppression of alpha-synuclein toxicity in a *Drosophila* model for Parkinson's disease. Science 2002;295:865-868.

33. Klucken J, Shin Y, Masliah E, et al: Hsp70 reduces alpha-synuclein aggregation and toxicity. J Biol Chem 2004;279:25497-25502.

34. Takayama S, Reed JC, Homma S: Heat-shock proteins as regulators of apoptosis. Oncogene 2003;22:9041-9047.

35. Auluck PK, Bonini NM: Pharmacological prevention of Parkinson disease in *Drosophila*. Nat Med 2002;8:1185-1186.

36. Yao D, Gu Z, Nakamura T, et al: Nitrosative stress linked to sporadic Parkinson's disease: S-nitrosylation of parkin regulates its E3 ubiquitin ligase activity. Proc Natl Acad Sci U S A 2004;101:10810-10814.

37. Kalia SK, Lee S, Smith PD, et al: BAG5 inhibits parkin and enhances dopaminergic neuron degeneration. Neuron 2004;44:931-945.

38. Gasser T: Update on the genetics of Parkinson's disease. Mov Disord 2007;22(Suppl 17):S343-S350.

39. Biskup S, Moore DJ, Celsi F, et al: Localization of LRRK2 to membranous and vesicular structures in mammalian brain. Ann Neurol 2006;60:557-569.

40. West AB, Moore DJ, Biskup S, et al: Parkinson's disease-associated mutations in leucine-rich repeat kinase 2 augment kinase activity. Proc Natl Acad Sci U S A 2005;102:16842-16847.

41. Smith WW, Pei Z, Jiang H, et al: Kinase activity of mutant LRRK2 mediates neuronal toxicity. Nat Neurosci 2006;9:1231-1233.

42. West AB, Moore DJ, Choi C, et al: Parkinson's disease-associated mutations in LRRK2 link enhanced GTP-binding and kinase activities to neuronal toxicity. Hum Mol Genet 2007;16:223-232.

43. MacLeod D, Dowman J, Hammond R, et al: The familial Parkinsonism gene LRRK2 regulates neurite process morphology. Neuron 2006;52:587-593.

44. Smith WW, Pei Z, Jiang H, et al: Leucine-rich repeat kinase 2 (LRRK2) interacts with parkin, and mutant LRRK2 induces neuronal degeneration. Proc Natl Acad Sci U S A 2005;102:18676-18681.

45. Moore DJ, Dawson VL, Dawson TM: Lessons from *Drosophila* models of DJ-1 deficiency. Sci Aging Knowledge Environ 2006;2:2.
46. Goldberg MS, Pisani A, Haburcak M, et al: Nigrostriatal dopaminergic deficits and hypokinesia caused by inactivation of the familial Parkinsonism-linked gene DJ-1. Neuron 2005;45:489-496.
47. Andres-Mateos E, Perier C, Zhang L, et al: DJ-1 gene deletion reveals that DJ-1 is an atypical peroxiredoxin-like peroxidase. Proc Natl Acad Sci U S A 2007;104:14807-14812.
48. Dodson MW, Guo M: PINK1, Parkin, DJ-1 and mitochondrial dysfunction in Parkinson's disease. Curr Opin Neurobiol 2007;17:331-337.
49. Clements CM, McNally RS, Conti BJ, et al: DJ-1, a cancer- and Parkinson's disease-associated protein, stabilizes the antioxidant transcriptional master regulator Nrf2. Proc Natl Acad Sci U S A 2006;103:15091-15096.
50. Zhong N, Kim CY, Rizzu P, et al: DJ-1 transcriptionally up-regulates the human tyrosine hydroxylase by inhibiting the sumoylation of pyrimidine tract-binding protein-associated splicing factor. J Biol Chem 2006;281:20940-20948.
51. Junn E, Taniguchi H, Jeong BS, et al: Interaction of DJ-1 with Daxx inhibits apoptosis signal-regulating kinase 1 activity and cell death. Proc Natl Acad Sci U S A 2005;102:9691-9696.
52. Valente EM, Abou-Sleiman PM, Caputo V, et al: Hereditary early-onset Parkinson's disease caused by mutations in PINK1. Science 2004;304:1158-1160.
53. Clark IE, Dodson MW, Jiang C, et al: *Drosophila* PINK1 is required for mitochondrial function and interacts genetically with parkin. Nature 2006;441:1162-1166.
54. Park J, Lee SB, Lee S, et al: Mitochondrial dysfunction in *Drosophila* PINK1 mutants is complemented by parkin. Nature 2006;441:1157-1161.
55. Exner N, Treske B, Paquet D, et al: Loss-of-function of human PINK1 results in mitochondrial pathology and can be rescued by parkin. J Neurosci 2007;27:12413-12418.
56. Tan JM, Dawson TM: Parkin blushed by PINK1. Neuron 2006;50:527-529.
57. Pridgeon JW, Olzmann JA, Chin LS, Li L: PINK1 protects against oxidative stress by phosphorylating mitochondrial chaperone TRAP1. PLoS Biol 2007;5:e172.
58. Plun-Favreau H, Klupsch K, Moisoi N, et al: The mitochondrial protease HtrA2 is regulated by Parkinson's disease-associated kinase PINK1. Nat Cell Biol 2007;9:1243-1252.
59. Strauss KM, Martins LM, Plun-Favreau H, et al: Loss of function mutations in the gene encoding Omi/HtrA2 in Parkinson's disease. Hum Mol Genet 2005;14:2099-2111.
60. Jones JM, Datta P, Srinivasula SM, et al: Loss of Omi mitochondrial protease activity causes the neuromuscular disorder of mnd2 mutant mice. Nature 2003;425:721-727.
61. Martins LM, Morrison A, Klupsch K, et al: Neuroprotective role of the Reaper-related serine protease HtrA2/Omi revealed by targeted deletion in mice. Mol Cell Biol 2004;24:9848-9862.
62. Alnemri ES: HtrA2 and Parkinson's disease: think PINK? Nat Cell Biol 2007;9:1227-1229.
63. Chan CS, Guzman JN, Ilijic E, et al: 'Rejuvenation' protects neurons in mouse models of Parkinson's disease. Nature 2007;447:1081-1086.
64. Sulzer D, Schmitz Y: Parkinson's disease: return of an old prime suspect. Neuron 2007;55:8-10.
65. Grace AA, Onn SP: Morphology and electrophysiological properties of immunocytochemically identified rat dopamine neurons recorded in vitro. J Neurosci 1989;9:3463-3481.
66. Striessnig J, Koschak A, Sinnegger-Brauns MJ, et al: Role of voltage-gated L-type Ca^{2+} channel isoforms for brain function. Biochem Soc Trans 2006;34:903-909.
67. Beal MF: Excitotoxicity and nitric oxide in Parkinson's disease pathogenesis. Ann Neurol 1998;44:S110-S114.
68. Bodner RA, Outeiro TF, Altmann S, et al: Pharmacological promotion of inclusion formation: a therapeutic approach for Huntington's and Parkinson's diseases. Proc Natl Acad Sci U S A 2006;103:4246-4251.
69. Outeiro TF, Kontopoulos E, Altmann SM, et al: Sirtuin 2 inhibitors rescue alpha-synuclein-mediated toxicity in models of Parkinson's disease. Science 2007;317:516-519.
70. Iwata A, Riley BE, Johnston JA, Kopito RR: HDAC6 and microtubules are required for autophagic degradation of aggregated huntingtin. J Biol Chem 2005;280:40282-40292.
71. Dillin A, Kelly JW: Medicine: the yin-yang of sirtuins. Science 2007;317:461-462.
72. Okawara M, Katsuki H, Kurimoto E, et al: Resveratrol protects dopaminergic neurons in midbrain slice culture from multiple insults. Biochem Pharmacol 2007;73:550-560.

11 | Imaging in Parkinson's Disease

DAVID JAMES BROOKS

Introduction

The definitive diagnosis of idiopathic Parkinson's disease (PD) requires demonstration of intracellular nigral Lewy body inclusions via histological examination of brain tissue and so is impractical during life. Clinicopathological studies suggest that at best 85% of patients diagnosed in life with standard Brain Bank criteria as having clinically probable PD subsequently show brainstem Lewy body disease.[1] The main differential diagnoses are severe tremors (essential and dystonic) and atypical parkinsonian disorders, such as multiple system atrophy (MSA), progressive supranuclear palsy (PSP), and corticobasal degeneration plus vascular parkinsonism. Although diagnostic specificity improves with disease duration and a knowledge of treatment response, patients with early disease, in which the full constellation of parkinsonian symptoms and signs are not yet manifest, can be difficult to diagnose. The ability to detect altered nigral structure or striatal dopamine terminal dysfunction noninvasively is a potentially valuable tool that can help increase diagnostic specificity for dopamine-deficient parkinsonian syndromes and rationalize management decisions at initial stages of disease.

Currently, it is unclear whether dementia with Lewy bodies (DLB), PD with later dementia (PDD), and PD without dementia all represent a spectrum of Lewy body disease. Nigral degeneration is a feature of all three of these conditions, but in most cases of PD without dementia it is possible to detect Lewy body inclusions at postmortem examination in the anterior cingulate cortex and other cortical association areas.[1] The dementia associated with DLB has overlapping clinical features with Alzheimer's disease (AD), although fluctuating confusion, hallucinations, and parkinsonism are added features. At postmortem examination, many cases of DLB show a mixture of cortical Lewy body inclusions and AD pathology.

Structural Imaging Approaches in Parkinsonian Disorders

MAGNETIC RESONANCE IMAGING

Magnetic resonance imaging (MRI) reveals brain structural changes as reductions in volume, alterations in water proton relaxation T1 and T2 signals or water diffusion, and changes in magnetic susceptibility or magnetization transfer. MRI also allows structural lesions, such as basal ganglia tumors and calcification, vascular disease, and hydrocephalus, to be excluded as causes of parkinsonism.

Using inversion recovery sequences designed to suppress gray or white matter signals, MRI has been reported to detect abnormal signal from the substantia nigra compacta in PD. The segmented inversion recovery ratio imaging (SIRRM) approach generates ratio images of these gray and white matter signal–suppressing inversion recovery sequences at a voxel level. In an initial series,[2] 6 PD cases all were reported to show altered nigral signal, although this was true of only 7 of 10 patients in a second series.[3] Minati and coworkers[4] generated subtraction rather than ratio images with gray and white matter–suppressing inversion recovery sequences, and detected significant hypointensity of the lateral nigra in PD. They noted a significant overlap between normal and PD ranges, however.

An alternative MRI approach uses T2-weighted sequences, which directly reflect the iron content of brain areas. With such an approach, Michaeli and colleagues[5] detected increased nigral magnetic susceptibility in PD, although midbrain relaxation times overlapped considerably with times of a normal group. Volumetric MRI studies so far have failed to detect a reduction in nigral volume in PD, possibly because of difficulties in accurately defining the border of the nigra compacta.[6] A reduction in putamen volume was reported in PD by these workers, however, even in early cases.

Although MRI approaches so far have failed to discriminate PD from normal subjects, they can play a valuable role in discriminating atypical parkinsonian syndromes, such as MSA and PSP, from typical PD. Volumetric MRI detects significant striatal, brainstem, and cerebellar atrophy in patients with MSA and PSP when present. Individual volumes of these structures show overlap, however, with the normal range with the possible exception of the reduced brainstem volumes in patients with MSA-cerebellar.[7,8] Diffusion-weighted and tensor MRI provide more sensitive modalities for discriminating atypical from typical parkinsonian disorders. Diffusion-weighted MRI has been reported to detect altered water apparent diffusion coefficients in the putamen of 90% to 100% of cases with clinically probable MSA and PSP in different reported series, whereas putamen apparent diffusion coefficients are normal in PD (Fig. 11–1).[9-11] MSA can be reliably

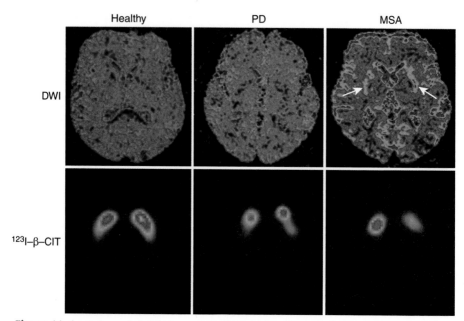

Healthy   PD   MSA

DWI

¹²³I–β–CIT

Figure 11–1   Color-coded diffusion-weighted MR images (DWI) and striatal β-CIT uptake for a healthy subject, a patient with Parkinson's disease (PD), and a case of the atypical parkinsonian syndrome multiple systems atrophy (MSA). In the *upper images,* the apparent diffusion coefficient is normal in the striatum of the PD case, but increased in MSA (*arrows*) because of the neuronal loss that targets the putamen. The *lower images* show that dopamine transporter binding is bilaterally reduced in the striata of the PD and MSA cases, but the caudate is relatively spared compared with putamen in PD. (*Upper images,* From Schocke MF, Seppi K, Esterhammer R, et al: Diffusion-weighted MRI differentiates the Parkinson variant of multiple system atrophy from PD. Neurology 2002;58:575-580; *Lower images,* courtesy of Gregor Wenning.)

discriminated from PSP by the presence of an altered water diffusion signal in the middle cerebral peduncle.[12] It remains to be seen how well diffusion-weighted MRI will perform with early gray cases in prospective series where clinical diagnostic uncertainty is still present.

TRANSCRANIAL SONOGRAPHY

Transcranial sonography (TCS) detects structural midbrain and striatal changes in parkinsonian disorders as hyperechogenic signals (Fig. 11–2). In an initial large series, 92% of cases with clinically established PD were reported to have increased midbrain echogenicity with TCS.[13] These workers used a threshold for abnormality of 1 standard deviation above the normal mean, however, to increase sensitivity, and 10% of their elderly normal subjects also showed hyperechogenicity. The increased TCS signal was more noticeable contralateral to the more clinically affected limbs, but did not correlate well with disability scores. In a more recent series, TCS was reported to have positive and negative predictive values of 86% and 83% for clinically probable PD.[14]

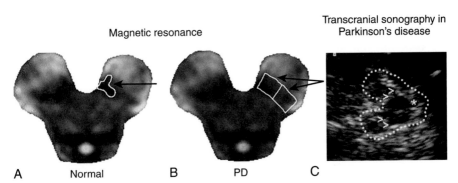

Magnetic resonance   Transcranial sonography in Parkinson's disease

A Normal   B PD   C

Figure 11–2   A-C, Midbrain structure in Parkinson's disease (PD) imaged using MRI (**A** and **B**) and transcranial sonography (**C**). **A** and **B,** MRI is a subtraction image of inversion recovery sequences designed to suppress gray and white matter signals and shows loss of nigral signal in PD. **C,** Transcranial sonography shows hyperechogenicity from the nigra in PD. (**A** and **B,** From Minati L, Grisoli M, Carella F, et al: Imaging degeneration of the substantia nigra in Parkinson disease with inversion-recovery MR imaging. AJNR Am J Neuroradiol 2007;28:309-313; **C,** from Berg D, Siefker C, Becker G. Echogenicity of the substantia nigra in Parkinson's disease and its relation to clinical findings. J Neurol 2001;248:684-689.)

Although TCS sensitively detects nigral hyperechogenicity in idiopathic PD, 15% of essential tremor patients[15] and 40% of depressed patients[16] have also been reported to show such nigral hyperechogenicity, raising questions about the specificity of this finding. In a 5-year follow-up study of PD cases, there was no significant change in TCS findings, while clinical disability progressed.[17] It has been suggested that the presence of midbrain hyperechogenicity is a trait rather than state marker for susceptibility to parkinsonism and may reflect the presence of midbrain iron deposition.[18] Abnormal nigral hyperechogenicity can also be detected in monogenic forms of parkinsonism, such as carriers of α-synuclein, *LRRK2, parkin,* and *DJ-1* mutations. Nigral hyperechogenicity does not seem to be associated with the atypical parkinsonian disorders MSA and PSP, although altered striatal signal can be detected in MSA.[19]

Imaging Presynaptic Dopaminergic Function in Parkinson's Disease

The function of dopamine terminals in PD can be examined in vivo in three main ways[20]:

1. The availability of presynaptic dopamine transporters (DATs) can be assessed with positron emission tomography (PET) and single photon emission computed tomography (SPECT) tracers, most of which are tropane based.
2. Terminal dopa decarboxylase activity and dopamine turnover can be measured with fluorodopa F 18 (^{18}F-dopa) PET.
3. Vesicle monoamine transporter (VMAT2) density in dopamine terminals can be examined with ^{11}C-dihydrotetrabenazine PET.

Early Hoehn and Yahr stage 1 hemiparkinsonian cases show bilaterally reduced putamen dopaminergic terminal function; activity is most depressed in the posterior putamen contralateral to the affected limbs. Head of caudate and ventral striatal function is relatively preserved. It has been estimated that clinical parkinsonism occurs when PD patients have lost approximately 50% of their posterior putamen dopamine terminal function.[21] Not all dopamine fibers degenerate in early PD—some seem to increase their dopamine turnover as an adaptive mechanism. Although posterior putamen ^{18}F-dopa uptake is reduced at the onset of parkinsonian rigidity and bradykinesia, globus pallidus interna uptake is increased by 50%.[22] As the disease advances, pallidal ^{18}F-dopa storage decreases, eventually becoming subnormal at a time when accelerated disability and treatment complications, such as fluctuating responses to levodopa, are evident. This observation suggests that putamen and globus pallidus interna require an intact dopaminergic input from the nigra to facilitate efficient and fluent limb movements, and when both sets of projections are damaged the "honeymoon period" in PD reaches an end.

In series where clinically probable PD and essential tremor cases have been compared, striatal DAT imaging with SPECT has been shown to differentiate these conditions with a sensitivity and specificity of approximately 90%.[23] An abnormal PET or SPECT scan of striatal DAT binding should be valuable for supporting a diagnosis of dopamine-deficient parkinsonism where there is diagnostic doubt. Three studies have examined the role of DAT imaging in aiding the diagnosis of gray parkinsonian cases. In the Query PD study, the standard of truth was the clinical impression of two movement disorder experts after 6 months of clinical follow-up.[24] Baseline clinical specificity for dopamine-deficient parkinsonism by referring clinicians and experts ranged from 30% to 40% compared with the gold standard, whereas baseline imaging specificity with β-CIT SPECT was greater than 80%.

The CUPS study followed the impact of knowledge of FP-CIT SPECT findings in the management of clinically uncertain parkinsonian syndromes. After imaging, the diagnosis of dopamine-deficient parkinsonian syndrome was revised in 52% of the 118 cases, and the management strategy changed in 72% of cases.[25] A 2-year follow-up of the CUPS study has confirmed its findings in that 90% of subjects still retained the diagnosis assigned by baseline FP-CIT SPECT imaging.[26] Based on these studies, including a measure of striatal dopaminergic function in the work-up of gray parkinsonian cases should help to rationalize and improve their management; however, the pathology of these patients still remains unclear because clinical follow-up was the ultimate standard of truth.

About 10% to 15% of early cases suspected of having a dopamine-deficient parkinsonian syndrome have normal dopamine terminal function when studied with PET or SPECT. The clinical significance of this finding remains uncertain, but a series by Marshall and colleagues[27] has helped to shed light on this by following over 2 years 150 cases with possible early parkinsonism but normal FP-CIT SPECT. Only four (3%) of these cases showed clinical progression, and they were still thought to have PD at follow-up; the rest were labeled as having either a tremulous disorder or nondegenerative parkinsonism. Given these findings, a SPECT or PET finding of normal presynaptic dopaminergic function in a case of suspected PD is likely to be associated with a good prognosis whatever the ultimate diagnosis.

Resting Glucose Metabolism in Typical and Atypical Parkinson's Disease

Flurodeoxyglucose F 18 ([18]FDG) PET studies have shown increased levels of resting cerebral glucose metabolism in the contralateral lentiform nucleus of hemiparkinsonian patients with early disease. Absolute lentiform nucleus resting cerebral glucose metabolism levels are usually normal in PD patients with established bilateral involvement[28]; however, covariance analysis reveals an abnormal profile of relatively increased resting lentiform nucleus and lowered frontal and parieto-temporal metabolism in nondemented PD patients with established disease.[29] The degree of expression of this PD-related profile correlates with clinical disease severity, providing a potential biomarker of disease progression, and normalizes after exposure to levodopa and deep brain stimulation.[30,31] Eckert and colleagues[32] performed [18]FDG PET on eight patients with suspected early parkinsonism but normal ^{18}F-dopa PET. None of these eight cases expressed a PD-related profile of glucose metabolism, and over 3 years none of them showed any clinical progression of their disorder. This finding reinforces the viewpoint that normal ^{18}F-dopa PET excludes the presence of a degenerative parkinsonian syndrome.

Evaluation of presynaptic dopamine terminal function with striatal DAT binding or ^{18}F-dopa PET has poor specificity (~70%) for discriminating typical and atypical PD,[33,34] although PSP patients show a more uniform and symmetrical pattern of nigrostriatal dysfunction compared with PD and MSA patients, where the pattern of loss is asymmetrical, and head of caudate tracer uptake is relatively preserved. In contrast, measurements of resting glucose metabolism can be very helpful. In PD lentiform nucleus, glucose metabolism is preserved, whereas it is reduced in 80% to 100% of MSA and PSP cases across different series.[28,35]

Detection of Preclinical Parkinson's Disease

It has been estimated that for every patient who presents with clinical PD there may be 10 to 15 subclinical cases with incidental brainstem Lewy body disease in the community.[36] Subjects at risk of developing PD include carriers of genes known to be associated with parkinsonism, relatives of patients with the disorder, elderly subjects with idiopathic hyposmia, and patients with rapid-eye-movement (REM) sleep behavior disorders.

Subclinical midbrain hyperechogenicity has been reported with TCS in 10% of elderly normal subjects, and this correlated with the presence of soft signs of parkinsonism.[37] Increased midbrain echogenicity has also been reported in asymptomatic *parkin* gene carriers, although only a minority of these had reduced striatal ^{18}F-dopa uptake.[38] In a third series, workers investigated hyposmic subjects with TCS. One third of idiopathic olfactory cases showed midbrain hyperechogenicity, and half of these had reduced striatal FP-CIT binding.[39] Overall, where increased nigral echogenicity has been detected in subjects at risk for PD, less than half of these cases have had impaired dopaminergic function. The alterations in nigral structure detected by TCS do not reflect dopamine cell function, as is emphasized by a study showing no correlation between midbrain hyperechogenicity in PD and striatal DAT binding measured with technetium 99m TRODAT SPECT.[40]

[18]F-dopa PET has been used to study asymptomatic adult relatives in familial PD kindreds.[41] Of the asymptomatic adult relatives scanned, 25% showed reduced levels of putamen ^{18}F-dopa uptake, and one third of these subsequently developed clinical parkinsonism over a 5-year follow-up period. ^{18}F-dopa PET has also been used to investigate *parkin* disease. Symptomatic compound heterozygote gene carriers show severe reductions of striatal ^{18}F-dopa uptake given their degree of disability, suggesting that adaptive processes to compensate for the dopamine deficiency may be taking place.[42,43] The pattern of dopaminergic deficit in symptomatic *parkin* patients can mimic PD, putamen being targeted, but the caudate and midbrain are relatively more involved in *parkin* disease.[44] Asymptomatic heterozygote *parkin* gene carriers show a significant but mild reduction in putamen ^{18}F-dopa uptake, which does not seem to progress over a 10-year period.[45] Whether carrying a single *parkin* mutation makes one more susceptible to late-onset PD is still being debated.

The most common known cause of dominantly inherited PD is carrying a mutation in the lysine-rich repeat kinase (*LRRK2*) gene (also known as PARK8). In a more recent series, 15 family members of an *LRRK2* kindred had ^{18}F-dopa, ^{11}C-DTBZ, and ^{11}C-MP PET to assess dopamine storage, VMAT2, and DAT binding.[46] Four clinically affected *LRRK2* members had imaging findings similar to PD with a typical gradient of loss of dopaminergic function targeting the putamen and sparing the head of caudate. Two asymptomatic mutation carriers had reduced putamen DAT binding measured with ^{11}C-MP PET. Another two had normal DAT binding, but this subsequently decreased over 4 years of follow-up. In these four asymptomatic individuals, ^{18}F-dopa uptake remained normal, although two of them had reduced ^{11}C-DTBZ binding. The authors concluded that the in vivo neurochemical phenotype of *LRRK2* mutations was indistinguishable from that of sporadic PD, and that compensatory changes, which included downregulation of DAT binding and upregulation of decarboxylase activity, may act to delay the onset of parkinsonian symptoms in carriers.

Elderly relatives of PD patients with hyposmia are likely to be at risk of PD. Ponsen and colleagues[47] collected 40 such relatives after screening 400 individuals for hyposmia and found that 7 of these showed reduced striatal ^{123}I-β-CIT uptake. Four of these seven individuals subsequently converted to clinical PD over a 2-year period.

REM sleep behavior disorder is commonly associated with PD. Eleven patients with isolated REM sleep behavior disorder have been investigated for the presence of dopamine deficiency with FP-CIT SPECT.[48] Three of these 11 cases showed reduced striatal DAT binding, one of whom had evidence of clinical parkinsonism.

Mechanisms Underlying Fluctuations and Dyskinesias

Although PD patients with fluctuating motor responses to levodopa show 20% lower mean putamen ^{18}F-dopa uptake than patients with sustained therapeutic responses, there is overlap of fluctuator and nonfluctuator ranges.[49] Loss of putamen dopamine terminal function alone cannot be the only factor responsible for determining the timing of onset of fluctuations, although it predisposes PD patients toward development of levodopa-associated complications.

^{123}I-IBZM SPECT studies have reported normal levels of striatal D2 binding in untreated PD patients, whereas ^{11}C-raclopride PET has shown 10% to 20% increases in putamen D2 site availability—although these subsequently normalize after repeated exposure to levodopa.[50,51] ^{11}C-SCH23390 PET, a marker of D1 site binding, reveals normal striatal uptake in de novo PD, whereas patients who have been chronically exposed to levodopa show a 20% reduction in striatal binding. Cohorts of levodopa-exposed dyskinetic and nondyskinetic PD patients with similar clinical disease duration, disease severity, and daily levodopa dosage have shown similar levels of striatal dopamine D1 and D2 receptor availability.[52] Putamen D1 and D2 binding are normal, whereas caudate D2 binding is mildly reduced. These findings suggest that onset of motor complications in PD is not primarily associated with alterations in striatal dopamine receptor availability.

In the last decade, it has become clear that changes in levels of dopamine in the synaptic cleft are paralleled by changes in D2 receptor availability to ^{11}C-raclopride PET. The higher the extracellular dopamine level, the lower the dopamine D2 site availability to the tracer. When PD patients are given an intravenous bolus of levodopa, they show a decrease in ^{11}C-raclopride binding, which is greater in the putamen of advanced cases with fluctuations compared with early cases.[53] Based on animal microdialysis studies, decreases in D2 receptor availability in sustained and fluctuating responders after levodopa were estimated to correspond to 4-fold and 10-fold increases in synaptic dopamine levels and indicate that, as loss of dopamine terminals in PD progresses, the striatum fails to buffer dopamine levels when exogenous levodopa is administered. Pavese and colleagues[54] have shown more recently that the response of bradykinesia and rigidity in PD to levodopa correlates with the associated increases in striatal dopamine levels detected with ^{11}C-raclopride PET.

This regulation failure reflects a combination of upregulation of striatal dopamine synthesis and release by the remaining terminals after administration of levodopa along with a severe loss of dopamine transporters impeding reuptake. This phenomenon, rather than changes in postsynaptic dopamine D1 and D2 receptor binding, is likely to be the explanation for the more rapid response of advanced PD patients to oral levodopa. The failure to buffer dopamine levels by the striatum in advanced PD also results in high nonphysiological swings in synaptic dopamine levels. This situation may promote excessive dopamine receptor internalization into neurons, the normal mechanism for dissociating dopamine from the receptor, leading to fluctuating and unpredictable treatment responses. In support of this viewpoint, De la Fuente-Fernandez and colleagues[55] measured striatal ^{11}C-raclopride binding in PD at 1 and 4 hours after oral levodopa challenges. These investigators found that fluctuators showed transiently increased synaptic dopamine levels, whereas sustained responders generated a progressive increase in striatal dopamine over 4 hours. They also noted that "off" episodes could coincide with apparently adequate synaptic dopamine levels, supporting the concept that excessive receptor internalization could lead sometimes to nonavailability of dopamine binding sites.

In their ^{11}C-raclopride PET study, Pavese and colleagues[54] noted that the severity of peak dose dyskinesias generated by levodopa administration correlated with striatal levels of dopamine. This finding implies that overstimulation of dopamine receptors is a factor in generating peak dose dyskinesias; however, it is known from animal studies that peptide transmitters also play a role. Medium spiny neurons in the caudate and putamen project to external and internal pallidum where, along with γ-aminobutyric acid (GABA), they release enkephalin (globus pallidus externa), dynorphin, and substance P (globus pallidus interna). Enkephalin binds mainly to δ opioid sites and inhibits GABA release in the globus pallidus externa. Dynorphin binds to κ opioid sites and inhibits glutamate release in the globus pallidus interna from subthalamic projections. Under normal physiological conditions, phasic firing of striatal projection neurons results primarily in GABA release in the pallidum, whereas sustained tonic firing causes additional modulatory opioid and substance P release. The caudate and putamen contain high densities of μ, κ, and δ opioid sites and NK1 sites, which bind substance P. Opioid receptors are located presynaptically on dopamine terminals, where they regulate dopamine release, and postsynaptically on interneurons and medium spiny projection neurons.

[11]C-diprenorphine PET is a nonselective marker of μ, κ, and δ opioid sites, and its binding is sensitive to levels of endogenous opioids. If increased basal ganglia levels of enkephalin and dynorphin are associated with levodopa-associated dyskinesias, PD patients with motor complications would be expected to show reduced binding of ^{11}C-diprenorphine. Piccini and coworkers[56] reported significant reductions in ^{11}C-diprenorphine binding in caudate, putamen, thalamus, and anterior cingulate in dyskinetic patients compared with sustained responders. Individual levels of putamen ^{11}C-diprenorphine uptake correlated inversely with severity of dyskinesia. ^{18}F-L829165 PET is a selective marker of NK1 site availability. In a preliminary study, thalamic NK1 availability was shown to be reduced in dyskinetic PD patients but normal in nondyskinetic cases.[57] These in vivo PET findings support the presence of elevated levels of endogenous peptides in the basal ganglia of dyskinetic PD patients. These elevated levels may lead to abnormal pallidal burst firing and involuntary movements when levodopa is administered because of a failure to regulate GABA and glutamate release in the globus pallidus interna.

Pharmacology of Depression in Parkinson's Disease

The prevalence of depression in PD depends on the criteria used for diagnosis and has been reported to vary from 10% to 45%.[58] Its functional substrate is still uncertain, but dysfunction of limbic dopaminergic neurotransmission along with serotoninergic and noradrenergic projections, all of which are known to be affected by Lewy body pathology, would seem reasonable candidates.

The role of noradrenergic and dopaminergic dysfunction in PD patients with depression has been investigated with ^{11}C-RTI 32 PET, a marker of dopamine (DAT) and norepinephrine transporters. In nondepressed PD patients, there is a reduced binding of ^{11}C-RTI 32 in the striatum. When ^{11}C-RTI 32 PET findings were compared in PD patients with and without depression who were matched for age, disability, disease duration, and doses of antiparkinsonian medications, patients with depression showed additional reductions of ^{11}C-RTI 32 binding in the noradrenergic locus caeruleus, the thalamus, and regions of the limbic system (amygdala, ventral striatum, and anterior cingulate).[59] Severity of anxiety in PD was inversely correlated with ^{11}C-RTI 32 binding in all these regions, whereas apathy was inversely correlated with the radiotracer binding in the ventral striatum. These results suggest that depression and anxiety in PD are associated with loss of norepinephrine innervation and dopaminergic projections to the limbic system.

It is common to treat depression in PD with selective serotonin reuptake inhibitors, although the rationale for this treatment remains unproven. ^{11}C-WAY 100635 PET is a marker of serotonin 5-HT$_{1A}$ receptors, which act presynaptically as autoreceptors on 5-HT cell bodies in the midbrain raphe nuclei, inhibiting serotonin release, and postsynaptically on cortical pyramidal neurons. Doder and colleagues[60] reported a 25% reduction of ^{11}C-WAY 100635 binding in midbrain raphe in PD patients compared with healthy controls; however, the magnitude of reduction was no different in PD patients with and without depression. ^{123}I-β-CIT binds with nanomolar affinity to dopamine, norepinephrine, and serotonin transporters, and midbrain uptake, 1 hour after intravenous injection, reflects serotonin transporter (SERT) availability.[61] Normal binding of ^{123}I-β-CIT binding in the brainstem of PD patients compared with normal subjects has been reported and no correlation between radiotracer uptake and Hamilton Depression Rating Scale scores.[62] The results from these ^{11}C-WAY 100635 PET and ^{123}I-β-CIT SPECT studies do not support the view that serotoninergic loss contributes to depression in PD. Based on current evidence, nonselective inhibitors of monoamine transporters would seem the most rational approach to treating depression in PD.

Mechanisms Underlying Dementia in Parkinson's Disease

The prevalence of dementia is approximately 40% in patients with PD across different series, and the incidence is six times higher than that in age-matched healthy individuals, increasing with age.[63] Possible factors contributing to cognitive dysfunction include involvement of the cortex by Lewy body pathology that targets the cingulate and association areas, cholinergic cell loss in the nucleus basalis of Meynert, incidental AD and vascular pathology, and degeneration of the medial substantia nigra and ventral tegmental area and subsequent loss of mesolimbic and mesocortical dopaminergic projections.

MAGNETIC RESONANCE IMAGING VOLUMETRY

Summerfield and colleagues[64] applied MRI with voxel-based morphometry to localize significant regional brain volume reductions in PD patients with (PDD) and without later dementia. These workers concluded that the structural correlate of dementia in PD is hippocampal, thalamic, and anterior cingulate atrophy, and that subclinical volume loss in these areas can be detected in PD. In a subsequent prospective series involving a 2-year follow-up, Ramirez-Ruiz and coworkers[65] noted that in PDD further volume loss occurred primarily in neocortical areas, whereas in PD volume loss occurred primarily in limbic and temporal association areas. Using the boundary shift integral approach, Burton and colleagues[66] compared whole-brain volume reductions over 1 year in PD and PDD cases. Loss of brain volume occurred at a normal rate in PD (0.31% per annum), whereas it was increased in PDD (1.12% per annum) approaching rates reported for AD

(2% per annum). These authors concluded that MRI may be a useful tool for following progression of PDD.

METABOLIC STUDIES

^{18}FDG PET is a marker of resting cerebral glucose metabolism and reveals a consistent pattern of reduced resting cerebral glucose metabolism in AD beginning in posterior cingulate, parietal, and temporal association regions spreading to prefrontal cortex.[67] In PD patients who develop dementia 1 or more years after onset of motor disability (PDD), ^{18}FDG PET has shown a similar pattern of reduced glucose metabolism affecting frontal and temporoparietal association areas.[68,69]

DLB is characterized by dementia, parkinsonism, visual hallucinations, psychosis, and fluctuating confusion. The dementia is present at onset or within the first year of parkinsonism. The pattern of reduced ^{18}FDG uptake resembles that seen in AD, although additional involvement of occipital areas has been reported.[70] Yong compared patterns of glucose metabolism in PD patients with and without dementia and patients fulfilling consensus criteria for DLB. A direct comparison between DLB and PDD showed a relative resting cerebral glucose metabolism decrease in anterior cingulate in patients with DLB.[71] These findings support the concept that PDD, DLB, and AD have overlapping patterns of cortical dysfunction, although anterior cingulate and occipital areas may be more involved in DLB. Temporoparietal cortical hypometabolism can also be observed in one third of PD patients without dementia and with established disease.[72] It remains to be determined whether the observed glucose hypometabolism in these subjects is a predictor of late-onset dementia.

DOPAMINERGIC STUDIES

Lewy body pathology targets the substantia nigra; whereas this is spared in AD. ^{123}I-FP-CIT SPECT, an in vivo marker of DAT binding, has been used to discriminate DLB from AD during life based on the detection of striatal dopamine terminal dysfunction. In an initial series, Walker and colleagues[73] assessed the integrity of nigrostriatal function in PD, AD, and DLB patients, and reported that DLB and PD patients had significantly lower striatal uptake of ^{123}I-FP-CIT than patients with AD and controls. Autopsy data subsequently became available for 10 of the dementia subjects investigated with SPECT. All four cases proven to have DLB at postmortem examination showed reduced striatal ^{123}I-FP-CIT uptake. Four of five autopsy-proven AD cases showed normal striatal ^{123}I-FP-CIT uptake, whereas the fifth, who had been diagnosed as having DLB in life, had concomitant small vessel disease and showed reduced DAT binding. SPECT provided a sensitivity of 100% and a specificity of 83% for DLB and performed better than clinical impression, which diagnosed only four of the nine DLB cases correctly in life. In a follow-up series gathered over 10 years, the same investigators workers reported correlations between clinical impression, pathology, and striatal ^{123}I-FP-CIT uptake in 20 cases (8 pathologically proven DLB, 9 AD [mostly with coexisting cerebrovascular disease], and 3 patients with other diagnoses [frontotemporal dementia, corticobasal degeneration, and nonspecific pathology]).[74] They found that the baseline sensitivity of an initial clinical diagnosis of DLB was 75%, and the specificity was 42%, whereas the baseline sensitivity of FP-CIT SPECT for the diagnosis of DLB was 88%, and the specificity was 100%.

^{123}I-FP-CIT SPECT has been used to assess the extent and pattern of dopamine transporter loss in patients with DLB compared with other dementias including PDD.[75] Striatal ^{123}I-FP-CIT uptake was normal in AD patients, whereas loss of DAT binding was of similar magnitude in DLB and PD. Compared with PD patients, in whom a selective involvement of putamen was observed, patients with DLB and PDD showed a more uniform striatal reduction in ^{123}I-FP-CIT binding with loss of the caudate-putamen gradient. There was a significant correlation between the mini-mental status examination scores and ^{123}I-FP-CIT binding in PDD, supporting the hypothesis that striatal dopaminergic loss may contribute to the cognitive impairment of these patients.

The role of the mesolimbic and mesocortical dopaminergic projections in PD dementia has been investigated with ^{18}F-dopa PET. Ito and colleagues[76] applied statistical parametric mapping to localize significant reductions in dopaminergic function in PD and PDD patients matched for age, disease duration, and disease severity. Compared with the PD patients, the PDD patients showed additional ^{18}F-dopa uptake reductions in the right caudate and bilaterally in the ventral striatum and the anterior cingulate. These findings add support to the concept that dementia in PD is associated with impaired mesolimbic, mesocortical, and caudate dopaminergic function. It has been previously reported that reductions in frontal ^{18}F-dopa uptake correlate with impaired performance on tests of verbal fluency, verbal recall, and digit span in PD.[77]

CHOLINERGIC STUDIES

[123]I-iodobenzovesamicol (^{123}I-BVM) SPECT is a marker of acetylcholine vesicle transporter binding, and has been employed to assess the association of cholinergic deficiency with dementia in PD. Reduced binding of ^{123}I-BVM can be seen in the parietal and occipital cortex of PD patients without dementia, and this becomes more severe and widespread in PDD and AD.[78] Acetylcholinesterase activity can be assessed with ^{11}C-MP4A and ^{11}C-PMP PET. In one series, cortical ^{11}C-MP4A binding was reduced by 11% in PD and by 30% in PDD, and tracer uptake correlated with striatal ^{18}F-dopa reduction, suggesting that the dementia of PDD is associated with a parallel reduction in dopaminergic and cholinergic function.[79] ^{11}C-PMP PET has revealed a significant correlation between cortical acetylcholinesterase activity and performance on tests of attentional and executive functions in a combined group of PD and PDD patients.[80] Cortical acetylcholinesterase deficiency did not correlate with motor symptoms. Taken together, these findings suggest that a deficiency of cholinergic transmission contributes to the dementia of PD and lends support for the use of acetylcholinesterase inhibitors.

MEASURING β-AMYLOID LOAD

The PET ligand ^{11}C-PIB is a neutral thioflavine that shows nanomolar affinity for neuritic β-amyloid plaques (Fig. 11–3) in AD brain slices, but low affinity for intracellular neurofibrillary tangles and Lewy bodies.[81] ^{11}C-PIB PET studies reveal twofold increases in tracer retention in the association cortex and cingulate of patients with AD compared with healthy controls.[82] Pathological studies

¹¹C–PIB PET

Amyloid load

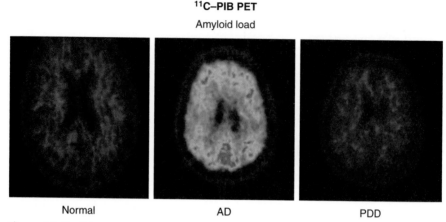

| Normal | AD | PDD |

Figure 11–3 ¹¹C-PIB PET images of β-amyloid plaque load. The elderly normal subject and Parkinson's disease patient with late dementia (PDD) show no significant plaque deposition in the brain compared with the patient with Alzheimer's disease (AD), in which amyloid deposition is extensive. (Courtesy of Paul Edison.)

have shown variable levels of β-amyloid deposition in DLB and PDD. Edison and colleagues[83] used ¹¹C-PIB PET to determine the association of an increased amyloid load with dementia in DLB and PDD. Although 11 of 13 DLB cases had significantly increased cortical amyloid levels, this was true of only 2 of 13 PDD cases. Ahmed and Brooks (unpublished observations) have used ¹¹C-PIB and ¹⁸F-FDG PET to correlate in vivo regional brain β-amyloid load with glucose metabolism in six patients with PDD. The PDD patients all had significant reduced glucose metabolism in frontal, temporal, parietal, and occipital association areas compared with controls, but none showed any increase in β-amyloid levels. These findings suggest that β-amyloid deposition does not contribute significantly to the pathogenesis of late dementia in PD, in accordance with pathological reports (Aarsland 2005).[84] Conversely, in patients with DLB, an increase in ¹¹C-PIB uptake is seen in most patients.[85]

Dementia in PD is multifactorial, being associated to varying degrees with cortical Lewy body disease, amyloid deposition, and loss of dopaminergic and cortical cholinergic transmission. Functional imaging can help determine the relative contributions of these factors in individual cases and potentially rationalize the use of antiamyloid strategies in PDD and DLB.

Microglial Activation in Parkinson's Disease

Microglia constitute 10% to 20% of white blood cells in the brain and are normally in a resting state, but local injury causes them to activate and swell expressing HLA antigens on the cell surface and to release cytokines such as tumor necrosis factor-α and interleukins. The mitochondria of activated but not resting microglia express peripheral benzodiazepine sites, which can be visualized with ¹¹C-PK11195 PET (Fig. 11–4).

Normal   PD

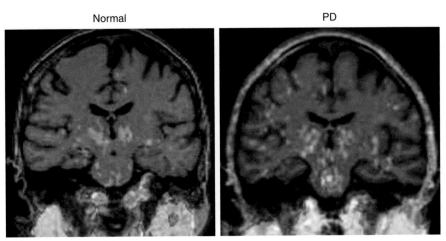

Figure 11–4 ¹¹C-PK11195 PET scans of a healthy subject and Parkinson's disease (PD) patient. Mild microglial activation is seen in the thalamus of the healthy control, whereas significantly increased activation is evident in the midbrain and striata of the PD patient along with the normal levels of thalamic activation. (Courtesy of Alex Gerhard.)

Loss of substantia nigra neurons in PD has been shown to be associated with microglial activation, and histochemical studies more recently have shown that microglial activation can also be seen in other basal ganglia, the cingulate, hippocampus, and cortical areas.[86] ¹¹C-PK11195 PET has been used to study microglial activation in PD, and increased midbrain signal has been reported to correlate inversely with levels of posterior putamen DAT binding measured with ¹¹C-CFT PET.[87] Gerhard and coworkers[88] subsequently reported additional microglial activation in the brainstem, striatum, pallidum, and frontal cortex, in accordance with the distribution of Lewy body pathology reported by Braak and colleagues in advanced PD.[89] There was little change in the level of microglial activation over a 2-year follow-up period, although the patients all deteriorated clinically. This could imply that microglial activation is merely an epiphenomenon in PD; however, postmortem studies have shown that these cells continue to express cytokine mRNA, suggesting that they could be driving disease progression.

Conclusions

Structural changes in PD nigra can be detected with TCS and MRI possibly reflecting increased iron levels. TCS may be valuable for revealing a susceptibility to PD and aiding diagnosis. PET and SPECT measurements of dopamine terminal function sensitively detect dopamine deficiency in symptomatic and at-risk subjects for parkinsonian syndromes, and provide biomarkers for monitoring disease progression. A normal scan in a patient suspected to have PD implies a good prognosis. Atypical PD can be most sensitively discriminated from PD with either diffusion-weighted MRI or ¹⁸FDG PET.

Depression in PD is associated with loss of noradrenergic and limbic monoaminergic function, but not serotoninergic dysfunction. DLB can be reliably discriminated from AD by detecting loss of striatal DAT binding. Most DLB patients also have a significant amyloid load, whereas this is uncommon in PD patients with later dementia. Microglial activation can be detected in PD with ^{11}C-PK11195 PET and provides a rationale for exploring the use of anti-inflammatory agents as potential neuroprotectants.

REFERENCES

1. Hughes AJ, Ben-Shlomo Y, Daniel SE, Lees AJ: What features improve the accuracy of clinical diagnosis in Parkinson's disease: a clinicopathological study. Neurology 1992;42:1142-1146.
2. Hutchinson M, Raff U: Structural changes of the substantia nigra in Parkinson's disease as revealed by MR imaging. AJNR Am J Neuroradiol 2000;21:697-701.
3. Hu MT, White SJ, Herlihy AH, et al: A comparison of (18)F-dopa PET and inversion recovery MRI in the diagnosis of Parkinson's disease. Neurology 2001;56:1195-1200.
4. Minati L, Grisoli M, Carella F, et al: Imaging degeneration of the substantia nigra in Parkinson disease with inversion-recovery MR imaging. AJNR Am J Neuroradiol 2007;28:309-313.
5. Michaeli S, Oz G, Sorce DJ, et al: Assessment of brain iron and neuronal integrity in patients with Parkinson's disease using novel MRI contrasts. Mov Disord 2007;22:334-340.
6. Geng DY, Li YX, Zee CS: Magnetic resonance imaging-based volumetric analysis of basal ganglia nuclei and substantia nigra in patients with Parkinson's disease. Neurosurgery 2006;58:256-262.
7. Schulz JB, Skalej M, Wedekind D, et al: Magnetic resonance imaging-based volumetry differentiates idiopathic Parkinson's syndrome from multiple system atrophy and progressive supranuclear palsy. Ann Neurol 1999;45:65-74.
8. Paviour DC, Price SL, Jahanshahi M, et al: Regional brain volumes distinguish PSP, MSA-P, and PD: MRI-based clinico-radiological correlations. Mov Disord 2006;21:989-996.
9. Schocke MF, Seppi K, Esterhammer R, et al: Diffusion-weighted MRI differentiates the Parkinson variant of multiple system atrophy from PD. Neurology 2002;58:575-580.
10. Seppi K, Schocke MF, Esterhammer R, et al: Diffusion-weighted imaging discriminates progressive supranuclear palsy from PD, but not from the parkinson variant of multiple system atrophy. Neurology 2003;60:922-927.
11. Nicoletti G, Lodi R, Condino F, et al: Apparent diffusion coefficient measurements of the middle cerebellar peduncle differentiate the Parkinson variant of MSA from Parkinson's disease and progressive supranuclear palsy. Brain 2006;129:2679-2687.
12. Paviour DC, Thornton JS, Lees AJ, Jager HR: Diffusion-weighted magnetic resonance imaging differentiates parkinsonian variant of multiple-system atrophy from progressive supranuclear palsy. Mov Disord 2007;22:68-74.
13. Berg D, Siefker C, Becker G: Echogenicity of the substantia nigra in Parkinson's disease and its relation to clinical findings. J Neurol 2001;248:684-689.
14. Prestel J, Schweitzer KJ, Hofer A, et al: Predictive value of transcranial sonography in the diagnosis of Parkinson's disease. Mov Disord 2006;21:1763-1765.
15. Stockner H, Sojer M, K KS, et al: Midbrain sonography in patients with essential tremor. Mov Disord 2007;22:414-417.
16. Walter U, Hoeppner J, Prudente-Morrissey L, et al: Parkinson's disease-like midbrain sonography abnormalities are frequent in depressive disorders. Brain 2007;130:1799-1807.
17. Berg D, Merz B, Reiners K, et al: Five-year follow-up study of hyperechogenicity of the substantia nigra in Parkinson's disease. Mov Disord 2005;20:383-385.
18. Berg D, Roggendorf W, Schroder U, et al: Echogenicity of the substantia nigra: association with increased iron content and marker for susceptibility to nigrostriatal injury. Arch Neurol 2002;59:999-1005.
19. Walter U, Dressler D, Probst T, et al: Transcranial brain sonography findings in discriminating between parkinsonism and idiopathic Parkinson disease. Arch Neurol 2007;64:1635-1640.
20. Brooks DJ, Frey KA, Marek KL, et al: Assessment of neuroimaging techniques as biomarkers of the progression of Parkinson's disease. Exp Neurol 2003;184:S68-S79.
21. Morrish PK, Sawle GV, Brooks DJ: Clinical and [18F]dopa PET findings in early Parkinson's disease. J Neurol Neurosurg Psychiatry 1995;59:597-600.
22. Whone AL, Moore RY, Piccini P, Brooks DJ: Plasticity in the nigropallidal pathway in Parkinson's disease: an 18F-dopa PET study. Ann Neurol 2003;53:206-213.

23. Benamer TS, Patterson J, Grosset DG, et al: Accurate differentiation of parkinsonism and essential tremor using visual assessment of [123I]-FP-CIT imaging: the [123I]-FP-CIT Study Group. Mov Disord 2000;15:503-510.
24. Jennings DL, Seibyl JP, Oakes D, et al: (123I) beta-CIT and single-photon emission computed tomographic imaging vs clinical evaluation in parkinsonian syndrome: unmasking an early diagnosis. Arch Neurol 2004;61:1224-1229.
25. Catafau AM, Tolosa E: Impact of dopamine transporter SPECT using 123I-Ioflupane on diagnosis and management of patients with clinically uncertain parkinsonian syndromes. Mov Disord 2004;19:1175-1182.
26. Tolosa E, Borght TV, Moreno E: Accuracy of DaTSCAN ((123)I-ioflupane) SPECT in diagnosis of patients with clinically uncertain parkinsonism: 2-year follow-up of an open-label study. Mov Disord 2007;22:2346-2351.
27. Marshall VL, Patterson J, Hadley DM, et al: Two-year follow-up in 150 consecutive cases with normal dopamine transporter imaging. Nucl Med Commun 2006;27:933-937.
28. Brooks DJ: Functional imaging in relation to parkinsonian syndromes. J Neurol Sci 1993;115: 1-17.
29. Eidelberg D, Moeller JR, Dhawan V, et al: The metabolic topography of parkinsonism. J Cereb Blood Flow Metab 1994;14:783-801.
30. Su PC, Ma Y, Fukuda M, et al: Metabolic changes following subthalamotomy for advanced Parkinson's disease. Ann Neurol 2001;50:514-520.
31. Feigin A, Fukuda M, Dhawan V, et al: Metabolic correlates of levodopa response in Parkinson's disease. Neurology 2001;57:2083-2088.
32. Eckert T, Feigin A, Lewis DE, et al: Regional metabolic changes in parkinsonian patients with normal dopaminergic imaging. Mov Disord 2007;22:167-173.
33. Burn DJ, Sawle GV, Brooks DJ: The differential diagnosis of Parkinson's disease, multiple system atrophy, and Steele-Richardson-Olszewski syndrome: discriminant analysis of striatal 18F-dopa PET data. J Neurol Neurosurg Psychiatry 1994;57:278-284.
34. Pirker W, Asenbaum S, Bencsits G, et al: [I-123]beta-CIT SPECT in multiple system atrophy, progressive supranuclear palsy, and corticobasal degeneration. Mov Disord 2000;15:1158-1167.
35. Eckert T, Barnes A, Dhawan V, et al: FDG PET in the differential diagnosis of parkinsonian disorders. Neuroimage 2005;26:912-921.
36. Golbe LI: The genetics of Parkinson's disease: a reconsideration. Neurology 1990;40;(Suppl 3): 7-16.
37. Berg D, Siefker C, Ruprecht-Dorfler P, Becker G: Relationship of substantia nigra echogenicity and motor function in elderly subjects. Neurology 2001;56:13-17.
38. Walter U, Klein C, Hilker R, et al: Brain parenchyma sonography detects preclinical parkinsonism. Mov Disord 2004;19:1445-1449.
39. Sommer U, Hummel T, Cormann K, et al: Detection of presymptomatic Parkinson's disease: combining smell tests, transcranial sonography, and SPECT. Mov Disord 2004;19:1196-1202.
40. Spiegel J, Hellwig D, Mollers MO, et al: Transcranial sonography and [123I]FP-CIT SPECT disclose complementary aspects of Parkinson's disease. Brain 2006;129:1188-1193.
41. Piccini P, Morrish PK, Turjanski N, et al: Dopaminergic function in familial Parkinson's disease: a clinical and 18F-dopa PET study. Ann Neurol 1997;41:222-229.
42. Hilker R, Klein C, Hedrich K, et al: The striatal dopaminergic deficit is dependent on the number of mutant alleles in a family with mutations in the parkin gene: evidence for enzymatic parkin function in humans. Neurosci Lett 2002;323:50-54.
43. Khan NL, Brooks DJ, Pavese N, et al: Progression of nigrostriatal dysfunction in a parkin kindred. Brain 2002;125:2248-2256.
44. Scherfler C, Khan NL, Pavese N, et al: Striatal and cortical pre- and postsynaptic dopaminergic dysfunction in sporadic parkin-linked parkinsonism. Brain 2004;127:1332-1342.
45. Khan NL, Scherfler C, Graham E, et al: Dopaminergic dysfunction in unrelated, asymptomatic carriers of a single parkin mutation. Neurology 2005;64:134-136.
46. Adams JR, van Netten H, Schulzer M, et al: PET in LRRK2 mutations: comparison to sporadic Parkinson's disease and evidence for presymptomatic compensation. Brain 2005;128:2777-2785.
47. Ponsen MM, Stoffers D, Booij J, et al: Idiopathic hyposmia as a preclinical sign of Parkinson's disease. Ann Neurol 2004;56:173-181.
48. Stiasny-Kolster K, Doerr Y, Moller JC, et al: Combination of 'idiopathic' REM sleep behaviour disorder and olfactory dysfunction as possible indicator for alpha-synucleinopathy demonstrated by dopamine transporter FP-CIT-SPECT. Brain 2005;128:126-137.

49. De La Fuente-Fernandez R, Pal PK, Vingerhoets FJG, et al: Evidence for impaired presynaptic dopamine function in parkinsonian patients with motor fluctuations. J Neural Transm 2000;107: 49-57.
50. Playford ED, Brooks DJ: In vivo and in vitro studies of the dopaminergic system in movement disorders. Cerebrovasc Brain Metab Rev 1992;4:144-171.
51. Antonini A, Schwarz J, Oertel WH, et al: [11C]raclopride and positron emission tomography in previously untreated patients with Parkinson's disease: influence of L-dopa and lisuride therapy on striatal dopamine D2-receptors. Neurology 1994;44:1325-1329.
52. Turjanski N, Lees AJ, Brooks DJ: PET studies on striatal dopaminergic receptor binding in drug naive and L-dopa treated Parkinson's disease patients with and without dyskinesia. Neurology 1997;49:717-723.
53. Torstenson R, Hartvig P, Långström B, et al: Differential effects of levodopa on dopaminergic function in early and advanced Parkinson's disease. Ann Neurol 1997;41:334-340.
54. Pavese N, Evans AH, Tai YF, et al: Clinical correlates of levodopa-induced dopamine release in Parkinson disease: a PET study. Neurology 2006;67:1612-1617.
55. De la Fuente-Fernandez R, Lu JQ, Sossi V, et al: Biochemical variations in the synaptic level of dopamine precede motor fluctuations in Parkinson's disease: PET evidence of increased dopamine turnover. Ann Neurol 2001;49:298-303.
56. Piccini P, Weeks RA, Brooks DJ: Opioid receptor binding in Parkinson's patients with and without levodopa-induced dyskinesias. Ann Neurol 1997;42:720-726.
57. Whone AL, Rabiner EA, Arahata Y, et al: Reduced substance P binding in Parkinson's disease complicated by dyskinesias: an F-18-L829165 PET study [Abstract]. Neurology 2002;58:(Suppl 3). A488.
58. Burn DJ: Beyond the iron mask: towards better recognition and treatment of depression associated with Parkinson's disease. Mov Disord 2002;17:445-454.
59. Remy P, Doder M, Lees AJ, et al: Depression in Parkinson's disease: loss of dopamine and noradrenaline innervation in the limbic system. Brain 2005;128:1314-1322.
60. Doder M, Rabiner EA, Turjanski N, et al: Brain serotonin HT1A receptors in Parkinson's disease with and without depression measured by positron emission tomography and 11C-WAY100635 [Abstract]. Mov Disord 2000;15(Suppl):213.
61. Laruelle M, Baldwin RM, Malison RT, et al: SPECT imaging of dopamine and serotonin transporters with [123I]beta-CIT: pharmacological characterization of brain uptake in nonhuman primates. Synapse 1993;13:295-309.
62. Kim SE, Choi JY, Choe YS, et al: Serotonin transporters in the midbrain of Parkinson's disease patients: a study with 123I-beta-CIT SPECT. J Nucl Med 2003;44:870-876.
63. Emre M: Dementia associated with Parkinson's disease. Lancet Neurol 2003;2:229-237.
64. Summerfield C, Junque C, Tolosa E, et al: Structural brain changes in Parkinson disease with dementia: a voxel-based morphometry study. Arch Neurol 2005;62:281-285.
65. Ramirez-Ruiz B, Marti MJ, Tolosa E, et al: Longitudinal evaluation of cerebral morphological changes in Parkinson's disease with and without dementia. J Neurol 2005;252:1345-1352.
66. Burton EJ, McKeith IG, Burn DJ, O'Brien JT: Brain atrophy rates in Parkinson's disease with and without dementia using serial magnetic resonance imaging. Mov Disord 2005;20:1571-1576.
67. Hoffman JM, Welsh-Bohmer KA, Hanson M, et al: FDG PET imaging in patients with pathologically verified dementia. J Nucl Med 2000;41:1920-1928.
68. Peppard RF, Martin WRW, Carr GD, et al: Cerebral glucose metabolism in Parkinson's disease with and without dementia. Arch Neurol 1992;49:1262-1268.
69. Vander-Borght T, Minoshima S, Giordani B, et al: Cerebral metabolic differences in Parkinson's and Alzheimer's disease matched for dementia severity. J Nucl Med 1997;38:797-802.
70. Albin RL, Minoshima S, D'Amato CJ, et al: Fluoro-deoxyglucose positron emission tomography in diffuse Lewy body disease. Neurology 1996;47:462-466.
71. Yong SW, Yoon JK, An YS J, et al: A comparison of cerebral glucose metabolism in Parkinson's disease, Parkinson's disease dementia and dementia with Lewy bodies. Eur J Neurol 2007;14(12):1357-1362.
72. Hu MTM, Taylor-Robinson SD, Chaudhuri KR, et al: Cortical dysfunction in non-demented Parkinson's disease patients: a combined 31Phosphorus MRS and 18FDG PET study. Brain 2000;123:340-352.
73. Walker Z, Costa DC, Walker RW, et al: Differentiation of dementia with Lewy bodies from Alzheimer's disease using a dopaminergic presynaptic ligand. J Neurol Neurosurg Psychiatry 2002;73:134-140.
74. Walker Z, Jaros E, Walker RW, et al: Dementia with Lewy bodies: a comparison of clinical diagnosis, FP-CIT SPECT imaging and autopsy. J Neurol Neurosurg Psychiatry 2007;78:1176-1181.

75. O'Brien JT, Colloby S, Fenwick J, et al: Dopamine transporter loss visualized with FP-CIT SPECT in the differential diagnosis of dementia with Lewy bodies. Arch Neurol 2004;61:919-925.
76. Ito K, Nagano-Saito A, Kato T, et al: Striatal and extrastriatal dysfunction in Parkinson's disease with dementia: a 6-[18F]fluoro-L-dopa PET study. Brain 2002;125:1358-1365.
77. Rinne JO, Portin R, Ruottinen H, et al: Cognitive impairment and the brain dopaminergic system in Parkinson disease: [18F]fluorodopa positron emission tomographic study. Arch Neurol 2000;57:470-475.
78. Kuhl DE, Minoshima S, Fessler JA, et al: In vivo mapping of cholinergic terminals in normal aging, Alzheimer's disease, and Parkinson's disease. Ann Neurol 1996;40:399-410.
79. Hilker R, Thomas AV, Klein JC, et al: Dementia in Parkinson disease: functional imaging of cholinergic and dopaminergic pathways. Neurology 2005;65:1716-1722.
80. Bohnen NI, Kaufer DI, Hendrickson R, et al: Cognitive correlates of cortical cholinergic denervation in Parkinson's disease and parkinsonian dementia. J Neurol 2006;253(2):242-247.
81. Bacskai BJ, Frosch MP, Freeman SH, et al: Molecular imaging with Pittsburgh Compound B confirmed at autopsy: a case report. Arch Neurol 2007;64:431-434.
82. Edison P, Archer HA, Hinz R, et al: Amyloid, hypometabolism, and cognition in Alzheimer disease—an [11C]PIB and [18F]FDG PET study. Neurology 2007;68:501-508.
83. Edison P, Rowe CC, Rinne J, et al: Amyloid load in Lewy body dementia (LBD), Parkinson's disease dementia (PDD) and Parkinson's disease (PD) measured with C-11-PIB PET. Neurology 2007;68:A98.
84. Aarsland D, Perry R, Brown A, et al: Neuropathology of dementia in Parkinson's disease: a prospective, community-based study. Ann Neurol 2005;58(5):773-776.
85. Rowe CC, Ng S, Ackermann U, et al: Imaging beta-amyloid burden in aging and dementia. Neurology 2007;68:1718-1725.
86. Imamura K, Hishikawa N, Sawada M, et al: Distribution of major histocompatibility complex class II-positive microglia and cytokine profile of Parkinson's disease brains. Acta Neuropathol (Berl) 2003;106:518-526.
87. Ouchi Y, Yoshikawa E, Sekine Y, et al: Microglial activation and dopamine terminal loss in early Parkinson's disease. Ann Neurol 2005;57:168-175.
88. Gerhard A, Pavese N, Hotton GR, et al: Microglial activation in Parkinson's disease—its longitudinal course and correlation with clinical parameters: an [11C](R)-PK11195 PET study. Neurology 2004;62(Suppl 5):A432.
89. Braak H, Ghebremedhin E, Rub U, et al: Stages in the development of Parkinson's disease-related pathology. Cell Tissue Res 2004;318(1):121-134.

12 Dementia in Parkinson's Disease

DAVID JOHN BURN

Introduction

In Parkinson's seminal description of the disorder that now bears his name, no mention is made of dementia, and he believed that "by the absence of any injury to the senses and to the intellect, we are taught that the morbid state does not extend to the encephalon." Later in the 19th century, however, Trousseau and Brazire noted, "The intellect ... gets weakened at last; the patient loses his memory and his friends notice soon that his mind is not as clear." In 1882, Ball commented that "paralysis agitans is accompanied more often than is thought by intellectual difficulties." Ball's insightful comments have proved to be accurate, and cognitive decline in Parkinson's disease (PD) is now recognized as a common complication of this neurodegenerative disease.

Dementia associated with PD (PDD) is associated with increased mortality,[1] reduced quality of life,[2] and increased caregiver distress,[3] and is a major risk factor for nursing home placement,[4] with important implications for costs of care. Neuropsychiatric symptoms, including psychotic features, accompany cognitive decline in PD in most cases and may be extremely troublesome. Dementia and psychosis constrain effective medical and surgical management of the movement disorder. These symptoms have serious social and health economic consequences, and pose unique therapeutic challenges.

This chapter discusses the epidemiology, clinical features, diagnosis, pathology, and management of dementia associated with PD. Areas of deficiency in our knowledge are highlighted. A practical approach to the topic has been maintained as far as possible throughout, with the clinician in mind.

Epidemiology of Dementia Associated with Parkinson's Disease

The incidence of dementia in patients with PD is 30 to 112.5 per 1000 person-years.[5] The variability almost certainly relates to methodological differences, including whether the patients were hospitalized or living in the community, and the definition of dementia employed. A patient with PD is five to six times more likely to have dementia than an age-matched control without PD.[6] Variations in point prevalence reflect methodological differences, with door-to-door studies generally yielding lower estimates than clinic-based studies. A comprehensive review determined the prevalence of dementia in PD to be 31.5% (95% confidence interval 29.3 to 33.5), and estimated that 3% to 4% of dementia cases in the general population were due to PDD.[7] With the secular increase in life expectancy for the whole population over the last 2 centuries, and the development of effective antiparkinsonian drugs, the cumulative incidence of dementia in PD may be 80%.[8,9] Time from the onset of PD to the development of PDD averages 10 years.

Lewy Body Dementia Spectrum

Confusion commonly arises when discussing *dementia associated with Parkinson's disease, dementia with Lewy bodies (DLB)*, and the *Lewy body dementias*. The currently accepted view is as follows: DLB is the most appropriate diagnosis when the patient develops dementia as the initial and dominant clinical feature or when dementia occurs in the context of parkinsonism that has been present for *less* than 12 months (Fig. 12–1). PDD is most apposite when dementia develops in the face of PD that has been present for *more* than 12 months. Lewy body dementia is a "catch-all" term that is inclusive of DLB and PDD.

Diagnostic criteria for DLB[10] and for PDD[11] (see later) adhere to this "12-month rule." These terms make many implicit assumptions that are incorrect. The first is that DLB and PDD are discrete conditions; this is highly improbable. Clinical, imaging, and pathological data tend to favor a "spectrum" approach, with DLB at one end and PD at the other.[12] Diagnostic labels do have use, however, in terms of patient management, relevant society support, and in regulatory and trial issues. A second assumption is that Lewy bodies are central to and necessary for

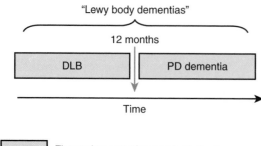

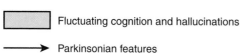

Fluctuating cognition and hallucinations

Parkinsonian features

Figure 12–1 The relationship between Parkinson's disease (PD) dementia, dementia with Lewy bodies (DLB), and the term "Lewy body dementias."

causing the dementia syndrome. The role of Lewy (i.e., synuclein protein–related) pathology and its relationship to PDD is discussed in more detail subsequently, but distribution of this pathology and the degree of coexisting Alzheimer's-like lesions can vary widely from patient to patient.

Predicting Dementia in Parkinson's Disease

Increasing age is the most important risk factor for PDD. Increasing motor disability is also predictive of dementia and is synergistic with current age.[13] A non–tremor-dominant motor phenotype is overrepresented in PDD,[14] and associated with a fourfold increased risk of dementia,[5] whereas conversion from a tremor-dominant to non–tremor-dominant phenotype is also predictive of dementia.[15] Longer disease duration and male gender have been associated with increased risk of PDD, with less well-established factors including low educational attainment and current smoking habit (contrasting with the well-established inverse association of smoking and PD).[16-18]

Differences in sustained attention occur between PD patients with and without orthostatic hypotension,[19] but it is unknown whether the autonomic abnormality is in some way causative, or simply associated with the cognitive deficit. Dementia *may* be associated with weight loss in PD,[20] but the predictive value of antecedent weight loss is unknown. Excessive daytime somnolence and rapid-eye-movement (REM) sleep behavior disorder may predict PDD, but the data to support both are weak at present. Anticholinergic drug use may be a risk factor for PDD, and prolonged use of these agents has been associated with an increased frequency of cortical plaques and tangles in PD patients without dementia.[21] Poor response to levodopa and hallucinations on dopaminergic treatment may also predict dementia.[22,23] Levodopa-induced elevation in plasma homocysteine could contribute to cognitive failure, whereas amantadine may delay and attenuate dementia.[24]

Deficits in auditory verbal learning and nonverbal reasoning, picture completion, Stroop interference, and verbal fluency all have been independently associated with an increased risk of cognitive failure in PD.[25] As simple bedside tests, pentagon copying and semantic fluency may predict cognitive decline.[5] It is uncertain whether depression is an independent risk factor for dementia in PD. There is an association between apathy and cognitive dysfunction, particularly executive impairment,[26] but it is unknown whether apathy is independently predictive of dementia.

Clinical Features of Dementia in Parkinson's Disease

MILD COGNITIVE IMPAIRMENT

Mild cognitive impairment (MCI) has not yet been defined for PD. It remains to be determined whether "MCI-PD" will prove to be a clinically useful concept. Loss of dopaminergic innervation of the caudate nucleus and functional deafferentation of the dorsolateral prefrontal cortex may produce cognitive deficits in PD sufficient to qualify for "MCI,"[27] but such deficits may be distinct from the pathophysiological processes underpinning frank dementia (see later).

Workers to date have generally applied modified Petersen criteria to define MCI-PD. In one study, using these criteria, 21% of 86 PD cases had MCI, with frontal/executive dysfunction being the most frequently abnormal cognitive domain, followed by amnestic deficit.[28] In another study involving 72 PD subjects initially without dementia,[29] the annual rate of progression from MCI-PD to PDD was 15% compared with a rate of 4% in cognitively intact PD subjects. Single-domain non–memory-related MCI and multiple-domain MCI were associated with later development of dementia, whereas amnestic MCI subtype was not, although small sample size limited the strength of this conclusion.

COGNITIVE FEATURES

The onset of PDD is insidious, with a mean annual decline in MMSE of approximately 2 to 3 points compared with 1 point in PD controls without dementia.[30,31] The cognitive profile of PDD has been mainly derived from the study of patients with mild or moderate dementia, with few data available for cases with more severe dementia. Differences with other dementias (e.g., Alzheimer's disease [AD]) are more likely to be evident in the earlier stages. A more recent study described a significantly different cognitive profile in PDD compared with AD, although the mean Mini-Mental State Examination (MMSE) score in each group was only 19 points.[32] Poor performance of AD patients on an orientation test best discriminated the groups, followed by poor attentional performance by PDD patients on the serial 7s subtraction test (a measure of attentional control).[32]

Impaired attention and executive and visuospatial dysfunction are typically prominent in PDD. Interpretation of abnormal neuropsychological results is, however, problematic because the tests frequently do not tap a pure domain. Deficits in one area may lead to secondary problems in another. Executive deficits, through difficulties in planning and the use of appropriate retrieval strategies, may lead to abnormal clock drawing and impaired mnemonic performance. In addition, this "typical" profile fails to capture what is undoubtedly a heterogeneous disorder, reflected by the work of Janvin and colleagues,[33] who determined that 56% of their patients with PDD had a so-called subcortical cognitive profile compared with only 33% of patients with AD, according to the Dementia Rating Scale. Conversely, 30% of patients with PDD were classified as having a cortical profile. Clinically, PDD patients may present with greater "instrumental" cortical deficits, and a more common subcortical profile.

Attention is a heterogeneous construct, comprising executive control functions, selective attention, and sustained attention. Selective attention implies being able to focus in on one aspect, despite extraneous distracters, whereas sustained attention is also described as vigilance. "Fluctuating attention" occurred in 29% of PDD and 42% of DLB patients in one study that used a computer-based mode of assessment and probably reflects impaired sustained attention.[34] Attentional deficits may be the strongest cognitive predictor of activities of daily living status in PDD,[35] so the assessment of this cognitive impairment should not be overlooked. In a retrospective analysis of 243 autopsy-confirmed cases of PDD and DLB, after adjusting for age, gender, and concomitant AD pathology, fluctuating cognition was identified as the best predictor of poor outcome.[36]

Regarding executive function, verbal fluency and concept formation are typically more impaired in PDD compared with AD. There is no evidence that PDD subjects show greater perseveration than AD, however, at least when assessed using the Wisconsin Card Sort Task.

Visual perception is globally more impaired in PDD patients than in PD patients without dementia.[37] Compared with AD, PDD patients perform worse in all perceptual scores (visual discrimination, space-motion, and object-form perception). Visuoconstructional skills are probably also defective in PDD, as evidenced by impaired clock drawing. This test draws on numerous cognitive and motor functions, however, and most studies have failed to control for these potential confounders.

Verbal and visual memory are impaired in PDD, and the degree of this impairment is probably less than that seen in AD. Recognition memory may be less affected than recall in mild to moderate PDD. Nevertheless, the differences previously proposed in memory deficits between PDD and AD patients, and in particular a mnemonic deficit in PDD characterized by retrieval rather than encoding deficits, have not been clearly shown in most studies to date.

Dysphasia is rare in PDD, and its presence would suggest an alternative, or secondary, diagnosis. Based on relatively few studies, patients with PDD seem to have less impairment in core language functions compared with patients with AD when formally assessed.

BEHAVIORAL AND NEUROPSYCHIATRIC SYMPTOMS

Behavioral and neuropsychiatric disturbances, termed *neuropsychiatric symptoms,* are extremely common in PDD and frequently predate the onset of dementia. In a study of 537 PDD patients, 89% presented with at least one symptom when assessed using the Neuropsychiatric Inventory; 77% had two or more symptoms.[38] Some evidence also indicates that neuropsychiatric symptoms may occur in clusters in PDD,[38] perhaps reflecting distinct underlying neurobiological changes.

Hallucinations occur in 45% to 65% of PDD patients, considerably more commonly than in AD (where typically <10% are affected) and less frequently than in DLB (60% to 80%). Visual hallucinations in PDD also predict more rapid cognitive deterioration.[39] Visual hallucinations are twice as frequent as auditory ones, and most are complex, formed hallucinations. Tactile hallucinations are uncommon. Initially, visual hallucinations may be simple and ill-defined—a feeling that someone is behind the patient ("presence"), or that someone has passed across their visual field ("passage"). Subsequently, the hallucinations become more formed and detailed, often in color, static, and centrally located. Anonymous people and family members (living or dead) are common, as are animals.

As insight is lost, delusional misinterpretation of the hallucinations may occur. Overall, delusions have a frequency in PDD of 25% to 30%. Paranoid ideation, such as spousal infidelity and "phantom boarder" (believing strangers are living in the house), are common themes.

When applying formal diagnostic criteria to a community-based sample, the rate of major depression in PDD was found to be 13% compared with 9% for PD patients without dementia.[40] Severity of depressed mood and prevalence of major depression may be higher in PDD than in AD. Anxiety is also common in PDD (30% to 50%) and tends to cluster with depressed mood. Elevated mood is rare in PDD. Irritability and aggression, common in AD, are not prominent features in PDD. Apathy affects more than 50% of patients with PDD, and in 70% this may be severe.[38] This finding contrasts with a previously reported frequency of 17% for patients with PD without dementia.

OTHER CLINICAL FEATURES OF DEMENTIA ASSOCIATED WITH PARKINSON'S DISEASE

A postural instability gait disorder phenotype is overrepresented in PDD compared with PD[41]; more severe cognitive failure is associated with significantly more impairment in motor and autonomic domains.[42] Falls are more common in PDD patients than PD patients without dementia, and are likely to be multifactorial in nature, resulting not only from cognitive and neuropsychiatric factors, but also from motor and autonomic elements.

There is no evidence that bedside clinical examination of eye movements can distinguish between PD, PDD, and AD, although electro-oculography has shown that PDD and DLB patients are similarly impaired on reflexive and complex saccades compared with AD patients, who show deficits only in complex saccades.[43] Using the Epworth Sleepiness Scale, 57% of PDD, 50% of DLB, and 41% of PD subjects were classified as having excessive daytime somnolence compared with 18% of AD subjects and 10% of controls.[44] Sleep quality was poorer in PDD, PD, and DLB patients compared with AD and normal controls.

A higher frequency of symptomatic orthostasis has been reported in association with cognitive impairment in PD.[45] In a cross-sectional study of cardiovascular autonomic function in patients with PDD, DLB, AD, and vascular dementia compared with elderly controls, significant differences were found in severity of cardiovascular autonomic dysfunction between the four dementias. PDD and DLB groups had considerable impairment, whereas the vascular dementia group showed limited evidence of autonomic dysfunction, and in the AD group, apart from orthostatic hypotension, autonomic functions were normal. PDD patients showed consistent impairment of parasympathetic and sympathetic function tests compared with controls and AD patients.[46] Higher autonomic symptom scores in PDD are associated with poorer outcomes in all measures of physical activity, activities of daily living, depression, and quality of life.[47]

Although some reports have suggested reduced levodopa responsiveness in PDD patients, this has not been formally established, particularly after controlling for confounders such as subcortical small vessel disease. In one study, no significant difference in mean improvement on Unified Parkinson Disease Rating Scale motor score to a single-dose 200-mg levodopa challenge was recorded, although more patients without dementia experienced greater than 20% improvement compared with patients with PDD (90% versus 65%).[48] Another study included patients with DLB, PD, and PDD, and failed to detect differences in levodopa responsiveness between PD and PDD groups.[49] Data are insufficient to infer differences in the occurrence of levodopa-induced motor complications in PDD patients compared with PD patients.

Diagnostic Criteria

Until more recently, there were no specific and operationalized criteria to diagnose PDD. The *Diagnostic and Statistical Manual of Psychiatric Disorders, Fourth Edition* (DSM-IV) criteria subsume PDD under "dementia due to other medical conditions"; the section specifically devoted to PDD is short and more descriptive. In the absence of other, more specific criteria, it has been common for investigators to apply DSM-IV criteria to define "PDD," even though these criteria fail to capture several core features of the condition.

After an extensive literature review, a Movement Disorder Society Task Force published clinical diagnostic criteria for PDD (Tables 12–1 and 12–2).[11] In contrast to DLB, the defining feature of PDD in these new criteria is that dementia develops in the context of *established* PD. The diagnosis of dementia is based on the presence of deficits in at least two of four core cognitive domains—attention, memory, executive, and visuospatial functions (see Table 12–1). These deficits should be elicited by clinical and cognitive examination, and should be severe enough to affect normal functioning. The criteria also take into account the fact that neuropsychiatric and behavioral symptoms are a frequent, but not invariable, accompaniment of PDD (see Table 12–1).

Clinical diagnostic criteria for levels of "probable" and "possible" PDD are proposed (see Table 12–2).[11] The sensitivity and specificity of the new criteria have not yet been determined in prospective studies, and further revision may be required. Nevertheless, they represent a useful starting point.

A second study, also commissioned by the Movement Disorder Society, proposed practical guidelines as to how the diagnostic criteria might be operationalized.[50] These guidelines are based on a two-level process, depending on the clinical scenario and the expertise of the evaluator. The level I assessment is aimed primarily at clinicians with no particular expertise in neuropsychological methods, but who require a simple, pragmatic set of tests that are not excessively time-consuming (Table 12–3). In addition to a clinical history and caregiver account, the MMSE,[51] supplemented by a clock drawing test and the four-item Neuropsychiatric Inventory,[52] would be sufficient to complete the level I assessment. Fluctuating attention, which, as described previously, is a dominant factor in determining disability in PDD, is examined by asking the patient to give the months of the year backward, starting from December, or by repeatedly subtracting 7, starting at 100. It remains to be seen whether these tests are sufficiently sensitive to detect this problem, or whether additional instruments, such as the Ferman four-item test, which has been shown to be highly discriminating of DLB from AD, may also be required.[53]

The level I assessment can be used alone or in combination with level II, which is more suitable when there is the need to specify the pattern and the severity of dementia associated with PD.[50] The level II assessment is suitable for detailed clinical monitoring, research studies, or pharmacologic trials. It requires neuropsychological expertise and is more time-consuming.

TABLE 12–1	Features of Dementia Associated with Parkinson's Disease

Core Features

Diagnosis of Parkinson's disease according to Queen Square Brain Bank criteria
A dementia syndrome with insidious onset and slow progression, developing within the context of established Parkinson's disease and diagnosed by history, clinical examination, and mental examination, defined as
    Impairment in more than one cognitive domain
    Representing a decline from premorbid level
    Deficits severe enough to impair daily life (social, occupational, or personal care), independent of the impairment ascribable to motor or autonomic symptoms

Associated Clinical Features

Cognitive features
    Attention: impaired. Impairment in spontaneous and focused attention, poor performance in attentional tasks; performance may fluctuate during the day and from day to day
    Executive functions: impaired. Impairment in tasks requiring initiation, planning, concept formation, rule finding, set shifting or set maintenance; impaired mental speed (bradyphrenia)
    Visuospatial functions: impaired. Impairment in tasks requiring visuospatial orientation, perception, or construction
    Memory: impaired. Impairment in free recall of recent events or in tasks requiring learning new material, memory usually improves with cueing, recognition is usually better than free recall
    Language: core functions largely preserved. Word-finding difficulties and impaired comprehension of complex sentences may be present
Behavioral features
    Apathy: decreased spontaneity; loss of motivation, interest, and effortful behavior
    Changes in personality and mood, including depressive features and anxiety
    Hallucinations: mostly visual, usually complex, formed visions of people, animals, or objects
    Delusions: usually paranoid, such as infidelity, or phantom boarder (unwelcome guests living in the home) delusions
    Excessive daytime sleepiness

Features that Do Not Exclude Dementia Associated with Parkinson's Disease, but Make the Diagnosis Uncertain

Coexistence of any other abnormality, which may by itself cause cognitive impairment, but judged not to be the cause of dementia (e.g., presence of relevant vascular disease on imaging)
Time interval between the development of motor and cognitive symptoms unknown

Features Suggesting Other Diseases as Cause of Mental Impairment, which When Present Make It Impossible to Diagnose Reliably Dementia Associated with Parkinson's Disease

Cognitive and behavioral symptoms appearing *solely* in the context of other conditions such as
    Acute confusion due to systemic diseases or abnormalities, or drug intoxication
    Major depression according to DSM-IV

Table continued on following page

TABLE 12–1	Features of Dementia Associated with Parkinson's Disease (Continued)

Features compatible with "probable vascular dementia" criteria according to NINDS-AIREN (dementia in the context of cerebrovascular disease as indicated by focal signs on neurological examination, such as hemiparesis, sensory deficits, and evidence of relevant cerebrovascular disease by brain imaging *and* a relationship between the two as indicated by the presence of one or more of the following: onset of dementia within 3 months after a recognized stroke; abrupt deterioration in cognitive functions; and fluctuating, stepwise progression of cognitive deficits)

DSM, Diagnostic and statistical manual of mental disorders; NINDS-AIREN, National Institute of Neurological Disorders and Stroke and Association Internationale pour la Recherche et l'Enseignement en Neurosciences.

TABLE 12–2	Criteria for the Diagnosis of Probable and Possible Dementia Associated with Parkinson's Disease

Probable Dementia Associated with Parkinson's Disease
Core features: both must be present
Associated clinical features
   Typical profile of cognitive deficits including impairment in at least two of the four core cognitive domains (impaired attention, which may fluctuate; impaired executive functions; impairment in visuospatial functions; and impaired free recall memory, which usually improves with cueing)
   The presence of at least one behavioral symptom (apathy, depressed or anxious mood, hallucinations, delusions, excessive daytime sleepiness) supports the diagnosis of probable dementia associated with Parkinson's disease; the lack of behavioral symptoms does not exclude the diagnosis
None of the group III criteria present
None of the group IV criteria present
Possible Dementia Associated with Parkinson's Disease
Core features: both must be present
Associated clinical features
   Atypical profile of cognitive impairment in one or more domains, such as prominent or receptive-type (fluent) aphasia, or pure storage-failure–type amnesia (memory does not improve with cueing or in recognition tasks) with preserved attention
Behavioral symptoms may or may not be present
or
One or more of the group III criteria present
None of the group IV criteria present

Investigation of Dementia and Its Predictors

SCREENING BLOOD TESTS FOR DEMENTIA

In the 2006 United Kingdom National Institute for Clinical Excellence Guidelines for dementia, it was concluded that there was no universal consensus on the appropriate diagnostic battery of blood tests that should be undertaken in patients

TABLE 12–3	Guidelines for Diagnosis of Dementia Associated with Parkinson's Disease at Level I

A diagnosis of PD based on the Queen's Square Brain Bank criteria
PD developed before the onset of dementia
MMSE score <26
Cognitive deficits severe enough to impact on daily living (elicited via caregiver
   interview or "Pill Questionnaire"*)
Impairment in at least two of the following cognitive domains
   Months reversed or seven backwards
   Lexical fluency or clock drawing
   MMSE pentagons
   MMSE 3-word recall

The presence of one of the following behavioral symptoms supports the diagnosis of probable dementia associated with Parkinson's disease: apathy or depressed mood or delusions or excessive daytime sleepiness†

The presence of major depression or delirium or any other abnormality that may by itself cause significant cognitive impairment makes the diagnosis uncertain‡

*This item, described in an appendix in reference 50, requires validation. In brief, patients are asked to describe verbally their treatment and its time schedule. Even if patients do not manage their own treatment, it is suggested that they have lost at least a part of their autonomy if they can no longer describe their treatment. The criterion of impairment is met if patients are no longer able to explain their daily PD medication, or if errors are made that are considered clinically significant.

†These can be assessed with the four-item Neuropsychiatric Inventory,[52] which includes hallucinations, depression, delusions, and apathy. A cutoff score of >3 for each item is proposed. Excessive daytime sleepiness may be assessed by specific questions.

‡Should be absent to permit diagnosis of probable dementia associated with Parkinson's disease.

MMSE, Mini-Mental State Examination; PD, Parkinson's disease.

with suspected dementia (http://guidance.nice.org.uk). In a review of 39 studies of more than 7000 cases, a potentially reversible cause was identified in 9%, but only 0.6% of cases *actually* reversed.[54] In the context of PDD, the selection of blood tests probably should be based on clinical grounds, according to individual patient history and clinical circumstances.

STRUCTURAL MAGNETIC RESONANCE IMAGING

The use of computed tomography and magnetic resonance imaging (MRI) is currently of limited diagnostic help in PDD; these techniques are primarily used when the clinical picture is atypical, or significant comorbid factors (e.g., vascular pathology) are suspected. Structural imaging also has been evaluated for its ability to predict incident dementia in PD. Changes shown to be predictive of AD (atrophy of the hippocampus and entorhinal cortex, perfusion changes in the posterior cingulate) may not be predictive of PDD (Fig. 12–2).[55] Using diffusion tensor MRI, Matsui and colleagues[56] showed that fractional anisotropy (a quantitative measure that reflects tissue organization) is significantly reduced in the bilateral posterior cingulate bundles of PDD patients compared with controls with PD without dementia. There is a nearly fourfold increased rate of whole-brain atrophy in PDD patients compared with PD patients without dementia and controls.[57] Rates of cerebral atrophy in PD correlate with global measures of cognitive

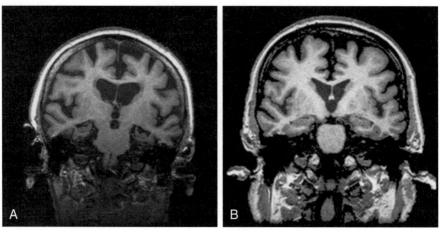

Figure 12–2 A and **B,** Comparable MRI coronal slices in Alzheimer's disease **(A)** and dementia associated with Parkinson's disease **(B),** showing hippocampal atrophy in Alzheimer's disease, but not in dementia associated with Parkinson's disease. (Courtesy of Professor John T. O'Brien.)

decline in some,[58] but not all, studies,[57] implying that MRI may be a useful technique in predicting preclinical onset of dementia in PD.

SINGLE PHOTON EMISSION COMPUTED TOMOGRAPHY AND POSITRON EMISSION TOMOGRAPHY

In subjects with PDD studied using cerebral fludeoxyglucose F 18 ([18]FDG) positron emission tomography (PET), early studies reported reduced glucose metabolism in frontal and temporoparietal association areas, a pattern similar to that seen in AD.[59] Using coregistration of single photon emission computed tomography (SPECT) images with MRI to account for changes owing to underlying atrophy, decreased blood flow has been described in posterior parieto-occipital regions, especially the precuneus (BA7), in PDD and DLB, but not in AD, where changes in posterior cingulate were observed instead (Fig. 12–3).[60] No decline in perfusion was seen over a 1-year period in established dementia, suggesting that perfusion changes may occur early in the disease before dementia develops.[61] In a small cross-sectional study of PD subjects without dementia, reduced glucose metabolism was shown on [18]FDG PET in posterior parietal and temporocortical gray matter.[62] The significance of this finding is unclear because no clinical follow-up was available, but because these subjects displayed abnormalities on formal neuropsychometric testing, it may be hypothesized that an abnormal [18]FDG PET scan, as a sensitive marker of cortical dysfunction, may be predictive of dementia in PD.

Although PD patients without dementia have moderate cholinergic dysfunction (assessed using N-[^{11}C] methyl-4-piperidyl acetate [MP4A] and PET), subjects with PDD exhibit severe cholinergic deficit in cortical regions.[63] Cortical cholinergic denervation in PD and PDD is associated with decreased performance on tests of attentional and executive functioning.[64]

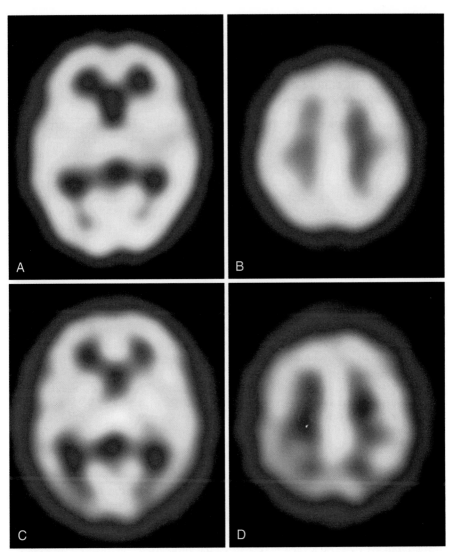

Figure 12–3 **A-D,** Blood flow SPECT studies in Parkinson's disease (**A** and **B**) and dementia associated with Parkinson's disease (**C** and **D**) at two different levels, showing relative hypoperfusion of occipital and precuneus cortex in dementia associated with Parkinson's disease, but not Parkinson's disease. (Courtesy of Professor John T. O'Brien.)

With the advent of PET ligands capable of binding to β-amyloid, it has become possible to study cortical amyloid burden in neurodegenerative dementias. As might be predicted, using ^{11}C-PIB PET, mean cortical levels of amyloid are increased twofold in AD[65] and by 60% in DLB.[66] Evidence so far for PDD, where motor disease duration preceded the onset of dementia by many years, suggests that group mean cortical amyloid load is not significantly elevated, although 20% of individuals showed an AD pattern of increased ^{11}C-PIB uptake.[67] Determining cortical amyloid burden in PDD and whether this protein affects the clinical phenotype is of vital importance in determining whether antiamyloid strategies may be beneficial in PDD.

GENETIC PREDICTORS OF DEMENTIA ASSOCIATED WITH PARKINSON'S DISEASE

The genetic and biological basis underlying the heterogeneity in cognitive profile, including the development of PDD, is largely unknown.[68] In contrast to AD, PDD is not clearly associated with apolipoprotein E polymorphisms.[69] Inherited genetic variation in tau (MAPT) may influence the rate of cognitive decline in PD, however, and the development of dementia.[70] The MAPT H1/H1 genotype has been associated with a greater rate of cognitive decline in 109 incident PD patients prospectively followed over a 3.5-year period. For 15% of H1/H1 homozygotes, but none of the H2 carriers, the rate of cognitive decline was sufficient to develop dementia within the follow-up period.[70]

OTHER BIOMARKER MEASURES

Elevated plasma homocysteine levels are associated in the general population with atherosclerosis, vascular disease, depression, and dementia. Levodopa may elevate plasma homocysteine. It is unknown whether increased plasma homocysteine is an independent risk factor for cognitive impairment in PD; some,[71,72] but not all,[73] studies have found an association. Generally, these studies have been small and cross-sectional in design.

More recent studies have shown that 18 signaling proteins in blood plasma can classify blinded samples from AD and controls with almost 90% accuracy.[74] This protein "signature" also correctly identified 91% patients with mild cognitive impairment that progressed to AD 2 to 6 years later.[74] It would be of great interest to know whether plasma testing in PD, using similar techniques, can predict the later development of dementia.

Although cerebrospinal fluid studies have been performed in PDD, they have been cross-sectional and mainly concerned with differentiating this dementia from DLB and AD.[75-77] A more recent study of cerebrospinal fluid biomarkers (β-amyloid$_{1-42}$, Aβ42, total tau, and phosphorylated tau) in patients with mild cognitive impairment yielded a sensitivity of 95% and specificity of 83% for detection of incipient AD.[78] Low levels of cerebrospinal fluid Aβ42 seem to predict cognitive decline over 8 years among older women without dementia.[79] It is unknown, however, whether cerebrospinal fluid analysis has predictive value for the development of PDD, or whether a cerebrospinal fluid profile can provide information regarding the pathological basis of the dementia and its clinical phenotype.

Regarding evoked potentials, the P300 latency is usually prolonged in PDD, but this may also occur in PD patients without dementia. Prepulse inhibition of the N1/P2 component of the auditory evoked potential may be reduced in DLB patients compared with controls and AD patients, with impairment of intermediate intensity in PDD patients.[80] Quantitative electroencephalography may have potential as a biomarker in the study of cognitive deterioration in PD.[81] Abnormal slow rhythm frequencies (delta, theta) were increasingly present with greater cognitive decline, a change that was independent of age and levodopa dose. These changes may be responsive to therapeutic intervention aimed at improving cognition, although further work is required to establish the sensitivity of this technique.

Pathological Basis of Dementia in Parkinson's Disease

Mixed brain pathologies, including Alzheimer's-type pathology, Lewy bodies, and vascular changes, probably account for most dementia cases in community-dwelling older individuals.[82] The relative admixture of these pathologies, the topography of the lesions (cortical and subcortical), and the potential for protein-protein synergy (i.e., the possibility of one protein influencing and enhancing aggregation of another) are important concepts when considering the pathophysiological basis for PDD (and DLB).[12] Such concepts may also help to reconcile seemingly disparate data regarding which protein aggregate is most crucial in causing dementia.

Cortical Lewy body density, especially in the temporal neocortex, correlates significantly with cognitive impairment in PD, independent of, or in addition to, Alzheimer's-type pathology, whereas high Lewy body densities in the amygdala and parahippocampus correlate with well-formed visual hallucinations (Fig. 12–4A-C).[83] Other authors have reported that cortical Lewy bodies are sensitive (91%) and specific (90%) neuropathological markers for PDD, and better indicators of dementia than neurofibrillary tangles, senile plaques, or dystrophic neurites.[84] Of patients in the latter series with neuropathological changes typical of PD and judged during life to be demented, however, 10% had no cortical pathology of note (i.e., no cortical Lewy bodies, neurofibrillary tangles, or senile plaques). Lewy body counts were increased nearly 10-fold in the neocortex, limbic cortex, and amygdala in demented compared with nondemented PD cases, according to Apaydin and colleagues.[23] High cortical Lewy body counts in one region correlated with high counts in other areas. Although Alzheimer's-type pathology was described as "modest," there were significant correlations between cortical Lewy body counts and senile plaque and (to a lesser extent) neurofibrillary tangle counts.

According to the influential Braak PD staging system, premortem MMSE scores correlate with neuropathological stages, and this association shows a linear trend.[85] Cognitively impaired individuals also have higher stages of AD-related neurofibrillary pathology and β-amyloid (Aβ) deposition than non–cognitively impaired individuals. In some individuals, cognitive decline can develop in the presence of mild PD-related cortical pathology, and, conversely, widespread cortical lesions do not always lead to cognitive decline.[85] In a prospective, community-based study, Lewy body disease was determined to be the main substrate driving the progression of cognitive impairment in PD.[86]

In contrast, the case for cortical Lewy bodies playing an exclusive role in the genesis of PDD is weakened by several lines of evidence. In one study, 17 PD cases were reported with no history of premortem cognitive impairment, yet pathologically these cases, which were typical of PD, also fulfilled diagnostic criteria for either limbic or neocortical types of DLB.[87] In another series, the distribution or load of α-synuclein pathology at postmortem examination did not reliably correlate with retrospective clinical records of extrapyramidal symptoms or cognitive impairment.[88] Others have linked PDD more closely with Alzheimer's-type

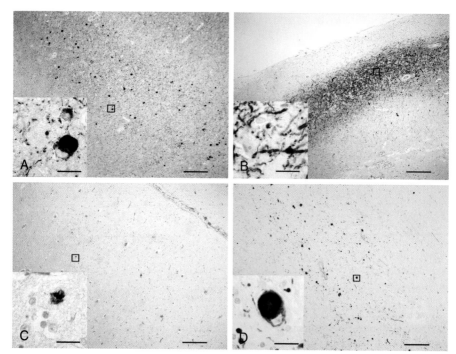

Figure 12–4 Pathology of dementia associated with Parkinson's disease. **A,** Transtentorhinal cortex, showing extensive α-synuclein pathology. Lewy bodies and neurites (*dark brown*); normal synaptic α-synuclein (*pale brown*); immunohistochemistry (IHC) for α-synuclein using clone KM51 monoclonal antibodies from Novocastra (Newcastle) on formalin-fixed, paraffin wax–embedded sections pretreated with formic acid; Vectastain Elite ABC peroxidase kit (Vector, Peterborough, UK); hematoxylin counterstain. *Scale bars in main image* = 400 μm, *in inset* = 30 μm. **B,** Hippocampal segment CA2. Lewy neurites (*dark brown*) at high density; normal synaptic α-synuclein (*pale brown*); IHC for α-synuclein and *scale bars* as in **A. C,** Transtentorhinal cortex showing sparse tangles and neurites; Gallyas silver stain; *scale bars* as in **A. D,** Nucleus of Meynert showing moderate neuronal loss and α-synuclein pathology. Lewy neurites (*dark brown*); normal synaptic α-synuclein (*pale brown*); IHC for α-synuclein and *scale bars* as in **A. (A-D,** Courtesy of Dr. Evelyn Jaros.)

pathology. In a series of 200 consecutive cases of pathologically confirmed PD cases, moderate to severe dementia was reported in 33%, and the degree of cognitive impairment was significantly correlated with Alzheimer's-type pathology.[89] The degree of Alzheimer's-type pathology was negatively correlated with survival. Regional neurofibrillary tangle counts have also been correlated with dementia in PD.[90]

It is unknown whether cortical deposition of amyloid protein is a time-dependent process, such that DLB and PDD with short duration of PD before dementia onset may behave similarly, displaying elevated cortical PIB binding on PET scanning, with tracer binding gradually reducing as motor disease duration increases before dementia onset. Amyloid may play a greater role the shorter the disease duration before dementia onset in PD. This hypothesis is supported by a more recent clinicopathological study,[91] in which cortical amyloid and α-synuclein burden was greater in DLB and PDD of shorter prior disease duration compared with PDD with a longer history of motor symptoms before dementia onset.

More recent observations suggest that processes involved in Lewy body formation and the accumulation of Aβ protein and metabolism of tau protein may not be entirely independent. The presence of Aβ deposits in the cerebral cortex is associated with extensive α-synuclein lesions and higher levels of insoluble α-synuclein, implying Aβ enhances development of cortical α-synuclein lesions in PD.[92] Regarding Aβ, double transgenic mice expressing the human form of this protein and α-synuclein develop severe memory and learning deficits in addition to motor problems.[93] Double transgenic mice also develop more α-synuclein immunoreactive inclusions than single transgenic α-synuclein mice. Aβ peptides can promote aggregation of α-synuclein in cell-free systems and intraneuronal accumulation of α-synuclein in cell culture.[93] Finally, tau immunostaining may be present at the periphery of Lewy bodies,[94] and interaction between tau and α-synuclein may facilitate protein aggregation.

In addition to the aforementioned predominantly cortical pathological changes, another notable feature of PDD is the profound loss of subcortical cholinergic neurons and resulting choline acetyltransferase activity compared with PD and AD.[95] Reduced neocortical presynaptic cholinergic activity reflects a marked loss of ascending cholinergic projections from basal forebrain nuclei (Fig. 12–4D). Loss of other cholinergic cells, such as cells within the pedunculopontine nucleus, may also influence the motor phenotype associated with PDD, and, through loss of projections to the thalamus, may play a role in fluctuating attention.

Management

GENERAL APPROACH

Having made the diagnosis of PDD, it is essential to consider what pharmacological and nonpharmacological measures (if any) are necessary. Nonpharmacological treatments for neuropsychiatric symptoms should always be considered, and may benefit depression, visual hallucinations, and apathy.[96] Attention to nutrition is often neglected. Sixty percent of demented residents in nursing homes in the United Kingdom may be malnourished (http://guidance.nice.org.uk). Improved nutrition is associated with reduced risk of infection and mortality.[97]

Several treatments used to manage behavioral and neuropsychiatric symptoms, in particular, may exacerbate parkinsonism, whereas effective treatment of the latter may worsen psychotic features. Management is usually a compromise, and a list of priorities is helpful, devised in consultation with the patient and caregiver. Figure 12–5 is a simple algorithm for a suggested pharmacological approach to the PD patient with neuropsychiatric or cognitive symptoms or both.

Regarding the control of parkinsonism, a gradual and systematic simplification of the drug regimen is essential, withdrawing anticholinergic drugs, selegiline, dopamine agonists, and catechol O-methyltransferase inhibitors one by one, aiming to maintain the patient on the lowest possible dose of levodopa monotherapy to preserve function. Anticholinergic drugs to control urinary urgency and frequency should be stopped if possible. Other medications to treat comorbid medical problems should also be reviewed and, if possible, discontinued.

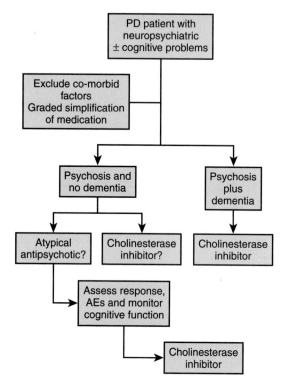

Figure 12–5 Algorithm for a suggested pharmacological approach to a Parkinson's disease (PD) patient with neuropsychiatric or cognitive symptoms or both. AEs, adverse events.

If depression is suspected, there should be a low threshold to treat, although there are no randomized controlled trial data to inform on choice of antidepressant in PDD. The choice by default is usually a selective serotonin reuptake inhibitor, although mixed reuptake inhibitors could theoretically benefit apathy and inattention. If excessive daytime drowsiness and inattention are problematic, reasons for nocturnal sleep fragmentation should be considered and treated if possible. REM sleep behavior disorder may respond to a small dose of clonazepam (starting dose 0.25 mg, increasing very gradually to avoid increasing risk of falls). Randomized controlled trial data are equivocal in supporting the use of modafinil for excessive daytime somnolence in PD, although no studies have focused specifically on PDD.[98-100]

ANTIPSYCHOTIC TREATMENT

Choice of atypical antipsychotic for troublesome visual hallucinations and delusions is limited by extrapyramidal side effects and increased risk of stroke with several of these agents in elderly patients. Severe neuroleptic sensitivity occurred in 40% of PDD patients in one study.[101] In practice, the choice usually is between quetiapine and clozapine, although trial data are far stronger for the latter. In the more recent PD Guidelines, the United Kingdom National Institute of Clinical Excellence suggested that clozapine may be used in the treatment of psychotic symptoms, but pointed out that registration with a mandatory monitoring scheme is required. Experience with this drug among specialists caring for patients with PD varies considerably throughout Europe and North America (http://guidance.nice. org.uk). In managing psychosis associated with PD, the American Academy of Neurology also recommended that clozapine should be considered (level B evidence), that quetiapine may be considered (level C evidence), but that olanzapine should not be used (level B evidence).[102] Finally, in a more recent structured review and meta-analysis, it was concluded that only clozapine could be fully recommended for the treatment of drug-induced psychosis in PD, and that olanzapine should be avoided for this indication.[103]

Studies involving newer atypical antipsychotic agents have been small and usually open-label. Eight of 14 PD subjects with drug-induced psychosis had to be withdrawn in an open-label study of the partial dopamine receptor agonist aripiprazole,[104] making it difficult to recommend the use of this agent. Ziprasidone, an antagonist at $5HT_{2A}$ and dopamine D_2 receptors, improved refractory drug-induced psychosis in three of four PD patients with psychosis, but resulted in worsening of extrapyramidal features in one subject and "pathological laughter" in two.[105] In a multicenter, randomized controlled phase II trial of 60 psychotic PD patients, pimavanserin (ACP-103), a $5\text{-}HT_{2A}$ inverse agonist/antagonist, did not lead to worsening of motor function and showed antipsychotic potential.[106] Further phase III trials are planned for this agent.

CHOLINESTERASE INHIBITORS

Multiple lines of evidence, including neuroimaging and neuropathological data, indicate a profound loss of ascending cholinergic projections in PDD, with relative preservation of postsynaptic muscarinic receptors, providing a strong rationale for the use of cholinesterase inhibitors in this disorder. Currently available cholinesterase inhibitors comprise donepezil (a reversible, noncompetitive, selective inhibitor of acetylcholinesterase), rivastigmine (a pseudoirreversible inhibitor of acetylcholinesterase and butyrylcholinesterase), and galantamine (a reversible inhibitor of acetylcholinesterase and allosteric modulator of nicotinic receptors). With two notable exceptions, clinical trials of cholinesterase inhibitors in PDD have been small, and there are no comparative trial data to indicate which, if any, of the drugs may be more efficacious or better tolerated.

A 6-month, multicenter, randomized, placebo-controlled trial reported the effects of rivastigmine in 541 patients with mild to moderate PDD, who were randomly assigned on a 2:1 basis to either active drug or placebo.[107] The primary end point for the study was the cognitive subscale of the Alzheimer's Disease Assessment Scale (ADAS-Cog, scored between 0 and 70). At 6 months, rivastigmine-treated subjects experienced a mean improvement of 2.1 points on this scale over a baseline score of 23.8 compared with the placebo group, who deteriorated by 0.7 point from a baseline mean score of 24.3. Other end points, including global clinical change, Neuropsychiatric Inventory, attentional measures, and MMSE, all also showed statistically significant changes in favor of the rivastigmine group. Of patients receiving rivastigmine, 72.7% completed the study compared with 82.1% of patients randomly assigned to placebo. The most common adverse events reported were nausea (29% of rivastigmine group versus 11.2% of placebo group) and vomiting (16.5% of rivastigmine group versus 1.7% of placebo group). Tremor worsened in 10.2% of the rivastigmine patients, although this was not reflected by any overall difference in mean Unified Parkinson Disease Rating Scale part III scores compared with placebo.

In an open-label extension to this study, long-term rivastigmine treatment was well tolerated and provided modest but sustained benefits in PDD patients for 48 weeks.[108] Based on this pivotal study, rivastigmine is now licensed for use in PDD in the European Union, the United States, and several other countries.

In the IDEAL study (Investigation of transDermal Exelon in ALzheimer's disease), 1195 patients with AD were randomly assigned to placebo or one of three active treatment target dose groups: a 10-cm^2 rivastigmine patch (delivering 9.5 mg/24 hours); 20-cm^2 rivastigmine patch (17.4 mg/24 hours); or 6-mg twice-a-day rivastigmine capsules.[109] All rivastigmine treatment groups showed significant improvement relative to placebo. The 10-cm^2 patch showed similar efficacy to capsules, with approximately two thirds fewer reports of nausea (7.2% versus 23.1%) and vomiting (6.2% versus 17%), incidences not significantly different from placebo (5% and 3.3% for nausea and vomiting). Although comparable data are not yet available for PDD, the transdermal mode of administering rivastigmine offers the hope that side effects may be reduced without loss of efficacy.

A randomized, double-blind, placebo-controlled crossover study of 22 PDD patients reported that donepezil was well tolerated, with modest benefits on some aspects of cognitive function.[110] Although reported only in abstract form to date, a 6-month, international multicenter, randomized controlled trial has also examined the effects of 5 mg or 10 mg of donepezil compared with placebo in 550 patients with mild to moderate PDD (MMSE 10 to 26), using the ADAS-Cog as a primary end point.[111] A dose-dependent improvement in cognition was observed, with mean (standard deviation) changes from baseline at week 24 of placebo –0.3 (6.49), donepezil 5 mg –2.45 (5.28), and donepezil 10 mg –3.72 (7.05), but because the *a priori* plan for analysis included controlling for between-country treatment effects, these differences did not reach statistical significance. Nevertheless, the size of effect on the ADAS-Cog was comparable to that reported by Emre and colleagues[107] for rivastigmine. Significant improvements were also noted in MMSE and measures of attention, but not in activities of daily living or Neuropsychiatric Inventory.

An American Academy of Neurology Practice Parameter concluded from a systematic literature review that donepezil or rivastigmine should be considered for the management of PDD.[102] A Cochrane review of the efficacy, safety, tolerability, and health economic data relating to the use of cholinesterase inhibitors in PDD concluded that rivastigmine improves cognition and activities of daily living, resulting in clinically meaningful benefit in about 15% of cases.[112] A need for more studies using pragmatic measures, such as time to residential care facility and patient and caregiver quality-of-life assessments, was highlighted, and the need to use tools to analyze data that limit bias and measure health economic factors.

OTHER AGENTS

It is unknown whether the N-methyl-D-aspartate glutamate receptor antagonist memantine is beneficial in the Lewy body dementias. In one open-label study, 7 of 11 DLB patients were "stable or improved" on memantine,[113] although 9 of these patients were also taking a cholinesterase inhibitor. Visual hallucinations worsened in two patients, one experienced excessive sedation, and lack of efficacy was reported in another patient. In a further case series, worsening delusions and visual hallucinations were associated with the use of memantine in three DLB patients, which significantly improved when treatment was discontinued.[114] In an open-label study reported in abstract form only, memantine was well tolerated in five PDD patients, with modest benefits to cognition and behavior in four patients.[115] A randomized, placebo-controlled, multicenter study of memantine in the Lewy body dementias (i.e., PDD and DLB) is ongoing, and it is hoped that this study will resolve whether this drug is tolerated by these patients, and if it is associated with significant improvements.

Modafinil may warrant further investigation to establish its effects on cognitive performance in PDD through improving alertness.[116] The highly selective norepinephrine reuptake inhibitor atomoxetine is also undergoing evaluation of its effects in improving executive dysfunction. A pilot open-label study of 25 to 100 mg of atomoxetine in 12 PD patients reported benefits in several end points relevant to executive problems.[117] Multifunctional antiparkinsonian drugs may offer combined benefits on motor and cognitive function. Ladostigil, which features monoamine oxidase B and acetylcholinesterase inhibitor moieties in its molecule, is one example of a multifunctional drug undergoing evaluation.[118] Safinamide, a promising new antiparkinsonian drug with multiple modes of action, including reversible monoamine oxidase B inhibition, glutamate release inhibition, and dopamine reuptake inhibition may also improve cognition in PD. Using a computerized cognitive test battery, safinamide improved executive function and verbal working memory in a phase III trial of 123 PD patients with relatively early disease.[119]

Ultimately, the "golden fleece" for managing PDD and its distressing features is the development of disease-modifying approaches. These could include generic disease-modifying approaches, targeting the primary pathophysiology of PD and retarding progression in all disease aspects. Dementia-specific disease-modifying approaches also could be considered, including techniques to reduce the protein-protein interaction and aggregation that are believed to be so deleterious in the pathophysiology of PDD. "Transferable" approaches from ongoing AD trials may also prove to be beneficial in PDD.

Conclusions

Dementia associated with PD is a common complication, affecting 80% of patients with PD during the course of their illness. Neuropsychiatric features, which may dominate clinical presentation and therapeutic prioritization, are an invariable feature of this dementia syndrome. It is hoped that new diagnostic criteria will assist in the accurate diagnosis and classification of PDD. In the clinic, a pragmatic but sensitive assessment of cognitive, neuropsychiatric, and motor deficits is essential to yield a baseline against which the effects of therapeutic interventions may be judged. Other than clozapine, which requires careful monitoring, atypical antipsychotics are currently of limited benefit in managing the psychotic features of PDD. Overall, cholinesterase inhibitors have modest effects on cognition and neuropsychiatric features, although some patients may respond extremely well, whereas others show no response. Further trials of these agents in PDD are needed to clarify their therapeutic impact and to guide clinical usage. There is also an urgent need for novel drug approaches in PDD, including the development of disease-modifying agents.

REFERENCES

1. Levy G, Tang MX, Louis ED, et al: The association of incident dementia with mortality in PD: Neurology 2002;59:1708-1713.
2. Playfer JR: Depression, cognition and quality of life in parkinsonian patients. Age Ageing 1999;28:333-334.
3. Aarsland D, Larsen JP, Karlsen K, et al: Mental symptoms in Parkinson's disease are important contributors to caregiver distress. Int J Geriatr Psychiatry 1999;14:866-874.
4. Aarsland D, Larsen JP, Tandberg E, Laake K: Predictors of nursing home placement in Parkinson's disease: a population-based, prospective study. J Am Geriatr Soc 2000;48:938-942.
5. Williams-Gray CH, Foltynie T, Brayne CEG, et al: Evolution of cognitive dysfunction in an incident Parkinson's disease cohort. Brain 2007;130:1787-1798.
6. Hobson P, Meara J: Risk and incidence of dementia in a cohort of older subjects with Parkinson's disease in the United Kingdom. Mov Disord 2004;19:1043-1049.
7. Aarsland D, Zaccai J, Brayne C: A systematic review of prevalence studies of dementia in Parkinson's disease. Mov Disord 2005;10:1255-1263.
8. Aarsland D, Andersen K, Larsen JP, et al: Prevalence and characteristics of dementia in Parkinson disease. Arch Neurol 2003;60:387-392.
9. Galvin JE, Pollack J, Morris JC: Clinical phenotype of Parkinson disease dementia. Neurology 2006;67:1605-1611.
10. McKeith I, Dickson D, Lowe J, et al: Diagnosis and management of dementia with Lewy bodies: third report of the DLB Consortium. Neurology 2005;65:1863-1872.
11. Emre M, Aarsland D, Brown R, et al: Clinical diagnostic criteria for dementia associated with Parkinson disease. Mov Disord 2007;22:1689-1707.
12. Lippa CF, Duda JE, Grossman M, et al: DLB and PDD boundary issues: diagnosis, treatment, molecular pathology and biomarkers. Neurology 2007;68:812-819.
13. Levy G, Schupf N, Tang MX, et al: Combined effect of age and severity on the risk of dementia in Parkinson's disease. Ann Neurol 2002;51:722-729.
14. Burn DJ, Rowan EN, Minett T, et al: Extrapyramidal features in Parkinson's disease with or without dementia and dementia with Lewy bodies: a cross-sectional comparative study. Mov Disord 2003;18:884-889.
15. Alves G, Larsen JP, Emre M, et al: Changes in motor subtype and risk for incident dementia in Parkinson's disease. Mov Disord 2006;21:1123-1130.
16. Glatt SL, Hubble JP, Lyons K, et al: Risk factors for dementia in Parkinson's disease: effect of education. Neuroepidemiology 1996;15:20-25.
17. Cohen OS, Vakil E, Tanne D, et al: Educational level as a modulator of cognitive performance and neuropsychiatric features in Parkinson disease. Cogn Behav Neurol 2007;20:68-72.
18. Levy G, Tang MX, Cote LJ, et al: Do risk factors for Alzheimer's disease predict dementia in Parkinson's disease? An exploratory study. Mov Disord 2002;17:250-257.
19. Allcock LM, Kenny RA, Tordoff S, et al: Orthostatic hypotension in Parkinson's disease: association with cognitive decline? Int J Geriatr Psychiatry 2006;21:778-783.
20. Uc EY, Struck LK, Rodnitzky RL, et al: Predictors of weight loss in Parkinson's disease. Mov Disord 2006;21:930-936.
21. Perry EK, Kilford L, Lees AJ, et al: Increased Alzheimer pathology in Parkinson's disease related to antimuscarinic drugs. Ann Neurol 2003;54:235-238.
22. Caparros-Lefebvre D, Pecheux N, Petit V, et al: Which factors predict cognitive decline in Parkinson's disease? J Neurol Neurosurg Psychiatry 1995;58:51-55.
23. Apaydin H, Ahlskog JE, Parisi JE, et al: Parkinson disease neuropathology: later-developing dementia and loss of the levodopa response. Arch Neurol 2002;59:102-112.
24. Inzelberg R, Bonuccelli U, Schechtman E, et al: Association between amantadine and the onset of dementia in Parkinson's disease. Mov Disord 2006;21:1375-1379.
25. Janvin CC, Aarsland D, Larsen JP: Cognitive predictors of dementia in Parkinson's disease: a community-based, 4-year longitudinal study. J Geriatr Psychiatry Neurol 2005;18:149-154.
26. Pluck GC, Brown RG: Apathy in Parkinson's disease. J Neurol Neurosurg Psychiatry 2002;73:636-642.

27. Carbon M, Ma Y, Barnes A, et al: Caudate nucleus: influence of dopaminergic input on sequence learning and brain activation in parkinsonism. Neuroimage 2004;21:1497-1507.
28. Caviness JN, Driver-Dunckley E, Connor DJ, et al: Defining mild cognitive impairment in Parkinson's disease. Mov Disord 2007;15:1272-1277.
29. Janvin CC, Larsen JP, Aarsland D, Hugdahl K: Subtypes of mild cognitive impairment in Parkinson's disease: progression to dementia. Mov Disord 2006;21:1343-1349.
30. Aarsland D, Andersen K, Larsen JP, et al: The rate of cognitive decline in Parkinson's disease. Arch Neurol 2004;61:1906-1911.
31. Burn D, Rowan E, Allan L, et al: Motor subtype and cognitive decline in Parkinson's disease, Parkinson's disease with dementia, and dementia with Lewy bodies. J Neurol Neurosurg Psychiatry 2006;77:585-589.
32. Bronnick K, Emre M, Lane R, et al: Profile of cognitive impairment in dementia associated with Parkinson's disease compared with Alzheimer's disease. J Neurol Neurosurg Psychiatry 2007;78:1064-1068.
33. Janvin C, Larsen J, Salmon D, et al: Cognitive profiles of individual patients with Parkinson's disease and dementia: comparison with dementia with Lewy bodies and Alzheimer's disease. Mov Disord 2006;21:337-342.
34. Ballard CG, Aarsland D, McKeith I, et al: Fluctuations in attention: PD dementia vs DLB with parkinsonism. Neurology 2002;59:1714-1720.
35. Bronnick K, Ehrt U, Emre M, et al: Attentional deficits affect activities of daily living in dementia-associated with Parkinson's disease. J Neurol Neurosurg Psychiatry 2006;77:1136-1142.
36. Jellinger KA, Wenning GK, Seppi K: Predictors of survival in dementia with Lewy bodies and Parkinson dementia. Neurodegener Dis 2007;4:428-430.
37. Mosimann UP, Mather G, Wesnes K, et al: Visual perception in Parkinson's disease dementia and dementia with Lewy bodies. Neurology 2004;63:2091-2096.
38. Aarsland D, Brønnick K, Ehrt U, et al: Neuropsychiatric symptoms in patients with Parkinson's disease and dementia: frequency, profile and associated care giver stress. J Neurol Neurosurg Psychiatry 2007;78:36-42.
39. Burn D, Emre M, McKeith I, et al: Effects of rivastigmine in patients with and without visual hallucinations in dementia associated with Parkinson's disease. Mov Disord 2006;21:1899-1907.
40. Aarsland D, Ballard CG, Larsen JP, McKeith IG: A comparative study of psychiatric symptoms in dementia with Lewy bodies and Parkinson's disease with and without dementia. Int J Geriatr Psychiatry 2001;16:528-536.
41. Burn DJ, Rowan EN, Minnett T, et al: Extrapyramidal features in Parkinson's disease with and without dementia and dementia with Lewy bodies: a cross-sectional comparative study. Mov Disord 2003;18:884-889.
42. Verbaan D, Marinus J, Visser M, et al: Cognitive impairment in Parkinson's disease. J Neurol Neurosurg Psychiatry 2007;78:1182-1187.
43. Mosimann UP, Müri RM, Burn DJ, et al: Saccadic eye movement changes in Parkinson's disease dementia and dementia with Lewy bodies. Brain 2005;128:1267-1276.
44. Boddy F, Rowan EN, Lett D, et al: Sleep quality and excessive daytime somnolence in Parkinson's disease with and without dementia, dementia with Lewy bodies and Alzheimer's disease: a comparative, cross-sectional study. Int J Geriatr Psychiatry 2007;22:529-535.
45. Graham JM, Sagar HJ: A data-driven approach to the study of heterogeneity in idiopathic Parkinson's disease: identification of three distinct subtypes. Mov Disord 1999;14:10-20.
46. Allan LM, Ballard CG, Allen J, et al: Autonomic dysfunction in dementia. J Neurol Neurosurg Psychiatry 2007;78:671-677.
47. Allan L, McKeith I, Ballard C, Kenny RA: The prevalence of autonomic symptoms in dementia and their association with physical activity, activities of daily living and quality of life. Dement Geriatr Cogn Disord 2006;22:230-237.
48. Bonelli SB, Ransmayr G, Steffelbauer M, et al: L-dopa responsiveness in dementia with Lewy bodies, Parkinson's disease with and without dementia. Neurology 2004;63:376-378.
49. Molloy S, McKeith IG, O'Brien JT, Burn DJ: The role of levodopa in the management of dementia with Lewy bodies. J Neurol Neurosurg Psychiatry 2005;76:1200-1203.
50. Dubois B, Burn D, Goetz C, et al: Diagnostic procedures for Parkinson's disease dementia recommendations from the Movement Disorder Society task force. Mov Disord 2007;22:2314-2324.
51. Folstein MF, Folstein SE, McHugh PR: "Mini-mental state": a practical method for grading the cognitive state of patients for the clinician. J Psychiatr Res 1975;12:189-198.

52. Bronnick K, Aarsland D, Larsen JP: Neuropsychiatric disturbances in Parkinson's disease clusters in five groups with different prevalence of dementia. Acta Psychiatr Scand 2005;112:201-207.

53. Ferman TJ, Smith GE, Boeve BF, et al: DLB fluctuations: specific features that reliably differentiate DLB from AD and normal aging. Neurology 2004;62:181-187.

54. Clarfield AM: The decreasing prevalence of reversible dementias: an updated meta-analysis. Arch Intern Med 2003;163:2219-2229.

55. Tam C, Burton E, McKeith I, et al: Temporal lobe atrophy on MRI in Parkinson disease with dementia: a comparison with Alzheimer disease and dementia with Lewy bodies. Neurology 2005;64:861-865.

56. Matsui H, Nishinaka K, Oda M, et al: Dementia in Parkinson's disease: diffusion tensor imaging. Acta Neurol Scand 2007;116:177-181.

57. Burton EJ, McKeith IG, Burn DJ, O'Brien JT: Brain atrophy rates in Parkinson's disease with and without dementia using serial magnetic resonance imaging. Mov Disord 2005;20:1571-1576.

58. Hu MTM, White SJ, Chaudhuri KR, et al: Correlating rates of cerebral atrophy in Parkinson's disease with measures of cognitive decline. J Neural Transm 2001;108:571-580.

59. Vander Borght T, Minoshima S, Giordani B, et al: Cerebral metabolic differences in Parkinson's and Alzheimer's diseases matched for dementia severity. J Nucl Med 1997;38:797-802.

60. Firbank MJ, Colloby SJ, Burn DJ, et al: Regional cerebral blood flow in Parkinson's disease with and without dementia. Neuroimage 2003;20:1309-1319.

61. Firbank M, Burn D, McKeith I, O'Brien J: Longitudinal study of cerebral blood flow SPECT in Parkinson's disease with dementia, and dementia with Lewy bodies. Int J Geriatr Psychiatry 2005;20:776-782.

62. Hu MTM, Taylor-Robinson SD, Ray Chaudhuri K, et al: Cortical dysfunction in non-demented Parkinson's disease patients: a combined ^{31}P-MRS and ^{18}FDG-PET study. Brain 2000;123:340-352.

63. Hilker R, Thomas AV, Klein JC, et al: Dementia in Parkinson disease: functional imaging of cholinergic and dopaminergic pathways. Neurology 2005;65:1716-1722.

64. Bohnen NI, Kaufer DI, Hendrickson R, et al: Cognitive correlates of cortical cholinergic denervation in Parkinson's disease and parkinsonian dementia. J Neurol 2006;253:242-247.

65. Edison P, Archer HA, Hinz R, et al: Amyloid, hypometabolism, and cognition in Alzheimer disease: an [11C]PIB and [18F]FDG PET study. Neurology 2007;68:501-508.

66. Rowe CC, Ng S, Ackermann U, et al: Imaging β-amyloid burden in aging and dementia. Neurology 2007;68:1718-1725.

67. Edison P, Rowe CC, Rinne J, et al: Amyloid load in Lewy body dementia, Parkinson's disease dementia and Parkinson's disease measured with ^{11}C-PIB PET. Neurology 2007;68(Suppl 1):A98.

68. Emre M: Dementia associated with Parkinson's disease. Lancet Neurol 2003;2:229-237.

69. Jasinska-Myga B, Opala G, Goetz CG, et al: Apolipoprotein E gene polymorphism, total plasma cholesterol level, and Parkinson disease dementia. Arch Neurol 2007;64:261-265.

70. Goris A, Williams-Gray CH, Clark GR, et al: Common variation in tau and alpha synuclein genes influences risk of developing idiopathic Parkinson disease and related cognitive impairment. Ann Neurol 2007;62:145-153.

71. O'Suilleabhain PE, Sung V, Hernandez C, et al: Elevated plasma homocysteine level in patients with Parkinson disease: motor, affective, and cognitive associations. Arch Neurol 2004;61:865-868.

72. Zoccolella S, Lamberti P, Iliceto G, et al: Plasma homocysteine levels in L-dopa-treated Parkinson's disease patients with cognitive dysfunctions. Clin Chem Lab Med 2005;43:1107-1110.

73. Hassin-Baer S, Cohen O, Vakil E, et al: Plasma homocysteine levels and Parkinson disease: disease progression, carotid intima-media thickness and neuropsychiatric complications. Clin Neuropharmacol 2006;29:305-311.

74. Ray S, Britschgi M, Herbert C, et al: Classification and prediction of clinical Alzheimer's diagnosis based on plasma signaling proteins. Nat Med 2007;13:1359-1362.

75. Gómez-Tortosa E, Gonzalo I, Fanjul S, et al: Cerebrospinal fluid markers in dementia with Lewy bodies compared with Alzheimer disease. Arch Neurol 2003;60:1218-1222.

76. Bibl M, Mollenhauer B, Esselmann H, et al: CSF amyloid-β-peptides in Alzheimer's disease, dementia with Lewy bodies and Parkinson's disease dementia. Brain 2006;129:1177-1187.

77. Wada-Isoe K, Kitayama M, Nakaso K, Nakashima K: Diagnostic markers for diagnosing dementia with Lewy bodies: CSF and MIBG scintigraphy study. J Neurol Sci 2007;260:33-37.

78. Hansson O, Zetterberg H, Buchhave P, et al: Association between CSF biomarkers and incipient Alzheimer's disease in patients with mild cognitive impairment: a follow-up study. Lancet Neurol 2006;5:228-234.

79. Gustafson DR, Skoog I, Rosengren L, et al: Cerebrospinal fluid beta-amyloid 1-42 concentration may predict cognitive decline in older women. J Neurol Neurosurg Psychiatry 2007;78:461-464.

80. Perriol M, Dujardin K, Derambure P, et al: Disturbance of sensory filtering in dementia with Lewy bodies: comparison with Parkinson's disease dementia and Alzheimer's disease. J Neurol Neurosurg Psychiatry 2005;76:106-108.

81. Caviness JN, Hentz JG, Evidente VG, et al: Both early and late cognitive dysfunction affects the electroencephalogram in Parkinson's disease. Parkinsonism Relat Disord 2007;13:348-354.

82. Schneider JA, Arvanitakis Z, Bang W, Bennett DA: Mixed brain pathologies account for most dementia cases in community-dwelling older persons. Neurology 2007;69:2197-2204.

83. Harding AJ, Broe GA, Halliday GM: Visual hallucinations in Lewy body disease relate to Lewy bodies in the temporal lobe. Brain 2002;125:391-403.

84. Hurtig HI, Trojanowski JQ, Galvin J, et al: Alpha-synuclein cortical Lewy bodies correlate with dementia in Parkinson's disease. Neurology 2000;54:1916-1921.

85. Braak H, Rüb U, Jansen Steur ENH, et al: Cognitive status correlates with neuropathologic stage in Parkinson's disease. Neurology 2005;64:1404-1410.

86. Aarsland D, Perry R, Brown A, et al: Neuropathology of dementia in Parkinson's disease: a prospective, community-based study. Ann Neurol 2005;58:773-776.

87. Colosimo C, Hughes AJ, Kilford L, Lees AJ: Lewy body cortical involvement may not always predict dementia in Parkinson's disease. J Neurol Neurosurg Psychiatry 2003;74:852-856.

88. Parkkinen L, Kauppinen T, Pirttila T, et al: Alpha-synuclein pathology does not predict extrapyramidal symptoms or dementia. Ann Neurol 2005;57:82-91.

89. Jellinger KA, Seppi K, Wenning GK, Poewe W: Impact of coexistent Alzheimer pathology on the natural history of Parkinson's disease. J Neural Transm 2002;109:329-339.

90. SantaCruz K, Pahwa R, Lyons K, et al: Lewy body, neurofibrillary tangle and senile plaque pathology in Parkinson's disease patients with and without dementia. Neurology 1999;52(Suppl 2): A476-A477.

91. Ballard C, Ziabreva I, Perry R, et al: Differences in neuropathologic characteristics across the Lewy body dementia spectrum. Neurology 2006;67:1931-1934.

92. Pletnikova O, West N, Lee MK, et al: Abeta deposition is associated with enhanced cortical alpha-synuclein lesions in Lewy body diseases. Neurobiol Aging 2005;26:1183-1192.

93. Masliah E, Rockenstein E, Veinbergs I, et al: β-amyloid peptides enhance α-synuclein accumulation and neuronal deficits in a transgenic mouse model linking Alzheimer's disease and Parkinson's disease. Proc Natl Acad Sci U S A 2001;98:12245-12250.

94. shizawa T, Mattila P, Davies P, et al: Colocalisation of tau and alpha-synuclein epitopes in Lewy bodies. J Neuropathol Exp Neurol 2003;62:389-397.

95. Francis PT, Perry EK: Cholinergic and other neurotransmitter mechanisms in Parkinson's disease, Parkinson's disease dementia, and dementia with Lewy bodies. Mov Disord 2007;22 Suppl 17:S351-357.

96. Cohen-Mansfield J, Mintzer JE: Time for change: the role of nonpharmacological interventions in treating behavior problems in nursing home residents with dementia. Alzheimer Dis Assoc Disord 2005;19:37-40.

97. Gil Gregorio P, Ramirez Diaz SP, Ribera Casado JM: group D: Dementia and nutrition: intervention study in institutionalized patients with Alzheimer disease. J Nutr Health Aging 2003;7:304-308.

98. Högl B, Saletu M, Brandauer E, et al: Modafinil for the treatment of daytime sleepiness in Parkinson's disease: a double-blind, randomized, crossover, placebo-controlled polygraphic trial. Sleep 2002;25:905-909.

99. Adler CH, Caviness JN, Hentz JG, et al: Randomized trial of modafinil for treating subjective daytime sleepiness in patients with Parkinson's disease. Mov Disord 2003;18:287-293.

100. Ondo WG, Fayle R, Atassi F, Jankovic J: Modafinil for daytime somnolence in Parkinson's disease: double blind, placebo controlled parallel trial. J Neurol Neurosurg Psychiatry 2005;76:1636-1639.

101. Aarsland D, Perry R, Larsen J, et al: Neuroleptic sensitivity in Parkinson's disease and parkinsonian dementias. J Clin Psychiatry 2005;66:633-637.

102. Miyasaki J, Shannon K, Voon V, et al: Practice Parameter: Evaluation and treatment of depression, psychosis, and dementia in Parkinson disease (an evidence-based review). Report of the Quality Standards Subcommittee of the American Academy of Neurology. Neurology 2006;66:996-1002.

103. Frieling H, Hillemacher T, Ziegenbein M, et al: Treating dopamimetic psychosis in Parkinson's disease: structured review and meta-analysis. Eur Neuropsychopharmacol 2007;17:165-171.

104. Friedman J, Berman RM, Goetz CG, et al: Open-label flexible-dose pilot study to evaluate the safety and tolerability of aripiprazole in patients with psychosis associated with Parkinson's disease. Mov Disord 2006;21:2078-2081.

105. Schindehütte J, Trenkwalder C: Treatment of drug-induced psychosis in Parkinson's disease with ziprasidone can induce severe dose-dependent off-periods and pathological laughing. Clin Neurol Neurosurg 2007;109:188-191.

106. Friedman J, Vanover KE, Taylor EM, et al: ACP-103 reduces psychosis without impairing motor function in Parkinson's disease. Mov Disord 2006;21:1546.

107. Emre M, Aarsland D, Albanese A, et al: Rivastigmine for dementia associated with Parkinson's disease. N Engl J Med 2004;351:2509-2518.

108. Poewe W, Wolters E, Emre M, et al: Long-term benefits of rivastigmine in dementia associated with Parkinson's disease: an active treatment extension study. Mov Disord 2006;21:456-461.

109. Winblad B, Grossberg G, Frölich L, et al: IDEAL: a 6-month, double-blind, placebo-controlled study of the first skin patch for Alzheimer disease. Neurology 2007;69(Suppl 1):S14-S22.

110. Ravina B, Putt M, Siderowf A, et al: Donepezil for dementia in Parkinson's disease: a randomised, double blind, placebo controlled, crossover study. J Neurol Neurosurg Psychiatry 2005;76:934-939.

111. Dubois B, Tolosa E, Kulisevsky J, et al: Efficacy and safety of donepezil in the treatment of Parkinson's disease patients with dementia. Neurodegener Dis 2007;4(Suppl 1): 90.

112. Maidment I, Fox C, Boustani M: Cholinesterase inhibitors for Parkinson's disease dementia. Cochrane Database Syst Rev 2006; CD004747.

113. Sabbagh MN, Hake AM, Ahmed S, Farlow MR: The use of memantine in dementia with Lewy bodies. J Alzheimers Dis 2005;7:285-289.

114. Ridha B, Josephs K, Rossor M: Delusions and hallucinations in dementia with Lewy bodies: worsening with memantine. Neurology 2005;65:481-482.

115. Fox CG, Umoh G, Samuel M, et al: Memantine in Parkinson's disease dementia: clinical experience. Mov Disord 2005;20(Suppl 10): S123.

116. Williams-Gray CH, Foltynie T, Lewis SJ, Barker RA: Cognitive deficits and psychosis in Parkinson's disease: a review of pathophysiology and therapeutic options. CNS Drugs 2006;20:477-505.

117. Marsh L, Bassett SS, Biglan K, et al: Atomoxetine for the treatment of executive dysfunction in Parkinson's disease: a pilot open-label study. Mov Disord 2007;22:1-2.

118. Youdim MB, Amit T, Bar-Am O, et al: Implications of co-morbidity for etiology and treatment of neurodegenerative diseases with multifunctional neuroprotective-neurorescue drugs: ladostigil. Neurotox Res 2006;10:181-192.

119. Sharma T, Stocchi F, Schapira AH, et al: Safinamide treatment improves cognition in Parkinson's disease. Mov Disord 2007;22:12-13.

13 Psychiatric Issues in Parkinson's Disease

DANIEL WEINTRAUB

Introduction

Although Parkinson's disease (PD) is diagnosed on the basis of neurological signs, the high prevalence of psychiatric complications suggests that it is more accurately conceptualized as a neuropsychiatric disease. Specific psychiatric disorders include affective disorders (depression and anxiety), psychosis, impulse control disorders (ICDs), disorders of sleep and wakefulness, apathy, and involuntary emotional expression disorder (IEED).

Psychiatric complications in PD are associated with a range of negative outcomes, including excess disability, worse quality of life, poorer motor and cognitive outcomes, and caregiver distress. Understanding of the epidemiology, phenomenology, risk factors, neuropathophysiology, and optimal treatment strategies for these disorders is incomplete, however. Psychiatric complications typically are associated with multiple morbidities, and there is significant intraindividual

213

and interindividual variability in presentation. Psychiatric disorders in PD are underrecognized and undertreated.

The neuropathophysiological changes that occur in PD, along with the association between a range of PD treatments and certain psychiatric disorders, suggest a neurobiological basis for many psychiatric symptoms, although psychological factors also contribute. Antidepressants, anxiolytics, and antipsychotics are commonly prescribed in routine clinical care, but controlled studies showing efficacy and tolerability are limited. Additional research in the psychiatric complications of PD is needed to determine if there are modifiable risk factors and to establish efficacious and effective treatments.

Depression

EPIDEMIOLOGY

Prevalence estimates for depression in PD are typically 20% to 40%, but range widely owing to differences in study populations, definitions of depression, and criteria for symptom attribution.[1-3] More recent research differentiating types of depression suggests that *major* depression may occur in 5% to 15% of patients, with an additional 10% to 25% experiencing *nonmajor* depression (e.g., minor depression or dysthymia).[4-7]

There is an increasing awareness that depression in PD may be more impairing than motor symptoms in many PD patients. Evidence from research shows an association between depression in PD and excess disability,[7,8] worse quality of life,[9,10] increased caregiver distress,[11] more rapid progression of motor impairment and disability,[12] and cognitive decline[12,13] or development of dementia.[14,15]

The most consistent risk factors for or correlates of depression in PD are female sex[4] and increasing severity of cognitive impairment,[4] with mixed evidence for a personal history of depression,[1] early-onset PD (i.e., before age 55),[6,16] predominantly right-sided motor symptoms,[1] and atypical parkinsonism (e.g., prominent akinesia-rigidity or extensive vascular disease).[5,17] Regarding other psychiatric symptoms, psychosis,[18,19] anxiety,[20] apathy,[21] fatigue,[22] and insomnia[10] frequently coexist with depression in PD, which can complicate assessment and treatment. Depression in PD and cognitive impairment likely have an adverse impact on each other.[13,17] Executive impairment, which in particular has been associated with depression in PD,[23,24] may be due to the additive effects of PD and depression.[13]

ETIOLOGY AND PATHOPHYSIOLOGY

Regarding psychosocial risk factors for depression in PD, the association between depression and early-onset PD reported in some studies[6,16] may be due to the fact that younger patients experience more significant career, family, and financial disruptions than patients with late-onset PD.[25] There is a growing appreciation of the neurobiological underpinnings of depression in PD. Research suggests that PD patients are more depressed than patients with other chronic disabling diseases.[26,27] Additionally, studies have found that PD patients have a higher lifetime prevalence of depressive disorders than non-PD controls,[28] and that non-PD patients with depression are at higher risk of subsequently developing PD than nondepressed controls.[29]

Biologically, the high frequency of depression in PD may be explained by dysfunction in (1) subcortical nuclei and the frontal lobes; (2) striatothalamic–frontal cortex circuits and the basotemporal limbic circuit; and (3) brainstem monoamine and indolamine systems (i.e., dopamine, serotonin, and norepinephrine). Neuroimaging studies have reported associations between depressive symptoms and either altered putaminal metabolism[30] or reduced basal limbic system echogenicity.[31] Functional brain imaging studies have reported simultaneous prefrontal cortex and striatal hypometabolism in depression in PD, reflecting disruption in frontostriatal pathways.[30,32] Regarding neurotransmitters, disproportionate degeneration of dopamine neurons in the ventral tegmental area has been reported in patients with a history of depression in PD.[33] In addition, imaging studies in depression in PD have found a decrease in signal intensity from neural pathways originating in monoaminergic brainstem nuclei,[31] and a negative correlation between depression scores and dorsal midbrain serotonin transporter (5-HTT) densities.[34] Other possible links between altered serotonin function and depression in PD include associations between depression in PD and a functional polymorphism (the short allele) in 5-HTT[35,36] and reduced cerebrospinal levels of the serotonin metabolite 5-hydroxyindoleacetic acid.[37]

PRESENTATION AND ASSESSMENT

On average, depression in PD may have a slightly different symptom profile than depression in the general population, including higher rates of anxiety, pessimism, suicide ideation without suicide behavior, and less guilt and self-reproach,[3,38,39] although there is significant interindividual variability. Core nonsomatic symptoms of depression (e.g., suicide thoughts, feelings of guilt, depressed mood, and anhedonia) discriminate best between depressed and nondepressed patients, whereas somatic symptoms correlate variably with depression.[40,41] Assessing depression in PD is challenging, partly because of symptom overlap between depression and PD symptoms (e.g., insomnia, psychomotor slowing, difficulty concentrating, and fatigue).

As mentioned previously, more recent research findings suggest that nonmajor (i.e., less severe) depression is more common than major depression in PD. Other experts state that atypical depressive disorders, such as recurrent brief depressive disorder, better capture the symptom variability that many PD patients experience.[42] Also, depressive symptoms can be specifically related to motor symptoms, as in patients who experience temporary dysphoria and anxiety during "off" periods.[43]

TREATMENT

Depression in PD is underrecognized and undertreated,[44] even in specialty care settings,[45] with two thirds of depressed patients going untreated.[46] Approximately 20% to 25% of PD patients in specialty care are taking an antidepressant at any given time, most commonly a selective serotonin reuptake inhibitor (SSRI).[46,47] Results of numerous open-label trials using SSRIs and other newer antidepressants in PD suggest a positive effect overall and good tolerability. Although concern has been raised via case reporting and physician surveys about SSRIs worsening parkinsonism,[47,48] clinical experience and open-label studies suggest that most PD patients tolerate SSRI treatment without worsening of their PD.[49]

There are only three published, placebo-controlled antidepressant studies for depression in PD. Although a small study found nortriptyline to be efficacious,[50] tricyclic antidepressants can be difficult for PD patients to tolerate because of worsening of orthostatic hypotension, constipation, and cognitive problems. Two SSRI studies[42,51] were underpowered and reported negative findings, and a more recent review and meta-analysis concluded that SSRIs may be less effective in PD patients than in the general, elderly population.[49]

Regarding PD medications, levodopa is not thought to have a consistent mood effect. Preliminary studies suggest that dopamine agonists have antidepressant properties in PD populations.[52,53] Selegiline has also been reported to have antidepressant properties in PD,[54] and in patch form is approved by the U.S. Food and Drug Administration for the treatment of major depression in the general population. Concern that the combination of selegiline and SSRIs might lead to serotonin syndrome has been allayed by clinical experience.[55]

Electroconvulsive therapy can be effective for severe depression in PD and temporarily improves parkinsonism.[56] Regarding nonpharmacological treatments, there is emerging evidence that psychotherapy (e.g., cognitive therapy) can be effective in treating depression in PD.[57] Anecdotally, many PD patients prefer talking therapy, do not respond to pharmacotherapy, or are reluctant to take another medication, so psychotherapy is an appropriate treatment option for depression in PD. In light of the fact that depressive symptoms in PD can be nonsevere and transient, it also may be appropriate initially to use watchful waiting as a treatment strategy, provided that the patient has regular follow-up.

CLINICAL RECOMMENDATIONS

PD patients should be screened regularly for depression. Given time constraints, a brief screening instrument that can be self-administered is recommended. The 15-item Geriatric Depression Rating Scale (GDS-15) is a brief, self-completed questionnaire that has good sensitivity and specificity for a diagnosis of depression in PD at a cutoff of 5.[58] Despite a lack of demonstrable efficacy, psychopharmacological treatment typically begins with an SSRI at a dosage recommended for geriatric patients,[59] but using dosages within the highest recommended range[59] if depressive symptoms persist and treatment is well tolerated. Other possible first-line or adjunctive antidepressants include venlafaxine, mirtazapine, and bupropion. A tricyclic antidepressant (e.g., nortriptyline) is a reasonable second-line treatment. A significant percentage of PD patients may not tolerate, respond to, or want antidepressant treatment, so it is important also to have access to and use nonpharmacological treatments when indicated.

Anxiety

Of PD patients, 40% may experience anxiety symptoms or disorders, including generalized anxiety disorder or panic attacks,[60,61] and anxiety symptoms are frequently comorbid with depression.[20] Clinical experience indicates that anxiety symptoms are often more upsetting and disabling than depressive symptoms in PD, perhaps because of their intensity, accompanying somatic complaints, and propensity to worsen parkinsonism.

Increasing levels of anxiety and discrete anxiety attacks have been associated with motor complications, particularly the onset of "off" periods, although this relationship is not apparent for all patients.[62] When it occurs, patients often describe a sensation of feeling "trapped" as they become increasingly immobilized, with symptoms resolving with improvement in motor symptoms.

Similar to depression, studies have reported an increased prevalence of anxiety disorders 20 years before PD onset.[28,63] This research underscores the biological underpinnings of anxiety in PD, and a neuropathophysiological link between anxiety and PD may be noradrenergic dysfunction.[60]

Regarding treatment, there are no published controlled anxiety treatment studies in PD to inform clinical decision making.[61] For patients who experience anxiety as part of an "off" state, PD medication adjustments may decrease the duration and severity of these episodes. Newer antidepressants (e.g., SSRIs) have variable antianxiety effects and are commonly used as first-line treatment for anxiety symptoms. Many patients require treatment with benzodiazepines (most commonly low-dose lorazepam, alprazolam, and clonazepam). Because PD patients commonly are physically and cognitively impaired, benzodiazepines must be used cautiously and at the lowest possible effective dosage.

Psychosis

EPIDEMIOLOGY

Hallucinations occur in less than 10% of *untreated* PD patients,[64] but in 15% to 40% of *treated* PD patients,[18,19,65,66] and approximately 5% of patients experience paranoid thinking (i.e., delusions) in addition to hallucinations.[18,67] As with other psychiatric disorders, persistent psychotic symptoms are associated with greater functional impairment, caregiver burden, and nursing home placement.[11,19,68] Reported risk factors for PD psychosis include exposure to PD medications,[69] older age,[18,70] greater cognitive impairment,[18,19,65,66] and increasing severity[18,19] and duration of PD.[65] Reported psychiatric risk factors include depression,[18,19,65,66] anxiety,[19] fatigue,[65] sleep disorders,[70] visual impairment,[71] and polypharmacy.[69]

ETIOLOGY AND PATHOPHYSIOLOGY

Exposure to dopaminergic therapy has been implicated as the major cause of psychosis in PD[72] because reports of psychosis in PD in the prelevodopa era were uncommon. Claims have been made that certain agents are less likely than others to induce psychosis, but evidence for this is anecdotal.[69] More recent studies have reported that the dosage and duration of antiparkinsonian treatment are not correlated with psychosis,[18,70] indicating that PD psychosis likely results from a complex interaction of medication exposure, PD neuropathology, and other risk factors, particularly cognitive impairment and visual disturbances.

Dopaminergic medication exposure may lead to excessive stimulation or hypersensitivity of mesocorticolimbic D2/D3 receptors and induce psychosis via this mechanism.[73] In addition, cholinergic deficits and a serotoninergic/dopaminergic imbalance have been implicated in the development of PD psychosis.[69,72-74]

PRESENTATION AND ASSESSMENT

Generally, one group of psychotic patients experiences visual illusions or hallucinations only, although hallucinations in other sensory modalities (auditory, olfactory, and tactile) can also occur.[65,69,75] Initially, patients typically retain insight into the hallucinations, do not find them troubling, and may not require treatment (i.e., "benign hallucinosis"). Another group experiences more complex psychotic symptoms, typically hallucinations plus persecutory delusions in the context of significant cognitive impairment. These patients typically do not have insight into their psychosis, may display behavioral changes (including agitation), and typically require treatment. Psychosis and cognitive impairment early in the course of parkinsonism suggests a diagnosis of dementia with Lewy bodies.[69]

The vivid dreaming and confused thinking that occurs as part of rapid-eye-movement (REM) sleep behavior disorder (RBD) should not be characterized as psychotic symptoms because they occur during the sleep state. Most psychotic PD patients also report sleep disturbances, however.[76-78]

TREATMENT

Treating PD psychosis is challenging because optimizing the management of motor symptoms with dopaminergic medication can worsen psychosis, whereas antipsychotic treatment can worsen parkinsonism. A thorough medical evaluation for reversible causes of psychosis (i.e., delirium) should be performed. Next, the risk-to-benefit ratio of each antiparkinsonian medication should be reviewed. Based on clinical experience, medications are usually discontinued (if tolerated from a motor standpoint) in the following order: anticholinergics, selegiline, amantadine, dopamine agonists (DAs), and catechol O-methyltransferase inhibitors. Finally, levodopa dosage is reduced.[69,79]

Antipsychotic treatment can be initiated for persistent and problematic psychosis. Typical antipsychotics are not recommended for use in PD patients because they have been reported to worsen parkinsonism significantly.[69] Clozapine has been shown to be efficacious for PD psychosis in placebo-controlled studies at much lower dosages (mean dosages of 25 to 36 mg/day) than typically used in psychiatric patients,[80,81] but is usually reserved for treatment-refractory patients because of its overall side-effect profile, and the need for frequent blood testing to monitor for agranulocytosis. Clinically, quetiapine has become the most commonly used antipsychotic, a preference based on clinical experience, the results of several positive open-label studies, and the adverse impact on parkinsonism reported with other atypical antipsychotics.[82] The two placebo-controlled quetiapine studies for PD psychosis have reported negative findings, however.[83,84]

Cholinesterase inhibitors may also have antipsychotic properties in PD. Initial evidence for this included the results of a rivastigmine study in dementia with Lewy bodies that showed improvement in cognition and psychosis.[85] Since then, several small open-label studies have found donepezil and rivastigmine to be beneficial for PD psychosis in the context of dementia.

CLINICAL RECOMMENDATIONS

Screening for psychosis can be done quickly by inquiring about perceptual changes, particularly visual disturbances. Treatment with an atypical antipsychotic should occur only if the symptoms are problematic, after acute medical conditions have been ruled out, and after the antiparkinsonian medications have been reviewed. Based on open-label studies and clinical experience, current first-line antipsychotic treatment is quetiapine (starting dosage 12.5 to 25 mg/day; mean maintenance dosage ~75 mg/day; dosage range 25 to 300 mg/day), with clozapine reserved for patients who do not respond to or tolerate quetiapine. Cholinesterase inhibitors may have antipsychotic effects in PD, and their cognitive-enhancing properties are likely to be beneficial to the large percentage of psychotic patients with comorbid cognitive impairment.

Impulse Control Disorders

EPIDEMIOLOGY

ICDs constitute a group of psychiatric disorders with the essential feature being a failure to resist an impulse, drive, or temptation to perform an act that is harmful to the individual or to others. Pathological gambling is an ICD with formal diagnostic criteria; disorders without formal diagnostic criteria include compulsive sexual behavior and compulsive buying. In addition, binge-eating disorder shares many of the clinical characteristics of ICDs.

Case reporting[86,87] and large-scale cross-sectional studies[88,89] suggest that ICDs, particularly compulsive gambling, are more common in PD patients than in the general population,[90,91] sometimes with devastating consequences. Although initial reporting in PD focused on compulsive gambling, more recent publications have reported the occurrence of compulsive sexual behavior,[89,92,93] compulsive buying,[89,94] and binge eating.[95] Ongoing epidemiological research and more recent literature suggest that 15% of PD patients may experience one or more ICDs at any time. Other related disorders reported to occur in PD and characterized by repetitive, or compulsive, behaviors include (1) dopamine dysregulation syndrome or hedonic homeostatic dysregulation,[96] an addiction-like state marked by excessive dopaminergic medication usage, particularly levodopa and short-acting DAs (e.g., subcutaneous apomorphine); (2) punding, an intense fascination with meaningless movements or activities (e.g., collecting, arranging, or taking apart objects)[97]; and (3) walkabout, defined as excessive, aimless wandering.[96]

ETIOLOGY AND PATHOPHYSIOLOGY

Dopamine receptor agonist (DA) treatment seems to be the primary risk factor for ICD development in PD because nearly all ICD patients have been reported to be taking a DA while symptomatic.[86-89] Other possible risk factors for ICD development include a previous history of ICD behaviors, a personal or family history of substance abuse, male sex (for compulsive sexual behavior), and early-onset PD.[98]

There are plausible explanations for an association between DA treatment and ICDs in PD. The dopamine depletion that occurs in PD affects distinct neural circuits subserving motor, cognitive, and limbic functions, perhaps leading to deficits in cognition (e.g., decision-making and response inhibition) and emotional state (e.g., the drive to engage in risk-reward behaviors) that may predispose to the development of ICDs. DAs, in addition to activating D1 and D2 receptors associated with their motor effects, also bind to the D3 receptor.[99] The D3 receptor is localized to limbic areas of the brain and may mediate psychiatric manifestations of dopamine receptor stimulation.[100] Excessive dopamine stimulation of an inherently vulnerable brain may lead to the development of ICDs in PD.

PRESENTATION AND ASSESSMENT

Patients may not spontaneously report ICD behaviors to their treating neurologist, either because of shame or not suspecting an association with PD pharmacotherapy. This situation leads to ICD behaviors being underrecognized in clinical practice.[89] Direct questioning about a range of ICD behaviors, including an informed other if possible, is necessary to ensure detection of these disorders.

When ICDs do occur, compulsive gambling and buying can be associated with significant financial losses, compulsive sexual behavior can be associated with significant health risks, compulsive eating can be associated with significant weight gain and medical comorbidity, and all of these ICDs can be associated with extensive damage to interpersonal relationships with significant others. One study reported a mean loss of $100,000 resulting from pathological gambling,[88] and cases series have reported significant adverse psychosocial effects with compulsive sexual behavior[93] or compulsive eating.[95]

TREATMENT

Anecdotally, there are reports of ICD symptom improvement or resolution with discontinuation of DA therapy, reducing the dose of the existing DA, or switching to a different DA.[86,87,93,95] More recent research suggests that a discontinuation or decrease in DA therapy is typically associated with a significant long-term improvement or resolution in ICD symptoms, with little change in motor symptoms.[101] Some patients do not experience remission of ICD symptoms with DA discontinuation, however, suggesting a multifactorial etiology in some cases. Other patients are reluctant to discontinue DA treatment because of motor benefits derived from taking the medication. The clinical management of ICD patients can be complicated. Case reports suggest that atypical antipsychotics,[93,102] antidepressants,[93] mood stabilizers,[86,93] and various psychosocial interventions[86] may be beneficial in the treatment of ICD behaviors in PD.

In a case series reporting on the outcomes of PD patients who underwent subthalamic nucleus deep brain stimulation (DBS) surgery, all patients who had pathological gambling before DBS surgery experienced a resolution of symptoms after DBS surgery.[103] The authors hypothesized that the physiological effects of DBS in conjunction with the concomitant decrease in overall dopaminergic treatment were responsible for the improvement in ICD symptoms.

CLINICAL RECOMMENDATIONS

Clinicians should be aware of certain demographic or clinical factors that may place patients at a higher risk for ICD development in the context of DA treatment, and patients should be notified about the possible risk of ICD development before initiating DA treatment. In addition, because there can be a long delay between initiation of DA treatment and onset of ICD behaviors, clinicians need to query patients routinely about a range of ICD behaviors. For patients who have clinically significant ICD behaviors, given the lack of demonstrable efficacy for psychiatric treatments for ICD behaviors, attempts should be made to discontinue, decrease, or change DA treatment. To help offset the loss of beneficial motor effects of DA treatment, a concomitant increase in levodopa treatment may be necessary.[101]

▌ Disorders of Sleep and Wakefulness

Disorders of sleep and wakefulness may be the most common nonmotor disorders in PD, with 90% of PD patients reporting insomnia, hypersomnia, sleep fragmentation, sleep terrors, nightmares, nocturnal movements, or RBD.[77,78,104,105] The last-mentioned disorder is characterized by loss of normal skeletal muscle atony during REM sleep, prominent motor activity, and dreams; RBD also may be a prodrome of PD.[106,107] Other sleep cycle–related disorders in PD include restless legs syndrome and periodic leg movements in sleep, which are overlapping but distinct disorders. In addition, patients with more advanced PD may have an increased frequency of obstructive or central apnea.[108]

RBD and other sleep disturbances have been attributed to progressive degeneration of the cholinergic pedunculopontine nucleus[109] and reduced striatal dopaminergic activity.[110] Clinical factors that can disrupt sleep are immobility secondary to core PD symptoms, dyskinesias, cramps, micturition, pain, and excessive sweating.[105,108,111] Sleep disturbances also are associated with other psychiatric disorders, including psychosis,[112] depression,[105] and cognitive impairment.[111]

Excessive daytime sleepiness (EDS) and fatigue, distinct but overlapping symptoms, occur in 15% to 50% of PD patients.[113,114] This clinical phenomenon has been attributed variably to impairments in the striatothalamic–frontal cortical system, exposure to dopaminergic medications (especially DAs), and nocturnal sleep disturbances.[108,111,115] In addition, advanced disease, depression, cognitive impairment, and psychosis are clinical correlates of EDS.[113,114,116] Daytime "sleep attacks" (i.e., sudden-onset REM sleep) have been reported rarely in PD patients, particularly in conjunction with DA treatment, although there is increasing evidence that this typically is medication-induced EDS.[108,117]

Regarding treatment, sleep disturbances that are due to nocturnal worsening of parkinsonism may respond to adjustments in bedtime or overnight PD medications. Restless legs syndrome and periodic leg movements in sleep are commonly treated with DAs, and RBD is typically treated with clonazepam.

Preliminary studies suggested that EDS could be treated successfully with modafinil,[118,119] but a more recent placebo-controlled study reported negative results.[120] Psychostimulants also are used in clinical practice for EDS and fatigue in PD, supported by positive results from a more recent double-blind study of methylphenidate for fatigue.[121]

Apathy

Apathy, succinctly defined as a decrease in goal-directed behavior, thinking, and mood, is reported to occur in 40% of PD patients.[21,122] Although there is overlap between apathy, depression and dementia, apathy also occurs independently of these syndromes.[21] Apathy usually is accompanied by diminished self-awareness, so changes typically are noticed and brought to the attention of clinicians by caregivers. A common assumption is that the patient is depressed, but a lack of endorsement of sad mood or the cognitive features of depression (e.g., guilt, helplessness, and hopelessness) suggest a diagnosis of apathy instead.

Goal-directed behavior is associated with dopaminergic and noradrenergic function, and with activation of the frontal cortex and basal ganglia.[123] Studies of apathy in PD have reported associations with executive and memory impairment.[21,122]

There are no published treatment studies for apathy in PD. Anecdotally, psychostimulants (e.g., methylphenidate) and stimulant-related compounds (e.g., modafinil) are used in clinical practice, but their effectiveness for this condition is unknown. It has been proposed that antidepressants and other medications that increase dopamine or norepinephrine activity may be beneficial.[124] In addition, it is important to educate patients and families on the distinction between apathy and depression, and to encourage patients to remain as physically and mentally active as possible.[125]

Involuntary Emotional Expression Disorder

IEED, also called pseudobulbar affect, emotional lability, and affective lability, can occur in various neurodegenerative diseases and neurological conditions, including PD. Clinically, IEED is characterized by repeated, brief episodes of involuntary expression of either crying or laughing with minimal provocation, with the expressed emotion typically incongruent with the patient's underlying mood and in excess of what would ordinarily be expected.[126] For some patients, the episodes are embarrassing and distressing, and family members may mistakenly attribute crying episodes for an underlying depression. A final common pathophysiological pathway for IEED seems to be disinhibition of brainstem bulbar nuclei that control the expression of crying and laughing, which in PD may result from impairment in neural pathways connecting the cortex and brainstem.[127]

Numerous small-scale studies in non-PD populations have found tricyclic antidepressants and SSRIs to be efficacious in the treatment of pseudobulbar affect.[128] In addition, it is important to educate patients and family members on the distinction between pseudobulbar affect and depression.

Impact of Deep Brain Stimulation

DBS, usually bilateral DBS of the subthalamic nucleus, is increasingly used as a treatment for PD. Its impact on nonmotor symptoms seems to be varied and complex, and to evolve over time.[129] Patients can experience transient abnormalities, such as confusional states, psychosis, and agitation, in the acute postoperative period.[130] Longer-term findings have included worsening in specific cognitive domains (e.g., executive abilities and verbal learning).[131,132] Psychiatric findings have included overall improvement[133] and occasional onset of or worsening in depression, anxiety, psychosis, mania, and emotional lability.[130,134] Overall, the full spectrum, prevalence, and permanence of neuropsychiatric sequelae of DBS remain unclear because of the uncontrolled nature of most follow-up study data and accompanying changes in PD medication postoperatively.

Generally, postsurgical neuropsychological decline seems most likely in patients with preexisting neuropsychiatric disorders,[134] a finding that emphasizes the need for a thorough presurgical evaluation, including a psychiatric history and neuropsychological evaluation. Postsurgical psychiatric monitoring also is warranted, especially given reports of suicide ideation[135] and attempted or completed suicides[129] after DBS surgery. Psychiatric intervention may take the form of adjusting DBS parameters, adjusting PD drugs, or initiating pharmacotherapy or psychotherapy.

Conclusions

A range of psychiatric complications, frequently comorbid or multimorbid, is common in PD. The etiology of these disorders is likely complex and includes the hallmark neuropathophysiological changes of PD, exposure to PD treatments, and psychosocial factors. Despite a growing awareness that psychiatric symptoms and disorders are a core aspect of PD and may have significant adverse effects, many unanswered questions remain regarding optimal assessment and treatment strategies for all of these disorders. Reducing the overall impact that PD has on patients and families depends in significant part on improving the management of psychiatric complications.

Acknowledgments

This chapter was supported, in part, by a grant from the National Institute of Mental Health (#067894).

REFERENCES

1. Starkstein SE, Preziosi TJ, Bolduc PL, et al: Depression in Parkinson's disease. J Nerv Ment Dis 1990;178:27-31.
2. Allain H, Schuck S, Manduit N: Depression in Parkinson's disease. BMJ 2000;320:1287-1288.
3. Cummings JL: Depression and Parkinson's disease: a review. Am J Psychiatry 1992;149: 443-454.
4. Tandberg E, Larsen JP, Aarsland D, et al: The occurrence of depression in Parkinson's disease: a community-based study. Arch Neurol 1996;53:175-179.

5. Starkstein SE, Petracca G, Chemerinski E, et al: Depression in classic versus akinetic-rigid Parkinson's disease. Mov Disord 1998;13:29-33.
6. Cole SA, Woodard JL, Juncos JL, et al: Depression and disability in Parkinson's disease. J Neuropsychiatry Clin Neurosci 1996;8:20-25.
7. Liu CY, Wang SJ, Fuh JL, et al: The correlation of depression with functional activity in Parkinson's disease. J Neurol 1997;244:493-498.
8. Weintraub D, Moberg PJ, Duda JE, et al: Effect of psychiatric and other non-motor symptoms on disability in Parkinson's disease. J Am Geriatr Soc 2004;52:784-788.
9. Kuopio A-M, Marttila RJ, Helenius H, et al: The quality of life in Parkinson's disease. Mov Disord 2000;15:4216-4223.
10. Caap-Ahlgren M, Dehlin O: Insomnia and depressive symptoms in patients with Parkinson's disease: relationship to health-related quality of life: an interview of patients living at home. Arch Gerontol Geriatr 2001;32:23-33.
11. Aarsland D, Larsen JP, Tandberg E, et al: Predictors of nursing home placement in Parkinson's disease: a population-based, prospective study. J Am Geriatr Soc 2000;48:938-942.
12. Starkstein SE, Mayberg HS, Leiguarda R, et al: A prospective longitudinal study of depression, cognitive decline, and physical impairments in patients with Parkinson's disease. J Neurol Neurosurg Psychiatry 1992;55:377-382.
13. Tröster AI, Stalp LD, Paolo AM, et al: Neuropsychological impairment in Parkinson's disease with and without depression. Arch Neurol 1995;52:1164-1169.
14. Marder K, Tang M-X, Cote L, et al: The frequency and associated risk factors for dementia in patients with Parkinson's disease. Arch Neurol 1995;52:695-701.
15. Stern Y, Marder K, Tang M-X, et al: Antecedent clinical features associated with dementia in Parkinson's disease. Neurology 1993;43:1690-1692.
16. Kostic VS, Filipovic SR, Lecic D, et al: Effect of age at onset of frequency of depression in Parkinson's disease. J Neurol Neurosurg Psychiatry 1994;57:1265-1267.
17. Tandberg E, Larsen JP, Aarsland D, et al: Risk factors for depression in Parkinson disease. Arch Neurol 1997;54:625-630.
18. Aarsland D, Larsen JP, Cummings JL, Laake K: Prevalence and clinical correlates of psychotic symptoms in Parkinson disease: a community-based study. Arch Neurol 1999;56:595-601.
19. Marsh L, Williams JR, Rocco M, et al: Psychiatric comorbidities in patients with Parkinson disease and psychosis. Neurology 2004;63:293-300.
20. Menza MA, Robertson-Hoffman DE, Bonapace AS: Parkinson's disease and anxiety: comorbidity with depression. Biol Psychiatry 1993;34:465-470.
21. Starkstein SE, Mayberg HS, Preziosi TJ, et al: Reliability, validity, and clinical correlates of apathy in Parkinson's disease. J Neuropsychiatry Clin Neurosci 1992;4:134-139.
22. Lou J-S, Kearns G, Oken B, et al: Exacerbated physical fatigue and mental fatigue in Parkinson's disease. Mov Disord 2001;16:190-196.
23. Kuzis G, Sabe L, Tiberti C, et al: Cognitive functions in major depression and Parkinson disease. Arch Neurol 1997;54:982-986.
24. Anguenot A, Loll PY, Neau JP, et al: Depression and Parkinson's disease: study of a series of 135 Parkinson's patients. Can J Neurol Sci 2002;29:139-146.
25. Brown RG, Maccarthy B, Gotham A-M, et al: Depression and disability in Parkinson's disease: a follow-up of 132 cases. Psychol Med 1988;18:49-55.
26. Ehmann TS, Beninger RJ, Gawel MJ, et al: Depressive symptoms in Parkinson's disease: a comparison with disabled control subjects. J Geriatr Psychiatry Neurol 1989;2:3-9.
27. Menza MA, Mark MH: Parkinson's disease and depression: the relationship to disability and personality. J Neuropsychiatry Clin Neurosci 1994;6:165-169.
28. Shiba M, Bower JH, Maraganore DM, et al: Anxiety disorders and depressive disorders preceding Parkinson's disease: a case-control study. Mov Disord 2000;15:669-677.
29. Schuurman AG, van den Akker M, Ensinck KTJL, et al: Increased risk of Parkinson's disease after depression. Neurology 2002;58:1501-1504.
30. Mentis MJ, McIntosh AR, Perrine K, et al: Relationships among the metabolic patterns that correlate with mnemonic, visuospatial, and mood symptoms in Parkinson's disease. Am J Psychiatry 2002;159:746-754.
31. Berg D, Supprian T, Hofmann E, et al: Depression in Parkinson's disease: brainstem midline alteration on transcranial sonography and magnetic imaging. J Neurol 1999;246:1186-1193.
32. Mayberg HS, Starkstein SE, Sadzot B, et al: Selective hypometabolism in the inferior frontal lobe in depressed patients with Parkinson's disease. Ann Neurol 1990;28:57-64.

33. Brown AS, Gershon S: Dopamine and depression. J Neural Transm Gen Sect 1993;91:75-109.
34. Murai T, Muller U, Werheid K, et al: In vivo evidence for differential association of striatal dopamine and midbrain serotonin systems with neuropsychiatric symptoms in Parkinson's disease. J Neuropsychiatry Clin Neurosci 2001;13:222-228.
35. Mössner R, Henneberg A, Schmitt A, et al: Allelic variation of serotonin transporter expression is associated with depression in Parkinson's disease. Mol Psychiatry 2001;6:350-352.
36. Menza MA, Palermo B, DiPaola R, et al: Depression and anxiety in Parkinson's disease: possible effect of genetic variation in the serotonin transporter. J Geriatr Psychiatry Neurol 1999;12:49-52.
37. Mayeux R, Stern Y, Sano M, et al: The relationship of serotonin to depression in Parkinson's disease. Mov Disord 1988;3:237-244.
38. Slaughter JR, Slaughter KA, Nichols D, et al: Prevalence, clinical manifestations, etiology, and treatment of depression in Parkinson's disease. J Neuropsychiatry Clin Neurosci 2001;13:187-196.
39. Leentjens AF: Depression in Parkinson's disease: conceptual issues and clinical challenges. J Geriatr Psychiatry Neurol 2004;17:120-126.
40. Leentjens AF, Marinus J, Van Hilten JJ, et al: The contribution of somatic symptoms to the diagnosis of depression in Parkinson's disease: a discriminant analytic approach. J Neuropsychiatry Clin Neurosci 2003;15:74-77.
41. Starkstein SE, Preziosi TJ, Forrester AW, Robinson RG: Specificity of affective and autonomic symptoms of depression in Parkinson's disease. J Neurol Neurosurg Psychiatry 1990;53:869-873.
42. Wermuth L, Sørensen PS, Timm S, et al: Depression in idiopathic Parkinson's disease treated with citalopram: a placebo-controlled trial. Nord J Psychiatry 1998;52:163-169.
43. Menza MA, Sage J, Marshall E, et al: Mood changes and "on-off" phenomena in Parkinson's disease. Mov Disord 1990;5:148-151.
44. Meara J, Mitchelmore E, Hobson P: Use of the GDS-15 geriatric depression scale as a screening instrument for depressive symptomatology in patients with Parkinson's disease and their carers in the community. Age Ageing 1999;28:35-38.
45. Shulman LM, Taback RL, Rabinstein AA, et al: Non-recognition of depression and other non-motor symptoms in Parkinson's disease. Parkinsonism Rel Disord 2002;8:193-197.
46. Weintraub D, Moberg PJ, Duda JE, et al: Recognition and treatment of depression in Parkinson's disease. J Geriatr Psychiatry Neurol 2003;16:178-183.
47. Richard IH, Kurlan R: Parkinson Study Group. A survey of antidepressant use in Parkinson's disease. Neurology 1997;49:1168-1170.
48. van de Vijver DA, Roos RA, Jansen PA, et al: Start of a selective serotonin reuptake inhibitor (SSRI) and increase of antiparkinsonian drug treatment in patients on levodopa. Br J Clin Pharmacol 2002;54:168-170.
49. Weintraub D, Morales KH, Moberg PJ, et al: Antidepressant studies in Parkinson's disease: a review and meta-analysis. Mov Disord 2005;20:1161-1169.
50. Andersen J, Aabro E, Gulmann N, et al: Anti-depressive treatment in Parkinson's disease: a controlled trial of the effect of nortriptyline in patients with Parkinson's disease treated with l-dopa. Acta Neurol Scand 1980;62:210-219.
51. Leentjens AF, Vreeling FW, Luijckx GJ, et al: SSRIs in the treatment of depression in Parkinson's disease. Int J Geriatr Psychiatry 2003;18:552-554.
52. Rektorova I, Rektor I, Bares M, et al: Pramipexole and pergolide in the treatment of depression in Parkinson's disease: a national multicentre prospective randomized study. Eur J Neurol 2003;10:399-406.
53. Barone P, Scarzella L, Marconi R, et al: the Depression/Parkinson Italian Study Group. Pramipexole versus sertraline in the treatment of depression in Parkinson's disease. J Neurol 2006;253:601-607.
54. Allain H, Cougnard J, Neukirch H-C, et al: Selegiline in de novo parkinsonian patients: the French Selegiline Multicenter Trial (FSMT). Acta Neurol Scand 1991;84(Suppl 136):73-78.
55. Richard IH, Kurlan R, Tanner C, et al: Serotonin syndrome and the combined use of deprenyl and an antidepressant in Parkinson's disease. Neurology 1997;48:1070-1077.
56. Moellentine C, Rummans T, Ahlskog JE, et al: Effectiveness of ECT in patients with parkinsonism. J Neuropsychiatry Clin Neurosci 1998;10:187-193.
57. Dobkin RD, Allen LA, Menza M: Cognitive-behavioral therapy for depression in Parkinson's disease: a pilot study. Mov Disord 2007;22:946-952.
58. Weintraub D, Oehlberg KA, Katz IR, Stern MB: Test characteristics of the 15-Item Geriatric Depression Scale and Hamilton Depression Rating Scale in Parkinson's disease. Am J Geriatr Psychiatry 2006;14:169-175.

59. Alexopoulos GS, Katz IR, Reynolds CF III, et al: The expert consensus guideline series: pharmacotherapy of depressive disorders in older patients. Postgrad Med 2001; Special Report:1-86.
60. Richard IH, Schiffer RB, Kurlan R: Anxiety and Parkinson's disease. J Neuropsychiatry Clin Neurosci 1996;8:383-392.
61. Walsh K, Bennett G: Parkinson's disease and anxiety. Postgrad Med J 2001;77:89-93.
62. Richard IH, Justus AW, Kurlan R: Relationship between mood and motor fluctuations in Parkinson's disease. J Neuropsychiatry Clin Neurosci 2001;13:35-41.
63. Gonera EG, van't Hof M, Berger HJC, et al: Symptoms and duration of the prodromal phase in Parkinson's disease. Mov Disord 1997;12:871-876.
64. Cummings JL: Neuropsychiatric complications of drug treatment in Parkinson's disease. In Huber S, Cummings JL, eds. *Parkinson's Disease: Neurobehavioral Aspects*. New York: Oxford University Press; 1992.
65. Fénelon G, Mahieux F, Huon R, Ziegler M: Hallucinations in Parkinson's disease: prevalence, phenomenology, and risk factors. Brain 2000;123:733-745.
66. Giladi N, Treves TA, Paleacu D, et al: Risk factors for dementia, depression and psychosis in long-standing Parkinson's disease. J Neural Transm 2000;107:59-71.
67. Wint DP, Okun MS, Fernandez HH: Psychosis in Parkinson's disease. J Geriatr Psychiatry Neurol 2004;17:127-136.
68. Goetz CG, Stebbins GT: Risk factors for nursing home placement in advanced Parkinson's disease. Neurology 1993;43:2227-2229.
69. Henderson MJ, Mellers JDC: Psychosis in Parkinson's disease: 'between a rock and a hard place.' Intl. Rev. Psychiatry 2000;12:319-334.
70. Sanchez-Ramos JR, Ortoll R, Paulson GW: Visual hallucinations associated with Parkinson disease. Arch Neurol 1996;53:1265-1268.
71. Diederich N, Goetz C, Raman R, et al: Primary deficits in visual discrimination is a risk factor for visual hallucinations in Parkinson's disease. Neurology 1997;48(3, Suppl 2):A181.
72. Wolters ECh: Intrinsic and extrinsic psychosis in Parkinson's disease. J Neurol 2001;248(Suppl 3):22-27.
73. Wolters ECh: Dopaminomimetic psychosis in Parkinson's disease patients: diagnosis and treatment. Neurology 1999;52(Suppl 3):S10-S13.
74. Perry E, Marshall E, Kerwin J: Evidence of monoaminergic-cholinergic imbalance related to visual hallucinations in Lewy body dementia. J Neurochem 1990;55:1454-1456.
75. Inzelberg R, Kipervasser S, Korczyn AD: Auditory hallucinations in Parkinson's disease. J Neurol Neurosurg Psychiatry 1998;64:533-535.
76. Moskovitz C, Moses H, Klawans HL: Levodopa-induced psychosis: a kindling phenomenon. Am J Psychiatry 1978;135:669-675.
77. Pappert E, Goetz C, Niederman F: Hallucinations, sleep fragmentation and altered dream phenomena in Parkinson's disease. Mov Disord 1999;14:117-121.
78. Arnulf I, Bonnet AM, Damier P, et al: Hallucinations, REM sleep, and Parkinson's disease: a medical hypothesis. Neurology 2000;55:281-288.
79. Olanow CW, Watts RL, Koller WC: An algorithm (decision tree) for the management of Parkinson's disease (2001): treatment guidelines. Neurology 2001;56(Suppl 5):S1-S88.
80. The Parkinson Study Group. Low-dose clozapine for the treatment of drug-induced psychosis in Parkinson's disease. N Engl J Med 1999;340:757-763.
81. The French Clozapine Parkinson Study Group. Clozapine in drug-induced psychosis in Parkinson's disease. Lancet 1999;353:2041-2042.
82. Friedman JH, Factor SA: Atypical antipsychotics in the treatment of drug-induced psychosis in Parkinson's disease. Mov Disord 2000;15:201-211.
83. Ondo WG, Tintner R, Voung KD, et al: Double-blind, placebo-controlled, unforced titration parallel trial of quetiapine for dopaminergic-induced hallucinations in Parkinson's disease. Mov Disord 2005;20:958-963.
84. Rabey JM, Prokhorov T, Miniovitz A, et al: Effect of quetiapine in psychotic Parkinson's disease patients: a double-blind labeled study of 3 months' duration. Mov Disord 2007;22:313-318.
85. McKeith I, Del Ser T, Spano PF, et al: Efficacy of rivastigmine in dementia with Lewy bodies: a randomised, double-blind, placebo-controlled international study. Lancet 2000;356:2031-2036.
86. Driver-Dunckley E, Samanta J, Stacy M: Pathological gambling associated with dopamine agonist therapy in Parkinson's disease. Neurology 2003;61:422-423.
87. Dodd ML, Klos KJ, Bower JH, et al: Pathological gambling caused by drugs used to treat Parkinson disease. Arch Neurol 2005;62:1-5.

88. Voon V, Hassan K, Zurowski M, et al: Prospective prevalence of pathological gambling and medication association in Parkinson disease. Neurology 2006;66:1750-1752.
89. Weintraub D, Siderowf AD, Potenza MN, et al: Association of dopamine agonist use with impulse control disorders in Parkinson disease. Arch Neurol 2006;63:969-973.
90. Avanzi M, Baratti M, Cabrini S, et al: Prevalence of pathological gambling in patients with Parkinson's disease. Mov Disord 2006;21:2068-2072.
91. Pietrzak RH, Morasco BJ, Blanco C, et al: Gambling level and psychiatric and medical disorders in older adults: results from the National Epidemiologic Survey on Alcohol and Related Conditions. Am J Geriatr Psychiatry 2007;15:301-313.
92. Voon V, Hassan K, Zurowski M, et al: Prevalence of repetitive and reward-seeking behaviors in Parkinson disease. Neurology 2006;67:1254-1257.
93. Klos KJ, Bower JH, Josephs KA, et al: Pathological hypersexuality predominantly linked to adjuvant dopamine agonist therapy in Parkinson's disease and multiple system atrophy. Parkinsonism Rel Disord 2005;11:381-386.
94. Pontone G, Williams JR, Bassett SS, Marsh L: Clinical features associated with impulse control disorders in Parkinson disease. Neurology 2006;67:1258-1261.
95. Nirenberg MJ, Waters C: Compulsive eating and weight gain related to dopamine agonist use. Mov Disord 2006;21:524-529.
96. Giovannoni G, O'Sullivan JD, Turner K, et al: Hedonistic homeostatic dysregulation in patients with Parkinson's disease on dopamine replacement therapies. J Neurol Neurosurg Psychiatry 2000;68:423-428.
97. Evans AH, Katzenschlager R, Paviour D, et al: Punding in Parkinson's disease: its relation to the dopamine dysregulation syndrome. Mov Disord 2004;19:397-405.
98. Voon V, Fox SH: Medication-related impulse control and repetitive behaviors in Parkinson disease. Arch Neurol 2007;64:1089-1096.
99. Gerlach M, Double K, Arzberger T, et al: Dopamine receptor agonists in current clinical use: comparative dopamine receptor binding profiles defined in the human striatum. J Neural Transm 2003;110:1119-1127.
100. Sokoloff P, Giros B, Martres MP, et al: Molecular cloning and characterization of a novel dopamine receptor (D3) as a target for neuroleptics. Nature 1990;347:146-151.
101. Mamikonyan E, Siderowf AD, Duda JE, et al: Long-term follow-up of impulse control disorders in Parkinson's disease. Mov Disord 2008;23:75-80.
102. Sevincok L, Akoglu A, Akyol A: Quetiapine in a case with Parkinson disease and pathological gambling [Letter]. J Clin Psychopharmacol 2007;27:107-108.
103. Ardouin C, Voon V, Worbe Y, et al: Pathological gambling in Parkinson's disease improves on chronic subthalamic nucleus stimulation. Mov Disord 2006;21:1941-1946.
104. Aarsland D, Larsen JP, Lim NG, et al: Range of neuropsychiatric disturbances in patients with Parkinson's disease. J Neurol Neurosurg Psychiatry 1999;67:492-496.
105. Smith MC, Ellgring H, Oertel WH: Sleep disturbances in Parkinson's disease patients and spouses. J Am Geriatr Soc 1997;45:194-199.
106. Schenck CH, Bundlie SR, Mahowald MW: Delayed emergence of a parkinsonian disorder in 38% of 29 older men initially diagnosed with idiopathic rapid eye movement sleep behaviour disorder. Neurology 1996;46:388-393.
107. Tan A, Salgado M, Fahn S: Rapid eye movement sleep behavior disorder preceding Parkinson's disease with therapeutic response to levodopa. Mov Disord 1996;11:214-216.
108. Stacy M: Sleep disorders in Parkinson's disease. Drugs Aging 2002;19:733-739.
109. Jellinger K: The pedunculopontine nucleus in Parkinson's disease. J Neurol Neurosurg Psychiatry 1988;51:540-543.
110. Eisensehr I, Linke R, Noachtar S, et al: Reduced striatal dopamine transporters in idiopathic rapid eye movement sleep behavior disorder: comparison with Parkinson's disease and controls. Brain 2000;123:1155-1160.
111. Phillips B: Movement disorders: a sleep specialist's perspective. Neurology 2004;62(Suppl 2): S9-S16.
112. Comella CL, Tanner CM, Ristanovic RK: Polysomnographic sleep measures in Parkinson's disease patients with treatment-induced hallucinations. Ann Neurol 1993;34:710-714.
113. Tandberg E, Larsen JP, Karlsen K: Excessive daytime sleepiness and sleep benefit in Parkinson's disease: a community-based study. Mov Disord 1999;14:922-927.
114. Friedman J, Friedman H: Fatigue in Parkinson's disease. Neurology 1993;43:2016-2018.
115. Chaudhuri A, Behan PO: Fatigue and basal ganglia. J Neurol Sci 2000;179:34-42.

116. Karlsen K, Larsen JP, Tandberg E, et al: Fatigue in patients with Parkinson's disease. Mov Disord 1999;14:237-241.
117. Hobson DE, Lang AE, Martin WR, et al: Excessive daytime sleepiness and sudden-onset sleep in Parkinson disease: a survey by the Canadian Movement Disorders Group. JAMA 2005;287:455-463.
118. Nieves AV, Lang AE: Treatment of excessive daytime sleepiness in patients with Parkinson's disease with modafinil. Clin Neuropharmacol 2002;25:111-114.
119. Adler CH, Caviness JN, Hentz JG, et al: Randomized trial of modafinil for treating subjective daytime sleepiness in patients with Parkinson's disease. Mov Disord 2003;18:287-293.
120. Ondo WG, Fayle R, Atassi F, Jankovic J: Modafinil for daytime somnolence in Parkinson's disease: double blind, placebo controlled parallel trial. J Neurol Neurosurg Psychiatry 2005;76:1636-1639.
121. Mendonça DA, Menezes K, Jog MS: Methylphenidate improves fatigue scores in Parkinson disease: a randomized controlled trial. Mov Disord 2007;22:2070-2076.
122. Isella V, Melzi P, Grimaldi M, et al: Clinical, neuropsychological, and morphometric correlates of apathy in Parkinson's disease. Mov Disord 2002;17:366-371.
123. Duffy JD: The neural substrates of motivation. Psychiatr Ann 1997;27:39-43.
124. Marin RS, Fogel BS, Hawkins J, et al: Apathy: a treatable syndrome. J Neuropsychiatry Clin Neurosci 1995;7:23-30.
125. Shulman LM: Apathy in patients with Parkinson's disease. Intl Rev Psychiatry 2000;12:298-306.
126. Cummings JL, Arciniegas DB, Brooks BR, et al: Defining and diagnosing involuntary emotional expression disorder. CNS Spectr 2006;11:1-7.
127. Green RL: Regulation of affect. Semin Clin Neuropsychiatry 1998;3:195-200.
128. Arciniegas DB, Topkoff J: The neuropsychiatry of pathologic affect: an approach to evaluation and treatment. Semin Clin Neuropsychiatry 2000;5:290-306.
129. Krack P, Batir A, Van Blercom N, et al: Five-year follow-up of bilateral stimulation of the subthalamic nucleus in advanced Parkinson's disease. N Engl J Med 2003;13:1925-1934.
130. Herzog J, Volkmann J, Krack P, et al: Two-year follow-up of subthalamic deep brain stimulation in Parkinson's disease. Mov Disord 2003;18:1332-1337.
131. Smeding HM, Speelman JD, Koning-Haanstra M, et al: Neuropsychological effects of bilateral STN stimulation in Parkinson disease: a controlled study. Neurology 2006;66:1830-1836.
132. Parsons TD, Rogers SA, Braaten AJ, et al: Cognitive sequelae of subthalamic nucleus deep brain stimulation in Parkinson's disease: a meta-analysis. Lancet Neurol 2006;5:578-588.
133. Voon V, Kubu C, Krack P, et al: Deep brain stimulation: neuropsychological and neuropsychiatric issues. Mov Disord 2006;21(Suppl 14):S305-S326.
134. Houeto JL, Mesnage V, Mallet L, et al: Behavioral disorders, Parkinson's disease and subthalamic stimulation. J Neurol Neurosurg Psychiatry 2002;72:701-707.
135. Berney A, Vingerhoets F, Perrin A, et al: Effect on mood of subthalamic DBS for Parkinson's disease: a consecutive series of 24 patients. Neurology 2002;59:1427-1429.

14 Nonmotor Aspects of Parkinson's Disease

EDUARDO TOLOSA • JOAN SANTAMARIA •
CARLES GAIG • YAROSLAU COMPTA

Introduction

Interest in nonmotor symptoms (NMS) in Parkinson's disease (PD) has increased in recent years. NMS are a major source of disability, and in contrast to the classic motor symptoms, they fail to improve with currently available treatments. Investigators are gaining additional insight into the underlying neuropathological substrate of these problems and the possible role that drugs used to treat the motor symptoms may play in their appearance. Finally, it has become evident that some NMS antedate the classic motor signs of PD, and investigations are being conducted worldwide to define the characteristics of this nonmotor, premotor, phase of PD (Table 14–1). Information on the nature of NMS in premotor PD may help in understanding the cause of PD and the study of drugs with neuroprotection potential independent of a symptomatic effect on motor symptoms.

Dementia and neuropsychiatric complications are perhaps the most disturbing NMS to patients and their families. They carry a poor prognosis and a higher risk for institutionalization. Their importance is highlighted by the fact that separate chapters in this book are devoted to each of these complications. The NMS reviewed in this chapter are nonetheless important because they are frequent, and they frequently have a negative impact on patients' quality of life.

TABLE 14-1	Nonmotor Symptoms in Parkinson's Disease: Neuropathological Substrate		
Nonmotor Symptoms	Presumed Underlying Brain Structures	Documented in Premotor Phase	Corresponding Braak Stage*
Smell loss*	Olfactory bulb; anterior olfactory nucleus; amygdala; perirhinal cortex	Hyposmia	1
Autonomic dysfunction*	Amygdala; dorsal nucleus of the vagus; intermediolateral column of the spinal cord; sympathetic ganglia; enteric plexus neurons	Constipation; genitourinary dysfunction	1
Sleep disturbances*	Nucleus subcaeruleus; pedunculopontine nucleus; thalamus; hypothalamus	REM behavior disorder Excessive daytime sleepiness	2 2-3
Behavioral/ emotional dysfunction	Locus caeruleus; raphe nuclei; amygdala; mesolimbic, mesocortical cortex	Depression; anxiety	2-3
Hallucinations, psychosis	Amygdala; limbic cortex	??†	4-5
Dementia and cognitive dysfunction	Frontal and ventral temporal lobe/neocortex, hippocampus, amygdala, nucleus basalis of Meynert, locus caeruleus	??†	5-6

*See the text for references.
†Hallucinations, psychosis, and dementia can be considered as possible premotor manifestations of Parkinson's disease. When occurring before parkinsonism (premotor), these are regarded, arbitrarily, as the early manifestation of dementia with Lewy bodies and not as a premotor manifestation of Parkinson's disease.

Most NMS are caused by lesions in the brain involving nondopaminergic structures (see Table 14–1). Consequently, they fail to respond adequately to dopaminergic medication. Examples of such nondopaminergic NMS include dementia, fatigue, smell loss, constipation, and rapid-eye-movement (REM) sleep behavior disorder (RBD). Another cause of NMS in PD is drug treatment. Numerous medications can produce or potentiate PD-related NMS, and acknowledgment of this is important because manipulation of the treatment regimen can alleviate some of these problems.

Examples of NMS induced or aggravated by medications in PD are orthostatic hypotension, hallucinations, excessive daytime sleepiness (EDS), and leg edema associated with dopaminergic treatment, and memory problems associated with anticholinergics. Although most NMS are thought not to be primarily dopaminergic, they may be influenced by dopaminergic drugs. Examples of such nonmotor nondopaminergic symptoms that may respond in part to dopaminergic drugs are insomnia and other nocturnal problems, urinary urgency, and depression and in general NMS occurring during "off" states. Investigations are still needed to clarify the role of dopamine in these symptoms.

TABLE 14–2	Other Nonmotor Symptoms in Parkinson's Disease

Sweating Disturbances

Can be localized or asymmetrical. May occur in association with "off" periods, "on" dyskinesias, or unrelated to motor fluctuations (related to autonomic dysfunction?)
    Hyperhidrosis (more frequent)
    Hypohidrosis

Cutaneous Disturbances

Facial seborrhea (seborrheic dermatitis) (related to autonomic dysfunction?)
Possible increased risk of skin cancer
    Malignant melanoma (unrelated to dopaminergic treatment)
    Keratosis and basal cell carcinoma
As adverse event of antiparkinsonian therapy
    Amantadine-induced livedo reticularis
    Leg edema (dopamine agonists)
    Erythromelalgia-like (dopamine agonists)
    Subcutaneous nodules related to apomorphine injections
    Skin erosion over implants in deep brain stimulation

Ocular Disturbances

Dry eyes (xerostomia; related to autonomic dysfunction)
Diplopia
Blurred vision

Other Disturbances

Weight loss
Weight gain (possibly drug induced)
Rhinorrhea
Hypersalivation (dysautonomia? swallowing difficulties?)
Ageusia

In this chapter, emphasis is placed on NMS considered to be an intrinsic part of the PD process, including smell disturbances, dysautonomia, pain and other sensory symptoms, sleep disturbances, and fatigue. Some less common or disabling NMS, such as seborrheic dermatitis or hyperhidrosis, and particularly NMS mostly related to treatment, such as skin erosions or skin nodules associated with deep brain stimulation or apomorphine, are listed in Table 14–2. The occurrence of NMS in premotor PD is briefly discussed at the end of the chapter.

Smell Loss

Smell loss occurs in 90% of PD patients and involves several functions, such as impairments of odor detection, identification, and discrimination. The olfactory deficit in PD is independent of the disease severity and duration—it is present in untreated new PD patients—and does not vary between "on" and "off" states. Hyposmia occurs bilaterally even when motor signs are asymmetrical or unilateral.[1,2] Smell loss causes little disability and is rarely mentioned spontaneously by the patient, but if it is specifically asked for, up to 70% of PD patients may indicate subjective olfactory loss.[3,4]

Hyposmia is a relevant issue because its presence can be useful in differentiating PD from other parkinsonian or tremor syndromes.[2] In addition, hyposmia has been considered an early marker for PD because it can antedate the classic motor signs of the disease.[5] Several inexpensive and noninvasive psychometric tests are available to assess smell, but they require patient's cooperation, and because of the culturally specific nature of some of the included odors, the results may be difficult to interpret in the setting of populations different from that where the smell test had been developed. Electrophysiological approaches, such as olfactory evoked potentials, do not require the patient's cooperation, and are not influenced by cultural background, but this method is technically demanding and remains a research tool.[2]

In PD, smell loss is generally pronounced, whereas olfactory function is preserved or mildly impaired in atypical parkinsonism, such as multiple system atrophy, progressive supranuclear palsy, or corticobasal degeneration,[3,6-10] or in secondary parkinsonism, such as vascular or drug-induced parkinsonism.[11,12] Smell also is preserved in essential tremor.[13] Olfactory function tends to remain intact in *parkin*-associated PD, which on neuropathological examination usually manifests with nigral degeneration without Lewy bodies.[14] Similarly to PD, dementia with Lewy bodies usually manifests with a severe loss of smell,[15] supporting the concept that dementia with Lewy bodies may be one end of the spectrum of disorders of Lewy bodies, which comprises PD and PD with dementia.

Dysautonomia

Dysautonomia has long been recognized as one of the nonmotor features of PD.[16-19] About 50% of PD patients complain of disabling dysautonomic symptoms, more commonly in advanced disease stages.[20] Dysautonomia may be caused by the disease itself or occur as a side effect of treatment. Genitourinary dysfunction and orthostatic hypotension are among the most common reasons for emergency admission of PD patients.[21] In some patients, dysautonomia may predate the cardinal motor signs of the disease (see later section for more details). Main dysautonomic symptoms and signs relate to gastrointestinal, genitourinary, and cardiovascular systems (Table 14–3).

Validated questionnaires to assess PD-related dysautonomia (NMSQuest, SCOPA-AUT) have been developed more recently[22,23] and show higher scores among patients than controls across all disease stages, mainly in the gastrointestinal and urinary domains. In PD, the presence of autonomic symptoms has been correlated to age, disease severity, and use of dopaminergic drugs, whereas dysautonomia severity has been associated with cognitive dysfunction, psychiatric symptoms, and sleep disturbances.[23,24] Dysautonomia does not seem to differ—neither in its presence nor in its severity—among the genetically determined PD variants, including α-synuclein point mutations and triplications[25,26]; mutations of *PINK-1* and *LRRK2* genes[27,28]; and *parkin* gene mutations, which usually lack Lewy body pathology.[29]

Severe, symptomatic dysautonomia mostly appears in advanced disease. Nevertheless, dysautonomia also occurs in early PD,[30] even mimicking pure autonomic failure or multiple system atrophy in some instances.[31,32] Trying to separate PD from multiple system atrophy on the bases of early dysautonomia alone may be misleading.

TABLE 14–3	Dysautonomic Features in Parkinson's Disease and Their Management	
Main Parkinson's Disease–related Dysautonomic Features	Diagnosis	Management
Gastrointestinal		
Constipation	Clinical history and examination	Diet, laxatives
Regurgitation, nausea	Clinical history and examination	Diet, postural recommendations, domperidone
Epigastric discomfort, heavy digestion (gastroparesis)	Clinical, x-ray	Domperidone, dopaminergic drug adjustment, erythromycin?
Anismus	Clinical, manometry, electromyogram	Botulinum toxin in pelvic musculature
Bowel pseudo-occlusion (Ogilvie's syndrome)	Clinical, x-ray	Nasogastric and rectal aspiration, intravenous hydration, erythromycin? ondansetron?
Sigmoid volvulus	Clinical, x-ray, ultrasound	Endoscopic reduction, surgery
Genitourinary		
Urinary dysfunction		
Frequency, urgency, and urge incontinence	Clinical, urodynamic studies	Avoid triggers; oxybutynin, amitriptyline, tolterodine, prazosin
Nocturia	Clinical, urodynamic studies	Desmopressin?
Urinary retention	Clinical, urodynamic studies	Bladder catheter (intermittent versus permanent)
Sexual dysfunction		
Erectile dysfunction	Clinical, urological evaluation	Sildenafil and derivatives; dopamine agonists
Cardiovascular		
Orthostatic hypotension	Clinical, tilt-table test, laboratory, 24-hour blood pressure monitoring	Diet, postural measures, avoiding triggers, dopaminergic drug adjustment, domperidone, midodrine, fludrocortisone, pyridostigmine
Postprandial hypotension	Clinical history and examination, 24-hour blood pressure monitoring	Diet, avoiding triggers, dopaminergic drug adjustment, octreotide?

GASTROINTESTINAL DYSFUNCTION

Constipation is present in 60% of PD patients, nearly three times the rate among age-matched controls.[33] Other gastrointestinal symptoms, such as regurgitation, nausea, and epigastric discomfort, all likely related to gastroparesis, are common in PD, ranging from 24% (nausea) to 45% (bloating), even in untreated patients.[34,35]

Gastroparesis in individuals with PD also has potentially relevant pharmacokinetic implications because delayed gastric emptying can cause increased exposure of levodopa to dopa-decarboxylase in the gastric mucosa resulting in erratic response owing to reduced absorption of the drug.

Patients with PD also may exhibit disturbances in defecation related to poor control of pelvic floor muscles during "on" and "off" periods, which can be detected on specific tests (anorectal videomanometry and electromyography), ranging from hypertonus in the perianal musculature, poor ability to contract the external anal sphincter voluntarily, and poor ability to activate pelvic muscles during "off" periods.[36-38] Constipation in PD may be aggravated by associated movement disorders, as puborectalis dystonia or anismus.[39,40] Overall, gastrointestinal motility dysfunction may worsen with disease progression, and eventually may become life-threatening, with some patients developing fatal gastroparesis,[41] Ogilvie's megacolon, and sigma volvulus.[42]

Lesions in the central and peripheral autonomic nervous systems seem to be the substrate of gastrointestinal dysfunction in PD because Lewy bodies and neuron loss have been found in dorsal nucleus of the vagus (a parasympathetic nucleus projecting prokinetic signals to the stomach, intestine, and all but the distal segment of the colon), in the intermediate ventrolateral column of the spinal cord, and within the enteric autonomic nervous system.[43-49] Treatment-related dysautonomia can contribute significantly to this nonmotor comorbidity.

GENITOURINARY DISTURBANCES

In PD patients, the prevalence of urinary symptoms has been found to 27% to 39%[50,51] using validated questionnaires and to be greater than 40% using a non-validated questionnaire.[52] Urinary symptoms correlate with age, duration and progression of motor symptoms, and presence of dementia.[53,54] Frequency, urgency, and urge incontinence, along with nocturia and bladder retention, are frequent in late-stage disease,[55] with a mean latency from disease onset to appearance of symptoms of about 144 months, in contrast to 12 months in multiple systems atrophy.[56] Urinary retention and incontinence may lead to recurrent urinary tract infections and sepsis, which account for nearly 30% of hospital admissions in PD patients.[21] Urodynamic testing may help in precisely identifying the type of urinary dysfunction and starting the appropriate treatment. The most common finding is detrusor hyperreflexia, present in 70% of PD patients with urinary symptoms[53,57,58]; detrusor-sphincter dyssynergia is rare.[53]

Sexual disturbances are common in PD[59-61] and mainly involve erectile and ejaculation dysfunction. Erectile dysfunction may be aggravated by motor disabilities ("off" dystonia, accompanying pain, difficulties in coital positioning), and can recur during "off" periods.[62,63] Decreased interest by the patient or the partner along with other affective disturbances may also play a role. Other consequences of generalized dysfunction of the autonomous nervous system, such as decreased mucosal lubrication in women and premature or delayed ejaculation, may occur. Less frequently, exaggerated penile erection can occur as a consequence of dopaminergic treatment.[62,63] Hypersexuality represents a behavioral disturbance generally linked to drug treatment, rather than a dysautonomic feature. Similarly to gastrointestinal dysfunction, brainstem and spinal autonomic nuclei derangement[43,44,64] and Onuf's nucleus involvement[32] along with side effects of drug treatment most likely underlie PD-related genitourinary disturbances.

CARDIOVASCULAR ABNORMALITIES

Orthostatic hypotension and much less frequently, postprandial hypotension are the main PD-related cardiovascular features, albeit other symptoms, such as dyspnea and palpitations, have been reported in PD. Orthostatic hypotension and postprandial hypotension are defined as a decrease in more than 20 mm Hg systolic pressure or 10 mm Hg diastolic pressure when changing position from lying to standing and after meals.[65,66] Except for the different circumstances in which they occur, clinically they present with similar symptoms, including somnolence, lightheadedness, "coat hanger" neck pain, and syncope.[67,68] Orthostatic hypotension and postprandial hypotension can also occur subclinically.

Diagnosis of orthostatic hypotension and postprandial hypotension is clinical, but may be strengthened by laboratory determinations (e.g., metanephrine plasma levels change from lying to standing)[69] or hemodynamic testing, such as the tilt-table test, the study of heart rate variability,[70] and 24-hour blood pressure monitoring.[71] Findings of reversal of the circadian rhythm, postprandial hypotension, and nocturnal hypertension are characteristic of PD.

The introduction of nuclear medicine techniques (mostly metaiodobenzyl-guanidine single photon emission computed tomography [SPECT] and meta-hydroxyephedrine positron emission tomography [PET]) measuring cardiac sympathetic innervation has represented an advance in the study of not only clinical, but also subclinical and premotor cardiovascular dysfunction in PD. A series of studies suggested that impaired sympathetic postganglionic function constitutes a marker of Lewy body disorders because other parkinsonisms without underlying Lewy bodies have normal or slightly decreased tracer uptake on SPECT.[72-74] The degree of tracer uptake seems to correlate with disease progression[75,76] and the rigid-akinetic phenotype,[77] but not with dysautonomic symptoms.[78-80] Nevertheless, some drugs altering adrenergic function (β-blockers) and certain comorbidities causing dysautonomia (diabetes) may limit the interpretation of the SPECT or PET results.[81,82]

Orthostatic hypotension is nowadays mostly recognized as a dysautonomic feature intrinsic to sympathetic neurocirculatory failure from generalized sympathetic denervation[19,68] secondary to PD pathology. Frequently, though, dopaminergic therapies may also induce or aggravate orthostatic hypotension.[83]

TREATMENT OF DYSAUTONOMIA

Despite the lack of strongly effective treatments, various nonpharmacological measures and drugs have proved to be helpful in the management of PD dysautonomia.[84,85]

Management of Gastrointestinal Dysfunction

Constipation is usually unresponsive to standard antiparkinsonian drug treatment, which can even worsen it in some instances. General measures for management of constipation include diet and laxatives, and reduction or discontinuation of anticholinergic drugs. In recent years, some laxatives (macrogol, dietary herbs extracts) and prokinetic drugs (tegaserod, mosapride) have been specifically tested in PD in double-blind controlled, randomized trials or observational short series with promising results.[86-90] Domperidone, a peripheral dopamine receptor blocker, increases gastric emptying and may reduce dopaminergic drug–related gastrointestinal symptoms.[91,92] Conversely, metoclopramide and clebopride, dopamine receptor blockers with central activity, must be avoided.[93] Other prokinetic drugs, such as erythromycin or ondansetron, have not been formally tested in PD. Treatment with botulinum toxin in pelvic musculature may show some benefit in cases with anismus.[94,95]

Management of Genitourinary Disturbances

Coffee and other natural diuretics, along with large water intake, are to be avoided, especially before bedtime, to minimize nocturia. Peripherally acting anticholinergic drugs (oxybutynin, amitriptyline), antispasmodic agents (propiverine, tolterodine), and α_1-agonists (prazosin and derived drugs) can be used for urinary urgency and incontinence, although these agents have not been specifically evaluated in PD. Evidence in support of intranasal desmopressin spray for nocturia is lacking.[96] Sildenafil has been found to be efficacious in the treatment of erectile dysfunction in PD.[97-99] Apomorphine, administered 30 minutes before sexual activity, and pergolide may also improve erectile function.[100-103]

Treatment of Orthostatic Hypotension and Postprandial Hypotension

Triggers of orthostatic hypotension and postprandial hypotension (alcohol, warm environment, antihypertensive drugs) must be avoided. Frequent small meals, increased salt intake, head-up tilt of bed at night, portable chairs, and elastic stockings are recommended.[104,105] In the particularly difficult setting of dopamine agonist–related orthostatic hypotension, in which reducing drug doses may lead to motor worsening, domperidone may be helpful.[106] Also helpful are the α-adrenergic agonist midodrine[107,108] and fludrocortisone, which induces tubular salt reuptake, normalizing daytime blood pressure, but favoring nocturnal hypertension.[109,110] Conversely, pyridostigmine (an anticholinesterase agent) has been shown to improve orthostatic hypotension with the advantage of not worsening supine hypertension.[111] Octreotide, a somatostatin agonist used for treating postprandial hypotension but not specifically studied in PD, may be helpful in this situation.[112,113] DBS does not seem to improve orthostatic hypotension directly, but may minimize its impact because it allows reduction in dopaminergic drug doses.[114,115]

❙ Sleep Disturbances

Sleep disturbances are 1.5 to 3.5 times more common in PD patients than in healthy controls or patients with other chronic disorders (Table 14–4). Symptoms of sleep disturbance may be underreported by patients. Lees and coworkers[116] reported that although 98% of a series of PD patients experienced problems with sleep of different types and severities, only 45% told their physicians about them, for unknown reasons. Perhaps patients consider the sleep problems as a

TABLE 14–4	Frequency of Sleep Disturbances in Parkinson's Disease (PD)*			
Author (yr)	PD Patients under Treatment with Sleep Disturbances	New PD Patients with Sleep Disturbances	Healthy Elderly with Sleep Disturbances	Patients with Chronic Disease with Sleep Disturbances
Factor (1990)	89% (78)	—	74% (43)	—
van Hilten (1993)	81% (90)	—	92% (71)	—
Tandberg (1998)	60.3% (245)	—	33% (100)	45% (100)
Lees (1988)	98% (220)	—	—	—
Oerlemans (2002)	82% (234)	—	—	—
Kumar (2002)	42% (149)	—	12% (115)	—
Fabrinni (2002)	80% (50)	60% (25)	56% (25)	—

*Numbers in parentheses indicate total number of subjects evaluated in each study.

part of the disease with less relevance than the diurnal motor symptoms. The most frequently reported problems are sleep fragmentation, nocturia, inability to turn over in bed, early awakening, or vivid dreams and nightmares.

Sleep disturbances do not occur early in the course of PD. When the disease advances, and probably as a result of a combination of factors, such as the involvement of systems other than the nigrostriatal pathway, increases in dopaminergic treatment, or worsening of motor performance, sleep disturbances become more common. One exception to this rule is RBD because in one fifth of patients with RBD and PD, the abnormal behavior during sleep was reported to start years before the appearance of the diurnal motor symptoms.[117]

INSOMNIA

Fragmentation of sleep can have a major impact on quality of life in PD. Many factors generally are responsible, and establishing relevant factors may be challenging. In early PD stages, use of selegiline or amantadine late in the day and excessive dopaminergic treatment may cause the patient to be too alert at night. Sleep apnea, with typical snoring, breathing pauses, broken sleep, and diurnal hypersomnia and fatigue, may occur in PD patients.[118] The fatigue and hypersomnia may erroneously be attributed to PD and remain undiagnosed and untreated. Restless legs syndrome (RLS) and depression may also produce insomnia in PD patients. In advanced PD stages, poor sleep at night may be due to lack of efficacy of dopaminergic agents with prolonged "off" periods during the night, difficulties in getting out of bed alone to pass urine,[116] nighttime hallucinations, and RBD, which may wake the patient up because of the abnormal dreaming or excessive movements in REM sleep.

RAPID-EYE-MOVEMENT SLEEP BEHAVIOR DISORDER

One of the most frequent parasomnias in PD is RBD. It consists of recurrent episodes of sudden, abnormally vigorous body, head, or limb movements that appear during REM sleep, usually associated with dreams in which the patient defends against a threat or aggression (e.g., by people or animals). The intensity of the abnormal behaviors and dreams may vary across the night (usually worst at the end of the night), across different nights, and from one patient to another. In the most severe form, the patient may injure himself or herself or his or her bed partner resulting in fractures, lacerations, or contusions of varying severity.

Some patients with milder forms of RBD may not mention the sleep problems to the physician if not specifically asked. Other patients, particularly individuals who sleep alone, may be unaware of the parasomnia.[119] Diagnostic confirmation of RBD requires polysomnography with audiovisual recording of the abnormal movements in REM sleep or excessive electromyographic activity during this sleep stage. In one study, at least 30% of the cases of PD had RBD clinically, or polysomnography detected suggestive findings,[120] but this figure is probably conservative because patients with antidepressant or hypnotic treatment or cognitive changes were excluded. There is no clear evidence that RBD is caused by the nigrostriatal dopaminergic dysfunction itself. It has been proposed that hallucinations are dreamlike phenomena that intrude into wakefulness.[121]

Although RBD was first reported in 1986, earlier reports described its typical symptoms in patients with PD as nightmares, night terrors, vivid dreams,[122] or altered dream events with nocturnal vocalizations and myoclonus.[123] These studies attributed the sleep symptoms to long-term levodopa use and suggested that the symptoms occurred during deep non-REM sleep. None of these suggestions has been proved. The presence of RBD in patients with PD has been proposed to represent a risk factor for the development of cognitive deterioration and possibly dementia.[124] RBD has been found to occur less often in the tremor-predominant subtype of PD.[125]

EXCESSIVE DAYTIME SLEEPINESS

EDS has been underrecognized in PD, and although initially considered a side effect of nonergot D2/D3 agonists,[126] it is not restricted to a specific class of dopaminomimetic agents. It has been reported with pramipexole, ropinirole, pergolide, bromocriptine, cabergoline, apomorphine, lisuride, piribedil, levodopa, tolcapone, and entacapone.[127,128] Sleepiness occurs either as a constant feeling that the patient is aware of or as episodes of "sudden, irresistible, overwhelming sleepiness without awareness of falling asleep" (sleep "attacks"). Sleep attacks usually occur in a background of relaxed wakefulness and mostly while doing sedentary activities. The frequency of EDS in PD depends on the studies, but ranges from 15% to 71% of patients (Table 14–5), or 1.5 to 15 times that found in healthy controls. This variability probably depends on the definition of sleepiness employed in the different studies.[129-137] Fabrinni and collaborators[138] did not find a significantly increased prevalence of EDS in untreated PD patients compared with an age-matched healthy control group, whereas EDS was more frequent in treated patients, suggesting that the progression of the disease, the treatment, or a combination of both may be crucial in the development

TABLE 14–5	Frequency of Excessive Daytime Sleepiness in Parkinson's Disease (PD)[*]			
Author (yr)	**PD Patients under Treatment with Sleepiness**	**New PD Patients with Sleepiness**	**Healthy Controls with Sleepiness**	**Chronic Disease with Sleepiness**
Factor (1990)	49% (78)	—	26% (43)	—
Van Hilten (1993)	44.4% (90)	—	31% (71)	—
Tandberg (1999)	15.5% (239)	—	1% (100)	4% (100)
Tan (2002)	19.9% (201)	—	9.8% (214)	—
Brodsky (2003)	76% (101)	—	47% (100)	—
Kumar (2003)	21% (149)	—	3% (115)	—
Hobson (2002)	51% (638)	—	—	—
Fabrinni (2002)	84% (50)	12% (25)	4% (25)	—
Verbaan (2008)	43% (418)	—	10% (149)	—

[*]Numbers in parentheses indicate total number of subjects evaluated in each study.

of this symptom. The degree of nocturnal sleep disruption does not seem to be related to EDS in most studies,[139-141] although other authors have found the opposite.[134]

Several factors have been associated with EDS in PD, including severity of motor impairment, amount of dopaminergic treatment (all the different drugs), cognitive impairment,[142] Epworth Sleepiness Scale score, or the Inappropriate Sleep Composite Score,[127] without universal agreement on which of them is more relevant. In addition, the presence of sleep attacks has been linked to an abnormally high Epworth Sleepiness Scale score, duration of the disease, and the use of dopaminergic drugs (mostly dopamine agonists) and a particular allele of the dopamine receptor subtype (D4 or D2),[143,144] and not associated with cognitive or motor impairment.

Gjerstad and coworkers[142] studied the development of EDS over time in a group of 142 PD patients followed during a 4-year period, and found that the 11 patients who had EDS at the beginning of the study continued to present at follow-up and showed more cognitive impairment than the rest, whereas 30 new patients developed EDS for the first time during the follow-up, suggesting that EDS correlates with more advanced disease and dementia. A decreased sleep latency and two or more REM sleep onset episodes in the multiple sleep latency test, typical of narcolepsy, have been described in 30%, 22%, and 29%[139,141,145] of PD patients evaluated because of EDS. This fact has created speculation about the presence of a subtype of PD patients with a narcoleptic phenotype, secondary to degeneration of specific brain areas. Hypocretin cell loss in the brain of patients with PD has been described in two different studies,[146,147] but studies measuring cerebrospinal fluid hypocretin-1 levels in PD have found low[148] or normal values.[149] Finally, a more recent epidemiological study has suggested that the presence of EDS in asymptomatic elderly men increases their risk of developing PD threefold.[150]

MANAGEMENT OF SLEEP DISORDERS IN PARKINSON'S DISEASE

Specific measures to treat insomnia in PD include (1) modification of antiparkinsonian treatment (e.g., reduction of selegiline or amantadine if present, particularly at night; increase in antiparkinsonian treatment or addition of an agent with a long half-life to avoid "off" periods during the night in advanced cases); (2) exclusion of RLS; (3) improvement of nocturia if possible; and (4) consideration of adding an hypnotic. RBD can respond to clonazepam at doses of 0.5 to 2 mg taken at night in one dose. For EDS, measures to improve nocturnal sleep, such as excluding and treating sleep apnea, may be necessary. Also, modifying dopaminergic treatment if there is a clear relationship with the introduction of one dopaminergic drug and the appearance of sleepiness is necessary. Addition of a stimulant drug, such as modafinil, 100 to 200 mg during the day, may be helpful.

Fatigue

PD patients often have greater physical and mental fatigue than normal controls. Fatigue can occur in 33% to 58% of PD patients; it is a major and disabling symptom in some patients.[151-157] Although fatigue may be a consequence of the motor impairment or secondary to NMS such as depression, anxiety, EDS, cognitive dysfunction, or apathy, fatigue also seems to be a primary symptom of PD, independent of these other comorbidities.[154,157-159] The extent of the overlap of these associated comorbidities in fatigue has not been well established. Despite its frequency, fatigue in PD is still a poorly understood symptom, and clinicians frequently do not recognize it.[156] Several scales have been developed to measure fatigue, but only one, the Parkinson Fatigue Scale, has been designed and validated specifically for PD.[160] Whether antidepressive or stimulant drugs have a beneficial effect on fatigue in PD is unclear, but two small controlled trials have shown that nortriptyline and methylphenidate can improve fatigue in PD.[161,162]

Pain and Sensory Symptoms

Pain and sensory complaints in PD are common, and in some patients can be severe enough to overshadow the motor deficits of the disease.[158,163,164] The precise mechanism underlying pain in PD is poorly understood, but some data support involvement of basal ganglia in pain perception[165] and consequently in PD. Pain in PD has been classified into five clinically different categories: musculoskeletal, radicular-neuropathic, dystonic, central primary, and akathisic discomfort (Table 14–6).[166,167]

Pain and sensory complaints often occur in the most bradykinetic or rigid limb, usually on the side where the motor symptoms first appeared, but sometimes they can be located in the neck or in peculiar body sites, such as intraoral (burning mouth syndrome), genital, or in the throat.[168,169] They can appear early in the course of the disease, and even antedate the motor symptoms or be the presenting symptom of the disease.[169,170] In the early stages, back and neck pain may result from stiff shoulders or neck rigidity, and leg pain may result from dystonia. In advanced stages, pain may also be caused by "on" dyskinesia, akathisia, or "off"

TABLE 14–6	**Pain and Sensory Symptoms in Parkinson's Disease**

Pain Categories

Musculoskeletal—aching, cramping, arthralgic, joint
Radicular-neuropathic—in the territory of a root or nerve
Dystonic—pain associated with dystonic movements and postures, usually during
  "off" states
Central primary—burning, tingling, formication, bizarre quality
Akathisia and akathisia-like symptoms/RLS and RLS-like symptoms

Continuous or Fluctuating Pain

Nonfluctuating pain—continuous, not related to timing of antiparkinson drugs
  Musculoskeletal or radicular-neuropathic types of neck, lower back or limb pain
  Central primary pain in a limb
  Akathisic discomfort
Fluctuating pain—related to "on" or "off" states
  "Off" states
    Central primary pain—limb; lower back; peculiar body sites (angina-like chest
      pain, burning mouth syndrome, genital pain)
    "Off" dystonia (usually in the foot)
    Akathisic discomfort
    RLS-like symptoms
  "On" states
    "On" dyskinesias
    Akathisic discomfort

RLS, restless legs syndrome.

period dystonia, and fluctuating pain can be related to "off" episodes.[167,171] Examples of "off" related pain are recurrent limb pain, angina-like chest pain, and lumbosacral or genital pain (see Table 14–6).[168]

Pain in PD is often due to PD itself, but evaluating for other pain etiologies is appropriate. Although rare, deep visceral pain may represent heart-valve, pleuropulmonary, or retroperitoneal fibrosis related to use of ergot dopamine agonists.[172] In addition, pain may be indirectly caused by PD. Radicular or nonradicular types of back pain occur in 59.6% to 74% of PD patients compared with 23% to 27% of control patients. Altered posture, abnormal muscle tone, and sometimes truncal dystonia may cause the increased frequency of back pain in PD, which seems to be often neglected and insufficiently treated.[173,174]

Treatment of painful sensations in PD is often difficult, and the effect of dopaminergic treatments varies. In cases of "off" state pain, minimizing "off" severity, when possible, is generally helpful. Painful "off" periods may require treatment with subcutaneous apomorphine.[175] Reduction of dopaminergic treatment is necessary to diminish severe painful "on" dyskinesias. Botulinum toxin has also been used for painful "off" dystonia.[176] Pain and sensory symptoms related to motor complications of dopaminergic drugs frequently improve remarkably after long-term deep brain stimulation to the pallidum or the subthalamus.[177,178] Many patients report pain that has no obvious relation to "on" or "off" states, however. In this setting, pain and sensory symptoms often respond poorly to dopaminergic treatment. The efficacy of analgesics, antidepressants, or other central pain suppressants in PD with pain is unknown, and larger double-blind, placebo-controlled trials are lacking.[179]

Akathisia or akathisia-like symptoms also occur commonly in PD. Patients may complain of tightness, raw nerves, or pain together with an inner tension ("restless inside") that forces them to move. In some patients, it may occur before levodopa treatment, but in others fluctuation akathisia occurs throughout the day, at the beginning of dose, wearing "off" or end of dose pattern, and during "on" periods such as a drug-induced dyskinesia. Akathisia symptoms are sometimes not clearly related to the timing of antiparkinson drugs, however.[180,181]

In some PD patients, sensory disturbances, especially during "off" periods, resemble RLS. It is unclear whether true RLS is more common in PD patients than in the general population,[182-183] and there is no clinical evidence that subjects initially diagnosed with idiopathic RLS eventually develop PD.[184,185] Although some PD patients can experience RLS symptoms before the onset of PD, parkinsonism usually precedes the onset of RLS by several years.[182,186] Classic RLS in PD patients may emerge after deep brain stimulation surgery, as a consequence of a reduction of the dopaminergic treatment,[187] but in some cases, RLS can improve with subthalamic stimulation, even when the dose of levodopa has been reduced.[188] The response to treatment of RLS in PD is often poorer than in idiopathic RLS.[185]

Nonmotor Symptoms in the Premotor Phase of Parkinson's Disease

In recent decades, epidemiological, pathological, and clinical studies all have provided data suggesting that various symptoms can precede the classic motor features of PD. Most of these early features are nonmotor, and the period when these symptoms arise can be referred to as the *premotor phase* of the disease.[189,190] Premotor symptoms in PD include constipation, loss of smell, sleep disturbances such as RBD, and mood disturbances such as depression (see Table 14–1). Other suggested premotor symptoms, although less well documented, are anxiety, RLS, pain, apathy, and fatigue. We review here several nonmotor disturbances such as dysautonomia, olfactory dysfunction, and sleep disorders known to occur in some patients in the premotor phase of PD.

Some autonomic disturbances are frequent in PD at the time of diagnosis,[191] and can precede the onset of motor symptoms.[192-194] In one study, diarrhea and hypertension were reported more frequently in PD patients antedating motor symptoms than in controls.[189] Several studies have shown that constipation can precede motor symptoms,[33,192,193,195] and more recent pathological studies have suggested that α-synuclein deposition at the dorsal nucleus of the vagus, and even more distally at the enteric plexus,[43,49] occurs before involvement of the substantia nigra. In a retrospective analysis in a large cohort of men, Gao and colleagues[196] observed that erectile dysfunction was associated with a higher risk of developing PD in the Health Professionals Follow-up Study. Urinary disturbances and orthostatic hypotension have been documented less commonly antedating PD, but Minguez-Castellanos and associates[197] determined the prevalence of α-synuclein aggregates in abdominopelvic autonomic plexuses in the general population and found such aggregates in autonomic plexuses in 9% of the whole sample, which were most common in vesicoprostatic plexuses.

Results of several studies support the notion that olfactory dysfunction is a premotor symptom of PD.[5,198-203] Ross and colleagues[201] assessed olfaction in 2263 elderly subjects included in the Honolulu Heart Program and found an association between impaired olfaction and the future development of PD. Olfactory dysfunction has also been observed in some asymptomatic relatives of patients with either familial or sporadic forms of PD.[5,204-206] One study found that 10% of a subgroup of relatives with hyposmia had developed PD, and another 12% had detectable presynaptic abnormalities on dopamine transporter SPECT, in contrast to none of the normosmic relatives of the cohort.[5]

RBD has been found to occur in the early stages of PD and to precede by several years the motor symptoms of PD in retrospective case reports and series, and more recently in a descriptive study with long-term follow-up.[117,119,207-209] Although it can evolve to diseases other than PD, RBD seems to be a premotor symptom at least in some PD patients. EDS is another sleep disturbance that also can be seen in untreated patients, suggesting that EDS constitutes another nonmotor feature of the disease. In a sample of Japanese patients from the Honolulu Heart Program followed from 1994 to 2001, EDS was found to be a risk factor for PD even when adjusted for other features, such as insomnia, depression, coffee drinking, or cigarette smoking.[150]

▌ Conclusions

NMS are common in PD and have an important impact on the quality of life of patients and caregivers. NMS are frequently a reflection of involvement of nondopaminergic nervous system structures by the pathological process causing PD. Treatment of NMS is often met with limited success, but nonetheless specific treatments available today can be remarkably helpful. Examples are clonazepam for the treatment of RBD and botulinum toxin for sialorrhea. Side effects of the various medical and surgical treatments currently used in PD can cause prominent nonmotor side effects, and many can be prevented or minimized if appropriately identified. Finally, it has become evident more recently that several NMS occur in the premotor phase of PD. The study of symptoms such as smell loss, constipation, and RBD in the premotor phase very likely provide important information on where and when PD will start, and may allow in the future the use of drugs with potential disease-modifying properties in the earliest stages of disease development.

REFERENCES

1. Doty RL, Stern MB, Pfeiffer C, et al: Bilateral olfactory dysfunction in early stage treated and untreated idiopathic Parkinson's disease. J Neurol Neurosurg Psychiatry 1992;55.138-142.
2. Katzenschlager R, Lees AJ: Olfaction and Parkinson's syndromes: its role in differential diagnosis. Curr Opin Neurol 2004;17:417-423.
3. Müller A, Müngersdorf M, Reichmann H, et al: Olfactory function in Parkinsonian syndromes. J Clin Neurosci 2002;9:521-524.
4. Henderson JM, Lu Y, Wang S, et al: Olfactory deficits and sleep disturbances in Parkinson's disease: a case-control survey. J Neurol Neurosurg Psychiatry 2003;74:956-958.
5. Ponsen MM, Stoffers D, Booij J, et al: Idiopathic hyposmia as a premotoral sign of Parkinson's disease. Ann Neurol 2004;56:173-181.
6. Doty RL, Golbe LI, McKeown DA, et al: Olfactory testing differentiates between progressive supranuclear palsy and idiopathic Parkinson's disease. Neurology 1993;43:962-965.

7. Wenning GK, Shephard B, Magalhaes M, et al: Olfactory function in multiple system atrophy. Neurodegeneration 1993;2:169-171.
8. Wenning GK, Shephard BC, Hawkes CH, et al: Olfactory function in progressive supranuclear palsy and corticobasal degeneration. J Neurol Neurosurg Psychiatry 1995;57:251-252.
9. Wenning GK, Shephard B, Hawkes C, et al: Olfactory function in atypical Parkinsonian syndromes. Acta Neurol Scand 1995;91:247-250.
10. Abele M, Riet A, Hummel T, et al: Olfactory dysfunction in cerebellar ataxia and multiple system atrophy. J Neurol 2003;250:1453-1455.
11. Katzenschlager R, Zijlmans J, Lees AJ: Olfactory function distinguishes vascular parkinsonism from Parkinson's disease. Eur J Neurol 2002;9(Suppl 2):27-28.
12. Lee PH, Yeo SH, Yong SW, Kim YJ: Odour identification test and its relation to cardiac 123I-metaiodobenzylguanidine in patients with drug induced parkinsonism. J Neurol Neurosurg Psychiatry 2007;78:1250-1252.
13. Louis ED, Bromley SM, Jurewicz EC, Watner D: Olfactory dysfunction in essential tremor. Neurology 2002;59:1631-1633.
14. Khan NL, Katzenschlager R, Watt H, et al: Olfaction differentiates parkin disease from early-onset parkinsonism and Parkinson disease. Neurology 2004;62:1224-1226.
15. McShane RH, Nagy Z, Esiri MM, et al: Anosmia in dementia is associated with Lewy bodies rather than Alzheimer's pathology. J Neurol Neurosurg Psychiatry 2001;70:739-743.
16. Parkinson J: *An Essay on the Shaking Palsy*. London: Sherwood, Neely, & Jones, 1817.
17. Gross M, Bannister R, Godwin-Austen R: Orthostatic hypotension in Parkinson's disease. Lancet 1972;1:174-176.
18. Goetz CG, Lutge W, Tanner CM: Autonomic dysfunction in Parkinson's disease. Neurology 1986;36:73-75.
19. Goldstein DS, Holmes CS, Dendi R, et al: Orthostatic hypotension from sympathetic denervation in Parkinson's disease. Neurology 2002;58:1247-1255.
20. Magerkurth C, Schnitzer R, Braune S: Symptoms of autonomic failure in Parkinson's disease: prevalence and impact on daily life. Clin Auton Res 2005;15:76-82.
21. Woodford H, Walker R: Emergency hospital admissions in idiopathic Parkinson's disease. Mov Disord 2005;20:1104-1108.
22. Chaudhuri KR, Martinez-Martin P, Schapira AHV, et al: An international multicentre pilot study of the first comprehensive self-completed non motor symptoms questionnaire for Parkinson's disease: the NMSQuest study. Mov Disord 2006;21:916-923.
23. Verbaan D, Marinus J, Visser M, et al: Patient-reported autonomic symptoms in Parkinson disease. Neurology 2007;69:333-341.
24. Allcock LM, Kenny RA, Mosimann UP, et al: Orthostatic hypotension in Parkinson's disease: association with cognitive decline? Int J Geriatr Psychiatry 2006;21:778-783.
25. Papapetropoulos S, Paschalis C, Athanassiadou A, et al: Clinical phenotype in patients with alpha-synuclein Parkinson's disease living in Greece in comparison with patients with sporadic Parkinson's disease. J Neurol Neurosurg Psychiatry 2001;70:662-665.
26. Singleton A, Gwinn-Hardy K, Sharabi Y, et al: Association between cardiac denervation and parkinsonism caused by alpha-synuclein gene triplication. Brain 2004;127:768-772.
27. Albanese A, Valente EM, Romito LM, et al: The PINK1 phenotype can be indistinguishable from idiopathic Parkinson disease. Neurology 2005;64:1958-1960.
28. Goldstein DS, Imrich R, Peckham E, et al: Neurocirculatory and nigrostriatal abnormalities in Parkinson disease from LRRK2 mutation. Neurology 2007;69:1580-1584.
29. Khan NL, Graham E, Critchley P, et al: Parkin disease: a phenotypic study of a large case series. Brain 2003;126:1279-1292.
30. Bonuccelli U, Lucetti C, Del Dotto P, et al: Orthostatic hypotension in de novo Parkinson disease. Arch Neurol 2003;60:1400-1404.
31. Kaufmann H, Nahm K, Purohit D, Wolfe D: Autonomic failure as the initial presentation of Parkinson disease and dementia with Lewy bodies. Neurology 2004;63:1093-1095.
32. O'Sullivan SS, Holton JL, Massey LA, et al: Parkinson's disease with Onuf's nucleus involvement mimicking multiple system atrophy. J Neurol Neurosurg Psychiatry 2008;79:232-234.
33. Kaye J, Gage H, Kimber A, et al: Excess burden of constipation in Parkinson's disease: a pilot study. Mov Disord 2006;21:1270-1273.
34. Edwards LL, Pfeiffer RF, Quigley EMM, et al: Gastrointestinal symptoms in Parkinson's disease. Mov Disord 1991;6:151-156..
35. Pfeiffer RF: Gastrointestinal dysfunction in Parkinson's disease. Lancet Neurol 2003;2:107-116.

36. Ashraf W, Wszolek ZK, Pfeiffer RF, et al: Anorectal function in fluctuating (on-off) Parkinson's disease: evaluation by combined anorectal manometry and electromyography. Mov Disord 1995;10:650-657.
37. Sakakibara R, Odaka T, Uchiyama T, et al: Colonic transit time and rectoanal videomanometry in Parkinson's disease. J Neurol Neurosurg Psychiatry 2003;74:268-272.
38. Bassotti G, Maggio D, Battaglia E, et al: Manometric investigation of anorectal function in early and late stage Parkinson's disease. J Neurol Neurosurg Psychiatry 2000;68:768-770.
39. Mathers SE, Kempster PA, Swash M, Lees AJ: Constipation and paradoxical puborectalis contraction in anismus and Parkinson's disease: a dystonic phenomenon. J Neurol Neurosurg Psychiatry 1988;51:1503-1507.
40. Ashraf W, Pfeiffer RF, Quigley EM: Anorectal manometry in the assessment of anorectal function in Parkinson's disease: a comparison with chronic idiopathic constipation. Mov Disord 1994;9:655-663.
41. Hermanowicz N: Fatal gastroparesis in a patient with Parkinson's disease. Mov Disord 2008;23:152-153.
42. Sonnenberg A, Tsou VT, Müller AD: The "institutional colon": a frequent colonic dysmotility in psychiatric and neurologic disease. Am J Gastroenterol 1994;89:62-66.
43. Braak H, Del Tredici K, Rub U, et al: Staging of brain pathology related to sporadic Parkinson's disease. Neurobiol Aging 2003;24:197-211.
44. Benarroch EE, Schmeichel AM, Parisi JE: Involvement of the ventrolateral medulla in parkinsonism with autonomic failure. Neurology 2000;54:963-968.
45. Qualman SJ, Haupt HM, Yang P, Hamilton SR: Esophageal Lewy bodies associated with ganglion cell loss in achalasia: similarity to Parkinson's disease. Gastroenterology 1984;87:848-856.
46. Jackson M, Lennox G, Balsitis M, Lowe J: Lewy body dysphagia. J Neurol Neurosurg Psychiatry 1995;58:756-758.
47. Singaram C, Ashraf W, Gaumnitz EA, et al: Dopaminergic defect of enteric nervous system in Parkinson's disease patients with chronic constipation. Lancet 1995;346:861-864.
48. Kupsky WJ, Grimes MM, Sweeting J, et al: Parkinson's disease and megacolon: concentric hyaline inclusions (Lewy bodies) in enteric ganglion cells. Neurology 1987;37:1253-1255.
49. Braak H, de Vos RA, Bohl J, Del Tredici K: Gastric alpha-synuclein immunoreactive inclusions in Meissner's and Auerbach's plexuses in cases staged for Parkinson's disease-related brain pathology. Neurosci Lett 2006;396:67-72.
50. Araki I, Kuno S: Assessment of voiding dysfunction in Parkinson's disease by the international prostate symptom score. J Neurol Neurosurg Psychiatry 2000;68:429-433.
51. Campos-Sousa RN, Quagliato E, da Silva BB, et al: Urinary symptoms in Parkinson's disease: prevalence and associated factors. Arq Neuropsiquiatr 2003;61:359-363.
52. Sakakibara R, Shinotoh H, Uchiyama T, et al: Questionnaire-based assessment of pelvic organ dysfunction in Parkinson's disease. Auton Neurosci 2001;92:76-85.
53. Araki I, Kitahara M, Oida T, Kuno S: Voiding dysfunction and Parkinson's disease: urodynamic abnormalities and urinary symptoms. J Urol 2000;164:1640-1643.
54. Uchiyama T, Sakakibara R, Hattori T, Yamanishi T: Short-term effect of a single levodopa dose on micturition disturbance in Parkinson's disease patients with the wearing-off phenomenon. Mov Disord 2003;18:573-578.
55. Fowler CJ: Neurological disorders of micturition and their treatment. Brain 1999;122:1213-1231.
56. Wenning GK, Scherfler C, Granata R, et al: Time course of symptomatic orthostatic hypotension and urinary incontinence in patients with postmortem confirmed parkinsonian syndromes: a clinicopathological study. J Neurol Neurosurg Psychiatry 1999;67:620-623.
57. Pavlakis AJ, Siroky MB, Goldstein I, Krane RJ: Neurourologic findings in Parkinson's disease. J Urol 1983;129:80-83.
58. Ransmayr GN, Holliger S, Schletterer K, et al: Lower urinary tract symptoms in dementia with Lewy bodies, Parkinson disease, and Alzheimer disease. Neurology 2008;70:299-303.
59. Bronner G, Royter V, Korczyn AD, Giladi N: Sexual dysfunction in Parkinson's disease. J Sex Marital Ther 2004;30:95-105.
60. Welsh M, Hung L, Waters CH: Sexuality in women with Parkinson's disease. Mov Disord 1997;12:923-927.
61. Wermuth L, Stenager E: Sexual problems in young patients with Parkinson's disease. Acta Neurol Scand 1995;91:453-455.
62. Jimenez-Jimenez FJ, Tallon-Barranco A, Cabrera-Valdivia F, et al: Fluctuating penile erection related with levodopa therapy. Neurology 1999;52:210.

63. Kanovsky P, Bares M, Pohanka M, Rektor I: Penile erections and hypersexuality induced by pergolide treatment in advanced, fluctuating Parkinson's disease. J Neurol 2002;249:112-114.

64. Wakabayashi K, Takahashi H: The intermediolateral nucleus and Clarke's column in Parkinson's disease. Acta Neuropathol 1997;94:287-289.

65. Schatz IJ, Bannister R, Freeman RL, et al: Consensus statement on the definition of orthostatic hypotension, pure autonomic failure, and multiple system atrophy. The Consensus Committee of the American Autonomic Society and the American Academy of Neurology. Neurology 1996;46:1470.

66. O'Mara G, Lyons D: Postprandial hypotension. Clin Geriatr Med 2002;18:307-321.

67. Bleasdale-Barr KM, Mathias CJ: Neck and other muscle pains in autonomic failure: their association with orthostatic hypotension. J R Soc Med 1998;91:355-359.

68. Oka H, Yoshioka M, Onouchi K, et al: Characteristics of orthostatic hypotension in Parkinson's disease. Brain 2007;130:2425-2432.

69. Goldstein DS, Holmes C, Sharabi Y, et al: Plasma levels of catechols and metanephrines in neurogenic orthostatic hypotension. Neurology 2003;60:1327-1332.

70. Holmberg B, Kallio M, Johnels B, Elam M: Cardiovascular reflex testing contributes to clinical evaluation and differential diagnosis of parkinsonian syndromes. Mov Disord 2001;16:217-225.

71. Ejaz AA, Sekhon IS, Munjal S: Characteristic findings on 24-h ambulatory blood pressure monitoring in a series of patients with Parkinson's disease. Eur J Intern Med 2006;17:417-420.

72. Hakusui S, Yasuda T, Yanagi T, et al: A radiological analysis of heart sympathetic functions with meta-(123I) iodobenzylguanidine in neurological patients with autonomic failure. J Auton Nerv Syst 1994;49:81-84.

73. Kashihara K, Ohno M, Kawada S, Okumura Y: Reduced cardiac uptake and enhanced washout of 123I-MIBG in pure autonomic failure occurs conjointly with Parkinson's disease and dementia with Lewy bodies. J Nucl Med 2006;47:1099-1101.

74. Orimo S, Oka T, Miura H, et al: Sympathetic cardiac denervation in Parkinson's disease and pure autonomic failure but not in multiple system atrophy. J Neurol Neurosurg Psychiatry 2002;73:776-777.

75. Li ST, Dendi R, Holmes C, Goldstein DS: Progressive loss of cardiac sympathetic innervation in Parkinson's disease. Ann Neurol 2002;52:220-223.

76. Hamada K, Hirayama M, Watanabe H, et al: Onset age and severity of motor impairment are associated with reduction of myocardial 123I-MIBG uptake in Parkinson's disease. J Neurol Neurosurg Psychiatry 2003;74:423-426.

77. Spiegel J, Hellwig D, Farmakis G, et al: Myocardial sympathetic degeneration correlates with clinical phenotype of Parkinson's disease. Mov Disord 2007;22:1004-1008.

78. Matsui H, Nishinaka K, Oda M, et al: Does cardiac metaiodobenzylguanidine (MIBG) uptake in Parkinson's disease correlate with major autonomic symptoms? Parkinsonism Relat Disord 2006;12:284-288.

79. Takatsu H, Nishida H, Matsuo H, et al: Cardiac sympathetic denervation from the early stage of Parkinson's disease: clinical and experimental studies with radiolabeled MIBG. J Nucl Med 2000;41:71-77.

80. Taki J, Nakajima K, Hwang EH, et al: Peripheral sympathetic dysfunction in patients with Parkinson's disease without autonomic failure is heart selective and disease specific. Eur J Nucl Med 2000;27:566-573.

81. de Milliano PA, van Eck-Smit BL, de Groot AC, Lie KI: Metoprolol-induced changes in myocardial (123)I-metaiodobenzylguanidine uptake in Parkinson's disease. Circulation 2001;102:2553-2554.

82. Schnell O, Kirsch CM, Stemplinger J, et al: Scintigraphic evidence for cardiac sympathetic dysinnervation in long-term IDDM patients with and without ECG-based autonomic neuropathy. Diabetologia 1995;38:1345-1352.

83. Kujawa K, Leurgans S, Raman R, et al: Acute orthostatic hypotension when starting dopamine agonists in Parkinson's disease. Arch Neurol 2000;57:1461-1463.

84. Goetz CG, Koller WC, Poewe W, et al: Management of Parkinson's disease: an evidence-based review. Mov Disord 2002;17:S1-S166.

85. Horstink M, Tolosa E, Bonuccelli U, et al: European Federation of Neurological Societies; Movement Disorder Society–European Section. Review of the therapeutic management of Parkinson's disease, part II: late (complicated) Parkinson's disease. Report of a joint task force of the European Federation of Neurological Societies (EFNS) and the Movement Disorder Society–European Section (MDS-ES). Eur J Neurol 2006;13:1186-1202.

86. Eichhorn TE, Oertel WH: Macrogol 3350/electrolyte improves constipation in Parkinson's disease and multiple system atrophy. Mov Disord 2001;16:1176-1177.
87. Zangaglia R, Martignoni E, Glorioso M, et al: Macrogol for the treatment of constipation in Parkinson's disease: a randomized placebo-controlled study. Mov Disord 2007;22:1239-1244.
88. Sullivan KL, Staffetti JF, Hauser RA, et al: Tegaserod (Zelnorm) for the treatment of constipation in Parkinson's disease. Mov Disord 2006;21:115-116.
89. Liu Z, Sakakibara R, Odaka T, et al: Mosapride citrate, a novel 5-HT4 agonist and partial 5-HT3 antagonist, ameliorates constipation in parkinsonian patients. Mov Disord 2005;20:680-686.
90. Sakakibara R, Odaka T, Lui Z, et al: Dietary herb extract dai-kenchu-to ameliorates constipation in parkinsonian patients (Parkinson's disease and multiple system atrophy). Mov Disord 2005;20:261-262.
91. Day JP, Pruitt RE: Diabetic gastroparesis in a patient with Parkinson's disease: effective treatment with domperidone. Am J Gastroenterol 1989;84:837-838.
92. Soykan I, Sarosiek I, Shifflett J, et al: Effect of chronic oral domperidone therapy on gastrointestinal symptoms and gastric emptying in patients with Parkinson's disease. Mov Disord 1997;12:952-957.
93. Jimenez-Jimenez FJ, Garcia-Ruiz PJ, Molina JA: Drug-induced movement disorders. Drug Saf 1997;16:180-204.
94. Cadeddu F, Bentivoglio AR, Brandara F, et al: Outlet type constipation in Parkinson's disease: results of botulinum toxin treatment. Aliment Pharmacol Ther 2005;22:997-1003.
95. Albanese A, Brisinda G, Bentivoglio AR, Maria G: Treatment of outlet obstruction constipation in Parkinson's disease with botulinum neurotoxin A. Am J Gastroenterol 2003;98:1439-1440.
96. Suchowersky O, Furtado S, Rohs G: Beneficial effect of intranasal desmopressin for nocturnal polyuria in Parkinson's disease. Mov Disord 1995;10:337-340.
97. Hussain IF, Brady CM, Swinn MJ, et al: Treatment of erectile dysfunction with sildenafil citrate in parkinsonism due to Parkinson's disease and multiple system atrophy with observations on orthostatic hypotension. J Neurol Neurosurg Psychiatry 2001;71:371-374.
98. Zesiewicz TA, Helal M, Hauser RA: Sildenafil citrate (Viagra) for the treatment of erectile dysfunction in men with Parkinson's disease. Mov Disord 2000;15:305-308.
99. Raffaele R, Vecchio I, Giammusso B, et al: Efficacy and safety of fixed-dose oral sildenafil in the treatment of sexual dysfunction in depressed patients with idiopathic Parkinson's disease. Eur Uroly 2002;41:382-386.
100. O'Sullivan JD, Hughes AJ: Apomorphine-induced penile erections in Parkinson's disease. Mov Disord 1998;13:536-539.
101. O'Sullivan JD: Apomorphine as an alternative to sildenafil in Parkinson's disease. J Neurol Neurosurg Psychiatry 2002;72:681.
102. Pohanka M, Kanovsky P, Bares M, et al: Pergolide mesylate can improve sexual dysfunction in patients with Parkinson's disease: the results of an open, prospective, 6-month follow-up. Eur J Neurol 2004;11:483-488.
103. Pohanka M, Kanovsky P, Bares M, et al: The long-lasting improvement of sexual dysfunction in patients with advanced, fluctuating Parkinson's disease induced by pergolide: evidence from the results of an open, prospective, one-year trial. Parkinsonism Relat Disord 2005;11:509-512.
104. Hasegawa Y, Hakusui S, Hirayama M, et al: Clinical effects of elastic bandage on neurogenic orthostatic hypotension. J Gravit Physiol 2000;7:159-160.
105. Smit AA, Wieling W, Opfer-Gehrking TL, et al: Patients' choice of portable folding chairs to reduce symptoms of orthostatic hypotension. Clin Auton Res 1999;9:341-344.
106. Lang AE: Acute orthostatic hypotension when starting dopamine agonist therapy in Parkinson disease: the role of domperidone therapy. Arch Neurol 2001;58:835.
107. Jankovic J, Gilden JL, Hiner BC, et al: Neurogenic orthostatic hypotension: a double-blind placebo-controlled study with midodrine. Am J Med 1993;95:38-48.
108. Low PA, Gilden FL, Freeman R, et al: Efficacy of midodrine vs placebo in neurogenic orthostatic hypotension: a randomized double-blind multicenter study. Midodrine study group. JAMA 1997;277:1046-1051.
109. Hakamaki T, Rajala T, Lehtonen A: Ambulatory 24-hour blood pressure recordings in patients with Parkinson's disease with or without fludrocortisone. Int J Clin Pharmacol Ther 1998;36:367-369.
110. Schoffer KL, Henderson RD, O'Maley K, O'Sullivan JD: Nonpharmacological treatment, fludrocortisone, and domperidone for orthostatic hypotension in Parkinson's disease. Mov Disord 2007;22:1543-1549.
111. Singer W, Sandroni P, Tonette L, et al: Pyridostigmine treatment trial in neurogenic orthostatic hypotension. Arch Neurol 2006;63:513-518.

112. Jansen RW, Lipsitz LA: Postprandial hypotension: epidemiology, pathophysiology, and clinical management. Ann Intern Med 1995;122:286-295.
113. Senard JM, Brefel-Courbon C, Rascol O, Montastruc JL: Orthostatic hypotension in patients with Parkinson's disease: pathophysiology and management. Drugs Aging 2001;18:495-505.
114. Holmberg B, Corneliusson O, Elam M: Bilateral stimulation of nucleus subthalamicus in advanced Parkinson's disease: no effects on, and of, autonomic dysfunction. Mov Disord 2005;20:976-981.
115. Ludwig J, Remien P, Guballa C, et al: Effects of subthalamic nucleus stimulation and levodopa on the autonomic nervous system in Parkinson's disease. J Neurol Neurosurg Psychiatry 2007;78: 742-745.
116. Lees AJ, Blackburn NA, Campbell VL: The nighttime problems of Parkinson's disease. Clin Neuropharmacol 1988;11:512-519.
117. Iranzo A, Molinuevo JL, Santamaria J, et al: Rapid-eye-movement sleep behaviour disorder as an early marker for a neurodegenerative disorder: a descriptive study. Lancet Neurol 2006;5: 572-577.
118. Basta M, Schiza S, Mauridis M, et al: Sleep breathing disorders in patients with idiopathic Parkinson's disease. Resp Med 2003;97:1151-1157.
119. Schenck C, Mahowald MW: REM sleep behavior disorder: clinical, developmental and neuroscience perspectives 16 years after its formal identification in SLEEP. Sleep 2002;55:281-288.
120. Gagnon JF, Bedard MA, Fantini MD, et al: REM sleep behavior disorder and REM sleep without atonia in Parkinson's disease. Neurology 2002;59:585-589.
121. Arnulf I, Bonnet MA, Damier P, et al: Hallucinations, REM sleep, and Parkinson's disease. Neurology 2000;55:281-288.
122. Scharf B: Moskowitz Ch, Lupton MD, Klawans HL: Dream phenomena induced by chronic levodopa therapy. J Neural Transm 1978;43:143-151.
123. Nausieda PA, Weiner WJ, Kaplan LR, et al: Sleep disruption in the course of chronic levodopa therapy: an early feature of the levodopa psychosis. Clin Neuropharmacol 1982;5:183-194.
124. Vendette M, Gagnon JF, Décary A, et al: REM sleep behavior disorder predicts cognitive impairment in Parkinson disease without dementia. Neurology 2007;69:1843-1849.
125. Kumru H, Santamaria J, Tolosa E, Iranzo A: Relation between subtype of Parkinson's disease and REM sleep behavior disorder. Sleep Med 2007;8:779-783.
126. Frucht S, Rogers MD, Greene PE, et al: Falling asleep at the wheel: motor vehicle mishaps in persons taking pramipexole and ropinirole. Neurology 1999;58:1908-1910.
127. Hobson DE, Lang AE, Martin WR, et al: Excessive daytime sleepiness and sudden-onset sleep in Parkinson disease: a survey by the Canadian movement disorder group. JAMA 2002;287:455-463.
128. Rascol O, Ferreira J, Montastruc JL: Somnolence diurne anormal, "attaques de sommeil" et médicaments antiparkinsoniens. Rev Neurol (Paris) 2001;157:1313-1315.
129. Tandberg E, Larsen JP, Karlsen KA: A community-based study of sleep disorders in patients with Parkinson's disease. Mov Disord 1998;13:895-899.
130. O'Suilleabhain PE, Dewey RB: Contributions of dopaminergic drugs and disease severity to daytime sleepiness in Parkinson disease. Arch Neurol 2002;59:986-989.
131. Tan EK, Lum SY, Fook-Chong SMC, et al: Evaluation of somnolence in Parkinson's disease: comparison with age and sex-matched controls. Neurology 2002;58:465-468.
132. Brodsky MA, Goldbold J, Roth T, Olanow WC: Sleepiness in Parkinson's disease: a controlled study. Mov Disord 2003;18:668-672.
133. Razmy A, Lang AE, Shapiro CM: Predictors of impaired daytime sleep and wakefulness in patients with Parkinson disease treated with older (Ergot) vs newer (nonergot) dopamine agonists. Arch Neurol 2004;61:97-102.
134. Stevens S, Comella CL, Stepanski EJ: Daytime sleepiness and alertness in patients with Parkinson disease. Sleep 2004;27:967-972.
135. Factor SA, McAlarney T, Sanchez-Ramos JR, Weiner WJ: Sleep disorders and sleep effect in Parkinson's disease. Mov Disord 1990;5:280-285.
136. Oerlemans WH, de Weerd AW: The prevalence of sleep disorders in patients with Parkinson's disease: a self-reported, community-based survey. Sleep Med 2002;3:147-149.
137. Verbaan D, van Rooden SM, Visser M, et al: Nighttime sleep problems and daytime sleepiness in Parkinson's disease. Mov Disord 2008;23:35-41.
138. Fabrinni G, Barbanti P, Aurilia C, et al: Excessive daytime sleepiness in de novo and treated Parkinson's disease. Mov Disord 2002;17:1026-1030.
139. Rye DB, Bliwise DL, Dihenia B, Gurecki P: Daytime sleepiness in Parkinson's disease. J Sleep Res 2000;9:63-69.

140. Young A, Horne M, Churchward T, et al: Comparison of sleep disturbance in mild versus severe Parkinson's disease. Sleep 2002;25:568-572.
141. Roth T, Rye DB, Borcher LD, et al: Assessment of sleepiness and unintended sleep in Parkinson's disease patients taking dopamine agonists. Sleep Med 2003;4:275-280.
142. Gjerstad MD, Aarsland D, Larsen JP: Development of daytime somnolence over time in Parkinson's disease. Neurology 2002;58:1544-1546.
143. Paus S, Seeger G, Brecht HM, et al: Association study of dopamine D2, D3, D4 receptor and serotonin transporter gene polymorphisms with sleep attacks in Parkinson's disease. Mov Disord 2004;19:705-707.
144. Rissling I, Geller F, Bandmann O, et al: Dopamine receptor gene polymorphisms in Parkinson's disease patients reporting "sleep attacks." Mov Disord 2004;19:1279-1284.
145. Arnulf I, Konofal E, Merino-Andreu M, et al: Parkinson's disease and sleepiness: an integral part of PD. Neurology 2002;58:1019-1024.
146. Fronczeck R, Overeem S, Lee SYY, et al: Hypocretin (orexin) loss in Parkinson's disease. Brain 2007;130:1577-1585.
147. Tannickal TC, Lai YY, Siegel JM: Hypocretin (orexin) cell loss in Parkinson's disease. Brain 2007;130:1586-1595.
148. Bauman C, Ferini-Strambi L, Waldvogel D, et al: Parkinsonism with excessive daytime sleepiness: a narcolepsy-like disorder? J Neurol 2005;252:139-145.
149. Drouot X, Moutereau S, Nguyen JP, et al: Low levels of ventricular CSF orexin/hypocretin in advanced PD. Neurology 2003;61:540-543.
150. Abbot RD, Ross GW, White LR, et al: Excessive daytime sleepiness and subsequent development of Parkinson disease. Neurology 2005;65:1442-1446.
151. Van Hilten JJ, Hoogland G, van der Velde EA, et al: Diurnal effects of motor activity and fatigue in Parkinson's disease. J Neurol Neurosurg Psychiatry 1993;56:874-877.
152. Friedman JH, Friedman H: Fatigue in Parkinson's disease. Neurology 1993;43:2016-2018.
153. Karlsen K, Larsen JP, Tandberg E, Jorgensen K: Fatigue in patients with Parkinson's disease. Mov Disord 1999;14:237-241.
154. Larsen JP, Karlsen K, Tandberg E: Clinical problems in nonfluctuating patients with Parkinson's disease: a community-based study. Mov Disord 2000;15:826-829.
155. Lou JS, Kearns G, Oken B, et al: Exacerbated physical fatigue and mental fatigue in Parkinson's disease. Mov Disord 2001;16:190-196.
156. Shulman LM, Taback R, Rabinstein AA, Weiner WJ: Non-recognition of depression and other non-motor symptoms in Parkinson's disease. Parkinsonism Relat Disord 2002;8:193-197.
157. Friedman JH, Brown RG, Comella C, et al: Fatigue in Parkinson's disease: a review. Mov Disord 2007;22:297-308.
158. Shulman LM, Taback RL, Bean J, Weiner WJ: Comorbidity of the non-motor symptoms of Parkinson's disease. Mov Disord 2001;16:507-510.
159. Alves G, Wentzel-Larsen T, Larsen JP: Is fatigue an independent and persistent symptom in patients with Parkinson disease? Neurology 2004;63:1908-1911.
160. Brown RG, Dittner A, Findley L, Wessely SC: The Parkinson fatigue scale. Parkinsonism Relat Disord 2005;11:49-55.
161. Andersen J, Aabro E, Gulmann N, et al: Anti-depressive treatment in Parkinson's disease: a controlled trial of the effect of nortriptyline in patients with Parkinson's disease treated with L-dopa. Acta Neurol Scand 1980;62:210-219.
162. Mendonça DA, Menezes K, Jog MS: Methylphenidate improves fatigue scores in Parkinson disease: a randomized controlled trial. Mov Disord 2007;22:2070-2076.
163. Quinn NP, Koller WC, Lang AE, et al: Painful Parkinson's disease. Lancet 1986;1:1366-1369.
164. Quittenbaum BH, Grahn B: Quality of life and pain in Parkinson's disease: a controlled cross-sectional study. Parkinsonism Relat Disord 2004;10:129-136.
165. Buzas B, Max MB: Pain in Parkinson disease. Neurology 2004;62:2156-2157.
166. Ford B: Pain in Parkinson's disease. Clin Neurosci 1998;5:63-72.
167. Tinazzi M, Del Vesco C, Fincati E, et al: Pain and motor complications in Parkinson's disease. J Neurol Neurosurg Psychiatry 2006;77:822-825.
168. Ford B, Louise P, Greene P, et al: Oral and genital pain syndromes in Parkinson's disease. Mov Disord 1996;11:421-426.
169. Djaldetti R, Shifrin A, Rogowski Z, et al: Quantitative measurement of pain sensation in patients with Parkinson's disease. Neurology 2004;62:2171-2175.

170. O'Sullivan SS, Williams DR, Gallagher DA, et al: Nonmotor symptoms as presenting complaints in Parkinson's disease: a clinicopathological study. Mov Disord 2008;23:101-106.
171. Hillen ME, Sage JI: Non-motor fluctuations in patients with Parkinson's disease. Neurology 1996;47:1180-1183.
172. Dhawan V, Medcalf P, Stegie F, et al: Retrospective evaluation of cardio-pulmonary fibrotic side effects in symptomatic patients from a group of 234 Parkinson's disease patients treated with cabergoline. J Neural Transm 2005;112:661-668.
173. Etchepare F, Rozenberg S, Mirault T, et al: Back problems in Parkinson's disease: an underestimated problem. Joint Bone Spine 2006;73:298-302.
174. Broetz D, Eichner M, Gasser T, et al: Radicular and nonradicular back pain in Parkinson's disease: a controlled study. Mov Disord 2007;22:853-856.
175. Factor SA, Brown DL, Molho ES: Subcutaneous apomorphine injections as a treatment for intractable pain in Parkinson's disease. Mov Disord 2000;15:167-169.
176. Panchetti C, Albani G, Martignoni E, et al: "Off" painful dystonia in Parkinson's disease treated with botulinum toxin. Mov Disord 1995;10:333-336.
177. Loher TJ, Burgunder JM, Weber S, et al: Effect of chronic pallidal deep brain stimulation on off period dystonia and sensory symptoms in advanced Parkinson's disease. J Neurol Neurosurg Psychiatry 2002;73:395-399.
178. Witjas T, Kaphan E, Régis J, et al: Effects of chronic subthalamic stimulation on nonmotor fluctuations in Parkinson's disease. Mov Disord 2007;22:1729-1734.
179. Djaldetti R, Yust-Katz S, Kolianov V, et al: The effect of duloxetine on primary pain symptoms in Parkinson disease. Clin Neuropharmacol 2007;30:201-205.
180. Lang AE, Johnson K: Akathisia in idiopathic Parkinson's disease. Neurology 1987;37:477-481.
181. Comella CL, Goetz CG: Akathisia in Parkinson's disease. Mov Disord 1994;9:545-549.
182. Ondo WG, Vuong KD, Jankovic J: Exploring the relationship between Parkinson disease and restless legs syndrome. Arch Neurol 2002;59:421-424.
183. Tan EK, Lum SY, Wong MC: Restless legs syndrome in Parkinson's disease. J Neurol Sci 2002;196:33-36.
184. Iranzo A, Comella CL, Santamaría J, Oertel W: Restless legs syndrome in Parkinson's disease and other neurodegenerative diseases of the central nervous system. Mov Disord 2007;22(Suppl 18): 424-430.
185. Nomura T, Inoue Y, Nakashima K: Clinical characteristics of restless legs syndrome in patients with Parkinson's disease. J Neurol Sci 2006;250:39-44.
186. Walters AS, LeBrocq C, Passi V, et al: A preliminary look at the percentage of patients with restless legs syndrome who also have Parkinson's disease, essential tremor or Tourette syndrome in a single practice. J Sleep Res 2003;12:343-345.
187. Kedia S, Moro E, Tagliati M, et al: Emergence of restless legs syndrome during subthalamic stimulation for Parkinson disease. Neurology 2004;63:2410-2412.
188. Driver-Dunckley E, Evidente VGH, Adler CH, et al: Restless legs syndrome in Parkinson's disease patients may improve with subthalamic stimulation. Mov Disord 2006;21:1287-1289.
189. Gonera EG, Van't Hof M, Berger HJC, et al: Symptoms and duration of the premotor phase in Parkinson's disease. Mov Disord 1997;12:871-876.
190. Becker G, Müller A, Braune S, et al: Early diagnosis of Parkinson's disease. J Neurol 2002;249(Suppl 3): 40-48.
191. Awerbuch GI, Sandyk R: Autonomic functions in the early stages of Parkinson's disease. Int J Neurosci 1994;74:9-16.
192. Abbott RD, Petrovitch H, White LR, et al: Frequency of bowel movements and the future risk of Parkinson's disease. Neurology 2001;57:456-462.
193. Ashraf W, Pfeiffer RF, Park F, et al: Constipation in Parkinson's disease: objective assessment and response to psyllium. Mov Disord 1997;12:946-951.
194. Camilleri M, Bharucha AE: Gastrointestinal dysfunction in neurologic disease. Semin Neurol 1996;16:203-216.
195. Ueki A, Otsuka M: Life style risks of Parkinson's disease: association between decreased water intake and constipation. J Neurol 2004;251(Suppl 7):18-23.
196. Gao X, Chen H, Schwarzschild M, et al: Erectile function and risk of Parkinson's disease. Am J Epidemiol 2007;166:1446-1450.
197. Minguez-Castellanos A, Chamorro CE, Escamilla-Sevilla F, et al: Do alpha-synuclein aggregates in autonomic plexuses predate Lewy body disorders? A cohort study. Neurology 2007;68:2012-2018.
198. Doty RL, Deems DA, Stellar S: Olfactory dysfunction in parkinsonism: a general deficit unrelated to neurologic signs, disease stage, or disease duration. Neurology 1988;38:1237-1244.

199. Tissingh G, Berendse HW, Bergmans P, et al: Loss of olfaction in de novo and treated Parkinson's disease: possible implications for early diagnosis. Mov Disord 2001;16:41-46.
200. Stern M, Doty RL, Dotti M, et al: Olfactory function in Parkinson's disease subtypes. Neurology 1994;44:266-268.
201. Ross W, Petrovitch H, Abbott RD, et al: Association of olfactory dysfunction with risk of future Parkinson's disease. Mov Disord 2005;20(Suppl 10):129-130.
202. Ross GW, Abbott RD, Petrovitch H, et al: Association of olfactory dysfunction with incidental Lewy bodies. Mov Disord 2006;21:2062-2067.
203. Sommer U, Hummel T, Cormann K, et al: Detection of presymptomatic Parkinson's disease: combining smell tests, transcranial sonography, and SPECT. Mov Disord 2004;19:1196-1202.
204. Markopoulou K, Larsen KW, Wszolek EK, et al: Olfactory dysfunction in familial parkinsonism. Neurology 1997;49:1262-1267.
205. Montgomery EB, Baker KB, Lyons K, Koller WC: Abnormal performance on the PD test battery by asymptomatic first degree relatives. Neurology 1999;52:757-762.
206. Berendse HW, Booij J, Francot GMJE, et al: Subclinical dopaminergic dysfunction in symptomatic Parkinson's disease patients' relatives with a decreased sense of smell. Ann Neurol 2001;50:34-41.
207. Boeve BF, Silber MH, Ferman TJ, et al: Association of REM sleep behavior disorder and neurodegenerative disease may reflect an underlying synucleopathy. Mov Disord 2001;16:622-630.
208. Postuma RB, Lang AE, Massicotte-Marquez J, Montplaisir J: Potential early markers of Parkinson's disease in idiopathic REM sleep behavior disorder. Neurology 2006;66:845-851.
209. Stiasny-Kolster K, Doerr Y, Möller JC, et al: Combination of 'idiopathic' REM sleep behaviour disorder and olfactory dysfunction as possible indicator for alfa-synucleinopathy demonstrated by dopamine transporter FP-CIT-SPECT. Brain 2005;128:126-137.

15 Therapy of the Motor Features of Parkinson's Disease

SUSAN FOX • ANTHONY E. T. LANG

Introduction

The motor symptoms of Parkinson's disease (PD) are manifold and include bradykinesia, resting tremor, rigidity, and postural instability owing in part to dopaminergic cell loss in the substantia nigra pars compacta. The modern pharmacological approach to treating such symptoms consists of polypharmacy using a combination of the "old," the dopamine precursor levodopa, and the "new," including dopamine receptor agonists, drugs to extend the duration of action of levodopa, drugs to reduce involuntary movements (dyskinesia), and drugs to reduce parkinsonian symptoms by targeting nondopaminergic systems with the aim of reducing the side effects of long-term levodopa therapy.

Despite 40 years since its first use in PD, levodopa remains the most effective treatment and cornerstone of good PD control. Evidence that the pathology of PD extends beyond the nigrostriatal system encourages the recognition that extranigral dopaminergic and nondopaminergic neurotransmitter systems are equally important, however. The increasing awareness of nonmotor symptoms, either as a consequence of disease or secondary to side effects of dopaminergic agents, is also affecting treatment choices for clinicians and patients. The future development of drugs capable of more selective targeting of specific neural pathways to improve motor symptoms without inducing side effects is encouraging.

Symptomatic Therapy of Early Parkinson's Disease

DELAYING TREATMENT WITH LEVODOPA

Investigators still debate the correct time to initiate symptomatic treatment for motor symptoms in the course of PD, and whether to use mild dopaminergic agents such as amantadine, monoamine oxidase B (MAOB) inhibitors, or dopamine receptor agonists (DAs), or to use levodopa immediately. The decision is a balance between the current need for symptomatic improvement to improve quality of life against avoidance of certain neuropsychiatric side effects more common with DAs and the potential motor complications associated with long-term levodopa therapy. These latter problems include various types of motor fluctuations, including wearing-off, "on-off" fluctuations, and dyskinesia. The risk factors for developing these motor complications include duration and dose of levodopa, early age of disease onset, and disease progression.[1,2] Despite awareness of the risks and attempts to reduce the onset, levodopa-induced motor complications remain common, affecting 40% to 50% of patients after 4 to 6 years of levodopa treatment.[3] In addition, dyskinesia has an impact on quality of life and can significantly increase health-related costs.[4,5]

More recent studies have raised some questions about the clinical importance of dyskinesia. In early PD, motor complications were shown not to have a significant negative effect on quality of life as measured by a visual analog scale.[6] In advanced PD, a survey found that although dyskinesia developed in nearly 60% of patients after 10 years, less than half of the patients required medication adjustments, and only 10% had dyskinesia that could not be controlled by drug adjustments.[7] The Sydney Multicentre study of Parkinson's Disease followed patients over 15 years and reported that although greater than 90% of patients experienced dyskinesia and wearing-off, 54% did not consider their dyskinesia bothersome.[8] In addition, a more recent study has shown a worse quality of life in PD patients who delayed starting treatment.[9]

THERAPEUTIC OPTIONS FOR TREATMENT OF MOTOR SYMPTOMS IN EARLY PARKINSON'S DISEASE

Many agents can be used in early PD to improve motor symptoms (Table 15-1). The MAOB inhibitors, selegiline and rasagiline, can potentially provide mild symptomatic benefit in early PD by inhibiting the metabolism of dopamine. Long-term follow-up of patients originally enrolled in the Deprenyl And Tocopherol Antioxidative Therapy Of Parkinsonism (DATATOP) study[10] showed that early selegiline use had beneficial effects on "on-off" motor fluctuations, freezing of gait, and motor parkinsonian scores, but with increased dyskinesia.[11] Rasagiline,

TABLE 15–1	Symptomatic Therapy for Motor Symptoms in Early Parkinson's Disease		
Class of Drug	**Name**	**Side Effects**	**Comments**
Monoamine oxidase B inhibitor	Selegiline; rasagiline	Nausea, hallucinations	Selegiline has amphetamine metabolites; earlier concerns of increased mortality with selegiline not shown in long-term follow-up[87,88]; rasagiline is also being investigated as a possible neuroprotectant (see Chapter 18)
Enhances dopamine neurotransmission	Amantadine	Hallucinations, livedo reticularis	Is also a nonselective NMDA antagonist and is used to treat peak dose dyskinesia (see Table 15–5)
Anticholinergic	Trihexyphenidyl, benztropine, orphenadrine, procyclidine	Dry mouth, blurred vision, confusion, urinary retention	Used primarily for tremor; no benefit on other Parkinson's disease symptoms
Dopamine receptor agonists	Ropinirole, pramipexole, pergolide, bromocriptine, cabergoline, rotigotine	See Table 15–3; rotigotine has application site reactions	Receptor profiles of dopamine (see Table 15–2)
Levodopa	Levodopa/carbidopa, levodopa/benserazide	Nausea, postural hypotension	

NMDA, N-methyl-D-aspartate.

an irreversible MAOB inhibitor, is 10 to 15 times more potent than selegiline, is not associated with amphetamine metabolites, and has been shown to have benefit in early PD.[12] The longer-term symptomatic benefits of rasagiline with respect to preventing motor complications are unclear.

Dopamine Receptor Agonists

Dopamine Receptor Agonists as Monotherapy for Motor Symptoms

Dopamine binds to two families of receptors, dopamine D1-like (D1 and D5) and dopamine D2-like (D2, D3, and D4) receptors; different locations and distributions suggest different functions. Dopamine D2 receptors are found presynaptically in the substantia nigra pars compacta and ventral tegmental area and postsynaptically colocalized with dopamine D1 receptors on medium spiny neurons in the striatum.

TABLE 15–2	Pharmacology of Clinically Available Dopamine Receptor Agonists: Relative Affinity of Clinically Available Dopamine Agonists				
Name of Drug	D1	D2	D3	D4	Nondopamine Receptors
Pergolide	+	++++	+++	++	5-HT1A, 5-HT2A; α1, α2
Bromocriptine	–	++	++	+	5-HT1A, 5-HT2B; α1A, α1B, α1D, α2A, β
Lisuride	++	++++	++++	+++	5-HT1A, 5-HT1D, 5-HT2A, 5-HT2B, 5-HT2C; H1; α1, α2, β
Apomorphine	++	+++	+++	+++	5-HT1A, 5-HT2A, 5-HT2B, 5-HT2C; α1B, α1D, α2C
Cabergoline	+	+++	++	+	5-HT1A, 5-HT1D, 5-HT2A, 5-HT2B; H1; α1A
Pramipexole	0	+++	++++	+++	5-HT1A; α2B
Ropinirole	0	+++	++++	+++	5-HT1A; α2B
Rotigotine	+	++	+++	+	5-HT1A; α2B

+, Agonist; –, antagonist; 0, no activity; + to ++++, increased potency; D, dopamine; 5-HT, 5-hydroxytryptamine; α, α-adrenoceptor; β, β-adrenoceptor; H, histamine.

The clinical benefit of dopamine replacement on motor symptoms in PD relates primarily to stimulation of the dopamine D2 receptor within the striatum and resultant inhibition of the overactive striatopallidal GABAergic input to the lateral globus pallidus, resulting in reversal of the overactivity of subthalamic nucleus and medial globus pallidus.[13] The clinically available DAs used in the treatment of PD all have significant binding to the dopamine D2 receptor, but also have a range of actions at other dopamine receptors (Table 15–2).[13,14] Randomized clinical trials of DAs have shown efficacy as monotherapy in all motor symptoms. Several systematic reviews have published evidence-based recommendations of therapy in PD and report similar benefits with all DAs.[15-17] Despite the variable dopamine receptor binding profile, the clinical efficacy of these agents seems similar. Specific DAs available only in selected countries are not discussed further, but include piribedil,[18] lisuride,[19] and α-dihydroergocryptine.[20]

Early Use of Dopamine Receptor Agonists to Prevent Long-term Motor Complications

The development of DAs was driven by the need to improve symptoms in PD without the long-term motor complications that occur with levodopa. In particular, the longer half-life of these agents is thought to reduce the propensity to induce motor fluctuations (by postsynaptic changes to neurotransmitter/modulatory basal ganglia pathways [see Chapter 1]), combined with a lack of interaction with dietary amino acids, avoiding erratic absorption and fluctuating dopamine levels. Several clinical studies have shown that ropinirole, pramipexole, cabergoline, and pergolide all have reduced propensity to induce dyskinesia and wearing-off, compared with levodopa, when assessed over a 4- to 5-year period.[21-24]

More recent re-evaluation has shown, however, that, after adjusting for disease duration and daily levodopa dosage, early use of pramipexole or ropinirole may delay only rather than prevent the onset of dyskinesia, and these benefits decline when levodopa therapy is started.[25,26] Studies evaluating the longer term (10-year) benefit of early initiation of DAs on development of motor complications have shown variable results: no difference in moderate to severe dyskinesia, or "on-off" fluctuations with bromocriptine,[27] or maintained benefit with ropinirole.[28] Interpretation of these studies is limited, however, because of high dropout rates resulting in small numbers and naturalistic study design inherent in such long follow-up.

Why Dopamine Agonists Are Less Effective Antiparkinsonian Agents than Levodopa

Despite the advantages outlined previously, all DAs have been shown to have less benefit on parkinsonian disability compared with levodopa. This has also been suggested to underlie the lower propensity to induce dyskinesia. Patients treated with bromocriptine, ropinirole, pramipexole, pergolide, and cabergoline all had significantly worse motor scores compared with levodopa in the first 5 years of follow-up.[21-24,27] At a time when patients may still be working and require optimal motor function, the early use of a DA as monotherapy may not provide optimal benefit to parkinsonian disability.

The reason for superior benefit on motor function with levodopa compared with DAs in early PD remains unclear. Many possibilities have been suggested, including levodopa conversion to dopamine activating dopamine D1-like and D2-like receptors, potentially resulting in more potent antiparkinsonian action. In addition, at least early in the disease, levodopa therapy results in a more physiological stimulation of dopamine receptors, owing to synthesis, vesicular transport, storage, and release of dopamine, providing a more regulated release of dopamine in response to requirements.[29,30] Levodopa is also converted into norepinephrine in adrenergic terminals, and can cause glutamate release and reduce γ-aminobutyric acid (GABA) release; these nondopaminergic effects may have added benefit, although the exact mechanisms remain unclear. Another major factor limiting use and potential efficacy of DAs in the treatment of motor symptoms of PD is the development of adverse effects (Table 15–3) that may prevent the ability to titrate to doses equivalent to those of levodopa used in comparative trials.

Improving Dopamine Receptor Agonist Efficacy

The clinical efficacy of DAs in PD probably relates to dopamine D2 receptor binding. As noted earlier, there may be a synergistic response to dopamine D2 and D1 receptor costimulation in the striatum, and DAs with mixed D1 and D2 receptor agonist effect may have greater efficacy.[31] The additional activity at dopamine D1 receptors of cabergoline, lisuride, pergolide, and apomorphine might suggest potential for greater therapeutic benefit than drugs purely selective for D2 receptors (e.g., sumanirole), although this has never been conclusively shown in clinical trials. Subtype selective D1 dopamine agonists have had limited study to date, showing equivalent benefit, but more potential to induce dyskinesia than nonselective D2 agonists.[32] Selective targeting of dopamine D3 receptors has been suggested to have reduced potential to develop dyskinesia,[33] although such selective D3 agents are not currently clinically available.

TABLE 15–3	Adverse Effects of Dopamine Receptor Agonists		
Adverse Effect	Incidence	Proposed Mechanism	Comments
Nausea	37.4-48.6%[15,21-24,45]	Dopamine D2 receptors in chemosensitive trigger zone	Can prevent/reduce with use of peripheral dopamine D2 antagonist (e.g., domperidone)
Dizziness, symptomatic postural hypotension	8.1-31.4%[15,21-24,45]	Dopamine D1 and D2 receptors in cardiovascular and renin-angiotensin systems	
Peripheral pedal edema	5.5-22.5%[15,21-24,45]	Unknown; higher risk associated with cardiac disease[89]	Peripheral, facial, and generalized edema reported in 42.4% patients using pramipexole compared with 14.7% with levodopa[22]
Somnolence, excessive daytime sleepiness, sudden sleep attacks	17.5-36.4%[15,21-24,45]	Presynaptic D2 receptors downregulate dopamine inputs to wakefulness-promoting systems in the brainstem, hypothalamus, and basal forebrain[90]	Unclear if this effect is secondary to dopaminergic stimulation per se or disease effect, as excessive daytime sleepiness is nearly as high among PD patients who have never used a dopamine[91]; all PD patients should be counseled, particularly if they drive or operate machinery
Visual hallucinations	3.4-17.3%[15,21-24,45]	Possible dopamine D2 mediated, combined with underlying pathology	Increased risk of inducing hallucinations with dopamine in patients with cognitive impairment[89,92]
ICDs: pathological gambling, compulsive shopping, hypersexuality; dopamine dysregulation syndrome[93]	5.6-6.6%[94,95]; 13.5% with dopamine, compared with levodopa alone 0.7%	Unknown—higher risk in young age and premorbidity of family history of ICD or substance abuse[96]	An association with any specific dopamine is unclear owing to variable prescribing habits of clinics and different methods of measuring prevalence rates[97]; ICDs may respond to reduction or stopping dopamine

Table continued on following page

TABLE 15–3	**Adverse Effects of Dopamine Receptor Agonists** (Continued)		
Adverse Effect	**Incidence**	**Proposed Mechanism**	**Comments**
Pleuropulmonary and retroperitoneal fibrosis	Rare case reports with ergot-derived agonists, bromocriptine, pergolide, lisuride, cabergoline[98]	Possible idiosyncratic immune reaction?; 5-HT mediated	ESR may be elevated; chest imaging required; fibrotic process may remit when the drug is stopped
Valvulopathy	Moderate-to-severe valvular changes in 23-28% of pergolide, cabergoline; 10% ropinirole, pramipexole (versus 10% of control patients; severe valvulopathy <1%[99]	5-HT2B agonist properties	True incidence is unclear owing to variable methods of measuring cardiac valve disease; there does not seem to be a consistent association with dose or duration of use of dopamine; FDA has announced that pergolide is being voluntarily withdrawn in US

ESR, erythrocyte sedimentation rate; FDA, U.S. Food and Drug Administration; ICDs, impulse control disorders; PD, Parkinson's disease.

Another approach to improve motor function without inducing dyskinesia and other extrastriatal dopamine D2 side effects may be to use partial dopamine D2 agonists. Such agents do not maximally stimulate D2, and stimulate D2 receptors at low levels of dopaminergic tone and act as antagonists when there is a high dopaminergic tone (Table 15–4). The reduced incidence of long-term motor complications with DAs also relates to the longer duration of action, which may be more critical than the selective dopamine receptor targeted.[34,35] Some DAs are being developed as longer acting formulations (see Table 15–4). To date, the advantages of these new formulations, apart from convenience and possibly better compliance as monotherapy, compared with levodopa or other DAs (including the standard formulations of the same agent) in early PD and in delaying onset of motor complications are unknown.

Levodopa

The use of the dopamine precursor levodopa, combined with a peripheral decarboxylase inhibitor, remains the key to good symptomatic benefit in early and advanced PD.[15,16,36] The first double-blind, placebo-controlled trial of levodopa was recently published (after 40 years of clinical use) showing the dose-dependent benefit of levodopa (dose range 150 to 600 mg/day) in early PD.[37] This study

TABLE 15–4	Dopamine Receptor Agonists in Development	
Dopamine Receptor	**Name of Drug**	**Clinical Effects**
Selective D2 agonist	Sumanirole	Less benefit compared with ropinirole in early PD,[100] but higher doses equivalent in advanced PD[101] (development has now stopped)
Partial D2/D3 agonist/ 5-HT1A agonist	SLV308	Phase III trials under way[102]
Partial D2 agonist/5HT1A agonist	Bifeprunox	Phase III trials under way[102]
D1/2/3 agonist—patch	Rotigotine	Improved motor scores compared with placebo[103]; marketed in some countries
D3/D2 agonist—long-acting	Ropinirole 24 hour	Improves "on" time in advanced PD[44]
D1/D2 agonist—patch	Lisuride patch	Phase III studies under way[104]
D3/D2 agonist—long-acting	Pramipexole ER	Phase III studies under way

PD, Parkinson's disease.

showed that in early PD, levodopa treatment may take several weeks before patients have a significant motor benefit. This is a key finding in clinical practice; patients should not expect a dramatic, quick response to levodopa initiation, particularly at lower doses. At the end of the 9-month study period, the influence of treatment on the underlying disease was evaluated using a 2-week study drug withdrawal. As expected, in patients treated with levodopa, PD disability increased, but did not reach the higher levels of disability seen in patients treated with placebo. The interpretation of this finding has been debated with explanations ranging from a clear disease-modifying effect to an inadequate washout of levodopa. Longer-term studies are needed to clarify this issue.

The issue of continuous dopaminergic stimulation as a means of delaying the onset of motor fluctuations has also been suggested by the early use of levodopa combined with a catechol O-methyltransferase (COMT) inhibitor (entacapone or tolcapone).[38] Clinical studies with levodopa and entacapone combination (Stalevo) are ongoing.

Treatment of Advanced Parkinson's Disease

The treatment of motor symptoms in advanced PD is determined by the development of fluctuations in motor symptoms related to drug dosing and worsening disability because of progression of the disease. Motor fluctuations are due to disease progression with loss of nigrostriatal dopaminergic terminals resulting in altered central pharmacokinetics of levodopa (presynaptic changes), combined with effects of long-term levodopa therapy resulting in changes to postsynaptic dopamine receptor signaling (central pharmacodynamic or postsynaptic changes). In addition, erratic absorption of levodopa because of gastrointestinal factors may play an important role in motor fluctuations. All these factors result in abnormal intrasynaptic dopamine concentrations with loss of normal constant stimulation of postsynaptic dopamine receptors (see Chapter 1).

Treatment of motor fluctuations is focused on smoothing out dopaminergic tone by using longer acting dopamine drugs such as DAs and prolonging the action of levodopa by combining it with agents that inhibit the breakdown of dopamine. Improving levodopa absorption by altering the solubility and improving delivery to the small bowel may also improve fluctuations in motor symptoms (Table 15–5).

DOPAMINE AGONISTS AS ADJUVANT THERAPY

All clinically available DAs improve "off" time in patients with motor fluctuations. There are few randomized prospective studies comparing efficacy between different DAs as add-on therapy for treating motor fluctuations. Systematic review and analysis of clinical trials comparing bromocriptine with ropinirole or pramipexole have shown no significant differences in efficacy.[39,40] The theoretical benefit of longer acting DAs in reducing "off" time has not been shown so far. Cabergoline (half-life 65 hours) is not superior to bromocriptine (half-life 6 hours).[41] The rotigotine patch, allowing nearly constant 24-hour delivery of drug, has been shown to be beneficial in reducing "off" time in PD compared with placebo.[42] In a study comparing oral pramipexole with rotigotine patch, there was no difference in benefit, however, and both were equally better than placebo in reducing "off" time in advanced PD.[43] The longer acting preparation of ropinirole (ropinirole 24 hour) has been shown to have benefit in reducing "off" time compared with placebo[44]; the benefit compared with shorter acting ropinirole is under investigation.

CATECHOL O-METHYLTRANSFERASE INHIBITORS

COMT inhibitors, by prolonging the duration of action of levodopa, are potentially useful in the treatment of wearing-off.[16,45] Many clinical trials have shown reduced "off" time, of 1 to 2 hours, with the addition of entacapone[46,47] or tolcapone[48,49] to levodopa. The clinical benefit is often minimal, however, and in practice such agents are often useful only in mildly fluctuating patients.[50] A 3-year follow-up study of 222 patients found that 122 (56%) had discontinued entacapone, 46% owing to lack of efficacy.[51] Tolcapone may have greater efficacy in controlling motor fluctuations than entacapone,[52] possibly in part owing to the central COMT inhibitor effects lacking in entacapone.

MONOAMINE OXIDASE B INHIBITORS

MAOB inhibition may prolong the duration of action of levodopa by inhibiting the metabolism of dopamine and increasing dopamine levels by 70% in the brain. Selegiline improves mild wearing-off, but not disabling motor fluctuations.[53] A new transmucosal preparation of selegiline (Zydis selegiline) is available that is absorbed directly into the systemic circulation, bypassing first-pass hepatic metabolism and production of theoretically toxic amphetamine-like metabolites.[54]

Studies have shown benefit in treating wearing-off.[55,56] To date, no comparisons have been made with conventional selegiline. Rasagiline, 0.5 mg/day and 1 mg/day, significantly reduced total daily "off" time by 1.41 hours and 1.85 hours,[57] and rasagiline, 1 mg, reduced "off" time by 1.18 hours.[58] There have been no comparative trials of rasagiline and selegiline.

Treatment of Unpredictable "Offs," "On-Off" Fluctuations, and Delayed "On" Responses

Patients can experience unpredictable "offs" that are fast, random, and unrelated to the timing of the last dose of levodopa. Unpredictable and sometimes rapid switching from being "on" and mobile with dyskinesia to being "off" and immobile is referred to as the "on-off" phenomenon. In addition, patients may experience an increase in the latency between taking a dose and experiencing benefit (delayed "on") or absence of benefit from a dose of levodopa (dose failure or no "on" response). These problems may relate to impaired levodopa absorption in the small intestine or across the blood-brain barrier because of competition with dietary amino acids. Taking levodopa on an empty stomach improves absorption and may reduce motor fluctuations. A more recent study has suggested an important role for *Helicobacter pylori* infection in altering levodopa adsorption, and eradication of the *H. pylori* infection may improve motor fluctuations.[59]

LEVODOPA FORMULATIONS

Soluble levodopa prodrug preparations, which are more rapidly and reliably absorbed compared with conventional levodopa, may be helpful for rapid reversal of "off" periods or increased speed of switching on (see Table 15–5).[60] A more recent double-blind randomized controlled trial comparing ethyl ester levodopa with standard levodopa failed, however, to show any significant difference in total daily time to turn-on or dose failures.[61] This trial suggests that such soluble preparations are probably useful only for intermittent as-needed use.

There have been several attempts at enteral delivery of levodopa directly into the duodenum as a way of circumventing the stomach to improve absorption and reduce "on-off" fluctuations.[62,63] An alternative stable suspension of levodopa and carbidopa in methylcellulose (Duodopa) has been developed for enteral administration that improves "on" time without an increase in dyskinesia in advanced PD.[64] This suspension agent may become a useful alternative for PD patients with disabling fluctuations who are not suitable candidates for surgery, although cost and practicality may prevent widespread use.

BEST STRATEGY FOR TREATING MOTOR FLUCTUATIONS IN ADVANCED PARKINSON'S DISEASE

There are very few randomized controlled comparator studies of different treatments for motor fluctuations in PD. Tolcapone has been compared with pergolide and bromocriptine in two short-term trials, but they were underpowered to

TABLE 15–5   Treatment of Motor Fluctuations in Advanced Parkinson's Disease

Motor Fluctuation	Class of Drug	Name	Side Effects	Comments
Predictable wearing-off	Dopamine receptor agonists[16,36,45]	Ropinirole, pramipexole, pergolide, bromocriptine, cabergoline, rotigotine	See Table 15–3	
	COMT inhibitor	Entacapone, tolcapone	Early—nausea, dizziness, increased dyskinesia (improves with levodopa reduction), urine discoloration; late—abdominal pain, severe diarrhea; tolcapone—elevation of liver transaminases (requires monitoring)	Long-term follow-up of effects of liver monitoring of tolcapone—mild increases in transaminases are common, but >3 times normal is rare (1-2%) with no mortality[105,106]
Dose failure, no "on" response, sudden "offs", "on-off" fluctuations	Monoamine oxidase B inhibitor	Selegiline, rasagiline, Zydis selegiline	See Table 15–1	Increased dyskinesia, may improve on reduction of levodopa dose
	Soluble levodopa	Levodopa/benserazide dispersible; levodopa/carbidopa—orally disintegrating tablets; levodopa methylester (melevodopa), levodopa ethylester (etilevodopa)		More reliable absorption than levodopa, but duration of action only 1-1.5 hr

Intraduodenal levodopa infusion pump	Levodopa/carbidopa (Duodopa)		Practical issues—cost, technical issues, and suitable community nursing support may limit use; infusions may also reduce dyskinesia[108,109]
Parenteral dopamine	Apomorphine—intermittent or subcutaneous infusion[107]; lisuride infusion	See Table 15–2 plus skin nodules	
Dyskinesia	Non–subtype selective NMDA receptor antagonist	Amantadine	See Table 15–1	Only a proportion of Parkinson's disease patients may respond well; benefit may last only a few months[110]
	Atypical antipsychotic	Clozapine	Requires blood monitoring for agranulocytosis	Clinical importance not clear because only dyskinesia measured at rest (not during activities) was reduced[77]

COMT, catecholamine O-methyl transferase; NMDA, N-methyl-D-aspartate.

detect clinically relevant differences between treatments.[65,66] In both studies, tolcapone was better tolerated than the DA. A study comparing entacapone with cabergoline also showed a similar reduction in wearing-off, of up to 2 hours, in both groups, but with a quicker onset and better tolerability in the entacapone group.[67] The LARGO study using rasagiline, 1 mg/day, showed similar efficacy to entacapone (200 mg per dose of levodopa) in reducing "off" time, with the one possible advantage of improved morning akinesia with rasagiline, possibly because of its longer duration of action.[58] To date, there seems to be little difference in efficacy for wearing-off between adding in a DA, MAOB inhibitor, or COMT inhibitor, but better tolerability of the last is an advantage. Little attention has been given to the potential additive or synergistic effects of these different treatment modalities.

Treatment of Dyskinesia

The most common form of dyskinesia occurs at the time of maximal improvement in motor symptoms in response to levodopa ("peak-dose dyskinesia"). Dyskinesia also occurs when the levels of levodopa are low, during "off" periods or wearing-off, and at the beginning and end of dose, when the levels of levodopa are increasing and decreasing, known as "diphasic dyskinesia." The decision regarding need for treatment of levodopa-induced dyskinesia is determined by the patient's perceived level of disability. Generally, peak or "on" period dyskinesia responds to a reduction in dopaminergic drugs, but frequently with an increase in parkinsonian disability. In contrast, "off" period and diphasic dyskinesia may respond to treating "off" periods by increasing dopaminergics (see earlier), particularly DAs. Specific pharmacological treatments for levodopa-induced dyskinesia are limited (see Table 15–5). Several agents are undergoing investigation, however; most are targeted at peak and "on" period dyskinesia (Table 15–6). To date, the most effective treatment for all disabling dyskinesia in advanced PD is functional neurosurgery (see Chapter 16).

GLUTAMATE ANTAGONISTS

Currently, the most effective drug in alleviating peak-dose dyskinesia is the non–subtype-selective N-methyl-D-aspartate (NMDA) receptor antagonist, amantadine. Long-term treatment with levodopa results in chronic stimulation of dopamine D1 receptors resulting in enhanced phosphorylation of NMDA and α-amino-3-hydroxy-5-methyl-4-poxazolepropionic acid (AMPA) receptor subunits within the striatum.[68,69] In clinical studies, amantadine significantly reduces dyskinesia, without exacerbating parkinsonism.[70,71] Other nonselective glutamatergic antagonists, such as memantine,[72] riluzole,[73] and remacemide,[74] have not shown efficacy in clinical trials, however. Subtype selective NMDA receptor antagonists may be more effective (see Table 15–6). Subtypes of AMPA receptors are also selectively localized within striatal neurons,[75] and targeting specific subtypes may improve efficacy without side effects. AMPA-selective antagonists reduce dyskinesia in animal models of PD[76]; however, clinical studies are limited (see Table 15–6).

TABLE 15–6	Drugs in Development for Treatment of Advanced Parkinson's Disease		
Class of Drug/ Mechanism of Action	**Drug Name**	**Clinical Effects**	**Comments**
Adenosine A2A receptor antagonists/ Blockade of A2a receptors on indirect striatopallidal pathway reduces GABA release in the globus pallidus; improves parkinsonism without causing dyskinesia[111]	Istradefylline, V2006, BIIB014, SCH 420814	Reduced "off" time (–1.2 hr compared with +0.5 hr with placebo), but with more dyskinesia[112]; phase I/II studies are under way	A2a antagonists are also being developed for neuroprotection (see Chapter ***)
Dopamine reuptake inhibitors/Sustain endogenous and exogenous synaptic dopamine	Tesofensine (NS 2330), O-1369, SEP-226330, SPD-451	Tesofensine ineffective in randomized controlled trial[113]; preclinical level of development[102]	Development of tesofensine has now halted
Reversible MAOB inhibition, modulation of dopamine function, inhibition of glutamate release/ Multiple proposed actions	Safinamide	Low dose (MAOB inhibitory effect?) was ineffective; high dose (affect glutamate release?) effective[114,115]; phase III trials under way	May also have neuroprotective properties[116]
Antiepileptic drug/Na+ channel–blocking; glutamate release inhibitor, MAOB inhibitor	Zonisamide	Improved "off" time by 1.6 hr— no change in dyskinesia[117]	May also be neuroprotective
NR2B-selective NMDA receptor antagonists/ Selective reduction in NMDA-mediated overactivity of glutamate neurotransmission— reduces peak-dose dyskinesia	CP-101, 606, Elipridil	Phase II studies are under way	Conflicting preclinical evidence as to which subtype of NMDA receptors involved in dyskinesia[118,119]
AMPA receptor antagonists/Reduce overactive glutamate neurotransmission— reduces peak dose dyskinesia	Talampanel, Perampanel (E-2007)	Phase II studies completed—no results[120]; phase II studies are under way	Studied for peak-dose dyskinesia; being studied for motor fluctuations

Table continued on following page

TABLE 15–6	**Drugs in Development for Treatment of Advanced Parkinson's Disease** (Continued)		
Class of Drug/ Mechanism of Action	**Drug Name**	**Clinical Effects**	**Comments**
Selective α_2- adrenoceptors antagonists/ Noradrenergic modulation of dopamine and GABAergic function, via α_2-receptors in the basal ganglia[121]	Fipamezole	Phase II study under way	Prior studies using idazoxan showed variable benefit[122]
5-HT1A agonist/5-HT modulates dopamine, GABA, and glutamate in the basal ganglia, via 5-HT1A, 2A, and 2C receptors[123]	Sarizotan	Phase III trial reported no significant benefit on dyskinesia, higher doses also increased "off" time[124]	Sarizotan also has mild D2 receptor blocking effects
Mild 5-HT2A receptor inverse agonist	ACP-103	Phase II study under way[125]	Also being studied as antipsychotic drug

AMPA, α-amino-3-hydroxy-5-methyl-4-poxazolepropionic acid; GABA, γ-aminobutyric acid; MAOB, monoamine oxidase B; NMDA, N-methyl-D-aspartate.

SEROTONINERGIC DRUGS

The atypical antipsychotic clozapine (39.4 ± 4.5 mg/day) has been shown to reduce the duration and the severity of dyskinesia without exacerbating parkinsonian disability (see Table 15–5).[77] In contrast, other so-called atypical antipsychotic drugs either have shown no benefit (e.g., quetiapine)[78] or have worsened parkinsonism (e.g., olanzapine and risperidone).[79,80] The unique pharmacological profile of clozapine may be key to reducing dyskinesia without worsening parkinsonism; this may relate to antagonism at serotonin 5-HT2A/2C receptors and relative affinity of cortical and striatal dopamine D2 receptors, and faster dissociation from the D2 receptor.[81] Other serotoninergic agents have also been investigated in dyskinesia (see Table 15–6).

CONTINUOUS DOPAMINERGIC STIMULATION: ENTERAL LEVODOPA AND PARENTERAL DOPAMINERGIC DRUGS

Continuous dopaminergic stimulation of striatal dopamine receptors in animal models of established motor fluctuations and dyskinesia results in changes within multiple neurotransmitter signaling pathways in the basal ganglia circuitry that are not seen with pulsatile administration of dopaminergics.[34,35,82] A "depriming" of the system results with a reduction in motor fluctuations and dyskinesia. This depriming may explain why continuous infusions using subcutaneous DAs (e.g., apomorphine, lisuride) or enteral levodopa (Duodopa) can be associated with a reduction in dyskinesia and "off" periods (see Table 15–5).[83,84]

Future Treatment Options for Advanced Parkinson's Disease

Table 15–6 provides information on many other drugs under development or recently studied for the treatment of advanced PD.

Nondopaminergic Motor Symptoms of Advanced Parkinson's Disease

The pathology of PD extends outside the nigrostriatal dopaminergic pathway, and as a consequence many symptoms of advanced PD become unresponsive to dopamine replacement. Most of these symptoms involve mood and nonmotor manifestations of the disease and are addressed elsewhere in this book. The predominant motor symptoms unresponsive to levodopa are "midline" or axial symptoms associated with bulbar function, gait, and balance. The neuropharmacology of many of these functions is complex, involving cholinergic, noradrenergic, and serotoninergic systems, and is unlikely to derive from dysfunction of one neurotransmitter system. To date, no effective drug treatments exist for most of these problems. One study that requires confirmation showed a beneficial effect of high doses of methylphenidate (1 mg/kg) for gait disorders that persisted in patients after long-term subthalamic nucleus deep brain stimulation.[85] The management of these drug-resistant motor symptoms relies primarily on nonpharmacological means, including speech pathology and physiotherapy.[86]

REFERENCES

1. Rajput AH, Fenton ME, Birdi S, et al: Clinical-pathological study of levodopa complications. Mov Disord 2002;17:289-296.
2. Kumar N, Van Gerpen JA, Bower JH, Ahlskog JE: Levodopa-dyskinesia incidence by age of Parkinson's disease onset. Mov Disord 2005;20:342-344.
3. Ahlskog JE, Muenter MD: Frequency of levodopa-related dyskinesias and motor fluctuations as estimated from the cumulative literature. Mov Disord 2001;16:448-458.
4. Dodel RC, Berger K, Oertel WH: Health-related quality of life and healthcare utilisation in patients with Parkinson's disease: impact of motor fluctuations and dyskinesias. Pharmacoeconomics 2001;19:1013-1038.
5. Pechevis M, Clarke CE, Vieregge P, et al: Effects of dyskinesias in Parkinson's disease on quality of life and health-related costs: a prospective European study. Eur J Neurol 2005;12:956-963.
6. Marras C, Lang A, Krahn M, et al: Parkinson Study Group. Quality of life in early Parkinson's disease: impact of dyskinesias and motor fluctuations. Mov Disord 2004;19:22-28.
7. Van Gerpen JA, Kumar N, Bower JH, et al: Levodopa-associated dyskinesia risk among Parkinson disease patients in Olmsted County, Minnesota 1976-1990. Arch Neurol 2006;63:205-209.
8. Hely MA, Morris JG, Reid WG, et al: Sydney Multicenter Study of Parkinson's disease: non-L-dopa-responsive problems dominate at 15 years. Mov Disord 2005;20:190-199.
9. Grosset D, Taurah L, Burn DJ, et al: A multicentre longitudinal observational study of changes in self reported health status in people with Parkinson's disease left untreated at diagnosis. J Neurol Neurosurg Psychiatry 2007;78:465-469.

10. Parkinson Study Group. Effect of deprenyl on the progression of disability in early Parkinson's disease. N Engl J Med 1989;321:1364-1371.

11. Shoulson I, Oakes D, Fahn S, et al: Parkinson Study Group. Impact of sustained deprenyl (selegiline) in levodopa-treated Parkinson's disease: a randomized placebo-controlled extension of the deprenyl and tocopherol antioxidative therapy of parkinsonism trial. Ann Neurol 2002;51:604-612.

12. Parkinson Study Group. A controlled trial of rasagiline in early Parkinson disease: the TEMPO Study. Arch Neurol 2002;59:1937-1943.

13. Jenner P: Pharmacology of dopamine agonists in the treatment of Parkinson's disease. Neurology 2002;58(Suppl 1):S1-S8.

14. Millan MJ, Maiofiss L, Cussac D, et al: Differential actions of antiparkinson agents at multiple classes of monoaminergic receptor, I: a multivariate analysis of the binding profiles of 14 drugs at 21 native and cloned human receptor subtypes. J Pharmacol Exp Ther 2002;303:791-804.

15. Miyasaki JM, Martin W, Suchowersky O, et al: Practice parameter: initiation of treatment for Parkinson's disease: an evidence-based review. Report of the Quality Standards Subcommittee of the American Academy of Neurology. Neurology 2002;58:11-17.

16. Goetz CG, Poewe W, Rascol O, Sampaio C: Evidence-based medical review update: pharmacological and surgical treatments of Parkinson's disease: 2001 to 2004. Mov Disord 2005;20:523-539.

17. Horstink M, Tolosa E, Bonuccelli U, et al: European Federation of Neurological Societies; Movement Disorder Society–European Section. Review of the therapeutic management of Parkinson's disease, part I: early (uncomplicated) Parkinson's disease. Report of a joint task force of the European Federation of Neurological Societies and the Movement Disorder Society–European Section. Eur J Neurol 2006;13:1170-1185.

18. Rondot P, Ziegler M: Activity and acceptability of piribedil in Parkinson's disease: a multicentre study. J Neurol 1992;239(Suppl 1):S28-S34.

19. Rinne UK: Lisuride a dopamine agonist in the treatment of early Parkinson's disease. Neurology 1989;39:336-339.

20. Bergamasco B, Frattola L, Muratorio A, et al: Alpha-dihydroergocryptine in the treatment of de novo parkinsonian patients: results of a multicentre, randomized, double-blind, placebo-controlled study. Acta Neurol Scand 2000;101:372-380.

21. Rascol O, Brooks DJ, Korczyn AD, et al: A five-year study of the incidence of dyskinesia in patients with early Parkinson's disease who were treated with ropinirole or levodopa. 056 Study Group. N Engl J Med 2000;342:1484-1491.

22. Parkinson Study Group. Pramipexole vs levodopa as initial treatment for Parkinson disease: a 4-year randomized controlled trial. Arch Neurol 2004;61:1044-1053.

23. Bracco F, Battaglia A, Chouza C, et al: PKDS009 Study Group. The long-acting dopamine receptor agonist cabergoline in early Parkinson's disease: final results of a 5-year, double-blind, levodopa-controlled study. CNS Drugs 2004;18:733-746.

24. Oertel WH, Wolters E, Sampaio C, et al: Pergolide versus levodopa monotherapy in early Parkinson's disease patients: the PELMOPET study. Mov Disord 2006;21:343-353.

25. Rascol O, Brooks DJ, Korczyn AD, et al: 056 Study Group. Development of dyskinesias in a 5-year trial of ropinirole and L-dopa. Mov Disord 2006;21:1844-1850.

26. Constantinescu R, Romer M, McDermott MP, et al: CALM-PD Investigators of the Parkinson Study Group. Impact of pramipexole on the onset of levodopa-related dyskinesias. Mov Disord 2007;22:1317-1319.

27. Lees AJ, Katzenschlager R, Head J, Ben-Shlomo Y: Ten-year follow-up of three different initial treatments in de-novo PD: a randomized trial. Neurology 2001;57:1687-1694.

28. Hauser RA, Rascol O, Korczyn AD, et al: Ten-year follow-up of Parkinson's disease patients randomized to initial therapy with ropinirole or levodopa. Mov Disord 2007;22(16):2409-2417.

29. Robinson S, Smith DM, Mizumori SJ, et al: Firing properties of dopamine neurons in freely moving dopamine-deficient mice: effects of dopamine receptor activation and anesthesia. Proc Natl Acad Sci U S A 2004;101:13329-13334.

30. Mercuri NB, Bernardi G: The "magic" of L-dopa: why is it the gold standard Parkinson's disease therapy? Trends Pharmacol Sci 2005;26:341-344.

31. Jenner P: Dopamine agonists, receptor selectivity and dyskinesia induction in Parkinson's disease. Curr Opin Neurol 2003;16(Suppl 1):S3-S37.

32. Rascol O, Nutt JG, Blin O, et al: Induction by dopamine D1 receptor agonist ABT-431 of dyskinesia similar to levodopa in patients with Parkinson disease. Arch Neurol 2001;58:249-254.

33. Bezard E, Ferry S, Mach U, et al: Attenuation of levodopa-induced dyskinesia by normalizing dopamine D3 receptor function. Nat Med 2003;9:762-767.
34. Goulet M, Grondin R, Blanchet PJ, et al: Dyskinesias and tolerance induced by chronic treatment with a D1 agonist administered in pulsatile or continuous mode do not correlate with changes of putaminal D1 receptors in drug-naive MPTP monkeys. Brain Res 1996;719(1-2):129-137.
35. Blanchet PJ, Calon F, Martel JC, et al: Continuous administration decreases and pulsatile administration increases behavioral sensitivity to a novel dopamine D2 agonist (U-91356A) in MPTP-exposed monkeys. J Pharmacol Exp Ther 1995;272:854-859.
36. Horstink M, Tolosa E, Bonuccelli U, et al: European Federation of Neurological Societies; Movement Disorder Society–European Section. Review of the therapeutic management of Parkinson's disease, part II: late (complicated) Parkinson's disease. Report of a joint task force of the European Federation of Neurological Societies (EFNS) and the Movement Disorder Society–European Section (MDS-ES). Eur J Neurol 2006;13:1186-1202.
37. Fahn S, Oakes D, Shoulson I, et al: Parkinson Study Group. Levodopa and the progression of Parkinson's disease. N Engl J Med 2004;351:2498-2508.
38. Smith LA, Jackson MJ, Al-Barghouthy G, et al: Multiple small doses of levodopa plus entacapone produce continuous dopaminergic stimulation and reduce dyskinesia induction in MPTP-treated drug-naive primates. Mov Disord 2005;20:306-314.
39. Clarke CE, Speller JM, Clarke JA: Pramipexole versus bromocriptine for levodopa-induced complications in Parkinson's disease. Cochrane Database Syst Rev 2000;CD002259.
40. Clarke CE, Deane K: Ropinirole versus bromocriptine for levodopa-induced complications in Parkinson's disease. Cochrane Database Syst Rev 2001;CD001517.
41. Clarke CE, Deane K: Cabergoline versus bromocriptine for levodopa-induced complications in Parkinson's disease. Cochrane Database Syst Rev 2001;CD001519.
42. LeWitt PA, Lyons KE, Pahwa R: SP 650 Study Group. Advanced Parkinson disease treated with rotigotine transdermal system: PREFER Study. Neurology 2007;68:1262-1267.
43. Poewe WH, Rascol O, Quinn N, et al: SP 515 Investigators. Efficacy of pramipexole and transdermal rotigotine in advanced Parkinson's disease: a double-blind, double-dummy, randomised controlled trial. Lancet Neurol 2007;6:513-520.
44. Pahwa R, Stacy MA, Factor SA, et al: EASE-PD Adjunct Study Investigators. Ropinirole 24-hour prolonged release: randomized, controlled study in advanced Parkinson disease. Neurology 2007;68:1108-1115.
45. Pahwa R, Factor SA, Lyons KE, et al: Quality Standards Subcommittee of the American Academy of Neurology. Practice Parameter: treatment of Parkinson disease with motor fluctuations and dyskinesia (an evidence-based review): report of the Quality Standards Subcommittee of the American Academy of Neurology. Neurology 2006;66:983-995.
46. Ruottinen HM, Rinne UK: Entacapone prolongs levodopa response in a one month double blind study in parkinsonian patients with levodopa related fluctuations. J Neurol Neurosurg Psychiatry 1996;60:36-40.
47. Parkinson Study Group. Entacapone improves motor fluctuations in levodopa-treated Parkinson's disease patients. Ann Neurol 1997;42:747-755.
48. Rajput AH, Martin W, Saint-Hilaire MH, et al: Tolcapone improves motor function in parkinsonian patients with the "wearing-off" phenomenon: a double-blind, placebo-controlled, multicenter trial. Neurology 1997;49:1066-1071.
49. Kurth MC, Adler CH, Hilaire MS, et al: Tolcapone improves motor function and reduces levodopa requirement in patients with Parkinson's disease experiencing motor fluctuations: a multicenter, double-blind, randomized, placebo-controlled trial. Tolcapone Fluctuator Study Group I: Neurology 1997;48:81-87.
50. Fénelon G, Giménez-Roldán S, Montastruc JL, et al: Efficacy and tolerability of entacapone in patients with Parkinson's disease treated with levodopa plus a dopamine agonist and experiencing wearing-off motor fluctuations: a randomized, double-blind, multicentre study. J Neural Transm 2003;110:239-251.
51. Parashos SA, Wielinski CL, Kern JA: Frequency, reasons, and risk factors of entacapone discontinuation in Parkinson disease. Clin Neuropharmacol 2004;27:119-123.
52. Entacapone to Tolcapone Switch Study Investigators. Entacapone to tolcapone switch: multicenter double-blind, randomized, active-controlled trial in advanced Parkinson's disease. Mov Disord 2007;22:14-19.
53. Lees AJ, Shaw KM, Kohout LJ, et al: Deprenyl in Parkinson's disease. Lancet 1977;15:791-795.
54. Clarke A, Brewer F, Johnson ES, et al: A new formulation of selegiline: improved bioavailability and selectivity for MAO-B inhibition. J Neural Transm 2003;110:1241-1255.

55. Waters CH, Sethi KD, Hauser RA, et al: Zydis Selegiline Study Group. Zydis selegiline reduces off time in Parkinson's disease patients with motor fluctuations: a 3-month, randomized, placebo-controlled study. Mov Disord 2004;19:426-432.

56. Lew MF, Pahwa R, Leehey M, et al: The Zydis Selegiline Study Group. Safety and efficacy of newly formulated selegiline orally disintegrating tablets as an adjunct to levodopa in the management of "off" episodes in patients with Parkinson's disease. Curr Med Res Opin 2007;23:741-750.

57. Parkinson Study Group. A randomized placebo-controlled trial of rasagiline in levodopa-treated patients with Parkinson disease and motor fluctuations: the PRESTO study. Arch Neurol 2005;62:241-248.

58. Rascol O, Brooks DJ, Melamed E, et al: LARGO study group. Rasagiline as an adjunct to levodopa in patients with Parkinson's disease and motor fluctuations (LARGO, Lasting effect in Adjunct therapy with Rasagiline Given Once daily, study): a randomised, double-blind, parallel-group trial. Lancet 2005;365:947-954.

59. Pierantozzi M, Pietroiusti A, Brusa L, et al: *Helicobacter pylori* eradication and l-dopa absorption in patients with PD and motor fluctuations. Neurology 2006;66:1824-1829.

60. Stocchi F, Fabbri L, Vecsei L, et al: Clinical efficacy of a single afternoon dose of effervescent levodopa-carbidopa preparation (CHF 1512) in fluctuating Parkinson disease. Clin Neuropharmacol 2007;30:18-24.

61. Blindauer K, Shoulson I, Oakes D, et al: Parkinson Study Group. A randomized controlled trial of etilevodopa in patients with Parkinson disease who have motor fluctuations. Arch Neurol 2006;63:210-216.

62. Kurlan R, Rubin AJ, Miller C, et al: Duodenal delivery of levodopa for on-off fluctuations in parkinsonism: preliminary observations. Ann Neurol 1986;20:262-265.

63. Kurth MC, Tetrud JW, Tanner CM, et al: Double-blind, placebo-controlled, crossover study of duodenal infusion of levodopa/carbidopa in Parkinson's disease patients with "on-off" fluctuations. Neurology 1993;43:1698-1703.

64. Nyholm D: Enteral levodopa/carbidopa gel infusion for the treatment of motor fluctuations and dyskinesias in advanced Parkinson's disease. Exp Rev Neurother 2006;6:1403-1411.

65. Tolcapone Study Group. Efficacy and tolerability of tolcapone compared with bromocriptine in levodopa-treated parkinsonian patients. Mov Disord 1999;14:38-44.

66. Koller W, Lees A, Doder M, et al: Tolcapone/Pergolide Study Group. Randomized trial of tolcapone versus pergolide as add-on to levodopa therapy in Parkinson's disease patients with motor fluctuations. Mov Disord 2001;16(5):858-866.

67. Deuschl G, Vaitkus A, Fox GC, et al: CAMP Study Group. Efficacy and tolerability of Entacapone versus Cabergoline in parkinsonian patients suffering from wearing-off. Mov Disord 2007;22:1550-1555.

68. Chase TN, Bibbiani F, Oh JD: Striatal glutamatergic mechanisms and extrapyramidal movement disorders. Neurotox Res 2003;5:139-146.

69. Hallett PJ, Dunah AW, Ravenscroft P, et al: Alterations of striatal NMDA receptor subunits associated with the development of dyskinesia in the MPTP-lesioned primate model of Parkinson's disease. Neuropharmacology 2005;48:503-516.

70. Verhagen Metman L, Del Dotto P, van den Munckhof P, et al: Amantadine as treatment for dyskinesias and motor fluctuations in Parkinson's disease. Neurology 1998;50:1323-1326.

71. Snow BJ, Macdonald L, McAuley D, et al: The effect of amantadine on levodopa-induced dyskinesias in Parkinson's disease: a double-blind, placebo-controlled study. Clin Neuropharmacol 2000;23:82-85.

72. Merello M, Nouzeilles MI, Cammarota A, et al: Effect of memantine (NMDA antagonist) on Parkinson's disease: a double-blind crossover randomized study. Clin Neuropharmacol 1999;22:273-276.

73. Braz CA, Borges V, Ferraz HB: Effect of riluzole on dyskinesia and duration of the on state in Parkinson disease patients: a double-blind, placebo-controlled pilot study. Clin Neuropharmacol 2004;27:25-29.

74. Parkinson Study Group. Evaluation of dyskinesias in a pilot, randomized, placebo-controlled trial of remacemide in advanced Parkinson disease. Arch Neurol 2001;58:1660-1668.

75. Deng YP, Xie JP, Wang HB, et al: Differential localization of the GluR1 and GluR2 subunits of the AMPA-type glutamate receptor among striatal neuron types in rats. J Chem Neuroanat 2007;33:167-192.

76. Konitsiotis S, Blanchet PJ, Verhagen L, et al: AMPA receptor blockade improves levodopa-induced dyskinesia in MPTP monkeys. Neurology 2000;54:1589-1595.

77. Durif F, Debilly B, Galitzky M, et al: Clozapine improves dyskinesias in Parkinson disease—a double-blind, placebo-controlled study. Neurology 2004;62:381-388.

78. Katzenschlager R, Manson AJ, Evans A, et al: Low dose quetiapine for drug induced dyskinesias in Parkinson's disease: a double blind cross over study. J Neurol Neurosurg Psychiatry 2004;75:295-297.
79. Goetz CG, Blasucci LM, Leurgans S, et al: Olanzapine and clozapine: comparative effects on motor function in hallucinating PD patients. Neurology 2000;26:789-794.
80. van de Vijver DA, Roos RA, Jansen PA, et al: Antipsychotics and Parkinson's disease: association with disease and drug choice during the first 5 years of antiparkinsonian drug treatment. Eur J Clin Pharmacol 2002;58:157-161.
81. Kapur S, Seeman P: Does fast dissociation from the dopamine d(2) receptor explain the action of atypical antipsychotics? A new hypothesis. Am J Psychiatry 2001;158:360-369.
82. Chase TN: The significance of continuous dopaminergic stimulation in the treatment of Parkinson's disease. Drugs 1998;55(Suppl 1):1-9.
83. Olanow CW, Obeso JA, Stocchi F: Continuous dopamine-receptor treatment of Parkinson's disease: scientific rationale and clinical implications. Lancet Neurol 2006;5:677-687.
84. Nutt J: Continuous dopaminergic stimulation: is it the answer to the motor complications of levodopa? Mov Disord 2007;22:1-9.
85. Devos D, Krystkowiak P, Clement F, et al: Improvement of gait by chronic, high doses of methylphenidate in patients with advanced Parkinson's disease. J Neurol Neurosurg Psychiatry 2007;78:470-475.
86. Fox SH, Lang AE: Treatment of motor complications in advanced Parkinson's disease. In: Hallett M, Peowe W, eds: Therapeutics of Parkinson's disease and other movement disorders. New York, John Wiley and Sons Ltd., 2008, 71-90.
87. Ives NJ, Stowe R, Marro J, et al: Monoamine oxidase type B inhibitors in early Parkinson's disease: meta-analysis of 17 randomised trials involving 3525 patients. BMJ 2004;329:593.
88. Marras C, McDermott MP, Rochon PA, et al: Parkinson Study Group. Survival in Parkinson disease: thirteen-year follow-up of the DATATOP cohort. Neurology 2005;64:87-93.
89. Biglan KM, Holloway RG Jr, McDermott MP, et al: Parkinson Study Group CALM-PD Investigators. Risk factors for somnolence, edema, and hallucinations in early Parkinson disease. Neurology 2007;69:187-195.
90. Monti JM, Monti D: The involvement of dopamine in the modulation of sleep and waking. Sleep Med Rev 2007;11:113-133.
91. Gjerstad MD, Alves G, Wentzel-Larsen T, et al: Excessive daytime sleepiness in Parkinson disease: is it the drug or the disease? Neurology 2006;67:853-858.
92. Fenelon G, Mahieux F, Huon R, Ziegler M: Hallucinations in Parkinson's disease: prevalence, phenomenology and risk factors. Brain 2000;123:733-745.
93. Evans AH, Katzenschlager R, Paviour D, et al: Punding in Parkinson's disease: its relation to the dopamine dysregulation syndrome. Mov Disord 2004;19:397-405.
94. Voon V, Hassan K, Zurowski M, et al: Prospective prevalence of pathologic gambling and medication association in Parkinson disease. Neurology 2006;66:1750-1752.
95. Weintraub D, Siderowf AD, Potenza MN, et al: Association of dopamine agonist use with impulse control disorders in Parkinson disease. Arch Neurol 2006;63:969-973.
96. Voon V, Thomsen T, Miyasaki JM, et al: Factors associated with dopaminergic drug-related pathological gambling in Parkinson disease. Arch Neurol 2007;64:212-216.
97. Gallagher DA, O'Sullivan SS, Evans AH, et al: Pathological gambling in Parkinson's disease: risk factors and differences from dopamine dysregulation. An analysis of published case series. Mov Disord 2007;22:1757-1763.
98. Agarwal P, Fahn S, Frucht SJ: Diagnosis and management of pergolide-induced fibrosis. Mov Disord 2004;19:699-704.
99. Simonis G, Fuhrmann JT, Strasser RH: Meta-analysis of heart valve abnormalities in Parkinson's disease patients treated with dopamine agonists. Mov Disord 2007;22:1936-1942.
100. Singer C, Lamb J, Ellis A, Layton G: Sumanirole for Early Parkinson's Disease Study Group. A comparison of sumanirole versus placebo or ropinirole for the treatment of patients with early Parkinson's disease. Mov Disord 2007;22:476-482.
101. Barone P, Lamb J, Ellis A, Clarke Z: Sumanirole versus placebo or ropinirole for the adjunctive treatment of patients with advanced Parkinson's disease. Mov Disord 2007;22:483-489.
102. Johnston TH, Brotchie JM: Drugs in development for Parkinson's disease: an update. Curr Opin Invest Drugs 2006;7:25-32.
103. Watts RL, Jankovic J, Waters C, et al: Randomized, blind, controlled trial of transdermal rotigotine in early Parkinson disease. Neurology 2007;68:272-276.
104. Woitalla D, Müller T, Benz S, et al: Transdermal lisuride delivery in the treatment of Parkinson's disease. J Neural Transm Suppl 2004;68:89-95.

105. Olanow CW, Watkins PB: Tolcapone: an efficacy and safety review (2007). Clin Neuropharmacol 2007;30:287-294.
106. Lees AJ, Ratziu V, Tolosa E, et al: Safety and tolerability of adjunctive tolcapone treatment in patients with early Parkinson's disease. J Neurol Neurosurg Psychiatry 2007;78:944.
107. Dewey RB Jr, Hutton JT, LeWitt PA, et al: A randomized, double-blind, placebo-controlled trial of subcutaneously injected apomorphine for parkinsonian off-state events. Arch Neurol 2001;58:1385-1392.
108. Katzenschlager R, Hughes A, Evans A, et al: Continuous subcutaneous apomorphine therapy improves dyskinesias in Parkinson's disease: a prospective study using single-dose challenges. Mov Disord 2005;20:151-157.
109. Stocchi F, Ruggieri S, Vacca L, et al: Prospective randomized trial of lisuride infusion versus oral levodopa in patients with Parkinson's disease. Brain 2002;125:2058-2066.
110. Thomas A, Iacono D, Luciano AL, et al: Duration of amantadine benefit on dyskinesia of severe Parkinson's disease. J Neurol Neurosurg Psychiatry 2004;75:141-143.
111. Ochi M, Koga K, Kurokawa M, et al: Systemic administration of adenosine A(2A) receptor antagonist reverses increased GABA release in the globus pallidus of unilateral 6-hydroxydopamine-lesioned rats: a microdialysis study. Neuroscience 2000;100:53-62.
112. Hauser RA, Hubble JP, Truong DD: Randomized trial of the adenosine A(2A) receptor antagonist istradefylline in advanced PD. Neurology 2003;61:297-303.
113. Hauser RA, Salin L, Juhel N, Konyago VL: Randomized trial of the triple monoamine reuptake inhibitor NS 2330 (tesofensine) in early Parkinson's disease. Mov Disord 2007;22:359-365.
114. Stocchi F, Arnold G, Onofrj M, et al: Safinamide Parkinson's Study Group. Improvement of motor function in early Parkinson disease by safinamide. Neurology 2004;63:746-748.
115. Stocchi F, Vacca L, Grassini P, et al: Symptom relief in Parkinson disease by safinamide: biochemical and clinical evidence of efficacy beyond MAO-B inhibition. Neurology 2006;67 (7 Suppl 2):S24-S29.
116. Caccia C, Maj R, Calabresi M, et al: Safinamide: from molecular targets to a new anti-Parkinson drug. Neurology 2006;67;(7 Suppl 2):S18-S23.
117. Murata M, Hasegawa K, Kanazawa I: The Japan Zonisamide on PD Study Group. Zonisamide improves motor function in Parkinson disease: a randomized, double-blind study. Neurology 2007;68:45-50.
118. Blanchet PJ, Konitsiotis S, Whittemore ER, et al: Differing effects of N-methyl-D-aspartate receptor subtype selective antagonists on dyskinesias in levodopa-treated 1-methyl-4-phenyl-tetrahydropyridine monkeys. J Pharmacol Exp Ther 1999;290:1034-1040.
119. Nash JE, Ravenscroft P, McGuire S, et al: The NR2B-selective NMDA receptor antagonist CP-101,606 exacerbates L-DOPA-induced dyskinesia and provides mild potentiation of anti-parkinsonian effects of L-DOPA in the MPTP-lesioned marmoset model of Parkinson's disease. Exp Neurol 2004;188:471-479.
120. Wu SS, Frucht SJ: Treatment of Parkinson's disease: what's on the horizon? CNS Drugs 2005;19:723-743.
121. Savola JM, Hill M, Engstrom M, et al: Fipamezole (JP-1730) is a potent alpha2 adrenergic receptor antagonist that reduces LID in the MPTP-lesioned primate model of Parkinson's disease. Mov Disord 2003;18:872-883.
122. Fox SH, Lang AE, Brotchie JM: Translation of nondopaminergic treatments for levodopa-induced dyskinesia from MPTP-lesioned nonhuman primates to phase IIa clinical studies: keys to success and roads to failure. Mov Disord 2006;21:1578-1594.
123. Nicholson SL, Brotchie JM: 5-hydroxytryptamine (5-HT, serotonin) and Parkinson's disease—opportunities for novel therapeutics to reduce the problems of levodopa therapy. Eur J Neurol 2002;9(Suppl 3):1-6.
124. Goetz CG, Damier P, Hicking C, et al: Sarizotan as a treatment for dyskinesias in Parkinson's disease: a double-blind placebo-controlled trial. Mov Disord 2007;22:179-186.
125. Roberts A: CACP-103, a 5-HT2A receptor inverse agonist. Curr Opin Invest Drugs 2006;7: 653-660.

16 Surgical Therapy for Parkinson's Disease

ADRIAN W. LAXTON • CLEMENT HAMANI •
ANDRES M. LOZANO

Introduction

Surgical therapy has become a standard adjunctive treatment option for patients with Parkinson's disease (PD).[1-3] This development, which represents a significant change in practice for movement disorder specialists, has arisen as a result of three main factors. First, although levodopa remains a first-line therapy for PD, a substantial percentage of patients, although still responsive to levodopa, experience motor fluctuations and adverse effects with long-term use.[4,5] These adverse effects can take several forms. Some patients experience prolonged or unpredictable "off" states in which disabling tremors, rigidity, akinesia, or painful dystonias predominate.[6] Most PD patients taking levodopa eventually develop levodopa-induced dyskinesias, which can be disabling dystonic or choreoathetotic movements during "on" periods.[7] Therapeutic alternatives, such as surgical therapy, are needed for a large proportion of PD patients who continue to be disabled despite best medical therapy. Second, although past surgical procedures involved the permanent ablation of brain regions and the associated possibility of permanent adverse side effects, deep brain stimulation (DBS) has emerged as a safe, modifiable, and reversible surgical procedure for the treatment of movement disorders. Finally, numerous studies have been published that show

TABLE 16–1	Ideal Candidates for Surgical Therapy in Parkinson's Disease

Patients with a diagnosis of idiopathic Parkinson's disease who
  Are responsive to dopaminergic medication, such as levodopa
  Have prolonged or unpredictable "off" periods *or* disabling levodopa-induced
    dyskinesias or motor fluctuations
  Are <70 years old
  Have no active psychiatric disorders or dementia
  Have no serious medical comorbidities that would preclude surgery

the ability of surgical therapy to optimize the medical management of PD.[4,8-22] For these reasons, surgical therapy is now used increasingly for patients with PD.

This chapter reviews the surgical options for treating PD, and summarizes the indications, anatomical targets, and surgical techniques. The relevant anatomy and pathophysiology and the proposed mechanisms of action of DBS are discussed. We also discuss the evidence supporting the use of surgical therapy for PD. The focus of this chapter is on DBS because it is currently the most commonly used modality in movement disorder surgery.

Surgical Indications

Surgical therapy may be considered for idiopathic PD patients who continue to respond to dopaminergic therapy, but whose response is of limited, unpredictable, or decreasing duration (i.e., patients with prolonged "off" periods), or who experience significant levodopa-induced side effects, including dyskinesias and psychiatric adverse effects (Table 16–1).[1,2,6,12,23-25] PD patients who are generally considered unsuitable for surgery are patients in whom the risk-to-benefit ratio is less favorable. This includes patients who are older than 70 years[12,26]; patients with atypical parkinsonism or Parkinson-plus syndromes, such as multiple system atrophy; patients who have an active psychiatric disorder or dementia; and patients who have serious medical comorbidities, such as unstable heart disease, advanced lung disease, active infection, or any condition that significantly limits their life expectancy such as cancer.[6,12]

Although PD patients are typically referred for surgical therapy many years after being diagnosed, when motor complications have significantly detracted from their quality of life, there is now evidence that earlier surgery may lead to better outcomes.[14,19,27] The primary goal of DBS is to re-establish the maximal benefit the patient previously achieved with levodopa, or to allow a levodopa dose reduction that would diminish drug-induced dyskinesias, while maintaining the patient in a good "on" state throughout the day.

Surgical Targets

For patients with PD, the most commonly used DBS target is the subthalamic nucleus (STN) (Fig. 16–1).[4,9,10,12,14,16,18] The internal segment of the globus pallidus (GPi) is another potential target.[8,9] STN and GPi DBS are used to improve the

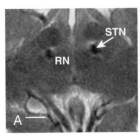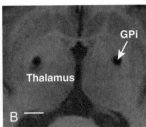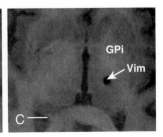

Figure 16–1 A-C, Magnetic resonance images of deep brain stimulation electrodes (*arrows*) implanted in the subthalamic nucleus (STN) **(A),** globus pallidus (GPi) **(B),** and ventral intermediate nucleus of the thalamus (Vim) **(C).** RN, red nucleus. *Scale bars* = 10 mm.

cardinal features of PD: bradykinesia, rigidity, and tremor.[28] For PD patients whose most disabling feature is tremor, the ventral intermediate nucleus of the thalamus (Vim) is a potential target,[29,30] although this is now much less commonly used than STN or GPi DBS for PD because it addresses only tremor.

Other potential surgical targets are now being investigated for patients with PD. DBS of the pedunculopontine nucleus has been reported in combination with STN DBS for PD patients.[20,31] Combining STN and pedunculopontine nucleus DBS may be more effective than STN DBS alone at improving gait disturbances and the axial symptoms of PD. Another investigational target is the caudal part of the zona incerta. In one report comparing PD patients who had undergone STN DBS with PD patients who had undergone zona incerta DBS, the authors found that improvements in contralateral motor scores (as measured by the Unified Parkinson's Disease Rating Scale) were greater after zona incerta DBS.[21]

Surgical Options

Before the development of DBS, lesioning procedures were the standard surgical approach to treat movement disorders.[11,15,17] Lesions are made with high-radiofrequency stimulation to the same targets used in DBS surgery. In ablative surgery, in contrast to DBS surgery, the STN is not the most commonly targeted structure. Desirable features of ablative surgery are that it involves a single procedure requiring less operating room time, requires no implanted hardware (meaning less infection risk), requires no ongoing adjustments, and has lower cost relative to DBS. Because ablative procedures involve the targeted creation of permanent brain lesions, however, they are also associated with unmodifiable treatment effects and potentially permanent adverse side effects. In particular, bilateral ablative procedures have generally been avoided because of the risk of unacceptable complications, leaving bilaterally affected patients inadequately treated.[2]

The adjustability and reversibility of DBS are two of its main advantages over lesioning procedures. With DBS therapy, stimulation parameters can be adjusted to enhance or maximize a positive effect, or to decrease unwanted side effects. Postoperative programming of the DBS system involves adjustments to the following parameters: choice of contact, type of stimulation (monopolar or bipolar), amplitude (voltage), frequency, and pulse width. The DBS system can be completely removed, returning the patient to his or her baseline level of function. Compared with ablative surgery, bilateral treatment with DBS is usually better tolerated. The major disadvantages of DBS include its expense; the need to replace internal pulse generators (IPGs) (i.e., the batteries) every 3 to 5 years, which involves minor surgery; and because it entails implanted foreign bodies, an increased infection risk relative to lesions.

Many alternative surgical treatment strategies are at the investigational stage, including intraventricular[32] and intraputaminal[33,34] injections of glial-derived neurotrophic factor, intrastriatal dopaminergic cell transplantation,[35,36] STN-targeted glutamic acid decarboxylase gene therapy,[37] motor cortex stimulation,[38,39] and intra-STN microinjections of lidocaine and muscimol.[40] For now, there is limited or preliminary evidence to support the use of these novel alternative strategies in PD. Because of its demonstrated therapeutic effects and its advantages over lesioning, DBS is presently the predominant surgical therapy used to treat PD.

Description of Deep Brain Stimulation

DBS involves the placement of electrode leads into desired brain regions to deliver targeted and adjustable electrical current. The electrode leads are connected to a programmable IPG, which is placed subcutaneously below the patient's clavicle (Fig. 16–2). Each DBS lead has four electrodes at its tip, typically 1.5 mm wide and 0.5 or 1.5 mm apart. The DBS leads are made out of polyurethane tubing, and the electrodes are made out of platinum and iridium. The IPG consists of a silver vanadium oxide or lithium ion cell and integrated circuits encased in titanium with an insulating coating.

Stimulation parameters are commonly set to a frequency of 130 to 185 Hz, a pulse width of 60 to 120 μsec, and an amplitude of 2 to 4 volts.[41] The typical wave shape of the delivered stimulation is square. Although stimulation can be delivered continuously or in cycles, the continuous mode is used most commonly. The longevity of the IPG battery depends on the stimulation parameters set for each patient. With typical stimulation parameters, the IPG needs to be replaced every 3 to 5 years.[42]

Anatomy and Pathophysiology

Surgical therapy for PD has developed from an understanding of the functional neuroanatomy of the cortical-basal ganglia–thalamic-cortical circuit and the pathophysiology of movement disorders.[2,3,43,44] A fundamental pathophysiological feature of PD is the degeneration of dopaminergic neurons in the (SNc) substantia nigra zona compacta.[2,43-46] Dopamine depletion leads to alterations in neuronal activity that are funneled to the output structures of the basal ganglia and conveyed to the thalamus and then to the corresponding cortical terminal fields to cause the widespread disturbance in function that is characteristic of PD. Several theories have been proposed for how the activity within this circuit is regulated. There is evidence for alterations in neuronal firing rates, changes in patterns of discharges and neuronal bursting behavior, the emergence of oscillatory behavior

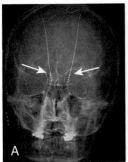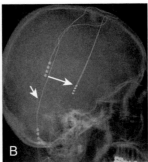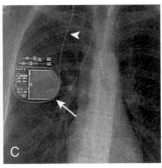

Figure 16–2 A-C, X-ray images showing a patient with subthalamic nucleus deep brain stimulation. Anteroposterior **(A)** and lateral **(B)** skull x-rays show the bilaterally implanted electrodes with four contacts each (*large arrows* are pointing at the most dorsal contacts). The *small arrow* in **B** is pointing to one of the extension cables that connect the electrodes to the internal pulse generator. **C,** Chest x-ray showing the extension cables (*arrowhead*) that connect the internal pulse generator (*arrow*) to the electrodes.

among specific groups of neurons, enhanced correlated activity across neurons, and the expansion of sensorimotor receptive fields as potential contributors to the pathophysiology of PD.[43,44,47,48] Points of surgical intervention include basal ganglia output structures such as the globus pallidus or the upstream regulatory nucleus, the STN, or thalamic nuclei that regulate cortical motor areas.

Mechanism of Action of Deep Brain Stimulation

The purpose of DBS is to disrupt the abnormal neuronal activity underlying PD and re-establish more normal motor function.[2] The specific mechanisms responsible for the effects of DBS are incompletely understood.[49-53] Electrical brain stimulation affects a broad range of neural elements, including neuronal cell bodies, axons, and glia. The electrophysiological properties associated with each of these elements vary depending on anatomical location. The effects of electrical stimulation on these elements are thought to vary with the intrinsic properties of the stimulated elements, with the stimulation parameters used (i.e., frequency, amplitude, and pulse width), and with the distance of the element from the stimulating electrode.[51,52]

Because high-frequency stimulation (HFS) of certain targets mimics some of the effects of lesions to those targets, it had been believed that stimulation produces a functional "lesion."[44] This simple view ignores the possibility of stimulation disrupting pathological activity through other mechanisms, however, including activating inhibitory afferents, the potential complex polysynaptic downstream effects of local activation, the possible differential effect of stimulation on cell bodies versus axons, and the possibility that HFS may lead to neurotransmitter depletion or synaptic failure.[24,50] To account better for the mechanisms of DBS, several explanations have been proposed.

It has been observed that single pulses in the vicinity of GPi neurons produce a cessation of spontaneous activity for 15 to 25 msec.[54] Because of the latency and duration of this effect, it has been suggested that stimulation near the GPi causes γ-aminobutyric acid (GABA) release from either pallidal (pars externa) or striatal axons projecting onto GPi neurons, or local dendritic release of GABA resulting in GPi neuronal inhibition. Although the GPi also receives glutamatergic afferents from the STN, the greater GABAergic input and the spatial topography of its synapses are believed to trump these excitatory signals. Further supporting the synaptic transmission proposal, studies have shown increased firing rates in the GPi after STN HFS,[55] and alterations in firing rates in the thalamus after GPi HFS.[56,57] Similarly, glutamate release in the STN[58] and in the downstream GPi and substantia nigra zona reticulata[59,60] has been found to be increased after STN HFS. These excitatory effects are thought to result from the activation of axonal fiber tracts, whereas stimulation of neuronal cell bodies is believed to be inhibitory.[24,49,61-63]

Computer modeling studies corroborate this perspective, showing that DBS may inhibit neuronal cell bodies and excite axons.[64-67] Functional imaging studies show alterations in cerebral cortical activity with STN and GPi DBS.[68,69] The effect of stimulation on axons also depends on the axons' proximity to the stimulating electrode, the amplitude of stimulation, and the orientation of the delivered current in relation to the stimulated axon.[24,70] The extent to which an axon is activated depends on the component of the voltage gradient parallel to the axon that provides an appropriate level of stimulation (dictated by the amplitude delivered by the electrode and the electrode's distance from the axon).[70] A variation on the synaptic transmission proposal states that although HFS is excitatory, the stores of neurotransmitter are soon depleted, resulting in functional inhibition.[24,71]

The ability of HFS to alter intrinsic membrane properties also has been posited as a potential mechanism of DBS.[72] Some in vitro studies suggest that HFS transiently depresses voltage-gated Ca^{2+} channels producing a "depolarization block."[73] Alternatively, HFS may help to replenish vesicle stores via calcium-dependent mechanisms.[74] HFS also may directly affect Na^+ channels, leading to initial depolarization and then slow inactivation.[61,75] The relevance of these in vitro findings awaits further investigation.

The varied and seemingly disparate explanations for DBS effects may actually be complementary. That is, the effect of DBS may depend on several mechanisms, and the effects may vary depending on what structures are being stimulated, and how far a structure is from the stimulating electrode.[24,49,50] The net effect of DBS seems, however, to be to disrupt the dysfunctional neuronal activity associated with PD.

▎ Operative Procedure

The specific details of DBS insertion and implantation vary depending on the preferences and expertise of the neurosurgical team performing the procedure. Some of the variations include the type of stereotactic frame used (e.g., Leksell, Cosman-Roberts-Wells, or, more recently, "frameless" systems), the timing of frame application and IPG implantation, the use of general versus local anesthetic, and the use of intraoperative microelectrode recordings.[25,28] Generally, DBS procedures involve the application of a stereotactic frame to the patient's skull, brain imaging with the applied frame, insertion of DBS electrodes, and implantation of the electrodes and IPG (Fig. 16–3).

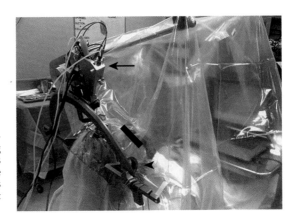

Figure 16–3 Intraoperative photograph of a patient undergoing deep brain stimulation. The *arrow* is pointing at the dual microelectrode recording stage. The *arrowhead* is pointing at the Leksell stereotactic frame.

In most centers, the identification of targets is based on the patient's preoperative MRI. Two general methods for determining the target location are used: *indirect*, based on standard target locations relative to the anterior and posterior commissure (AC-PC) coordinates,[28] or the red nucleus,[76] and *direct*, based on the identification of the target structure on the patient's MRI. Because a "one-size-fits-all" approach is inappropriate, direct targeting is usually preferred. In contrast to the STN and GPi, the Vim currently can be targeted only using indirect methods and electrophysiology. Typical indirect targets are as follows: for the STN—12 mm lateral to midline, 3 to 4 mm posterior to the midcommissural point, and 3 to 4 mm ventral to the intercommissural or AC-PC line; for the GPi—20 to 21 mm lateral to midline, 3 mm anterior to the midcommissural point, and 5 mm ventral to the AC-PC line; and for the Vim—11 to 12 mm lateral to the wall of the third ventricle and 4 to 6 mm anterior to the posterior commissure at the level of the AC-PC line. The insertion of the electrode leads is done through burr holes, commonly located 20 to 30 mm lateral to midline and 5 to 10 mm anterior to the coronal suture. Typical trajectory angles for the electrode leads are 50 to 70 degrees in the sagittal plane and 15 to 30 degrees in the coronal plane.[77]

Intraoperative Electrophysiological Mapping

Intraoperative electrophysiological mapping is used to characterize and confirm the location of the recording electrode in relation to the desired target, to assess the therapeutic effect of an electrode in a particular location, and to identify the potential unwanted side effects associated with stimulation in a given location.[77] Various approaches may be used, which may involve one or more microelectrodes (single unit recording; local field potentials; microstimulation)[78] or macroelectrodes (usually, the DBS electrode itself; local field potentials; macrostimulation). Most DBS centers that have published their experience use some combination of these techniques.[3,77] Neurosurgeons at most academic centers believe that electrophysiological mapping helps to localize targets accurately and improve outcomes.[25,77] Nevertheless, some functional neurosurgeons forego intraoperative microelectrode recordings.[79,80]

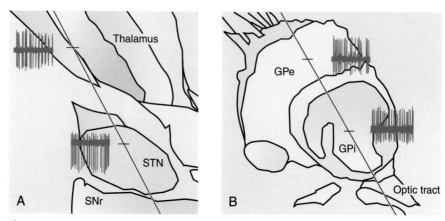

Figure 16–4 A and **B,** Schematic representations of sagittal sections of the brain that are 12 mm **(A)** and 20 mm **(B)** from the midline. The oblique line in the center of each image represents a typical microelectrode trajectory during intraoperative mapping of the subthalamic nucleus (STN) **(A)** and globus pallidus (GPi) **(B)**. **A,** During STN mapping, neuronal activity may be recorded from the thalamus, STN, and substantia nigra zona reticulata (SNr). Examples of a thalamic bursting cell and an irregularly firing STN cell are shown on the left side of the trajectory line. **B,** Neuronal activity recorded from the globus pallidus externus (GPe) and GPi. Stimulation of the optic tract often induces phosphenes, and identifies the bottom of the trajectory. Details on the neuronal firing characteristics in each of these regions can be found in the text.

Standard mapping of the STN begins with microelectrode recordings starting 10 to 15 mm above the chosen target.[81] The single unit activity recorded depends on the specific trajectory chosen, but may include the following structures in order (Fig. 16–4): the thalamus (with its characteristic bursting cells), the zona incerta (exhibiting a low firing rate), the STN (with its characteristic dense cellular activity ranging from 30 to 50 Hz, and occasional 4- to 6-Hz bursting activity synchronized to the patient's tremor), and the substantia nigra zona reticulata (characterized by a more regular firing rate in the 50- to 70-Hz range, without bursting or tremor cells).[77,81,82] When the STN has been reached, testing begins to determine if the cellular activity changes in response to the patient's active or passive limb movements. The presence of movement-related activity identifies the sensorimotor target territory.

Stimulation may then be performed within the STN to check for clinical benefits, including improvement in bradykinesia, decreased rigidity, and tremor arrest, or to detect the presence of paresthesias, muscle contractions, diplopia, or other unwanted side effects. The microelectrodes may be repositioned to sample other STN areas, and to identify the STN motor territory better. The microelectrodes are removed and replaced by the DBS electrode. In some centers, this insertion is done using x-ray guidance to ensure that the electrode is placed in the desired location. When in place, each contact of the DBS electrode is stimulated with incrementally increasing voltage to check the threshold for stimulation-induced clinical benefit and unwanted side effects. The DBS electrode position can be adjusted if necessary to minimize adverse effects.

The general procedure and rationale for intraoperative electrophysiological mapping of the GPi and Vim is similar to that described for the STN except for differences in regional anatomy and associated cellular characteristics. The microelectrode trajectory to the GPi traverses through the striatum, the globus pallidus externus (firing activity ~50 Hz), the GPi (high frequency activity ~80 Hz with occasional 4- to 6-Hz tremor-associated bursts), and either the optic tract (inferiorly) or the internal capsule (medial and posteriorly).[77,83] As with the STN, movement-related cells are sought within the GPi, and stimulation is used to identify side effects, such as muscle contractions (posterior limb of the internal capsule) or visual phosphenes (optic tract).

To reach the Vim, the microelectrode may traverse the following thalamic nuclei depending on trajectory: ventral oralis anterior/posterior (tonic firing rate ~20 Hz; movement-responsive activity), Vim (~25 Hz; movement-responsive activity), ventral caudalis (similar cellular activity to Vim, but displays tactile/sensory-responsive activity), and finally beyond the thalamus into the medial lemniscus.[77,83] Stimulation of the Vim should produce tremor suppression; stimulation of the ventral caudalis and medial lemniscus elicits paresthesias.

Complications and Adverse Effects of Deep Brain Stimulation Surgery

SURGICAL AND HARDWARE-RELATED COMPLICATIONS

The risk of intracranial hemorrhage during DBS procedures is 2% to 5%, with 0.5% to 2% being symptomatic.[4,9,12,84,85] Hypertension is a consistent modifiable risk factor for DBS-related intracranial hemorrhage,[85] and should be carefully monitored and controlled intraoperatively. Approximately 0.5% to 2% of PD patients undergoing DBS procedures experience a serious adverse event, such as persistent neurological deficits or death (most often caused by pulmonary embolism or myocardial infarction).[12,84,85] Perioperative confusion has been reported in approximately 15% of patients undergoing STN DBS for PD.[4,12,86] It is usually transient and may be related to perioperative changes in medications, particularly levodopa.[87,88] Advanced age, cognitive compromise, and the duration of the procedure may be contributing factors. Seizures occur in about 1% of DBS patients.[12,84] Hardware complications after DBS surgery include infection (6%), lead migration (5%), lead fractures (5%), and skin erosions (1% to 2%).[89,90] When infection occurs, a trial of antibiotics alone may be warranted because greater than 20% of infections are likely to clear without removal of the DBS system.[90] Overall, DBS procedures have an acceptable safety profile.[12,84]

STIMULATION-INDUCED ADVERSE EFFECTS

STN DBS has been associated with weight gain, dyskinesias, postural instability, gait akinesia, speech dysfunction (dysarthria and hypophonia), muscle contractions, paresthesias, eye movement abnormalities (eyelid apraxia and ocular deviation leading to diplopia), neuropsychiatric disturbances (depression, apathy, hypomania, mania, hypersexuality, and hallucinations), and cognitive changes (decreases in verbal fluency and memory changes).[4,86,91] Particular attention should be paid to patients' neuropsychiatric condition because suicide attempts and completed suicides have been reported after STN DBS.[4,86] After GPi DBS, weight gain, postural instability, gait akinesia, muscle contractions, eyelid apraxia, and phosphenes have been reported.[91] Speech dysfunction is the most common adverse effect after Vim DBS.[91] Postural instability, gait akinesia, muscle contractions, and paresthesias also have been reported after Vim DBS.[86,91] Adverse stimulation effects usually can be reduced or abolished with adjustments to stimulation settings.[12,86,91]

Deep Brain Stimulation Outcomes

STN DBS for PD patients off medication has been found to improve motor function and activities of daily living for at least 5 years after surgery.[4,9,10,14,16,18] Stimulation-associated improvements in the off medication state vary across the various motor domains of PD as follows: tremor 90%, rigidity 75%, gait 60%, akinesia 50%, and postural instability 40%.[12,14,18] The early benefits of STN DBS on gait, akinesia, and postural stability are not maintained beyond 1 year.[14] The variable and short-lived improvement in gait and postural stability with STN DBS represents a major limitation of the therapy, and has prompted the examination of alternative targets, such as the pedunculopontine nucleus.[20,31] PD patients receiving STN DBS and medication report greater satisfaction in quality of life than patients taking medication alone.[10] STN DBS is associated with a greater than 50% reduction in levodopa dosage and a 70% reduction in levodopa-induced dyskinesias 5 years after surgery.[4,14]

GPi DBS for PD patients off medication is associated with a 40% improvement in motor function 4 years after surgery.[8,9,18] Bradykinesia may be more likely to improve with STN DBS than with GPi DBS.[8] STN DBS is more likely to enable a levodopa dose reduction than GPi DBS.[13,18] STN and GPi DBS decrease levodopa-induced dyskinesias. STN DBS decreases levodopa-induced dyskinesias secondary to levodopa dose reductions, whereas GPi DBS seems to have a direct antidyskinetic effect.[13] Although STN DBS is currently the favored target for PD, its superiority over GPi DBS, with respect to effectiveness or adverse effect profile, has not been shown.

Vim stimulation is associated with 90% tremor reduction in PD patients.[29,30] Compared with STN and GPi stimulation, however, Vim DBS does not improve the bradykinesia, postural instability, gait disturbances, and rigidity associated with PD.

To achieve optimal results for PD patients, surgical therapy should be provided in the context of a multidisciplinary team of movement disorder specialists, including neurologists with expertise in PD diagnosis, pharmacotherapy, and DBS parameter adjustment; nurse specialists with expertise in functional assessments, patient education, and community support; and neurosurgeons with subspecialty training in stereotactic movement disorder surgery.[3,28,91]

Surgical therapy for PD has made significant advances with the emergence of DBS. A substantial proportion of levodopa-responsive PD patients may benefit from adjunctive therapy with DBS. The primary DBS targets for PD are the STN, GPi, and Vim. Because of its adjustability and reversibility, DBS can be tailored to optimize its effects for each patient. To realize the potential benefits of DBS for PD, an experienced and knowledgeable team of movement disorder specialists is necessary.

REFERENCES

1. Volkmann J: Update on surgery for Parkinson's disease. Curr Opin Neurol 2007;20:465-469.
2. Lang AE, Lozano AM: Parkinson's disease: second of two parts. N Engl J Med 1998;339: 1130-1143.
3. Eskandar EN, Cosgrove GR, Shinobu LA: Surgical treatment of Parkinson disease. Jama 2001;286:3056-3059.
4. Kleiner-Fisman G, Herzog J, Fisman DN, et al: Subthalamic nucleus deep brain stimulation: summary and meta-analysis of outcomes. Mov Disord 2006;21;(Suppl 14):S290-S304.
5. Ahlskog JE, Muenter MD: Frequency of levodopa-related dyskinesias and motor fluctuations as estimated from the cumulative literature. Mov Disord 2001;16:448-458.
6. Lang AE, Houeto JL, Krack P, et al: Deep brain stimulation: preoperative issues. Mov Disord 2006;21(Suppl 14):S171-S196.
7. Fabbrini G, Brotchie JM, Grandas F, et al: Levodopa-induced dyskinesias. Mov Disord 2007;22: 1379-1389.
8. Anderson VC, Burchiel KJ, Hogarth P, et al: Pallidal vs subthalamic nucleus deep brain stimulation in Parkinson disease. Arch Neurol 2005;62:554-560.
9. Obesso JA, Olanow CW, Rodriguez-Oroz MC, et al: Deep-brain stimulation of the subthalamic nucleus or the pars interna of the globus pallidus in Parkinson's disease. N Engl J Med 2001;345: 956-963.
10. Deuschl G, Schade-Brittinger C, Krack P, et al: A randomized trial of deep-brain stimulation for Parkinson's disease. N Engl J Med 2006;355:896-908.
11. Fine J, Duff J, Chen R, et al: Long-term follow-up of unilateral pallidotomy in advanced Parkinson's disease. N Engl J Med 2000;342:708-714.
12. Hamani C, Richter E, Schwalb JM, Lozano AM: Bilateral subthalamic nucleus stimulation for Parkinson's disease: a systematic review of the clinical literature. Neurosurgery 2005;56:1313-1321.
13. Krack P, Pollack P, Limousin P, et al: Subthalamic nucleus or internal pallidal stimulation in young onset Parkinson's disease. Brain 1998;121(Pt 3):451-457.
14. Krack P, Batir A, Van Blercom N, et al: Five-year follow-up of bilateral stimulation of the subthalamic nucleus in advanced Parkinson's disease. N Engl J Med 2003;349:1925-1934.
15. Lang AE, Lozano AM, Montgomery E, et al: Posteroventral medial pallidotomy in advanced Parkinson's disease. N Engl J Med 1997;337:1036-1042.
16. Limousin P, Krack P, Pollack P, et al: Electrical stimulation of the subthalamic nucleus in advanced Parkinson's disease. N Engl J Med 1998;339:1105-1111.
17. Lozano AM, Lang AE, Galvez-Jimenez N, et al: Effect of GPi pallidotomy on motor function in Parkinson's disease. Lancet 1995;346:1383-1387.
18. Rodriguez-Oroz MC, Obeso JA, Lang AE, et al: Bilateral deep brain stimulation in Parkinson's disease: a multicentre study with 4 years follow-up. Brain 2005;128:2240-2249.
19. Schupbach WM, Maltete D, Houeto JL, et al: Neurosurgery at an earlier stage of Parkinson disease: a randomized, controlled trial. Neurology 2007;68:267-271.
20. Stefani A, Lozano AM, Peppe A, et al: Bilateral deep brain stimulation of the pedunculopontine and subthalamic nuclei in severe Parkinson's disease. Brain 2007;130:1596-1607.
21. Plaha P, Ben-Shlomo Y, Patel NK, Gill SS: Stimulation of the caudal zona incerta is superior to stimulation of the subthalamic nucleus in improving contralateral parkinsonism. Brain 2006;129:1732-1747.
22. Tir M, Devos D, Blond S, et al: Exhaustive, one-year follow-up of subthalamic nucleus deep brain stimulation in a large, single-center cohort of parkinsonian patients. Neurosurgery 2007;61:297-304.
23. Abosch A, Lozano A: Stereotactic neurosurgery for movement disorders. Can J Neurol Sci 2003;30(Suppl 1):S72-S82.
24. Perlmutter JS, Mink JW: Deep brain stimulation. Annu Rev Neurosci 2006;29:229-257.
25. Rezai AR, Kopell BH, Gross RE, et al: Deep brain stimulation for Parkinson's disease: surgical issues. Mov Disord 2006;21(Suppl 14):S197-S218.
26. Derost PP, Ouchchane L, Morand D, et al: Is DBS-STN appropriate to treat severe Parkinson disease in an elderly population? Neurology 2007;68:1345-1355.
27. Riley D, Lozano A: The fourth dimension of stereotaxis: timing of neurosurgery for Parkinson disease. Neurology 2007;68:252-253.
28. Machado A, Rezai AR, Kopell BH, et al: Deep brain stimulation for Parkinson's disease: surgical technique and perioperative management. Mov Disord 2006;21(Suppl 14):S247-S258.
29. Putzke JD, Wharen RE, Wszolek ZK, et al: Thalamic deep brain stimulation for tremor-predominant Parkinson's disease. Parkinson Rel Disord 2003;10:81-88.

30. Schuurman PR, Bosch DA, Bossuyt PM, et al: A comparison of continuous thalamic stimulation and thalamotomy for suppression of severe tremor. N Engl J Med 2000;342:461-468.

31. Plaha P, Gill SS: Bilateral deep brain stimulation of the pedunculopontine nucleus for Parkinson's disease. Neuroreport 2005;16:1883-1887.

32. Nutt JG, Burchiel KJ, Comella CL, et al: Randomized, double-blind trial of glial cell line-derived neurotrophic factor (GDNF) in PD. Neurology 2003;60:69-73.

33. Gill SS, Patel NK, Hotton GR, et al: Direct brain infusion of glial cell line-derived neurotrophic factor in Parkinson disease. Nat Med 2003;9:89-95.

34. Lang AE, Gill S, Patel NK, et al: Randomized controlled trial of intraputamenal glial cell line-derived neurotrophic factor infusion in Parkinson disease. Ann Neurol 2006;59:459-466.

35. Minguez-Castellanos A, Escamilla-Sevilla F, Hotton GR, et al: Carotid body autotransplantation in Parkinson disease: a clinical and positron emission tomography study. J Neurol Neurosurg Psychiatry 2007;78:825-831.

36. Freed CR, Greene PE, Breeze RE, et al: Transplantation of embryonic dopamine neurons for severe Parkinson's disease. N Engl J Med 2001;344:710-719.

37. Kaplitt MG, Feigin A, Tang C, et al: Safety and tolerability of gene therapy with an adeno-associated virus (AAV) borne GAD gene for Parkinson's disease: an open label, phase I trial. Lancet 2007;369:2097-2105.

38. Strafella AP, Lozano AM, Lang AE, et al: Subdural motor cortex stimulation in Parkinson's disease does not modify movement-related rCBF pattern. Mov Disord 2007;22:2113-2116.

39. Pagni CA, Altibrandi MG, Bentivoglio A, et al: Extradural motor cortex stimulation (EMCS) for Parkinson's disease. History and first results by the study group of the Itlian neurosurgical society. Acta Neurochirurgica Supplementa 2005:113-119.

40. Levy R, Lang AE, Dostrovsky JO, et al: Lidocaine and muscimol microinjections in subthalamic nucleus reverse Parkinsonian symptoms. Brain 2001;124:2105-2118.

41. Volkmann J, Moro E, Pahwa R: Basic algorithms for the programming of deep brain stimulation in Parkinson's disease. Mov Disord 2006;21(Suppl 14):S284-S289.

42. Bin-Mahfoodh M, Hamani C, Sime E, Lozano AM: Longevity of batteries in internal pulse generators used for deep brain stimulation. Stereotact Funct Neurosurg 2003;80:56-60.

43. DeLong MR, Wichmann T: Circuits and circuit disorders of the basal ganglia. Arch Neurol 2007;64:20-24.

44. Kopell BH, Rezai AR, Chang JW, Vitek JL: Anatomy and physiology of the basal ganglia: implications for deep brain stimulation for Parkinson's disease. Mov Disord 2006;21(Suppl 14):S238-S246.

45. Moore DJ, West AB, Dawson VL, Dawson TM: Molecular pathophysiology of Parkinson's disease. Annu Rev Neurosci 2005;28:57-87.

46. Hamani C, Lozano AM: Physiology and pathophysiology of Parkinson's disease. Ann N Y Acad Sci 2003;991:15-21.

47. Plenz D, Kital ST: A basal ganglia pacemaker formed by the subthalamic nucleus and external globus pallidus. Nature 1999;400:677-682.

48. Wichmann T, Delong MR: Deep brain stimulation for neurologic and neuropsychiatric disorders. Neuron 2006;52:197-204.

49. Kringelbach ML, Jenkinson N, Owen SLF, Aziz TZ: Translational principles of deep brain stimulation. Nat Rev Neurosci 2007;8:623-635.

50. Benabid AL, Benazzous A, Pollak P: Mechanisms of deep brain stimulation. Mov Disord 2002;17(Suppl 3):S73-S74.

51. Dostrovsky JO, Lozano AM: Mechanisms of deep brain stimulation. Mov Disord 2002;17 (Suppl 3):S63-S68.

52. Vitek JL: Mechanisms of deep brain stimulation: excitation or inhibition. Mov Disord 2002;17;(Suppl 3):S69-S72.

53. McIntyre CC, Savasta M, Walter BL, Vitek JL: How does deep brain stimulation work? Present understanding and future questions. J Clin Neurophysiol 2004;21:40-50.

54. Dostrovsky JO, Levy R, Wu JP, et al: Microstimulation-induced inhibition of neuronal firing in human globus pallidus. J Neurophysiol 2000;84:570-574.

55. Hashimoto T, Elder CM, Okun MS, et al: Stimulation of the subthalamic nucleus changes the firing pattern of pallidal neurons. J Neurosci 2003;(23):1916-1923.

56. Anderson ME, Postupna N, Ruffo M: Effects of high-frequency stimulation in the internal globus pallidus on the activity of thalamic neurons in the awake monkey. J Neurophysiol 2003;89:1150-1160.

57. Montgomery J, Erwin B: Effects of GPi stimulation on human thalamic neuronal activity. Clin Neurophysiol 2006;117:2691-2702.
58. Lee KH, Kristic K, van Hoff R, et al: High-frequency stimulation of the subthalamic nucleus increases glutamate in the subthalamic nucleus of rats as demonstrated by in vivo enzyme-linked glutamate sensor. Brain Res 2007;1162:121-129.
59. Windels F, Bruet N, Poupard A, et al: Effects of high frequency stimulation of subthalamic nucleus on extracellular glutamate and GABA in substantia nigra and globus pallidus in the normal rat. Eur J Neurosci 2000;12:4141-4146.
60. Boulet S, Lacombe E, Carcenac C, et al: Subthalamic stimulation-induced forelimb dyskinesias are linked to an increase in glutamate levels in the substantia nigra pars reticulata. J Neurosci 2006;26:10768-10776.
61. Magarinos-Ascone C, Pazo JH, Macadar O, Buno W: High-frequency stimulation of the subthalamic nucleus silences subthalamic neurons: a possible cellular mechanism in Parkinson's disease. Neuroscience 2002;115:1109-1117.
62. Windels F, Carcenac C, Poupard A, Savasta M: Pallidal origin of GABA release within the substantia nigra pars reticulata during high-frequency stimulation of the subthalamic nucleus. J Neurosci 2005;25:5079-5086.
63. Ashby P, Kim YJ, Kumar R, et al: Neurophysiological effects of stimulation through electrodes in the human subthalamic nucleus. Brain 1999;(122):1919-1931.
64. Miocinovic S, Parent M, Butson CR, et al: Computational analysis of subthalamic nucleus and lenticular fasciculus activation during therapeutic deep brain stimulation. J Neurophysiol 2006;96:1569-1580.
65. Grill WM, Snyder AN, Miocinovic S: Deep brain stimulation creates an informational lesion of the stimulated nucleus. Neuroreport 2004;15:1137-1140.
66. McIntyre CC, Grill WM, Sherman DL, Thakor NV: Cellular effects of deep brain stimulation: model-based analysis of activation and inhibition. J Neurophysiol 2004;91:1457-1469.
67. McIntyre CC, Mori S, Sherman DL, et al: Electric field and stimulating influence generated by deep brain stimulation of the subthalamic nucleus. Clin Neurophysiol 2004;115:589-595.
68. Davis KD, Taub E, Houle S, et al: Globus pallidus stimulation activates the cortical motor system during alleviation of parkinsonian symptoms. Nat Med 1997;3:671-674.
69. Limousin P, Greene J, Pollack P, et al: Changes in cerebral activity pattern due to subthalamic nucleus or internal pallidum stimulation in Parkinson's disease. Ann Neurol 1997;42:283-291.
70. Ranck Jr JB: Which elements are excited in electrical stimulation of mammalian central nervous system: a review. Brain Res 1975;98:417-440.
71. Iremonger KJ, Anderson TR, Hu B, Kiss ZHT: Cellular mechanisms preventing sustained activation of cortex during subcortical high-frequency stimulation. J Neurophysiol 2006;96:613-621.
72. Chang J-Y, Shi L-H, Luo F, et al: Studies of the neural mechanisms of deep brain stimulation in rodent models of Parkinson's disease. Neurosci Biobehav Rev 2007;31:643-657.
73. Beurrier C, Bioulac B, Audin J, Hammond C: High-frequency stimulation produces a transient blockade of voltage-gated currents in subthalamic neurons. J Neurophysiol 2001;85:1351-1356.
74. Wang L-Y, Kaczmarek LK: High-frequency firing helps replenish the readily releasable pool of synaptic vesicles. Nature 1998;394:384-388.
75. Do MTH, Bean BP: Subthreshold sodium currents and pacemaking of subthalamic neurons: modulation by slow inactivation. Neuron 2003;39:109-120.
76. Andrade-Souza YM, Schwalb JM, Hamani C, et al: Comparison of three methods of targeting the subthalamic nucleus for chronic stimulation in Parkinson's disease. Neurosurgery 2005;56:360-368.
77. Gross RE, Krack P, Rodriguez-Oroz MC, et al: Electrophysiological mapping for the implantation of deep brain stimulators for Parkinson's disease and tremor. Mov Disord 2006;21(Suppl 14): S259-S283.
78. Levy R, Lozano AM, Hutchison WD, Dostrovsky JO: Dual microelectrode technique for deep brain stereotactic surgery in humans. Neurosurgery 2007;60:277-283.
79. Tabbal SD, Revilla FJ, Mink JW, et al: Safety and efficacy of subthalamic nucleus deep brain stimulation performed with limited intraoperative mapping for treatment of Parkinson's disease. Neurosurgery 2007;61:119-127.
80. Palur RS, Berk C, Schulzer M, Honey CR: A metaanalysis comparing the results of pallidotomy performed using microelectrode recording or macroelectrode stimulation. J Neurosurg 2002;96:1058-1062.
81. Abosch A, Hutchison WD, Saint-Cyr JA, et al: Movement-related neurons of the subthalamic nucleus in patients with Parkinson disease. J Neurosurg 2002;97:1167-1172.

82. Benazzouz A, et al: Intraoperative microrecordings of the subthalamic nucleus in Parkinson's disease. Mov Disord 2002;17(Suppl 3):S145-S149.
83. Magnin M, Morel A, Jeanmonod D: Single-unit analysis of the pallidum, thalamus and subthalamic nucleus in parkinsonian patients. Neuroscience 2000;96:549-564.
84. Kenney C, Simpson R, Hunter C, et al: Short-term and long-term safety of deep brain stimulation in the treatment of movement disorders. J Neurosurg 2007;106:621-625.
85. Sansur CA, Frysinger RC, Pouratian N, et al: Incidence of symptomatic hemorrhage after stereotactic electrode placement. J Neurosurg 2007;107:998-1003.
86. Voon V, Kubu C, Krack P, et al: Deep brain stimulation: neuropsychological and neuropsychiatric issues. Mov Disord 2006;21(Suppl 14):S305-S327.
87. Berney A, Vingerhoets F, Perrin A, et al: Effect on mood of subthalamic DBS for Parkinson's disease: a consecutive series of 24 patients. Neurology 2002;59:1427-1429.
88. Lang AE, Kleiner-Fisman G, Saint-Cyr JA, et al: Subthalamic DBS replaces levodopa in Parkinson's disease: two-year follow-up. Neurology 2003;60:154-155; author reply 154–155.
89. Oh MY, Abosch A, Kim SH, et al: Long-term hardware-related complications of deep brain stimulation. Neurosurgery 2002;50:1268-1274.
90. Hamani C, Lozano AM: Hardware-related complications of deep brain stimulation: a review of the published literature. Stereotact Funct Neurosurg 2006;84:248-251.
91. Deuschl G, Herzog J, Kleiner-Fisman G, et al: Deep brain stimulation: postoperative issues. Mov Disord 2006;21(Suppl 14):S219-S237.

17 Cell-Based and Gene-Based Therapy for Parkinson's Disease

C. WARREN OLANOW

Introduction

Degeneration of dopaminergic nerve cells represents the pathological hallmark of Parkinson's disease (PD), and modern therapy is primarily based on a dopamine replacement strategy.[1] Although dopaminergic therapies have provided benefit to millions of PD patients, particularly for patients in the early stages of the disease, long-term levodopa treatment is associated with the development of motor complications in 90% of patients.[2] Further, features such as falling, freezing, and dementia emerge, which are not adequately controlled with dopaminergic therapies. These nonresponsive features represent the primary source of disability in advanced PD and the primary reason that patients require placement in nursing homes.[3] There has been an intensive search for new treatments and treatment strategies that might provide additional benefit for PD patients. The ideal therapy would have disease-modifying effects that slow or stop disease progression.

Despite major advances in molecular genetics, however, no therapy has as yet been shown to provide neuroprotective benefits in PD.[4,5] In an attempt to address this important need, interest has focused on cell-based and gene-based therapies that could replace, restore function, or obviate the consequences of damaged dopamine neurons in PD. Such treatments offer the potential of restoring dopamine innervation to the striatum and other brain regions in a more physiological manner than can be accomplished with standard levodopa therapy, providing enhanced benefits without motor complications. These types of therapies might provide the maximal benefits of levodopa without motor complications, and might theoretically have downstream effects on nondopaminergic areas that are affected in PD. Substantial basic science supports the potential value of cell-based and gene-based therapies, and clinical trials have been performed with each of these classes of therapies. This chapter considers the existing state of information with regard to cell-based and gene-based therapies, the results of existing clinical trials, and the likelihood of future success.

Cell-based Therapies

The concept underlying cell-based therapies is that implantation of dopaminergic cells into the denervated striatum of a PD patient might compensate for the loss of cells that occur as a part of the disease process. Table 17–1 lists cell-based therapies that have been tested in animal or human trials. Initial trials examined implantation of cells derived from the adrenal medulla and reported dramatic success in a few patients.[6] These results were not replicated in subsequent clinical trials,[7] and there was substantial morbidity related to the need for intracranial and intra-abdominal surgeries, however, and the procedure was soon abandoned.

FETAL NIGRAL TRANSPLANTATION

Interest soon began to focus on the greater potential of fetal nigral mesencephalic neurons to replace degenerated dopamine neurons in PD. In the laboratory, implanted fetal dopaminergic neurons were shown to be able to survive, reinnervate the striatum, autoregulate, and provide motor benefits to dopamine-lesioned rodents and primates.[8] In PD patients, open-label studies reported significant clinical benefits accompanied by increased striatal fluorodopa F 18 (^{18}F-dopa) uptake on positron emission tomography (PET).[9-15] Postmortem studies showed robust graft survival with extensive reinnervation of the striatum in an organotypic manner.[16,17] The clinical results in these studies varied, possibly reflecting the many transplant variables and different evaluation techniques (Table 17–2).[8]

Based on the promising laboratory data and initial open-label clinical trials, two prospective, randomized, double-blind clinical trials funded by the National Institutes of Health were performed.[18,19] In both studies, patients with advanced PD who could not be satisfactorily controlled with medical therapy were randomly assigned to receive bilateral fetal nigral transplant procedures or a sham control consisting of a burr hole without direct invasion of the brain. In the first study,[18] 40 patients had solid grafts (noodles) of mesencephalic tissue derived from two donors per side implanted bilaterally into the putamen and caudate nucleus using two needle tracts per side. Immunosuppression was not employed. Patients were followed for 1 year. The primary end point was a measure of quality of life, and was not significantly improved in transplant versus placebo patients. Quality-of-life score changed by 0.0 ± 2.1 among the 19 transplanted patients and by 0.4 ± 1.7 in the sham surgery group ($P = .62$). Unified Parkinson's Disease Rating Scale (UPDRS) scores were a secondary end point and were not significantly changed between groups, although modest benefits in motor scores were detected, particularly in patients younger than 60 years. There was a mean $40\% \pm 42\%$ increase in striatal ^{18}F-dopa uptake compared with baseline in transplanted patients ($P < .001$), whereas patients in the sham-surgery group improved by only $2\% \pm 17\%$ ($P = .40$). Postmortem studies were performed in two patients and

TABLE 17–1	Cell-based Therapies

Adrenal medulla
Fetal mesencephalon
Fetal porcine mesencephalon
Retinal pigmented epithelial cells
Carotid body cells
Stem cells
Embryonic
Autologous

TABLE 17–2	Transplant Variables

Patient selection
Donor age
Number of donors
Type of transplant—solid versus suspension
Site of transplantation—posterior putamen, anterior putamen, caudate nucleus,
    substantia nigra pars compacta
Number of tracts and number of deposits per tract
Use of immunosuppression

showed 6840 to 38,392 tyrosine hydroxylase (TH)–positive cells per striatum. Some inflammatory cells were noted, which stained positively for CD3 and HLA class II antigen.

In the second trial,[19] 34 patients were randomly assigned to receive bilateral transplantation with one or four donors per side or a sham procedure and followed for 2 years. Solid grafts of tissue derived from donors aged 6 to 9.5 weeks post conception were implanted exclusively into the postcommissural putamen (the area that is most affected in PD), using four needle tracts per side and four donor sites per tract. Care was taken to ensure that deposits were separated by no more than 5 mm throughout the target area. All patients received immunosuppression with cyclosporine beginning 2 weeks before the transplant procedure and ending after 6 months. The primary end point was the change from baseline to final visit at 2 years. Transplantation was associated with a significant increase in striatal ^{18}F-dopa uptake on PET ($P < .001$ on each side) with significantly increased uptake observed bilaterally for patients in the one-donor and four-donor groups. Postmortem studies were performed on four transplanted patients, and showed robust graft survival with survival of approximately 70,000 to 120,000 cells per striatum in the four-donor group and 30,000 cells per striatum in the one-donor group. Fibers extended from the graft into the striatum to provide extensive organotypic innervation. There was virtually no TH staining in the striatum of patients in the sham group or in the nontransplanted regions of patients in the one-donor and four-donor groups.

Despite a significant transplant-induced improvement in striatal ^{18}F-dopa uptake on PET (Fig. 17–1) and robust graft survival at postmortem examination (Fig. 17–2), there was no statistical difference in the primary end point or in any of the secondary end points between patients in any of the three treatment groups. Post hoc analyses showed that patients with relatively mild disease (baseline UPDRS motor score <49) had significant benefits from transplantation, particularly in the four-donor group. Transplanted patients showed an apparent improvement at 6 months that deteriorated thereafter. The timing of this loss of benefit coincided with the discontinuation of immunosuppression and was associated with activation of microglia at postmortem examination as evidenced by prominent CD45 staining.[17] These findings raise the possibility that some degree of immune rejection may have occurred and limited potential benefit (see further discussion later).

Although the results of the double-blind trials were disappointing, post hoc analyses suggested that a different transplant protocol might provide superior clinical results. Patient selection seems to be most important. In these two trials, patients were chosen based on having advanced disease that was not adequately controlled with medical therapy. In the first clinical trial, patients younger than 60 years had the best results,[18] whereas in the second trial, patients with milder PD scores at baseline had the best outcome.[19] These results make sense because these groups of patients would be most likely to have dominant dopaminergic lesions, and it is unreasonable to expect that dopaminergic transplants would have a positive influence on the nondopaminergic features of the disease.

Other investigators have similarly remarked that the best results were obtained in patients who had the best preoperative response to levodopa and the most restricted changes on ^{18}F-dopa PET.[20] It would seem reasonable to select patients for dopamine transplantation who have relatively little disability resulting from nondopaminergic degeneration that is not likely to benefit from a dopamine transplant. Additionally, it is reasonable to reconsider the manner in which immunosuppression was employed (in study 2) or not employed at all (in study 1). As mentioned earlier, patients in the second study seemed to deteriorate after withdrawal of immunosuppression, and activated microglia with T and B cells were observed in grafted regions at postmortem examination.[16,19] Better results might be obtained with longer-term immunosuppression. It has been considered that solid grafts might be more immunogenic than grafts comprising dissociated cells, and this warrants further investigation as well. It is also possible that enhanced results could be obtained with transplant of larger numbers of cells, and with different target sites, such as the substantia nigra pars compacta.[21]

The decision of whether to pursue fetal nigral transplantation in further clinical trials has been complicated by the issue of off-medication dyskinesia. Although the procedure itself is generally well tolerated, a new and previously unreported form of dyskinesia has been observed in 50% of transplanted patients. In contrast to classic peak dose dyskinesias, off-medication dyskinesias persist after reduction of or even stopping the levodopa dose.[18,19,22] In some instances, these dyskinesias were so severe and disabling as to warrant an additional surgical procedure (deep brain stimulation). There is some debate as to the nature of off-medication dyskinesia, and there have been few descriptions of this problem in the literature even though it remains an obstacle to further clinical trials. Classic dyskinesias associated with levodopa occur at peak dose and maximal clinical effect, and are primarily choreiform in nature. The pathophysiological basis of

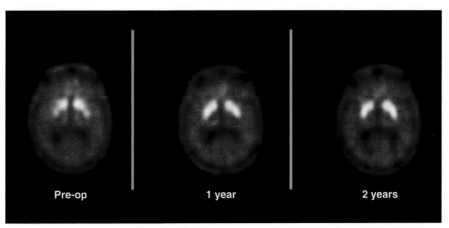

Figure 17–1 Representative PET scans at baseline, 1 year, and 2 years from a patient receiving transplantation with four donors per side. (From Olanow CW, Goetz CG, Kordower JH, et al. A double blind controlled trial of bilateral fetal nigral transplantation in Parkinson's disease. *Ann Neurol.* 2003;54:403-414.)

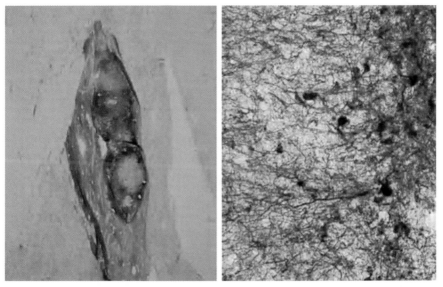

Figure 17–2 *Left panel,* Representative tyrosine hydroxylase–stained graft deposit from patient transplanted with four donors per side. *Right panel,* Higher power view of graft interface with host striatum. Note the extensive innervation of the host striatum.

levodopa-induced dyskinesias is unknown, but is thought to relate to restoration of striatal dopamine in a pulsatile and nonphysiological manner.[23] The possibility that off-medication dyskinesias are related to this mechanism has been considered based on the possibility that inhomogeneous transplant deposits might lead to intermittent or pulsatile stimulation of dopamine receptors.

[18]F-dopa PET studies in patients with off-medication dyskinesias have been reported to show "hot spots,"[24] and dyskinesias have been reported in animal models in which graft deposits were widely separated.[25] It has also been postulated that off-medication dyskinesias may be a prolonged form of diphasic dyskinesias.[19] In contrast to peak dose dyskinesias, diphasic dyskinesias are associated with low levels of plasma levodopa and tend to occur as the patient begins to turn "on" and wear "off" from the levodopa dose.[26,27] Diphasic dyskinesias are characterized by stereotypic, patterned repetitive movements that preferentially affect the lower extremities and are associated with parkinsonian features in other body regions. Off-medication dyskinesias have been reported to resemble diphasic dyskinesias, and it has been considered that they might arise from a continuous release of dopamine from grafts in levels that are insufficient to induce a complete "on" response, but sufficient to produce these dyskinesias.[19] It is also possible that graft-induced dyskinesias somehow relate to the site of implantation, nonphysiological restoration of the nigrostriatal system, or terminal damage induced by an immune response. At present, the precise cause of off-medication dyskinesia is unknown, and methods to prevent its occurrence have not yet been developed. These factors constitute a hurdle toward further clinical trials testing new transplant protocols.

More recently, there have been stunning reports indicating that grafted neurons contain Lewy bodies and may not function normally.[26,27] Two independent autopsy studies, performed in patients who had received transplantation procedures approximately 14 years earlier, showed the presence of classic-appearing Lewy bodies and Lewy neurites within grafted neurons (Fig. 17–3). These Lewy bodies stained for α-synuclein and ubiquitin and were identical to Lewy bodies found in the host substantia nigra pars compacta neurons. Their significance is unknown, but these findings raise the possibility that the implanted neurons (which are only ~13 years of age) have been affected by the PD pathological process even though they are in a non-nigral location. The possibility that they do not function normally as a consequence is supported by the finding of reduced staining for dopamine transporter despite normal TH staining.[28] These findings raise the possibility that any benefit observed with transplantation may be self-limited, and represent another potential obstacle to the utility of transplantation as a viable therapeutic option for PD.

STEM CELLS AND OTHER CELL-BASED THERAPIES

Other forms of dopaminergic cell-based therapy have been tested in PD. Fetal nigral porcine cells have been studied based on the potential of this approach to provide large numbers of cells (large numbers of litters), and the idea that this might address regulatory, societal, and logistical issues associated with the use of human fetal nigral cells. Preliminary studies showed modest benefit in animal studies and in PD patients with survival of a few dopaminergic cells at postmortem examination.[30,31] No benefit was observed, however, in a double-blind, placebo-controlled study,[32] and this procedure is not currently being investigated further. Retinal pigmented epithelial cells have been studied in PD based on their potential to produce levodopa and possibly trophic factors. Retinal pigmented epithelial cells are administered attached to microcarriers (Spheramine) and have shown benefit in animal models of PD.[33] Improvement in motor scores and daily "on" time has also been reported in an

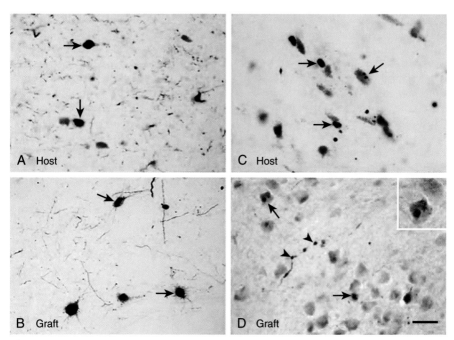

Figure 17–3 A-D, Ubiquitin-stained sections from host (**A** and **B**) and graft (**C** and **D**) showing inclusion bodies within melanized neurons and Lewy neurites (note also higher power in *inset* of graft in **D**). These are present in neurons in both locations.

open-label study involving a few PD patients.[34] A prospective randomized, double-blind study was recently completed and failed to show any benefit in comparison to placebo. These study illustrate that open label trials are not reliable and that clinical determinations can only be made based on double blind controlled studies.

Most attention in this category has focused on stem cells because of their potential to provide an unlimited supply of optimized dopamine neurons. Dopamine neurons make up only about 5% of cells in mesencephalic grafts, and these include cells that project to the nucleus accumbens and are not normally targeted to the striatum. Stem cells offer the potential to provide numerous relatively pure dopamine neurons, which can theoretically be induced further to differentiate into specific dopamine nerve cell subtypes, such as A9 cells.

Most basic research has focused on embryonic stem cells, which are derived from the blastocyst and can be plated, expanded, and induced to differentiate into dopamine neurons.[37] The potential of embryonic stem cells to form dopamine nerve cells has been shown in mice, primates, and humans. Direct transplant of embryonic stem cells into 6-hydroxydopamine–lesioned rats has been shown to result in the formation of a few TH-positive dopaminergic neurons and motor benefits coupled with increases in dopaminergic activity on PET.[38] Many of these animals developed intracerebral teratomas, however. Motor benefits have also been reported with transplant of dopamine neurons derived from embryonic stem cells in dopamine-lesioned rodents and monkeys.[39,40] The benefits achieved in these models are relatively limited, however, and there is only modest long-term cell survival.

Specifically, benefits in laboratory models have not been shown to be superior to what can be achieved with fetal nigral transplant, which so far has failed to provide significant benefits in double-blind trials in PD patients. No off-medication dyskinesias have been observed in animal models, but there remains considerable concern about unanticipated long-term adverse events, particularly tumor formation, and safety issues have to be resolved before clinical trials can be initiated. There has also been considerable interest in the potential to generate dopamine neurons from autologous stem cells that are derived from bone marrow, umbilical matrix, or reprogrammed fibroblasts.[41-43] This approach would avoid immunological and ethical concerns related to the use of embryonic tissue. Results to date have been even less impressive, however, than the results obtained with embryonic stem cells. Partially differentiated neural progenitor cells can also be found in the nervous system, particularly in the subventricular and olfactory regions. There has been interest in the potential of inducing these cells to differentiate into dopamine neurons and migrate to the substantia nigra pars compacta, but to date this has not proved easy to accomplish.[44] Overall, stem cells have great potential for providing dopamine cells for transplantation, but many issues remain to be resolved before they can be considered for clinical testing in PD patients.[45]

CELL-BASED THERAPY CONCLUSIONS

The concept of cell-based therapy has attracted considerable attention, but clinical studies that have been performed to date have been disappointing. Although open-label trials with several techniques have been positive, all double-blind trials that have been performed to date have been negative. This emphasizes the importance of employing double-blind, placebo-controlled trials when assessing cell-based therapies to control for placebo effect and physician bias.[46] Off-medication dyskinesia is a potentially disabling complication of transplant procedures that remains an important obstacle to further trials, and tumors remain an important theoretical problem, particularly with the use of stem cells.

It is also hard to envision how dopamine cell transplantation will address the nondopaminergic features of PD, which constitutes the major source of disability in patients with advanced PD. The more recent finding of Lewy bodies in implanted neurons further complicates the potential value of cell-based therapeutic strategies in PD. These problems might be overcome, at least in part. It is possible that enhanced results could be obtained with refined transplant protocols. Physiological restoration of the nigrostriatal dopaminergic system might have downstream consequences on nondopaminergic pathology in the cerebral cortex and brainstem that are not currently anticipated. Finally, it is possible that dopamine or other cells could be used to transport novel molecules, such as trophic factors, to the nervous system and extend on dopaminergic benefits. These concepts are theoretical, however, and remain to be established.

Gene-based Therapy

An alternative approach to treat patients with advanced PD involves the use of gene delivery techniques to introduce therapeutic proteins into specific brain targets (Table 17–3). This concept involves the use of a viral vector to deliver the

TABLE 17–3	**Gene Therapy for Parkinson's Disease**	
AAV2	Aromatic acid decarboxylase	Striatum
AAV2	Glutamic acid decarboxylase	Subthalamic nucleus
AAV2	Neurturin	Striatum

AAV2, adeno-associated virus serotype 2.

TABLE 17–4	**Issues in Gene Therapy**
Viral vector	
Therapeutic protein	
Brain target site	
Distribution of virus and protein throughout target	
Anterograde transmission	
Retrograde transmission	
Persistence of transgene	
Safety profile	
Efficacy	
Regulator	

DNA or RNA of the therapeutic protein. The construct can be injected into a specific brain target site, such as the striatum, and include a targeting sequence, such as a TH promoter, so that only a specific subset of nerve cells are affected. When the desired cell is infected, an integrase incorporates the transgene into the host genome, which begins to manufacture the desired protein. Important issues in gene therapy are listed in Table 17–4.

Most gene therapy studies have used the adeno-associated virus serotype 2 (AAV2) as the vector because it is not immunogenic is relatively localized, and it is associated with prolonged persistence of the transgene (at least 4 years). Three different clinical studies have used gene delivery techniques in PD. The first used the AAV-2 viral vector to deliver aromatic amino acid decarboxylase (AADC) to the striatum based on the concept that this would facilitate conversion of levodopa to dopamine and provide more continuous availability of dopamine. Benefits with this approach have been reported in 1-methyl-4-phenyl-1,2,3,6-tetrahydropyridine (MPTP)-lesioned primates,[47] and clinical trials in PD patients are ongoing. An alternative approach uses the same vector to deliver glutamic acid decarboxylase to the subthalamic nucleus with the intention of increasing γ-aminobutyric acid formation and inhibiting subthalamic nucleus excitatory neurons, which are overactive in PD. There is only limited preclinical information using this approach. An open-label clinical trial was performed in six PD patients and was reported to show improvement in motor features with reduced motor complications.[48] No patient was reported to have hemiballismus, a potential consequence of excess inhibition of the subthalamic nucleus.

Gene therapy has been most widely studied as a means of delivering trophic factors to the striatum and possibly other brain targets. Trophic factors enhance the growth and development of cultured dopamine neurons and protect them against various toxins. Among these, glial-derived neurotrophic factor (GDNF) seems to be the most effective. GDNF has been shown to be able to protect dopamine neurons in MPTP monkeys and restore function even when administered weeks after the toxin.[49] Open-label studies reported benefits with direct catheter administration into the putamen of four of five patients with advanced PD.[50] No benefit was detected, however, with catheter delivery of GDNF into the putamen in a double-blind, placebo-controlled trial.[51] This lack of benefit may have related to the inability of point source delivery to provide adequate distribution of the trophic factor throughout the target region.[52]

Gene delivery offers an opportunity to provide more complete distribution of the trophic factor. Studies in primates confirm that gene delivery can provide diffuse delivery of GDNF throughout the putamen and provide motor benefits in MPTP monkeys.[53] Neurturin is a member of the GDNF family of trophic factors[54] and has been shown to enhance TH staining in aged monkeys[55] and to improve motor function and protect dopamine neurons in MPTP monkeys.[56] In these studies, AAV2-neurturin was shown to provide diffuse distribution throughout the striatum, anterograde and retrograde transmission, and persistent expression of the transgene. Based on these trials, AAV2-neurturin was tested in 12 patients with advanced PD in an open label study. Significant improvements were observed in UPDRS motor score in the practically defined "off" state and "on" time without troublesome dyskinesia.[57] The procedure was well tolerated, and no patient experienced off-medication dyskinesia or other unanticipated side effects. Based on these results, a double-blind, placebo-controlled study is now being performed.

GENE-BASED THERAPY CONCLUSIONS

Initial studies show the feasibility of performing these procedures, and to date no serious adverse events have been encountered. Gene therapy is in an early stage of development, and it is likely that there will be many additional procedures testing different therapeutic molecules and target sites that may be more effective than those that have been tested to date. Gene therapy may be particularly helpful for forms of PD in an open label study that are associated with mutations or defects in specific proteins. Insight into the cause of cell death in hereditary forms of PD and more specifically in the forms that occur sporadically is likely to provide new targets for a gene therapy. At present, no major side effects have been associated with gene therapy for PD, and specifically no patient has experienced off-medication dyskinesia, new-onset tumor formation, or immune reactions directed at the virus or the therapeutic protein.

Only a few patients have been studied, however, and they have been followed for a relatively short time, so long-term safety is not yet ensured. Regulator vectors have been proposed to help address these unforeseen problems. A regulator DNA is inserted into the construct, and when activated can turn on or turn off production of the transgene. Examples are the tet, steroid, or ecosyd (an insect steroid) systems, which can be activated by introduction of tetracycline or a steroid. This system has never been tested in a human patient. Although the concept is appealing, there is no assurance that suppression of manufacture of the therapeutic protein after the onset of toxicity would be effective, and it is possible that there might be immune reactions directed against the regulatory protein.[58] As stated, none of the clinical trials that have been initiated to date have used a regulatory system, and it is likely to be several years before such a system is available for human trial. Finally, as with cell-based therapies, it is important to consider that current approaches to gene therapy are not likely to improve the nondopaminergic features of PD, and long-term success may depend on developing approaches that can accomplish this goal.

Conclusions

New therapies are urgently required for PD. Current therapies provide benefit for the classic motor features of the illness, but patients continue to experience disability despite these accomplishments. Cell-based and gene-based therapies offer novel opportunities to provide additional benefits for PD patients, and have attracted enormous scientific and public enthusiasm. There is still a long way to go, however, before any of these therapies can be seriously considered as a standard therapy for PD. Although cell transplant and gene-based therapies have provided benefit in open-label trials, none has been confirmed yet to be effective in a double-blind trial.

It is also important to consider whether any of these therapies can provide benefits that exceed those that can be achieved with levodopa. They each offer the potential of restoring nigrostriatal function in a more physiological manner than levodopa, which might reduce the risk of motor complications, but modifications of levodopa formulations may allow similar benefits to be attained without the need for a surgical intervention.[59,60]

The great unanswered question is whether a cell-based or gene-based therapy can provide benefits with respect to the nondopaminergic features of PD. Early restoration of dopaminergic tone to the brainstem and cortex theoretically might improve nondopaminergic features. Alternatively, dopamine-mediated inhibition of subthalamic nucleus may diminish overactivity and prevent excitotoxic damage in target neurons. Implanted cells or gene therapies also may be able to influence PD through means that are independent of the dopamine system by way of trophic factors, by replacement of dysfunctional or mutant proteins, and by enhancing or inhibiting systems that are critical to cell death or neuroprotection. These issues remain theoretical and seem far from the clinic at the present time. For now clinicians need to determine why some patients develop off-medication dyskinesia and how to prevent this problem, to proceed with carefully assessing preclinical safety and methods of optimizing transplant and gene therapy protocols, and to determine why implanted neurons develop Lewy bodies and if an ongoing PD pathological process would limit the potential of cell-based and gene-based therapies.

REFERENCES

1. Olanow CW: The scientific basis for the current treatment of Parkinson's disease. Ann Rev Med 2004;55:41-60.
2. Ahlskog JE, Muenter MD: Frequency of levodopa-related dyskinesias and motor fluctuations as estimated from the cumulative literature. Mov Disord 2001;16:448-458.

3. Hely MA, Morris JG, Reid WG, Trafficante R: Sydney Multicenter Study of Parkinson's disease: non-L-dopa-responsive problems dominate at 15 years. Mov Disord 2005;20:190-199.
4. Schapira AHV, Olanow CW: Neuroprotection in Parkinson's disease: myths, mysteries, and misconceptions. Jama 2004;291:358-364.
5. Olanow CW, Kieburtz K, Schapira AH: Why have we failed to achieve neuroprotection in Parkinson's disease? Ann Neurol 2008;64 Suppl 2:S101-S110.
6. Madrazo I, Drucker-Colín R, Díaz V, et al: Open microsurgical autograft of adrenal medulla to the right caudate nucleus in two patients with intractable Parkinson's disease. N Engl J Med 1987;316:831–814.
7. Goetz CG, Olanow CW, Koller WC, et al: Multicenter study of autologous adrenal medullary transplantation to the corpus striatum of patients with advanced Parkinson's disease. N Eng J Med 1989;320:337-341.
8. Olanow CW, Freeman TB, Kordower JH: Fetal nigral transplantation as a therapy for Parkinson's disease. Trends Neurosci 1996;19:102-109.
9. Lindvall O, Brundin P, Widner H, et al: Grafts of fetal dopamine neurons survive and improve motor function in Parkinson's disease. Science 1990;247:574-577.
10. Freed CR, Breeze RE, Rosenberg NL, et al: Survival of implanted fetal dopamine cells and neurologic improvement 12 to 46 months after transplantation for Parkinson's disease. N Engl J Med 1992;327:1549-1555.
11. Peschanski M, Defer G, N'Guyen J, et al: Bilateral motor improvement and alteration of L-dopa effect in two patients with Parkinson's disease following intrastriatal transplantation of fetal ventral mesencephalon. Brain 1994;117:487-499.
12. Freeman TB, Olanow CW, Hauser RA, et al: Bilateral fetal nigral transplantation into the postcommissural putamen in Parkinson's disease. Ann Neurol 1995;38:379-388.
13. Hauser RA, Freeman TB, Snow BJ, et al: Long-term evaluation of bilateral fetal nigral transplantation in Parkinson's disease. Arch Neurol 1999;56:179-187.
14. Sawle GV, Bloomfield PM, Bjorklund A, et al: Transplantation of fetal dopamine neurons in Parkinson's disease: PET [18F]-6-L-fluorodopa studies in two patients with putaminal implants. Ann Neurol 1992;31:166-173.
15. Remy P, Samson Y, Hantraye P, et al: Clinical correlates of [18F] fluorodopa uptake in five grafted Parkinsonian patients. Ann Neurol 1995;38:580-588.
16. Kordower JH, Freeman TB, Snow BJ, et al: Neuropathological evidence of graft survival and striatal reinnervation after the transplantation of fetal mesencephalic tissue in a patient with Parkinson's disease. N Engl J Med 1995;332:1118-1124.
17. Kordower JH, Rosenstein JM, Collier TM, et al: Functional fetal nigral grafts in a patient with Parkinson's disease: chemoanatomic, ultrastructural, and metabolic studies. J Comp Neurol 1996;370:203-230.
18. Freed CR, Greene PE, Breeze RE, et al: Transplantation of embryonic dopamine neurons for severe Parkinson's disease. N Engl J Med 2001;344:710-719.
19. Olanow CW, Goetz CG, Kordower JH, et al: A double blind controlled trial of bilateral fetal nigral transplantation in Parkinson's disease. Ann Neurol 2003;54:403-414.
20. Piccini P, Pavese N, Hagell P, et al: Factors affecting the clinical outcome after neural transplantation in Parkinson's disease. Brain 2005;128:2977-2986.
21. Mendez I, Dagher A, Hong M, et al: Simultaneous intrastriatal and intranigral fetal dopaminergic grafts in patients with Parkinson disease: a pilot study. Report of three cases. J Neurosurg 2002;96:589-596.
22. Hagell P, Piccini P, Bjorklund A, et al: Dyskinesias following neural transplantation in Parkinson's disease. Nat Neurosci 2002;5:627-628.
23. Olanow CW, Obeso JA, Stocchi F: Continuous dopamine receptor stimulation in the treatment of Parkinson's disease: scientific rationale and clinical implications. Lancet Neurol 2006;5:677-687.
24. Ma Y, Feigin A, Dhawan V, et al: Dyskinesia after fetal cell transplantation for parkinsonism: a PET study. Ann Neurol 2002;52:628-634.
25. Carlsson T, Winkler C, Lundblad M, et al: Graft placement and uneven pattern of reinnervation in the striatum is important for development of graft-induced dyskinesia. Neurobiol Dis 2006;21:657-668.
26. Muenter MD, Sharpless NS, Tyce GM, Darley FL: Patterns of dystonia ("I-D-I" and "D-I-D") in response to l-dopa therapy for Parkinson's disease. Mayo Clin Proc 1977;52:163-174.
27. Luquin MR, Scipioni O, Vaamonde J, et al: Levodopa-induced dyskinesias in Parkinson's disease: clinical and pharmacological classification. Mov Disord 1992;7:117-122.

28. Kordower JH, Chu Y, Hauser RA, et al: Lewy body-like pathology in long-term embryonic nigral transplants in Parkinson's disease. Nat Med 2008;14:504-506.
29. Li JY, Englund E, Holton JL, et al: Lewy bodies in grafted neurons in subjects with Parkinson's disease suggest host-to-graft disease propagation. Nat Med 2008;14(5):501-503.
30. Fink JS, Schumacher JM, Ellias SL, et al: Porcine xenografts in Parkinson's disease and Huntington's disease patients: preliminary results. Cell Transplant 2000;9:273-278.
31. Deacon T, Schumacher J, Dinsmore J, et al: Histological evidence of fetal pig neural cell survival after transplantation into a patient with Parkinson's disease. Nat Med 1997;3:350-353.
32. Watts RL, Freeman TB, Hauser RA, et al: A double-blind, randomized, controlled, multicenter clinical trial of the safety and efficacy of stereotaxic intrastriatal implantation of fetal porcine ventral mesencephalic tissue (Neurocelltm-PD) vs imitation surgery in patients with Parkinson disease (PD). Parkinson Rel Disord 2001;7(Suppl):S87.
33. Subramanian T, Marchionini D, Potter EM, Cornfeldt ML: Striatal xenotransplantation of human retinal pigment epithelial cells attached to microcarriers in hemiparkinsonian rats ameliorates behavioral deficits without provoking a host immune response. Cell Transplant 2002;11:207-214.
34. Stover NP, Bakay RA, Subramanian T, et al: Intrastriatal implantation of human retinal pigmented epithelial cells attached to microcarriers in advanced Parkinson's disease. Arch Neurol 2005;62:1833-1837.
35. Itakura T, Uematsu Y, Nakao N, et al: Transplantation of autologous sympathetic ganglion into the brain with Parkinson's disease: long-term follow-up of 35 cases. Stereotact Funct Neurosurg 1997;69:112-115.
36. Minguez-Castellanos A, Escamilla-Sevilla F, Hotton GR, et al: Carotid body autotransplantation in Parkinson's disease: a clinical and positron emission tomography study. J Neurol Neurosurg Psychiatry 2007;78:825-831.
37. Lindvall O, Kokaia Z, Martinez-Serrano A: Stem cell therapy for human neurodegenerative disorders—how to make it work. Nat Med 2004;10:542-550.
38. Bjorklund LM, Sanchez-Pernaute R, Chung S, et al: Embryonic stem cells develop into functional dopaminergic neurons after transplantation in a Parkinson rat model. Proc Natl Acad Sci U S A 2002;99:2344-2349.
39. Kim JH, Auerbach JM, Rodriguez-Gomez JA, et al: Dopamine neurons derived from embryonic stem cells function in an animal model of Parkinson's disease. Nature 2002;418:50-56.
40. Takagi Y, Takahashi J, Saiki H: Dopaminergic neurons generated from monkey embryonic stem cells function in a Parkinson primate model. J Clin Invest 2005;115:102-109.
41. Weiss ML, Medicetty S, Bledsoe AR, et al: Human umbilical cord matrix stem cells: preliminary characterization and effect of transplantation in a rodent model of Parkinson's disease. Stem Cells 2006;24:781-792.
42. Bouchez G, Sensebe L, Vourc'h P, et al: Partial recovery of dopaminergic pathway after graft of adult mesenchymal stem cells in a rat model of Parkinson's disease. Neurochem Int 2008;5:1332-1342.
43. Wernig M, Zhao JP, Pruszak J, et al: Neurons derived from reprogrammed fibroblasts functionally integrate into the fetal brain and improve symptoms of rats with Parkinson's disease. Proc Natl Acad Sci U S A 2008;15:5856-5861.
44. Zhao C, Deng W, Gage FH: Mechanisms and functional implications of adult neurogenesis. Cell 2008;22:645-660.
45. Morizame A, Li JY, Brundin P: From bench to bed: the potential of stem cells for the treatment of Parkinson's disease. Cell Tissue Res 2008;331:323-336.
46. Freeman TB, Vawter DE, Leaverton PE, et al: Use of placebo surgery in a controlled trial of a cellular-based therapy for Parkinson's disease. N Engl J Med 1999;341:988-992.
47. Bankiewicz KS, Forsayeth J, Eberling JL, et al: Long-term clinical improvement in MPTP-lesioned primates after gene therapy with AAV-hAADC. Mol Ther 2006;14:564-570.
48. Kaplitt MG, Feigin A, Tang C, et al: Safety and tolerability of gene therapy with an adeno-associated virus (AAV) borne GAD gene for Parkinson's disease: an open label, phase I trial. Lancet 2007;369:2097-2105.
49. Gash DM, Zhang Z, Ovadia A, et al: Functional recovery in parkinsonian monkeys treated with GDNF. Nature 1996;380:252-255.
50. Gill SS, Patel NK, Hotton GR, et al: Direct brain infusion of glial cell line-derived neurotrophic factor in Parkinson disease. Nat Med 2003;9:589-595.
51. Lang AE, Gill S, Patel NK, et al: Randomized controlled trial of intraputamenal glial cell line-derived neurotrophic factor infusion in Parkinson disease. Ann Neurol 2006;59:459-466.

52. Salvatore MF, Ai Y, Fischer B, et al: Point source concentration of GDNF may explain failure of phase II clinical trial. Exp Neurol 2006;202:497-505.
53. Kordower JH, Emborg ME, Bloch J, et al: Neurodegeneration prevented by lentiviral vector delivery of GDNF in primate models of Parkinson's disease. Science 2000;290:767-773.
54. Kotzbauer PT, Lampe PA, Heuckeroth RO, et al: Neurturin, a relative of glial-cell-line-derived neurotrophic factor. Nature 1996 Dec 5;384:467-470.
55. Herzog CD, Dass B, Holden JE, et al: Striatal delivery of CERE-120, an AAV2 vector encoding human neurturin, enhances activity of the dopaminergic nigrostriatal system in aged monkeys. Mov Disord 2007;22:1124-1132.
56. Kordower JH, Herzog CD, Dass B, et al: Delivery of neurturin by AAV2 (CERE-120)-mediated gene transfer provides structural and functional neuroprotection and neurorestoration in MPTP-treated monkeys. Ann Neurol 2006;60:706-715.
57. Marks WJ Jr, Ostrem JL, Verhagen L, et al: Gene transfer of a trophic factor for Parkinson's disease: initial clinical trial with AAV2-neurturin (CERE-120). Lancet Neurol 2008;7:400-408.
58. Kordower J, Olanow CW: Regulatable promoters and gene therapy for Parkinson's disease: is the only thing to fear, fear itself? Exp Neurol 2008;209:34-40.
59. Olanow CW. Levodopa/dopamine replacement strategies in Parkinson's disease–future directions. Mov Disord 2008;23 Suppl 3:S613-S622.
60. Olanow CW, Kordower JH, Lang AE, Obeso JA: Dopaminergic transplantation for Parkinson's Disease: current status and future prospects. Ann Neurol (in press).

18 Neuroprotection in Parkinson's Disease

ANTHONY H.V. SCHAPIRA

Introduction

Parkinson's disease (PD) is the second most common progressive neurodegenerative disease. PD produces significant morbidity and impairment of quality of life. Although the predominant early clinical features of PD are motor and result from loss of nigral dopaminergic neurons, other neurotransmitter pathways are involved. The nonmotor symptoms progress, become more evident with advanced disease, and are relatively refractory to treatment. Perhaps the most important challenge for treatment in PD is a mechanism to delay or prevent further loss of dopaminergic and nondopaminergic neurons. This delaying or preventive treatment would in effect be a "cure" for PD if the intervention were able to prevent progression of motor and nonmotor symptoms. In this context, neuroprotection is discussed.

Neuroprotection is defined as the ability for a therapy to prevent neuronal cell death by intervening in and inhibiting the pathogenetic cascade that results in cell dysfunction and eventual death. *Neurorescue* might be considered slightly differently: an ability to intervene in the same pathogenetic pathways and prevent cell death, but also restore function to damaged and malfunctioning neurons. Neurorescue would have the capacity to reverse some of the clinical symptoms of PD.

Neurorestoration implies a treatment that can increase the number of neurons in a pathway and reverse clinical features; this might be by the use of cell implants or growth factors.

To develop any of these disease-modifying therapies, researchers must have a sound understanding of the causes of PD and the pathways to cell damage and death. Other chapters in this section have dealt with the etiology and pathogenesis of PD, and these are not considered in detail any further. The development and trial of neuroprotective agents in PD have for the most part derived from our understanding of pathogenesis (Fig. 18–1). The range of drugs evaluated is substantial and includes several different mechanisms of action: promitochondrial, antioxidant, and antiapoptotic. Some drugs have shown more than one property that could be classified as neuroprotective, however. This chapter focuses on the better studied drugs and groups of compounds and only the agents that have entered clinical trials.

Monoamine Oxidase B Inhibitors

SELEGILINE

Monoamine oxidase B (MAOB) metabolizes dopamine and is implicated in the generation of free radicals by dopamine. Inhibition of this enzyme reduces dopamine turnover and oxidative stress. MAOB inhibition also increases the half-life of dopamine in the synaptic cleft, and enhances receptor stimulation and reuptake of dopamine into the presynaptic bulb. MAOB inhibitors would be anticipated to have a dual action: (1) improvement of symptoms related to dopamine deficiency and (2) potentially antioxidant properties. MAOB is required for the conversion of the protoxin 1-methyl-4-phenyl-1,2,3,6-tetrahydropyridine (MPTP) to the neurotoxin 1-methyl-4-phenylpyridinium (MPP$^+$). There is the additional possible benefit that the drug also might interfere with a putative endogenous or exogenous toxin using the same pathway.

Against this background, selegiline was considered for trial as a drug that might slow the progression of PD. At the time of trial design, however, it was not thought that the drug would have a symptomatic effect. The DATATOP (Deprenyl [selegiline] And Tocopherol Antioxidant Therapy Of PD) study was a prospective double-blind, placebo-controlled trial that evaluated the antioxidant vitamin E in a total daily dose of 2000 IU and selegiline (deprenyl) in a dose of 5 mg twice daily as putative neuroprotective therapies.[1] The time until the randomly assigned PD patients required the initiation of levodopa was the primary end point. No beneficial effect of vitamin E was detected, although it is possible that there was poor brain penetration or inadequate dosing. In contrast, selegiline significantly delayed the need for levodopa compared with placebo by 9 to 12 months. Levodopa treatment was required in 26% of selegiline recipients compared with 47% of subjects who received placebo. This result was consistent with slowing of disease progression. Selegiline was also found to exert a mild symptomatic effect, however, which confounded interpretation of the study. It was impossible to determine if the delay in the need for levodopa was because the drug slowed neuronal degeneration, or because symptomatic effects masked ongoing disease progression.

A second study was performed to try to circumvent this confound. Selegiline was compared with placebo using as the primary end point the change in motor

NEUROPROTECTION IN PARKINSON'S DISEASE –
CLUES AND TARGETS

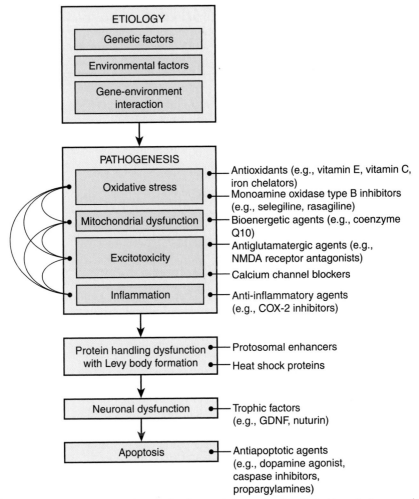

Figure 18–1   Summary of etiologic and pathogenetic factors involved in Parkinson's disease and the potential targets for neuroprotection drugs. COX-2, cyclooxygenase-2; GDNF, glial-derived neurotrophic factor; NMDA, N-methyl-d-aspartate. (Adapted from Schapira AH, Olanow CW. Neuroprotection in Parkinson disease: mysteries, myths, and misconceptions. *JAMA*. 2004;291:358-364.)

score between an untreated baseline visit and an untreated final visit performed after 12 months of treatment and 2 months of study drug withdrawal.[2] Patients treated with selegiline had less deterioration from baseline than placebo patients, suggesting that the drug might be neuroprotective. This study may also have been confounded, however, by the potential of selegiline to have long-lasting symptomatic effects.

These studies generated considerable interest and debate. The symptomatic action of selegiline was not anticipated, and the most parsimonious explanation for the DATATOP results was that patients had a delay in levodopa introduction simply because of selegiline's symptomatic effect. The study by Olanow and colleagues[2] had a 2-month washout period for selegiline, and although some may consider this sufficient, there is evidence to indicate that the irreversible inhibition of MAOB by this compound is not fully overcome (by new protein synthesis) after this period. Neither the DATATOP study nor the Olanow study was able to provide a definitive answer to the potential for selegiline to offer a neuroprotective effect.

Two long-term follow-up studies of PD patients initiated on selegiline as opposed to placebo have shown effects that could still be construed as neuroprotective. In a long-term follow-up study of the original DATATOP cohort, levodopa patients who had been taking selegiline for 7 years compared with patients who were changed to placebo after 5 years had a significantly slower decline, and less wearing-off, "on-off," and freezing, but more dyskinesias occurred in the patients on selegiline.[3]

Another long-term follow-up of patients initiated on selegiline as opposed to placebo showed that after 6 to 7 years, the patients started on this MAOB inhibitor were better off in terms of motor function and activities of daily living, and required a smaller levodopa dose.[4] Both long-term follow-up studies indicate that early initiation of selegiline may have lasting benefits, at least over 7 years. The mechanisms underlying this effect are unknown, but could include a true neuroprotective action. These long-term studies were confounded, however, by high dropout rates over the years of follow-up. There were some concerns that selegiline may be associated with excess mortality, but a large meta-analysis indicated that no such effect is evident.[5]

LAZABEMIDE

Lazabemide is a short-acting and reversible MAOB inhibitor.[6] A randomized, placebo-controlled, double-blind trial assigned 321 untreated patients with early PD to placebo or one of four treatment arms (25 mg/day, 50 mg/day, 100 mg/day, or 200 mg/day of lazabemide) with follow-up for up to 1 year.[7] The risk of reaching the primary end point (the onset of disability sufficient to require levodopa therapy) was reduced by 51% for the patients who received lazabemide compared with placebo-treated subjects ($P < .001$). This effect was consistent among all dosages with a similar magnitude and pattern of benefit as seen in the DATATOP trial. As with selegiline, lazabemide also has symptomatic effects, however, and there were similar concerns as to whether or not the results were due to a neuroprotective or symptomatic action.[8]

RASAGILINE

Similar to selegiline, rasagiline is a propargylamine, but is a more potent irreversible inhibitor of MAOB.[9] Rasagiline has shown neuroprotective properties similar to selegiline in several laboratory models of dopamine neurotoxicity and PD.[10] This action seems to be related to numerous actions, including antiapoptosis and growth factor induction.[11]

In cultures of neonatal rat cerebellar granule cells, the increase in cell death by glutamate-induced excitotoxicity was significantly reduced by the presence of rasagiline in a wide range of concentrations (1 mM to 1 nM).[12] The neuroprotective properties of rasagiline were evaluated in cultured rat adrenal pheochromocytoma PC-12 cells and dopaminergic human neuroblastoma SH-SY5Y cells subjected to serum and nerve growth factor withdrawal.[13] In the absence of serum or nerve growth factor, these cells die via an apoptotic process, with significant loss of cell viability within 24 hours. Pretreatment of cells with rasagiline or selegiline significantly reduced cell death, with rasagiline showing a greater efficacy than selegiline. The neuroprotective activity of rasagiline and selegiline was blocked by the addition of the selegiline metabolite, methamphetamine, but not by the rasagiline metabolite, aminoindan.

In vitro studies suggest that the antiapoptotic, neuroprotective activity of rasagiline resides in the propargyl moiety and is not related to monoamine oxidase inhibition. TVP1022, the *S*-enantiomer of rasagiline, has 1000-fold weaker monoamine oxidase inhibitory activity but exhibits similar neuroprotective effects in vitro.[11,14,15] Some of the neuroprotective effects of rasagiline have been seen in cell lines and primary neurons that express only the monoamine oxidase A isoenzyme. The neuroprotective effects of rasagiline are independent of its inhibition of MAOB. By activating antiapoptotic molecules such as Bcl-2 and Bcl-xL and the protein kinase C/mitogen-activated protein kinase pathway, and downregulating proapoptotic molecules such as Bax and Bad, the propargylamine moiety protects mitochondrial viability and prevents opening of the mitochondrial permeability transition pore, caspase activation, and the apoptotic cascade.[16,17]

Glial cell line–derived neurotrophic factor (GDNF) is known to promote the survival of dopaminergic neurons in vivo and in vitro. Treatment of SH-SY5Y cells with rasagiline (100 nM) produced a sixfold increase in GDNF protein.[18] This study also showed that rasagiline activated nuclear factor κB (NF-κB), a common transcription factor for GDNF and for brain-derived neurotrophic factor, superoxide dismutase, and Bcl-2. These authors suggested that part of the pharmacological activity of rasagiline and related propargylamines may be due to induction of prosurvival genes such as *GDNF* and *Bcl-2* through NF-κB activation.

Two studies, one a blinded extension of the other, have been published on the use of rasagiline in patients with early PD.[19,20] The initial study randomly assigned 404 patients with early untreated PD to placebo or rasagiline (1 mg/day or 2 mg/day). At the end of the 6-month trial period, the 1-mg rasagiline group had an improved Unified Parkinson's Disease Rating Scale (UPDRS) score compared with the placebo group of 4.2 units ($P < .001$), and this was 3.56 ($P < .001$) for the 2-mg group. The degree of motor improvement over the 6-month period was comparable to that seen for selegiline in the DATATOP study. At 6 months, the two treatment arms were almost back to their respective baseline UPDRS scores.

This study was extended for a further 6 months with 380 of the original 404 patients entering the treatment phase.[20] Patients were continued on their original dose of rasagiline or, if on placebo, were given 2 mg/day of rasagiline. Patients requiring additional dopaminergic therapy were prescribed either levodopa or a dopamine agonist. The UPDRS was assessed at baseline and various time points 52 weeks from initiation. The primary end point was the change in total UPDRS from baseline to week 52. For the whole 12-month period, deterioration from baseline scores was 3.01, 1.97, and 4.17 UPDRS units for the 1-mg, 2-mg, and delayed 2-mg cohorts. Patients given 1 mg/day of rasagiline for 12 months compared with patients given the 2-mg dose for only the last 6 months maintained

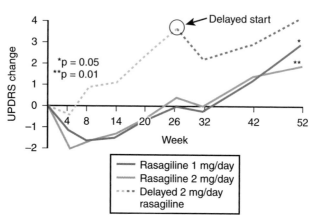

12-MONTH RESULTS: MEAN CHANGE IN TOTAL UPDRS

Figure 18–2 TEMPO delayed start study design for rasagiline in early Parkinson's disease. UPDRS, Unified Parkinson's Disease Rating Scale. (Adapted from Parkinson's Disease Study Group. A controlled, randomized, delayed-start study of rasagiline in early Parkinson disease. *Arch Neurol.* 2004;61:561-566.)

a total UPDRS improvement of 1.82 UPDRS units (P = .05). The 12-month 2-mg rasagiline group had a 2.29 unit (P = .01) improvement over the 6-month 2-mg rasagiline group (Fig. 18–2).

This long-term study was the first "delayed start" trial in PD, and provides several important clinical insights not only into the potential for rasagiline use in early PD, but also in trial interpretation (see later). The fact that all treatment groups had been taking rasagiline for 6 months before the final clinical assessment makes it highly unlikely that the positive results were due to a symptomatic effect. The benefit of beginning the rasagiline 6 months earlier may indicate a true neuroprotective action of this drug, in line with its preclinical data. Alternatively, the benefit of simply beginning symptomatic therapy earlier rather than later could account for the effect seen. This explanation is discussed in more detail subsequently in relation to when to begin therapy.

Dopamine Agonists

Dopamine agonists were developed for the symptomatic treatment of PD. There are several reasons, however, for considering dopamine agonists as potential neuroprotective agents in PD. Their activation of presynaptic autoreceptors reduces the turnover of dopamine and the production of reactive oxygen species in the nigrostriatal neurons.[21,22] Their inhibition of the output of the subthalamic nucleus could reduce the excitotoxic input into the substantia nigra. Their hydroxylated benzene ring structure implies inherent antioxidant activity.

Several in vitro and in vivo experiments have shown that dopamine agonists can prevent cell death induced by several toxins that are relevant to PD.[23-25] Bromocriptine protects against 6-hydroxydopamine, MPTP, and 3-acetylpyridine toxicity in rodents[26-28] and scavenges free radicals in vitro.[29] Apomorphine and pergolide attenuated 6-hydroxydopamine induced cell death in PC12 cells and mice.[30,31] Pramipexole reduces the toxicity of 6-hydroxydopamine and MPTP in vivo and in vitro.[32-34] Ropinirole, a D2/D3, agonist has been shown in vitro to scavenge hydroxyl radicals with an inhibitory concentration (IC_{50}) of 1.5 mM, a concentration significantly greater than that of pergolide or bromocriptine.[35] Similarly, ropinirole was able to scavenge nitric oxide, but not superoxide, radicals, but at relatively high concentration. Ropinirole did increase mouse striatal reduced glutathione, catalase, and superoxide dismutase levels, however, when administered intraperitoneally. These effects on the striatum were blocked by prior administration of the dopamine receptor blocker sulpiride. Pretreatment with ropinirole ameliorated the effects of 6-hydroxydopamine toxicity in mouse striatum, and this effect was blocked by sulpiride. These results suggest that ropinirole exerts its protective effect via interaction with D2 receptors.

The mechanism of action of dopamine agonist–mediated neuroprotection is uncertain. Although these drugs can act as free radical scavengers, this property seems to depend on relatively high concentrations. Whether dopamine agonists reach such levels in the central nervous system is unknown, and possible selective concentration into certain cell types or organelles is a further complication in this interpretation.

An important consideration is whether dopamine agonists mediate their protective action through dopamine receptors. The available data are conflicting, perhaps relating to the use of different agonists and concentrations, cell types, and incubation protocols. As discussed earlier, there is evidence that ropinirole-mediated protection is via the D2 receptor.[35] In the case of pramipexole, in vitro studies have shown that dopamine receptor blockade with sulpiride or clozapine does not prevent or diminish the protective action of this drug against MPP+ toxicity.[36,37] The receptor inactive enantiomer of pramipexole is protective.[37,38] Using rodent mesencephalic cultures, D3 receptor blockade prevented protection by pramipexole, however.[32] Another group using rat PC12 cells showed that protection by bromocriptine depended on expression of the dopamine D2 receptor.[39] It may be that different dopamine agonists may exert their protective effects via different routes. Pramipexole has shown that it can increase the expression of GDNF and brain-derived neurotrophic factor in primary mesencephalic cultures.[40]

Based on these encouraging preclinical data, two clinical trials to evaluate the neuroprotective action of dopamine agonists were undertaken. Both trials used imaging as a marker for nigrostriatal cell loss; this was in large part an attempt to overcome the confounding effect of the symptomatic action of these drugs on any clinical end point. Striatal fluorodopa F 15 (^{15}F-dopa) uptake on position emission tomography (PET) and striatal β-CIT uptake on single photon emission computed tomography (SPECT) were taken to provide surrogate markers of the integrity of the nigrostriatal system.

The first of the studies (CALM-PD-CIT) randomly assigned newly diagnosed PD patients to initiate treatment with either the dopamine agonist pramipexole or levodopa.[41] Striatal β-CIT uptake on SPECT to determine dopamine transporter density was performed at baseline and at various time points over the course of the 4-year trial. Patients in either group requiring additional symptomatic therapy could be supplemented with open-label levodopa if deemed necessary. In this study, patients randomly assigned to receive pramipexole had a significant

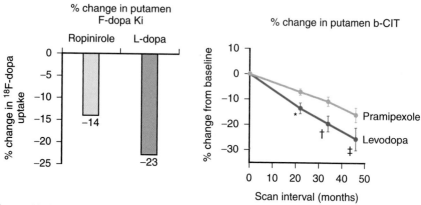

PD PROGRESSION: DA vs L-DOPA

Figure 18–3 Results of imaging end points in dopamine agonist (DA) neuroprotection trials in early Parkinson's disease (PD). (Adapted from Parkinson's Disease Study Group. Dopamine transporter brain imaging to assess the effects of pramipexole vs levodopa on Parkinson disease progression. *JAMA.* 2002;287:1653-1661; and Whone AL, Watts RL, Stoessl AJ, et al. Slower progression of Parkinson's disease with ropinirole versus levodopa: the REAL-PET study. *Ann Neurol.* 2003;54:93-101.)

36% reduction in the rate of decline of β-CIT uptake compared with patients initiated on levodopa (Fig. 18–3). In the second study (REAL-PET), untreated PD patients were randomly assigned to begin therapy with the dopamine agonist ropinirole or levodopa.[42] In this study, patients randomly assigned to initiate treatment with the agonist had a significant 35% reduction in the rate of decline in striatal [15]F-dopa uptake on PET compared with patients on levodopa (see Fig. 18–3). Neither study showed any clinical benefit in favor of the dopamine agonists to go along with these imaging findings.

A placebo group was not included in either study, and so these results cannot confirm a neuroprotective effect of either dopamine agonist. Alternative explanations include a deleterious effect of levodopa or manipulation of the imaging signal by the drug. The similarity of the results obtained using two different but complementary techniques and the in vitro and in vivo laboratory data available provide some support that agonists can exert a neuroprotective action. Even if these imaging findings do reflect an agonist-induced slowing in the rate of neuronal degeneration, neither of these studies detected any corresponding clinical benefit. The studies were relatively short-term, however, and benefits may have been masked by the symptomatic effects of the dopaminergic agents.

To establish that these drugs have neuroprotective properties, it likely will be necessary to perform longer term studies that are designed to capture differences in quality of life that correlate with imaging changes. A randomized early-start trial of pramipexole versus placebo completed recruitment in early 2008, and a report is expected in 2009. Patients received either pramipexole or placebo for 9 months, and then all patients were randomly assigned again to pramipexole. The end point measured the difference from baseline at 15 months in UPDRS. There was also a SPECT substudy that compared baseline and 15-month dopamine transporter levels.

Mitochondrial Function Enhancers

The discovery of mitochondrial complex I deficiency and the subsequent identification of genetic causes that involved mitochondrial proteins has focused attention on the potential for enhancing bioenergetics to treat PD.[43,44] Coenzyme Q10 (CoQ10) functions as a component of the respiratory chain in shuttling electrons between complexes I and III, and as an antioxidant. In a double-blind randomized placebo-controlled study, 16 to 23 patients were recruited per treatment arm to assess the efficacy of three doses of CoQ10 (300 mg/day, 600 mg/day, and 1200 mg/day) in patients with early PD.[45] Over a 16-month period, the highest dose group progressed at a slower rate in terms of worsening of motor function and activities of daily living (UPDRS parts II and III) compared with the control group, although much of this benefit was related to the activities of daily living component and was established very early in the trial.

A futility analysis assessed CoQ10 using historic control data and the total score of the UPDRS and failed to show futility (i.e., suggested that the compound was worthy of future study).[46] The authors called into question the validity of their historic control data, however, in the light of more recent placebo progression rates in the UPDRS, and with these, CoQ10 did suggest futility. A small study of 28 treated PD patients supplemented with 360 mg daily of CoQ10 showed a mild symptomatic motor effect over 4 weeks.[47] However, A larger study of 300 mg daily (which produced the same plasma levels as 1200 mg daily in the Shults study[45]) found no symptomatic effect on the UPDRS.[48]

Creatine is converted to phosphocreatine and can transfer a phosphoryl group to adenosine diphosphate to synthesize adenosine triphosphate and so enhance energy production. Creatine can reduce dopaminergic cell loss in the MPTP rodent model of PD.[49] Creatine is a dietary supplement and is well tolerated in high doses for short periods. It is one of the drugs investigated in the NINDS NET-PD futility studies of compounds for neuroprotection in PD. At a dose of 10 g daily, creatine was well tolerated, and satisfied the predetermined criterion for nonfutility based on time to requirement for symptomatic therapy for 66 patients with early PD.[50] Another blinded placebo-controlled study of 2 g daily for 6 months (after a loading dose of 20 g for 6 days) then 4 g daily for 18 months in 31 PD patients compared with 17 patients given placebo showed no significant difference in UPDRS scores or SPECT dopamine transporter density.[51] There was a significantly lower requirement for dopaminergic symptomatic treatment in the creatine arm, however, which could be indicative of a positive effect of creatine.

Levodopa

Levodopa is considered the most potent oral medication for PD. Its benefits include good control of motor symptoms and a consequent improvement in quality of life and life expectancy. Over time, however, there have been concerns regarding the potential toxicity of levodopa. These concerns relate mainly to its potential to generate free radicals and induce cell death in cultured cells. Depending on the concentration, levodopa can have no effect in these in vitro systems, however, or even exert protective effects through alterations in reduced glutathione levels or through increased production of neurotrophic factors.[52,53] These observations are consistent with the fact that levodopa can act as a pro-oxidant and antioxidant molecule depending on circumstance. Low concentrations of levodopa can induce an upregulation in reduced glutathione and in other neuroprotective molecules possibly because the drug acts as a "minimal stressor" that enhances the production of protective molecules.

An important and relevant difference between in vitro culture conditions and conditions in vivo is that ascorbate concentrations are typically high in tissues but low in culture. One report suggests that much of the in vitro evidence for a toxic effect of dopamine on neuronal cells may be artifactual and a consequence of the culture medium employed.[54] Many of the studies showing levodopa toxicity in culture used high concentrations (>50 µM/L) of levodopa, whereas peak plasma concentrations in patients are 10 to 20 µM/L, and only approximately 12% of an oral dose appears in the cerebrospinal fluid.[55] The incorporation of glial cells into the cell culture models and the addition of ascorbate, situations that more closely mimic the substantia nigra, significantly diminish or abolish levodopa toxicity.[56,57]

The ELLDOPA study investigated the effect of levodopa versus placebo on disease progression using as a primary end point the change in motor score between untreated baseline and an untreated final visit performed after 9 months of study drug treatment and 2 weeks of drug withdrawal.[58] At the completion of the trial, patients who had been randomly assigned to receive levodopa had less deterioration from baseline than patients receiving placebo showing no evidence of toxicity, a result consistent with neuroprotection (Fig. 18–4A). As part of this study, a subgroup of patients underwent β-CIT SPECT scans at baseline and at 9 months. Patients treated with levodopa had a greater rate of decline in this imaging marker than patients in the placebo group, consistent with levodopa having a toxic effect (Fig. 18–4B).

The results of the study are in part difficult to reconcile. The clinical improvement in the levodopa arms after 2 weeks of washout could relate to a long duration benefit of levodopa that persists after the washout period. Alternatively, the sustained clinical benefit after washout could be interpreted as a neuroprotective effect of levodopa. At the clinical level, these results do not suggest that levodopa is toxic. In contrast, the imaging results could suggest a toxic effect of levodopa on nigrostriatal cells, or, alternatively, a downregulation of the transporter such as was suggested for the dopamine agonist neuroprotection trials. A further possibility is that earlier treatment in itself had a protective effect, which would be consistent with the results from many other studies.[59] The ELLDOPA study established the dose-response effectiveness of levodopa in these patients with early PD, but also showed that motor complications were dose-related and could develop within 6 months of initiation of levodopa, reaching levels of 30% for wearing-off and 16.5% for dyskinesias in the high-dose group.

N-Methyl-D-Aspartate Receptor Antagonists

There is some evidence that excitotoxicity may be important in the pathogenesis of PD. N-methyl-D-aspartate (NMDA) receptor antagonists can protect dopamine neurons from glutamate-mediated toxicity in tissue culture and in rodent and

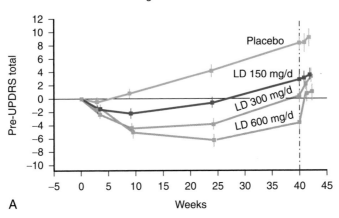

ELLDOPA
Change in UPDRS total score

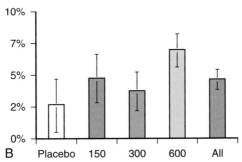

ELLDOPA
% change striatal β-CIT at 9 months

Figure 18–4 **A** and **B,** Results of the ELLDOPA trial showing maintenance of clinical response after washout (**A**), but a greater loss of dopamine transporter in the levodopa-treated patients (**B**). LD, levodopa; UPDRS, Unified Parkinson's Disease Rating Scale. (Adapted from Fahn S, Oakes D, Shoulson I, et al. Levodopa and the progression of Parkinson's disease. *N Engl J Med.* 2004;351:2498-2508.)

primate models of PD.[60-62] A retrospective analysis suggested that early use of the NMDA receptor antagonist amantadine might slow the rate of progression in PD patients.[63] On the basis of limited laboratory data, a double-blind placebo-controlled dosing study was undertaken to assess the safety and tolerability of remacemide hydrochloride, a low-affinity NMDA channel blocker.[64] There were more adverse events with daily doses of 150 mg, 300 mg, and 600 mg of the drug compared with placebo. There was no obvious symptomatic effect, although only small numbers of patients were studied.

Riluzole is another antiglutamate drug that acts by inhibiting sodium channels and prevents the release of glutamate. The drug is approved for use in the treatment of motor neuron disease (amyotrophic lateral sclerosis).[65,66] Laboratory studies showed the capacity of riluzole to protect dopamine neurons in rodent and primate models of PD.[67,68] A small open-label pilot study in PD patients showed that riluzole was well tolerated at doses of 100 mg/day and did not provide any symptomatic benefit.[69] This finding prompted a multicenter placebo-controlled trial to investigate the potential neuroprotective effect of riluzole in patients with early untreated and more advanced PD. As in the DATATOP study, the primary end point was the need for supplemental dopaminergic therapy. The final results of the trial have not yet been published, but it is known that the trial was aborted after an interim futility analysis showed no potential of detecting a neuroprotective effect. A study to determine whether riluzole could reduce dyskinesias in PD patients was similarly negative.[70]

Immunophilins

Immunophilins are small proteins and function as cytosolic receptors for immunosuppressant drugs. Some agonists of these cytosolic receptor proteins may have a protective action and can have a nerve growth factor–like effect, increasing sprouting after MPTP or 6-hydroxydopamine toxicity.[71-73] Other studies of immunophilins in animal models have been negative, however.[74,75] Two immunophilin agents have been tested in PD patients, but the results have been disappointing, and no evidence of a neuroprotective or restorative effect has been observed.[76]

Antiapoptotic Agents

Several different compounds exhibit antiapoptotic properties, including selegiline, rasagiline, and the dopamine agonists, specifically pramipexole. These were discussed in detail earlier. One promising antiapoptotic agent for study in PD was TCH346 (N-methyl-N-propargyl-10-aminomethyl-dibenzo[b,f]-oxepin), or CGP3466. This was a propargylamine drug and resembled selegiline, but did not inhibit MAOB. It was predicted to have no symptomatic effects in PD. TCH346 had been shown to prevent degeneration of dopaminergic neurons in various in vitro models of apoptosis,[77-82] and to protect against neurodegeneration in animal models of PD.[83] TCH346 was active at picomolar concentrations and was thought to exhibit potent antiapoptotic activity. TCH346 interacted with glyceraldehyde-3-phosphate dehydrogenase[79] and prevented its translocation from cytoplasm to nucleus and its initiation of the apoptotic cascade.[77,78]

After appropriate safety studies, TCH346 entered a phase II/III trial in early PD.[84] This trial randomly assigned 301 patients with early PD to one of three doses of TCH346 (0.5 mg, 2.5 mg, or 10 mg) or placebo. The primary end point was predetermined as the time to require intervention with a dopaminergic agent as judged by a blinded rater. There were no significant differences between any of the TCH346 dose arms and placebo in the primary end point or in any of the secondary analyses.

This disappointing result may have been the consequence of several different factors. The most parsimonious is that the drug has no neuroprotective action in PD patients. If so, it must be accepted that the preclinical models are not an accurate reflection of PD pathogenesis and neuroprotection and have to be used with caution in the prediction of clinical effects. Alternatively, it may be that the wrong dose of drug was used. Translating an effective dose from animals to humans, especially in testing for neuroprotection, is complicated. The dose effect may be directly related to increasing concentrations, or have a U-shaped curve with only a small range of concentrations being effective. Other considerations include the selection of end point and the cohort of patients recruited. Although time to dopaminergic therapy is an important event in the progression of PD, it can be a blunt instrument, and a trial may miss a subtle effect. If a neuroprotective drug is to have maximum effect, it could be argued that it should be given at the earliest opportunity. Although the patients in the TCH346 study had early disease, it is known that even at this time, dopaminergic neuronal cell degeneration is well advanced and may be beyond the effectiveness of anything but the most potent drugs.

CEP1347 is a mixed lineage kinase inhibitor of apoptosis that also showed promise in preclinical studies of PD models. The drug entered a pivotal phase II/III trial in early PD with 806 patients with early PD randomly assigned to placebo or one of three doses of CEP1347 (10 mg, 25 mg, or 50 mg).[85] In addition, patients had a dopamine transporter SPECT scan at baseline and conclusion of the study. There was no significant difference between any of the treatment arms and placebo. The SPECT marker declined more in the drug arms than placebo. It seems that this antiapoptotic agent is not an effective neuroprotective drug for PD. The interpretations and limitations of this study are directly comparable to those of TCH346.

Anti-inflammatory Drugs

There is evidence for inflammatory cell activation in the nigra in PD.[86] Animal models suggest that this may occur early in the course of cell damage and death. The debate about whether the inflammation is primary or secondary is unresolved, but in the context of an anti-inflammatory strategy for neuroprotection in PD, the answer may be irrelevant. It seems likely that inflammation at least contributes to cell damage, and limiting its effect would seem logical.

Preclinical studies have shown some benefit for anti-inflammatory drugs. Acetylsalicylic acid is an inhibitor of cyclooxygenase-1 and cyclooxygenase-2, whereas meloxicam is a cyclooxygenase-2 inhibitor. In the MPTP mouse model of nigrostriatal cell loss, cell death and dopamine depletion were significantly protected by both drugs when given before the toxin.

Epidemiological studies have sought to determine whether the use of anti-inflammatory drugs can protect against the development of PD. A study in PD has shown that use of a nonsteroidal anti-inflammatory drug two or more times per week can produce a 45% lower risk for PD.[87] Minocycline is an anti-inflammatory agent and has antiapoptotic action. In a futility analysis, the use of minocycline was considered suitable for further study as a drug for neuroprotection in PD.[88] The adverse event profile was unfavorable, however, and the dropout rate was high. A study of minocycline in anterior horn cell disease not only showed no benefit, but also some worsening in patient outcome.[89]

Adenosine Antagonists

Adenosine A2A receptors are abundant in the striatum and modulate the neurotransmission of γ-aminobutyric acid, acetylcholine, and glutamate transmission. There has been interest in developing A2A antagonists for the symptomatic treatment of PD. There is also interest in the part that adenosine receptors may play in mediating neuroprotection in PD.

A case-control study compared the past dietary habits of PD patients and found that they drank less coffee than controls.[90] A prospective study of 8004 Japanese-American men (45 to 68 years old) enrolled in the Honolulu Heart Program found that higher coffee and caffeine intake was associated with a significantly lower incidence of PD.[91] In another study, the relative risk for PD was 0.42 (95% confidence interval 0.23 to 0.78; P for trend < .001) for men in the top one fifth of caffeine intake compared with men in the bottom one fifth, after adjustment for age and smoking.[92] This association was maintained with caffeine from noncoffee sources and tea. Among women, the relationship between caffeine or coffee intake and risk of PD was U-shaped, with the lowest risk observed at moderate intakes (one to three cups of coffee per day, or the third quintile of caffeine consumption). They concluded that moderate doses of caffeine might have a protective effect on the risk of PD.

Calcium Channel Blockers

Adult nigral dopaminergic cells are calcium-dependent autonomous pacemakers, driven by voltage-dependent L-type calcium channels, probably $Ca_v1.3$-type.[93] This dependence increases with age, and together with other pathogenetic factors in PD might contribute to pathogenesis. Blockade of the $Ca_v1.3$-type channel might lead to a less calcium-dependent phenotype, which is more prevalent in less mature dopaminergic neurons.[94] Preclinical studies have shown that calcium channel blockers (e.g., nimodipine) and angiotensin-converting enzyme blockers can protect against MPTP toxicity.[95,96] A retrospective case-control analysis of individuals taking antihypertensives long-term showed a modest but significant reduction in risk for developing PD, particularly for individuals older than 80 years.[97]

Timing of Treatment and Compensatory Mechanisms

An alternative strategy for disease modification in PD that is based not on a specific neuroprotective agent, but rather the support of intrinsic compensatory mechanisms and basal ganglia plasticity, has been proposed.[59] It is suggested that early correction of the basal ganglia functional abnormalities caused by dopaminergic cell loss and dopamine deficiency is a means to support the intrinsic physiological compensatory mechanisms, and limit and delay the circuitry changes that evolve as PD progresses. Review of the outcomes of the DATATOP, ELLDOPA, and TEMPO studies may support such a proposition.

In the DATATOP, ELLDOPA, and TEMPO studies (see earlier), patients who received effective symptomatic treatment earlier in the course of their disease fared significantly better clinically than patients initiated on placebo even when, as in the case of TEMPO, they were switched to the active drug after only 6 months. The failure of trials of nonsymptomatic drugs (e.g., TCH346 or CEP1347) to show any benefit over placebo may be a consequence not only of their lack of neuroprotective effects, but also of their inability to "reset" the defective basal ganglia system by dopaminergic compensation.

The "normalization" of basal ganglia function by early dopaminergic therapy would have benefits in terms of symptomatic improvements and longer term effects in delaying clinical progression. The interpretation of the DATATOP, ELLDOPA, and TEMPO data as evidence to support early symptomatic intervention does not preclude any potential disease-modifying beneficial effects of these and other dopaminergic drugs by alternative, additional protective mechanisms. Initiation of dopaminergic treatment can be associated with unwanted side effects, which may include gastrointestinal disturbances, cognitive problems, and sedation. These side effects need to be weighed against the symptomatic improvement that the patient would experience and the hypothetical long-term benefit outlined here.

Prospects for the Future

There are signs that some compounds, such as MAOB inhibitors and dopamine agonists, may truly have a neuroprotective role. Two trials recently completed may reinforce this view. The ADAGIO and PROUD studies are randomized start design trials; the first with rasagiline, and the second with pramipexole. This particular trial design (Fig. 18–5) recruits patients with early untreated PD and randomly assigns them to placebo or an active arm. Because both drugs involved in these studies improve symptoms, the active arms will be improved compared with placebo. After 9 months, the patients are randomly assigned again so that all will be on active treatment. After a further 6 to 9 months the patients are assessed by a blinded rater with a primary end point of change in UPDRS clinical score from baseline. The symptomatic effect will be balanced by all arms being on active therapy for the last 6 to 9 months. Any change in clinical score should be a consequence of the drug given to patients during the first period of the trial.

A positive result could be interpreted as showing a neuroprotective effect. An alternative, and as explained earlier not mutually exclusive, explanation would be that earlier treatment itself provided longer term benefit. The PROUD study is supplemented by an imaging arm using SPECT to quantify the dopamine transporter. Patients will have had imaging at baseline and at the end of the study. The results of this secondary end point may help explain any effect, and should provide insight into the interpretation of the CALM-PD study described earlier. Preliminary data from ADAGIO indicated that the 1mg dose of rasagiline produced a significant improvement in outcome at 15 months in UPDRS when initiated earlier as apposed to later. The 2mg dose failed to reach significance.

Trial design for neuroprotection studies has also advanced as a result of experience over the past 20 years. The selection of end points remains a complex issue, however. Ultimately, retarding the progress of nonmotor, predominantly nondopaminergic problems, such as cognitive decline and autonomic features, is a major goal of therapy.[98] A true neuroprotective agent might be expected to slow nondopaminergic and dopaminergic cell loss. The use of these as an end point, perhaps combined with motor scores, would also be valid. The identification of

TESTING THE DELAYED-START HYPOTHESIS

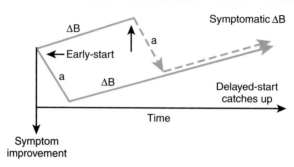

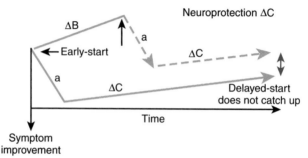

Figure 18–5   The randomized start (or early start) design. Patients with early untreated Parkinson's disease are randomly assigned to placebo or a putative neuroprotective drug that also has symptomatic action. In placebo patients, there is a rate of deterioration—ΔB. In the patients receiving the symptomatic treatment without neuroprotective action, there is improvement—a—followed by deterioration—ΔB. At some time point (e.g., 6 to 9 months), patients are randomly assigned again for all to receive the active drug. Patients on placebo in the first phase now experience symptomatic improvement—a. In the case of a drug with no neuroprotective action, both groups now merge, and continue to progress at ΔB. In the case of a drug with protective action, the rate of progression is slowed to ΔC. Patients who received this drug in the first phase will now always be at an advantage, and patients in the early placebo group will never catch up.

biomarkers that advance with disease as a consequence of neurodegeneration would be an important contribution to this field.

REFERENCES

1. Parkinson's Disease Study Group: Effects of tocopherol and deprenyl on the progression of disability in early Parkinson's disease. The Parkinson Study Group. N Engl J Med 1993;328:176-183.
2. Olanow CW, Hauser RA, Gauger L, et al: The effect of deprenyl and levodopa on the progression of Parkinson's disease. Ann Neurol 1995;38:771-777.
3. Shoulson I, Oakes D, Fahn S, et al: Impact of sustained deprenyl (selegiline) in levodopa-treated Parkinson's disease: a randomized placebo-controlled extension of the deprenyl and tocopherol antioxidative therapy of parkinsonism trial. Ann Neurol 2002;51:604-612.
4. Palhagen S, Heinonen E, Hagglund J, et al: Selegiline slows the progression of the symptoms of Parkinson disease. Neurology 2006;66:1200-1206.
5. Ives NJ, Stowe RL, Marro J, et al: Monoamine oxidase type B inhibitors in early Parkinson's disease: meta-analysis of 17 randomised trials involving 3525 patients. BMJ 2004;329:593.
6. Cesura AM, Galva MD, Imhof R, et al: [3H]Ro 19-6327: a reversible ligand and affinity labelling probe for monoamine oxidase-B. Eur J Pharmacol 1989;162:457-465.

7. Parkinson's Disease Study Group: Effect of lazabemide on the progression of disability in early Parkinson's disease. The Parkinson Study Group. Ann Neurol 1996;40:99-107.
8. LeWitt PA, Segel SA, Mistura KL, Schork MA: Symptomatic anti-parkinsonian effects of monoamine oxidase-B inhibition: comparison of selegiline and lazabemide. Clin Neuropharmacol 1993;16:332-337.
9. Schapira A, Bate G, Kirkpatrick P: Rasagiline. Nat Rev Drug Discov 2005;4:625-626.
10. Schapira AH, Bezard E, Brotchie J, et al: Novel pharmacological targets for the treatment of Parkinson's disease. Nat Rev Drug Discov 2006;5:845-854.
11. Youdim MB, Weinstock M: Molecular basis of neuroprotective activities of rasagiline and the anti-Alzheimer drug TV3326 [(N-propargyl-(3R)aminoindan-5-YL)-ethyl methyl carbamate]. Cell Mol Neurobiol 2001;21:555-573.
12. Bonneh-Barkay D, Ziv N, Finberg JP: Characterization of the neuroprotective activity of rasagiline in cerebellar granule cells. Neuropharmacology 2005;48:406-416.
13. Bar AO, Amit T, Youdim MB: Contrasting neuroprotective and neurotoxic actions of respective metabolites of anti-Parkinson drugs rasagiline and selegiline. Neurosci Lett 2004;355:169-172.
14. Maruyama W, Weinstock M, Youdim MB, et al: Anti-apoptotic action of anti-Alzheimer drug, TV3326 [(N-propargyl)-(3R)-aminoindan-5-yl]-ethyl methyl carbamate, a novel cholinesterase-monoamine oxidase inhibitor. Neurosci Lett 2003;341:233-236.
15. Youdim MB, Wadia A, Tatton W, Weinstock M: The anti-Parkinson drug rasagiline and its cholinesterase inhibitor derivatives exert neuroprotection unrelated to MAO inhibition in cell culture and in vivo. Ann N Y Acad Sci 2001;939:450-458.
16. Mandel S, Weinreb O, Amit T, Youdim MB: Mechanism of neuroprotective action of the anti-Parkinson drug rasagiline and its derivatives. Brain Res Brain Res Rev 2005;48:379-387.
17. Youdim MB, Bar AO, Yogev-Falach M, et al: Rasagiline: neurodegeneration, neuroprotection, and mitochondrial permeability transition. J Neurosci Res 2005;79:172-179.
18. Maruyama W, Nitta A, Shamoto-Nagai M, et al: N-Propargyl-1 (R)-aminoindan, rasagiline, increases glial cell line-derived neurotrophic factor (GDNF) in neuroblastoma SH-SY5Y cells through activation of NF-kappaB transcription factor. Neurochem Int 2004;44:393-400.
19. Parkinson's Disease Study Group: A controlled trial of rasagiline in early Parkinson disease: the TEMPO Study. Arch Neurol 2002;59:1937-1943.
20. Parkinson's Disease Study Group: A controlled, randomized, delayed-start study of rasagiline in early Parkinson disease. Arch Neurol 2004;61:561-566.
21. Carter AJ, Muller RE: Pramipexole, a dopamine D2 autoreceptor agonist, decreases the extracellular concentration of dopamine in vivo. Eur J Pharmacol 1991;200:65-72.
22. Piercey M, Camacho-Ochoa M, Smith M: Functional roles for dopamine receptor subtypes. Clin Neuropharmacol 1995;18:34-42.
23. Schapira AH: Neuroprotection in PD—a role for dopamine agonists? Neurology 2003;61:S34-S42.
24. Schapira AH, Olanow CW: Rationale for the use of dopamine agonists as neuroprotective agents in Parkinson's disease. Ann Neurol 2003;53(Suppl 3):S149-S157.
25. Le WD, Jankovic J: Are dopamine receptor agonists neuroprotective in Parkinson's disease? Drugs Aging 2001;18:389-396.
26. Ogawa N, Tanaka K, Asanuma M, et al: Bromocriptine protects mice against 6-hydroxydopamine and scavenges hydroxyl free radicals in vitro. Brain Res 1994;657:207-213.
27. Muralikrishnan D, Mohanakumar KP: Neuroprotection by bromocriptine against 1-methyl-4-phenyl-1,2,3,6-tetrahydropyridine-induced neurotoxicity in mice. FASEB J 1998;12:905-912.
28. Sethy VH, Wu H, Oostveen JA, Hall ED: Neuroprotective effects of the dopamine agonists pramipexole and bromocriptine in 3-acetylpyridine-treated rats. Brain Res 1997;754:181-186.
29. Takashima H, Tsujihata M, Kishikawa M, Freed WJ: Bromocriptine protects dopaminergic neurons from levodopa-induced toxicity by stimulating D(2)receptors. Exp Neurol 1999;159:98-104.
30. Gassen M, Gross A, Youdim MB: Apomorphine enantiomers protect cultured pheochromocytoma (PC12) cells from oxidative stress induced by H2O2 and 6-hydroxydopamine. Mov Disord 1998;13:242-248.
31. Asanuma M, Ogawa N, Nishibayashi S, et al: Protective effects of pergolide on dopamine levels in the 6-hydroxydopamine-lesioned mouse brain. Arch Int Pharmacodyn Ther 1995;329:221-230.
32. Kitamura Y, Kohno Y, Nakazawa M, Nomura Y: Inhibitory effects of talipexole and pramipexole on MPTP-induced dopamine reduction in the striatum of C57BL/6N mice. Jpn J Pharmacol 1997;74:51-57.
33. Zou L, Xu J, Jankovic J, et al: Pramipexole inhibits lipid peroxidation and reduces injury in the substantia nigra induced by the dopaminergic neurotoxin 1-methyl-4-phenyl-1,2,3,6-tetrahydropyridine in C57BL/6 mice. Neurosci Lett 2000;281:167-170.

34. Vu TQ, Ling ZD, Ma SY, et al: Pramipexole attenuates the dopaminergic cell loss induced by intraventricular 6-hydroxydopamine. J Neural Transm 2000;107:159-176.
35. Iida M, Miyazaki I, Tanaka K, et al: Dopamine D2 receptor-mediated antioxidant and neuroprotective effects of ropinirole, a dopamine agonist. Brain Res 1999;838:51-59.
36. Kitamura Y, Kosaka T, Kakimura JI, et al: Protective effects of the antiparkinsonian drugs talipexole and pramipexole against 1-methyl-4-phenylpyridinium-induced apoptotic death in human neuroblastoma SH-SY5Y cells. Mol Pharmacol 1998;54:1046-1054.
37. Gu M, Iravani MM, Cooper JM, et al: Pramipexole protects against apoptotic cell death by non-dopaminergic mechanisms. J Neurochem 2004;91:1075-1081.
38. Cassarino DS, Fall CP, Smith TS, Bennett JP Jr: Pramipexole reduces reactive oxygen species production in vivo and in vitro and inhibits the mitochondrial permeability transition produced by the parkinsonian neurotoxin methylpyridinium ion. J Neurochem 1998;71:295-301.
39. Nair VD, Olanow CW, Sealfon SC: Activation of phosphoinositide 3-kinase by D2 receptor prevents apoptosis in dopaminergic cell lines. Biochem J 2003;373:25-32.
40. Du F, Li R, Huang Y, et al: Dopamine D3 receptor-preferring agonists induce neurotrophic effects on mesencephalic dopamine neurons. Eur J Neurosci 2005;22:2422-2430.
41. Parkinson's Disease Study Group: Dopamine transporter brain imaging to assess the effects of pramipexole vs levodopa on Parkinson disease progression. JAMA 2002;287:1653-1661.
42. Whone AL, Watts RL, Stoessl AJ, et al: Slower progression of Parkinson's disease with ropinirole versus levodopa: the REAL-PET study. Ann Neurol 2003;54:93-101.
43. Schapira AH: Mitochondrial disease. Lancet 2006;368:70-82.
44. Schapira AH: Mitochondria in the aetiology and pathogenesis of Parkinson's disease. Lancet Neurol 2008;7:97-109.
45. Shults CW, Oakes D, Kieburtz K, et al: Effects of coenzyme Q10 in early Parkinson disease: evidence of slowing of the functional decline. Arch Neurol 2002;59:1541-1550.
46. NINDS NET-PD Investigators: A randomized clinical trial of coenzyme Q10 and GPI-1485 in early Parkinson disease. Neurology 2007;68:20-28.
47. Muller T, Buttner T, Gholipour AF, Kuhn W: Coenzyme Q10 supplementation provides mild symptomatic benefit in patients with Parkinson's disease. Neurosci Lett 2003;341:201-204.
48. Storch A, Jost WH, Vieregge P, et al: Randomized, double-blind, placebo-controlled trial on symptomatic effects of coenzyme Q(10) in Parkinson disease. Arch Neurol 2007;64:938-944.
49. Matthews RT, Ferrante RJ, Klivenyi P, et al: Creatine and cyclocreatine attenuate MPTP neurotoxicity. Exp Neurol 1999;157:142-149.
50. NINDS NET-PD Investigators: A randomized, double-blind, futility clinical trial of creatine and minocycline in early Parkinson disease. Neurology 2006;66:664-671.
51. Bender A, Koch W, Elstner M, et al: Creatine supplementation in Parkinson disease: a placebo-controlled randomized pilot trial. Neurology 2006;67:1262-1264.
52. Mytilineou C, Han SK, Cohen G: Toxic and protective effects of L-dopa on mesencephalic cell cultures. J Neurochem 1993;61:1470-1478.
53. Mena MA, Davila V, Sulzer D: Neurotrophic effects of L-DOPA in postnatal midbrain dopamine neuron/cortical astrocyte cocultures. J Neurochem 1997;69:1398-1408.
54. Clement MV, Long LH, Ramalingam J, Halliwell B: The cytotoxicity of dopamine may be an artefact of cell culture. J Neurochem 2002;81:414-421.
55. Olanow CW, Gauger LL, Cedarbaum JM: Temporal relationships between plasma and cerebrospinal fluid pharmacokinetics of levodopa and clinical effect in Parkinson's disease. Ann Neurol 1991;29:556-559.
56. Mena MA, Casarejos MJ, Carazo A, et al: Glia protect fetal midbrain dopamine neurons in culture from L-DOPA toxicity through multiple mechanisms. J Neural Transm 1997;104:317-328.
57. Mytilineou C, Walker RH, Baptiste R, Olanow CW: Levodopa is toxic to dopamine neurons in an in vitro but not an in vivo model of oxidative stress. J Pharmacol Exp Ther 2003;304:792-800.
58. Fahn S, Oakes D, Shoulson I, et al: Levodopa and the progression of Parkinson's disease. N Engl J Med 2004;351:2498-2508.
59. Schapira AH, Obeso J: Timing of treatment initiation in Parkinson's disease: a need for reappraisal? Ann Neurol 2006;59:559-562.
60. Doble A: The role of excitotoxicity in neurodegenerative disease: implications for therapy. Pharmacol Ther 1999;81:163-221.
61. Turski L, Bressler K, Rettig KJ, et al: Protection of substantia nigra from MPP+ neurotoxicity by N-methyl-D-aspartate antagonists. Nature 1991;349:414-418.

62. Greenamyre JT, Eller RV, Zhang Z, et al: Antiparkinsonian effects of remacemide hydrochloride, a glutamate antagonist, in rodent and primate models of Parkinson's disease. Ann Neurol 1994;35:655-661.
63. Uitti RJ, Rajput AH, Ahlskog JE, et al: Amantadine treatment is an independent predictor of improved survival in Parkinson's disease. Neurology 1996;46:1551-1556.
64. Parkinson's Disease Study Group: A multicenter randomized controlled trial of remacemide hydrochloride as monotherapy for PD. Parkinson Study Group. Neurology 2000;54:1583-1588.
65. Lacomblez L, Bensimon G, Leigh PN, et al: Dose-ranging study of riluzole in amyotrophic lateral sclerosis. Amyotrophic Lateral Sclerosis/Riluzole Study Group II. Lancet 1996;347:1425-1431.
66. Bensimon G, Lacomblez L, Meininger V: A controlled trial of riluzole in amyotrophic lateral sclerosis. ALS/Riluzole Study Group. N Engl J Med 1994;330:585-591.
67. Araki T, Kumagai T, Tanaka K, et al: Neuroprotective effect of riluzole in MPTP-treated mice. Brain Res 2001;918:176-181.
68. Obinu MC, Reibaud M, Blanchard V, et al: Neuroprotective effect of riluzole in a primate model of Parkinson's disease: behavioral and histological evidence. Mov Disord 2002;17:13-19.
69. Jankovic J, Hunter C: A double-blind, placebo-controlled and longitudinal study of riluzole in early Parkinson's disease. Parkinsonism Relat Disord 2002;8:271-276.
70. Braz CA, Borges V, Ferraz HB: Effect of riluzole on dyskinesia and duration of the on state in Parkinson disease patients: a double-blind, placebo-controlled pilot study. Clin Neuropharmacol 2004;27:25-29.
71. Steiner JP, Hamilton GS, Ross DT, et al: Neurotrophic immunophilin ligands stimulate structural and functional recovery in neurodegenerative animal models. Proc Natl Acad Sci U S A 1997;94:2019-2024.
72. Ross DT, Guo H, Howorth P, et al: The small molecule FKBP ligand GPI 1046 induces partial striatal re-innervation after intranigral 6-hydroxydopamine lesion in rats. Neurosci Lett 2001;297:113-116.
73. Zhang C, Steiner JP, Hamilton GS, et al: Regeneration of dopaminergic function in 6-hydroxydopamine-lesioned rats by neuroimmunophilin ligand treatment. J Neurosci 2001;21. RC156.
74. Bocquet A, Lorent G, Fuks B, et al: Failure of GPI compounds to display neurotrophic activity in vitro and in vivo. Eur J Pharmacol 2001;415:173-180.
75. Emborg ME, Shin P, Roitberg B, et al: Systemic administration of the immunophilin ligand GPI 1046 in MPTP-treated monkeys. Exp Neurol 2001;168:171-182.
76. Gold BG, Nutt JG: Neuroimmunophilin ligands in the treatment of Parkinson's disease. Curr Opin Pharmacol 2002;2:82-86.
77. Carlile GW, Chalmers-Redman RM, Tatton NA, et al: Reduced apoptosis after nerve growth factor and serum withdrawal: conversion of tetrameric glyceraldehyde-3-phosphate dehydrogenase to a dimer. Mol Pharmacol 2000;57:2-12.
78. Tatton WG, Chalmers-Redman RM, Ju WJ, et al: Propargylamines induce antiapoptotic new protein synthesis in serum- and nerve growth factor (NGF)-withdrawn, NGF-differentiated PC-12 cells. J Pharmacol Exp Ther 2002;301:753-764.
79. Kragten E, Lalande I, Zimmermann K, et al: Glyceraldehyde-3-phosphate dehydrogenase, the putative target of the antiapoptotic compounds CGP 3466 and R-(-)-deprenyl. J Biol Chem 1998;273:5821-5828.
80. Waldmeier PC, Spooren WP, Hengerer B: CGP 3466 protects dopaminergic neurons in lesion models of Parkinson's disease. Naunyn Schmiedebergs Arch Pharmacol 2000;362:526-537.
81. Matarredona ER, Meyer M, Seiler RW, Widmer HR: CGP 3466 increases survival of cultured fetal dopaminergic neurons. Restor Neurol Neurosci 2003;21:29-37.
82. Waldmeier PC, Boulton AA, Cools AR, et al: Neurorescuing effects of the GAPDH ligand CGP 3466B. J Neural Transm Suppl 2000;60:197-214.
83. Andringa G, van Oosten RV, Unger W, et al: Systemic administration of the propargylamine CGP 3466B prevents behavioural and morphological deficits in rats with 6-hydroxydopamine-induced lesions in the substantia nigra. Eur J Neurosci 2000;12:3033-3043.
84. Olanow CW, Schapira AH, LeWitt PA, et al: TCH346 as a neuroprotective drug in Parkinson's disease: a double-blind, randomised, controlled trial. Lancet Neurol 2006;5:1013-1020.
85. Parkinson Study Group PRECEPT Investigators: Mixed lineage kinase inhibitor CEP1347 fails to delay disability in early Parkinson's disease. Neurology 2007;69:1476-1477.
86. Boka G, Anglade P, Wallach D, et al: Immunocytochemical analysis of tumor necrosis factor and its receptors in Parkinson's disease. Neurosci Lett 1994;172:151-154.

87. Chen H, Zhang SM, Hernan MA, et al: Nonsteroidal anti-inflammatory drugs and the risk of Parkinson disease. Arch Neurol 2003;60:1059-1064.
88. NINDS NET-PD Investigators: A randomized, double-blind, futility clinical trial of creatine and minocycline in early Parkinson disease. Neurology 2006;66:664-671.
89. Gordon PH, Moore DH, Miller RG, et al: Efficacy of minocycline in patients with amyotrophic lateral sclerosis: a phase III randomised trial. Lancet Neurol 2007;6:1045-1053.
90. Hellenbrand W, Seidler A, Boeing H, et al: Diet and Parkinson's disease, I: a possible role for the past intake of specific foods and food groups: results from a self-administered food-frequency questionnaire in a case-control study. Neurology 1996;47:636-643.
91. Ross GW, Abbott RD, Petrovitch H, et al: Association of coffee and caffeine intake with the risk of Parkinson disease. JAMA 2000;283:2674-2679.
92. Ascherio A, Zhang SM, Hernan MA, et al: Prospective study of caffeine consumption and risk of Parkinson's disease in men and women. Ann Neurol 2001;50:56-63.
93. Chan CS, Guzman JN, Ilijic E, et al: 'Rejuvenation' protects neurons in mouse models of Parkinson's disease. Nature 2007;447:1081-1086.
94. Surmeier DJ: Calcium, ageing, and neuronal vulnerability in Parkinson's disease. Lancet Neurol 2007;6:933-938.
95. Kupsch A, Sautter J, Schwarz J, et al: MPTP-induced neurotoxicity in non-human primates is antagonised by pre-treatment with nimodipine at the nigral, but not at the striatal level. Brain Res 1996;741:185-196.
96. Jenkins TA, Wong JY, Howells DW, et al: Effect of chronic ACE inhibition on striatal dopamine content in the MPTP treated mouse. J Neurochem 1999;73:214-219.
97. Becker C, Jick SS, Meier CR: Use of anti-hypertensives and the risk of Parkinson's disease. Neurology 2008;70:1438-1444.
98. Chaudhuri KR, Healy DG, Schapira AH: Non-motor symptoms of Parkinson's disease: diagnosis and management. Lancet Neurol 2006;5:235-245.

19 Etiology, Pathology, and Pathogenesis

FELIX GESER • KURT JELLINGER •
MARTIN KÖLLENSPERGER • NADIA STEFANOVA •
GREGOR K. WENNING

Introduction

Multiple system atrophy (MSA) is a rapidly progressive neurodegenerative disease of unknown etiology that manifests clinically with autonomic failure, parkinsonism, cerebellar ataxia, and pyramidal signs in various combinations. The presence of α-synuclein–positive glial cytoplasmic inclusions (GCIs) in multiple regions of the brain and spinal cord represents the unique neuropathological hallmark of MSA. The significance of GCIs in the pathogenesis of this neuronal multisystem degeneration remains to be established. This chapter reviews the currently available evidence on the etiopathogenesis and pathology of MSA. This may guide future research efforts in these poorly understood areas.

Etiology

Although many studies report a possible role of environmental toxins in Parkinson's disease (PD), such a role is even more likely in MSA because this is usually considered to be a sporadic disease.[1] Only a few studies have addressed environmental risk factors in MSA to date, however.[2-5] A case-control study in North America showed an increased risk of MSA associated with occupational exposure to organic solvents, plastic monomers and additives, pesticides, and metal dusts and fumes.[2] A multicenter case-control study in Europe showed a significantly higher risk of developing MSA in subjects having worked in agriculture.[5] Smoking habits seem to be less frequent in MSA cases (as in PD cases) than in healthy controls.[4] The finding that an inverse association with smoking previously shown in PD patients is shared by MSA patients, but not by progressive supranuclear palsy patients, lends epidemiologic support to the notion that different smoking habits are associated with different parkinsonian disorders. No single environmental factor has been clearly established, however, as conferring increased or reduced risks to develop MSA.[6]

A definite role of genetic factors in the pathogenesis of MSA has not been established so far. Similar to other degenerative movement disorders, monogenic disease may rarely occur. Wullner and colleagues[7] described a family with phenotypic MSA and probable autosomal dominant inheritance. There were only two affected family members, however, and postmortem examination was not performed. Of 157 Japanese patients with MSA, one was found to have a family history of MSA.[8] More recently, eight MSA patients in four Japanese families were reported with two siblings affected by this condition in each family, suggesting the presence of familial MSA with autosomal recessive inheritance; no mutations in the α-synuclein gene were detected.[9]

In 1996, Gilman and colleagues[10] reported an MSA-like phenotype including GCIs in one spinocerebellar ataxia type 1 family. The significance of α-synuclein as a major component of GCIs in MSA was unknown at that time, however, and hence no data on α-synuclein staining were reported. More recently, a patient with the typical features of MSA associated with cerebellar ataxia (MSA-C) on clinical and pathological grounds (including α-synuclein–positive inclusions) was found to exhibit an abnormal expansion of the spinocerebellar ataxia type 3 allele.[11] Further, MSA-C seems to be a frequent form of sporadic late-onset cerebellar ataxia. Of patients with sporadic adult-onset ataxia, 29% have MSA.[12] This finding corresponds well with data of a study of patients with sporadic olivopontocerebellar atrophy who were followed for 3 months to 10 years.[13] Within this period, 17 of 51 patients developed autonomic failure or parkinsonism, indicating a diagnosis of MSA.

There is significant overlap in the clinical features between the fragile X–associated tremor/ataxia syndrome (FXTAS) and atypical parkinsonism, in particular MSA-C. Numerous cases with FXTAS have already been described in male carriers of the fragile X mental retardation 1 gene (FMR1) premutation.[14,15] In a large European study, 4 patients carrying FMR1 premutations (55 to 200 CGG repeats) were identified among 426 clinically diagnosed MSA cases (within the subgroup probable MSA-C: 3 of 76);[16] no premutation carriers among 81 patients with pathologically proven MSA and only 1 carrier among 622 controls were found. Another European group found 1 MSA patient out of 77 studied to be a carrier of an FMR1 premutation.[17] A study of 77 Japanese MSA patients did not show any association between FMR1 premutations,[18] and a North American study of 65 MSA patients yielded similar results.[19] Taken together, FMR1 premutations do not play a major role in the pathogenesis of MSA, and FXTAS is only rarely found in MSA. More recently, two patients with a diagnosis of early-onset ataxia with ocular motor apraxia and hypoalbuminemia were reported to present with clinical features resembling MSA-C. Each patient had a different nucleotide transition in the aprataxin gene and did not show ocular motor apraxia and hypoalbuminemia, illustrating the diagnostic challenge in each patient.[20]

A spectrum of genetic susceptibility factors may underlie MSA, increasing the risk of developing the disease. A possibly effective strategy for determining the genetic susceptibility spectrum is to perform association studies of important genes for neurodegenerative diseases that are prevalent in a population by using linkage disequilibrium mapping in MSA patients with well-characterized morphological phenotypes.[21] Initial screening studies for candidate genes revealed no risk factors, however.[21-23]

While it has been shown that α-synuclein plays a role in the pathogenesis of some types of familial (but not sporadic) PD,[24] no mutations in the entire coding region of the α-synuclein gene have been found in MSA.[25] However, α-synuclein gene variants have been related to an increased risk of MSA in a multi-centre whole genomic association study recently.[26] This important finding has been replicated by other consortia (N. Leigh, personal communication). Although multiple mutations in the leucine-rich repeat kinase 2 gene are associated with parkinsonian disorders, no MSA patient carried the most common G2019S mutation.[27] The reported association between alcohol dehydrogenase 1C gene stop mutation and MSA in a British population, but not in a German population, needs further substantiation.[28] The apolipoprotein E e4 allele frequency of MSA cases was not significantly different from that of control subjects.[29] Similarly, others have reported no effect of apolipoprotein E tau, α-synuclein, or synphilin gene variability on the development of MSA.[21,30] Genotyping of a functional polymorphism in the dopamine β-hydroxylase gene showed no association between the dopamine β-hydroxylase -1021C → T polymorphism and MSA.[31] The cytochrome P-450-2D6 R296C polymorphism has been reported to be present in MSA according to one group of investigators,[32] but not to another.[33] In a large European study comprising 257 MSA patients, no genetic variation in the ubiquitin carboxyl-terminal esterase L1 gene was found.[34]

Further search for polymorphisms, in particular for proteins that interact with α-synuclein, is required to identify genetic risk factors for MSA. The finding of polymorphisms in various proinflammatory pathways is a promising step in further elucidating the pathogenesis of MSA. Reported polymorphisms associated with an elevated risk for MSA include the following genes: interleukin (IL)-1A,[35] IL-1β,[36] IL-8, intercellular adhesion molecule-1,[37] tumor necrosis factor-1031C,[38] and α1-antichymotrypsin.[39] The actual pathogenetic link between inclusion pathology and the proinflammatory processes is not yet understood, however.

Pathology

In 1998, MSA was recognized as α-synucleinopathy with distinctive GCIs (Fig. 19–1).[40-44] GCIs are faintly eosinophilic and erythrophilic, sickle-shaped, oval, or conical cytoplasmic inclusions, ultrastructurally composed of a meshwork of randomly aggregated, loosely packed filaments with cross-sectional diameters of 15 to 30 nm, in addition to granulated material that often entraps cytoplasmic organelles such as mitochondria and secretory vesicles.[45-47] Further immunoelectron microscopic analysis of GCIs has revealed the presence of different types of α-synuclein filaments whose width may be uniform or show periodic variation.[41]

Diffuse neuronal cytoplasmic α-synuclein immunoreactivity is often referred to as "preinclusions,"[48] and may reflect incipient inclusion or Lewy body–like formation enhanced in sympathetic ganglia in MSA patients.[49] Clusters of neuronal inclusions and abnormal neurons have been shown to be spatially correlated,

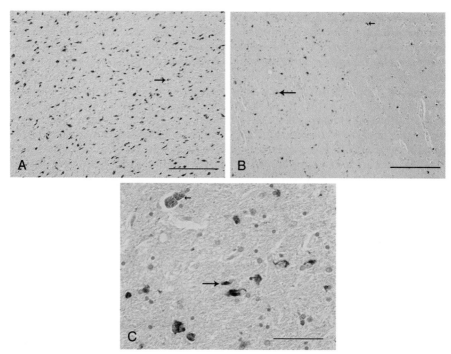

Figure 19–1 Glial inclusion pathology in multiple system atrophy. **A-C,** Anti-α-synuclein immunohistochemistry. **A,** Pons with glial inclusions (*arrow*) (bar = 200 μm). **B,** Cingulate gyrus with glial inclusions in white matter (*large arrow*) and grey matter (*short arrow*) (bar = 200 μm). **C,** Substantia nigra with glial inclusions (*large arrow*). Neuromelanin granules containing neuron (*short arrow*) (bar = 50 μm).

whereas GCIs were not spatially correlated with either neuronal inclusions or abnormal neurons, suggesting that neuronal pathology evolves secondary to glial pathology consistent with the concept of "gliodegeneration."[50,51] The distribution of GCIs is widespread, diffuse rather than topographical, and involves—among others—the basal ganglia. including the internal and external capsule, frontal or supplementary/primary motor cortex, reticular formation, basis pontis, middle cerebellar peduncles, and cerebellar white matter.[52-54]

More recently, the multisystem character of MSA was underpinned at an international workshop supported by the National Institute of Neurological Disorders, and neuropathological criteria for MSA were revised by the Working Group for MSA: "A definite neuropathological diagnosis of MSA is established when there is evidence of widespread and abundant CNS alpha-synuclein-positive CGIs in association with neurodegenerative changes in striatonigral or olivopontocerebellar systems."[51] GCIs may originate from cytoskeletal proteins, as evidenced by ubiquitin, α-tubulin and β-tubulin, and tau immunoreactivity.[55] In most MSA cases, tau seems to be seen only in a subset of GCIs, however, and when present, it is in a hypophosphorylated state.[56]

Although MSA is now widely accepted as a single multisystem disease, there is evidence of clinicopathological heterogeneity. Indeed, MSA associated with parkinsonism (i.e., MSA-P) is characterized by pathology mainly in the striatonigral system, and conversely, in MSA with ataxia (i.e., MSA-C) shows a predominant involvement of the olivopontocerebellar system.[55,57]

Macroscopically, the putamen of MSA-P patients may be atrophic, the caudate nucleus and pallidum are less frequently affected. There is loss of pigment of the substantia nigra and often of the locus coeruleus.[55,58] Semiquantitative grading of striatonigral degeneration (SND) is captured by a novel scale ranging from SND I (degeneration widely restricted to the substantia nigra—"minimal change MSA")[59,61] to SND III (with pathology extending from the posterior dorsolateral putamen to the anterior ventromedial parts of the striatum.[62] Indeed, in MSA-P associated with SND, the degenerative process affects nigrostriatal dopaminergic transmission at presynaptic and postsynaptic sites.[59,63] Pathologically, the loss of dopaminergic neurons in MSA-P is comparable to that found in PD.[64] Only a few patients with MSA exhibit a presynaptic pattern with minimal neurodegenerative putaminal changes.[60,61,64] Several postmortem immunohistochemical and autoradiographical studies suggest that both striatal outflow pathways are affected: encephalin-containing striatal neurons projecting to the external globus pallidus that carry dopamine D2 receptors (indirect pathway) and substance P–containing cells projecting to internal globus pallidus and substantia nigra pars reticulata that carry D1 receptors (direct pathway).[65-71] As a result of striatal degeneration, the posterolateral portions of the external and internal globus pallidus and the ventrolateral substantia nigra pars reticulata are deafferented.[72] Churchyard and colleagues,[70] in a postmortem binding study of two MSA brains, found loss of putaminal D2 receptors in both, but loss of D1 receptors in only one brain. Because the duration of the disease was shorter, and histopathological changes were less severe in the latter case, they suggested the possibility that the disease may initially affect striatal cells expressing D2 receptors (indirect pathway), and only subsequently D1 receptor–expressing neurons (direct pathway). This assumption remains contentious, however. The evidence considered so far suggests that the pathology of parkinsonism in MSA-P incorporates variable combinations of loss of dopaminergic nigrostriatal transmission and impairment of the indirect and direct striatal outflow pathways at the striatal level, with relative preservation of subthalamic nucleus, globus pallidus, and thalamus. Progressive loss of striatal dopamine receptors and striatal output systems might explain levodopa unresponsiveness in most MSA-P patients.[64,71,73,74]

In cases with MSA-C, the paleocerebellum and neocerebellum, middle cerebellar peduncles, basis pontis, and inferior olives may show varying degrees of atrophy (see Fig. 19–2).[55,57,58,75] Histologically, oligodendroglial pathology is present in particular in the projections from the precerebellar nuclei to the cerebellum (i.e., pontocerebellar, olivocerebellar, and reticulocerebellar tracts) and in descending or ascending fiber tracts of the motor system (i.e., corticopontine, corticobulbar, corticospinal, spinoreticular, spino-olivary, and spinocerebellar tracts).[76] A disproportionate depletion of transverse pontocerebellar fibers from the middle cerebellar peduncles compared with the loss of pontine neurons is often observed in the context of a "dying back" process.[55,77]

Based on the presence of neuronal cytoplasmic inclusions and the abnormalities of the neuronal Golgi apparatus in the inferior olivary nucleus in MSA, however, it has been suggested that the degeneration of the inferior olivary nucleus may not be the result of secondary retrograde transsynaptic degeneration after

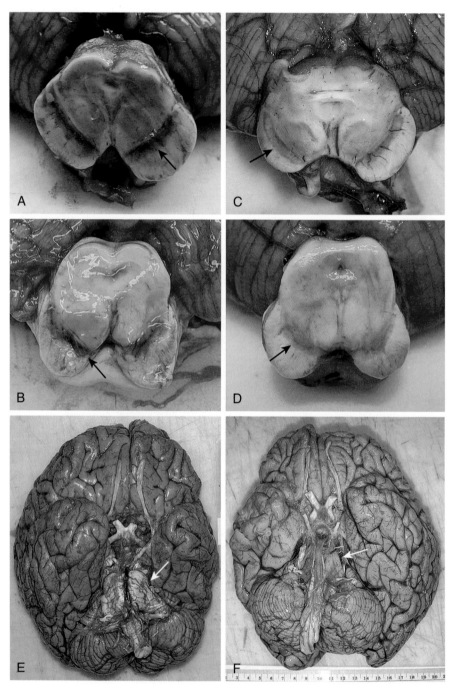

Figure 19–2   A-F, Macroscopic findings in multiple system atrophy (MSA). Cross-section through upper (**A** and **C**) and lower midbrain (**B** and **D**) showing pallor of the substantia nigra in patients with MSA associated with parkinsonism (**C** and **D**), but not in controls (**A** and **B**) (*arrows*). Basal surface of the brain including brainstem and cerebellum of a normal subject (**E**) and patient with MSA associated with cerebellar ataxia showing a pontocerebellar atrophy (*arrow*) (**F**).

Purkinje cell loss, but a primary degenerative mechanism.[78] This suggestion is also supported by a poor topographic correlation between neuronal cell loss in inferior olives and cerebellar cortex.[57] As to the Purkinje cells in the cerebellum, it has been suggested that their function is impaired from the peripheral dendrites toward the cell bodies, and that the presence of aberrant phosphorylation of neurofilament proteins, synaptophysin and alphaB-crystallin, may be related to their degeneration.[79] The Bergman glia also occasionally may be the target of α-synuclein pathology in MSA.[80]

The morphological semiquantitative grading of SND[62] was more recently supplemented by an olivopontocerebellar atrophy scale (OPCA 0-III), and both grading systems were shown to correlate well with initial symptoms and clinical key features of MSA-C and MSA-P (Fig. 19–3).[81] Analogous to *minimal change MSA* in the striatonigral system, the term *minimal change olivopontocerebellar atrophy* has been proposed more recently for the combination of neuronal loss restricted to the olivopontocerebellar system and widespread glial α-synuclein–positive inclusions denoting an early stage in the disease.[82]

Autonomic failure in MSA is caused by dysfunction of (1) central and preganglionic efferent autonomic activity, (2) neuronal networks in the brainstem that control cardiovascular and respiratory function, and (3) the neuroendocrine component of the autonomic regulation via the hypothalamopituitary axis. The morphological substrate of autonomic failure has been reviewed in detail elsewhere.[55,83] The supraspinal lesion sites include the cholinergic neurons in dorsal vagal nucleus and ventrolateral nucleus ambiguus,[84,85] catecholaminergic neurons of ventrolateral medulla,[86] neurokinin-1 receptor–like immunoreactive neurons in ventrolateral medulla,[87] serotoninergic neurons of the medulla,[88] Edinger-Westphal nucleus and posterior hypothalamus[89] (including the tuberomammillary nucleus[90]), and brainstem pontomedullary reticular formation.[52,55]

In the hypothalamus, loss of arginine-vasopressin neurons in the posterior portion of the paraventricular nucleus may contribute to sympathetic failure, whereas loss of catecholaminergic input from the brainstem to the magnocellular arginine-vasopressin neurons may contribute to impaired arginine-vasopressin secretion in response to orthostatic stress. Loss of arginine-vasopressin neurons in the suprachiasmatic nucleus may contribute to impaired circadian regulation of endocrine and autonomic functions.[91] Degeneration of sympathetic preganglionic neurons in the intermediolateral column of the thoracolumbar spinal cord (contributory to orthostatic hypotension), including neuronal loss or gliosis, is present in more than two thirds of MSA cases (Table 19–1).[92] There is not always a strong correlation between nerve cell depletion or gliosis and the clinical degree of autonomic failure.[55,93]

Sympathetic ganglia have also been shown to be affected by neuronal cytoplasmic α-synuclein immunoreactivity or inclusion in MSA.[48,49] Neuronal dropout coupled with reactive astrogliosis in parasympathetic preganglionic neurons of the spinal cord is followed by autonomic disturbances, such as urogenital and rectal dysfunction, and an involvement of Onuf's nucleus is well established—also in terms of possible diagnostic implications using sphincter electromyography.[83,94,95]

Given the multisystem character of this disease, other than the above-mentioned neuronal populations may show varying degrees of neuronal dropout associated with gliosis (Table 19–2). Of particular interest is the involvement of cortical areas because established dementia is considered as an exclusion criterion for the

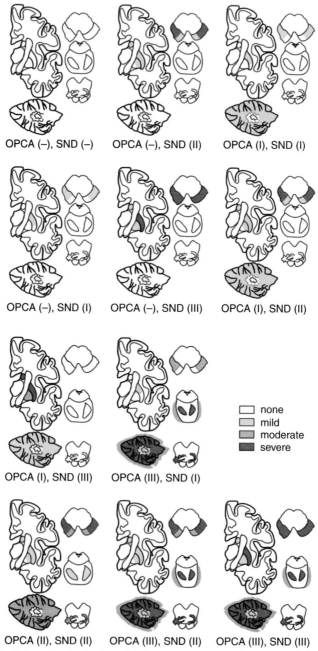

OPCA (–), SND (–) OPCA (–), SND (II) OPCA (I), SND (I)

OPCA (–), SND (I) OPCA (–), SND (III) OPCA (I), SND (II)

OPCA (I), SND (III) OPCA (III), SND (I)

☐ none
☐ mild
☐ moderate
☐ severe

OPCA (II), SND (II) OPCA (III), SND (II) OPCA (III), SND (III)

Figure 19–3 Schematic distribution of lesions in various combinations of SND and OPCA. [From Jellinger KA, Seppi K, Wenning GK. Grading of neuropathology in multiple system atrophy: proposal for a novel scale. *Mov Disord.* 2005;20(Suppl 12):S29-S36. Wiley Liss, Inc., a subsidiary of John Wiley & Sons, Inc. Reprinted with permission of John Wiley & Sons, Inc. SND, striatonigral degeneration; OPCA, olivopontocerebellar atrophy.]

TABLE 19–1	Main Pathological Abnormalities in 203 Multiple System Atrophy Cases									
	SN	Putamen	Caudate	Pallidum	Inferior Olive	Pons	PC	Dentate nucleus	ILCC	AHC	Pyramidal Tract
Normal (%)	8.6	14.6	45.2	25.5	22.1	30.2	16.9	68.8	31.7	51.9	45.2
Mild (%)	6.5	6.7	24.5	36.6	17.7	9.5	22.4	16.1	6.9	16	26.9
Moderate (%)	29.6	16.3	27.7	30.4	21.5	21.9	30.1	11.6	34.7	28.3	25.8
Severe (%)	55.4	62.4	2.6	7.5	38.7	38.5	30.6	3.6	26.7	3.8	2.2
Total No.	186	178	155	161	181	169	183	112	101	106	93

AHC, anterior horn cells; ILCC, intermediolateral cell column; PC, Purkinje cells; SN, substantia nigra.
Modified from Wenning GK, Tison F, Ben Shlomo Y, et al. Multiple system atrophy: a review of 203 pathologically proven cases. *Mov Disord.* 1997;12:133-147.
Wiley Liss, Inc., a subsidiary of John Wiley & Sons, Inc. Reprinted with permission of John Wiley & Sons, Inc.

TABLE 19–2	Other Pathological Abnormalities in 203 Multiple System Atrophy Cases							
	Cortex	Thalamus	STN	Ceruleus	Vestibularis	DVN	Ambiguous Nucleus	Onuf Nucleus
Normal (%)	78.4	77.6	59.4	12.8	43.6	29.6	58.3	35.7
Mild (%)	12.7	11.2	18.8	11.2	21.8	22.2	25	0
Moderate (%)	6.9	8.4	15.6	45.6	32.7	33.3	8.3	14.3
Severe (%)	2	2.8	6.3	30.4	1.8	14.8	8.3	50
Total No.	102	107	32	125	55	504	12	14

DVN, dorsal vagal nucleus X; STN, subthalamic nucleus.
Modified from Wenning GK, Tison F, Ben Shlomo Y, et al. Multiple system atrophy: a review of 203 pathologically proven cases. *Mov Disord.* 1997;12:133-147.
Wiley Liss, Inc., a subsidiary of John Wiley & Sons, Inc. Reprinted with permission of John Wiley & Sons, Inc.

clinical diagnosis of MSA according to the Consensus criteria.[96] Mild, moderate, and severe mental deterioration in autopsy-proven cases of MSA has been reported in 22%, 2%, and 0.5%.[92] In the more recent Neuroprotection and Natural History in Parkinson Plus Syndromes study, cognitive dysfunction occurred in both PSP and MSA patients, although at a higher rate in the former as compared to the latter.[97] The cognitive impairment has been largely regarded as a result of subcortical dysfunction.[98] Alzheimer's-related cortical pathology has been reported in only a few autopsy-proven cases of MSA. In a study of Alzheimer's-related pathological features in synucleinopathies, tauopathies, and frontotemporal degeneration, Josephs and colleagues[99] found concomitant Alzheimer's-type lesions in 79% of synucleinopathies (inlcuding 95 patients with diffuse Lewy body disease and 12 MSA cases with a mean age at death of 77.5 years) versus only 24% and 35% in tauopathies (mean age at death: 74.0) and frontotemporal degeneration (mean age at death: 71.2 years) without differences in the frequency of ApoE e4 allele among these groups. More recently, two patients at the age of 71 or 72 years were reported to show combined MSA and Alzheimer's disease (Braak stages III and VI) with only a few neurons showing coexisting of α-synuclein and tau pathology.[100] In a study of 44 MSA cases (mean age 61 years), Lewy bodies were found in 22.7%, and Alzheimer's-type lesions in 14%.[101] Only a few reports have described the coexistence of GCIs and Lewy bodies.[53,102,103] In the MSA cohort (i.e., 35 cases with a mean age at death of 62.8 years) examined by Wenning and associates[104] the total prevalence of Lewy bodies was 20.3% (including 5 patients with nigral and 3 cases with neocortical Lewy bodies), whereas Ozawa and coworkers[53] reported Lewy bodies in the brainstem in 7 of 94 cases (10.6%). Various degrees of other abnormalities in the cerebral hemispheres, including Betz cell loss and astrocytosis, were detected in pathologically proven MSA cases.[105-108] More recently, it was shown that there is profound degeneration of the frontal and temporal neocortices in MSA with the lower cortical laminae being affected more significantly than the upper laminae.[109] The upper and lower motor neuron may also show some degree of neuronal loss, rarely severely.[55,94,110]

Pathogenesis

The correlation of subregional GCI density and neuronal loss[53] suggests that α-synuclein aggregation is tightly linked to selective neurodegeneration in MSA. How oligodendroglial dysfunction could lead to regional neuronal loss remains unknown. There is no evidence that oligodendrocytes can be subtyped according to the neuronal systems they subserve. GCIs involve all types of oligodendrocytes (perivascular, perifascicular, and perineuronal), illustrating that there is no selective vulnerability of a specific oligodendrocyte.[111] Because GCIs and oligodendroglial loss show pronounced preponderance over neuronal pathology, however, it has been suggested that oligodendroglial pathology may be the primary lesion of MSA, rather than an epiphenomenon.[111] This assumption is supported by the more recent description of early MSA-specific oligodendroglial changes affecting the p25a protein before the development of the α-synuclein–containing GCIs,[112-114] highlighting the importance of oligodendroglia-axon interactions in the pathogenesis of MSA, and leading to its definition as a specific oligodendrogliopathy.[115,116]

Because α-synuclein represents a major component of oligodendroglial and neuronal inclusions in MSA, other authors have discussed two degenerative processes in this disease: one resulting from the widespread occurrence of GCIs associated with oligodendrogliopathy in the central nervous system, and the other resulting from the filamentous aggregation of α-synuclein in the neurons in several brain regions.[117] Although the widespread involvement and functional disturbance of oligodendroglia in the former contrasts with restricted neuronal loss, particularly in the early stages of MSA,[60,62] a subgroup of MSA with severe temporal atrophy shows numerous GCIs, particularly in the limbic system, suggesting that primary nonfibrillar and fibrillar α-synuclein aggregation also occurs in neurons. The oligo-myelin-axon-neuron complex mechanisms, along with direct involvement of neurons themselves, may synergistically accelerate the neurodegenerative process in MSA.[118] α-Synuclein levels are increased, however, even in brain areas that do not contain many, or any, GCIs.[119] In conjunction with the fact that myelin degeneration in MSA is far more widespread than are GCIs, it seems likely that underlying oligodendroglial degenerative mechanisms play a key role in MSA pathogenesis.[120]

In adult human brain, α-synuclein is a protein characteristically found in neuronal cells and not in normal glial cells.[121,122] The expression of α-synuclein is exclusively found in the soluble fraction of the cytoplasm, whereas in brains of patients with MSA it gets pathologically redistributed into insoluble aggregates, in particular in oligodendroglial cells.[42] This redistribution could be due to either an accumulation of α-synuclein normally produced at low levels, owing to insufficient cellular degradation mechanisms, or abnormal α-synuclein expression.[42,47,123] A couple of studies show no differential expression levels of α-synuclein mRNA in MSA brain samples,[114,124] however, suggesting that the transcriptional regulation of the α-synuclein gene is unlikely to be affected in MSA brains. A more recent screening study on genomic multiplication of α-synuclein in MSA was negative.[125]

In an attempt to measure global changes in gene expression on pons tissue of MSA patients, a microarray study revealed significant changes in expression of 254 genes (180 downregulated and 74 upregulated), 86 (73 downregulated and 13 upregulated) of which were associated with the amount of α-synuclein aggregation, suggesting that regional expression changes may occur in MSA.[126] Based on immunohistochemical and biochemical analyses, it was suggested that *DJ-1* is upregulated in various neurodegenerative diseases and inclusions, including GCIs.[127] This was not the case with *PINK-1*, another gene that has been identified to play a role in autosomal recessive PD.[128] Hashida and colleagues[129] showed an increased expression of a brain-specific gene, neuronal double zinc finger protein (*ZNF231*), in cerebellar neurons that might represent a nuclear protein or transcription regulator. How the above-mentioned expression changes ultimately contribute to neurodegeneration is not yet elucidated, however.

In vitro and in vivo experimental models of MSA have been introduced to study the pathogenesis of the disease. To investigate the consequence of α-synuclein overexpression in glia, Stefanova and colleagues[130,131] transfected glial cells with vectors encoding wild-type or C-terminally truncated α-synuclein fused to red fluorescent protein. α-Synuclein immunocytochemistry showed diffuse cytoplasmic labeling associated with discrete inclusions within cell bodies and processes. Immunoelectron microscopy of the inclusions showed α-synuclein–immunoreactive amorphous dense core and a predominantly filamentous halo around.[132] Overexpression of α-synuclein induced apoptotic death of glial cells and increased susceptibility to oxidative stress, especially in the presence of cytoplasmic inclusions.[130]

In a follow-up study on glial cells overexpressing α-synuclein, tumor necrosis factor-α treatment was shown to lead to an increased susceptibility to apoptotic cell death with induction of caspase activation, significant cytoskeletal changes, and elevation of high-molecular-weight α-synuclein species indicating the possible role of neuroinflammatory cytokines in MSA type of neurodegeneration.[133] Oligodendrocytic progenitor cells overexpressing human α-synuclein exhibited impaired adhesion to fibronectin and increased cell death, suggesting the role of GCI-like pathology in alterations of cell–extracellular matrix interactions.[134]

Further information about the pathogenesis of MSA has been garnered by the development of transgenic mouse models by targeted overexpression of human α-synuclein driven by specific oligodendroglial promoters (Fig. 19–4). Kahle and coworkers[135] used the proteolipid protein promoter to generate transgenic mice with human wild-type α-synuclein in oligodendrocytes. The diagnostic

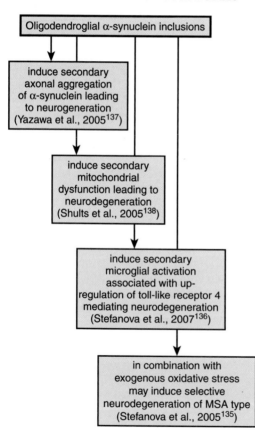

LESSONS ON THE PATHOGENESIS OF MSA
FROM THE TRANSGENIC MOUSE MODELS

Oligodendroglial α-synuclein inclusions

induce secondary axonal aggregation of α-synuclein leading to neurogeneration (Yazawa et al., 2005[137])

induce secondary mitochondrial dysfunction leading to neurodegeneration (Shults et al., 2005[138])

induce secondary microglial activation associated with up-regulation of toll-like receptor 4 mediating neurodegeneration (Stefanova et al., 2007[136])

in combination with exogenous oxidative stress may induce selective neurodegeneration of MSA type (Stefanova et al., 2005[135])

Figure 19–4 Possible mechanisms of neurodegeneration associated with oligodendroglial α-synucleinopathy as observed in three different transgenic mouse models. MSA, multiple system atrophy.

hyperphosphorylation at S129 of α-synuclein was reproduced, and a significant proportion of the transgenic α-synuclein was detergent insoluble, as is the case in MSA brains. The biochemical abnormalities were found to be specific for α-synuclein because control green fluorescent protein was fully soluble and evenly distributed throughout oligodendrocyte cell bodies and processes.[135] The proteolipid protein-α-synuclein transgenic mouse model was characterized further by widespread microglial activation and mild dopaminergic neuronal loss in substantia nigra pars compacta, correlating with shortened stride length.[136]

Suppression of activated microglia by early minocycline treatment protected nigral neurons in proteolipid protein-α-synuclein mice supporting the idea of neuroinflammation as a mediator of MSA-like neurodegeneration.[137] The same study revealed for the first time the possible role of toll-like receptor 4 upregulation for neuroinflammation in the transgenic mouse model and the human disease MSA. Targeted overexpression of human wild-type α-synuclein in oligodendrocytes driven by the 2,′ 3′-cyclic nucleotide 3′-phosphodiesterase promoter[138] or the myelin basic protein promoter[139] was associated with neuronal degeneration in the spinal cord and brain atrophy; however, the striatonigral and olivopontocerebellar pathways typically affected in human MSA were spared in these transgenic mice. The transgenic models of oligodendroglial α-synucleinopathy supported the idea, however, that GCI-like pathology plays a crucial role in the pathogenesis of the disease, and may induce neurodegeneration associated with either secondary aggregation of α-synuclein in axons or mitochondrial dysfunction.

Finally, overexpression of oligodendroglial α-synuclein in transgenic mice combined with exposure to mitochondrial inhibition by 3-nitropropionic acid generated the first model of MSA replicating glial and neuronal pathology (with SND and olivopontocerebellar atrophy) of the human disease suggesting the possible role of genetic predisposition and environmental stress for the pathogenesis of the disease.[131] A double transgenic mouse model expressing α-synuclein and tau suggests synergistic fibrillation of those two proteins, providing an animal model for the common finding of concomitant synucleinopathy and tauopathy in oligodendrocytes.[140]

Conclusions

Oligodendrocytes and myelin may serve as early indicators of neurodegenerative disease processes, and glial involvement in neurodegeneration seems to represent an intrinsic part of disease-specific pathogenesis in various neurodegenerative diseases (e.g., α-synucleinopathies and tauopathies). Critical analysis of the hitherto available data supports the concept of *gliodegeneration,* which has been proposed to represent an essential, although largely disregarded, component of the spectrum of various types of "neurodegeneration" with MSA representing a specific form of oligodendrogliopathy associated with α-synucleinopathy.

Acknowledgment

We gratefully acknowledge Dr. John Q. Trojanowski, the Center of Neurodegenerative Disease Research, Philadelphia, PA, for kindly providing us with the MSA postmortem tissues depicted in Figures 19–1 and 19–2.

REFERENCES

1. Wenning GK, Wagner S, Daniel S, Quinn NP: Multiple system atrophy: sporadic or familial? Lancet 1993;342:681.
2. Nee LE, Gomez MR, Dambrosia J, et al: Environmental-occupational risk factors and familial associations in multiple system atrophy: a preliminary investigation. Clin Auton Res 1991;1:9-13
3. Hanna PA, Jankovic J, Kirkpatrick JB: Multiple system atrophy: the putative causative role of environmental toxins. Arch Neurol 1999;56:90-94.
4. Vanacore N, Bonifati V, Fabbrini G, et al: Smoking habits in multiple system atrophy and progressive supranuclear palsy. European Study Group on Atypical Parkinsonisms. Neurology 2000;54:114-119.
5. Vanacore N, Bonifati V, Fabbrini G, et al: Case-control study of multiple system atrophy. Mov Disord 2005;20:158-163.
6. Brown RC, Lockwood AH, Sonawane BR: Neurodegenerative diseases: an overview of environmental risk factors. Environ Health Perspect 2005;113:1250-1256.
7. Wullner U, Abele M, Schmitz-Huebsch T, et al: Probable multiple system atrophy in a German family. J Neurol Neurosurg Psychiatry 2004;75:924-925.
8. Soma H, Yabe I, Takei A, et al: Heredity in multiple system atrophy. J Neurol Sci 2006;240(1-2): 107-110.
9. Hara K, Momose Y, Tokiguchi S, et al: Multiplex families with multiple system atrophy. Arch Neurol 2007;64:545-551.
10. Gilman S, Sima AA, Junck L, et al: Spinocerebellar ataxia type 1 with multiple system degeneration and glial cytoplasmic inclusions. Ann Neurol 1996;39:241-255.
11. Nirenberg MJ, Libien J, Vonsattel JP, Fahn S: Multiple system atrophy in a patient with the spinocerebellar ataxia 3 gene mutation. Mov Disord 2007;22:251-254.
12. Abele M, Burk K, Schols L, et al: The aetiology of sporadic adult-onset ataxia. Brain 2002; 125(Pt 5):961-968.
13. Gilman S, Little R, Johanns J, et al: Evolution of sporadic olivopontocerebellar atrophy into multiple system atrophy. Neurology 2000;55:527-532.
14. Hagerman RJ, Leehey M, Heinrichs W, et al: Intention tremor, parkinsonism, and generalized brain atrophy in male carriers of fragile X. Neurology 2001;57:127-130.
15. Jacquemont S, Hagerman RJ, Leehey M, et al: Fragile X premutation tremor/ataxia syndrome: molecular, clinical, and neuroimaging correlates. Am J Hum Genet 2003;72:869-878.
16. Kamm C, Healy DG, Quinn NP, et al: The fragile X tremor ataxia syndrome in the differential diagnosis of multiple system atrophy, data from the EMSA Study Group. Brain 2005; 128(Pt 8):1855-1860.
17. Biancalana V, Toft M, Le Ber I, et al: FMR1 premutations associated with fragile X-associated tremor/ataxia syndrome in multiple system atrophy. Arch Neurol 2005;62:962-966.
18. Yabe I, Soma H, Takei A, et al: No association between FMR1 premutations and multiple system atrophy. J Neurol 2004;251:1411-1412.
19. Garland EM, Vnencak-Jones CL, Biaggioni I, et al: Fragile X gene premutation in multiple system atrophy. J Neurol Sci 2004;227:115-118.
20. Baba Y, Uitti RJ, Boylan KB, et al: Aprataxin (APTX) gene mutations resembling multiple system atrophy. Parkinsonism Relat Disord 2007;13:139-142.
21. Ozawa T, Healy DG, Abou-Sleiman PM, et al: The alpha-synuclein gene in multiple system atrophy. J Neurol Neurosurg Psychiatry 2006;77:464-467.
22. Bandmann O, Sweeney MG, Daniel SE, et al: Multiple-system atrophy is genetically distinct from identified inherited causes of spinocerebellar degeneration. Neurology 1997;49:1598-1604.
23. Nicholl DJ, Bennett P, Hiller L, et al: A study of five candidate genes in Parkinson's disease and related neurodegenerative disorders. European Study Group on Atypical Parkinsonism. Neurology 1999;53:1415-1421.
24. Gasser T: Update on the genetics of Parkinson's disease. Mov Disord 2007;22(Suppl 17):S343-S350.
25. Ozawa T, Takano H, Onodera O, et al: No mutation in the entire coding region of the alpha-synuclein gene in pathologically confirmed cases of multiple system atrophy. Neurosci Lett 1999;270:110-112.
26. Scholz SW, Houlden H, Schulte C, et al: SNCA variants are associated with increased risk for multiple system atrophy. Ann Neurol 2009;65:610-614.
27. Ozelius LJ, Foroud T, May S, et al: G2019S mutation in the leucine-rich repeat kinase 2 gene is not associated with multiple system atrophy. Mov Disord 2007;22:546-549.

28. Schmitt I, Wullner U, Healy DG, et al: The ADH1C stop mutation in multiple system atrophy patients and healthy probands in the United Kingdom and Germany. Mov Disord 2006;21:2034.
29. Cairns NJ, Atkinson PF, Kovacs T, et al: Apolipoprotein E e4 allele frequency in patients with multiple system atrophy. Neurosci Lett 1997;221(2-3):161-164.
30. Morris HR, Vaughan JR, Datta SR, et al: Multiple system atrophy/progressive supranuclear palsy: alpha-Synuclein, synphilin, tau, and APOE Neurology 2000;55:1918-1920.
31. Healy DG, Abou-Sleiman PM, Ozawa T, et al: A functional polymorphism regulating dopamine beta-hydroxylase influences against Parkinson's disease. Ann Neurol 2004;55:443-446.
32. Iwahashi K, Miyatake R, Tsuneoka Y, et al: A novel cytochrome P-450IID6 (CYPIID6) mutant gene associated with multiple system atrophy. J Neurol Neurosurg Psychiatry 1995;58:263-264.
33. Bandmann O, Wenning GK, Quinn NP, Harding AE: Arg296 to Cys296 polymorphism in exon 6 of cytochrome P-450-2D6 (CYP2D6) is not associated with multiple system atrophy. J Neurol Neurosurg Psychiatry 1995;59:557.
34. Healy DG, Abou-Sleiman PM, Quinn N, et al: UCHL-1 gene in multiple system atrophy: a haplotype tagging approach. Mov Disord 2005;20:1338-1343.
35. Combarros O, Infante J, Llorca J, Berciano J: Interleukin-1A (-889) genetic polymorphism increases the risk of multiple system atrophy. Mov Disord 2003;18:1385-1386.
36. Nishimura M, Kawakami H, Komure O, et al: Contribution of the interleukin-1beta gene polymorphism in multiple system atrophy. Mov Disord 2002;17:808-811.
37. Infante J, Llorca J, Berciano J, Combarros O: Interleukin-8, intercellular adhesion molecule-1 and tumour necrosis factor-alpha gene polymorphisms and the risk for multiple system atrophy. J Neurol Sci 2005;228:11-13.
38. Nishimura M, Kuno S, Kaji R, Kawakami H: Influence of a tumor necrosis factor gene polymorphism in Japanese patients with multiple system atrophy. Neurosci Lett 2005;374:218-221.
39. Furiya Y, Hirano M, Kurumatani N, et al: Alpha-1-antichymotrypsin gene polymorphism and susceptibility to multiple system atrophy (MSA). Brain Res Mol Brain Res 2005;138:178-181.
40. Lantos PL: The definition of multiple system atrophy: a review of recent developments. J Neuropathol Exp Neurol 1998;57:1099-1111.
41. Spillantini MG, Crowther RA, Jakes R, et al: Filamentous alpha-synuclein inclusions link multiple system atrophy with Parkinson's disease and dementia with Lewy bodies. Neurosci Lett 1998;251:205-208.
42. Tu PH, Galvin JE, Baba M, et al: Glial cytoplasmic inclusions in white matter oligodendrocytes of multiple system atrophy brains contain insoluble alpha-synuclein. Ann Neurol 1998;44: 415-422.
43. Wakabayashi K, Yoshimoto M, Tsuji S, Takahashi H: Alpha-synuclein immunoreactivity in glial cytoplasmic inclusions in multiple system atrophy. Neurosci Lett 1998;249(2-3):180-182.
44. Wakabayashi K, Hayashi S, Kakita A, et al: Accumulation of alpha-synuclein/NACP is a cytopathological feature common to Lewy body disease and multiple system atrophy. Acta Neuropathol 1998;96:445-452.
45. Kato S, Nakamura H, Hirano A, et al: Argyrophilic ubiquitinated cytoplasmic inclusions of Leu-7-positive glial cells in olivopontocerebellar atrophy (multiple system atrophy). Acta Neuropathol 1991;82:488-493.
46. Arima K, Murayama S, Mukoyama M, Inose T: Immunocytochemical and ultrastructural studies of neuronal and oligodendroglial cytoplasmic inclusions in multiple system atrophy, 1: neuronal cytoplasmic inclusions. Acta Neuropathol 1992;83:453-460.
47. Burn DJ, Jaros E: Multiple system atrophy: cellular and molecular pathology. Mol Pathol 2001;54:419-426.
48. Nishie M, Mori F, Fujiwara H, et al: Accumulation of phosphorylated alpha-synuclein in the brain and peripheral ganglia of patients with multiple system atrophy. Acta Neuropathol 2004;107:292-298.
49. Sone M, Yoshida M, Hashizume Y, et al: alpha-Synuclein-immunoreactive structure formation is enhanced in sympathetic ganglia of patients with multiple system atrophy. Acta Neuropathol 2005;110:19-26.
50. Armstrong RA, Cairns NJ, Lantos PL: Multiple system atrophy (MSA): topographic distribution of the alpha-synuclein-associated pathological changes. Parkinsonism Relat Disord 2006;12:356-362.
51. Trojanowski JQ, Revesz T: Proposed neuropathological criteria for the post mortem diagnosis of multiple system atrophy. Neuropathol Appl Neurobiol 2007;33:615-620.
52. Papp MI, Lantos PL: The distribution of oligodendroglial inclusions in multiple system atrophy and its relevance to clinical symptomatology. Brain 1994;117(Pt 2):235-243.

53. Ozawa T, Paviour D, Quinn NP, et al: The spectrum of pathological involvement of the striato-nigral and olivopontocerebellar systems in multiple system atrophy: clinicopathological correlations. Brain 2004;127(Pt 12):2657-2671.

54. Armstrong RA, Cairns NJ, Lantos PL: A quantitative study of the pathological changes in white matter in multiple system atrophy. Neuropathology 2007;27:221-227.

55. Daniel S: The neuropathology and neurochemistry of multiple system atrophy. In Mathias CJ, Bannister R, eds: Autonomic Failure: A Textbook of Clinical Disorders of the Autonomic Nervous System. Oxford: Oxford University Press 1999, pp 321-328.

56. Giasson BI, Mabon ME, Duda JE, et al: Tau and 14-3-3 in glial cytoplasmic inclusions of multiple system atrophy. Acta Neuropathol 2003;106:243-250.

57. Wenning GK, Tison F, Elliott L, et al: Olivopontocerebellar pathology in multiple system atrophy. Mov Disord 1996;11:157-162.

58. Dickson DW: Neuropathology of parkinsonian disorders. In Jankovic J, Tolosa E, eds: Parkinson's Disease and Movement Disorders. Philadelphia: Lippincott Williams & Wilkins 2007, pp 271-283.

59. Kume A, Takahashi A, Hashizume Y: Neuronal cell loss of the striatonigral system in multiple system atrophy. J Neurol Sci 1993;117(1-2):33-40.

60. Wenning GK, Quinn N, Magalhaes M, et al: "Minimal change" multiple system atrophy. Mov Disord 1994;9:161-166.

61. Berciano J, Valldeoriola F, Ferrer I, et al: Presynaptic parkinsonism in multiple system atrophy mimicking Parkinson's disease: a clinicopathological case study. Mov Disord 2002;17:812-816.

62. Wenning GK, Seppi K, Tison F, Jellinger K: A novel grading scale for striatonigral degeneration (multiple system atrophy). J Neural Transm 2002;109:307-320.

63. Fearnley JM, Lees AJ: Striatonigral degeneration: a clinicopathological study. Brain 1990; 113(Pt 6):1823-1842.

64. Tison F, Wenning GK, Daniel SE, Quinn NP: The pathophysiology of parkinsonism in multiple system atrophy. Eur J Neurol 1995;2:435-444.

65. Quik M, Spokes EG, Mackay AV, Bannister R: Alterations in [3H]spiperone binding in human caudate nucleus, substantia nigra and frontal cortex in the Shy-Drager syndrome and Parkinson's disease. J Neurol Sci 1979;43:429-437.

66. Cortes R, Camps M, Gueye B, et al: Dopamine receptors in human brain: autoradiographic distribution of D1 and D2 sites in Parkinson syndrome of different etiology. Brain Res 1989;483: 30-38.

67. Goto S, Hirano A, Matsumoto S: Subdivisional involvement of nigrostriatal loop in idiopathic Parkinson's disease and striatonigral degeneration. Ann Neurol 1989;26:766-770.

68. Goto S, Hirano A, Rojas-Corona RR: Immunohistochemical visualization of afferent nerve terminals in human globus pallidus and its alteration in neostriatal neurodegenerative disorders. Acta Neuropathol (Berl) 1989;78:543-550.

69. Goto S, Matsumoto S, Ushio Y, Hirano A: Subregional loss of putaminal efferents to the basal ganglia output nuclei may cause parkinsonism in striatonigral degeneration. Neurology 1996;47:1032-1036.

70. Churchyard A, Donnan GA, Hughes A, et al: Dopa resistance in multiple-system atrophy: loss of postsynaptic D2 receptors. Ann Neurol 1993;34:219-226.

71. Ito H, Kusaka H, Matsumoto S, Imai T: Striatal efferent involvement and its correlation to levodopa efficacy in patients with multiple system atrophy. Neurology 1996;47:1291-1299.

72. Brooks DJ, Ibanez V, Sawle GV, et al: Striatal D2 receptor status in patients with Parkinson's disease, striatonigral degeneration, and progressive supranuclear palsy, measured with 11C-raclopride and positron emission tomography. Ann Neurol 1992;31:184-192.

73. Rajput AH, Rozdilsky B, Rajput A, Ang L: Levodopa efficacy and pathological basis of Parkinson syndrome. Clin Neuropharmacol 1990;13:553-558.

74. Parati EA, Fetoni V, Geminiani GC, et al: Response to L-DOPA in multiple system atrophy. Clin Neuropharmacol 1993;16:139-144.

75. Tsuchiya K, Watabiki S, Sano M, et al: Distribution of cerebellar cortical lesions in multiple system atrophy: a topographic neuropathological study of three autopsy cases in Japan. J Neurol Sci 1998;155:80-85.

76. Braak H, Rub U, Del Tredici K: Involvement of precerebellar nuclei in multiple system atrophy. Neuropathol Appl Neurobiol 2003;29:60-76.

77. Oppenheimer D: Diseases of the basal ganglia, cerebellum and motor neurons. In Adams JH, Corsellis JAN, Duchen LW, eds: Greenfield's Neuropathology. New York: Wiley 1984, pp 699-747.

78. Sakurai A, Okamoto K, Yaguchi M, et al: Pathology of the inferior olivary nucleus in patients with multiple system atrophy. Acta Neuropathol 2002;103:550-554.
79. Kato S, Hayashi H, Mikoshiba K, et al: Purkinje cells in olivopontocerebellar atrophy and granule cell-type cerebellar degeneration: an immunohistochemical study. Acta Neuropathol 1998;96:67-74.
80. Piao YS, Mori F, Hayashi S, et al: Alpha-synuclein pathology affecting Bergmann glia of the cerebellum in patients with alpha-synucleinopathies. Acta Neuropathol 2003;105:403-409.
81. Jellinger KA, Seppi K, Wenning GK: Grading of neuropathology in multiple system atrophy: proposal for a novel scale. Mov Disord 2005;20(Suppl 12):S29-S36.
82. Wakabayashi K, Mori F, Nishie M, et al: An autopsy case of early ("minimal change") olivopontocerebellar atrophy (multiple system atrophy-cerebellar). Acta Neuropathol 2005;110:185-190.
83. Ozawa T: Morphological substrate of autonomic failure and neurohormonal dysfunction in multiple system atrophy: impact on determining phenotype spectrum. Acta Neuropathol 2007;114:201-211.
84. Sung JH, Mastri AR, Segal E: Pathology of Shy-Drager syndrome. J Neuropathol Exp Neurol 1979;38:353-368.
85. Benarroch EE, Schmeichel AM, Sandroni P, et al: Involvement of vagal autonomic nuclei in multiple system atrophy and Lewy body disease. Neurology 2006;66:378-383.
86. Benarroch EE, Smithson IL, Low PA, Parisi JE: Depletion of catecholaminergic neurons of the rostral ventrolateral medulla in multiple systems atrophy with autonomic failure. Ann Neurol 1998;43:156-163.
87. Benarroch EE, Schmeichel AM, Low PA, Parisi JE: Depletion of ventromedullary NK-1 receptor-immunoreactive neurons in multiple system atrophy. Brain 2003;126(Pt 10):2183-2190.
88. Benarroch EE, Schmeichel AM, Low PA, Parisi JE: Involvement of medullary serotonergic groups in multiple system atrophy. Ann Neurol 2004;55:418-422.
89. Shy GM, Drager GA: A neurological syndrome associated with orthostatic hypotension: a clinical-pathological study. Arch Neurol 1960;2:511-527.
90. Nakamura S, Ohnishi K, Nishimura M, et al: Large neurons in the tuberomammillary nucleus in patients with Parkinson's disease and multiple system atrophy. Neurology 1996;46:1693-1696.
91. Benarroch EE, Schmeichel AM, Sandroni P, et al: Differential involvement of hypothalamic vasopressin neurons in multiple system atrophy. Brain 2006;129(Pt 10):2688-2696.
92. Wenning GK, Tison F, Ben Shlomo Y, et al: Multiple system atrophy: a review of 203 pathologically proven cases. Mov Disord 1997;12:133-147.
93. Oppenheimer DR: Lateral horn cells in progressive autonomic failure. J Neurol Sci 1980;46:393-404.
94. Konno H, Yamamoto T, Iwasaki Y, Iizuka H: Shy-Drager syndrome and amyotrophic lateral sclerosis: cytoarchitectonic and morphometric studies of sacral autonomic neurons. J Neurol Sci 1986;73:193-204.
95. Vodusek DB: How to diagnose MSA early: the role of sphincter EMG. J Neural Transm 2005;112:1657-1668.
96. Gilman S, Low P, Quinn N, et al: Consensus statement on the diagnosis of multiple system atrophy. American Autonomic Society and American Academy of Neurology. Clin Auton Res 1998;8:359-362.
97. Bensimon G, Ludolph A, Agid Y, et al: Riluzole treatment, survival and diagnostic criteria in Parkinson plus disorders: the NNIPPS study. Brain 2009;132:156-171.
98. Burk K, Daum I, Rub U: Cognitive function in multiple system atrophy of the cerebellar type. Mov Disord 2006;21:772-776.
99. Josephs KA, Tsuboi Y, Cookson N, et al: Apolipoprotein E epsilon 4 is a determinant for Alzheimer-type pathologic features in tauopathies, synucleinopathies, and frontotemporal degeneration. Arch Neurol 2004;61:1579-1584.
100. Terni B, Rey MJ, Boluda S, et al: Mutant ubiquitin and p62 immunoreactivity in cases of combined multiple system atrophy and Alzheimer's disease. Acta Neuropathol (Berl) 2007;113:403-416.
101. Jellinger KA: More frequent Lewy bodies but less frequent Alzheimer-type lesions in multiple system atrophy as compared to age-matched control brains. Acta Neuropathol (Berl) 2007;114:299-303.
102. Mochizuki A, Komatsuzaki Y, Shoji S: Association of Lewy bodies and glial cytoplasmic inclusions in the brain of Parkinson's disease. Acta Neuropathol (Berl) 2002;104:534-537.
103. Sikorska B, Papierz W, Preusser M, et al: Synucleinopathy with features of both multiple system atrophy and dementia with Lewy bodies. Neuropathol Appl Neurobiol 2007;33:126-129.

104. Wenning GK, Ben-Shlomo Y, Magalhaes M, et al: Clinicopathological study of 35 cases of multiple system atrophy. J Neurol Neurosurg Psychiatry 1995;58:160-166.

105. Fujita T, Doi M, Ogata T, et al: Cerebral cortical pathology of sporadic olivopontocerebellar atrophy. J Neurol Sci 1993;116:41-46.

106. Wakabayashi K, Ikeuchi T, Ishikawa A, Takahashi H: Multiple system atrophy with severe involvement of the motor cortical areas and cerebral white matter. J Neurol Sci 1998;156: 114-117.

107. Konagaya M, Konagaya Y, Sakai M, et al: Progressive cerebral atrophy in multiple system atrophy. J Neurol Sci 2002;195:123-127.

108. Konagaya M, Sakai M, Matsuoka Y, et al: Multiple system atrophy with remarkable frontal lobe atrophy. Acta Neuropathol 1999;97:423-428.

109. Armstrong RA, Lantos PL, Cairns NJ: Multiple system atrophy: laminar distribution of the pathological changes in frontal and temporal neocortex—a study in ten patients. Clin Neuropathol 2005;24:230-235.

110. Sima AA, Caplan M, D'Amato CJ, et al: Fulminant multiple system atrophy in a young adult presenting as motor neuron disease. Neurology 1993;43:2031-2035.

111. Lantos PL, Papp MI: Cellular pathology of multiple system atrophy: a review. J Neurol Neurosurg Psychiatry 1994;57:129-133.

112. Otzen DE, Lundvig DM, Wimmer R, et al: p25alpha is flexible but natively folded and binds tubulin with oligomeric stoichiometry. Protein Sci 2005;14:1396-1409.

113. Kovacs GG, Gelpi E, Lehotzky A, et al: The brain-specific protein TPPP/p25 in pathological protein deposits of neurodegenerative diseases. Acta Neuropathol 2007;113:153-161.

114. Song YJ, Lundvig DM, Huang Y, et al: p25alpha relocalizes in oligodendroglia from myelin to cytoplasmic inclusions in multiple system atrophy. Am J Pathol 2007;171:1291-1303.

115. Wenning GK, Jellinger KA: The role of alpha-synuclein in the pathogenesis of multiple system atrophy. Acta Neuropathol (Berl) 2005;109:129-140.

116. Croisier E, Graeber MB: Glial degeneration and reactive gliosis in alpha-synucleinopathies: the emerging concept of primary gliodegeneration. Acta Neuropathol 2006;112:517-530.

117. Wakabayashi K, Takahashi H: Cellular pathology in multiple system atrophy. Neuropathology 2006;26:338-345.

118. Yoshida M: Multiple system atrophy: alpha-synuclein and neuronal degeneration. Neuropathology 2007;27:484-493.

119. Dickson DW, Liu W, Hardy J, et al: Widespread alterations of alpha-synuclein in multiple system atrophy. Am J Pathol 1999;155:1241-1251.

120. Matsuo A, Akiguchi I, Lee GC, et al: Myelin degeneration in multiple system atrophy detected by unique antibodies. Am J Pathol 1998;153:735-744.

121. Solano SM, Miller DW, Augood SJ, et al: Expression of alpha-synuclein, parkin, and ubiquitin carboxy-terminal hydrolase L1 mRNA in human brain: genes associated with familial Parkinson's disease. Ann Neurol 2000;47:201-210.

122. Miller DW, Johnson JM, Solano SM, et al: Absence of alpha-synuclein mRNA expression in normal and multiple system atrophy oligodendroglia. J Neural Transm 2005;112:1613-1624.

123. Arima K, Ueda K, Sunohara N, et al: NACP/alpha-synuclein immunoreactivity in fibrillary components of neuronal and oligodendroglial cytoplasmic inclusions in the pontine nuclei in multiple system atrophy. Acta Neuropathol (Berl) 1998;96:439-444.

124. Ozawa T, Okuizumi K, Ikeuchi T, et al: Analysis of the expression level of alpha-synuclein mRNA using postmortem brain samples from pathologically confirmed cases of multiple system atrophy. Acta Neuropathol (Berl) 2001;102:188-190.

125. Lincoln SJ, Ross OA, Milkovic NM, et al: Quantitative PCR-based screening of alpha-synuclein multiplication in multiple system atrophy. Parkinsonism Relat Disord 2007;13:340-342.

126. Langerveld AJ, Mihalko D, DeLong C, et al: Gene expression changes in postmortem tissue from the rostral pons of multiple system atrophy patients. Mov Disord 2007;22:766-777.

127. Neumann M, Muller V, Gorner K, et al: Pathological properties of the Parkinson's disease-associated protein DJ-1 in alpha-synucleinopathies and tauopathies: relevance for multiple system atrophy and Pick's disease. Acta Neuropathol 2004;107:489-496.

128. Gandhi S, Muqit MM, Stanyer L, et al: PINK1 protein in normal human brain and Parkinson's disease. Brain 2006;129(Pt 7):1720-1731.

129. Hashida H, Goto J, Zhao N, et al: Cloning and mapping of ZNF231, a novel brain-specific gene encoding neuronal double zinc finger protein whose expression is enhanced in a neurodegenerative disorder, multiple system atrophy (MSA). Genomics 1998;54:50-58.

130. Stefanova N, Klimaschewski L, Poewe W, et al: Glial cell death induced by overexpression of alpha-synuclein. J Neurosci Res 2001;65:432-438.
131. Stefanova N, Reindl M, Poewe W, Wenning GK: In vitro models of multiple system atrophy. Mov Disord 2005;20(Suppl 12):S53-S56.
132. Stefanova N, Emgard M, Klimaschewski L, et al: Ultrastructure of alpha-synuclein-positive aggregations in U373 astrocytoma and rat primary glial cells. Neurosci Lett 2002;323:37-40.
133. Stefanova N, Schanda K, Klimaschewski L, et al: Tumor necrosis factor-alpha-induced cell death in U373 cells overexpressing alpha-synuclein. J Neurosci Res 2003;73:334-340.
134. Tsuboi K, Grzesiak JJ, Bouvet M, et al: Alpha-synuclein overexpression in oligodendrocytic cells results in impaired adhesion to fibronectin and cell death. Mol Cell Neurosci 2005;29:259-268.
135. Kahle PJ, Neumann M, Ozmen L, et al: Hyperphosphorylation and insolubility of alpha-synuclein in transgenic mouse oligodendrocytes. EMBO Rep 2002;3:583-588.
136. Stefanova N, Reindl M, Neumann M, et al: Oxidative stress in transgenic mice with oligodendroglial alpha-synuclein overexpression replicates the characteristic neuropathology of multiple system atrophy. Am J Pathol 2005;166:869-876.
137. Stefanova N, Reindl M, Neumann M, et al: Microglial activation mediates neurodegeneration related to oligodendroglial alpha-synucleinopathy: implications for multiple system atrophy. Mov Disord 2007;22:2196-2203.
138. Yazawa I, Giasson BI, Sasaki R, et al: Mouse model of multiple system atrophy alpha-synuclein expression in oligodendrocytes causes glial and neuronal degeneration. Neuron 2005;45:847-859.
139. Shults CW, Rockenstein E, Crews L, et al: Neurological and neurodegenerative alterations in a transgenic mouse model expressing human alpha-synuclein under oligodendrocyte promoter: implications for multiple system atrophy. J Neurosci 2005;25:10689-10699.
140. Fillon G, Kahle PJ: Alpha-synuclein transgenic mice: relevance to multiple system atrophy. Mov Disord 2005;20(Suppl 12):S64-S66.

20 | Multiple System Atrophy: Clinical Features and Management

WERNER POEWE • KLAUS SEPPI

Introduction

Multiple system atrophy (MSA) is a sporadic and progressive neurodegenerative disorder characterized by abnormal α-synuclein aggregation in oligodendroglia and neuronal loss in multiple areas of the central nervous system. Major sites of pathology include the nigrostriatal system, cerebellum, and inferior olives, and the intramediolateral cell columns of the spinal cord and other parts of the central autonomic nervous system. Depending on the predominant site of pathology, clinical presentations of MSA differ, with 80% of patients presenting with parkinsonian features (MSA-P subtype, striatonigral degeneration type) and 30% presenting with cerebellar signs (MSA-C subtype, olivopontocerebellar atrophy type). The exact prevalence of MSA is unknown, but available data suggest that at least 4 to 6 per 100,000 population are affected. Onset is usually in the sixth decade followed by relentless progression with death occurring after an average of 9 years of disease.[1]

MSA-P may be strikingly similar to Parkinson's disease (PD) in the first years after symptom onset causing a high rate of clinical diagnostic errors early in the disease.[2] This chapter summarizes the clinical features of MSA, emphasizing useful clinical differential diagnostic clues versus PD and a review of diagnostic tests that have been found useful in diagnosing MSA. In addition, the chapter provides an overview of currently available treatment options for MSA.

Clinical Features

The salient clinical features of MSA include autonomic failure, parkinsonism, cerebellar ataxia, and pyramidal signs in any combination. The disease is usually classified along two major motor presentations, however: Parkinsonian features predominate in 80% of white MSA patients, characterizing the MSA-P subtype, whereas cerebellar ataxia is the presenting feature in about 20% (MSA-C subtype).[1,3] In Japanese patients, the MSA-C subtype seems to be more common with a reported ratio of MSA-C to MSA-P of 70% to 30%. Such differences between ethnic groups suggest that genetic or environmental factors or both may influence the clinical phenotype of MSA.[4,5]

Previous studies suggest that 29% to 33% of patients with isolated late-onset cerebellar ataxia and 8% of patients presenting with pure bradykinetic parkinsonism eventually develop MSA.[1,6-8] MSA is a rapidly and relentlessly progressive disorder with a mean disease duration until death of 9 years or less, but there is considerable variation of disease progression in MSA among individuals with survival of more than 15 years in some instances. Patients with MSA-P tend to show more rapid functional deterioration than patients with MSA-C,[1,4] but both motor presentations of MSA are associated with similar survival times.[9] Most MSA patients ultimately die from bronchopneumonia or respiratory insufficiency during sleep.

AUTONOMIC DYSFUNCTION

Dysautonomia is characteristic of both MSA motor presentations, primarily comprising urogenital and orthostatic dysfunction. Some degree of dysautonomia develops in virtually all patients with MSA. Erectile dysfunction is often the earliest symptom of MSA and affects virtually all male patients. Preserved erectile function makes a diagnosis of MSA unlikely.[1,10] Reduced genital sensitivity is a frequent clinical sign in female MSA patients, and it shows a close temporal relation to the onset of the disease.[11] Urinary incontinence and retention are common early in the course or as presenting symptoms.[12] Disorders of micturition in MSA are caused by changes in the complex peripheral and central innervation of the bladder[13] and commonly appear earlier and are more severe than in PD. By contrast, constipation occurs equally in PD and MSA, and fecal incontinence occurs only occasionally.

Orthostatic hypotension may indicate autonomic failure and can be asymptomatic or symptomatic. Symptoms of orthostatic hypotension result from hypoperfusion and include postural faintness and instability, blurred vision, dizziness, lightheadedness, pain in the back of the neck and shoulders (coat-hanger pain) eventually on rising in the morning, and syncope. Symptomatic orthostatic hypotension is present in 68% of clinically diagnosed patients, but recurrent syncopes emerge in only 15%.[1] When symptomatic, orthostatic hypotension frequently occurs after the onset of erectile dysfunction and urinary symptoms.[10,14,15] Levodopa or dopamine agonists may provoke or worsen orthostatic hypotension.

PARKINSONISM

MSA-P–associated parkinsonism is characterized by progressive akinesia and rigidity, with jerky postural tremor and, less commonly, tremor at rest. Many patients have orofacial or craniocervical dystonia[16,17] associated with a characteristic quivering high-pitched dysarthria. Postural stability is compromised early on in the disease course; however, recurrent falls at disease onset are unusual in contrast to progressive supranuclear palsy (PSP). Differential diagnosis of MSA-P and PD may be very difficult in the early stages owing to several overlapping features, such as rest tremor or asymmetrical akinesia and rigidity. Levodopa-induced improvement of parkinsonism may be seen in 30% to 50% of patients with MSA-P.[1,18,19]

The benefit of levodopa is transient in most patients, however, and 90% of MSA-P patients are unresponsive to levodopa in the long-term. Fifty percent of patients with MSA-P have levodopa-induced dyskinesia affecting orofacial and neck muscles, sometimes without motor benefit.[17] Dysphagia is common in more advanced disease stages of the disorder.[20] Laryngeal stridor is another serious manifestation of the disease, which usually occurs with nocturnal stridor,[21] and which may result from laryngeal dystonia or from vocal cord abductor paralysis.[22-24] In most cases, a fully developed clinical picture of MSA-P evolves within 5 years of disease onset, allowing a clinical diagnosis during follow-up.[25]

CEREBELLAR FEATURES

The cerebellar disorder of MSA-C comprises gait ataxia, and scanning dysarthria and cerebellar oculomotor disturbances. MSA-C generally manifests clinically as a midline cerebellar disorder that progresses more rapidly than other late-onset sporadic ataxias; typically, a patient becomes wheelchair-dependent by 5 years after onset.[26,27] Limb ataxia may be seen, but is generally less prominent than gait or speech disturbances. Patients with MSA-C usually develop additional noncerebellar symptoms and signs, but, before doing so, may be indistinguishable from other patients with idiopathic late-onset cerebellar ataxia, many of whom have disease restricted clinically to cerebellar signs and pathologically to degeneration of the cerebellum and olives.[6]

MISCELLANEOUS FEATURES

Sleep disorders are almost universal in MSA and include insomnia with difficulties falling asleep, frequent awakenings, and overall reduced sleep efficiency, and excessive daytime sleepiness. Sleep problems in MSA are due to a multitude of factors, including primary dysfunction of sleep-wake cycle regulation and rapid-eye movement (REM) sleep behavior disorder, and secondary effects of PD medications and comorbid conditions such as sleep-disordered breathing.[28,29] Often occurring with sleep apnea, nocturnal stridor is an inspiratory sound produced by complex vocal cord muscle dysfunction, and it is associated with respiratory failure and sudden death during sleep and with decreased survival.[21,24,30] Polysomnographic abnormalities associated with REM sleep behavior disorder in the setting of MSA are more pronounced than in PD.[31] Levodopa may induce sleepiness in MSA.[32]

The core cognitive dysfunction in MSA is characterized by deficits in frontal executive function.[33,34] Half of MSA patients may develop frontal dysfunction within 1 year after the onset of cerebellar or parkinsonian symptoms.[35] As the disease progresses, cognitive dysfunction in MSA may include deficits in memory, attention, and visuospatial and visuoconstructive capabilities.[35-37] Language and praxic functions may rarely be compromised in patients with MSA.[33-35]

Depressive symptoms occur in approximately 80% of patients with MSA, with 40% endorsing symptoms consistent with moderate to severe depression.[12,38,39] Peripheral neuropathy is usually subtle or subclinical in patients with MSA, but rarely it may be the initial symptom in MSA involving large myelinated fibers of the sensory nerves.[40,41]

DIAGNOSTIC "RED FLAGS"

Besides the poor response to levodopa, and the additional presence of pyramidal or cerebellar signs or autonomic failure as major diagnostic clues, certain other features known as "red flags," or warning signs, such as "cold hands sign" (i.e., changes in skin color or temperature with cold, dusky, violaceous hands, with poor circulatory return after blanching by pressure), orofacial dystonia, or stridor, may raise suspicion of MSA.[20,42-44] The European MSA Study Group has evaluated the frequencies and the diagnostic role of "red flags" in patients with MSA-P compared with patients with PD. The prevalence of the diagnostic "red flags" that have been found to be very specific (>95%) compared with PD are listed in Table 20–1.[45] A combination of two out of the six "red flag" categories proposed by the European MSA Study Group is highly specific with good sensitivity when comparing MSA-P and PD patients. Indeed, approximately three quarters of the patients diagnosed as possible MSA-P could have been correctly diagnosed as probable MSA-P more than 1 year earlier in the disease course than with the Consensus criteria alone.

Clinical Diagnostic Criteria

The clinical diagnosis of MSA rests largely on history and physical examination. The original Consensus criteria are now widely used for a clinical diagnosis of MSA.[3] The criteria used separate features and criteria for diagnosis, however, which were complex and difficult to keep in mind, particularly for clinicians in a busy clinic setting. The Consensus criteria were revised retaining the fundamental structure of the previous Consensus criteria.[27] Two diagnostic categories refer to the predominant motor feature at the time the patient is evaluated: MSA with predominant parkinsonism (parkinsonian variant of MSA, MSA-P) and MSA with predominant cerebellar ataxia (cerebellar variant of MSA, MSA-C). The Consensus criteria specify three diagnostic categories of increasing certainty: possible, probable, and definite (Table 20–2). Definite MSA requires neuropathological demonstration of central nervous system α-synuclein–positive glial cytoplasmic

TABLE 20–1	"Red Flags": Warning Features of Multiple System Atrophy	
"Red Flag"	**Frequency in MSA-P (%)**	**Definition**
Early instability with recurrent falls[1]*	67.9	Within 3 yr of disease onset
Rapid progression[2]	66.7	"Wheelchair sign": dependent <10 yr from disease onset
Pisa syndrome[3]	42.1	Prolonged episodes of lateral trunk flexion
Disproportionate antecollis[3]	36.8	Severe neck flexion, minor flexion elsewhere
Contractures of hands or feet[3]	15.8	Excluding Dupuytren's or contracture from other known cause
Severe dysphonia[4]	50.9	Based on clinical judgment
Severe dysarthria[4]	49.1	Based on clinical judgment
Severe dysphagia[4]	33.3	Based on clinical judgment
Diurnal inspiratory stridor[5]	22.8	Based on clinical judgment
Nocturnal inspiratory stridor[5]	37.7	Based on clinical judgment
Inspiratory sighs[5]	43.6	Involuntary deep inspiratory sighs/gasps
Emotional incontinence— crying without sadness[6]	26.3	Inappropriate crying without sadness
Emotional incontinence— laughing without mirth[6]	14	Inappropriate laughing without mirth

MSA-P, multiple system atrophy associated with parkinsonism.
*Superscript numbers represent "red flag" categories: 1 = early instability; 2 = rapid progression; 3 = abnormal postures; 4 = bulbar dysfunction; 5 = respiratory dysfunction; 6 = emotional incontinence.
From Köllensperger M, Geser F, Seppi K, et al. Red flags for multiple system atrophy. *Mov Disord* 2008; 23(8):1093-1099.

inclusions with neurodegenerative changes in striatonigral or olivopontocerebellar structures. Probable MSA requires a sporadic, progressive adult-onset disorder including rigorously defined autonomic failure and poorly levodopa-responsive parkinsonism or cerebellar ataxia. Possible MSA requires a sporadic, progressive adult-onset disease including parkinsonism or cerebellar ataxia, and at least one feature suggesting autonomic dysfunction plus one other feature that may be a clinical or a neuroimaging abnormality (Table 20–3). Features supporting ("red flags") and not supporting MSA (Table 20–4) and differential diagnoses for possible MSA-C (Table 20–5) were defined.

Differential Diagnostic Tests for Multiple System Atrophy

Although the clinical diagnosis of MSA rests largely on history and physical examination, additional investigations, such as autonomic function tests, sphincter electromyography, pharmacological tests, neuroimaging, and different blood

TABLE 20–2	**Second Consensus Statement: Diagnostic Categories of Multiple System Atrophy**

I. Definite MSA

Neuropathological findings of widespread and abundant CNS α-synuclein-positive glial cytoplasmic inclusions (Papp-Lantos inclusions) in association with neurodegenerative changes in striatonigral or olivopontocerebellar structures

II. Probable MSA

Sporadic, progressive, adult-onset (>30 yr old) disease characterized by:
(1) Autonomic failure involving an orthostatic decrease of blood pressure within 3 min of standing by at least 30 mm Hg systolic or 15 mm Hg diastolic or urinary incontinence (with ED in men) *and*
(2a) Poorly levodopa-responsive parkinsonism (bradykinesia with rigidity, tremor, or postural instability) (MSA-P) *or*
(2b) A cerebellar syndrome (gait ataxia with cerebellar dysarthria, limb ataxia, or cerebellar oculomotor dysfunction) (MSA-C)

III. Possible MSA

Sporadic, progressive adult-onset (>30 yr old) disease characterized by:
(1a) Parkinsonism (bradykinesia with rigidity or tremor) *or*
(1b) A cerebellar syndrome with gait ataxia plus at least one of the following: cerebellar dysarthria, limb ataxia, and cerebellar oculomotor dysfunction, *and*
(2) At least one feature suggesting autonomic dysfunction (otherwise unexplained urinary urgency, frequency, or incomplete bladder emptying; ED in men; or significant orthostatic blood pressure decline that does not meet the level required in probable MSA), *and*
(3) At least one of the additional features for possible MSA

CNS, central nervous system; ED, erectile dysfunction; MSA, multiple system atrophy; MSA-C, multiple system atrophy associated with cerebellar ataxia; MSA-P, multiple system atrophy associated with parkinsonism.

and cerebrospinal fluid tests, may be used to support the diagnosis or to exclude other diseases. The abnormalities described subsequently have been observed in patients with defined and usually advanced rather than early disease, when diagnosis of the disease is unclear.

In early disease stages, investigations may give equivocal results. Atrophy of putamen, middle cerebellar peduncle, pons, or cerebellum on structural magnetic resonance imaging (MRI) and hypometabolism in putamen, brainstem, or cerebellum on positron emission tomography with fludeoxyglucose F 18 ([18]FDG PET) have been consistently found in patients with MSA and were implemented as features of possible MSA-P in the revised Consensus criteria. The same is true for atrophy of putamen, middle cerebellar peduncle, or pons on structural MRI; hypometabolism in the putamen, brainstem, or cerebellum on [18]FDG PET; and presynaptic nigrostriatal dopaminergic denervation on single photon emission computed tomography (SPECT) or PET. The latter were implemented as features of possible MSA-C in the revised Consensus criteria.[46]

TABLE 20–3	Second Consensus Statement: Additional Features of Possible Multiple System Atrophy

Features of Possible MSA-P	Features of Possible MSA-C
Rapidly progressive parkinsonism Poor response to levodopa Postural instability within 3 yr of motor onset Gait ataxia, cerebellar dysarthria, limb ataxia, or cerebellar oculomotor dysfunction Babinski's sign with hyperreflexia Stridor Dysphagia within 5 yr of motor onset Atrophy on MRI of putamen, middle cerebellar peduncle, pons, or cerebellum Hypometabolism on ¹⁸FDG PET in putamen, brainstem, or cerebellum	Parkinsonism (Bradykinesia and rigidity) Babinski's sign with hyperreflexia Stridor Atrophy on MRI of putamen, middle cerebellar peduncle, or pons Hypometabolism on ¹⁸FDG PET in putamen Presynaptic nigrostriatal dopaminergic denervation on SPECT or PET

¹⁸FDG PET, positron emission tomography with fludeoxyglucose F 18; MRI, magnetic resonance imaging; MSA-C, multiple system atrophy with predominant cerebellar ataxia; MSA-P, multiple system atrophy associated with parkinsonism; SPECT, single photon emission computed tomography.

TABLE 20–4	Second Consensus Statement: Features Supporting ("Red Flags") and Not Supporting Multiple System Atrophy

Supporting Features	Non supporting Features
Orofacial dystonia Disproportionate antecollis Camptocormia (severe anterior flexion of the spine) and/or Pisa syndrome (severe lateral flexion of the spine) Contractures of hands or feet Inspiratory sighs Severe dysphonia Severe dysarthria New or increased snoring Cold hands and feet Pathological laughter or crying Jerky, myoclonic postural/action tremor	Classic pill-rolling rest tremor Clinically significant neuropathy Hallucinations not induced by drugs Onset >75 yr old Family history of ataxia or parkinsonism Dementia (on DSM IV) White matter lesions suggesting multiple sclerosis

DSM IV, Diagnostic and Statistical Manual of Mental Disorders, fourth edition.

AUTONOMIC FUNCTION TESTS

Cardiovascular and Sudomotor Function

The clinical diagnosis of probable MSA requires a reduction of systolic blood pressure by at least 30 mm Hg or of diastolic blood pressure by at least 15 mm Hg after 3 minutes of standing from a previous 3-minute interval in the recumbent

TABLE 20–5	Differential Diagnoses for Possible MSA-C	
Disorder	**Test**	**Result**
MSA-C	MRI ^{18}FDG PET PET or SPECT with a dopamine presynaptic ligand	Atrophy of putamen or pons Putaminal hypometabolism Abnormal striatal dopamine binding
Paraneoplastic cerebellar degeneration	Paraneoplastic antibodies, and consider searching for primary	Positive paraneoplastic antibody test
SCAs	Genetic testing for dominantly inherited SCAs	Positive test, frequently SCA 1, 2, 3, 6, 7, 12, or 17
Fragile X–associated tremor/ataxia syndrome	Genetic testing for fragile X mental retardation syndrome (*FMR1*) gene	Moderate expansion of CGG trinucleotide repeats
Friedreich's ataxia	Genetic testing	Homozygous abnormal GAA expansion on chromosome 9 or point mutations in compound heterozygous subjects with one expanded allele

MRI, magnetic resonance imaging; ^{18}FDG PET, PET with $^{F-18}$fludeoxyglucose; MSA-C, multiple system atrophy associated with cerebellar ataxia; PET, positron emission tomography; SCA, spinocerebellar ataxia; SPECT, single photon emission computed tomography.

position. In MSA, cardiovascular dysregulation seems to be caused by central rather than peripheral autonomic failure. During supine rest, norepinephrine levels (representing postganglionic sympathetic efferent activity) are normal,[47] and there is no denervation hypersensitivity.[48] In contrast, mainly postganglionic sympathetic dysfunction is thought to account for autonomic failure associated with PD. More recent studies showed, however, that abnormal cardiovascular autonomic function tests to study sympathetic and parasympathetic function, such as orthostatism, head-up tilt, cold pressor test, deep breathing, Valsalva maneuver, and hyperventilation, failed to differentiate autonomic failure associated with PD versus MSA.[49,50] Similarly, an abnormal sympathetic skin response is not only frequently seen in patients with MSA, but also can be detected in patients with PD.[51,52] Although such abnormalities may be nonspecific, their presence within the first 3 to 5 years of disease onset make a diagnosis of MSA more likely than PD.

Urogenital Function and Sphincter Electromyography

Assessment of bladder function is mandatory in MSA and usually provides evidence of involvement of the autonomic nervous system already at an early stage of the disease (when bladder function is still normal in most PD patients). The nature of bladder dysfunction is different in MSA and PD.[13,15] Although frequency and urgency are common in both disorders, marked urge or stress incontinence with continuous leakage is not a feature of PD apart from very advanced cases. Urodynamic studies show a characteristic pattern of abnormality in MSA patients.[53] In the early stages, there is often detrusor hyperreflexia, often with bladder neck incompetence owing to abnormal urethral sphincter function, which results in early frequency and urgency followed by urge incontinence. Later on, the ability to initiate a voluntary micturition reflex and the strength of the hyperreflexic detrusor contractions diminish, and the bladder may become atonic, accounting for increasing postmicturition residual urine volumes. Postvoid residual volume needs to be determined sonographically or via catheterization to initiate intermittent self-catheterization in due course.

External anal sphincter electromyography (EMG) frequently shows spontaneous activity and increased polyphasia of motor unit potentials consistent with deinnervation and reinnervation of voluntary sphincter muscles in patients with MSA.[13] Neurogenic changes of external anal sphincter muscle have also been shown in patients in advanced stages of PD, however, and in constipated patients. A normal sphincter EMG is unlikely in pathologically proven MSA, at least in cases with a symptom duration of more than 5 years when the test is performed.[54,55]

PHARMACOLOGICAL TESTS

An acute dopaminergic challenge using oral levodopa (single dose ≤250 mg) or subcutaneous apomorphine (a single injection of 50 µg/kg [usually 3 mg] or repeated challenges with a starting dose of 25 µg/kg [usually 1.5 mg] followed by stepwise increments of 25-50 µg/kg [usually 1.5-3 mg], up to 150 µg/kg [usually 9 mg], once every 30 minutes) performed in a standardized manner allows a rapid enhancement of brain dopaminergic transmission.[56] A systematic review revealed that overall diagnostic accuracy of acute dopaminergic challenge tests referring patients with PD versus patients with atypical parkinsonian disorders (APDs) including MSA is suboptimal.[57] The negative predictive value in de novo patients with parkinsonism is 60% at maximum,[58,59] and several patients with MSA, PSP, and vascular parkinsonism may initially show a good or even marked response to levodopa.[60-62] Similar diagnostic accuracies were shown for acute dopaminergic challenge tests and long-term dopaminergic therapies, suggesting that an acute dopaminergic challenge adds nothing for the differential diagnosis of neurodegenerative parkinsonism.[57]

Activation of hypothalamic α_2-adrenoceptors and muscarinic cholinergic receptors induces growth hormone release.[63] Similar to healthy individuals, the response to the growth hormone secretagogues clonidine, an α_2-adrenoceptor agonist, and arginine, an amino acid activating the cholinergic system, is normal (i.e., increase of growth hormone) in patients with PD and patients with idiopathic late-onset cerebellar ataxia,[64,65] whereas it is abnormal in patients with MSA. Diagnostic accuracy of the growth hormone stimulation test using arginine in differentiating MSA-P from PD is about 90%, and in differentiating MSA-P from PSP slightly lower.[65,66]

STRUCTURAL IMAGING WITH MAGNETIC RESONANCE IMAGING AND TRANSCRANIAL SONOGRAPHY

Numerous studies have consistently found that increased hyperechogenicity in the substantia nigra region of the midbrain as assessed by transcranial sonography is an almost universal feature of PD, occurring in about 80% to 90% of patients with PD, but also present in about 10% of healthy adult controls and patients with APDs including patients with MSA.[67-70] Unilateral or bilateral hyperechogenicity of the lentiform nucleus can be detected in at least two thirds of patients with APDs including MSA and in around one quarter of patients with PD.[71,72] Combining a hyperechogenic lentiform nucleus with a nonmarked echogenic substantia nigra is quite specific for APDs, although sensitivity seems to be suboptimal.[70,72]

Conventional MRI including standard T2-, T1-weighted and proton-density sequences at 1.5 Tesla machines is believed to be usually normal in patients with PD, whereas it frequently shows characteristic abnormalities in patients with APD, offering the potential for objective criteria in the differential diagnosis of neurodegenerative parkinsonism. In patients with MSA, atrophy and signal changes in the putamen and in infratentorial structures may occur. These changes include putaminal abnormalities, such as putaminal atrophy, T2 hypointensity, and T2 "slitlike" marginal hyperintensity (putaminal rim); atrophy of the lower brainstem, middle cerebellar peduncles, and cerebellum; and hyperintensities in the pons, middle cerebellar peduncles, and cerebellum. Overall, specificity of these abnormal findings compared with PD is considered quite high, whereas sensitivity seems to be suboptimal, especially in the early disease stages.[73,74] The role of signal changes for the differential diagnosis of MSA from PD on T2 weighted sequences at 3.0 Tesla is unclear. Indeed, a T2 hyperintense putaminal rim is a nonspecific, normal finding at 3.0 Tesla.[75]

Several more recent studies have shown that diffusion-weighted imaging (DWI) permits discrimination between MSA-P in early disease stages and PD and healthy humans on the basis of putaminal diffusivity measures.[76-78] Although putaminal diffusivity changes overlap in MSA-P and PSP patients, diffusivity changes in the middle cerebellar peduncle in patients with MSA and diffusivity changes in the superior cerebellar peduncle in patients with PSP may be helpful to differentiate between MSA and PSP.[77,79]

Voxel-based morphometry showed basal ganglia and infratentorial volume loss and prominent cortical volume loss in MSA-P mainly comprising the cortical targets of striatal projections, such as the primary sensorimotor and lateral premotor cortices, and the prefrontal cortex.[80,81] MRI-based volumetry is a helpful tool to investigate the progression of cortical and subcortical atrophy patterns in MSA[82] compared with other disorders; however, at this time, it cannot be applied for routine diagnostic work-up of individual patients.

FUNCTIONAL IMAGING (SINGLE PHOTON EMISSION COMPUTED TOMOGRAPHY AND POSITRON EMISSION TOMOGRAPHY)

Functional imaging methods for the differential diagnosis of parkinsonian disorders can be divided into investigations of receptor binding and the investigation of glucose metabolism. Studies of receptor binding in disorders with parkinsonism examine the presynaptic nigrostriatal neurons by evaluating the dopa decarboxylase activity and the dopamine transporter (DAT), and the postsynaptic dopaminergic function evaluating the dopamine D2 receptor. More recently, SPECT and PET ligands have become available to study cardiac sympathetic innervation as well.

SPECT targeting the DAT on the dopamine neuronal terminals and quantifying the loss of these terminals and positron emission tomography (PET) using fluorodopa F 18 (^{18}F-dopa) have been proposed as diagnostic tools to help differentiate neurodegenerative parkinsonian disorders including PD and APDs from other non-neurodegenerative parkinsonian or tremor disorders by identifying presynaptic nigrostriatal terminal dysfunction based on reduced tracer binding in the caudate and putamen.[83] Although ^{18}F-dopa PET is a reliable biomarker for the determination of presynaptic dopaminergic terminal function by quantifying the reduction of levodopa metabolism caused by dopaminergic neuronal death or dysfunction, its use in routine clinical practice is limited by high hardware costs and a short radioactive half-life of ^{18}F.[84]

Although resolution and interscan variability are less accurate, radioligands with affinity to DAT, such as [^{123}I]2-β-carbomethoxy-3β-(4-iodophenyl) tropane ([^{123}I]β-CIT) or [^{123}I]N-w-fluoropropyl-2β-carbomethoxy-3β-(4-iodophenyl) nortropane ([^{123}I]FP-CIT), and detected by SPECT have emerged as a less expensive alternative.[85] Several studies have shown that DAT ligand uptake is reduced severely even in the early stages of neurodegenerative parkinsonian disorders compared with age-matched healthy subjects.[84,86] Because striatal dopaminergic terminals are affected in all APDs, evaluation of striatal DAT binding or dopa decarboxylase activity has limited value to discriminate between patients with PD and APDs.[87-89] In addition to reductions in striatal DAT activity in early MSA-P, PSP, and PD, statistical parametric mapping, a technique that objectively localizes focal changes of the radiotracer throughout the entire brain volume without having to make an a priori hypothesis as to their location, and [^{123}I]β-CIT SPECT detected focal reductions of DAT uptake in brainstem regions in MSA-P and PSP compared with controls and PD patients.[90,91] Adding the brainstem analysis to the routinely performed striatal analysis may have a high potential of [^{123}I]β-CIT SPECT to discriminate between APDs and PD, but remain in an exploratory phase of development.

Functional imaging studies using PET or SPECT have employed dopamine D2 receptor ligands ([^{11}C]raclopride for PET and [^{123}I]iodobenzamide or [^{123}I] iodobenzofuran for SPECT) to detect differences in striatal binding in MSA versus PD patients. Reduced tracer binding has been consistently found in MSA, in line with the degeneration of striatal projection neurons and decreased postsynaptic dopamine D2 receptor density in the striatum of patients with MSA-P as revealed by a postmortem study.[92] Dopamine D2 receptor binding between MSA and PD may overlap, however, limiting diagnostic accuracy.[93-96]

^{18}FDG PET can be helpful for discriminating PD from APDs, particularly when combined with computer-assisted statistical parametric mapping, which increases the sensitivity relative to visual analysis from 80% to 95%. MSA cases show striatal, brainstem, and cerebellar hypometabolism, whereas putamen metabolism is elevated and frontotemporal metabolism is reduced in PD.[97]

The basal ganglia are rich in opioid peptides and binding sites, and these are differentially affected in striatonigral degeneration and PD. ^{11}C-diprenorphine is a nonspecific opioid antagonist binding with equal affinity to μ, κ, and δ sites. In nondyskinetic PD patients, caudate and putamen ^{11}C-diprenorphine uptake is preserved, but becomes reduced in dyskinetic cases,[98] whereas putamen uptake is reduced in 50% of patients thought to have striatonigral degeneration.[99] ^{11}C-PK11195 PET, an in vivo marker of microglial activation, has been used to study neuroinflammatory changes in MSA.[100] Widespread subcortical increases in ^{11}C-PK11195 uptake were seen, particularly in substantia nigra, putamen, globus pallidum, thalamus, and brainstem. Similar changes were evident in PD, although to a reduced extent.[101] Given this, neither ^{11}C-diprenorphine nor ^{11}C-PK11195 PET provides sensitive discriminators of MSA from PD.

Imaging of sympathetic cardiac innervation with scintigraphic visualization and [^{123}I]metaiodobenzylguanidine (MIBG) and with ^{18}F-dopa or [^{11}C]hydroxyephedrine PET in many reports has shown preserved sympathetic postganglionic neurons in MSA, in contrast to PD.[102-105] PD patients also may have normal cardiac MIBG binding, however, and some sympathetic cardiac denervation has been shown in MSA using MIBG scintigraphy and [^{11}C]hydroxyephedrine and PET.[105-110]

BLOOD AND CEREBROSPINAL FLUID TESTS

In patients with sporadic adult-onset progressive ataxia (see Table 20-5), which may develop into MSA-C, screening test for antigliadin antibodies and anti-glutamic acid decarboxylase (anti-GAD) antibodies (a diagnosis of paraneoplastic disease should be considered in patients with an aggressive clinical course with or without general systemic malaise), as well as screening tests for Friedreich's ataxia mutation, or the fragile X–associated tremor/ataxia syndrome (FXTAS), which results from a premutation (moderate expansions of 55 to 200 repeats) of a CGG trinucleotide in the fragile X mental retardation 1 (*FMR1*) gene, and the dominantly inherited spinocerebellar ataxias (SCAs) should be considered, because even with a negative family history, there is a 15% to 20% chance of a mutation in one of the polyglutamine SCAs, notably SCA 1, 2, 3, 6 and 7.[6,110-112] Increased levels of neurofilament light chain and tau and decreased levels of 3-methoxy-4-hydroxyphenylethyleneglycol in the cerebrospinal fluid were associated with high accuracy levels in differentiating MSA-C from idiopathic late-onset cerebellar ataxia.[113] The cerebrospinal fluid neurofilament light chain and tau tests have been found to differentiate MSA from PD, but remain in an exploratory phase of development.[114]

Management

Similar to PD, there is currently no treatment that has proven efficacy in slowing the progression of MSA or otherwise significantly modifying disease course. Available symptomatic therapies are limited by poor responsiveness of parkinsonism in MSA to levodopa, a lack of effective therapies for cerebellar ataxia, and a limited armamentarium to treat autonomic failure. Treatment of MSA is largely palliative, but affected patients require care by a specialist to ensure that potential benefits of available symptomatic measures for the different domains are fully exploited.

TREATMENT OF PARKINSONISM

Levodopa is the gold standard of symptomatic efficacy in treating the motor symptoms of PD, and assessing responsiveness to levodopa is essential in the clinical diagnostic work-up of MSA-P in particular. Although a poor or absent response to levodopa is part of the diagnostic criteria for MSA, about 30-50% of patients may show at least a partial and transient response.[1,18,115] This response sometimes may last for several years, but approximately 90% of patients with MSA-P lose a clinically meaningful response to levodopa in the long-term.[116] Levodopa responsiveness in MSA-P should be assessed by escalating doses to at least 1000 mg/day if needed and tolerated, and clinical response should be assessed over a 3-month period.[27] Even in patients who eventually fail to gain significant motor benefit from levodopa, this drug may still produce dyskinesias, which have been shown to be predominantly dystonic and to affect the face and neck in approximately 50% of patients.[17]

There is no evidence that treatment with dopamine agonists offers any greater benefit over that observed with levodopa. Although there are some anecdotal reports on partial efficacy of the older ergot dopamine agonists lisuride and bromocriptine,[117-119] there are no reports on the efficacy and tolerability of the newer ergot or nonergot dopamine agonists in MSA. Because of the greater propensity of dopamine agonists to induce postural hypotension compared with levodopa, their use in MSA is usually not recommended.

Because of the small effect size compared with levodopa in PD, there is also no rationale to use monoamine oxidase B inhibitors for the control of motor symptoms in MSA-P. Similarly, there is generally no role for anticholinergics or amantadine to treat parkinsonism in MSA. While reports on the open-label use of the latter drug in MSA suggest no or variable antiparkinsonian efficacy,[1,120] amantadine was found ineffective in a randomized placebo-controlled trial.[121] Another more recent randomized placebo-controlled study[122] has reported beneficial motor effects of the serotonin reuptake inhibitor paroxetine (up to 30 mg three times daily) on upper limb motor function and speech in 19 patients with MSA. Paroxetine treatment was well tolerated despite the high doses used. To date, there have been no confirmatory reports of this effect.

Although there have been occasional reports on beneficial effects of bilateral subthalamic nucleus stimulation in patients with MSA-P,[123] most cases reported did not benefit from this procedure.[124,125] There is currently no role for deep brain stimulation procedures in the routine management of MSA patients.

Nonpharmacological treatments including physiotherapy and speech and occupational therapy may be beneficial in improving parkinsonian motor features.[126] These should be an obligatory part of the palliative management program in all patients with MSA.

TREATMENT OF AUTONOMIC FAILURE

Autonomic failure is a clinical diagnostic pointer and a major source of disability in MSA. Autonomic dysfunction has been associated with reduced quality of life,[50,127] and can give rise to serious complications, such as injury from syncope-related falls.

Orthostatic Hypotension

Management of orthostatic hypotension and syncope in MSA usually requires combinations of antihypotensive drugs, but care must be taken to exploit nonpharmacological options fully. These options include sufficient fluid intake, high-salt diet, and the use of compression stockings or, rarely, custom-made elastic body garments. Patients should also be instructed to change their dietary habits towards more frequent, but smaller meals, if postprandial hypotension is a problem. Tilting the head up during the night can increase intravasal volume, and may help to improve early morning hypotension.

There are no randomized controlled trials of antihypotensive agents specifically in MSA, but the α-adrenergic agonist midodrine was efficacious in randomized placebo-controlled trials in patients with neurogenic hypotension of different etiologies, including MSA.[128,129] Two more recent double-blind, placebo-controlled trials of the norepinephrine precursor drug L-threo-DOPS (Droxidopa, L-threo-dihydroxy-phenylserine) have included patients with MSA and shown overall efficacy.[130-132] Although specific trials in MSA are lacking, the adrenergic agents phenylpropanolamine and yohimbine can be used to treat orthostatic hypotension in MSA.[133] The somatostatin analogue octreotide may improve postprandial hypotension in patients with pure autonomic failure[134] via an action believed to involve release inhibition of vasodilatory gastrointestinal peptides. The mineralocorticoid fludrocortisone can be beneficial via increasing intravasal volume.

Urogenital Dysfunction

Similar to PD, but usually more pronounced, detrusor hyperreflexia and sphincter detrusor dyssynergy are key components of urinary urgency and incontinence in MSA. These conditions may be helped by anticholinergic drugs such as oxybutynin or tolterodine. Trospium chloride differs from the aforementioned agents by its exclusively peripheral mode of action, and has equal efficacy without the risk of central anticholinergic side effects.[15,135,136]

α-Adrenergic receptor antagonists, such as prazosin, have been shown to reduce residual volumes in MSA patients and to improve voiding function.[137] Desmopressin, a vasopressin analogue, reduces nocturnal polyuria, and may improve morning postural hypotension.[138]

When postmicturition volumes are greater than 150 mL despite optimized pharmacological therapy, intermittent self-catheterization (three to four times daily) is usually required. Permanent transcutaneous suprapubic catheter implantation may become necessary if intermittent self-catheterization is impractical or impossible.

Male erectile dysfunction in MSA has been shown to respond to sildenafil in a placebo-controlled randomized trial including patients with MSA.[139] In this particular study, there was, however, a serious exacerbation of orthostatic hypotension in several patients such that sildenafil or other phosphodiesterase inhibitors should be prescribed with great caution to patients with MSA, and never without prior measurement of lying and standing blood pressure. Erectile dysfunction may also be improved by oral yohimbine or—as a last resort—by intracavernosal injection of papaverine.[13]

MANAGEMENT OF CEREBELLAR ATAXIA

Ataxia of gait, postural instability, and falls and dysarthria are among the symptoms least amenable to symptomatic therapies in MSA. Although it is generally believed that speech therapy and physiotherapy are helpful in cerebellar disorders, there is little evidence from controlled trials to support this notion.[140] Nevertheless, such treatment should be offered in concert with symptomatic therapies for the other symptom domains of MSA in an attempt to maintain independent ambulation or communication for as long as possible. Most patients require walking aids, however, and eventually become wheelchair-bound after an average of 5 years.[4]

DYSTONIA AND OTHER MOTOR PROBLEMS

Local injections of botulinum toxin have been shown to be effective in cranial and limb dystonia associated with MSA.[141] Attempts to alleviate antecollis posturing in MSA via botulinum toxin injections into neck flexors have been associated with severe dysphagia, and this type of treatment is not recommended.[142] Dysarthria in MSA can be alleviated by speech therapy, and palliative care for severe dysarthria should include the use of communication aids.[126] Dysphagia, in less severe stages, can also profit from appropriate training, but may require feeding via percutaneous endoscopic gastrostomy tubes in advanced cases.

MANAGEMENT OF SLEEP-RELATED DISORDERS

Although there is a paucity of sleep studies using polysomnography in MSA, approximately 60% of patients are believed to have REM sleep behavior disorder.[143,144] If self-injuries or injurious behavior toward bed partners occurs, treatment with clonazepam (0.25-1 mg at bedtime) would be beneficial in most patients.

Approximately 30% of patients with MSA have nocturnal inspiratory stridor, which may seriously disrupt sleep of caregivers, even if not sleeping in the same room with the patient. Some reports have suggested positive effects of non-invasive ventilation approaches inclucding continuous positive airway pressure or non-invasive positive pressure ventilation such as biphasic positive airway pressure in MSA patients with inspiratory stridor.[145-147] These non-invasive ventilation approaches are not always possible, however, and may be associated with worsening of respiration in sleep in some patients.[21,28] In advanced cases of severe insufficiency of vocal cord opening, a tracheostomy may be required as a last resort.

REFERENCES

1. Wenning GK, Ben Shlomo Y, Magalhaes M, et al: Clinical features and natural history of multiple system atrophy: sn analysis of 100 cases. Brain 1994;117(Pt 4):835-845.
2. Hughes AJ, Daniel SE, Ben Shlomo Y, Lees AJ: The accuracy of diagnosis of parkinsonian syndromes in a specialist movement disorder service. Brain 2002;125(Pt 4):861-870.
3. Gilman S, Low PA, Quinn N, et al: Consensus statement on the diagnosis of multiple system atrophy. J Auton Nerv Syst 1998;74(2-3):189-192.
4. Watanabe H, Saito Y, Terao S, et al: Progression and prognosis in multiple system atrophy: an analysis of 230 Japanese patients. Brain 2002;125(Pt 5):1070-1083.
5. Yabe I, Soma H, Takei A, et al: MSA-C is the predominant clinical phenotype of MSA in Japan: analysis of 142 patients with probable MSA. J Neurol Sci 2006;249:115-121.
6. Abele M, Burk K, Schols L, et al: The aetiology of sporadic adult-onset ataxia. Brain 2002;125 (Pt 5):961-968.
7. Gilman S, Little R, Johanns J, et al: Evolution of sporadic olivopontocerebellar atrophy into multiple system atrophy. Neurology 2000;55:527-532.
8. Schwarz J, Tatsch K, Gasser T, et al: 123I-IBZM binding compared with long-term clinical follow up in patients with de novo parkinsonism. Mov Disord 1998;13:16-19.
9. Ben Shlomo Y, Wenning GK, Tison F, Quinn NP: Survival of patients with pathologically proven multiple system atrophy: a meta-analysis. Neurology 1997;48:384-393.
10. Kirchhof K, Apostolidis AN, Mathias CJ, Fowler CJ: Erectile and urinary dysfunction may be the presenting features in patients with multiple system atrophy: a retrospective study. Int J Impot Res 2003;15:293-298.
11. Oertel WH, Wachter T, Quinn NP, et al: Reduced genital sensitivity in female patients with multiple system atrophy of parkinsonian type. Mov Disord 2003;18:430-432.
12. Geser F, Seppi K, Stampfer-Kountchev M, et al: The European Multiple System Atrophy-Study Group (EMSA-SG). J Neural Transm 2005;112(12):1677-1686.
13. Beck RO, Betts CD, Fowler CJ: Genitourinary dysfunction in multiple system atrophy: clinical features and treatment in 62 cases. J Urol 1994;151:1336-1341.
14. Sakakibara R, Hattori T, Uchiyama T, et al: Urinary dysfunction and orthostatic hypotension in multiple system atrophy: which is the more common and earlier manifestation? J Neurol Neurosurg Psychiatry 2000;68:65-69.
15. Fowler CJ, O'Malley KJ: Investigation and management of neurogenic bladder dysfunction. J Neurol Neurosurg Psychiatry 2003;74(Suppl 4):iv-27-iv-31.
16. Wenning GK, Geser F, Poewe W: The 'risus sardonicus' of multiple system atrophy. Mov Disord 2003;18:1211.
17. Boesch SM, Wenning GK, Ransmayr G, Poewe W: Dystonia in multiple system atrophy 24. J Neurol Neurosurg Psychiatry 2002;72:300-303.
18. Seppi K, Yekhlef F, Diem A, et al: Progression of parkinsonism in multiple system atrophy. J Neurol 2005;252:91-96.

19. Bensimon G, Ludolph A, Agid Y, Vidailhet M, et al: NNIPPS Study Group. Riluzole treatment, survival and diagnostic criteria in Parkinson plus disorders: the NNIPPS study. Brain 2009;132(Pt 1): 156-171. Epub 2008 Nov 23.
20. Muller J, Wenning GK, Verny M, et al: Progression of dysarthria and dysphagia in postmortem-confirmed parkinsonian disorders. Arch Neurol 2001;58:259-264.
21. Silber MH, Levine S: Stridor and death in multiple system atrophy. Mov Disord 2000;15:699-704.
22. Benarroch EE, Schmeichel AM, Sandroni P, et al: Involvement of vagal autonomic nuclei in multiple system atrophy and Lewy body disease. Neurology 2006;66:378-383.
23. Merlo IM, Occhini A, Pacchetti C, Alfonsi E: Not paralysis, but dystonia causes stridor in multiple system atrophy. Neurology 2002;58:649-652.
24. Shimohata T, Shinoda H, Nakayama H, et al: Daytime hypoxemia, sleep-disordered breathing, and laryngopharyngeal findings in multiple system atrophy. Arch Neurol 2007;64:856-861.
25. Wenning GK, Ben Shlomo Y, Hughes A, et al: What clinical features are most useful to distinguish definite multiple system atrophy from Parkinson's disease? J Neurol Neurosurg Psychiatry 2000;68:434-440.
26. Klockgether T, Ludtke R, Kramer B, et al: The natural history of degenerative ataxia: a retrospective study in 466 patients. Brain 1998;121(Pt 4):589-600.
27. Gilman S, Wenning G, Low P, et al: Second consensus statement on the diagnosis of multiple system atrophy. Neurology 2008;71(9):670-676.
28. Ghorayeb I, Bioulac B, Tison F: Sleep disorders in multiple system atrophy. J Neural Transm 2005;112:1669-1675.
29. Boeve BF, Silber MH, Ferman TJ, et al: Association of REM sleep behavior disorder and neurodegenerative disease may reflect an underlying synucleinopathy. Mov Disord 2001;16:622-630.
30. Iranzo A: Sleep and breathing in multiple system atrophy. Curr Treat Options Neurol 2007;9:347-353.
31. Iranzo A, Santamaria J, Rye DB, et al: Characteristics of idiopathic REM sleep behavior disorder and that associated with MSA and PD. Neurology 2005;65:247-252.
32. Seppi K, Hogl B, Diem A, et al: Levodopa-induced sleepiness in the Parkinson variant of multiple system atrophy. Mov Disord 2006;21:1281-1283.
33. Monza D, Soliveri P, Radice D, et al: Cognitive dysfunction and impaired organization of complex motility in degenerative parkinsonian syndromes. Arch Neurol 1998;55:372-378.
34. Leiguarda RC, Pramstaller PP, Merello M, et al: Apraxia in Parkinson's disease, progressive supranuclear palsy, multiple system atrophy and neuroleptic-induced parkinsonism. Brain 1997;120(Pt 1):75-90.
35. Lyoo CH, Jeong Y, Ryu YH, et al: Effects of disease duration on the clinical features and brain glucose metabolism in patients with mixed type multiple system atrophy. Brain 2008;131 (Pt 2):438-446.
36. Bak TH, Crawford LM, Hearn VC, et al: Subcortical dementia revisited: similarities and differences in cognitive function between progressive supranuclear palsy (PSP), corticobasal degeneration (CBD) and multiple system atrophy (MSA). Neurocase 2005;11:268-273.
37. Kawai Y, Suenaga M, Takeda A, et al: Cognitive impairments in multiple system atrophy: MSA-C vs MSA-P. Neurology 2008;70(16 Pt 2):1390-1396.
38. Benrud-Larson LM, Sandroni P, Schrag A, Low PA: Depressive symptoms and life satisfaction in patients with multiple system atrophy. Mov Disord 2005;20:951-957.
39. Gilman S, May SJ, Shults CW, et al: The North American Multiple System Atrophy Study Group. J Neural Transm 2005;112:1687-1694.
40. Rodolico C, Toscano A, De Luca G, et al: Peripheral neuropathy as the presenting feature of multiple system atrophy. Clin Auton Res 2001;11:119-121.
41. Wu YR, Chen CM, Ro LS, et al: Sensory neuropathy as the initial manifestation of multiple system atrophy. J Formos Med Assoc 2004;103:727-730.
42. Gouider-Khouja N, Vidailhet M, Bonnet AM, et al: "Pure" striatonigral degeneration and Parkinson's disease: a comparative clinical study. Mov Disord 1995;10:288-294.
43. Quinn N: Multiple system atrophy—the nature of the beast. J Neurol Neurosurg Psychiatry 1989;52:78-89.
44. Quinn NP: How to diagnose multiple system atrophy. Mov Disord 2005;20(Suppl 12):S5-S10.
45. Köllensperger M, Geser F, Seppi K, et al: Red flags for multiple system atrophy. Mov Disord 2008;23(8):1093-1099.
46. Brooks DJ, Seppi K: Neuroimaging Working Group on MSA. Proposed neuroimaging criteria for the diagnosis of multiple system atrophy. Mov Disord 2009;24(7):949-964.

47. Ziegler MG, Lake CR, Kopin IJ: The sympathetic-nervous-system defect in primary orthostatic hypotension. N Engl J Med 1977;296:293-297.
48. Polinsky RJ, Kopin IJ, Ebert MH, Weise V: Pharmacologic distinction of different orthostatic hypotension syndromes. Neurology 1981;31:1-7.
49. Riley DE, Chelimsky TC: Autonomic nervous system testing may not distinguish multiple system atrophy from Parkinson's disease. J Neurol Neurosurg Psychiatry 2003;74:56-60.
50. Kollensperger M, Stampfer-Kountchev M, Seppi K, et al: Progression of dysautonomia in multiple system atrophy: a prospective study of self-perceived impairment. Eur J Neurol 2007;14:66-72.
51. Schestatsky P, Ehlers JA, Rieder CR, Gomes I: Evaluation of sympathetic skin response in Parkinson's disease. Parkinsonism Relat Disord 2006;12:486-491.
52. De Marinis M, Stocchi F, Gregori B, Accornero N: Sympathetic skin response and cardiovascular autonomic function tests in Parkinson's disease and multiple system atrophy with autonomic failure. Mov Disord 2000;15:1215-1220.
53. Kirby R, Fowler C, Gosling J, Bannister R: Urethro-vesical dysfunction in progressive autonomic failure with multiple system atrophy. J Neurol Neurosurg Psychiatry 1986;49:554-562.
54. Giladi N, Simon ES, Korczyn AD, et al: Anal sphincter EMG does not distinguish between multiple system atrophy and Parkinson's disease. Muscle Nerve 2000;23:731-734.
55. Paviour DC, Williams D, Fowler CJ, et al: Is sphincter electromyography a helpful investigation in the diagnosis of multiple system atrophy? A retrospective study with pathological diagnosis. Mov Disord 2005;20:1425-1430.
56. Albanese A, Bonuccelli U, Brefel C, et al: Consensus statement on the role of acute dopaminergic challenge in Parkinson's disease. Mov Disord 2001;16:197-201.
57. Clarke CE, Davies P: Systematic review of acute levodopa and apomorphine challenge tests in the diagnosis of idiopathic Parkinson's disease. J Neurol Neurosurg Psychiatry 2000;69:590-594.
58. Gasser T, Schwarz J, Arnold G, et al: Apomorphine test for dopaminergic responsiveness in patients with previously untreated Parkinson's disease. Arch Neurol 1992;49:1131-1134.
59. Hughes AJ, Lees AJ, Stern GM: Challenge tests to predict the dopaminergic response in untreated Parkinson's disease. Neurology 1991;41:1723-1725.
60. Williams DR, de Silva R, Paviour DC, et al: Characteristics of two distinct clinical phenotypes in pathologically proven progressive supranuclear palsy: Richardson's syndrome and PSP-parkinsonism. Brain 2005;128(Pt 6):1247-1258.
61. Colosimo C, Pezzella FR: The symptomatic treatment of multiple system atrophy. Eur J Neurol 2002;9:195-199.
62. Zijlmans JC, Katzenschlager R, Daniel SE, Lees AJ: The L-dopa response in vascular parkinsonism. J Neurol Neurosurg Psychiatry 2004;75:545-547.
63. Pellecchia MT, Pivonello R, Colao A, Barone P: Growth hormone stimulation tests in the differential diagnosis of Parkinson's disease. Clin Med Res 2006;4:322-325.
64. Pellecchia MT, Pivonello R, Salvatore E, et al: Growth hormone response to arginine test distinguishes multiple system atrophy from Parkinson's disease and idiopathic late-onset cerebellar ataxia. Clin Endocrinol (Oxf) 2005;62:428-433.
65. Pellecchia MT, Longo K, Pivonello R, et al: Multiple system atrophy is distinguished from idiopathic Parkinson's disease by the arginine growth hormone stimulation test. Ann Neurol 2006;60:611-615.
66. Pellecchia MT, Longo K, Manfredi M, et al: The arginine growth hormone stimulation test in bradykinetic-rigid parkinsonisms. Mov Disord 2008;23:190-194.
67. Berg D, Behnke S, Walter U: Application of transcranial sonography in extrapyramidal disorders: updated recommendations. Ultraschall Med 2006;27:12-19.
68. Berg D: Transcranial sonography in the early and differential diagnosis of Parkinson's disease. J Neural Transm Suppl 2006;70:249-254.
69. Stockner H, Seppi K, Kiechl S, et al: Midbrain transcranial sonography findings in a population-based study [Abstract]. Mov Disord 2006;21(Suppl 15):S634.
70. Gaenslen A, Unmuth B, Godau J, et al: The specificity and sensitivity of transcranial ultrasound in the differential diagnosis of Parkinson's disease: a prospective blinded study. Lancet Neurol 2008;7(5):417-424. Epub 2008 Apr 3.
71. Walter U, Niehaus L, Probst T, et al: Brain parenchyma sonography discriminates Parkinson's disease and atypical parkinsonian syndromes. Neurology 2003;60:74-77.
72. Behnke S, Berg D, Naumann M, Becker G: Differentiation of Parkinson's disease and atypical parkinsonian syndromes by transcranial ultrasound. J Neurol Neurosurg Psychiatry 2005;76:423-425.

73. Seppi K, Schocke MF, Wenning GK, Poewe W: How to diagnose MSA early: the role of magnetic resonance imaging. J Neural Transm 2005;112:1625-1634.
74. Seppi K, Schocke MF: An update on conventional and advanced magnetic resonance imaging techniques in the differential diagnosis of neurodegenerative parkinsonism. Curr Opin Neurol 2005;18:370-375.
75. Lee WH, Lee CC, Shyu WC, et al: Hyperintense putaminal rim sign is not a hallmark of multiple system atrophy at 3T. AJNR Am J Neuroradiol 2005;26(9):2238-2242.
76. Seppi K, Schocke MF, Esterhammer R, et al: Diffusion-weighted imaging discriminates progressive supranuclear palsy from PD, but not from the parkinson variant of multiple system atrophy. Neurology 2003;60:922-927.
77. Nicoletti G, Lodi R, Condino F, et al: Apparent diffusion coefficient measurements of the middle cerebellar peduncle differentiate the Parkinson variant of MSA from Parkinson's disease and progressive supranuclear palsy. Brain 2006;129(Pt 10):2679-2687.
78. Schocke MF, Seppi K, Esterhammer R, et al: Trace of diffusion tensor differentiates the Parkinson variant of multiple system atrophy and Parkinson's disease. Neuroimage 2004;21:1443-1451.
79. Nicoletti G, Tonon C, Lodi R, et al: Apparent diffusion coefficient of the superior cerebellar peduncle differentiates progressive supranuclear palsy from Parkinson's disease. Mov Disord 2008;23(16):2370-2376.
80. Brenneis C, Seppi K, Schocke MF, et al: Voxel-based morphometry detects cortical atrophy in the Parkinson variant of multiple system atrophy. Mov Disord 2003;18:1132-1138.
81. Minnerop M, Specht K, Ruhlmann J, et al: Voxel-based morphometry and voxel-based relaxometry in multiple system atrophy—a comparison between clinical subtypes and correlations with clinical parameters. Neuroimage 2007;36:1086-1095.
82. Brenneis C, Egger K, Scherfler C, et al: Progression of brain atrophy in multiple system atrophy. A longitudinal VBM study. J Neurol 2007;254:191-196.
83. Brooks DJ: Neuroimaging in Parkinson's disease. NeuroRx 2004;1:243-254.
84. Poewe W, Scherfler C: Role of dopamine transporter imaging in investigation of parkinsonian syndromes in routine clinical practice. Mov Disord 2003;18(Suppl 7):S16-S21.
85. Scherfler C, Schwarz J, Antonini A, et al: Role of DAT-SPECT in the diagnostic work up of parkinsonism. Mov Disord 2007;22:1229-1238.
86. Seibyl J, Jennings D, Tabamo R, Marek K: The role of neuroimaging in the early diagnosis and evaluation of Parkinson's disease. Minerva Med 2005;96:353-364.
87. Pirker W, Asenbaum S, Bencsits G, et al: [123I]beta-CIT SPECT in multiple system atrophy, progressive supranuclear palsy, and corticobasal degeneration. Mov Disord 2000;15:1158-1167.
88. Varrone A, Marek KL, Jennings D, et al: [(123)I]beta-CIT SPECT imaging demonstrates reduced density of striatal dopamine transporters in Parkinson's disease and multiple system atrophy. Mov Disord 2001;16:1023-1032.
89. Brooks DJ, Ibanez V, Sawle GV, et al: Differing patterns of striatal 18F-dopa uptake in Parkinson's disease, multiple system atrophy, and progressive supranuclear palsy. Ann Neurol 1990;28:547-555.
90. Scherfler C, Seppi K, Donnemiller E, et al: Voxel-wise analysis of [123I]β-CIT SPECT differentiates the Parkinson variant of multiple system atrophy from idiopathic Parkinson's disease. Brain 2005 Jul;128(Pt 7):1605-1612.
91. Seppi K, Scherfler C, Donnemiller E, et al: Topography of dopamine transporter availability in progressive supranuclear palsy: a voxelwise [123I]beta-CIT SPECT analysis. Arch Neurol 2006;63:1154-1160.
92. Churchyard A, Donnan GA, Hughes A, et al: Dopa resistance in multiple-system atrophy: loss of postsynaptic D2 receptors. Ann Neurol 1993;34:219-226.
93. Seppi K, Schocke MF, Donnemiller E, et al: Comparison of diffusion-weighted imaging and [(123)I]IBZM-SPECT for the differentiation of patients with the Parkinson variant of multiple system atrophy from those with Parkinson's disease. Mov Disord 2004;19:1438-1445.
94. Schwarz J, Tatsch K, Arnold G, et al: 123I-iodobenzamide-SPECT in 83 patients with de novo parkinsonism. Neurology 1993;43(12 Suppl 6):S17-S20.
95. Brooks DJ, Ibanez V, Sawle GV, et al: Striatal D2 receptor status in patients with Parkinson's disease, striatonigral degeneration, and progressive supranuclear palsy, measured with 11C-raclopride and positron emission tomography. Ann Neurol 1992;31:184-192.
96. Kim YJ, Ichise M, Ballinger JR, et al: Combination of dopamine transporter and D2 receptor SPECT in the diagnostic evaluation of PD, MSA, and PSP. Mov Disord 2002;17(2):303-312.

97. Eckert T, Barnes A, Dhawan V, et al: FDG PET in the differential diagnosis of parkinsonian disorders. Neuroimage 2005;26:912-921.

98. Piccini P, Weeks RA, Brooks DJ: Alterations in opioid receptor binding in Parkinson's disease patients with levodopa-induced dyskinesias. Ann Neurol 1997;42:720-726.

99. Burn DJ, Rinne JO, Quinn NP, et al: Striatal opioid receptor binding in Parkinson's disease, striatonigral degeneration and Steele-Richardson-Olszewski syndrome, A [11C]diprenorphine PET study. Brain 1995;118(Pt 4):951-958.

100. Gerhard A, Banati RB, Goerres GB, et al: [11C](R)-PK11195 PET imaging of microglial activation in multiple system atrophy. Neurology 2003;61:686-689.

101. Gerhard A, Pavese N, Hotton G, et al: In vivo imaging of microglial activation with [11C](R)-PK11195 PET in idiopathic Parkinson's disease. Neurobiol Dis 2006;21:404-412.

102. Iwasa K, Nakajima K, Yoshikawa H, et al: Decreased myocardial 123I-MIBG uptake in Parkinson's disease. Acta Neurol Scand 1998;97:303-306.

103. Braune S, Reinhardt M, Schnitzer R, et al: Cardiac uptake of [123I]MIBG separates Parkinson's disease from multiple system atrophy. Neurology 1999;53:1020-1025.

104. Courbon F, Brefel-Courbon C, Thalamas C, et al: Cardiac MIBG scintigraphy is a sensitive tool for detecting cardiac sympathetic denervation in Parkinson's disease. Mov Disord 2003;18:890-897.

105. Hirayama M, Hakusui S, Koike Y, et al: A scintigraphical qualitative analysis of peripheral vascular sympathetic function with meta-[123I]iodobenzylguanidine in neurological patients with autonomic failure. J Auton Nerv Syst 1995;53(2-3):230-234.

106. Yoshita M, Hayashi M, Hirai S: [Iodine 123-labeled meta-iodobenzylguanidine myocardial scintigraphy in the cases of idiopathic Parkinson's disease, multiple system atrophy, and progressive supranuclear palsy]. Rinsho Shinkeigaku 1997;37:476-482.

107. Nagayama H, Hamamoto M, Ueda M, et al: Reliability of MIBG myocardial scintigraphy in the diagnosis of Parkinson's disease. J Neurol Neurosurg Psychiatry 2005;76:249-251.

108. Raffel DM, Koeppe RA, Little R, et al: PET measurement of cardiac and nigrostriatal denervation in Parkinsonian syndromes. J Nucl Med 2006;47:1769-1777.

109. Kollensperger M, Seppi K, Liener C, et al: Diffusion weighted imaging best discriminates PD from MSA-P: a comparison with tilt table testing and heart MIBG scintigraphy. Mov Disord 2007;22:1771-1776.

110. Kamm C, Healy DG, Quinn NP, et al: The fragile X tremor ataxia syndrome in the differential diagnosis of multiple system atrophy: data from the EMSA Study Group. Brain 2005;128(Pt 8):1855-1860.

111. Burk K, Bosch S, Muller CA, et al: Sporadic cerebellar ataxia associated with gluten sensitivity. Brain 2001;124(Pt 5):1013-1019.

112. Abele M, Weller M, Mescheriakov S, et al: Cerebellar ataxia with glutamic acid decarboxylase autoantibodies. Neurology 1999;52:857-859.

113. Abdo WF, van de Warrenburg BP, Munneke M, et al: CSF analysis differentiates multiple-system atrophy from idiopathic late-onset cerebellar ataxia. Neurology 2006;67:474-479.

114. Abdo WF, Bloem BR, Van Geel WJ, et al: CSF neurofilament light chain and tau differentiate multiple system atrophy from Parkinson's disease. Neurobiol Aging 2007;28:742-747.

115. Wenning GK, Colosimo C, Geser F, Poewe W: Multiple system atrophy. Lancet Neurol 2004;3:93-103.

116. Geser F, Wenning GK, Seppi K, et al: Progression of multiple system atrophy (MSA): a prospective natural history study by the European MSA Study Group (EMSA SG). Mov Disord 2006;21:179-186.

117. Goetz CG, Tanner CM, Klawans HL: Bupropion in Parkinson's disease. Neurology 1984;34:1092-1094.

118. Heinz A, Suchy I, Klewin I, et al: Long-term observation of chronic subcutaneous administration of lisuride in the treatment of motor fluctuations in Parkinson's disease. J Neural Transm Park Dis Dement Sect 1992;4:291-301.

119. Lees AJ, Bannister R: The use of lisuride in the treatment of multiple system atrophy with autonomic failure (Shy-Drager syndrome). J Neurol Neurosurg Psychiatry 1981;44:347-351.

120. Colosimo C, Merello M, Pontieri FE: Amantadine in parkinsonian patients unresponsive to levodopa: a pilot study. J Neurol 1996;243:422-425.

121. Wenning GK: Placebo-controlled trial of amantadine in multiple-system atrophy. Clin Neuropharmacol 2005;28:225-227.

122. Friess E, Kuempfel T, Modell S, et al: Paroxetine treatment improves motor symptoms in patients with multiple system atrophy. Parkinsonism. Relat Disord 2006;12(7):432-437.

123. Visser-Vandewalle V, Temel Y, Colle H, van der LC: Bilateral high-frequency stimulation of the subthalamic nucleus in patients with multiple system atrophy–parkinsonism: report of four cases. J Neurosurg 2003;98:882-887.

124. Lezcano E, Gomez-Esteban JC, Zarranz JJ, et al: Parkinson's disease-like presentation of multiple system atrophy with poor response to STN stimulation: a clinicopathological case report. Mov Disord 2004;19:973-977.
125. Santens P, Vonck K, De Letter M, et al: Deep brain stimulation of the internal pallidum in multiple system atrophy. Parkinsonism Relat Disord 2006;12:181-183.
126. Jain S, Dawson J, Quinn NP, Playford ED: Occupational therapy in multiple system atrophy: a pilot randomized controlled trial. Mov Disord 2004;19:1360-1364.
127. Schrag A, Geser F, Stampfer-Kountchev M, et al: Health-related quality of life in multiple system atrophy. Mov Disord 2006;21:809-815.
128. Jankovic J, Gilden JL, Hiner BC, et al: Neurogenic orthostatic hypotension: a double-blind, placebo-controlled study with midodrine 2746. Am J Med 1993;95:38-48.
129. Low PA, Gilden JL, Freeman R, et al: Efficacy of midodrine vs placebo in neurogenic orthostatic hypotension: s randomized, double-blind multicenter study. Midodrine Study Group. JAMA 1997;277:1046-1051.
130. Kaufmann H, Biaggioni I: Autonomic failure in neurodegenerative disorders. Semin Neurol 2003;23:351-363.
131. Mathias CJ, Senard JM, Braune S, et al: L-threo-dihydroxyphenylserine (L-threo-DOPS; droxidopa) in the management of neurogenic orthostatic hypotension: a multi-national, multi-center, dose-ranging study in multiple system atrophy and pure autonomic failure. Clin Auton Res 2001;11:235-242.
132. Mathias CJ: L-dihydroxyphenylserine (Droxidopa) in the treatment of orthostatic hypotension: the European experience. Clin Auton Res 2008;18(Suppl 1):25-29. Epub 2008 Mar 27.
133. Jordan J, Shannon JR, Biaggioni I, et al: Contrasting actions of pressor agents in severe autonomic failure. Am J Med 1998;105:116-124.
134. Senard JM, Brefel-Courbon C, Rascol O, Montastruc JL: Orthostatic hypotension in patients with Parkinson's disease: pathophysiology and management. Drugs Aging 2001;18:495-505.
135. Apostolidis AN, Fowler CJ: Evaluation and treatment of autonomic disorders of the urogenital system. Semin Neurol 2003;23:443-452.
136. Fowler CJ: Update on the neurology of Parkinson's disease. Neurourol Urodyn 2007;26:103-109.
137. Sakakibara R, Hattori T, Uchiyama T, et al: Are alpha-blockers involved in lower urinary tract dysfunction in multiple system atrophy? A comparison of prazosin and moxisylyte. J Auton Nerv Syst 2000;79(2-3):191-195.
138. Mathias CJ, Fosbraey P, da Costa DF, et al: The effect of desmopressin on nocturnal polyuria, overnight weight loss, and morning postural hypotension in patients with autonomic failure. Br Med J (Clin Res Ed) 1986;293:353-354.
139. Hussain IF, Brady CM, Swinn MJ, et al: Treatment of erectile dysfunction with sildenafil citrate (Viagra) in parkinsonism due to Parkinson's disease or multiple system atrophy with observations on orthostatic hypotension. J Neurol Neurosurg Psychiatry 2001;71:371-374.
140. Klockgether T. Ataxia. In Hallett M, Poewe W, eds. Therapeutics of Parkinson's Disease and Other Movement Disorders; chapter 27, pp 407-415. Chichester: John Wiley & Sons Ltd, 2008.
141. Muller J, Wenning GK, Wissel J, et al: Botulinum toxin treatment in atypical parkinsonian disorders associated with disabling focal dystonia. J Neurol 2002;249:300-304.
142. Thobois S, Broussolle E, Toureille L, Vial C: Severe dysphagia after botulinum toxin injection for cervical dystonia in multiple system atrophy. Mov Disord 2001;16:764-765.
143. Iranzo A, Molinuevo JL, Santamaria J, et al: Rapid-eye-movement sleep behaviour disorder as an early marker for a neurodegenerative disorder: a descriptive study. Lancet Neurol 2006;5:572-577.
144. Schenck CH, Bundlie SR, Mahowald MW: Delayed emergence of a parkinsonian disorder in 38% of 29 older men initially diagnosed with idiopathic rapid eye movement sleep behaviour disorder. Neurology 1996;46:388-393.
145. Iranzo A: Sleep and breathing in multiple system atrophy. Curr Treat Options Neurol 2007;9:347-353.
146. Nonaka M, Imai T, Shintani T, et al: Non-invasive positive pressure ventilation for laryngeal contraction disorder during sleep in multiple system atrophy. J Neurol Sci 2006;247:53-58.
147. Iranzo A, Santamaria J, Tolosa E: Continuous positive air pressure eliminates nocturnal stridor in multiple system atrophy. Barcelona Multiple System Atrophy Study Group. Lancet 2000;356(9238):1329-1330.

21 Progressive Supranuclear Palsy

HUW R. MORRIS

Introduction	Pathology
Clinical Features	Treatment
Molecular Genetics	

Introduction

Progressive supranuclear palsy (PSP) was described by Steele and colleagues in 1963 and 1964,[1] and at the time seemed to be a "new" clinical syndrome. Research into the early accounts of movement disorders indicates that the syndrome predated their description, and patients with PSP appear in the film archive of Denny-Brown dating from the 1950s, a photograph taken by Duteil in the 1890s, and probably in the work of Charles Dickens, published in 1857.[2-4] The seminal description of the clinicopathological syndrome was needed, however, to galvanize clinical research, and once described, PSP became increasingly widely recognized through the 1970s and 1980s.[5,6] The precise clinicopathological definition of PSP has been followed over the last 10 years by new insights into the molecular pathology, genetics, and epidemiology of the disease. Among patients diagnosed in life to have Parkinson's disease (PD), PSP was the most common pathological diagnosis in the Queen Square Brain Bank series after PD itself.[7]

PSP is an age-dependent neurodegenerative condition, and patients typically present in their early 60s. The incidence of PSP in Olmsted County, Minnesota, is 1.1 per 100,000 per year.[8] Two epidemiological studies in the United Kingdom have shown that the age-adjusted prevalence of probable PSP is 5 per 100,000.[9,10] PSP is a malignant neurodegenerative condition with median survival of 5 to 7 years.[5,8,11,12] The clinical progression of PSP has similarities to amyotrophic lateral sclerosis—with progressive loss of speech, swallowing, and ambulation in the setting of largely intact cognitive function. The classic form of PSP has distinctive clinical features that enable rapid bedside or office diagnosis: a staring expression, related to a decreased blink rate and frontalis overactivity; an extended neck and erect posture; and an unsteady or lurching gait with an uncontrolled descent into the chair when sitting. After the diagnosis of PSP, effective symptomatic treatments are very limited, and the mainstay of treatment is supportive and palliative care.

Over the last decade, great progress has occurred in understanding the clinico-pathological basis of PSP and in understanding the molecular and genetic setting in which the disease occurs. These developments have been driven by increasing clinical interest in PSP, mendelian neurodegenerative disease genetics, the advo-cacy of patient support groups in the United States and Europe, and the active participation of patients and caregivers in clinical studies and in making blood and postmortem brain donations. This increased interest is likely to lead to the development of new trials of disease-modifying treatments for patients with PSP over the next decade.

Clinical Features

The core features of PSP are well established and have been formulated in the Na-tional Institute for Neurological Disorders and Stroke–Society for Progressive Su-pranuclear Palsy (NINDS-SPSP) clinical criteria initially published in 1996, with an updated version proposed in 2003 (Table 21–1).[13,14] Following the initial in-clusion criteria (a progressive disorder, with age at onset >40 years), the presence of a vertical supranuclear gaze palsy and prominent postural instability with falls in the first year of symptoms leads to a diagnosis of *clinically probable PSP*, and the presence of the balance disorder with slowing of vertical saccades or an isolated supranuclear gaze palsy leads to a diagnosis of *clinically possible PSP*.[14,15] In the proposed revised criteria, "postural instability with falls in the first year of symp-toms" is revised to "postural instability with a tendency to fall in the first year of symptoms," and the designation of *clinically probable PSP* is revised to *clinically definite PSP*, and *clinically possible PSP* is revised to *clinically probable*. A third cate-gory with a progressive balance disorder lasting for more than 12 months without an eye movement disorder is designated *clinically possible PSP*.[14,15]

The proposed revision of the diagnostic criteria reflect the facts that although a balance and gait disorder is ubiquitous in PSP, it may not involve falls in the first 12 months of symptoms, and that the first iteration of the NINDS-SPSP criteria have had a very high specificity and positive predictive value for a postmortem-confirmed diagnosis of PSP.[14] The exclusion criteria help to rule out frontotemp-oral dementia (FTD), Alzheimer's disease (AD), corticobasal degeneration (CBD), and multiple system atrophy (MSA).

Impairment of postural reflexes in PSP seems to be exacerbated by axial rigidity and by the extended neck posture. Formal analyses of balance in early PSP suggest that there is a defect in central vestibular processing with an overreliance on vi-sual input, meaning that the supranuclear gaze palsy further impairs balance with disease progression.[16] The progression of the balance disorder is a major cause of disability in PSP and correlates with survival, and has been related to involvement of the pedunculopontine nucleus.[11,17] Patients with PSP often present with visual symptoms that are unexplained until the identification of the correct underlying disease. A decrease in blink rate (~4/min) and frontalis overactivity together with frequent square wave jerks (>20/min) are common features.[18,19] Levator inhibi-tion and blepharospasm are also common in PSP, and many patients touch their eyelids or forehead to initiate or sustain eye opening.[19]

TABLE 21–1	Proposed Revision of NINDS-SPSP Criteria
Inclusion Criteria	**Exclusion Criteria***
Progressive disorder, age at onset >40 yr *Clinically definite PSP*: (1) postural instability with falls or tendency to fall in first year of symptoms and (2) vertical supranuclear gaze palsy *Clinically probable PSP*: vertical supranuclear gaze palsy or (1) slowing of vertical saccades and (2) postural instability with falls or the tendency to fall in the first year of symptoms *Clinically possible PSP*: postural instability with falls or tendency to fall in first year of symptoms; >1 yr of disease duration; no evidence of CJD	History of encephalitis lethargica; alien hand syndrome/cortical sensory loss; frontal or temporoparietal atrophy; hallucinations or delusions unrelated to dopaminergic therapy; cortical dementia of AD type; early cerebellar features; unexplained autonomic failure; relevant radiological abnormality; evidence of Whipple's disease; evidence of other disease that could explain symptoms

*Must not be present for any PSP diagnosis.

AD, Alzheimer's disease; CJD, Creutzfeldt-Jakob disease; NINDS-SPSP, National Institute for Neurological Disorders and Stroke–Society for Progressive Supranuclear Palsy; PSP, progressive supranuclear palsy.

(From Litvan I, Bhatia KP, Burn DJ, et al. Movement Disorders Society Scientific Issues Committee Report: SIC task force appraisal of clinical diagnostic criteria for parkinsonian disorders. *Mov Disord*. 2003;18:467-486.)

The eye movement disorder of PSP progresses and deteriorates with time.[20] The earliest phases involve slowing of downward saccadic eye movement velocity. Later, there is limitation in the range of vertical eye movements to command, which can be improved by presenting a visual target. Following this phase, the restriction in vertical movement can be overcome only by using the doll's head maneuver to activate the vestibulo-ocular response, and the finding of restriction of vertical gaze with full horizontal gaze is a striking and characteristic physical finding. The latter stages of the disease involve a complete paralysis of eye movements, often accompanied by profound blepharospasm. The preferential involvement of the vertical over the horizontal eye movement system is thought to relate to neurofibrillary degeneration involving midbrain structures, which probably include the rostral interstitial nucleus of the medial longitudinal fasciculus, interstitial nucleus of Cajal, and central mesencephalic reticular formation.[21]

In addition to frontalis overactivity, patients with PSP often have a degree of facial dystonia with deep nasolabial folds and an impassive facial expression. Patients develop a progressive bulbar syndrome that causes difficulties with recurrent respiratory tract infections and aspiration as the disease progresses. The speech disorder of PSP is usually not hypophonic in the early stages, in contrast to MSA and PD, but involves a gruff, growling dysarthria. The changes in cognition and behavior in early PSP are often thought to be subtle, but a more recent population-based study of PSP suggested that 20% of clinically diagnosed PSP patients may have a significant behavioral syndrome at presentation.[22]

As PSP progresses, a frontal dysexecutive syndrome with profound slowing in response time and reduction in verbal fluency emerges. Bedside testing with the Addenbrooke's Cognitive Examination or the Dementia Rating Scale shows that patients with PSP have a more severe impairment of initial letter verbal fluency than patients with AD, CBD, and MSA, and this can be a useful distinguishing test.[23] Patients with PSP often have striking generalized akinesia with extreme slowness of spontaneous and associative movement and accompanying bradyphrenia with a prolonged delay in making verbal or motor responses to command. Although there may be some distal bradykinesia and difficulty with repeated finger taps, patients usually do not have the typical decrement in speed and amplitude seen in patients with PD. Many other signs are common in PSP, including prolonged inspiratory or expiratory sighs and intermittent involuntary leg extension.

Initial work with PSP patients has commandeered PD rating scales such as the Unified Parkinson's Disease Rating Scale. Experience with the clinical profile of PSP has led to the development by Golbe and Ohman-Strickland[24] of a specific PSP clinical rating scale and by Schrag and coworkers[25] of a specific PSP quality-of-life scale. These scales focus on the gait, bulbar function, and visual disturbances of PSP, and will be useful tools for future clinical trials.

PSP manifests with a distinctive clinical picture; three quarters of patients given the diagnosis of PSP in life are confirmed to have PSP at postmortem examination.[26,27] Alternative diagnoses at autopsy include cortical Lewy body disease, MSA, AD, and vascular parkinsonism.[26,27] Numerous rarer, non-tau conditions have been mistaken for PSP, including neurosyphilis; Whipple's disease; cerebral autosomal dominant arteriopathy with subcortical leukoencephalopathy (CADASIL); Creutzfeldt-Jakob disease; FTD with ubiquitin inclusions (either sporadic motor neuron inclusion dementia or FTD with parkinsonism linked to chromosome 17 with ubiquitin-only inclusions [FTDP-17U]); some spinocerebellar ataxias, particularly SCA 3; and structural midbrain lesions, including tectal and pineal tumors.[28-31] The more recently identified FTDP-17U, caused by progranulin mutations, has also been reported rarely to manifest with a PSP-like picture.[32]

The overlap between PSP, CBD, and FTDP-17 with tau inclusions (FTDP-17T) is particularly noteworthy because of the genetic and pathological similarities between these disorders (see later). It may be impossible to distinguish between PSP and FTDP-17T clinically, although patients with FTDP-17T are likely to have a younger age at onset, are likely to have disabling disinhibition and/or apathy and usually, but not always have a concordant family history.[33-35] CBD patients usually have signs of asymmetrical parietal degeneration and slowing of initiation of saccadic eye movements. Some CBD patients also have a progressive and severe balance and saccadic eye movement disorder, however, sometimes leading to a clinical diagnosis of a PSP-CBD overlap syndrome,[36] and some PSP patients may present with an asymmetrical CBD-like phenotype. Postmortem series indicate that many patients given a diagnosis of CBD during life have PSP at postmortem examination, and vice versa.[27,37]

Magnetic resonance imaging (MRI) is helpful in excluding structural lesions and in established PSP often shows midbrain and superior cerebellar peduncular atrophy, which can be used to distinguish PSP from PD and MSA associated with parkinsonism (Fig. 21–1).[38,39] Serial MRI evaluating progressive midbrain

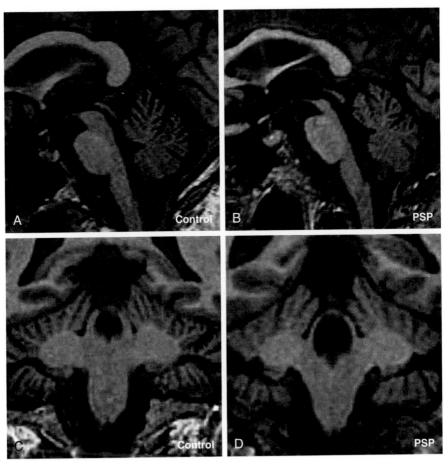

Figure 21–1 MRI in progressive supranuclear palsy. **A-D,** Sagittal (**A** and **B**) and axial (**C** and **D**) T1-weighted MR images show atrophy of the midbrain (**B**) and superior cerebellar peduncles (**D**) in patients with progressive supranuclear palsy compared with controls (**A** and **C**). (Courtesy of Dr. Dominic Paviour.)

atrophy in PSP has the potential to be a useful biomarker for future trials of neuroprotective agents.[40]

Numerous other clinical presentations are now recognized to occur in patients who are identified to have PSP at postmortem examination. Daniel and colleagues[41] initially identified a series of patients with pathologically diagnosed PSP who did not have a supranuclear gaze palsy, suggesting that this may not be an obligate clinical feature.[42] The individual clinical features of patients with pathologically defined PSP have been systematically analyzed by Williams and colleagues at the Queen Square Brain Bank.[43] They identify three main presentations: (1) classic PSP, which they suggest is described as Richardson's syndrome; (2) parkinsonism without a supranuclear gaze palsy, which may be asymmetrical and levodopa responsive, which they term PSP-parkinsonism; and (3) pure akinesia, also known as primary progressive freezing of gait.

Pure akinesia has easily identifiable features, and Williams and colleagues[44] suggested diagnostic criteria including a gradual onset of freezing of gait or speech, absent limb rigidity and tremor, no levodopa response, and no dementia or ophthalmoplegia in the first 5 years of disease. In seven cases identified meeting these criteria at the Queen Square Brain Bank, six had a pathological diagnosis of PSP.[44] PSP-parkinsonism is harder to identify because it may initially be indistinguishable from PD, with the subsequent appearance of a progressive balance disorder and gaze palsy. There may be some overlap between PSP-parkinsonism and other causes of neurofibrillary tangle parkinsonism reported to have a PD-like presentation.[45] Four of six PSP cases identified by Hughes and associates[7] as having been given the diagnosis of PD in life were diagnosed to have atypical PSP, and these cases may have had what is now recognized as PSP-parkinsonism. A few patients have been described more recently with progressive spasticity and a syndrome resembling primary lateral sclerosis who have had PSP pathology with spinal cord involvement at autopsy, further widening the clinical spectrum associated with pathologically defined PSP.[46,47]

Molecular Genetics

PSP is usually a sporadic disorder. In 1997, Conrad and colleagues[48] showed that one allele (A0) of a microsatellite marker located in an intronic segment of the tau gene (*MAPT*) was associated with PSP. Although this was originally based on a small study of 22 PSP cases, this finding has been replicated many times, and the association between PSP and tau is robust (see Chapter 5 for a discussion of the similar relationship between tau and corticobasal ganglionic degeneration).[49-52] *MAPT* encodes tau protein, which normally promotes the formation and stabilization of microtubules.[53] Tau has four imperfectly repeated microtubule binding domains encoded by exons 9, 10, 11, and 12 of *MAPT*.[54] *MAPT* exon 10 is alternatively spliced forming either four-repeat (4R) or three-repeat (3R) forms of tau mRNA and protein (Fig. 21–2).

Abnormally hyperphosphorylated and aggregated tau forms neurofibrillary tangles (NFTs) in the NFT disorders, including AD and PSP.[54] The initial tau microsatellite marked a raft of variation across *MAPT* (the H1 haplotype) associated with PSP and occurring on 78% of control chromosomes and 94% of PSP chromosomes.[52] Further work on the region indicated that there was an extensive area of linkage disequilibrium around *MAPT*, implicated in the PSP-*MAPT* or PSP-17q21 association, raising the possibility that variation in other genes and regulatory regions might play a role in the susceptibility to the development of PSP.[55-58] It has been shown more recently that this area of linkage disequilibrium is due to a 900-kb inversion on 17q21, and that the rarer H2 haplotype is associated with Northern European ancestry.[59-61] This ethnic variation predicts that nonwhite populations have a slightly higher prevalence of PSP, although an epidemiological study in Japan did not identify an increased disease prevalence.[62]

Following the initial work on susceptibility to PSP, *MAPT* was identified as the gene responsible for FTDP-17 (now FTDP-17T, to denote that there are two forms of FTDP17, one with tau inclusions—FTDP-17T—and one with ubiquitin inclusions—FTDP-17U).[63,64] There are major clinical and pathological similarities between PSP and FTDP-17T suggesting that there may be convergent pathogenic

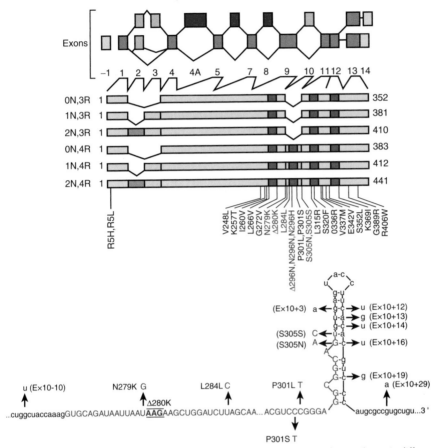

Figure 21-2 *MAPT* gene structure and mutations. Alternative splicing of tau to form six different isoforms with or without exon 10 (4R or 3R tau). Some coding sequence mutations in FTDP-17T shown under the longest 441 amino acid isoforms of tau. Mutations that alter the alternative splicing of tau are shown in purple. *Lower panel* shows intron-exon boundary of tau and stem loop structure with the location of mutations thought to disrupt stem loop and alter the alternative splicing of exon 10 coding mutations that alter the alternative splicing of tau are shown in purple. (Courtesy of Drs. Alan Pittman and Rohan de Silva, modified from a figure by Goedert.[53])

mechanisms in the sporadic and the dominant disease. FTDP-17T mutations that have been reported to have a PSP-like phenotype include an exon 1 mutation R5L, and the exon 10 mutations N279K, S305S, exon 10+1 (*MAPT*, IVS10, G-A, +1), and exon 10+16 (*MAPT*, IVS10, C-U, +16).[33,34,65-68] Some of these families have been referred to as having familial PSP, although it is also reasonable to describe them as FTDP-17T families with a PSP-like phenotype, particularly because some of these mutations can have a variable phenotypic presentation. Exon 10+16 (*MAPT*, IVS10, C-U, +16) can manifest with a PSP-like or frontal behavioral illness.

FTDP-17T mutations have various effects, including an alteration in the 4R-to-3R tau ratio, accelerated filament and aggregate formation, and loss of microtubule binding with destabilization of microtubules.[53] Mutations in *MAPT* are either nonsynonymous single nucleotide polymorphisms, which lead to an alteration in the amino acid sequence, or splicing mutations, which affect the 4R-to-3R ratio by altering the exon 10 splice site or by affecting the sequence of exonic splice enhancers or inhibitors. Further refinement of the *MAPT/PSP* association has established that one subhaplotype of *MAPT* designated H1c by Pittman and colleagues[69] and H1b by Rademakers and coworkers[70] is primarily responsible for disease risk, with disease protection conferred by the rarer H2 haplotype.

Currently, genetic tests do not play a role in the diagnostic assessment of patients with PSP—the *MAPT* A0 allele and H1 and H1c haplotypes are common in the general population and the possession of the risk haplotype has a low predictive value for a diagnosis of PSP, even among patients with a parkinsonian syndrome. A family history of a neurodegenerative disease or an early age at onset (age at onset <45 years) should prompt consideration that a patient with a PSP-like syndrome may have a form of FTDP-17T, and sequence analysis of *MAPT* or occasionally progranulin may be informative. Neuroimaging normally provides a pointer to an underlying diagnosis of CADASIL.

The development of genome-wide assays that allow the simultaneous analysis of greater than 100,000 single nucleotide polymorphisms in cases and controls will lead to the further definition of genetic risk factors for PSP. To date, one study has been published that provides some preliminary evidence for the involvement of a region containing the DNA damage-binding protein 2 (*DDB2*) and lysosomal acid phosphatase 2 (*ACP2*) genes.[71] A further genetic lead in PSP is linkage in a Spanish family with autosomal dominant PSP on chromosome 1q34.[72] No further families have been identified linked to that locus, there is clinical heterogeneity within the 1q-linked family, and the causative gene mutation has not been identified.

Pathology

PSP was originally defined on the basis of its clinicopathological phenotype. The detailed analysis of the molecular pathology and comparison with FTDP-17 has the potential to define the basic pathogenic process. Pathologically, PSP involves the deposition of NFTs, gliosis, and cell loss in a specific distribution, particularly affecting the subthalamic nucleus, globus pallidus, substantia nigra (pars compacta and reticulata), pretectal area of the midbrain, and basis pontis.[73] The NFTs are best seen with silver staining or tau immunocytochemistry. The NFTs of PSP are usually globose NFTs, and at the electron microscopic level are composed of straight filaments with a diameter of 15 to 18 nm (Fig. 21–3).[74,75]

The pathological differential diagnosis of PSP includes FTDP-17T, CBD, and other neurodegenerative tauopathies. The disease distribution and glial pathology are useful in defining and distinguishing these disorders. In FTDP-17T, there is frontotemporal atrophy, and in CBD, there is asymmetrical frontoparietal atrophy, whereas in PSP, there is usually no macroscopic cortical involvement. In PSP, tufted astrocytes are found in the striatum and motor cortex with coiled oligodendroglial inclusions predominantly in the subcortical white matter (see Fig. 21–3). CBD (see Chapter 5) is characterized by astrocytic plaques with cortical white matter tau-positive threads.[76] In addition to the characteristic glial changes, CBD involves the deposition of frequent α-B crystallin–positive ballooned neurons.

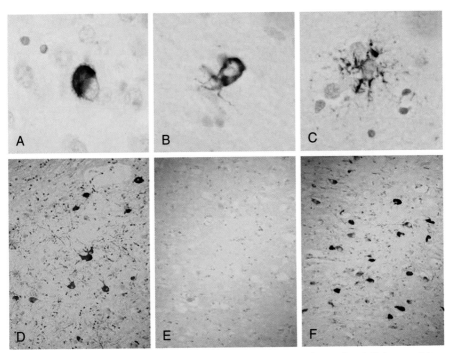

Figure 21–3 Tau immunohistochemistry in progressive supranuclear palsy. **A-F,** Immunohisto-chemical analysis of progressive supranuclear palsy using antibody AT-8 (**A, C,** and **D**) three-repeat specific antibody RD-3 (**E**), and four-repeat specific antibody RD-4 (**B** and **F**). Typical tau-positive neurofibrillary tangle in the granule cell layer (**A**). Glial pathology includes oligodendroglial coiled bodies (**B**) and tufted astrocytes (**C**). Neurofibrillary tangles in the griseum pontis stain positively for tau with antibody AT-8 and the four-repeat antibody (**D** and **F**), but not with a three-repeat antibody (**E**). (Courtesy of Dr. Rohan de Silva.)

Tau in PSP is abnormally hyperphosphorylated, as in AD. In AD, there are three major bands on Western blot at 68 kD, 64 kD, and 60 kD, whereas in PSP there are two major bands at 64 kD and 60 kD.[77] The tau deposited in PSP is predominantly 4R tau, which can be identified either using Western blot analysis of dephos-phorylated protein or using specific four-repeat antibodies (see Fig. 21–3).[78,79] In FTDP-17T, splicing mutations, which increase the 4R-to-3R ratio without altering the amino acid sequence, are sufficient to cause early-onset neurodegeneration. Many families with these mutations, listed earlier, have clinical phenotypes that are very similar to PSP. In these families, analyses of RNA and protein show an excess of 4R species. Coding mutations of exon 10 of *MAPT* also lead to preferential deposition of 4R tau protein, however, without altering the alternative splicing of tau, or altering the 4R-to-3R RNA ratios.

A possible link between the *MAPT* risk genotypes and PSP is suggested by the observation by some groups that there is an excess of transcription of tau encoded by the H1 compared with H2 haplotype, and this effect is increased for 4R tau.[80,81] Some groups have also reported that the H1 and the H1c risk haplotype may have a specific effect in upregulating tau transcription and the synthesis of 4R tau iso-forms.[80] The occurrence of α-synuclein and APP duplications and triplications causing familial PD and AD indicates that an increase in the amount of protein synthesis can lead to neurodegeneration, and this may be relevant to PSP.[82]

Two other sporadic conditions are also 4R predominant tauopathies—CBD and argyrophilic grain disease.[83] Both of these conditions also show an association with *MAPT* H1, whereas the 3R tauopathy Pick's disease does not.[84,85] The molecular pathology of PSP and the link between FTDP-17T and PSP give an insight into disease processes that may be amenable to disease-modifying treatment. Potentially, therapies that alter the expression, alternative splicing, or phosphorylation of tau may be useful agents. To date, analysis of tau levels in cerebrospinal fluid has not proved to be a useful test in PSP because total cerebrospinal fluid tau levels overlap with many other conditions. There is some preliminary evidence, however, that the ratio of different tau isoforms in cerebrospinal fluid may distinguish PSP from other conditions.[86] Cerebrospinal fluid tau analysis may become a biomarker, which might be useful in the diagnosis of PSP or in tracking the response to disease-modifying therapies.

Treatment

Supportive and palliative care is the most important part of treatment of patients with PSP. Regular swallowing and dietetic assessment and advice are essential to avoid the complications of aspiration pneumonia and poor nutritional intake. Feeding often becomes very prolonged and laborious for patients with PSP, and increasing numbers of patients choose to receive nutrition via percutaneous gastrostomy feeding when oral intake becomes difficult. Blepharospasm and sometimes cervical dystonia can respond well to local botulinum toxin injection treatment. Review by physiotherapy and occupational therapy helps to preserve mobility and to minimize the risk of injury in falls and accidents. Further aspects of supportive care that may be helpful include artificial tears for eye irritation, prism glasses, talking books, antidepressants, and topical or systemic anticholinergics for drooling.[15] Patient organizations in the United States and Europe are a useful source of advice and information for patients and their families (www.pspeur.org, www.psp.org).

There are no proven symptomatic drug treatments for PSP. Most neurologists recommend a trial of levodopa, and many clinicians recommend a trial of amantadine and amitriptyline, but there are no large-scale randomized trials supporting the use of these treatments, and patients usually derive modest and unsustained benefit. Cholinergic systems are particularly damaged in patients with PSP, but randomized trials of donepezil have not shown any benefit from cholinesterase inhibitors.[87-89] Available surgical therapies including subthalamic nucleus deep brain stimulation are ineffective. The more recent interest in deep brain stimulation of the pedunculopontine nucleus for ambulatory disturbances in PD[90] may extend to PSP; however, this should be considered only in the setting of a carefully developed clinical research trial.

Large-scale trials to assess neuroprotection in rare conditions such as PSP may be difficult to organize and carry out. The European Neuroprotection and Natural History in Parkinson Plus Syndromes consortium have successfully completed a trial of riluzole in 766 subjects (363 with PSP, and 403 with MSA). Although the administration of riluzole did not confer any survival benefit at

36 months, the successful completion of this trial has shown that it is possible to organize large-scale trials for PSP, using the collaborative efforts of neurologists, patients, and research staff working at many sites.[91] It is likely that future therapies for PSP will involve trials of further agents that modulate tau expression and phosphorylation.[92] Our hope is that the insights derived from molecular genetics, development of new clinical assessment tools, and successes in trial design and organization will translate into effective new treatments for this neurodegenerative condition.

REFERENCES

1. Steele JC, Richardson JC, Olszewski J: Progressive supranuclear palsy: a heterogeneous degeneration involving the brain stem, basal ganglia and cerebellum with vertical gaze and pseudobulbar palsy, nuchal dystonia and dementia. Arch Neurol 1964;10:333-359.
2. Goetz CG: An early photographic case of probable progressive supranuclear palsy. Mov Disord 1996;11:617-618.
3. Larner AJ: Did Charles Dickens describe progressive supranuclear palsy in 1857? Mov Disord 2002;17:832-833.
4. Robertson WM, Gilman S, Vilensky JA: The Denny-Brown collection: recognition of progressive supranuclear palsy as a unique disorder in the decade before the clinico-pathological description. Neurology 1997;48(3):A145.
5. Brusa A, Mancardi GL, Bugiani O: Progressive supranuclear palsy 1979: an overview. Ital J Neurol Sci 1980;1:205-222.
6. Maher ER, Lees AJ: The clinical features and natural history of the Steele-Richardson-Olszewski syndrome (progressive supranuclear palsy). Neurology 1986;36:1005-1008.
7. Hughes AJ, Daniel SE, Kilford L, Lees AJ: Accuracy of clinical diagnosis of idiopathic Parkinson's disease: a clinico-pathological study of 100 cases. J Neurol Neurosurg Psychiatry 1992;55:181-184.
8. Bower JH, Maraganore DM, McDonnell SK, Rocca WA: Incidence of progressive supranuclear palsy and multiple system atrophy in Olmsted County, Minnesota, 1976 to 1990. Neurology 1997;49:1284-1288.
9. Nath U, Ben-Shlomo Y, Thomson RG, et al: The prevalence of progressive supranuclear palsy (Steele-Richardson-Olszewski syndrome) in the UK. Brain 2001;124(Pt 7):1438-1449.
10. Schrag A, Ben-Shlomo Y, Quinn NP: Prevalence of progressive supranuclear palsy and multiple system atrophy: a cross-sectional study. Lancet 1999;354:1771-1775.
11. Nath U, Ben-Shlomo Y, Thomson RG, et al: Clinical features and natural history of progressive supranuclear palsy: a clinical cohort study. Neurology 2003;60:910-916.
12. Nath U, Thomson R, Wood R, et al: Population based mortality and quality of death certification in progressive supranuclear palsy (Steele-Richardson-Olszewski syndrome). J Neurol Neurosurg Psychiatry 2005;76:498-502.
13. Litvan I, Agid Y, Jankovic J, et al: Accuracy of clinical criteria for the diagnosis of progressive supranuclear palsy (Steele-Richardson-Olszewski syndrome). Neurology 1996;46:922-930.
14. Litvan I, Bhatia KP, Burn DJ, et al: Movement Disorders Society Scientific Issues Committee report: SIC task force appraisal of clinical diagnostic criteria for parkinsonian disorders. Mov Disord 2003;18:467-486.
15. Litvan I: Diagnosis and management of progressive supranuclear palsy. Semin Neurol 2001;21:41-48.
16. Ondo W, Warrior D, Overby A, et al: Computerized posturography analysis of progressive supranuclear palsy: A case-control comparison with Parkinson's disease and healthy controls. Arch Neurol 2000;57:1464-1469.
17. Zweig RM, Whitehouse PJ, Casanova MF, et al: Loss of pedunculopontine neurons in progressive supranuclear palsy. Ann Neurol 1987;22:18-25.
18. Altiparmak UE, Eggenberger E, Coleman A, Condon K: The ratio of square wave jerk rates to blink rates distinguishes progressive supranuclear palsy from Parkinson disease. J Neuro-ophthalmol 2006;26:257-259.
19. Golbe LI, Davis PH, Lepore FE: Eyelid movement abnormalities in progressive supranuclear palsy. Mov Disord 1989;4:297-302.

20. Golbe LI: Progressive supranuclear palsy. In Jankovic J, Tolosa E, eds: Parkinson's Disease and Movement Disorders. Philadelphia: Lippincott Williams & Wilkins, 2007, pp 161-174.
21. Bhidayasiri R, Riley DE, Somers JT, et al: Pathophysiology of slow vertical saccades in progressive supranuclear palsy. Neurology 2001;57:2070-2077.
22. Kaat LD, Boon AJ, Kamphorst W, et al: Frontal presentation in progressive supranuclear palsy. Neurology 2007;69:723-729.
23. Bak TH, Crawford LM, Hearn VC, et al: Subcortical dementia revisited: Similarities and differences in cognitive function between progressive supranuclear palsy (PSP), corticobasal degeneration (CBD) and multiple system atrophy (MSA). Neurocase 2005;11:268-273.
24. Golbe LI, Ohman-Strickland PA: A clinical rating scale for progressive supranuclear palsy. Brain 2007;130(Pt 6):1552-1565.
25. Schrag A, Selai C, Quinn N, et al: Measuring quality of life in PSP: The PSP-QOL. Neurology 2006;67:39-44.
26. Josephs KA, Dickson DW: Diagnostic accuracy of progressive supranuclear palsy in the Society for Progressive Supranuclear Palsy Brain Bank. Mov Disord 2003;18:1018-1026.
27. Osaki Y, Ben-Shlomo Y, Lees AJ, et al: Accuracy of clinical diagnosis of progressive supranuclear palsy. Mov Disord 2004;19:181-189.
28. Magherini A, Pentore R, Grandi M, et al: Progressive supranuclear gaze palsy without parkinsonism: A case of neuro-Whipple. Parkinsonism Relat Disord 2007;13:449-452.
29. Van Gerpen JA, Ahlskog JE, Petty GW: Progressive supranuclear palsy phenotype secondary to CADASIL. Parkinsonism Relat Disord 2003;9:367-369.
30. Paviour DC, Schott JM, Stevens JM, et al: Pathological substrate for regional distribution of increased atrophy rates in progressive supranuclear palsy. J Neurol Neurosurg Psychiatry 2004;75:1772-1775.
31. Morris HR, Wood NW, Lees AJ: Progressive supranuclear palsy (Steele-Richardson-Olszewski disease). Postgrad Med J 1999;75:579-584.
32. Josephs KA, Ahmed Z, Katsuse O, et al: Neuropathologic features of frontotemporal lobar degeneration with ubiquitin-positive inclusions with progranulin gene (PGRN) mutations. J Neuropathol Exp Neurol 2007;66:142-151.
33. Morris HR, Osaki Y, Holton J, et al: Tau exon 10 +16 mutation FTDP-17 presenting clinically as sporadic young onset PSP. Neurology 2003;61:102-104.
34. Murrell JR, Koller D, Foroud T, et al: Familial multiple-system tauopathy with presenile dementia is localized to chromosome 17. Am J Hum Genet 1997;61:1131-1138.
35. Reed LA, Wszolek ZK, Hutton M: Phenotypic correlations in FTDP-17. Neurobiol Aging 2001;22:89-107.
36. Kertesz A, Munoz D: Relationship between frontotemporal dementia and corticobasal degeneration/progressive supranuclear palsy. Dement Geriatr Cogn Disord 2004;17:282-286.
37. Josephs KA, Petersen RC, Knopman DS, et al: Clinicopathologic analysis of frontotemporal and corticobasal degenerations and PSP. Neurology 2006;66:41-48.
38. Paviour DC, Price SL, Jahanshahi M, et al: Regional brain volumes distinguish PSP, MSA-P, and PD: MRI-based clinico-radiological correlations. Mov Disord 2006;21:989-996.
39. Tsuboi Y, Slowinski J, Josephs KA, et al: Atrophy of superior cerebellar peduncle in progressive supranuclear palsy. Neurology 2003;60:1766-1769.
40. Paviour DC, Price SL, Lees AJ, Fox NC: MRI derived brain atrophy in PSP and MSA-P: determining sample size to detect treatment effects. J Neurol 2007;254:478-481.
41. Daniel SE, de Bruin VM, Lees AJ: The clinical and pathological spectrum of Steele-Richardson-Olszewski syndrome (progressive supranuclear palsy): a reappraisal. Brain 1995;118(Pt 3):759-770.
42. Morris HR, Gibb G, Katzenschlager R, et al: Pathological, clinical and genetic heterogeneity in progressive supranuclear palsy. Brain 2002;125(Pt 5):969-975.
43. Williams DR, de Silva R, Paviour DC, et al: Characteristics of two distinct clinical phenotypes in pathologically proven progressive supranuclear palsy: Richardson's syndrome and PSP-parkinsonism. Brain 2005;128(Pt 6):1247-1258.
44. Williams DR, Holton JL, Strand K, et al: Pure akinesia with gait freezing: A third clinical phenotype of progressive supranuclear palsy. Mov Disord 2007;22:2235-2241.
45. Morris HR, Lees AJ, Wood NW: Neurofibrillary tangle parkinsonian disorders—tau pathology and tau genetics. Mov Disord 1999;14:731-736.
46. Josephs KA, Katsuse O, Beccano-Kelly DA, et al: Atypical progressive supranuclear palsy with corticospinal tract degeneration. J Neuropathol Exp Neurol 2006;65:396-405.

47. Papapetropoulos S, Scaravilli T, Morris H, et al: Young onset limb spasticity with PSP-like brain and spinal cord NFT-tau pathology. Neurology 2005;64:731-733.
48. Conrad C, Andreadis A, Trojanowski JQ, et al: Genetic evidence for the involvement of tau in progressive supranuclear palsy. Ann Neurol 1997;41:277-281.
49. Bennett P, Bonifati V, Bonuccelli U, et al: Direct genetic evidence for involvement of tau in progressive supranuclear palsy. European Study Group on Atypical Parkinsonism Consortium. Neurology 1998;51:982-985.
50. Oliva R, Tolosa E, Ezquerra M, et al: Significant changes in the tau A0 and A3 alleles in progressive supranuclear palsy and improved genotyping by silver detection. Arch Neurol 1998;55:1122-1124.
51. Morris HR, Janssen JC, Bandmann O, et al: The tau gene A0 polymorphism in progressive supranuclear palsy and related neurodegenerative diseases. J Neurol Neurosurg Psychiatry 1999;66:665-667.
52. Baker M, Litvan I, Houlden H, et al: Association of an extended haplotype in the tau gene with progressive supranuclear palsy. Hum Mol Genet 1999;8:711-715.
53. Goedert M: Tau gene mutations and their effects. Mov Disord 2005;20(Suppl 12):S45-S52.
54. Lee VM, Goedert M, Trojanowski JQ: Neurodegenerative tauopathies. Annu Rev Neurosci 2001;24:1121-1159.
55. Pastor P, Ezquerra M, Perez JC, et al: Novel haplotypes in 17q21 are associated with progressive supranuclear palsy. Ann Neurol 2004;56:249-258.
56. Pastor P, Ezquerra M, Tolosa E, et al: Further extension of the H1 haplotype associated with progressive supranuclear palsy. Mov Disord 2002;17:550-556.
57. Ezquerra M, Pastor P, Valldeoriola F, et al: Identification of a novel polymorphism in the promoter region of the tau gene highly associated to progressive supranuclear palsy in humans. Neurosci Lett 1999;275:183-186.
58. de Silva R, Weiler M, Morris HR, et al: Strong association of a novel tau promoter haplotype in progressive supranuclear palsy. Neurosci Lett 2001;311:145-148.
59. Stefansson H, Helgason A, Thorleifsson G, et al: A common inversion under selection in Europeans. Nat Genet 2005;37:129-137.
60. Hardy J, Pittman A, Myers A, et al: Evidence suggesting that Homo Neanderthalensis contributed the H2 MAPT haplotype to Homo Sapiens. Biochem Soc Trans 2005;33(Pt 4):582-585.
61. Evans W, Fung HC, Steele J, et al: The tau H2 haplotype is almost exclusively caucasian in origin. Neurosci Lett 2004;369:183-185.
62. Kawashima M, Miyake M, Kusumi M, et al: Prevalence of progressive supranuclear palsy in Yonago, Japan. Mov Disord 2004;19:1239-1240.
63. Hutton M, Lendon CL, Rizzu P, et al: Association of missense and 5'-splice-site mutations in tau with the inherited dementia FTDP-17. Nature 1998;393:702-705.
64. Hardy J, Momeni P, Traynor BJ: Frontal temporal dementia: Dissecting the aetiology and pathogenesis. Brain 2006;129(Pt 4):830-831.
65. Poorkaj P, Muma NA, Zhukareva V, et al: An R5L tau mutation in a subject with a progressive supranuclear palsy phenotype. Ann Neurol 2002;52:511-516.
66. Delisle MB, Murrell JR, Richardson R, et al: A mutation at codon 279 (N279K) in exon 10 of the tau gene causes a tauopathy with dementia and supranuclear palsy. Acta Neuropathol (Berl) 1999;98:62-77.
67. Stanford PM, Halliday GM, Brooks WS, et al: Progressive supranuclear palsy pathology caused by a novel silent mutation in exon 10 of the tau gene: expansion of the disease phenotype caused by tau gene mutations. Brain 2000;123(Pt 5):880-893.
68. Spillantini MG, Murrell JR, Goedert M, et al: Mutation in the tau gene in familial multiple system tauopathy with presenile dementia. Proc Natl Acad Sci U S A 1998;95:7737-7741.
69. Pittman AM, Myers AJ, Abou-Sleiman P, et al: Linkage disequilibrium fine mapping and haplotype association analysis of the tau gene in progressive supranuclear palsy and corticobasal degeneration. J Med Genet 2005;42:837-846.
70. Rademakers R, Melquist S, Cruts M, et al: High-density SNP haplotyping suggests altered regulation of tau gene expression in progressive supranuclear palsy. Hum Mol Genet 2005;14:3281-3292.
71. Melquist S, Craig DW, Huentelman MJ, et al: Identification of a novel risk locus for progressive supranuclear palsy by a pooled genomewide scan of 500,288 single-nucleotide polymorphisms. Am J Hum Genet 2007;80:769-778.
72. Ros R, Gómez Garre P, Hirano M, et al: Genetic linkage of autosomal dominant progressive supranuclear palsy to 1q31.1. Ann Neurol 2005;57:634-641.

73. Hauw JJ, Daniel SE, Dickson D, et al: Preliminary NINDS neuropathologic criteria for Steele-Richardson-Olszewski syndrome (progressive supranuclear palsy). Neurology 1994;44:2015-2019.
74. Buée L, Delacourte A: Comparative biochemistry of tau in progressive supranuclear palsy, corticobasal degeneration, FTDP-17 and pick's disease. Brain Pathol 1999;9:681-693.
75. Roy S, Datta CK, Hirano A, et al: Electron microscopic study of neurofibrillary tangles in Steele-Richardson-Olszewski syndrome. Acta Neuropathol (Berl) 1974;29:175-179.
76. Dickson DW, Rademakers R, Hutton ML: Progressive supranuclear palsy: Pathology and genetics. Brain Pathol 2007;17:74-82.
77. Mailliot C, Sergeant N, Bussière T, et al: Phosphorylation of specific sets of tau isoforms reflects different neurofibrillary degeneration processes. FEBS Lett 1998;433:201-204.
78. de Silva R, Lashley T, Gibb G, et al: Pathological inclusion bodies in tauopathies contain distinct complements of tau with three or four microtubule-binding repeat domains as demonstrated by new specific monoclonal antibodies. Neuropathol Appl Neurobiol 2003;29:288-302.
79. Liu WK, Le TV, Adamson J, et al: Relationship of the extended tau haplotype to tau biochemistry and neuropathology in progressive supranuclear palsy. Ann Neurol 2001;50:494-502.
80. Myers AJ, Pittman AM, Zhao AS, et al: The MAPT h1c risk haplotype is associated with increased expression of tau and especially of 4 repeat containing transcripts. Neurobiol Dis 2007;25:561-570.
81. Caffrey TM, Joachim C, Paracchini S, et al: Haplotype-specific expression of exon 10 at the human MAPT locus. Hum Mol Genet 2006;15:3529-3537.
82. Singleton A, Myers A, Hardy J: The law of mass action applied to neurodegenerative disease: a hypothesis concerning the etiology and pathogenesis of complex diseases. Hum Mol Genet 2004;13(Spec No 1):R123-R126.
83. Togo T, Sahara N, Yen SH, et al: Argyrophilic grain disease is a sporadic 4-repeat tauopathy. J Neuropathol Exp Neurol 2002;61:547-556.
84. Morris HR, Baker M, Yasojima K, et al: Analysis of tau haplotypes in Pick's disease. Neurology 2002;59:443-445.
85. Houlden H, Baker M, Morris HR, et al: Corticobasal degeneration and progressive supranuclear palsy share a common tau haplotype. Neurology 2001;56:1702-1706.
86. Borroni B, Gardoni F, Parnetti L, et al: Pattern of Tau forms in CSF is altered in progressive supranuclear palsy. Neurobiol Aging 2007;30(1):34-40. Published: 2009.
87. Warren NM, Piggott MA, Lees AJ, Burn DJ: The basal ganglia cholinergic neurochemistry of progressive supranuclear palsy and other neurodegenerative diseases. J Neurol Neurosurg Psychiatry 2007;78:571-575.
88. Fabbrini G, Barbanti P, Bonifati V, et al: Donepezil in the treatment of progressive supranuclear palsy. Acta Neurol Scand 2001;103:123-1255.
89. Litvan I, Phipps M, Pharr VL, et al: Randomized placebo-controlled trial of donepezil in patients with progressive supranuclear palsy. Neurology 2001;57:467-473.
90. Stefani A, Lozano AM, Peppe A, et al: Bilateral deep brain stimulation of the pedunculopontine and subthalamic nuclei in severe Parkinson's disease. Brain 2007;130(Pt 6):1596-1607.
91. Leigh PN, Ludolph A, Agid Y, Bensimon G: NNIPPS Consortium. Neuroprotection and natural history in Parkinson plus syndromes (NNIPPS): Results of a randomized placebo-controlled trial of riluzole in PSP and MSA. Mov Disord 2007;22(S16):S3-S4.
92. Burn DJ, Warren NM: Toward future therapies in progressive supranuclear palsy. Mov Disord 2005;20(Suppl 12):S92-S98.

22 Corticobasal Ganglionic Degeneration

KEITH A. JOSEPHS, JR.

Introduction

In 1968, Rebeiz and colleagues[1] published a series of three patients with unusual neurological features characterized by abnormalities of posture, gait, and movement, and involuntary movements. Because all three patients had died with homogeneous pathological findings of frontoparietal atrophy, and neuronal loss and gliosis of substantia nigra and cerebellar dentate nuclei, they proposed the term *corticodentatonigral degeneration with neuronal achromasia*. One of the characteristic histological findings of all cases was the presence of achromatic swollen neurons, and corticodentatonigral degeneration with neuronal achromasia was proposed as a distinct clinicopathological entity.

Subsequent to the original description, there were few reports of additional cases, mainly in abstract form, until a large series of 15 patients was described by Riley and colleagues in 1990.[2] In that series, it became clear that the cardinal clinical features included cortical sensory loss, focal reflex myoclonus, alien limb phenomena, apraxia, rigidity and akinesia, postural and action tremor, limb dystonia, and postural instability. It became more apparent that the symptoms, signs, and brain imaging characteristics were asymmetrical, affecting one side of the body and one hemisphere more than the other. Since 1990, there has been a significant increase in the recognition of this asymmetrical Parkinson-plus syndrome, and there have been major advances in understanding of the disease.

A review of the literature shows that this disease has also been called corticobasal ganglionic degeneration[2] and, more recently, corticobasal degeneration (CBD).[3] Clinical criteria for the diagnosis of CBD have been proposed[4]; however, clinicopathological studies have shown that although there are characteristic clinical features associated with the pathological findings of CBD, many other neurodegenerative and non-neurodegenerative disorders may have similar clinical features. The term *corticobasal syndrome* (CBS)[5] has been introduced to characterize the clinical features suggestive of the pathological diagnosis of CBD. The term CBD is now reserved only for cases meeting the proposed consensus pathological criteria.[6]

Epidemiology and Demographics

There have been many case reports of CBS and CBD; however, there have been fewer large clinicopathological series.[7-10] These large series have shown that the mean age of symptom onset of subjects with CBD is approximately 62 years old (standard deviation approximately 7 years). The mean disease duration is around 6 years, although survival can range from 2 to 13 years. Men and women seem to be equally affected. The exact cause of CBD is unknown, and although CBD is considered a sporadic disease, there have been a few reports of families with CBD-like pathology[11,12] or mutations within the microtubule-associated protein tau (*MAPT*) gene linked to pathological findings similar to CBD.[13,14] It is unclear whether these familial cases truly represent CBD.

CBD is a relatively rare neurodegenerative disease. Prevalence and incidence studies are limited by the lack of good correlation between the clinical diagnosis of CBS and the pathological findings of CBD. The exact incidence and prevalence of CBD is unknown. In one community-based prevalence study looking at cases of parkinsonian disorders, no cases of CBD were identified among 121,628 subjects.[15] It has been estimated, however, that CBD may account for approximately 5% of parkinsonism, which would translate into an incidence of 0.62 to 0.92 per 100,000 and a prevalence of 4.9 to 7.3 per 100,000.[16]

Clinical Features

The clinical features associated with CBD consist of any combination of the following signs and symptoms: action and postural tremor, rarely rest tremor, bradykinesia, myoclonus, ideomotor apraxia, alien limb phenomena, limb dystonia, gait impairment, dysarthria, aphasia, apraxia of speech, and dementia.[7] There have been increasing reports more recently showing that cognitive impairment,[17] especially impairment in speech and language,[18-20] and less so visuospatial and perceptual deficits,[21,22] is a presentation of CBD and should be a feature of the CBS. The features of CBD, regardless of whether they are predominantly motor or predominantly cognitive, tend to be strongly asymmetrical, although there are autopsy-confirmed cases of CBD that had symmetrical features (personal experience).

PARKINSONISM

The most common motor feature is asymmetrical parkinsonism, which usually affects the upper extremity first. Rigidity, bradykinesia, postural instability, and tremor, in order of decreasing frequency, have been reported.[23] In contrast to Parkinson's disease, in which the tremor is typically approximately 4 Hz, the tremor in CBD is faster at 6 to 8 Hz, and appears more irregular and jerky.[24] In addition, very early reports suggested that the tremor tends to be seen with posture or action, rather than at rest.[2] Postural instability may lead to falls, and eventually the patient becomes wheelchair bound. Falls tend to be later in onset, however, compared with the very early falls that are more typical of progressive supranuclear palsy (PSP).

DYSTONIA

Dystonia is a common feature of CBS. In one study during the course of the disease, 95% of patients with CBS had dystonia affecting one or more limbs; 92% developed arm dystonia, whereas only 28% developed leg dystonia.[25] Approximately one third of the patients in that study also developed dystonia of the head, neck, or trunk. Less than 5% of patients had blepharospasm, which seems to be more common in PSP. Dystonia can be one of the most disabling features in CBD rendering the affected limb or limbs immobile and essentially useless. Most patients with dystonia later develop contractures and associated pain. Pain may accompany dystonia in almost 50% of patients.[25]

APRAXIA

One of the most studied features of CBD and the CBS is apraxia.[26-33] Of all the neurodegenerative disorders, apraxia is most commonly associated with CBD, although it is not pathognomonic for CBD. Apraxia has been a consistent feature across all the proposed diagnostic criteria for CBD.[5,24,34,35] In CBD, limb-kinetic apraxia and ideomotor apraxia have been well described, although ideational apraxia clearly also occurs. Ideomotor limb apraxia tends to be bilateral, but typically asymmetrical, particularly early in the disease course. It has been reported that ideomotor apraxia in CBD consists of spatial, temporal, and sequencing errors.[36] One study showed that imitative transitive and intransitive limb nonrepresentational gestures are abnormal; however, intransitive limb representational gestures are not.[28]

In addition to limb apraxia, truncal apraxia[31] and orofacial apraxia[30] can occur in CBD. A few studies have compared apraxia occurring in CBS with apraxia in patients with PSP.[26,27,29] It has been suggested that apraxia in PSP is of the ideomotor type, but tends to be less severe than in CBS.[27,29] It has been suggested that limb kinetic apraxia is a feature of CBD, not PSP, which accounts for distal to proximal differences in limb praxis in CBD.[26]

A subset of patients with limb apraxia develop what is termed an *alien limb phenomenon*. Alien limb phenomenon refers to the development of movements of a limb that are involuntary and uncontrollable, with the limb acting as though it has a mind of its own. It can affect the arms or the legs.[37] Patients with an alien limb may personify the limb, referring to it as "my little friend," or "this thing." Alien limb phenomenon is not specific to CBD and has been described in Creutzfeldt-Jakob disease[38] and Alzheimer's disease.[39]

MYOCLONUS

Myoclonus occurs in about half of all cases with CBS. The myoclonus is usually focal and confined to one limb, usually one arm, and less commonly a leg. Electrophysiological studies have shown the presence of action and reflex myoclonus.[40-42] The phenomenon is predominantly distal, but can extend to involve the entire arm.[40] Although myoclonus seems to be present at rest, electromyographic recordings reveal that myoclonus occurs on a background of continuous muscle activity. The action myoclonus tends to repeat at an interval of 70 to 90 ms and may resemble tremor, but usually is not preceded by an identifiable cortical wave in the electroencephalogram back averaged before each jerk.[40] Focal reflex myoclonus is characterized by bursts of 24 brief (25 to 50 ms) spikes separated by 60- to 80-ms intervals.[43] Myoclonus in CBD is strongly suspected to be of cortical origin because of the presence of long-latency reflex response.[44] Giant somatosensory evoked potentials are absent[40,44,45]; the latency of reflex myoclonus is about 10 ms shorter than that seen in cortical reflex myoclonus[40,42]; and, as mentioned earlier, there is a lack of a back-averaged prejerk focal cortical electroencephalogram activity.[40-42]

COGNITIVE IMPAIRMENT

Although initial reports of CBD focused on motor phenomena, more recent evidence suggests that cognitive impairment is as common and may even be a more common presentation. Aphasia is the most common type of cognitive impairment, although frontal dysexecutive features and posterior cortical dysfunction have also been described. Language impairment usually takes the form of a nonfluent aphasia with agrammatical and telegraphic speech, superimposed on apraxia of speech.[18-20] It has been suggested that if the apraxia of speech is the dominant feature, PSP is more likely the underlying pathology, whereas a predominance of linguistic abnormalities is more suggestive of CBD.[19] Dysarthria, dysphasia, and orofacial apraxia may accompany aphasia.[19,46,47]

Executive dysfunction is common in CBD and can be shown on bedside testing,[48] and confirmed with neuropsychological testing.[49-51] Neuropsychological testing cannot differentiate CBD from atypical presentations of PSP with features of CBS.[50]

Posterior cortical dysfunction is less common, but has been described in CBD[22,52] and in patients presenting with CBS.[53] Although features of Balint's syndrome[53] are not a part of CBS, the combination of posterior cortical dysfunction and extrapyramidal features should result in the consideration of a diagnosis of CBD, especially because visuospatial dysfunction is much more pronounced in CBS compared with other atypical parkinsonian syndromes.[21]

NEUROPSYCHIATRIC FEATURES

Neuropsychiatric features are present in patients with CBD.[54] The most common neuropsychiatric features in one study with 36 autopsy-confirmed cases of CBD included depression and compulsive behavior, which were present in 22% of patients, whereas psychosis was absent. In contrast, another study showed that 73% of patients with CBS had depression, 40% had apathy, and 20% had irritability and agitation.[55] These differences may be due to the fact that one study was clinically based, whereas the other was autopsy-confirmed.

OTHER FEATURES

Other, less common features have also been described in CBS. It is unclear, however, whether these features are associated with CBD because none of these cases have had autopsy confirmation. Rapid-eye movement (REM) sleep behavior disorder, which has been reported to suggest underlying synucleinopathy,[56] has been reported in CBS.[57-59] Vertical supranuclear gaze palsy is typical of PSP, but does occur in CBD, although studies have suggested that in PSP oculomotor impairment affects velocity and amplitude, whereas increased saccadic latency is a feature of CBD.[60,61] Another feature classic for PSP, frontalis hyperactivity, or the procerus sign, has also been described in CBS.[62] Primitive reflexes, or frontal release signs, typically associated with frontal lobe dysfunction and the frontotemporal lobar degenerations (FTLD) have been found to occur in CBS. In 13 patients with CBS, 61% had a glabellar, 54% had a snout, and 15% had a palmomental reflex.[63] Progressive frontal gait disturbances have been described in a case with CBD.[64]

Differential Diagnoses

Presenting clinical features suggestive of CBD in the absence of pathological confirmation are now referred to as CBS,[5] or the corticobasal degeneration syndrome.[65] The most common pathological diagnosis that underlies CBS is CBD.[66] Although neurodegenerative diseases such as Alzheimer's disease,[39,66] Pick's disease with Pick bodies,[66] Creutzfeldt-Jakob disease,[66-70] and atypical PSP[71,72] are other common causes of the CBS, less common causes include FTLD with ubiquitin/TDP-43 immunoreactive inclusions,[8,73] dementia lacking distinctive histology,[66] neurofilament inclusion body disease,[74] and hereditary diffuse leukoencephalopathy with spheroids.[75] In addition, there have been single case reports or small case series of non-neurodegenerative diseases causing CBS, including thalamic tuberculoma,[76] neurosyphilis,[77] primary antiphospholipid syndrome,[78] Fahr's disease,[79] central pontine myelinolysis,[80] and progressive multifocal leukoencephalopathy.[81]

It has been shown more recently that there is significant clinicopathological overlap between CBD, PSP, and FTLD.[8,82,83] The overlap can occur clinically or pathologically (i.e., clinical features suggestive of CBD, PSP, or FTLD may be due to any of the underlying pathological diseases, CBD, PSP, or FTLD). Given the significant overlap, some authors advocate lumping CBD, PSP, and FTLD under the rubric of "Pick's complex"[84]; not everyone agrees with this recommendation.

DIAGNOSTIC CRITERIA

There have been many proposed diagnostic criteria for CBD.[5,24,34,35] None of them have been formally validated in a large prospective clinicopathological series, however, and none seem very sensitive or specific. Almost all of the proposed criteria for CBD have focused on the presence of motor abnormalities, while neglecting cognitive deficits. In the most recent iteration, with the recognition of the overlap of CBD and FTLD, apraxia of speech and nonfluent aphasia were added to the CBS criteria.[5]

CORTICOBASAL GANGLIONIC DEGENERATION VERSUS PROGRESSIVE SUPRANUCLEAR PALSY

Differentiating CBD from PSP can be very difficult because both diseases can have overlapping clinical features: both can manifest with CBS.[72] False-negative misdiagnoses of CBD mainly occur with PSP,[85] and CBD is the most likely cause for a misdiagnosis of PSP.[86] Many studies have tried to determine whether there are any clinical features or laboratory findings specific to either pathology, without success. The presence of photophobia in PSP has been suggested as a possible feature distinguishing PSP from CBD.[87]

Diagnostic Investigations

There is no specific test for the diagnosis of CBD; however, ancillary testing is important to rule out other diagnoses that can cause CBS and mimic CBD. Cerebrospinal fluid (CSF) evaluations are important to exclude infectious and inflammatory etiologies. Abnormalities in the neuron-specific enolase, 14-3-3 protein and S-100 protein, may be suggestive of Creutzfeldt-Jakob disease. CSF studies have also been performed to determine whether increased levels of certain proteins could be used as biomarkers in CBD. CSF tau has been shown to be increased in CBS patients compared with controls in one study,[88] but not in another.[89] Total tau and phospho-tau were increased compared with controls and with patients with PSP in one study,[90] in keeping with reports of differences in CSF tau between PSP and CBD.[91,92] CSF levels of β-amyloid,[93] neurofilament heavy chain,[94] and orexin[95] have been assessed in CBS and compared with other neurodegenerative diseases, with conclusions suggesting that these markers may have diagnostic utility. Further studies on these CSF proteins are needed.

Electroencephalography may be useful in distinguishing patients with CBS and Creutzfeldt-Jakob disease from patients with CBS and CBD. Utility of electroencephalography in CBD is limited, however. Focal slow wave patterns occur in approximately 80% of patients with CBS, but in less than 15% of patients with PSP.[96]

Substantia nigra hyperechogenicity measured by the use of brain parenchyma sonography is increased in CBS, but not PSP, and may be a useful measure in differentiating these two diseases.[97] Because of the common misdiagnosis of PSP as CBS, however, the utility of this finding requires confirmation.

Myoclonus in CBD, as stated earlier, may be cortically mediated, but has characteristic features, such as absent cortical spikes preceding myoclonic jerks, absent giant evoked potentials, and enhanced long latency reflex. Electrophysiological studies, especially in early stages of CBD, may have clinical utility.[98,99]

Somatosensory evoked potentials,[100] visual event–related potentials,[101] and motor evoked potentials[102] measured by transcranial magnetic stimulation of the cortex have been assessed in patients with CBS, with assessment of transcallosal pathways in particular.[103,104] These studies are rarely performed in clinical practice, but may be useful in differentiating CBD from other neurodegenerative diseases.[105,106] Pathological data are needed to determine the sensitivity and specificity of these electrophysiological tests.

Neuroimaging

STRUCTURAL

Magnetic resonance imaging (MRI) studies in CBS show predominantly posterior frontal and superior parietal neocortical atrophy (Fig. 22–1). This atrophy tends to be asymmetrical, being more severe in the hemisphere that is contralateral to the more affected limb.[107] Atrophy of the corpus callosum has been reported in CBS.[108] In cases in which there is significant behavioral dyscontrol, atrophy may spread into premotor and prefrontal areas correlating with the clinical presentation. Similarly in cases with predominantly visuospatial and perceptual deficits, atrophy may extend into more posterior parietal and occipital regions.[22] Mesial temporal lobe structures are generally preserved except for rare reports.[109] The basal ganglia may show atrophy with corresponding dilation of the lateral and third ventricles.

Decreased T2 and fluid-attenuated inversion recovery (FLAIR) signal changes can also be seen in the basal ganglia (Fig. 22–2), indicative of possibly increased iron deposition versus gliosis. Increased T2 and FLAIR signal abnormalities immediately beneath atrophic cortices can be seen especially in primary motor and sensory cortices (see Fig. 22–1), and may be associated with apraxia and alien limb phenomenon.[37,110]

A more recent study showed that these imaging characteristics are not specific to the underlying pathology of CBD, however, and are more indicative of CBS.[111] Although these patterns are characteristic of CBD, they can also be seen in other pathological processes causing CBS. Many imaging studies have tried to differentiate CBD from other pathological entities, especially PSP. These studies lack autopsy confirmation.[107,112-115]

A technique called voxel-based morphometry, which uses statistical comparisons across groups of subjects, has been applied to subjects with CBS (Fig. 22–3) and PSP, with similar results to those reported in more descriptive analysis.[116] This is not surprising because the results of this study are also affected by the lack of autopsy confirmation. A single study using voxel-based morphometry has compared autopsy-confirmed subjects with CBD with subjects with PSP.[117] In this study, CBD subjects had frontoparietal atrophy, whereas PSP subjects had mainly white matter tract degeneration including superior cerebellar peduncle,

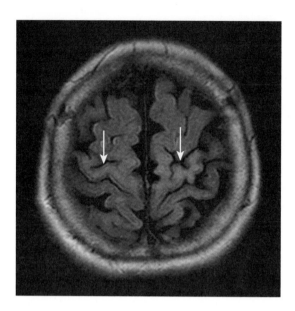

Figure 22–1 Axial FLAIR MRI shows asymmetrical left > right posterior frontal lobe atrophy with increased signal noted in bilateral precentral gyri (left > right) (*arrows*) in a 66-year-old man with corticobasal syndrome, left alien limb phenomenon, and illness duration of 2 years.

and midbrain atrophy. The authors also showed that the pattern of atrophy in the CBD patients differed depending on whether the predominant presenting symptom was dementia versus an extrapyramidal syndrome.[117] Differences also have been observed between CBD and PSP, and other degenerative diseases, in the rate of whole-brain atrophy over time.[118] The rate of brain atrophy in CBD was significantly greater than in patients with PSP.

FUNCTIONAL

Positive emission tomography (PET), single photon emission computed tomography (SPECT), proton magnetic resonance spectroscopy, and functional MRI all have been performed in patients with CBS. fludeoxyglucose F 18 ([18]FDG) PET scans have shown hypometabolism in frontal and parietal lobes, and in basal ganglia and thalamus (see Fig. 22–2).[119-123] Similar to MRI studies, hypometabolism tends to be asymmetrical and worse in the hemisphere contralateral to the more affected side of the body.[124] [18]FDG PET studies have also been applied to try to differentiate PSP from CBS. These studies tend to show more hypometabolism in parietal cortex in CBS,[125,126] whereas PSP subjects tend to show more hypometabolism in deep gray and midbrain regions.[125,127]

Frontal lobe hypometabolism has not always differed between CBS and PSP in these studies. One study showed that there was very good correlation between [18]FDG PET diagnosis and clinical diagnosis.[128] In cases with significant atrophy on MRI, it is unclear whether corresponding hypometabolism on [18]FDG PET merely reflects the pattern of atrophy (see Fig. 22–2). In such cases, it is better to compare the subject's PET data with a database of normal controls (Fig. 22–4). Many such software programs currently exist.

In addition, to [18]FDG PET, PET studies using [^{11}C]PK 11195, a marker of peripheral benzodiazepine binding sites expressed by activated microglia, have shown increased [^{11}C]PK 11195 binding in striatum; substantia nigra;

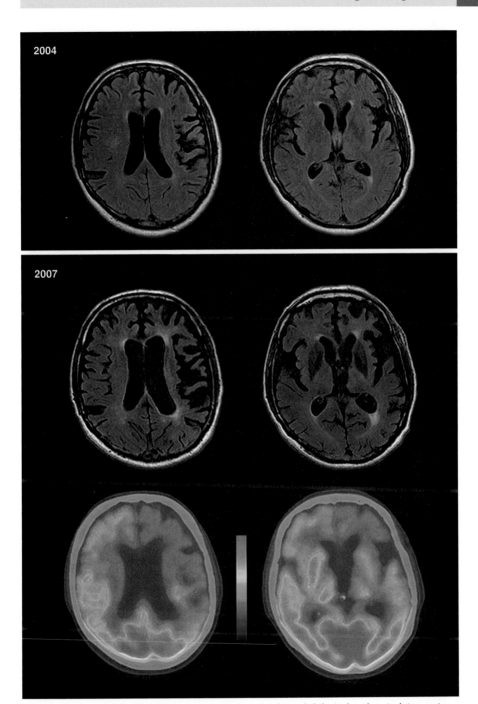

Figure 22–2   Axial FLAIR MRI shows progressive atrophy in left frontal and perisylvian regions, and enlargement of the lateral and third ventricles and decreased signal in basal ganglia, over 3 years (2004-2007) in a 64-year-old man who first presented with a progressive nonfluent aphasia, but later developed corticobasal syndrome. In 2007, PET scan shows hypometabolism in left > right frontoparietal regions, and left basal ganglia and thalamus.

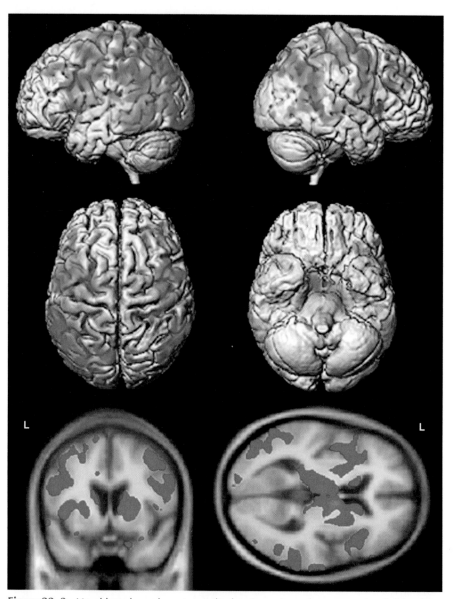

Figure 22–3 Voxel-based morphometry results showing regions of gray matter loss in 25 patients with either corticobasal syndrome or corticobasal degeneration (*n* = 11) compared with 24 healthy controls. The three-dimensional surface renders show cortical gray matter loss in the posterior frontal lobes and the parietal lobes, with relative sparing of the temporal lobe and frontal pole. The axial and coronal slices show loss in the basal ganglia. L, left. (Courtesy of Jennifer L. Whitwell, PhD, Mayo Clinic, Rochester, MN.)

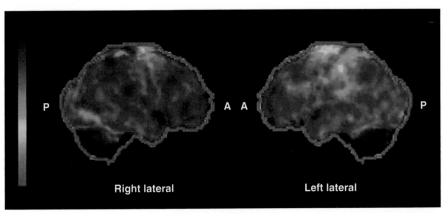

Figure 22–4 ^{18}FDG PET with CT fusion shows decreased metabolism of the left sensorimotor strip greater than 2 standard deviations from the norm compared with an age-matched normal database (subject from Fig. 22–1).

and frontal, temporal, and parietal cortex suggesting that microglial activation is involved in the pathogenesis of CBS.[129,130] Fluorodopa F 18 PET has shown reduced, asymmetrical uptake in striatum in CBS.[131] PET studies also lack autopsy confirmation.

Studies using SPECT have produced similar findings to those reported with PET, showing predominantly frontoparietal and striatal hypoperfusion.[132,133] SPECT studies have also been used to try to differentiate between CBS and PSP and other neurodegenerative disorders.[134-141] Results have been similar to those reported in PET studies.

Proton magnetic resonance spectroscopy studies have shown a significant reduction in the N-acetyl aspartate (NAA)/creatine ratio in frontal cortex and putamen in CBS patients compared with patients with Parkinson's disease, multiple system atrophy, and vascular parkinsonism. Although PSP subjects showed a similar reduction in the putamen, no reduction was noted in frontal cortex, and in contrast to in CBS, there was no asymmetry.[142] Another study found significantly reduced NAA/choline ratio in parietal cortex in CBS, whereas reduced NAA/choline ratio in the lentiform nucleus was noted in PSP.[143] Functional MRI studies are limited in CBS.[144,145]

Pathology

Macroscopic and microscopic findings consistent with CBD were first reported in 1968 by Rebeiz and colleagues.[1] Since the original report, many neuropathological studies have been done on the morphology, distribution, biochemistry, and ultrastructure of the typical lesions of CBD. Consensus neuropathological criteria for CBD[6] form the basis for current pathological diagnosis, and are the gold standard for making a diagnosis of CBD. Definitive diagnosis of CBD requires neuropathological examination as described in the consensus criteria.[6]

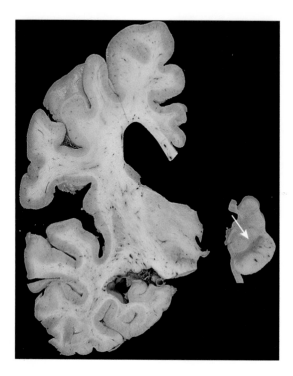

Figure 22–5 Coronal section on gross examination shows evidence of enlargement of the lateral ventricles with enlarged frontal horns and depigmentation of the substantia nigra (*arrow*) in a patient with corticobasal degeneration. (Courtesy of Dennis W. Dickson, MD, Mayo Clinic, Jacksonville, FL.)

MACROSCOPY

In CBD, cortical atrophy is often focal and asymmetrical affecting parasagittal, perisylvian, and perirolandic regions. The superior frontal gyrus is more affected than middle and inferior frontal gyri.[6] On sectioning the brain, cerebral white matter volume loss and thinning of the corpus callosum may be observed.[108] The ventricular system may be enlarged (Fig. 22–5). The anterior limb of the internal capsule can be affected. The substantia nigra tends to be severely affected with evidence of depigmentation (see Fig. 22–5). Regions of the basal ganglia, including globus pallidus, striatum, and subthalamic nuclei, and thalamic nuclei and brainstem regions are variably affected.

MICROSCOPY

Microscopic findings include neuronal loss and gliosis predominantly affecting frontal and parietal neocortex and substantia nigra; other neocortical, basal ganglia, brainstem, and cerebellar regions are affected, but usually to a lesser degree. Spinal cord involvement has also been described.[146] The cardinal lesions typical of CBD include balloon neurons, neuronal inclusions, coiled bodies, threads, and astrocytic plaques. Balloon neurons are swollen achromatic neurons that can be seen with routine hematoxylin and eosin stain (Fig. 22–6), but are not specific to CBD, being observed in other neurodegenerative diseases such as argyrophilic grain disease and PSP, although in PSP balloon neurons may be secondary to the presence of argyrophilic grain disease.[147] The other lesions (neuronal inclusions,

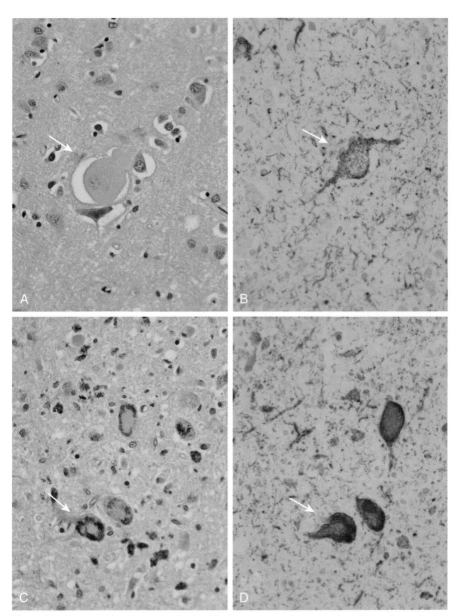

Figure 22–6   A-D, Photomicrographs show balloon neurons in cortex (**A** and **B**) and a corticobasal body in substantia nigra (**C** and **D**). (**A** and **C,** Hematoxylin and eosin, ×400; **B** and **D,** phospho-
tau, ×400.) (Courtesy of Dennis W. Dickson, MD, Mayo Clinic, Jacksonville, FL.)

coiled bodies, threads, and astrocytic plaques) are best identified with silver stain or tau immunohistochemistry.

Tau is a microtubule-associated protein whose function is to promote assembly and stabilization of microtubules. Based on alternative RNA splicing of exon 10, six tau isoforms exist with either three or four conserved repeat sequences. Tau immunoreactive neurodegenerative diseases can be separated into diseases in which exon 10 is spliced in (4R tau) versus diseases in which exon 10 is spliced out (3R tau). Insoluble tau in CBD is predominantly 4R tau. Neuronal inclusions tend to be found in small neurons in the upper lamina of the cortex, or may be seen in brainstem nuclei such as substantia nigra or locus caeruleus, and are immunoreactive to 4R tau. In original descriptions, neuronal inclusions in substantia nigra were referred to as corticobasal bodies (see Fig. 22–6).[3] Coiled bodies are also immunoreactive to 4R tau and are oligodendroglial in origin (Fig. 22–7). Threads are neuronal and glial in origin and tend to be numerous in gray and white matter in CBD (see Fig. 22–7). The astrocytic plaques are probably the most specific lesion to CBD and are astrocytic in origin—hence the term astrocytic plaques (see Fig. 22–7). Here tau is found in the terminal processes of astrocytes.

In addition to these tau immunoreactive lesions, there is evidence for microglial activation that parallels system degeneration in CBD.[148] Ultrastructure studies are not a part of routine neuropathological investigation of CBD; however, they have identified features that can be helpful in differentiating CBD from other neurodegenerative disorders.[149,150]

The disease that can be most difficult to distinguish from CBD is PSP. In contrast to in CBD, where astrocytic plaques are found, PSP is characterized by tufts of astrocytes (tufted astrocytes). In contrast to astrocytic plaques, tau accumulates in proximal processes of tufted astrocytes. Tufted astrocytes and astrocytic plaques do not coexist in CBD and PSP.[151] The distribution of these two lesions is different, with astrocytic plaques being most abundant in prefrontal and premotor cortices in CBD, whereas tufted astrocytes are most prominent in precentral and premotor areas in PSP. Tufted astrocytes are typical in globus pallidus, subthalamic nucleus, and thalamus in PSP—regions that are typically not affected by astrocytic plaques in CBD.[152] One recent study has also reported that amino-terminally cleaved tau fragments distinguish PSP from CBD.[153] Although PSP, CBD, and Pick's disease may have some overlapping neuropathological features, there are morphological and biochemical features and differences in the distribution of the pathological lesions that can help to differentiate CBD from PSP, and CBD from other neurodegenerative disorders.[154-156]

Genetics

There is no evidence that CBD has any genetic underpinning, but CBD is associated with the protein tau. The chromosomal region containing the *MAPT* gene has been shown to involve two major haplotypes, H1 and H2, which are defined by linkage disequilibrium between several polymorphisms over the entire *MAPT* gene. Similar to PSP, studies have shown that there is an association between the CBS and the *MAPT* H1 haplotype,[157] which was confirmed in a large pathological series of 57 CBD subjects.[158] Linkage disequilibrium fine mapping analysis have shown further an association for PSP and a trend for an association between CBS and the

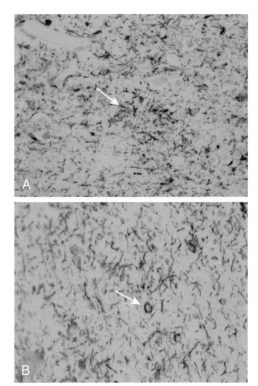

Figure 22–7 A and **B,** Photomicrographs show numerous threads in gray matter and white matter, and an astrocytic plaque (**A**) and a coiled body (**B**). (**A** and **B,** Phospho-tau ×400.) (Courtesy of Dennis W. Dickson, MD, Mayo Clinic, Jacksonville, FL.)

MAPT H1c haplotype, which is a variant of the H1 haplotype.[159] These findings suggest that patients with PSP and CBD share a common genetic predisposition.

Two genes on chromosome 17 are associated with familial FTLD: the *MAPT* gene[160] and the gene coding for the protein progranulin (*PGRN*).[161,162] There have been reported families with mutations in the *MAPT* gene in which autopsy has shown pathological features similar to those of CBD.[13,14] It is unclear, however, whether these cases are truly CBD. There have been many reports of families associated with mutations in the *PGRN* gene that has been associated with CBS, and this seems to be the most common cause of familial CBS.[163-165] To date, however, all of these subjects have had pathological characteristics of FTLD with abnormal TDP-43-positive lesions and an absence of tau-immunoreactive pathology. In contrast to in Alzheimer's disease, in which there is a clear association with the apolipoprotein E ε4 allele, neither of two studies showed convincingly that there is an association between CBD and the apolipoprotein E ε4 allele.[10,166]

Management

No treatment is available at present that halts progression or significantly improves dysfunction in CBD. Some patients with CBD may obtain some benefit, however, from certain types of therapies targeting one or more specific signs or symptoms. As mentioned earlier, CBD is characterized by the emergence of signs and symptoms involving many different systems. The treatment approach is complex and tailored to the different symptoms.

One of the most disabling features of CBD is parkinsonism. Consideration of high-dose levodopa therapy, preferably with greater than 1000 mg of levodopa per day, on an empty stomach, if tolerated, is warranted. A rare patient without any response to levodopa at lower doses may experience mild to moderate benefit at doses greater than 1000 mg. A study assessing the efficacy of levodopa treatment in CBS showed that although a few patients may have some improvement in parkinsonism, the benefit tends to be at best modest and transient.[23] In another study, only one of four patients treated with levodopa had any response.[7] Levodopa side effects can occur, and levodopa-induced dyskinesias are extremely rare, but have been reported.[167]

Dystonia and myoclonus are also very disabling, and require pharmacological intervention to try to ameliorate the primary symptom or secondary symptoms, such as pain, that may be associated with the dystonia. Benzodiazepines, primarily clonazepam, may improve myoclonus and dystonia in CBD.[23] In a retrospective study, 23% of patients with myoclonus and 9% with dystonia experienced some benefit from clonazepam therapy.[23] Anticholinergics and baclofen were rarely beneficial, but are still worth considering, although anticholinergic side effects may limit usage. Dystonia treatment with botulinum toxin injections has been studied.[168] Of three patients with CBS and a dystonic clenched fist treated with botulinum toxin A, all had significant pain relief, and two had marked improvement of posture; however, no patient had any functional improvement.[168] Another study reported that six of nine patients experienced improvement of dystonia with botulinum toxin injections.[23]

Deep brain stimulation was inadvertently completed in one patient with CBS without significant improvement.[169] To date, deep brain stimulation has not been reported to be effective in ameliorating dystonia or pain associated with dystonia in CBD.

Palliative therapies for CBS are extremely important to obtain the best possible quality of life. Symptoms causing significant concern to patients should be individually addressed with appropriate intervention. Physical therapy should be completed, and wheelchair use should be considered in patients with moderate to severe gait and postural instability, especially if the patient is falling. Subjects with dysphagia should undergo swallowing evaluations, and adaptive feeding techniques should be implemented depending on performance. Speech and language therapy are very important for patients with significant dysarthria and aphasia. Depression and emotional lability may respond to serotonin specific reuptake inhibitors. Patient and family support should be addressed, and information regarding diagnosis, prognosis, and support groups should be provided.

REFERENCES

1. Rebeiz JJ, Kolodny EH, Richardson EP Jr: Corticodentatonigral degeneration with neuronal achromasia. Arch Neurol 1968;18:20-33.
2. Riley DE, Lang AE, Lewis A, et al: Cortical-basal ganglionic degeneration. Neurology 1990;40:1203-1212.
3. Gibb WR, Luthert PJ, Marsden CD: Corticobasal degeneration. Brain 1989;112(Pt 5):1171-1192.
4. Litvan I, Bhatia KP, Burn DJ, et al: Movement Disorders Society Scientific Issues Committee report: SIC Task Force appraisal of clinical diagnostic criteria for Parkinsonian disorders. Mov Disord 2003;18:467-486.

5. Boeve BF, Lang AE, Litvan I: Corticobasal degeneration and its relationship to progressive supranuclear palsy and frontotemporal dementia. Ann Neurol 2003;54(Suppl 5):S15-S19.
6. Dickson DW, Bergeron C, Chin SS, et al: Office of Rare Diseases neuropathologic criteria for corticobasal degeneration. J Neuropathol Exp Neurol 2002;61:935-946.
7. Wenning GK, Litvan I, Jankovic J, et al: Natural history and survival of 14 patients with corticobasal degeneration confirmed at postmortem examination. J Neurol Neurosurg Psychiatry 1998;64:184-189.
8. Josephs KA, Petersen RC, Knopman DS, et al: Clinicopathologic analysis of frontotemporal and corticobasal degenerations and PSP. Neurology 2006;66:41-48.
9. Rinne JO, Lee MS, Thompson PD, Marsden CD: Corticobasal degeneration: a clinical study of 36 cases. Brain 1994;117(Pt 5):1183-1196.
10. Schneider JA, Watts RL, Gearing M, et al: Corticobasal degeneration: neuropathologic and clinical heterogeneity. Neurology 1997;48:959-969.
11. Uchihara T, Nakayama H: Familial tauopathy mimicking corticobasal degeneration an autopsy study on three siblings. J Neurol Sci 2006;246:45-51.
12. Brown J, Lantos PL, Roques P, et al: Familial dementia with swollen achromatic neurons and corticobasal inclusion bodies: a clinical and pathological study. J Neurol Sci 1996;135:21-30.
13. Mirra SS, Murrell JR, Gearing M, et al: Tau pathology in a family with dementia and a P301L mutation in tau. J Neuropathol Exp Neurol 1999;58:335-345.
14. Spillantini MG, Yoshida H, Rizzini C, et al: A novel tau mutation (N296N) in familial dementia with swollen achromatic neurons and corticobasal inclusion bodies. Ann Neurol 2000;48:939-943.
15. Schrag A, Ben-Shlomo Y, Quinn NP: Prevalence of progressive supranuclear palsy and multiple system atrophy: a cross-sectional study. Lancet 1999;354:1771-1775.
16. Togasaki DM, Tanner CM: Epidemiologic aspects. Adv Neurol 2000;82:53-59.
17. Bergeron C, Davis A, Lang AE: Corticobasal ganglionic degeneration and progressive supranuclear palsy presenting with cognitive decline. Brain Pathol 1998;8:355-365.
18. Frattali CM, Grafman J, Patronas N, et al: Language disturbances in corticobasal degeneration. Neurology 2000;54:990-992.
19. Josephs KA, Duffy JR, Strand EA, et al: Clinicopathological and imaging correlates of progressive aphasia and apraxia of speech. Brain 2006;129:1385-1398.
20. McMonagle P, Blair M, Kertesz A: Corticobasal degeneration and progressive aphasia. Neurology 2006;67:1444-1451.
21. Bak TH, Caine D, Hearn VC, Hodges JR: Visuospatial functions in atypical parkinsonian syndromes. J Neurol Neurosurg Psychiatry 2006;77:454-456.
22. Tang-Wai DF, Josephs KA, Boeve BF, et al: Pathologically confirmed corticobasal degeneration presenting with visuospatial dysfunction. Neurology 2003;61:1134-1135.
23. Kompoliti K, Goetz CG, Boeve BF, et al: Clinical presentation and pharmacological therapy in corticobasal degeneration. Arch Neurol 1998;55:957-961.
24. Watts RL, Mirra SS, Richardson EP Jr, Corticobasal ganglionic degeneration. In Marsden CD & Fahn S, ed: Movement Disorders 3. Oxford: Butterworths-Heinemann, 1994, pp 282–299.
25. Vanek Z, Jankovic J: Dystonia in corticobasal degeneration. Mov Disord 2001;16:252-257.
26. Soliveri P, Piacentini S, Paridi D, et al: Distal-proximal differences in limb apraxia in corticobasal degeneration but not progressive supranuclear palsy. Neurol Sci 2003;24:213-214.
27. Soliveri P, Piacentini S, Girotti F: Limb apraxia in corticobasal degeneration and progressive supranuclear palsy. Neurology 2005;64:448-453.
28. Salter JE, Roy EA, Black SE, et al: Gestural imitation and limb apraxia in corticobasal degeneration. Brain Cogn 2004;55:400-402.
29. Pharr V, Uttl B, Stark M, et al: Comparison of apraxia in corticobasal degeneration and progressive supranuclear palsy. Neurology 2001;56:957-963.
30. Ozsancak C, Auzou P, Dujardin K, et al: Orofacial apraxia in corticobasal degeneration, progressive supranuclear palsy, multiple system atrophy and Parkinson's disease. J Neurol 2004;251:1317-1323.
31. Okuda B, Tanaka H, Kawabata K, et al: Truncal and limb apraxia in corticobasal degeneration. Mov Disord 2001;16:760-762.
32. Leiguarda R, Lees AJ, Merello M, et al: The nature of apraxia in corticobasal degeneration. J Neurol Neurosurg Psychiatry 1994;57:455-459.
33. Jacobs DH, Adair JC, Macauley B, et al: Apraxia in corticobasal degeneration. Brain Cogn 1999;40:336-354.

34. Lang AE, Riley DE, Bergeron C: Cortico-basal ganglionic degeneration. In Calne D, ed: Neurodegenerative Diseases. Philadelphia: Saunders, 1994, pp 877–894.
35. Watts RL, Brewer RP, Schneider JA, Mirra SS: Corticobasal degeneration. In Watts RL & Koller WC, ed: Movement Disorders: Neurologic Principles and Practice. New York: McGraw Hill, 1997, pp 611–621.
36. Leiguarda R, Merello M, Balej J: Apraxia in corticobasal degeneration. Adv Neurol 2000;82:103-121.
37. Hu WT, Josephs KA, Ahlskog JE, et al: MRI correlates of alien leg-like phenomenon in corticobasal degeneration. Mov Disord 2005;20:870-873.
38. Fogel B, Wu M, Kremen S, et al: Creutzfeldt-Jakob disease presenting with alien limb sign. Mov Disord 2006;21:1040-1042.
39. Chand P, Grafman J, Dickson D, et al: Alzheimer's disease presenting as corticobasal syndrome. Mov Disord 2006;21:2018-2022.
40. Thompson PD, Day BL, Rothwell JC, et al: The myoclonus in corticobasal degeneration: evidence for two forms of cortical reflex myoclonus. Brain 1994;117(Pt 5):1197-1207.
41. Carella F, Scaioli V, Franceschetti S, et al: Focal reflex myoclonus in corticobasal degeneration. Funct Neurol 1991;6:165-170.
42. Thompson PD: Myoclonus in corticobasal degeneration. Clin Neurosci 1995;3:203-208.
43. Caviness JN: Myoclonus and neurodegenerative disease—what's in a name? Parkinsonism Relat Disord 2003;9:185-192.
44. Carella F, Ciano C, Panzica F, Scaioli V: Myoclonus in corticobasal degeneration. Mov Disord 1997;12:598-603.
45. Brunt ER, van Weerden TW, Pruim J, Lakke JW: Unique myoclonic pattern in corticobasal degeneration. Mov Disord 1995;10:132-142.
46. Muller J, Wenning GK, Verny M, et al: Progression of dysarthria and dysphagia in postmortem-confirmed parkinsonian disorders. Arch Neurol 2001;58:259-264.
47. Ozsancak C, Auzou P, Hannequin D: Dysarthria and orofacial apraxia in corticobasal degeneration. Mov Disord 2000;15:905-910.
48. Bak TH, Rogers TT, Crawford LM, et al: Cognitive bedside assessment in atypical parkinsonian syndromes. J Neurol Neurosurg Psychiatry 2005;76:420-422.
49. Pillon B, Blin J, Vidailhet M, et al: The neuropsychological pattern of corticobasal degeneration: comparison with progressive supranuclear palsy and Alzheimer's disease. Neurology 1995;45:1477-1483.
50. Vanvoorst WA, Greenaway MC, Boeve BF, et al: Neuropsychological findings in clinically atypical autopsy confirmed corticobasal degeneration and progressive supranuclear palsy. Parkinsonism Relat Disord 2008;14:376-378.
51. Murray R, Neumann M, Forman MS, et al: Cognitive and motor assessment in autopsy-proven corticobasal degeneration. Neurology 2007;68:1274-1283.
52. Renner JA, Burns JM, Hou CE, et al: Progressive posterior cortical dysfunction: a clinicopathologic series. Neurology 2004;63:1175-1180.
53. Mendez MF: Corticobasal ganglionic degeneration with Balint's syndrome. J Neuropsychiatry Clin Neurosci 2000;12:273-275.
54. Geda YE, Boeve BF, Negash S, et al: Neuropsychiatric features in 36 pathologically confirmed cases of corticobasal degeneration. J Neuropsychiatry Clin Neurosci 2007;19:77-80.
55. Litvan I, Cummings JL, Mega M: Neuropsychiatric features of corticobasal degeneration. J Neurol Neurosurg Psychiatry 1998;65:717-721.
56. Boeve BF, Silber MH, Parisi JE, et al: Synucleinopathy pathology and REM sleep behavior disorder plus dementia or parkinsonism. Neurology 2003;61:40-45.
57. Kimura K, Tachibana N, Aso T, et al: Subclinical REM sleep behavior disorder in a patient with corticobasal degeneration. Sleep 1997;20:891-894.
58. Thomas A, Bonanni L, Onofrj M: Symptomatic REM sleep behaviour disorder. Neurol Sci 2007;28(Suppl 1):S21-S36.
59. Gatto EM, Uribe Roca MC, Martinez O, et al: Rapid eye movement (REM) sleep without atonia in two patients with corticobasal degeneration (CBD). Parkinsonism Relat Disord 2007;13:130-132.
60. Vidailhet M, Rivaud S, Gouider-Khouja N, et al: Eye movements in parkinsonian syndromes. Ann Neurol 1994;35:420-426.
61. Rivaud-Pechoux S, Vidailhet M, Gallouedec G, et al: Longitudinal ocular motor study in corticobasal degeneration and progressive supranuclear palsy. Neurology 2000;54:1029-1032.
62. Shibasaki Warabi Y, Nagao M, Bandoh M, et al: Procerus sign in corticobasal degeneration. Intern Med 2002;41:1217-1218.

63. Borroni B, Broli M, Costanzi C, et al: Primitive reflex evaluation in the clinical assessment of extrapyramidal syndromes. Eur J Neurol 2006;13:1026-1028.
64. Rossor MN, Tyrrell PJ, Warrington EK, et al: Progressive frontal gait disturbance with atypical Alzheimer's disease and corticobasal degeneration. J Neurol Neurosurg Psychiatry 1999;67: 345-352.
65. Kertesz A, Davidson W, Munoz DG: Clinical and pathological overlap between frontotemporal dementia, primary progressive aphasia and corticobasal degeneration: the Pick complex. Dement Geriatr Cogn Disord 1999;10(Suppl 1):46-49.
66. Boeve BF, Maraganore DM, Parisi JE, et al: Pathologic heterogeneity in clinically diagnosed corticobasal degeneration. Neurology 1999;53:795-800.
67. Vandenberghe W, Sciot R, Demaerel P, Van Laere K: Sparing of the substantia nigra in sporadic Creutzfeldt-Jakob disease presenting as an acute corticobasal syndrome. Mov Disord 2007;22:1668-1669.
68. Moreaud O, Monavon A, Brutti-Mairesse MP, et al: Creutzfeldt-Jakob disease mimicking corticobasal degeneration clinical and MRI data of a case. J Neurol 2005;252:1283-1284.
69. Magherini A, Pentore R, Galassi G, et al: MV2 subtype of sporadic Creutzfeldt-Jakob disease presenting as corticobasal syndrome. Mov Disord 2007;22:898-899.
70. Avanzino L, Marinelli L, Buccolieri A, et al: Creutzfeldt-Jakob disease presenting as corticobasal degeneration: a neurophysiological study. Neurol Sci 2006;27:118-121.
71. Josephs KA, Katsuse O, Beccano-Kelly DA, et al: Atypical progressive supranuclear palsy with corticospinal tract degeneration. J Neuropathol Exp Neurol 2006;65:396-405.
72. Tsuboi Y, Josephs KA, Boeve BF, et al: Increased tau burden in the cortices of progressive supranuclear palsy presenting with corticobasal syndrome. Mov Disord 2005;20:982-988.
73. Grimes DA, Bergeron CB, Lang AE: Motor neuron disease-inclusion dementia presenting as cortical-basal ganglionic degeneration. Mov Disord 1999;14:674-680.
74. Josephs KA, Holton JL, Rossor MN, et al: Neurofilament inclusion body disease: a new proteinopathy? Brain 2003;126:2291-2303.
75. Baba Y, Ghetti B, Baker MC, et al: Hereditary diffuse leukoencephalopathy with spheroids: clinical, pathologic and genetic studies of a new kindred. Acta Neuropathol 2006;111:300-311.
76. Mridula KR, Alladi S, Varma DR, et al: Corticobasal syndrome due to a thalamic tuberculoma and focal cortical atrophy. J Neurol Neurosurg Psychiatry 2008;79:107-108.
77. Benito-Leon J, Alvarez-Linera J, Louis ED: Neurosyphilis masquerading as corticobasal degeneration. Mov Disord 2004;19:1367-1370.
78. Morris HR, Lees AJ: Primary antiphospholipid syndrome presenting as a corticobasal degeneration syndrome. Mov Disord 1999;14:530-532.
79. Warren JD, Mummery CJ, Al-Din AS, et al: Corticobasal degeneration syndrome with basal ganglia calcification: Fahr's disease as a corticobasal look-alike? Mov Disord 2002;17:563-567.
80. Shamim A, Siddiqui BK, Josephs KA: The corticobasal syndrome triggered by central pontine myelinolysis. Eur J Neurol 2006;13:82-84.
81. Van Zanducke M, Dehaene I: A "cortico-basal degeneration"-like syndrome as first sign of progressive multifocal leukoencephalopathy. Acta Neurol Belg 2000;100:242-245.
82. Kertesz A, McMonagle P, Blair M, et al: The evolution and pathology of frontotemporal dementia. Brain 2005;128:1996-2005.
83. Hodges JR, Davies RR, Xuereb JH, et al: Clinicopathological correlates in frontotemporal dementia. Ann Neurol 2004;56:399-406.
84. Kertesz A, Hudson L, Mackenzie IR, Munoz DG: The pathology and nosology of primary progressive aphasia. Neurology 1994;44:2065-2072.
85. Litvan I, Agid Y, Goetz C, et al: Accuracy of the clinical diagnosis of corticobasal degeneration: a clinicopathologic study. Neurology 1997;48:119-125.
86. Josephs KA, Dickson DW: Diagnostic accuracy of progressive supranuclear palsy in the Society for Progressive Supranuclear Palsy brain bank. Mov Disord 2003;18:1018-1026.
87. Cooper AD, Josephs KA: Photophobia, visual hallucinations, and REM sleep behavior disorder in progressive supranuclear palsy and corticobasal degeneration: a prospective study. Parkinsonism Relat Disord 2009;15:59-61.
88. Mitani K, Furiya Y, Uchihara T, et al: Increased CSF tau protein in corticobasal degeneration. J Neurol 1998;245:44-46.
89. Arai H, Morikawa Y, Higuchi M, et al: Cerebrospinal fluid tau levels in neurodegenerative diseases with distinct tau-related pathology. Biochem Biophys Res Commun 1997;236:262-264.
90. Borroni B, Gardoni F, Parnetti L, et al: Pattern of Tau forms in CSF is altered in progressive supranuclear palsy. Neurobiol Aging 2009;30:34-40.

91. Urakami K, Mori M, Wada K, et al: A comparison of tau protein in cerebrospinal fluid between corticobasal degeneration and progressive supranuclear palsy. Neurosci Lett 1999;259:127-129.

92. Urakami K, Wada K, Arai H, et al: Diagnostic significance of tau protein in cerebrospinal fluid from patients with corticobasal degeneration or progressive supranuclear palsy. J Neurol Sci. 2001;183:95-98.

93. Noguchi M, Yoshita M, Matsumoto Y, et al: Decreased beta-amyloid peptide 42 in cerebrospinal fluid of patients with progressive supranuclear palsy and corticobasal degeneration. J Neurol Sci 2005;237:61-65.

94. Brettschneider J, Petzold A, Sussmuth SD, et al: Neurofilament heavy-chain NfH(SMI35) in cerebrospinal fluid supports the differential diagnosis of Parkinsonian syndromes. Mov Disord 2006;21:2224-2227.

95. Yasui K, Inoue Y, Kanbayashi T, et al: CSF orexin levels of Parkinson's disease, dementia with Lewy bodies, progressive supranuclear palsy and corticobasal degeneration. J Neurol Sci 2006;250:120-123.

96. Tashiro K, Ogata K, Goto Y, et al: EEG findings in early-stage corticobasal degeneration and progressive supranuclear palsy: a retrospective study and literature review. Clin Neurophysiol 2006;117:2236-2242.

97. Walter U, Dressler D, Wolters A, et al: Sonographic discrimination of corticobasal degeneration vs progressive supranuclear palsy. Neurology 2004;63:504-509.

98. Lu CS, Ikeda A, Terada A, et al: Electrophysiological studies of early stage corticobasal degeneration. Mov Disord 1998;13:140-146.

99. Grosse P, Kuhn A, Cordivari C, Brown P: Coherence analysis in the myoclonus of corticobasal degeneration. Mov Disord 2003;18:1345-1350.

100. Monza D, Ciano C, Scaioli V, et al: Neurophysiological features in relation to clinical signs in clinically diagnosed corticobasal degeneration. Neurol Sci 2003;24:16-23.

101. Wang L, Kuroiwa Y, Kamitani T, et al: Visual event-related potentials in progressive supranuclear palsy, corticobasal degeneration, striatonigral degeneration, and Parkinson's disease. J Neurol 2000;247:356-363.

102. Frasson E, Bertolasi L, Bertasi V, et al: Paired transcranial magnetic stimulation for the early diagnosis of corticobasal degeneration. Clin Neurophysiol 2003;114:272-278.

103. Wolters A, Classen J, Kunesch E, et al: Measurements of transcallosally mediated cortical inhibition for differentiating parkinsonian syndromes. Mov Disord 2004;19:518-528.

104. Trompetto C, Buccolieri A, Marchese R, et al: Impairment of transcallosal inhibition in patients with corticobasal degeneration. Clin Neurophysiol 2003;114:2181-2187.

105. Takeda M, Tachibana H, Okuda B, et al: Electrophysiological comparison between corticobasal degeneration and progressive supranuclear palsy. Clin Neurol Neurosurg 1998;100:94-98.

106. Kuhn AA, Grosse P, Holtz K, et al: Patterns of abnormal motor cortex excitability in atypical parkinsonian syndromes. Clin Neurophysiol 2004;115:1786-1795.

107. Soliveri P, Monza D, Paridi D, et al: Cognitive and magnetic resonance imaging aspects of corticobasal degeneration and progressive supranuclear palsy. Neurology 1999;53:502-507.

108. Yamauchi H, Fukuyama H, Nagahama Y, et al: Atrophy of the corpus callosum, cortical hypometabolism, and cognitive impairment in corticobasal degeneration. Arch Neurol 1998;55:609-614.

109. Kobayashi K, Fukutani Y, Miyazu K, Arai N: Corticobasal degeneration with hippocampal involvement. Clin Neuropathol 1999;18:106-108.

110. Winkelmann J, Auer DP, Lechner C, et al: Magnetic resonance imaging findings in corticobasal degeneration. Mov Disord 1999;14:669-673.

111. Josephs KA, Tang-Wai DF, Edland SD, et al: Correlation between antemortem magnetic resonance imaging findings and pathologically confirmed corticobasal degeneration. Arch Neurol 2004;61:1881-1884.

112. Savoiardo M: Differential diagnosis of Parkinson's disease and atypical parkinsonian disorders by magnetic resonance imaging. Neurol Sci 2003;24(Suppl 1):S35-S37.

113. Savoiardo M, Girotti F, Strada L, Ciceri E: Magnetic resonance imaging in progressive supranuclear palsy and other parkinsonian disorders. J Neural Transm Suppl 1994;42:93-110.

114. Schrag A, Good CD, Miszkiel K, et al: Differentiation of atypical parkinsonian syndromes with routine MRI. Neurology 2000;54:697-702.

115. Yekhlef F, Ballan G, Macia F, et al: Routine MRI for the differential diagnosis of Parkinson's disease, MSA, PSP, and CBD. J Neural Transm 2003;110:151-169.

116. Boxer AL, Geschwind MD, Belfor N, et al: Patterns of brain atrophy that differentiate corticobasal degeneration syndrome from progressive supranuclear palsy. Arch Neurol 2006;63:81-86.

117. Josephs KA, Whitwell JL, Dickson DW, et al: Voxel-based morphometry in autopsy proven PSP and CBD. Neurobiol Aging 2008;29:280-289.
118. Whitwell JL, Jack CR Jr, Parisi JE, et al: Rates of cerebral atrophy differ in different degenerative pathologies. Brain 2007;130:1148-1158.
119. Coulier IM, de Vries JJ, Leenders KL: Is FDG-PET a useful tool in clinical practice for diagnosing corticobasal ganglionic degeneration? Mov Disord 2003;18:1175-1178.
120. Laureys S, Salmon E, Garraux G, et al: Fluorodopa uptake and glucose metabolism in early stages of corticobasal degeneration. J Neurol 1999;246:1151-1158.
121. Nagasawa H, Tanji H, Nomura H, et al: PET study of cerebral glucose metabolism and fluorodopa uptake in patients with corticobasal degeneration. J Neurol Sci 1996;139:210-217.
122. Hirono N, Ishii K, Sasaki M, et al: Features of regional cerebral glucose metabolism abnormality in corticobasal degeneration. Dement Geriatr Cogn Disord 2000;11:139-146.
123. Garraux G, Salmon E, Peigneux P, et al: Voxel-based distribution of metabolic impairment in corticobasal degeneration. Mov Disord 2000;15:894-904.
124. Blin J, Vidailhet MJ, Pillon B, et al: Corticobasal degeneration: decreased and asymmetrical glucose consumption as studied with PET. Mov Disord 1992;7:348-354.
125. Hosaka K, Ishii K, Sakamoto S, et al: Voxel-based comparison of regional cerebral glucose metabolism between PSP and corticobasal degeneration. J Neurol Sci 2002;199:67-71.
126. Nagahama Y, Fukuyama H, Turjanski N, et al: Cerebral glucose metabolism in corticobasal degeneration: comparison with progressive supranuclear palsy and normal controls. Mov Disord 1997;12:691-696.
127. Juh R, Pae CU, Kim TS, et al: Cerebral glucose metabolism in corticobasal degeneration comparison with progressive supranuclear palsy using statistical mapping analysis. Neurosci Lett 2005;383:22-27.
128. Eckert T, Barnes A, Dhawan V, et al: FDG PET in the differential diagnosis of parkinsonian disorders. Neuroimage 2005;26:912-921.
129. Gerhard A, Watts J, Trender-Gerhard I, et al: In vivo imaging of microglial activation with [11C](R)-PK11195 PET in corticobasal degeneration. Mov Disord 2004;19:1221-1226.
130. Henkel K, Karitzky J, Schmid M, et al: Imaging of activated microglia with PET and [11C]PK 11195 in corticobasal degeneration. Mov Disord 2004;19:817-821.
131. Sawle GV, Brooks DJ, Marsden CD, Frackowiak RS: Corticobasal degeneration: a unique pattern of regional cortical oxygen hypometabolism and striatal fluorodopa uptake demonstrated by positron emission tomography. Brain 1991;114(Pt 1B):541-556.
132. Koyama M, Yagishita A, Nakata Y, et al: Imaging of corticobasal degeneration syndrome. Neuroradiology 2007;49:905-912.
133. Okuda B, Tachibana H, Takeda M, et al: Focal cortical hypoperfusion in corticobasal degeneration demonstrated by three-dimensional surface display with 123I-IMP: a possible cause of apraxia. Neuroradiology 1995;37:642-644.
134. Okuda B, Tachibana H, Kawabata K, et al: Cerebral blood flow in corticobasal degeneration and progressive supranuclear palsy. Alzheimer Dis Assoc Disord 2000;14:46-52.
135. Okuda B, Tachibana H, Kawabata K, et al: Comparison of brain perfusion in corticobasal degeneration and Alzheimer's disease. Dement Geriatr Cogn Disord 2001;12:226-231.
136. Plotkin M, Amthauer H, Klaffke S, et al: Combined 123I-FP-CIT and 123I-IBZM SPECT for the diagnosis of parkinsonian syndromes: study on 72 patients. J Neural Transm 2005;112:677-692.
137. Lai SC, Weng YH, Yen TC, et al: Imaging early-stage corticobasal degeneration with [99mTc]TRODAT-1 SPET. Nucl Med Commun 2004;25:339-345.
138. Markus HS, Lees AJ, Lennox G, et al: Patterns of regional cerebral blood flow in corticobasal degeneration studied using HMPAO SPECT: comparison with Parkinson's disease and normal controls. Mov Disord 1995;10:179-187.
139. Kreisler A, Defebvre L, Lecouffe P, et al: Corticobasal degeneration and Parkinson's disease assessed by HmPaO SPECT: the utility of factorial discriminant analysis. Mov Disord 2005;20:1431-1438.
140. Pirker W, Asenbaum S, Bencsits G, et al: [123I]beta-CIT SPECT in multiple system atrophy, progressive supranuclear palsy, and corticobasal degeneration. Mov Disord 2000;15:1158-1167.
141. Zhang L, Murata Y, Ishida R, et al: Differentiating between progressive supranuclear palsy and corticobasal degeneration by brain perfusion SPET. Nucl Med Commun 2001;22:767-772.
142. Abe K, Terakawa H, Takanashi M, et al: Proton magnetic resonance spectroscopy of patients with parkinsonism. Brain Res Bull 2000;52:589-595.

143. Tedeschi G, Litvan I, Bonavita S, et al: Proton magnetic resonance spectroscopic imaging in progressive supranuclear palsy, Parkinson's disease and corticobasal degeneration. Brain 1997;120 (Pt 9):1541-1552.

144. Moretti R, Ukmar M, Torre P, et al: Cortical-basal ganglionic degeneration: a clinical, functional and cognitive evaluation (1-year follow-up). J Neurol Sci 2000;182:29-35.

145. Ukmar M, Moretti R, Torre P, et al: Corticobasal degeneration: structural and functional MRI and single-photon emission computed tomography. Neuroradiology 2003;45:708-712.

146. Iwasaki Y, Yoshida M, Hattori M, et al: Widespread spinal cord involvement in corticobasal degeneration. Acta Neuropathol 2005;109:632-638.

147. Togo T, Dickson DW: Ballooned neurons in progressive supranuclear palsy are usually due to concurrent argyrophilic grain disease. Acta Neuropathol (Berl) 2002;104:53-56.

148. Ishizawa K, Dickson DW: Microglial activation parallels system degeneration in progressive supranuclear palsy and corticobasal degeneration. J Neuropathol Exp Neurol 2001;60:647-657.

149. Ksiezak-Reding H, Morgan K, Mattiace LA, et al: Ultrastructure and biochemical composition of paired helical filaments in corticobasal degeneration. Am J Pathol 1994;145:1496-1508.

150. Yang L, Ksiezak-Reding H: Ubiquitin immunoreactivity of paired helical filaments differs in Alzheimer's disease and corticobasal degeneration. Acta Neuropathol (Berl) 1998;96:520-526.

151. Komori T, Arai N, Oda M, et al: Astrocytic plaques and tufts of abnormal fibers do not coexist in corticobasal degeneration and progressive supranuclear palsy. Acta Neuropathol 1998;96:401-408.

152. Hattori M, Hashizume Y, Yoshida M, et al: Distribution of astrocytic plaques in the corticobasal degeneration brain and comparison with tuft-shaped astrocytes in the progressive supranuclear palsy brain. Acta Neuropathol 2003;106:143-149.

153. Arai T, Ikeda K, Akiyama H, et al: Identification of amino-terminally cleaved tau fragments that distinguish progressive supranuclear palsy from corticobasal degeneration. Ann Neurol 2004;55:72-79.

154. Buee Scherrer V, Hof PR, Buee L, et al: Hyperphosphorylated tau proteins differentiate corticobasal degeneration and Pick's disease. Acta Neuropathol (Berl) 1996;91:351-359.

155. Dickson DW: Neuropathologic differentiation of progressive supranuclear palsy and corticobasal degeneration. J Neurol 1999;246(Suppl 2):II-6-II-15.

156. Feany MB, Mattiace LA, Dickson DW: Neuropathologic overlap of progressive supranuclear palsy, Pick's disease and corticobasal degeneration. J Neuropathol Exp Neurol 1996;55:53-67.

157. Di Maria E, Tabaton M, Vigo T, et al: Corticobasal degeneration shares a common genetic background with progressive supranuclear palsy. Ann Neurol 2000;47:374-377.

158. Houlden H, Baker M, Morris HR, et al: Corticobasal degeneration and progressive supranuclear palsy share a common tau haplotype. Neurology 2001;56:1702-1706.

159. Pittman AM, Myers AJ, Abou-Sleiman P, et al: Linkage disequilibrium fine mapping and haplotype association analysis of the tau gene in progressive supranuclear palsy and corticobasal degeneration. J Med Genet 2005;42:837-846.

160. Hutton M, Lendon CL, Rizzu P, et al: Association of missense and 5'-splice-site mutations in tau with the inherited dementia FTDP-17. Nature 1998;393:702-705.

161. Baker M, Mackenzie IR, Pickering-Brown SM, et al: Mutations in progranulin cause tau-negative frontotemporal dementia linked to chromosome 17. Nature 2006;442:916-919.

162. Cruts M, Gijselinck I, van der Zee J, et al: Null mutations in progranulin cause ubiquitin-positive frontotemporal dementia linked to chromosome 17q21. Nature 2006;442:920-924.

163. Kelley BJ, Haidar W, Boeve BF, et al: Prominent phenotypic variability associated with mutations in Progranulin. Neurobiol Aging 2009;30:739-751.

164. Masellis M, Momeni P, Meschino W, et al: Novel splicing mutation in the progranulin gene causing familial corticobasal syndrome. Brain 2006;129:3115-3123.

165. Benussi L, Binetti G, Sina E, et al: A novel deletion in progranulin gene is associated with FTDP-17 and CBS. Neurobiol Aging 2008;29:427-435.

166. Schneider JA, Gearing M, Robbins RS, et al: Apolipoprotein E genotype in diverse neurodegenerative disorders. Ann Neurol 1995;38:131-135.

167. Frucht S, Fahn S, Chin S, et al: Levodopa-induced dyskinesias in autopsy-proven cortical-basal ganglionic degeneration. Mov Disord 2000;15:340-343.

168. Cordivari C, Misra VP, Catania S, Lees AJ: Treatment of dystonic clenched fist with botulinum toxin. Mov Disord 2001;16:907-913.

169. Okun MS, Tagliati M, Pourfar M, et al: Management of referred deep brain stimulation failures: a retrospective analysis from 2 movement disorders centers. Arch Neurol 2005;62:1250-1255.

23 Frontotemporal Dementia

CHRISTIAN W. WIDER • DENNIS W. DICKSON •
ROSA RADEMAKERS • ZBIGNIEW K. WSZOLEK

Introduction

In his classic monograph published in 1892, Pick[1] described patients with dementia
and severe atrophy of the frontal and temporal lobes. In 1911, Alzheimer reported
the cellular inclusions (later named Pick bodies) found in neurons of patients
with the condition that soon became known as Pick's disease.

Frontotemporal lobar degeneration (FTLD) refers to a group of neurodegenerative diseases in which patients display behavioral or language impairment, with
atrophy of the frontal and temporal lobes.[2,3] The most common clinical presentation of FTLD is the behavioral variant referred to as *frontotemporal dementia* (FTD);
language impairment predominates in progressive nonfluent aphasia (PNFA) and
semantic dementia (SD). The nomenclature is confusing because some authors
refer to the same group of disorders by the term FTD and to its behavioral variant

TABLE 23–1	Terminology Commonly Used in Frontotemporal Lobar Degeneration
Overall clinical	Frontotemporal lobar degeneration (FTLD)
	Frontotemporal dementia (FTD)
	Pick's disease
	Pick complex
Behavioral variant	FTD
	Behavioral variant of frontotemporal dementia (bvFTD)
	Frontal lobe dementia
	Primary progressive behavioral disorder
Nonfluent aphasia	Progressive nonfluent aphasia (PNFA)
	Primary progressive aphasia (PPA)
	Progressive language disorder
Fluent aphasia	Semantic dementia (SD)
	Semantic aphasia
	Temporal variant of FTD
Overall pathology	FTLD
	FTD
	Pick complex
	Focal atrophy

by bvFTD (Table 23–1). In this chapter, FTLD refers to a group of neurodegenerative diseases comprising the clinical and pathological entities FTD, PNFA, and SD.[2]

In addition to the behavioral and language symptoms, many FTLD patients present with associated clinical and pathological features of motor neuron disease (FTD-MND).[4,5] FTLD also shows distinct clinical and pathological similarities with the motor syndromes corticobasal degeneration (CBD) and progressive supranuclear gaze palsy (PSP), which are considered to be part of the same disease spectrum.[6] PSP and CBD are discussed in detail in Chapters 21 and 22.

FTLD is the second most common cause of early-onset dementia (<65 years old) after Alzheimer's disease, accounting for 10% to 20% of the cases. It also represents the third most common cause of overall cortical dementia. The disease starts in individuals in their 50s or 60s and has a relentless progression. Cognitive and motor impairment rapidly become a burden to the patients and their families, requiring increasing levels of care, particularly in end-stage disease.

Although most cases are sporadic, a positive family history is found in 35% to 50% of patients. This applies mainly to FTD and PNFA; only about 10% of SD patients reported a positive family history in one large study.[7] Two genes account for most familial FTLD cases: the tau gene (*MAPT*) and the most recently described progranulin gene (*PGRN*). Rare mutations in the charged multivesicular body protein 2B (*CHMP2B*) and the valosin-containing protein (*VCP*) have also been identified.

This chapter discusses the most relevant and recent advances in clinical diagnosis, imaging, pathology, genetics, and treatment strategies in FTLD. A special emphasis is on the genetically determined forms of FTLD because the past decade has witnessed tremendous progress in this area.

Epidemiology

FTLD is an early-onset dementia that occurs in men and women with a fairly similar incidence. In a series from the United Kingdom, the prevalence of FTLD was found to be 15 per 100,000 among subjects 45 to 64 years old.[8] Prevalence rates were comparable in a study from The Netherlands, with a prevalence rate of 3.6 per 100,000 between ages 50 and 59, 9.4 per 100,000 between ages 60 and 69, and 3.8 per 100,000 between ages 70 and 79.[9]

The incidence of FTLD (new patients per 100,000 person-years) in Rochester, Minnesota, was found to be 2.2 for ages 40 to 49, 3.3 for ages 50 to 59, and 8.9 for ages 60 to 69.[10] In comparison, the incidence of Alzheimer's disease in the same series was expectedly lower for ages 40 to 49, similar for ages 50 to 59, and higher for ages 60 to 69.

Diagnostic Criteria and Clinical Features

DIAGNOSTIC CRITERIA

The consensus diagnostic criteria published by Neary and colleagues[2] in 1998 are presented in Table 23–2. Although these criteria are mainly clinical, a relationship between the symptoms and the predominantly affected areas exists with FTD mainly affecting the frontal lobes, PNFA affecting the left frontal lobe, and SD affecting the left temporal lobe. Although these criteria have greatly improved the diagnosis of FTLD for clinical and research purposes, several drawbacks have emerged. Most of them relate to the highly dynamic nature of FTLD, and to the poor sensitivity of the criteria in the early stages of the disease.[6] The aphasic and behavioral symptoms may overlap, or patients may present with nonfluent aphasia and later develop behavioral difficulties. Conversely, patients may present with a FTD phenotype and later evolve into SD or PNFA. In this regard, studies have confirmed that although the initial presentation may suggest one type of FTLD, the diagnosis often changes over time.[6,11,12]

Although a large prospective validation is still lacking, several studies have looked at the applicability and accuracy of the Neary criteria. In one study, the positive predictive value of the clinical criteria was 85%, with a specificity of 99%[13]; however in another study, only one third of the patients with FTD fulfilled all of the five core diagnostic criteria early in the disease.[14] Finally, although anterograde amnesia is an exclusion criterion for all types of FTLD, memory complaints were the dominant symptom in 3 of 29 pathologically verified FTD patients.[13]

Other diagnostic criteria have been proposed, in particular by McKhann and coworkers (Table 23–3).[15] The McKhann clinical criteria for FTLD aim at improving and facilitating the diagnosis by general neurologists, to ensure adequate referral. Although they have not been prospectively evaluated, they are easy to use in daily clinical practice. These criteria are prone to miss patients with SD, however.

No consensus criteria have been established for the genetically determined forms of FTLD (including FTDP-17 secondary to mutations in MAPT and PGRN). Table 23–4 presents useful clinical features that should alert the clinician to the possibility of one of these familial forms.

TABLE 23–2	Diagnostic Criteria for Frontotemporal Lobar Degeneration

Frontotemporal dementia

Core Criteria

Insidious onset, gradual progression
Early decline in social interpersonal conduct
Early impairment in regulation of personal conduct
Early emotional blunting
Early loss of insight

Supportive Criteria

Behavioral disorder
    Decline in personal hygiene and grooming
    Mental rigidity and inflexibility
    Distractibility and impersistence
    Hyperorality and dietary changes
    Perseverative and stereotyped behavior
    Utilization behavior
Speech and language
    Altered speech output (aspontaneity and economy of speech, or press of speech), stereotypy, echolalia, perseveration, mutism
Physical signs
    Primitive reflexes, incontinence, parkinsonsim

Progressive Nonfluent Aphasia

Core Criteria

Insidious onset, gradual progression
Nonfluent spontaneous speech, with at least one of the following: agrammatism, phonemic paraphasia, anomia

Supportive Criteria

Speech and language
    Stuttering, oral apraxia, impaired repetition, alexia or agraphia
    Early preservation of word meaning, late mutism
Behavior
    Early preservation of social skills, late behavioral changes similar to frontotemporal dementia
Physical signs
    Late contralateral primitive reflexes, parkinsonism

Semantic Dementia

Core Criteria

Insidious onset, gradual progression
Language disorder
    At least one of the following: fluent empty spontaneous speech, loss of word meaning (impaired naming and comprehension)
Perceptual disorder
    Prosopagnosia (impaired recognition of familiar faces) or agnosia (impaired object recognition)
    Preserved drawing reproduction
    Preserved single word repetition
    Preserved ability to read aloud and write to dictation orthographically regular words

TABLE 23–2	Diagnostic Criteria for Frontotemporal Lobar Degeneration (Continued)

Supportive Criteria
Speech and language
Press of speech, idiosyncratic word usage, no phonemic paraphasia, preserved
  calculation, surface dyslexia
Behavior
  Loss of sympathy and empathy, narrowed preoccupation, parsimony
Physical signs
  Absent of late primitive reflexes, parkinsonism

Adapted from Neary D, Snowden JS, Gustafson L, et al. Frontotemporal lobar degeneration: a consensus on clinical diagnostic criteria. *Neurology.* 1998;51:1546-1554.

TABLE 23–3	Clinical Diagnostic Criteria for Frontotemporal Lobar Degeneration

Behavioral or cognitive deficits
  (*either*) Early progressive personality changes with difficulty in modulating behavior,
    inappropriate responses or activities
  (*or*) Early progressive language difficulties, with expression impairment or severe
    naming difficulties and problems with words meaning
Behavioral or cognitive deficits cause significant social or occupational functioning
  impairment, and clearly represent a decline
Gradual onset, progression
No other cause identified including psychiatric
Deficits do not occur exclusively during a delirium

Adapted from McKhann GM, Albert MS, Grossman M, et al. Clinical and pathological diagnosis of frontotemporal dementia: report of the Work Group on Frontotemporal Dementia and Pick's Disease. *Arch Neurol.* 2001;58:1803-1809.

CLINICAL FEATURES

Kertesz and associates[12] performed a large prospective study involving 319 FTLD patients followed for more than 3 years. At presentation, the proportion of the different FTLD clinical syndromes was 37.6% FTD, 31.6% PNFA, 10.6% possible PNFA, 8.1% corticobasal syndrome (CBS) and PSP, 6.6% SD, and 5.3% possible FTD. Age of onset was significantly younger in the FTD and SD groups compared with the others. At follow-up, two thirds of the patients presented with additional FTLD syndromes. During the course of the disease, FTLD patients present with worsening and more widespread dementia, ultimately dying of end-stage disease.

Frontotemporal Dementia

Early symptoms in FTD patients are dominated by impairment in social behavior and character changes (see Table 23–2). Patients present with a lack of insight, mental inflexibility, inertia, loss of volition, emotional blunting, and impulsive

TABLE 23–4	Useful Clinical Features That Support the Diagnosis of Familial Frontotemporal Lobar Degeneration	
	FTDP-17 (Mutation in *MAPT*)	FTDP-17 (Mutation in *PGRN*)
Inheritance	Autosomal dominant	
Mean age at onset (yr)	Usually earlier than sporadic FTLD	
	49 (range 25-76)	59 (range 37-84)
Mean duration (yr)	7 (range 2-30)	
Presentation	Personality or behavioral changes, language impairment (mostly *PGRN*), parkinsonism (mostly *MAPT*)	
Other symptoms	Cognitive impairment, parkinsonism, corticobasal syndrome, amyotrophy	
	Supranuclear gaze palsy	Motor neuron disease (rare)
Treatment	Levodopa ineffective but may have a limited effect for some time	

and inappropriate behavior. Major changes in their religious or political beliefs may occur, and family members often suspect mental illness in early stages. Additional symptoms include a wide range of frontal-type behaviors, mostly of the disinhibited form, along with speech alterations without true aphasia. Dietary changes including binge eating are common among FTD patients.[16] Frontal release signs and parkinsonism are common; parkinsonism has a predominance of akinesia and rigidity, with rest tremor virtually absent. Clinical exclusion criteria include severe amnesia, aphasia, and spatial perceptual alterations.

Progressive Nonfluent Aphasia

PNFA is mostly an expressive language disorder, in which patients present with a nonfluent aphasia that usually remains the main symptom throughout the disease (see Table 23–2). Aphasia comprises anomia, agrammatism, phonemic paraphasias, alexia, and agraphia. At least in the early stages, the significance of words remains unaltered, which is in contrast to SD. Mutism or frontal behavioral impairment are commonly seen in later stages. Akinesia, rigidity, and tremor can also be seen.

Semantic Dementia

In SD, aphasia is mainly characterized by the early loss of the meaning of words, along with retained fluency (see Table 23–2). Naming and comprehension are affected. The speech is empty and contains numerous semantic paraphasias. Prosopagnosia (impaired face recognition) and agnosia (impaired object recognition) are common. Patients often retain the ability to read aloud and write to dictation, without understanding the content. Parkinsonism with akinesia, rigidity, and tremor is commonly seen.

Frontotemporal Dementia Associated with Motor Neuron Disease

MND symptoms occur in about 10% of FTLD patients, most commonly in patients with FTD.[4,5] Patients may present with FTD and more or less subtle MND signs, with FTD and amyotrophic lateral sclerosis, or with amyotrophic lateral sclerosis with FTD features. The clinical observation linking these two diseases is supported by pathology, in which similar inclusions are found in FTLD, FTD-MND, and amyotrophic lateral sclerosis. Also, a locus has been found to be linked to familial FTD-MND (see later).

FAMILIAL FORMS

Useful clinical features of the most common familial forms of FTLD are summarized in Table 23–4.

FTDP-17 Tau-Positive Families

In patients with autosomal dominant FTLD and parkinsonism linked to chromosome 17 (FTDP-17) owing to a mutation in the tau gene (*MAPT*), the cardinal clinical features are behavioral and personality changes, cognitive impairment, and motor symptoms (Fig. 23–1).[17-19] The mean age of onset (49 years, range 25 to 76 years) is younger than that of the overall FTLD population. Parkinsonism consists of bradykinesia, tremor (most often of the postural type), rigidity, and postural instability.[20] In some patients, FTD is the predominant feature, whereas it is parkinsonism in others.[21] The variability of symptoms is high not only between, but also within families. The phenotype may include pyramidal signs, vertical gaze palsy, anosmia, myoclonus, autonomic dysfunction, dystonia, and rarely epileptic seizures.[22-26] In one family, a phenotype suggesting Alzheimer's disease has been described.[27]

FTDP-17 Tau-Negative, Ubiquitin-Positive Families

Among families with a progranulin gene (*PGRN*) mutation, the most common clinical phenotype is FTD with prominent language difficulties.[28] The mean age of onset was 59 years in one study, with a wide range (48 to 83 years).[28] The penetrance of FTLD in *PGRN* mutation carriers is age-dependent with more than 90% of the subjects affected after the age of 70. In about 70% of patients, the initial diagnosis is FTD, followed by language impairment of the PNFA type in 10% to 20%.[28,29] Also, a more recent study showed that language was significantly more impaired among *PGRN* mutation carriers compared with noncarriers.[30] Parkinsonism, mainly of the akinetic-rigid type, tends to occur later in the disease in approximately 50% of *PGRN* mutation carriers, whereas the association with MND is distinctly rare.[28,31,32]

Hallucinations were described in 30% of patients in one study.[33] Families have been described with a corticobasal syndrome (CBS) similar to that seen in CBD.[28,34-36] Other diagnoses include Parkinson's disease and dementia with Lewy bodies. In a clinicopathological study of *PGRN* mutation carriers, the initial diagnoses were FTD in 44%, Alzheimer's-type dementia in 22%, PNFA in 17%,

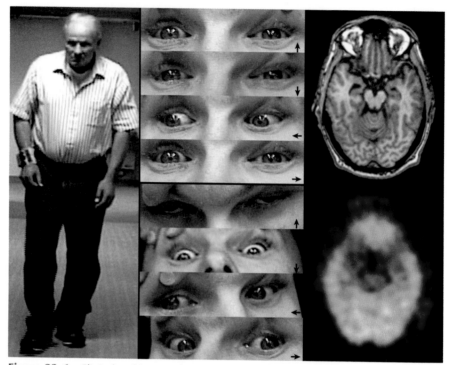

Figure 23–1 Clinical and imaging features of three FTDP-17 patients from the PPND family (N279K *MAPT* mutation). *Left,* Hypomimia and flexed posture of the trunk and of the right arm in a 57-year-old man who, 1 year after developing stiffness, had parkinsonism with postural tremor, emotional lability, and mild cognitive impairment. *Middle,* Supranuclear gaze palsy in a 48-year-old man 7 years into the disease who also had cognitive impairment, emotionality, parkinsonism, and pyramidal signs leading to major motor limitations; the patient was instructed to look in the directions indicated by *arrows* (*upper part,* movement amplitude incomplete); alternatively, the movement was elicited by the doll's head maneuver (*lower part,* movement amplitude almost normal). *Right,* Structural MRI showing bilateral temporal atrophy (*upper panel*); [18]FDG PET showing bilateral frontal and temporal hypometabolism (*lower panel*). This patient was a 47-year-old man who had developed left leg stiffness at age 41, and who displayed parkinsonism, pyramidal signs, vertical gaze palsy, dysphagia, dystonia, personality and cognitive dysfunction, and mutism.

and parkinsonism in 17% .[37] Of the patients, 82% eventually developed language impairment.

Imaging

STRUCTURAL IMAGING

The diagnosis of FTLD historically has been made in patients showing normal morphological imaging, and it remains true that in many cases, no significant atrophy can be seen at least in the early stages of the disease. As the disease progresses, however, atrophy can often be identified by standard computed tomography and magnetic resonance imaging (MRI) scans. In accordance with the anatomy, atrophy usually predominates in the frontal and temporal lobes in FTD, in the left frontal lobe in PNFA, and in the left temporal lobe in SD. This pattern displays wide variability and overlap, however; atrophy may occur in frontal or temporal lobes with or without asymmetry, or can extend to the parietal lobes. In SD patients, using voxel-based morphometry, a good correlation was found between left-predominant temporopolar cortex atrophy and severity of the semantic deficit.[38] Atrophy did not correlate with the type of FTLD in a volumetric study, however, in which frontal, limbic, and temporal cortices were affected early in the disease, and posterior and white matter involvement occurred later.[39] In FTDP-17 patients, frontotemporal atrophy can be seen (see Fig. 23–1). In a prospective study, Davies and coworkers[40] found that FTD patients with a normal or borderline MRI scan had a longer survival than patients with frontal and temporal atrophy. Age, cognitive performance, and behavioral impairment did not predict a better outcome.

In a detailed study of a patient with a strong family history of FTLD, MRI showed regional frontal atrophy before the onset of symptoms.[41] Later, asymmetrical frontal and parietal atrophy occurred and paralleled clinical progression. In a more recent voxel-based morphometric MRI study, investigators examined FTLD patients with or without binge eating behavioral change.[42] They found that binge eaters, who all had FTD, had significantly greater atrophy in the right ventral insula, striatum, and orbitofrontal cortex compared with non–binge eaters.

FUNCTIONAL IMAGING

Hypometabolism on fludeoxyglucose F 18 positron emission tomography ([18]FDG PET) and hypoperfusion on single photon emission computed tomography (SPECT) have proven useful in the early diagnosis of FTLD.[43,44] In a longitudinal [18]FDG PET study, Diehl-Schmied and colleagues[45] found hypometabolism in the lateral and medial prefrontal cortices, caudate nucleus, insula, and thalamus, which later involved temporal and parietal cortices. In a European [18]FDG PET study involving 41 FTD patients, abnormalities were found in the ventromedial and orbital prefrontal cortex, in the dorsolateral prefrontal cortex, and in the left anterior insula.[46]

The severity of apathy and disinhibition correlated with the degree of hypometabolism in the posterior orbitofrontal cortex. In another study involving 61 FTD patients who underwent detailed clinical examination and SPECT, a correlation was found between ventromedial prefrontal and temporal hypoperfusion and disinhibition.[47] In a study comparing SPECT results between patients fulfilling the core criteria for FTD at baseline evaluation with patients fulfilling the criteria only after 2 years of follow-up, McMurtray and coworkers[14] found right frontal hypoperfusion to be more common among patients not fulfilling all the criteria at baseline. Right frontal hypoperfusion correlated with apathy and loss of insight, whereas left temporal hypoperfusion correlated with hypomanic-type behavior.[14]

In a presymptomatic carrier of an *MAPT* mutation, frontal hypoperfusion was shown in a SPECT study with statistical parametric mapping.[48] SPECT and [18]FDG PET studies of FTDP-17 patients have shown consistently frontal and temporal hypoperfusion and hypometabolism of the frontotemporal regions (see Fig. 23–1).[26] In addition, a predominantly presynaptic dopaminergic deficit can be found, which accounts for parkinsonian symptoms early in the disease and for the response to levodopa.[19,26,49] A mild postsynaptic component has also been described, which may explain why the response to levodopa is limited in time.[26] In other fluorodopa F 18 PET studies of the pallido-ponto-nigral degeneration (PPND) family carrying the N279K mutation in *MAPT,* reduced striatal tracer uptake was shown in a presymptomatic mutation carrier, although of lesser magnitude than in symptomatic patients.[49,50] These functional imaging techniques are valuable tools to study the presymptomatic phases of the disease, and may help define surrogate end points for the prospective evaluation of neuroprotective treatments.

Genetics

Familial forms of FTLD have been associated with numerous mutations, which are primarily found in two genes on chromosome 17q21, *MAPT* and *PGRN* (Fig. 23–2). These discoveries provide valuable insight into the pathophysiology of FTLD, generating potential targets for future therapeutic strategies aiming at halting the progression of the disease or at preventing its occurrence. In addition, such knowledge allows clinicians to provide patients with better counseling when faced with familial FTLD cases, particularly regarding prognosis, and the possibility to perform prenatal testing.

MICROTUBULE-ASSOCIATED PROTEIN TAU (*MAPT*)

Linkage to a locus on chromosome 17q21 was first reported in 1994 in a family with disinhibition-dementia-parkinsonism-amyotrophy complex.[51] At a consensus conference 2 years later, 12 additional families were reported, and the term *FTDP-17* was coined, recapitulating the main clinical characteristics found in these patients.[52] Mutations in the *MAPT* gene were subsequently identified in 9 of the 13 FTDP-17 families.[53] More than 40 mutations have since been identified in more than 100 families worldwide (see Fig. 23–2) (FTLD mutation database, available at: http://www.molgen.ua.ac.be/FTDMutations).[54] They account for approximately one third of familial FTLD cases, and 5% to 10% of all FTLD cases.[54-57]

MAPT codes for tau, a protein implicated in microtubule assembly and stabilization. In humans, six tau isoforms are produced from a single gene by alternative mRNA splicing of exons 2, 3, and 10 (see Fig. 23–2). These tau isoforms differ by the number of microtubule binding domains and can be divided in two groups—isoforms with three (3R) and isoforms with four (4R) microtubule binding repeats. It has been shown that the 4R tau isoform has better binding and assembling properties with respect to its interaction with microtubules.[58] In human disease, the tau protein becomes hyperphosphorylated and assembles into filaments.[59] Several diseases display tau-positive inclusions, including Pick's disease, Alzheimer's disease, PSP, CBD, argyrophilic grain disease, and familial FTLD with a mutation in *MAPT.*

Mutations in *MAPT* include missense mutations, single-codon deletions, silent mutations, and intronic mutations (see Fig. 23–2). The two most common mutations are P301L and IVS10+16C>T. Most mutations influence the expression of all six isoforms, whereas mutations in exon 10 affect only the expression of 4R tau.[57] Pathogenic *MAPT* mutations are generally divided into mutations that alter the interaction with microtubules or fibril formation, and mutations that affect exon

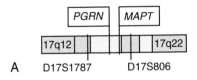

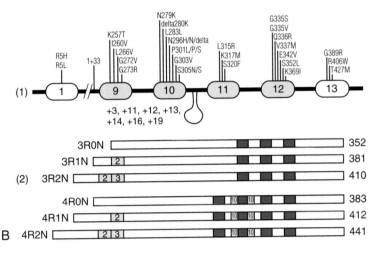

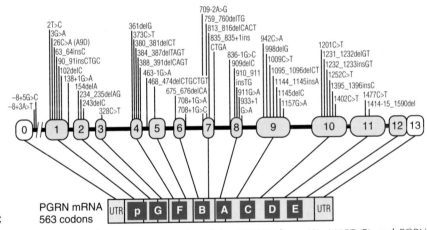

Figure 23–2 A-C, Schematic representation of the FTDP-17 locus (**A**), *MAPT* (**B**), and *PGRN* (**C**). **A,** The FTDP-17 locus on chromosome 17q, illustrating the physical proximity of the two genes *MAPT* and *PGRN*. **B,** The *MAPT* gene with exons numbered, displaying known mutations (*1*). The six tau isoforms, with three or four microtubule-binding domains, and alternative splicing of exons 2, 3, and 10 (*2*). **C,** The *PGRN* gene with exons numbered, displaying known mutations. The mRNA is shown with the granulin domains labeled with capital letters.

10 splicing. Most of the mutations in exons 9, 11, 12, and 13 reduce the ability of the mutant protein to promote microtubule assembly, and some display profibrillogenic properties.[60,61] Intronic mutations, which all are located in the introns flanking the alternatively spliced exon 10, act on exon 10 splicing, increasing the relative proportion of 4R tau isoforms. Several coding *MAPT* mutations also increase the 4R/3R tau isoform ratio by affecting splicing regulating elements in exon 10. It has been suggested that 4R is more fibrillogenic than 3R tau.[59]

It has been observed that mutations in exons 9 and 13 are usually associated with a phenotype devoid of motor symptoms, whereas mutations altering *MAPT* splicing are more commonly found in patients with FTD and parkinsonism.[62] Similarly, mutations altering the first two microtubule binding domains seem to be associated with an earlier age of onset and a shorter disease duration than other mutations.[63]

PROGRANULIN *(PGRN)*

In many families with a phenotype similar to that found in FTDP-17 and linkage to the same locus, mutations in *MAPT* could not be identified. The explanation for this puzzling finding came from the discovery of mutations in *PGRN*, a gene located only 1.7 Mb centromeric of *MAPT* on chromosome 17q21 (see Fig. 23–2).[64,65] A year after the discovery of PGRN, 44 pathogenic mutations were described (see Fig. 23–2) (FTLD mutation database, available at: http://www.molgen.ua.ac.be/FTDMutations).

These mutations account for approximately 5% to 10% of FTLD cases and 20% of familial FTLD cases.[66] Mutations have been identified in rare, apparently sporadic cases, raising the issue of incomplete penetrance.[33] Proven pathogenic mutations include insertions, deletions, out-of-frame splice site mutations, nonsense mutations, and a missense mutation in the signal peptide sequence. These mutations all create functional null alleles resulting in a reduced amount of normal *PGRN* protein production (haploinsufficiency); in most of the mutations, this is due to the introduction of a premature stop codon inducing mRNA degradation by nonsense mediated decay.[28]

PGRN codes for a precursor protein that can be proteolytically cleaved in a family of granulins. Although the precise role of *PGRN* in the brain remains unknown, it is thought to act as a mitogenic factor in various tissues, regulating cell cycle and cell migration, wound repair and inflammation, and tumorigenesis.[67]

The three most common mutations are Arg493X, IVS0+5G>C, and IVS6-1G.A.[32,65,68] In a more recent international study on families with the Arg493X mutation, clinical diagnoses included FTD, PNFA, CBS, and Alzheimer's disease, and the age at onset ranged from 44 to 69 years.[68] Haplotype analysis showed that the mutation occurred twice, with a single founder for 27 of the families.[68] A more recent report suggests IVS6-1G>A may be associated with the CBS phenotype.[32]

CHARGED MULTIVESICULAR BODY PROTEIN 2B *(CHMP2B)*

The first mutation in *CHMP2B* was described in a Danish FTD family in 2004.[69] Since then, a few more mutations have been identified in FTD cases and in one patient with amyotrophic lateral sclerosis, although their pathogenicity remains controversial, especially since the discovery of a mutation in two unaffected members of a FTD family and not in their affected relatives. This discovery has led to the thought that mutations in *CHMP2B* are a rare cause of FTLD, which was supported by a study that found no *CHMP2B* mutations in 141 familial FTLD cases.[70] Although the exact role of the protein remains unknown, overexpression of the two Danish and of one Belgian *CHMP2B* mutant proteins led to dysmorphic organelles, suggesting a role at the level of endosomal trafficking.[69,71]

VALOSIN-CONTAINING PROTEIN (*VCP*)

FTD with inclusion body myopathy and Paget's disease of the bone (IBMPFD) is a rare autosomal dominant disease with adult-onset muscle weakness, Paget's disease of the bone, and early-onset FTD in approximately 30% of the patients.[72] Since the initial *VCP* mutations were reported in 13 IBMPFD families,[73] several new mutations and families have been reported.[74,75] *VCP* acts as a molecular chaperone in cellular activities including cell cycle regulation, protein degradation, and apoptosis. It is currently thought that *VCP* mutations cause disease by an altered ubiquitin-proteasome system activity, leading to the accumulation of ubiquitinated proteins in the cell.

LOCUS FOR FRONTOTEMPORAL DEMENTIA ASSOCIATED WITH MOTOR NEURON DISEASE ON CHROMOSOME 9

A growing number of families have been reported in the past few years with linkage to a locus on chromosome 9p13.3-p21.3.[76,66] Although the various studies have narrowed down the region to approximately 8.1 cM, the gene remains to be found.

Pathology

Although FTLD is pathologically heterogeneous, the common underlying finding is cortical degeneration of the frontal and temporal lobes (Figs. 23–3 and 24–4).[15,78] The pathology of FTLD can be separated in two major categories based on the immunohistochemical profile: FTLD with tau-positive pathology (tau-positive FTLD) (see Fig. 23–3), and FTLD with tau-negative, ubiquitin-positive inclusions (FTLD-U) (see Fig. 23–4).[55] A third category consists of dementia lacking distinctive histopathology (DLDH), but further evaluation of most of these cases with better immunohistochemical techniques has reclassified them as FTLD-U, which has emerged as the major pathology found in FTLD.[79] This reappraisal began with the finding of neuronal cytoplasmic inclusions and neurites in the frontotemporal cortex and hippocampus of patients with MND and dementia, which displayed immunoreactivity for ubiquitin, but not for tau and α-synuclein.[80] Approximately 45% of FTLD cases display tau-positive pathology, whereas in about 50% of the patients, ubiquitin-positive inclusions can be shown.[79,81,82] More recently, TAR DNA-binding protein 43 (TDP-43) was identified as the key component of the ubiquitin-positive inclusions in FTLD-U and MND.[83] This finding has prompted a revision of the consensus criteria for pathological diagnosis of FTLD, which now includes TDP-43 proteinopathy as a distinct

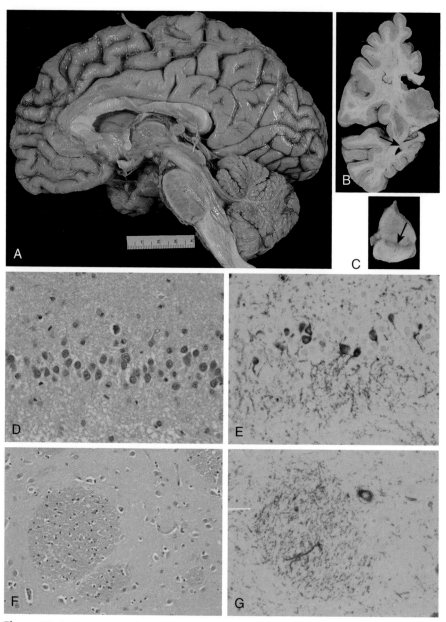

Figure 23–3 Tau-positive frontotemporal lobar degeneration. **A,** Sagittal view of the brain of a patient with the N279K mutation in *MAPT*. There is mild frontal atrophy, more marked medial temporal atrophy, and atrophy of the midbrain. **B,** Coronal section at the level of the thalamus shows marked hippocampal atrophy (*arrow*). **C,** Transverse section of the midbrain shows loss of neuromelanin pigment in the substantia nigra (*arrow*). **D,** The dentate gyrus of the hippocampus shows neuronal loss and gliosis. **E,** Tau immunohistochemistry in the dentate gyrus shows tau immunoreactivity in neuronal perikarya and apical dendrites. **F** and **G,** The striatum is histologically unremarkable (**F**), but tau immunohistochemistry (**G**) reveals neuronal inclusions and numerous threadlike processes, and glial inclusions in the pencil fibers.

category that encompasses FTLD-U with or without MND, FTLD-U caused by *PGRN* or *VCP* mutations, and FTD-MND linked to chromosome 9p.[83]

FTLD with tau-positive pathology includes classic Pick's disease with Pick cells (tau-positive swollen achromatic neurons) and Pick bodies (round argyrophilic inclusions), CBD, PSP, argyrophilic grain disease, and familial cases of FTLD with a mutation in *MAPT*. Tau-positive pathology is marked by neuronal loss, gliosis, and accumulation of hyperphosphorylated tau protein in the cytoplasm of neurons and glial cells (see Fig. 23–3). Patterns have emerged in terms of the tau isoforms preferentially found in those conditions. PSP and CBD show predominant deposition of 4R tau isoforms, whereas 3R tau isoforms accumulate in Pick's disease.[78,83]

Although FTLD-U patients share common neuropathological staining characteristics (see Fig. 23–4), heterogeneity exists that may have clinical relevance.[84,85] Mackenzie and colleagues[84] have identified three main subtypes of FTLD-U pathology, based on the distribution, morphology, and relative proportion of neuronal cytoplasmic inclusions and neurites. In type 1, numerous neuronal cytoplasmic inclusions and short neurites are found mainly in the upper cortical layers. In type 2, elongated neurites and relatively few neuronal cytoplasmic inclusions are found in upper neocortical layers. Type 3 is subdivided in 3a, with neurites widely distributed throughout cortical layers, and 3b where neurites are restricted to the hippocampal dentate fascia. Although imperfect, a clinicopathological correlation was found: most of the type 1 patients had FTD or PNFA, type 2 was associated with SD, and all cases with FTD-MND had type 3 pathology.[84]

In families with *PGRN* mutations, atrophy not only occurs in the frontotemporal lobes, but also in the caudate nucleus, medial thalamus, substantia nigra, and CA1 sector of the hippocampus (see Fig. 23–4).[86] Apart from neuronal cytoplasmic inclusions, a second type of ubiquitin-positive inclusion is found consistently, neuronal intranuclear inclusions. Although not specific to *PGRN* mutation carriers, these lentiform inclusions are highly characteristic and have been described in only rare sporadic FTLD cases. Neuronal intranuclear inclusions are also found in familial FTLD cases caused by *VCP* mutations and in FTD-MND linked to chromosome 9p.[83,87]

CLINICOPATHOLOGICAL CORRELATION

In a large prospective study involving 60 patients with FTD, PNFA, CBS, and PSP, Kertesz and associates[6] looked at the correlation between clinical diagnoses and histology type. FTLD-U type pathology was the most common (18 patients), followed by CBD (12 patients), Pick's disease (6 patients), DLDH (6 patients), and PSP (3 patients). Other types included Alzheimer's pathology, Lewy body variant, prion disease, and vascular dementia. Among the tau-negative cases (FTLD-U and DLDH), FTD was the predominant clinical diagnosis, sometimes evolving into PNFA, CBS, or SD. In the tau-positive patients, PNFA dominated along with CBS and PSP, although behavioral symptoms were common. In another study based on 34 pathological FTLD cases, 29 patients had been clinically diagnosed with FTLD, and the specificity of the clinical diagnosis was 99%.[13] Of the patients, 79% had a clinical history of FTLD; these figures decreased to 62% for the neuropsychological profile and to 50% for MRI. Three of the five patients with a clinical incorrect diagnosis were diagnosed with Alzheimer's disease.

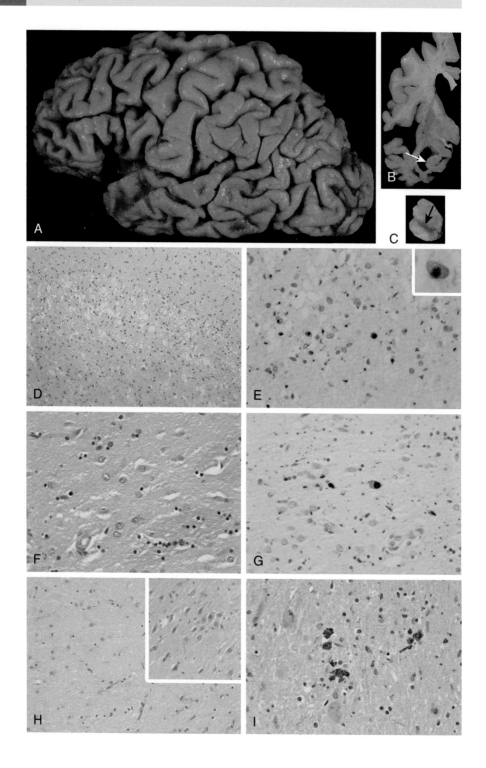

Figure 23–4 Frontotemporal lobar degeneration with tau-negative, ubiquitin-positive inclusions. **A,** External view of the cerebrum of a patient with a *PGRN* mutation shows marked atrophy of the frontal and temporal poles, with sparing of the perirolandic gyri. **B,** Coronal section at the level of the amygdala shows marked temporal lobe atrophy and relative sparing of the hippocampus (*arrow*). The caudate is also flattened. **C,** Transverse section of the midbrain shows loss of neuromelanin pigment in the substantia nigra (*arrow*). **D,** The cortex has spongiosis in superficial cortical lamina. **E,** Ubiquitin immunohistochemistry in frontal cortex shows neuronal cytoplasmic and intranuclear (*inset*) inclusions, and neuritic processes. **F** and **G,** The striatum has mild gliosis (**F**), and ubiquitin immunohistochemistry (**G**) reveals neuronal inclusions. **H,** The CA1 sector of the hippocampus has severe neuronal loss, whereas CA3 (*inset*) is spared, consistent with so-called hippocampal sclerosis. **I,** The substantia nigra has neuronal loss with extraneuronal neuromelanin in macrophages.

Treatment

Treatment currently consists of symptomatic measures because no specific pharmacological treatment is approved for FTLD. Some clinicians may try off-label use of acetylcholinesterase inhibitors or memantine, but no benefit has been established for cognitive symptoms. Atypical antipsychotics and antidepressants should be considered in patients displaying significant behavioral or mood alterations.

Patients with language impairment may benefit from speech therapy. Physical therapy may help for gait impairment, and to improve activities of daily living. Finally, as in other types of dementias, driving ability should be assessed, and driving should be discouraged in patients with significant cognitive impairment.

Acknowledgments

C.W.W. is supported by the Swiss National Science Foundation and the Swiss Parkinson's Disease Foundation. C.W.W. and R.R. are supported by the Robert and Clarice Smith Fellowship program. Z.K.W. and D.W.D. are supported by the Morris K. Udall Center for Excellence in Parkinson's Disease Research (P50-NS40256). D.W.D. and R.R. are supported by the Mayo Clinic ADRC grant P50-AG16574. Z.K.W., R.R., and D.W.D. are supported by the Pacific Alzheimer Research Foundation (PARF) grant C06-01.

REFERENCES

1. Pick A: Uber die Beziehungen der senilen Hirnatrophie zur Aphasie. Prager Med Wochenschr 1892;17:165-167.
2. Neary D, Snowden JS, Gustafson L, et al: Frontotemporal lobar degeneration: a consensus on clinical diagnostic criteria. Neurology 1998;51:1546-1554.
3. Clinical and neuropathological criteria for frontotemporal dementia. The Lund and Manchester Groups. J Neurol Neurosurg Psychiatry 1994;57:416-418.
4. Neary D, Snowden JS, Mann DM, et al: Frontal lobe dementia and motor neuron disease. J Neurol Neurosurg Psychiatry 1990;53:23-32.
5. Lomen-Hoerth C: Characterization of amyotrophic lateral sclerosis and frontotemporal dementia. Dement Geriatr Cogn Disord 2004;17:337-341.
6. Kertesz A, McMonagle P, Blair M, et al: The evolution and pathology of frontotemporal dementia. Brain 2005;128(Pt 9):1996-2005.

7. Snowden J, Neary D, Mann D: Frontotemporal lobar degeneration: clinical and pathological relationships. Acta Neuropathol (Berl) 2007;114:31-38.
8. Ratnavalli E, Brayne C, Dawson K, et al: The prevalence of frontotemporal dementia. Neurology 2002;58:1615-1621.
9. Rosso SM, Donker Kaat L, Baks T, et al: Frontotemporal dementia in The Netherlands: patient characteristics and prevalence estimates from a population-based study. Brain 2003;126 (Pt 9):2016-2022.
10. Knopman DS, Petersen RC, Edland SD, et al: The incidence of frontotemporal lobar degeneration in Rochester, Minnesota, 1990 through 1994. Neurology 2004;62:506-508.
11. Le Rhun E, Richard F, Pasquier F: Natural history of primary progressive aphasia. Neurology 2005;65:887-891.
12. Kertesz A, Blair M, McMonagle P, et al: The diagnosis and course of frontotemporal dementia. Alzheimer Dis Assoc Disord 2007;21:155-163.
13. Knopman DS, Boeve BF, Parisi JE, et al: Antemortem diagnosis of frontotemporal lobar degeneration. Ann Neurol 2005;57:480-488.
14. McMurtray AM, Chen AK, Shapira JS, et al: Variations in regional SPECT hypoperfusion and clinical features in frontotemporal dementia. Neurology 2006;66:517-522.
15. McKhann GM, Albert MS, Grossman M, et al: Clinical and pathological diagnosis of frontotemporal dementia: report of the Work Group on Frontotemporal Dementia and Pick's Disease. Arch Neurol 2001;58:1803-1809.
16. Miller BL, Darby AL, Swartz JR, et al: Dietary changes, compulsions and sexual behavior in frontotemporal degeneration. Dementia 1995;6:195-199.
17. Wszolek ZK, Tsuboi Y, Ghetti B, et al: Frontotemporal dementia and parkinsonism linked to chromosome 17 (FTDP-17). Orphanet J Rare Dis 2006;1:30.
18. Reed LA, Wszolek ZK, Hutton M: Phenotypic correlations in FTDP-17. Neurobiol Aging 2001;22:89-107.
19. Wszolek ZK, Pfeiffer RF, Bhatt MH, et al: Rapidly progressive autosomal dominant parkinsonism and dementia with pallido-ponto-nigral degeneration. Ann Neurol 1992;32:312-320.
20. Tsuboi Y, Uitti RJ, Delisle MB, et al: Clinical features and disease haplotypes of individuals with the N279K tau gene mutation: a comparison of the pallidopontonigral degeneration kindred and a French family. Arch Neurol 2002;59:943-950.
21. Baba Y, Baker MC, Le Ber I, et al: Clinical and genetic features of families with frontotemporal dementia and parkinsonism linked to chromosome 17 with a P301S tau mutation. J Neural Transm 2007;114:947-950.
22. Slowinski J, Dominik J, Uitti RJ, et al: Frontotemporal dementia and Parkinsonism linked to chromosome 17 with the N279K tau mutation. Neuropathology 2007;27:73-80.
23. Arvanitakis Z, Witte RJ, Dickson DW, et al: Clinical-pathologic study of biomarkers in FTDP-17 (PPND family with N279K tau mutation). Parkinsonism Relat Disord 2007;13:230-239.
24. Lossos A, Reches A, Gal A, et al: Frontotemporal dementia and parkinsonism with the P301S tau gene mutation in a Jewish family. J Neurol 2003;250:733-740.
25. Tsuboi Y, Baker M, Hutton ML, et al: Clinical and genetic studies of families with the tau N279K mutation (FTDP-17). Neurology 2002;59:1791-1793.
26. Sperfeld AD, Collatz MB, Baier H, et al: FTDP-17: an early-onset phenotype with parkinsonism and epileptic seizures caused by a novel mutation. Ann Neurol 1999;46:708-715.
27. Doran M, du Plessis DG, Ghadiali EJ, et al: Familial early-onset dementia with tau intron 10 + 16 mutation with clinical features similar to those of Alzheimer disease. Arch Neurol 2007;64:1535-1539.
28. Gass J, Cannon A, Mackenzie IR, et al: Mutations in progranulin are a major cause of ubiquitin-positive frontotemporal lobar degeneration. Hum Mol Genet 2006;15:2988-3001.
29. Mesulam M, Johnson N, Krefft TA, et al: Progranulin mutations in primary progressive aphasia: the PPA1 and PPA3 families. Arch Neurol 2007;64:43-47.
30. Bruni AC, Momeni P, Bernardi L, et al: Heterogeneity within a large kindred with frontotemporal dementia: a novel progranulin mutation. Neurology 2007;69:140-147.
31. Schymick JC, Yang Y, Andersen PM, et al: Progranulin mutations and amyotrophic lateral sclerosis or amyotrophic lateral sclerosis-frontotemporal dementia phenotypes. J Neurol Neurosurg Psychiatry 2007;78:754-756.
32. Lopez de Munain A, Alzualde A, Gorostidi A, et al: Mutations in progranulin gene: clinical, pathological, and ribonucleic acid expression findings. Biol Psychiatry 2007.
33. Le Ber I, van der Zee J, Hannequin D, et al: Progranulin null mutations in both sporadic and familial frontotemporal dementia. Hum Mutat 2007;28:846-855.
34. Masellis M, Momeni P, Meschino W, et al: Novel splicing mutation in the progranulin gene causing familial corticobasal syndrome. Brain 2006;129(Pt 11):3115-3123.

35. Benussi L, Binetti G, Sina E, et al: A novel deletion in progranulin gene is associated with FTDP-17 and CBS. Neurobiol Aging 2006.
36. Spina S, Murrell JR, Huey ED, et al: Corticobasal syndrome associated with the A9D progranulin mutation. J Neuropathol Exp Neurol 2007;66:892-900.
37. Josephs KA, Ahmed Z, Katsuse O, et al: Neuropathologic features of frontotemporal lobar degeneration with ubiquitin-positive inclusions with progranulin gene (PGRN) mutations. J Neuropathol Exp Neurol 2007;66:142-151.
38. Williams GB, Nestor PJ, Hodges JR: Neural correlates of semantic and behavioural deficits in frontotemporal dementia. Neuroimage 2005;24:1042-1051.
39. Kril JJ, Macdonald V, Patel S, et al: Distribution of brain atrophy in behavioral variant frontotemporal dementia. J Neurol Sci 2005;232(1-2):83-90.
40. Davies RR, Kipps CM, Mitchell J, et al: Progression in frontotemporal dementia: identifying a benign behavioral variant by magnetic resonance imaging. Arch Neurol 2006;63:1627-1631.
41. Janssen JC, Schott JM, Cipolotti L, et al: Mapping the onset and progression of atrophy in familial frontotemporal lobar degeneration. J Neurol Neurosurg Psychiatry 2005;76:162-168.
42. Woolley JD, Gorno-Tempini ML, Seeley WW, et al: Binge eating is associated with right orbitofrontal-insular-striatal atrophy in frontotemporal dementia. Neurology 2007;69:1424-1433.
43. Pasquier F, Fukui T, Sarazin M, et al: Laboratory investigations and treatment in frontotemporal dementia. Ann Neurol 2003;54(Suppl 5):S32-S35.
44. Salmon E, Kerrouche N, Herholz K, et al: Decomposition of metabolic brain clusters in the frontal variant of frontotemporal dementia. Neuroimage 2006;30:871-878.
45. Diehl-Schmid J, Grimmer T, Drzezga A, et al: Decline of cerebral glucose metabolism in frontotemporal dementia: a longitudinal 18F-FDG-PET-study. Neurobiol Aging 2007;28:42-50.
46. Peters F, Perani D, Herholz K, et al: Orbitofrontal dysfunction related to both apathy and disinhibition in frontotemporal dementia. Dement Geriatr Cogn Disord 2006;21(5-6):373-379.
47. Le Ber I, Guedj E, Gabelle A, et al: Demographic, neurological and behavioural characteristics and brain perfusion SPECT in frontal variant of frontotemporal dementia. Brain 2006;129 (Pt 11):3051-3065.
48. Alberici A, Gobbo C, Panzacchi A, et al: Frontotemporal dementia: impact of P301L tau mutation on a healthy carrier. J Neurol Neurosurg Psychiatry 2004;75:1607-1610.
49. Pal PK, Wszolek ZK, Kishore A, et al: Positron emission tomography in pallido-ponto-nigral degeneration (PPND) family (frontotemporal dementia with parkinsonism linked to chromosome 17 and point mutation in tau gene). Parkinsonism Relat Disord 2001;7:81-88.
50. Kishore A, Wszolek ZK, Snow BJ, et al: Presynaptic nigrostriatal function in genetically tested asymptomatic relatives from the pallido-ponto-nigral degeneration family. Neurology 1996;47:1588-1590.
51. Wilhelmsen KC, Lynch T, Pavlou E, et al: Localization of disinhibition-dementia-parkinsonism-amyotrophy complex to 17q21-22. Am J Hum Genet 1994;55:1159-1165.
52. Foster NL, Wilhelmsen K, Sima AA, et al: Frontotemporal dementia and parkinsonism linked to chromosome 17: a consensus conference. Conference Participants. Ann Neurol 1997;41:706-715.
53. Hutton M, Lendon CL, Rizzu P, et al: Association of missense and 5'-splice-site mutations in tau with the inherited dementia FTDP-17. Nature 1998;393:702-705.
54. Rademakers R, Cruts M, van Broeckhoven C: The role of tau (MAPT) in frontotemporal dementia and related tauopathies. Hum Mutat 2004;24:277-295.
55. Morris HR, Khan MN, Janssen JC, et al: The genetic and pathological classification of familial frontotemporal dementia. Arch Neurol 2001;58:1813-1816.
56. Poorkaj P, Grossman M, Steinbart E, et al: Frequency of tau gene mutations in familial and sporadic cases of non-Alzheimer dementia. Arch Neurol 2001;58:383-387.
57. van Swieten J, Spillantini MG: Hereditary frontotemporal dementia caused by Tau gene mutations. Brain Pathol 2007;17:63-73.
58. Goedert M, Jakes R: Expression of separate isoforms of human tau protein: correlation with the tau pattern in brain and effects on tubulin polymerization. Embo J 1990;9:4225-4230.
59. Lee VM, Goedert M, Trojanowski JQ: Neurodegenerative tauopathies. Annu Rev Neurosci 2001;24:1121-1159.
60. Hasegawa M, Smith MJ, Goedert M: Tau proteins with FTDP-17 mutations have a reduced ability to promote microtubule assembly. FEBS Lett 1998;437:207-210.
61. Rizzini C, Goedert M, Hodges JR, et al: Tau gene mutation K257T causes a tauopathy similar to Pick's disease. J Neuropathol Exp Neurol 2000;59:990-1001.
62. Ingram EM, Spillantini MG: Tau gene mutations: dissecting the pathogenesis of FTDP-17. Trends Mol Med 2002;8:555-562.

63. Heutink P: Untangling tau-related dementia. Hum Mol Genet 2000;9:979-986.
64. Baker M, Mackenzie IR, Pickering-Brown SM, et al: Mutations in progranulin cause tau-negative frontotemporal dementia linked to chromosome 17. Nature 2006;442:916-919.
65. Cruts M, Gijselinck I, van der Zee J, et al: Null mutations in progranulin cause ubiquitin-positive frontotemporal dementia linked to chromosome 17q21. Nature 2006;442:920-924.
66. Rademakers R, Hutton M: The genetics of frontotemporal lobar degeneration. Curr Neurol Neurosci Rep 2007;7:434-442.
67. He Z, Ong CH, Halper J, et al: Progranulin is a mediator of the wound response. Nat Med 2003;9:225-229.
68. Rademakers R, Baker M, Gass J, et al: Phenotypic variability associated with progranulin haploinsufficiency in patients with the common 1477C→T (Arg493X) mutation: an international initiative. Lancet Neurol 2007;6:857-868.
69. Skibinski G, Parkinson NJ, Brown JM, et al: Mutations in the endosomal ESCRTIII-complex subunit CHMP2B in frontotemporal dementia. Nat Genet 2005;37:806-808.
70. Cannon A, Baker M, Boeve B, et al: CHMP2B mutations are not a common cause of frontotemporal lobar degeneration. Neurosci Lett. 2006;398(1-2):83-84.
71. van der Zee J, Urwin H, Engelborghs S, et al: CHMP2B C-truncating mutations in frontotemporal lobar degeneration are associated with an aberrant endosomal phenotype in vitro. Hum Mol Genet 2007.
72. Kovach MJ, Waggoner B, Leal SM, et al: Clinical delineation and localization to chromosome 9p13.3-p12 of a unique dominant disorder in four families: hereditary inclusion body myopathy, Paget disease of bone, and frontotemporal dementia. Mol Genet Metab 2001;74:458-475.
73. Watts GD, Wymer J, Kovach MJ, et al: Inclusion body myopathy associated with Paget disease of bone and frontotemporal dementia is caused by mutant valosin-containing protein. Nat Genet 2004;36:377-381.
74. Watts GD, Thomasova D, Ramdeen SK, et al: Novel VCP mutations in inclusion body myopathy associated with Paget disease of bone and frontotemporal dementia. Clin Genet 2007;72: 420-426.
75. Bersano A, Del Bo R, Lamperti C, et al: Inclusion body myopathy and frontotemporal dementia caused by a novel VCP mutation. Neurobiol Aging 2007.
76. Vance C, Al-Chalabi A, Ruddy D, et al: Familial amyotrophic lateral sclerosis with frontotemporal dementia is linked to a locus on chromosome 9p13.2-21.3. Brain 2006;129(Pt 4):868-876.
77. Valdmanis PN, Dupre N, Bouchard JP, et al: Three families with amyotrophic lateral sclerosis and frontotemporal dementia with evidence of linkage to chromosome 9p. Arch Neurol 2007;64: 240-245.
78. Trojanowski JQ, Dickson D: Update on the neuropathological diagnosis of frontotemporal dementias. J Neuropathol Exp Neurol 2001;60:1123-1126.
79. Josephs KA, Holton JL, Rossor MN, et al: Frontotemporal lobar degeneration and ubiquitin immunohistochemistry. Neuropathol Appl Neurobiol 2004;30:369-373.
80. Okamoto K, Murakami N, Kusaka H, et al: Ubiquitin-positive intraneuronal inclusions in the extramotor cortices of presenile dementia patients with motor neuron disease. J Neurol 1992;239:426-430.
81. Shi J, Shaw CL, Du Plessis D, et al: Histopathological changes underlying frontotemporal lobar degeneration with clinicopathological correlation. Acta Neuropathol (Berl) 2005;110:501-512.
82. Mackenzie IR, Shi J, Shaw CL, et al: Dementia lacking distinctive histology (DLDH) revisited. Acta Neuropathol (Berl) 2006;112:551-559.
83. Cairns NJ, Bigio EH, Mackenzie IR, et al: Neuropathologic diagnostic and nosologic criteria for frontotemporal lobar degeneration: consensus of the Consortium for Frontotemporal Lobar Degeneration. Acta Neuropathol (Berl) 2007;114:5-22.
84. Mackenzie IR, Baborie A, Pickering-Brown S, et al: Heterogeneity of ubiquitin pathology in frontotemporal lobar degeneration: classification and relation to clinical phenotype. Acta Neuropathol (Berl) 2006;112:539-549.
85. Sampathu DM, Neumann M, Kwong LK, et al: Pathological heterogeneity of frontotemporal lobar degeneration with ubiquitin-positive inclusions delineated by ubiquitin immunohistochemistry and novel monoclonal antibodies. Am J Pathol 2006;169:1343-1352.
86. Mackenzie IR, Baker M, Pickering-Brown S, et al: The neuropathology of frontotemporal lobar degeneration caused by mutations in the progranulin gene. Brain 2006;129(Pt 11):3081-3090.
87. Forman MS, Mackenzie IR, Cairns NJ, et al: Novel ubiquitin neuropathology in frontotemporal dementia with valosin containing protein gene mutations. J Neuropathol Exp Neurol 2006;65:571-581.

24 Etiology, Pathology, and Pathogenesis

PATRICK WEYDT •
G. BERNHARD LANDWEHRMEYER •
ALBERT C. LUDOLPH

Introduction

Huntington's disease (HD) is the most common autosomal dominant inherited adult-onset neurodegenerative disease.[1] It is encountered worldwide and affects 4 to 10 per 100,000. This amounts to roughly 30,000 to 40,000 people in the United States or Europe, and more than three times as many if one includes people at risk (i.e., first-degree relatives of patients with manifest HD).

Clinically, HD is characterized by a classic triad of symptoms consisting of movement disorder (chorea/dystonia) associated with psychiatric abnormalities and cognitive decline.[1] The onset of symptoms is insidious and typically occurs in midlife (i.e., between 30 and 40 years of age).[2] The range of age of onset is very wide, however, with individual patients becoming symptomatic as early as 1 year old and as late more than 80 years old. The disease course is invariably devastating; HD progresses relentlessly and is always fatal, typically within 15 to 20 years, and marked by severe incapacitation and suffering for patients and their families.[1]

HD shares many salient clinical and pathological features with the major sporadic neurodegenerative diseases, such as Alzheimer's disease, Parkinson's disease, and amyotrophic lateral sclerosis, which suggests that similar pathogenic mechanisms are involved.[3] Because of its clear-cut genetic basis, the study of HD has allowed researchers to dissect the pathways leading to neurodegeneration in unprecedented detail.

Despite steady and important progress in the understanding of the molecular underpinnings of HD, the exact pathological mechanisms remain incompletely understood.[4,5] As a result, there is still no efficient curative treatment for HD, and therapeutic options are limited to symptom management and palliative measures. This chapter reviews the more recent advances in understanding of HD etiology, pathology, and pathogenesis and discusses therapeutic implications.

Etiology

HUNTINGTON'S DISEASE MUTATION

HD is caused by the unstable expansion of a trinucleotide (CAG) repeat tract within the coding region of a gene of ill-defined functions located on the short arm of chromosome 4 (4p16.3).[6] The CAG repeat is translated into a polyglutamine stretch in the cognate protein, huntingtin (htt). This places HD prominently among a group of eight other heritable neurodegenerative diseases, which are also characterized by mutated proteins harboring abnormal polyglutamine stretches and are termed *polyglutamine disorders*.[7] In addition to HD, these are X-linked spinal and bulbar muscular atrophy (Kennedy's disease), dentatorubral-pallidoluysian atrophy, and six forms of spinocerebellar ataxia (SCA 1, 2, 3, 6, 7, and 17).[7]

The identification of the HD mutation in 1993 was the seminal event in modern HD research, and represents an important milestone in molecular medicine.[6,8] Drawing on the analysis of a pedigree comprising more than 15,000 individuals, an international consortium of researchers identified the cause of HD as the mutation as the abnormal expansion of a CAG repeat tract in a novel gene, termed *IT15* (for *interesting transcript 15*) at the time and now commonly referred to as the huntingtin (*htt*) gene. The gene is unusually large and consists of 67 exons. The CAG repeat is located in the first exon. It is polymorphous and normally between 8 and 35 repeats long with a peak at 16 repeats. If the expansion exceeds 39 repeats, the HD phenotype is fully penetrant; the range between 36 and 39 represents a transition zone with incomplete penetrance of the HD phenotype.[9] The age of onset is inversely correlated with the CAG repeat length. In mutated alleles, the repeat length tends to expand from one generation to the next, leading to increasingly earlier symptom onset and a more severe disease course. This effect seems to be more pronounced in paternal transmission and is called *anticipation*.[10]

NORMAL HUNTINGTIN: STRUCTURE AND POSSIBLE FUNCTIONS

Normal huntingtin (htt) is a protein of 3144 amino acids and is 348 kD.[11] Despite its size, native htt is completely soluble in the cell; it localizes to the nucleus, the endoplasmic reticulum, and the Golgi apparatus. In neurons, it is also found in neurites and at the synapses. htt is expressed ubiquitously throughout the body, with particularly high levels in neurons, testes, muscle, liver, and lymphocytes.

htt has no significant sequence homology with other known proteins, and its secondary and tertiary structure remains to be determined.

The function of normal htt is only beginning to be elucidated.[11] Normal htt expression is essential for development in mice; htt knockout mice are embryogenically lethal.[12-14] In humans, deletions have never been observed, suggesting that this is also not compatible with life. Some clues to the disease-relevant functions of htt are suggested by its binding partners, especially because many of these protein-protein interactions are mediated by the polyglutamine tract itself.[15] Polyglutamine stretches are found in several different transcription factors, and they mediate interactions with regulatory proteins.[16] The deletion of the CAG tract in the murine HD gene homolog produces only a mild phenotype, suggesting that it is a weak modulator of htt function.[17] The pathways in which normal huntingtin function has been implicated include gene transcription, vesicular trafficking, axonal transport, and synaptic transmission.[11]

GENETIC AND ENVIRONMENTAL MODIFIERS

Despite the clear monogenetic nature of HD, it is evident from the considerable heterogeneity of the complex disease phenotype even among patients with similar repeat lengths that many factors other than the size of CAG tract expansion exert a significant impact on the manifestations of the disease.[10] This idea is borne out by statistical analysis of HD pedigrees, the largest now comprising more than 18,000 individuals spanning 10 generations.[18] Quantification of these results reveals that the CAG repeat size accounts for approximately 66% of the variability in age of onset.[19] Other genes and environmental factors account for the remaining differences.[18] Because every modifier, whether genetic or environmental, represents a potential therapeutic target, the search for disease modifiers of HD has become a field of intense investigation, and the focus has so far been on genetic modifiers.

Conventional candidate gene approaches have led to the identification of several potential genetic modifiers, including neurotrophic factors and neurotransmitters (Table 24–1). To date, two of these have been reproduced in more than one population: *GRIK2* is the gene for a subunit of the kainate-type glutamate receptor, and *UCHL1* encodes for ubiquitin C-terminal esterase L1.[20-24] Both modifier genes account for only a small portion (<10%) of the genetically determined variation in disease onset.

The first example of an unbiased screening approach is a more recent 10-cM density genome-wide scan in 629 affected sibling pairs.[25] This study suggested evidence for linkage of modifiers of age of onset at 4p16, 6p21-2, and 6q24-24, and more marginal evidence for linkage at positions on chromosomes 1, 2, 5, and 18. With the rapid advances in genomics, much more detailed unbiased genome-wide scans for genetic modifiers are now feasible and promise to stimulate further progress.

Nongenetic modifiers of HD are less well studied. Environmental enrichment is beneficial in animal models of HD.[26,27] Caloric restriction can delay symptom onset and prolongs survival in the N171-82Q model of HD.[28] Other bona fide environmental modifiers have not been identified, but our own more recent work suggests that ambient temperature can modulate symptom onset and survival in several transgenic mouse models of HD.[29] In this study, high temperatures

TABLE 24-1		Potential Genetic Modifiers		
Gene	Polymorphism	Function	Effect Size (%)	References
BDNF	V66M	Growth factor	5.9-8.2	Alberch et al, 2005
			—	Kishikawa et al, 2006
			—	Metzger et al, 2006
			—	Mai et al, 2006
GRIK2	$(TAA)_n$	GluR subunit	4.1	Rubinsztein et al, 1997
			0.6	MacDonald et al, 1999
			2	Chattopadhyay et al, 2003
			—	Naze et al, 2002
			—	Cannella et al, 2004
			—	Metzger et al, 2006
			—	Andresen et al, 2007
GRIN2B	C/T SNP	GluR subunit	3.8	Arning et al, 2005
			—	Andresen et al, 2007
TP53	R72P	Transcription factor	4	Chattopadhyay et al, 2003
			—	Andresen et al, 2007
			—	Arning et al, 2005
UCHL1	S18Y	Ubiquitin thiolesterase	4.2%	Naze et al, 2002
			1.1%	Metzger et al, 2006
			—	Andresen et al, 2007

(30° C) were protective, and low temperatures (4° C) were deleterious compared with room temperature (20° C). Although these findings cannot be extrapolated directly to human HD patients, they represent a noteworthy proof of principle pointing to the power of nonpharmacological therapeutic interventions.

TRANSGENIC MODEL ORGANISMS

HD or other polyglutamine diseases do not occur naturally in nonhuman animal species. Transgenic expression of the mutant *htt* gene or its fragments (but not of the human wild-type gene) in model organisms is toxic, however. In rodents, expression of the *htt* transgene can produce a phenotype that recapitulates crucial aspects of the human disease—motor abnormalities, wasting, and premature death, and histopathological features such as neurodegeneration and inclusion body formation.[30,31] These mouse models have become powerful and widely used tools in HD research.[30] The available transgenic mouse models are commonly categorized into three broad groups: (1) mice that express only the first exon of the mutant huntingtin (commonly termed *fragment* or *truncated* or *exon 1 models*),[32,33] (2) mice with the CAG expansion inserted into the murine *htt* homolog (*knock-in models*),[34] and (3) mice that express the full-length mutant huntingtin (*full-length models*).[35] In addition, more recently a transgenic rat model has been generated that offers the advantage of a much more differentiated behavioral phenotype and a significantly larger body size, with benefits for imaging studies and surgical interventions.[36]

Therapeutic animal trials are done almost exclusively in the exon 1 models—the R6/2[33] and the N171[32] lines—because they develop a severe disease phenotype with clear end points (i.e., weight loss, overt motor deficits, and premature death).[30] Although many interventions have yielded promising results in these models, translation to the clinic has unsuccessful so far.[37] The results of published therapeutic mouse trials can be monitored at the website www.hdbase.org. The Huntington Project offers a systematic evaluation of treatments for Huntington's disease (SET-HD) that can be accessed at their website (www.huntingtonproject.org).

Pathology

Although conventional pathologic investigations were effectively limited to the analysis of postmortem brain specimens from HD patients, advances in imaging techniques and the advent of transgenic model organisms have opened new avenues for systematically studying HD pathology in the presymptomatic and early symptomatic phases. These approaches were complemented by the development of specific antibodies against the expanded polyglutamine, which allowed researchers to identify polyglutamine-specific hallmarks of HD pathology.

GROSS PATHOLOGY

At autopsy, HD brains are typically severely atrophic with a weight reduced by about 10% to 20%.[38] The atrophy is most obvious in the basal ganglia, especially the caudate nucleus and the putamen. Brain atrophy is accompanied by secondary enlargement of the ventricles. A reduction in size also occurs in other areas of the brain, including the cerebral hemispheres, the diencephalons, the cerebellum, and the brainstem and spinal cord.[38]

Because of its noninvasive and objectively quantifiable nature, structural magnetic resonance imaging (MRI) of the HD brain has a great appeal as a biomarker of disease progression and as a surrogate end point of therapeutic interventions.[39] Volumes of caudate, putamen, and total basal ganglia significantly decrease over time and have the potential to be used as biomarkers.[40,41] The hypothalamus is another topographical region that might be useful in this respect.[42]

NEURONAL PATHOLOGY

In the HD brain, pathology is most pronounced in, but not limited to, the striatum and the cerebral cortex. Progressive striatal atrophy is the basis for staging the severity of the disease.[43] The medium spiny neurons, which make up 95% of the neurons of the striatum, and their GABAergic striatal efferents are most severely hit. These cell types have become the focus of most investigations.[44,45] Other brain regions, including thalamus, substantia nigra, the subthalamic nucleus, and the cerebellum, are affected much later in the disease course.[31]

Important clues suggest that the hypothalamus is involved already in the early stages of HD, and that changes in hypothalamic structure and function represent promising makers of disease.[46] Structural changes can be detected in vivo using voxel-based MRI.[42] This finding likely foreshadows the severe cell loss that is found in postmortem HD brains.[47,48]

The development of antibodies specific for the expanded polyglutamine tract shed new light on the pathology.[49] The detection of intranuclear inclusion bodies in neurons from HD patient brain specimens and the observation that the development of these inclusion bodies precedes the onset of symptoms in HD transgenic mice made pharmacological dissolution of intracellular protein aggregates an attractive therapeutic target.[50] This idea was reinforced by the finding that conditional shutdown of mutant *htt* expression in transgenic mice led to reversal of inclusion body formation and clinical symptoms.[51] More recent evidence from in vitro studies tracking the inclusion body formation in individual cells over their lifetime suggests that, quite to the contrary, aggregate formation is protective (see later).[52]

NON-NEURONAL PATHOLOGY AND PROJECTING NEURONS

Although gliosis is a prominent hallmark of HD pathology, this has long been dismissed as reactive. The understanding that toxic effects of mutant *htt* are not limited to neurons is more recent.[53] This important insight has emerged mainly from the study of transgenic mouse models of neurodegenerative diseases in general and of HD in particular. Several such studies show that the degeneration of neurons can be *noncell autonomous* (i.e., cell populations other than the dying neurons themselves are critically involved in the degenerative process).[53]

In HD, there is now compelling evidence that projecting neurons and surrounding glial cells, the support cells of the nervous system, are mediators of mutant *htt* toxicity. Studies with conditional transgene expression using the Cre-LoxP system revealed that a widespread expression of mutant *htt* in the brain, extending well beyond the primarily affected cortical and striatal neurons, is necessary to produce either brain pathology or motor dysfunction in transgenic mice.[35,54] Because mutant *htt* expression results in reduced *BDNF* gene transcription,[55] one specific noncell autonomous effect of the HD mutation could be to deprive the medium spiny neurons of the striatum of their trophic input from cortical neurons. The plausibility of this mechanism is underscored by a study from Strand and colleagues,[56] in which they show that targeted knockdown of *BDNF* expression in the forebrain results in gene expression changes in the striatum that closely resemble the gene expression changes in human HD striata. Conversely, targeted overexpression of *BDNF* in the forebrain reduces pathology in the striatum and ameliorates the motor phenotype.[57]

Non-neuronal cells are also affected by the expression of mutant *htt*. The best evidence here is available for astrocytes. Shin and associates[58] showed that mutant *htt* expression in astrocytes reduces their ability to clear glutamate from the extracellular space, and compounds the excitotoxic burden on vulnerable neurons in vitro. In *Drosophila*, the presence of polyglutamine-expanded peptides inhibits the reactive upregulation of glial glutamate transporters.[59] The ability of polyglutamine expansions to impair the glutamate transport capacity of astrocytes in vivo has been shown for SCA 7, another polyglutamine disorder.[60] The observation of deficient in vivo glycolysis, a predominantly astrocytic function, in the striata of patients with early HD highlights the clinical relevance of non-neuronal effects of mutant *htt* expression.[61]

Neuroinflammation

The term *neuroinflammation* refers to the cellular and biochemical processes that are initiated in the central nervous system in response to noxious stimuli.[62] Depending on the circumstances, the net effect of the neuroinflammatory response can be beneficial or detrimental for the central nervous system.[62]

The cellular substrate of inflammation in the brain are the microglia.[63] The last 2 decades have brought compelling evidence that microglia are important determinants of the microenvironment of the brain and involved in many acute and chronic neurological diseases, including neurodegeneration.[62] In the unperturbed adult brain, microglia exist as so-called resting or quiescent microglia.[63,64] In this state, they have a small cell body with fine, ramified processes and minimal expression of surface antigens. Far from what the terminology of "quiescent" and "resting" would suggest, microglia in the healthy central nervous system are quite busy "patrolling" the brain tissue for lesions and intruders.[65] In the event of central nervous system injury, these cells are swiftly "activated," and they are involved in the pathology of nearly any neurological disorder. The net effect of neuroinflammation is the result of a delicate balance between the neurotoxic and neuroprotective factors that microglia release into their immediate environment.[62]

Pathological and imaging studies in HD show that neuroinflammation is an integral and remarkably early event in the disease process.[66,67] Postmortem studies have revealed activated microglia mainly in the striatum and cortex of HD brains.[67] The level of activation is a function of the degree of neuronal pathology. As the distribution of the activated microglia extends well into the white matter, axonal pathology rather than neuronal loss is thought to be triggering and sustaining the neuroinflammatory response in HD.

The pathology findings are corroborated and expanded by functional imaging studies. Microglial activation involves the upregulation of the peripheral benzodiazepine-binding site on the outer mitochondrial membrane. Through advances in brain imaging, it is now possible to detect and visualize this process in vivo in experimental animals and in humans using the C 11–labeled benzodiazepine receptor ligand PK-1195.[68] Such studies show that microglial activation can be detected not only in symptomatic HD patients, but also in presymptomatic gene carriers.[66,69] In the small cohort of presymptomatic gene carriers, microglial activation as measured by PK-11195 binding positron emission tomography (PET) was closely associated anatomically with subclinical striatal dysfunction as measured by raclopride C 11 PET. Striatal PK-11195 binding was also significantly correlated with a shorter "predicted time to symptomatic onset" of HD. In a gene array study of HD brain, mRNA expression revealed a generalized activation of inflammatory pathways.[70] Using proteomics approaches, a systemic inflammatory response is also detectable in plasma and cerebrospinal fluid of HD patients,[71] whereas the transcriptome of peripheral blood did not show consistent inflammation.[72]

Although microglial activation is also a feature of transgenic mouse models of HD at the histological level,[73,74] experimental treatments with putative inhibitors of microglial activation, such as minocycline, have so far yielded conflicting results.[75-78] This highlights the urgent need to understand better the neuroinflammatory pathways activated in HD. An important step in this direction was the discovery that mutant *htt* expression induces the activity of the macrophage-specific and microglia-specific enzyme KMO in the kynurenine pathway leading to the generation of neurotoxic metabolites.[79] A more recent follow-up study now suggests that histone deacetylase (HDAC) inhibitors can mitigate the neurotoxic activities of mutant *htt* expressing microglia in vitro and in vivo.[80]

White Matter Pathology

White matter changes are a subtle but consistent feature of HD pathology. In postmortem HD brains, oligodendrocyte densities are increased independent of the presence of manifest astrocytosis.[81,82] Also, white matter changes are found in imaging studies of presymptomatic HD patients.[83,84] PGC-1a$^{-/-}$ mice, which recapitulate many aspects of the mouse HD phenotype, also display significant oligodendrocyte abnormalities.[85,86] Studies of the effect of mutant *htt* expression on oligodendrocyte function and their interactions with neurons are lacking. It is impossible at the present time to evaluate whether and how oligodendrocyte abnormalities contribute to HD pathogenesis, and further research is necessary.

Pathogenesis

The identification of CAG tract expansion in the *htt* gene as the cause of HD has brought HD research to the forefront of molecular medicine and spawned a wealth of studies into the molecular pathogenesis. A wide range of possible pathogenetic pathways have emerged from this research, a selection of which is discussed here.

PROTEIN MISFOLDING

Accurate folding of proteins is essential for the proper functioning of every cell.[87] Chaperones are a class of specialized proteins that have evolved to ensure proper protein folding.[88] Misfolded proteins are eliminated through the ubiquitin-proteosome system.[87]

The expansion of the polyglutamine tract alters the proper conformation of the huntingtin protein,[89,90] and this triggers the formation of abnormal aggregations of mutant *htt*.[91] Although initially it was thought that the microscopically visible aggregates were the effectors of polyglutamine toxicity, a more detailed understanding of the misfolded protein aggregation pathway suggests that specific intermediates, the protofibrils and annular oligomers, are the toxic conformers of mutant *htt*.[92] As mentioned previously, the aggregates may represent a mechanism to neutralize the potentially toxic misfolded proteins.[4] This view is supported by the in vitro observation that formation of microscopically visible aggregate is protective rather than deleterious for neurons.[52]

Three broad strategies are currently being pursued to target protein misfolding in HD therapeutically:[92] (1) pharmacological modulation of the endogenous chaperone system, (2) administration of direct inhibitors of protein aggregation (chemical chaperones), and (3) RNA interference as a means to prevent selectively the expression of mutated proteins in the first place.

TRANSCRIPTIONAL DYSREGULATION

The polyglutamine tract is a common motif in transcription factors and their interacting partners.[16] Conversely, several of the proteins harboring expanded polyglutamine tracts are established transcription factors, most prominently the androgen receptor associated with spinal and bulbar muscular atrophy and the TATA-box binding protein associated with SCA 17.[7] Finally, mutant *htt* can exert its full toxicity only when it localizes to the nucleus.[93] This constellation suggests that toxicity of the polyglutamine tract expansion is played out at least in part through alteration of gene transcription. Huntingtin interferes in a polyglutamine length–dependent fashion with the function of the transcription factor Sp1 and its coactivator TAF_{II} 130 (also termed TAF4).[94]

Candidate gene expression studies further support the concept that transcription of specific pathways and genes is suppressed in HD. A broad range of pharmacologically targetable genes are downregulated in tissue from HD patients and transgenic mouse models. These include neurotransmitters and growth factors, such as *BDNF* and enkephalin, and neurotransmitter receptors or transcriptional coregulators.[95] More recently, the advent of microarray technology allowed for unbiased analysis of gene expression changes in tissue from HD patients and transgenic animals, and this approach is being validated as a therapeutic readout.[95]

Two more recent reports suggest that transcriptional dysregulation in HD prominently involves the targets of the transcriptional coactivator PGC-1α.[29,96] Cui and colleagues[96] showed that mutant *htt* leads to the suppression of the expression of PGC-1α and its target genes in the striatum, whereas Weydt and associates[29] showed that mutant *htt* interferes with the expression of PGC-1α-regulated genes. Because PGC-1α regulates its own transcription, these two scenarios are not mutually exclusive.[97] Determining their relative importance in HD pathogenesis has significant implications, however, for devising therapeutic strategies. In any case, because PGC-1α regulates the expression of nuclearly encoded mitochondrial genes, these findings suggest an unexpected molecular link between transcriptional and mitochondrial abnormalities in HD.[98]

AXONAL TRANSPORT

Several observations suggest that disturbed axonal transport plays a role in HD pathogenesis. Wild-type huntingtin involvement in axonal transport is mediated through the huntingtin-associated protein 1 (HAP1), which interacts with p150^{glu}, an integral part of the dynein-based axonal transport machinery. The polyglutamine expansion increases the interaction between *htt*, HAP1, and p150^{glu}—inhibiting the interaction of HIP1/p150^{glu} with microtubules and so inhibiting axonal transport.[7] This inhibition impairs the intracellular transport of mitochondria and growth factors such as brain-derived neurotrophic factor.[99]

METABOLIC AND MITOCHONDRIAL ABNORMALITIES

In addition to the neurological and psychiatric symptoms, the clinical course of HD is marked by severe weight loss and emaciation, especially during the late stages of the disease (Fig. 24–1).[100,101] This observation is not new. The first mention of emaciation as a feature of HD can be traced back to George Huntington.

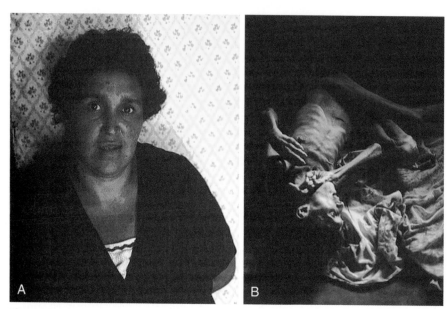

Figure 24–1 Huntington's disease is a devastating inherited neurodegenerative disorder that is always fatal, typically within 15 to 20 years. These two pictures of the same patient were taken 13 years apart. Note the severe emaciation caused by the disease. (Courtesy of the Hereditary Disease Foundation.)

In 1910, he recalled how in 1858, at the age of 8, he met for the first time patients with the disease that was later to carry his name: "... Driving with my father through a wooded road leading from East Hampton to Amagansett we suddenly came upon two women, mother and daughter, both tall and thin, almost cadaverous, both bowing, twisting, grimacing...."[102]

For a long time, the clinical focus remained on the motor symptoms, and the "cadaverous" weight loss and emaciation were seen as secondary to increased energy expenditure owing to chorea, possibly exacerbated by reduced energy intake as a result of dysphagia and general incapacitation.[101] More recent evidence has led to modifications of this view. It was shown that subtle weight loss is a very early hallmark of HD in humans, occurring well before onset of motor symptoms.[103] There is now a consensus that weight loss in HD has a multifactorial etiology, and probably includes energy failure at the cellular level.[104] Metabolite profiling of serum samples using gas chromatography/mass spectrometry found a procatabolic constellation in HD patients versus controls.[105] Analogous changes have been observed in transgenic mouse models of HD.[105] Recent and more detailed metabolic studies have revealed that these animals also have an increased baseline metabolism before onset of overt motor symptoms.[29,106] These findings suggest that transgenic mouse represents a reasonable model of the metabolic abnormalities of HD. Animal studies indicate that manipulation of the metabolic system (e.g., through caloric restriction) represents a promising therapeutic target in HD.[28,104]

Toxicological studies have long established that striatal neurons are exquisitely vulnerable to mitochondrial dysfunction.[107,108] Mutant *htt* can affect mitochondrial function directly and indirectly.[109] Mutant *htt* directly alters the calcium signaling at the mitochondrial membrane and leads to calcium in the cytoplasm, which is a potent apoptotic signal.[110,111] As mentioned earlier, mutant htt also has a direct specific inhibitory effect on PGC-1α, a master regulator of mitochondrial biogenesis and activity.[29,96]

Conclusions

The identification of the *htt* mutation as the cause of HD in 1993 put researchers very early in a position to take full advantage of the advances in molecular biology, such as the development of transgenic model organisms, gene array techniques, and RNA interference. This situation has led to the identification of a wide range of molecular and cellular pathways through which mutant *htt* plays out its toxicity. At the subcellular level, this includes disruption of mitochondrial function, calcium homeostasis, protein degradation, and gene transcription. The cellular effects of the *htt* mutation are not limited to the vulnerable cell populations, such as the medium spiny neurons of the striatum or the projecting cortical neurons. It is now clear that other cell compartments of the central nervous system—astrocytes, oligodendrocytes, and microglia—are also impaired in their functions. What is needed urgently is a better understanding of the relative importance of these effects for the development of the disease phenotype.

REFERENCES

1. Walker FO: Huntington's disease. Lancet 2007;369:218-228.
2. Zoghbi HY, Orr HT: Glutamine repeats and neurodegeneration. Annu Rev Neurosci 2000;23:217-247.
3. Martin JB: Molecular basis of the neurodegenerative disorders. N Engl J Med 1999;340:1970-1980.
4. Finkbeiner S, Cuervo AM, Morimoto RI, Muchowski PJ: Disease-modifying pathways in neurodegeneration. J Neurosci 2006;26:10349-10357.
5. Li S, Li XJ: Multiple pathways contribute to the pathogenesis of Huntington disease. Mol Neurodegener 2006;1:19.
6. A novel gene containing a trinucleotide repeat that is expanded and unstable on Huntington's disease chromosomes. The Huntington's Disease Collaborative Research Group. Cell 1993;72:971-983.
7. Orr HT, Zoghbi HY: Trinucleotide repeat disorders. Annu Rev Neurosci 2007;30:575-621.
8. Bates GP: History of genetic disease: the molecular genetics of Huntington disease—a history. Nat Rev Genet 2005;6:766-773.
9. Rubinsztein DC, Leggo J, Coles R, et al: Phenotypic characterization of individuals with 30-40 CAG repeats in the Huntington disease (HD) gene reveals HD cases with 36 repeats and apparently normal elderly individuals with 36-39 repeats. Am J Hum Genet 1996;59:16-22.
10. Gusella JF, MacDonald ME: Molecular genetics: unmasking polyglutamine triggers in neurodegenerative disease. Nat Rev Neurosci 2000;1:109-115.
11. Cattaneo E, Zuccato C, Tartari M: Normal huntingtin function: an alternative approach to Huntington's disease. Nat Rev Neurosci 2005;6(12):919-930.
12. Zeitlin S, Liu JP, Chapman DL, et al: Increased apoptosis and early embryonic lethality in mice nullizygous for the Huntington's disease gene homologue. Nat Genet 1995;11:155-163.
13. Duyao MP, Auerbach AB, Ryan A, et al: Inactivation of the mouse Huntington's disease gene homolog Hdh. Science 1995;269:407-410.
14. Nasir J, Floresco SB, O'Kusky JR, et al: Targeted disruption of the Huntington's disease gene results in embryonic lethality and behavioral and morphological changes in heterozygotes. Cell 1995;81:811-823.

15. Harjes P, Wanker EE: The hunt for huntingtin function: interaction partners tell many different stories. Trends Biochem Sci 2003;28:425-433.

16. Freiman RN,Tjian R: Neurodegeneration: a glutamine-rich trail leads to transcription factors. Science 2002;296:2149-2150.

17. Clabough EB, Zeitlin SO: Deletion of the triplet repeat encoding polyglutamine within the mouse Huntington's disease gene results in subtle behavioral/motor phenotypes in vivo and elevated levels of ATP with cellular senescence in vitro. Hum Mol Genet 2006;15:607-623.

18. Wexler NS, Lorimer J, Porter J, et al: Venezuelan kindreds reveal that genetic and environmental factors modulate Huntington's disease age of onset. Proc Natl Acad Sci U S A 2004;101:3498-3503.

19. Gusella JF, Macdonald ME: Huntington's disease: seeing the pathogenic process through a genetic lens. Trends Biochem Sci 2006;31:533-540.

20. Chattopadhyay B, Ghosh S, Gangopadhyay PK, et al: Modulation of age at onset in Huntington's disease and spinocerebellar ataxia type 2 patients originated from eastern India. Neurosci Lett 2003;345:93-96.

21. Naze P, Vuillaume I, Destee A, et al: Mutation analysis and association studies of the ubiquitin carboxy-terminal hydrolase L1 gene in Huntington's disease. Neurosci Lett 2002;328:1-4.

22. Metzger S, Bauer P, Tomiuk J, et al: The S18Y polymorphism in the UCHL1 gene is a genetic modifier in Huntington's disease. Neurogenetics 2006;7:27-30.

23. Rubinsztein DC, Leggo J, Chiano M, et al: Genotypes at the GluR6 kainate receptor locus are associated with variation in the age of onset of Huntington disease. Proc Natl Acad Sci U S A 1997;94:3872-3876.

24. Zeng W, Gillis T, Hakky M, et al: Genetic analysis of the GRIK2 modifier effect in Huntington's disease. BMC Neurosci 2006;7:62.

25. Li JL, Hayden MR, Almqvist EW, et al: A genome scan for modifiers of age at onset in Huntington disease: the HD MAPS study. Am J Hum Genet 2003;73:682-687.

26. Spires TL, Grote HE, Garry S, et al: Dendritic spine pathology and deficits in experience-dependent dendritic plasticity in R6/1 Huntington's disease transgenic mice. Eur J Neurosci 2004;19:2799-2807.

27. Hockly E, Cordery PM, Woodman B, et al: Environmental enrichment slows disease progression in R6/2 Huntington's disease mice. Ann Neurol 2002;51:235-242.

28. Duan W, Guo Z, Jiang H, et al: Dietary restriction normalizes glucose metabolism and BDNF levels, slows disease progression, and increases survival in huntingtin mutant mice. Proc Natl Acad Sci U S A 2003;100:2911-2916.

29. Weydt P, Pineda VV, Torrence AE, et al: Thermoregulatory and metabolic defects in Huntington's disease transgenic mice implicate PGC-1alpha in Huntington's disease neurodegeneration. Cell Metab 2006;4:349-362.

30. Beal MF, Ferrante RJ: Experimental therapeutics in transgenic mouse models of Huntington's disease. Nat Rev Neurosci 2004;5:373-384.

31. Vonsattel JP: Huntington disease models and human neuropathology: similarities and differences. Acta Neuropathol (Berl) 2008;115(1):55-69.

32. Schilling G, Becher MW, Sharp AH, et al: Intranuclear inclusions and neuritic aggregates in transgenic mice expressing a mutant N-terminal fragment of huntingtin. Hum Mol Genet 1999;8:397-407.

33. Mangiarini L, Sathasivam K, Seller M, et al: Exon 1 of the HD gene with an expanded CAG repeat is sufficient to cause a progressive neurological phenotype in transgenic mice. Cell 1996;87:493-506.

34. Menalled LB, Sison JD, Dragatsis I, et al: Time course of early motor and neuropathological anomalies in a knock-in mouse model of Huntington's disease with 140 CAG repeats. J Comp Neurol 2003;465:11-26.

35. Gu X, Li C, Wei W, et al: Pathological cell-cell interactions elicited by a neuropathogenic form of mutant Huntingtin contribute to cortical pathogenesis in HD mice. Neuron 2005;46:433-444.

36. von Horsten S, Schmitt I, Nguyen HP, et al: Transgenic rat model of Huntington's disease. Hum Mol Genet 2003;12:617-624.

37. Hughes RE,Olson JM: Therapeutic opportunities in polyglutamine disease. Nat Med 2001;7:419-423.

38. Gutekunst CA, Norflus F, Hersch S: In Bates G, Harper P, Jones L, eds: Huntington's Disease. Oxford: Oxford University Press, 2002, pp 256-275.

39. Aylward EH: Change in MRI striatal volumes as a biomarker in preclinical Huntington's disease. Brain Res Bull 2007;72:152-158.
40. Aylward EH, Li Q, Stine OC, et al: Longitudinal change in basal ganglia volume in patients with Huntington's disease. Neurology 1997;48:394-399.
41. Aylward EH, Codori AM, Rosenblatt A, et al: Rate of caudate atrophy in presymptomatic and symptomatic stages of Huntington's disease. Mov Disord 2000;15:552-560.
42. Kassubek J, Juengling FD, Kioschies T, et al: Topography of cerebral atrophy in early Huntington's disease: a voxel based morphometric MRI study. J Neurol Neurosurg Psychiatry 2004;75:213-220.
43. Vonsattel JP, Myers RH, Stevens TJ, et al: Neuropathological classification of Huntington's disease. J Neuropathol Exp Neurol 1985;44:559-577.
44. Graveland GA, Williams RS, DiFiglia M: Evidence for degenerative and regenerative changes in neostriatal spiny neurons in Huntington's disease. Science 1985;227:770-773.
45. Trettel F, Rigamonti D, Hilditch-Maguire P, et al: Dominant phenotypes produced by the HD mutation in STHdh(Q111) striatal cells. Hum Mol Genet 2000;9:2799-2809.
46. Petersen A, Bjorkqvist M: Hypothalamic-endocrine aspects in Huntington's disease. Eur J Neurosci 2006;24:961-967.
47. Kremer HP, Roos RA, Dingjan GM, et al: The hypothalamic lateral tuberal nucleus and the characteristics of neuronal loss in Huntington's disease. Neurosci Lett 1991;132:101-104.
48. Petersen A, Gil J, Maat-Schieman ML, et al: Orexin loss in Huntington's disease. Hum Mol Genet 2005;14:39-47.
49. Ross CA, Poirier MA: Protein aggregation and neurodegenerative disease. Nat Med 2004;10(Suppl):S10-S17.
50. DiFiglia M, Sapp E, Chase KO, et al: Aggregation of huntingtin in neuronal intranuclear inclusions and dystrophic neurites in brain. Science 1997;277:1990-1993.
51. Yamamoto A, Lucas JJ, Hen R: Reversal of neuropathology and motor dysfunction in a conditional model of Huntington's disease. Cell 2000;101:57-66.
52. Arrasate M, Mitra S, Schweitzer ES, et al: Inclusion body formation reduces levels of mutant huntingtin and the risk of neuronal death. Nature 2004;431:805-810.
53. Lobsiger CS, Cleveland DW: Glial cells as intrinsic components of non-cell-autonomous neurodegenerative disease. Nat Neurosci 2007;10:1355-1360.
54. Gu X, Andre VM, Cepeda C, et al: Pathological cell-cell interactions are necessary for striatal pathogenesis in a conditional mouse model of Huntington's disease. Mol Neurodegener 2007;2:8.
55. Zuccato C, Ciammola A, Rigamonti D, et al: Loss of huntingtin-mediated BDNF gene transcription in Huntington's disease. Science 2001;293:493-498.
56. Strand AD, Baquet ZC, Aragaki AK, et al: Expression profiling of Huntington's disease models suggests that brain-derived neurotrophic factor depletion plays a major role in striatal degeneration. J Neurosci 2007;27:11758-11768.
57. Gharami K, Xie Y, An JJ, et al: Brain-derived neurotrophic factor over-expression in the forebrain ameliorates Huntington's disease phenotypes in mice. J Neurochem 2008;105(2):369-379.
58. Shin JY, Fang ZH, Yu ZX, et al: Expression of mutant huntingtin in glial cells contributes to neuronal excitotoxicity. J Cell Biol 2005;171:1001-1012.
59. Lievens JC, Rival T, Iche M, et al: Expanded polyglutamine peptides disrupt EGF receptor signaling and glutamate transporter expression in Drosophila. Hum Mol Genet 2005;14:713-724.
60. Custer SK, Garden GA, Gill N, et al: Bergmann glia expression of polyglutamine-expanded ataxin-7 produces neurodegeneration by impairing glutamate transport. Nat Neurosci 2006;9:1302-1311.
61. Powers WJ, Videen TO, Markham J, et al: Selective defect of in vivo glycolysis in early Huntington's disease striatum. Proc Natl Acad Sci U S A 2007;104:2945-2949.
62. Wyss-Coray T, Mucke L: Inflammation in neurodegenerative disease—a double-edged sword. Neuron 2002;35:419-432.
63. Hanisch UK, Kettenmann H: Microglia: active sensor and versatile effector cells in the normal and pathologic brain. Nat Neurosci 2007;10:1387-1394.
64. Kreutzberg GW: Microglia: a sensor for pathological events in the CNS. Trends Neurosci 1996;19:312-318.
65. Nimmerjahn A, Kirchhoff F, Helmchen F: Resting microglial cells are highly dynamic surveillants of brain parenchyma in vivo. Science 2005;308:1314-1318.

66. Tai YF, Pavese N, Gerhard A, et al: Microglial activation in presymptomatic Huntington's disease gene carriers. Brain 2007;130:1759-1766.
67. Sapp E, Kagel KB, Aronin N, et al: Early and progressive accumulation of reactive microglia in the Huntington disease brain. J Neuropathol Exp Neurol 2001;60:161-172.
68. Banati RB: Visualising microglial activation in vivo. Glia 2002;40:206-217.
69. Pavese N, Gerhard A, Tai YF, et al: Microglial activation correlates with severity in Huntington disease: a clinical and PET study. Neurology 2006;66:1638-1643.
70. Hodges A, Strand AD, Aragaki AK, et al: Regional and cellular gene expression changes in human Huntington's disease brain. Hum Mol Genet 2006;15(6):965-977.
71. Dalrymple A, Wild EJ, Joubert R, et al: Proteomic profiling of plasma in Huntington's disease reveals neuroinflammatory activation and biomarker candidates. J Proteome Res 2007;6:2833-2840.
72. Runne H, Kuhn A, Wild EJ, et al: Analysis of potential transcriptomic biomarkers for Huntington's disease in peripheral blood. Proc Natl Acad Sci U S A 2007;104:14424-14429.
73. Simmons DA, Casale M, Alcon B, et al: Ferritin accumulation in dystrophic microglia is an early event in the development of Huntington's disease. Glia 2007;55:1074-1084.
74. Ma L, Morton AJ, Nicholson LF: Microglia density decreases with age in a mouse model of Huntington's disease. Glia 2003;43:274-280.
75. Hersch S, Fink K, Vonsattel JP, Friedlander RM: Minocycline is protective in a mouse model of Huntington's disease. Ann Neurol 2003;54:841. author reply 842–843.
76. Smith DL, et al: Minocycline and doxycycline are not beneficial in a model of Huntington's disease. Ann Neurol 2003;54:186-196.
77. Chen M, Ona VO, Li M, et al: Minocycline inhibits caspase-1 and caspase-3 expression and delays mortality in a transgenic mouse model of Huntington disease. Nat Med 2000;6:797-801.
78. Stack EC, Smith KM, Ryu H, et al: Combination therapy using minocycline and coenzyme Q10 in R6/2 transgenic Huntington's disease mice. Biochim Biophys Acta 2006;1762:373-380.
79. Giorgini F, Guidetti P, Nguyen Q, et al: A genomic screen in yeast implicates kynurenine 3-monooxygenase as a therapeutic target for Huntington disease. Nat Genet 2005;37:526-531.
80. Giorgini F, Moller T, Kwan W, et al: Histone deacetylase inhibition modulates kynurenine pathway activation in yeast, microglia, and mice expressing a mutant huntingtin fragment. J Biol Chem 2008:283(12):7390-7400.
81. Myers RH, Vonsattel JP, Paskevich PA, et al: Decreased neuronal and increased oligodendroglial densities in Huntington's disease caudate nucleus. J Neuropathol Exp Neurol 1991;50:729-742.
82. Gomez-Tortosa E, MacDonald ME, Friend JC, et al: Quantitative neuropathological changes in presymptomatic Huntington's disease. Ann Neurol 2001;49:29-34.
83. Thieben MJ, Duggins AJ, Good CD, et al: The distribution of structural neuropathology in pre-clinical Huntington's disease. Brain 2002;125:1815-1828.
84. Ciarmiello A, Cannella M, Lastoria S, et al: Brain white-matter volume loss and glucose hypometabolism precede the clinical symptoms of Huntington's disease. J Nucl Med 2006;47:215-222.
85. Lin J, Wu PH, Tarr PT, et al: Defects in adaptive energy metabolism with CNS-linked hyperactivity in PGC-1alpha null mice. Cell 2004;119:121-135.
86. Leone TC, Lehman JJ, Finck BN, et al: PGC-1alpha deficiency causes multi-system energy metabolic derangements: muscle dysfunction, abnormal weight control and hepatic steatosis. PLoS Biol 2005;3:e101.
87. Bukau B, Weissman J, Horwich A: Molecular chaperones and protein quality control. Cell 2006;125:443-451.
88. Muchowski PJ, Wacker JL: Modulation of neurodegeneration by molecular chaperones. Nat Rev Neurosci 2005;6:11-22.
89. Gatchel JR, Zoghbi HY: Diseases of unstable repeat expansion: mechanisms and common principles. Nat Rev Genet 2005;6:743-755.
90. Perutz MF, Johnson T, Suzuki M, Finch JT: Glutamine repeats as polar zippers: their possible role in inherited neurodegenerative diseases. Proc Natl Acad Sci U S A 1994;91:5355-5358.
91. Scherzinger E, Lurz R, Turmaine M, et al: Huntingtin-encoded polyglutamine expansions form amyloid-like protein aggregates in vitro and in vivo. Cell 1997;90:549-558.
92. Weydt P, La Spada AR: Targeting protein aggregation in neurodegeneration—lessons from polyglutamine disorders. Expert Opin Ther Targets 2006;10:505-513.
93. Saudou F, Finkbeiner S, Devys D, Greenberg ME: Huntingtin acts in the nucleus to induce apoptosis but death does not correlate with the formation of intranuclear inclusions. Cell 1998;95:55-66.

94. Dunah AW, Jeong H, Griffin A, et al: Sp1 and TAFII130 transcriptional activity disrupted in early Huntington's disease. Science 2002;296:2238-2243.
95. Cha JH: Transcriptional signatures in Huntington's disease. Prog Neurobiol 2007;83:228-248.
96. Cui L, Jeong H, Borovecki F, et al: Transcriptional repression of PGC-1alpha by mutant huntingtin leads to mitochondrial dysfunction and neurodegeneration. Cell 2006;127:59-69.
97. Soyal S, Krempler F, Oberkofler H, Patsch W: PGC-1alpha: a potent transcriptional cofactor involved in the pathogenesis of type 2 diabetes. Diabetologia 2006;49:1477-1488.
98. Ross CA, Thompson LM: Transcription meets metabolism in neurodegeneration. Nat Med 2006;12:1239-1241.
99. Gauthier LR, Charrin BC, Borrell-Pages M, et al: Huntingtin controls neurotrophic support and survival of neurons by enhancing BDNF vesicular transport along microtubules. Cell 2004;118:127-138.
100. Stoy N, McKay E: Weight loss in Huntington's disease. Ann Neurol 2000;48:130-131.
101. Pratley RE, Salbe AD, Ravussin E, Caviness JN: Higher sedentary energy expenditure in patients with Huntington's disease. Ann Neurol 2000;47:64-70.
102. Huntington G: Recollections of Huntington's chorea, as I saw it at East Hampton, Long Island, during my boyhood. J Nerv Mental Dis 1910;37:5.
103. Djousse L, Knowlton B, Cupples LA, et al: Weight loss in early stage of Huntington's disease. Neurology 2002;59:1325-1330.
104. Walker FO, Raymond LA: Targeting energy metabolism in Huntington's disease. Lancet 2004;364:312-313.
105. Underwood BR, Broadhurst D, Dunn WB, et al: Huntington disease patients and transgenic mice have similar pro-catabolic serum metabolite profiles. Brain 2006;129:877-886.
106. van der Burg JM, Bacos K, Wood NI, et al: Increased metabolism in the R6/2 mouse model of Huntington's disease. Neurobiol Dis 2008;29(1):41-51.
107. Ludolph AC, He F, Spencer PS, et al: 3-Nitropropionic acid-exogenous animal neurotoxin and possible human striatal toxin. Can J Neurol Sci 1991;18:492-498.
108. Beal MF, Brouillet E, Jenkins BG, et al: Neurochemical and histologic characterization of striatal excitotoxic lesions produced by the mitochondrial toxin 3-nitropropionic acid. J Neurosci 1993;13:4181-4192.
109. Lin MT, Beal MF: Mitochondrial dysfunction and oxidative stress in neurodegenerative diseases. Nature 2006;443:787-795.
110. Panov AV, Gutekunst CA, Leavitt BR, et al: Early mitochondrial calcium defects in Huntington's disease are a direct effect of polyglutamines. Nat Neurosci 2002;5:731-736.
111. Tang TS, Slow E, Lupu V, et al: Disturbed Ca2+ signaling and apoptosis of medium spiny neurons in Huntington's disease. Proc Natl Acad Sci U S A 2005;102:2602-2607.

25 Clinical Features and Care

IRA SHOULSON

Introduction

The clinical phenotype of Huntington disease (HD) has been extensively examined and elaborated on since this hereditary chorea was described lucidly by Huntington in 1872.[1] Expanding knowledge of phenotype-genotype relationships and how best to care for patients and families affected by this disabling neurological disorder is largely a consequence of remarkable scientific advances in genetics, neuroscience, and experimental therapeutics. Genetic discoveries have enabled individuals at risk for having inherited HD to choose to learn of their gene-carrier status and the robust "dosage" relationship between the trinucleotide repeat expansion on the HD gene and the clinical onset of emerging signs and symptoms. Pathogenetic discoveries have implicated cellular mechanisms in HD that have prompted rational approaches to ameliorating the progressive neurodegeneration and resulting impairments. Large population-based studies and clinical trials have characterized the natural history of this devastating disorder and set the stage for rational interventions aimed at delaying the clinical onset of premanifest HD and slowing the disability of manifest HD. Although these scientific advances hold great promise, the present reality of HD challenges clinicians to care for the manifold unmet needs of patients and families.

Population Characteristics, Genetic Basis, and Natural History

HD is the most common inherited form of chorea and occurs worldwide, perhaps a consequence of multiple introductions of the gene from European migrations.[2] Because of its autosomal dominant mode of inheritance, family histories usually reveal other individuals in the family who are or have been affected by this progressively disabling disease.

It is now recognized that HD results from an expanded cytosine-adenine-guanine (CAG) trinucleotide repeat of the *IT15* (*interesting transcript 15*) gene that is located near the telomere of the short arm of chromosome 4. The expanded CAG repeat (CAGn), occurring in the first exon of the 5′ region of the gene, codes for an expanded polyglutamine region within the mutant protein named *huntingtin*.[3] The functions of the wild-type and mutant *huntingtin* proteins are unknown, but *huntingtin* seems to be involved in intracellular protein handling, including trafficking between cytoplasm and the nucleus.

What seem to be new mutations are rare and may represent expansion of the unstable trinucleotide repeat from an intermediate range (30 to 35 repeats) in the parent to a pathological range (≥36 repeats) in the offspring.[3] This tendency for expansion, especially when passed on from an affected father, and the phenotypic variation within families and between generations are examples of the "dynamic mutation" of the trinucleotide repeat underlying HD.

HD is found throughout Europe, North America, South America, and Australia, especially in white populations, with prevalence rates relatively uniform, ranging from 2 to 8 per 100,000.[4] Prevalence rates are highest around Lake Maracaibo in Venezuela and the Moray Firth region of Scotland, and HD is relatively rare in Asian countries and among African blacks.[4,5] Regions of the world largely populated by individuals of European descent show a similar prevalence as Europe.[4,6,7]

On average, about two thirds of the life of an HD gene carrier is lived in a relatively healthy premanifest phase, whereas the last one third is characterized by the onset and progression of illness. At any point in time, HD gene carriers, who represent about 50% of the offspring of an affected parent, include one third who are manifest and two thirds who are not (yet). For the other 50% who did not inherit the HD gene, all (three thirds) never manifest HD. A prevalence snapshot of HD shows that for every individual who has manifest disease, there are five individuals at risk (two of whom are gene carriers and three of whom are not). In this context, approximately 30,000 people in the United States are estimated to have clinical manifestations of HD, and an additional 150,000 healthy people are at risk of developing HD.[8,9]

The HD gene is highly penetrant such that clinical features emerge eventually in HD gene carriers who live long enough to manifest illness. Individuals who

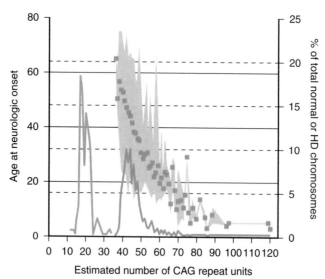

Figure 25–1 CAG repeat (CAGn) length on normal and Huntington's disease (HD) chromosomes and age at onset in HD. The CAGn length distribution of alleles found on normal (*blue line*) and HD (*dark pink line*) chromosomes is expressed as a percentage of each type of chromosome (*right axis*). The mean age at onset associated with each CAGn length is plotted as a *dark pink square* (against the *left axis*). The *light pink area* surrounding the mean age at onset denotes the range of ages at onset associated with any given repeat length, with deviations presumably being due to the effects of genetic, environmental, or stochastic modifiers. (From Gusella JF. Huntington's disease: two decades from mystery to models. *NeuroScience News.* 2000;3(2-3):15-22.)

have inherited the HD gene are very likely to show clinical features of illness in their lifetime. Illness usually becomes manifest between 35 and 40 years of age,[10] but there is considerable variation that depends largely on the length of the CAGn expansion, with onset varying from childhood to ninth decade of life. The average age of death for HD patients in the United States is approximately 60 years.[11] Very early age of onset seems to portend a short duration of illness, especially in juvenile-onset patients.[12,13] Other investigators have failed to confirm the association between age of onset and disease duration, however.[14]

Clinical expressivity varies, largely related to age at clinical onset, which is heavily influenced by the extent of CAGn expansion (Fig. 25–1). On average, the longer the CAGn expansion, the earlier the clinical onset of HD. Longitudinal observation of the extensive Venezuela HD cohort showed a slightly younger mean age of onset of 33 years in this population compared with a North American population.[15] Overall, CAGn accounts for 60% to 70% of the variance in clinical age at onset, representing a powerful biological effect of the HD gene mutation.[3] CAGn accounts for only about 45% of the variance among HD patients with a CAGn in the 40 to 50 range, however, which is the most common CAGn range, and the most variable with respect to age at onset.

As powerful as the CAGn expansion length is in influencing age at onset, it exerts much weaker effects in determining the course or pace of illness progression and disability.[16] It is as if CAGn is the major trigger of clinical onset, but then plays a less influential role in shaping the course of progressive functional decline and disability. This phenomenon suggests the interplay of genetic factors other than CAGn and environmental factors that affect the course of illness after HD has become manifest.

The Huntington Study Group (HSG) (www.huntington-study-group.org) is an international consortium of clinical investigators who are committed to developing better treatments for HD. The Unified Huntington Disease Rating Scale (UHDRS), developed by HSG, measures disease severity in manifest HD across four domains: motor, cognition, behavior, and functional capacity.[17] The UHDRS has been shown to have a high degree of internal consistency and inter-rater reliability.[18] Over time, HD patients generally show a worsening of motor function with increasing dystonia and stable chorea scores, worsening cognitive performance, increased occurrence of behavioral disorders, and worsening functional status.[19] The UHDRS has been used extensively in research to evaluate the impact of experimental therapies on disease progression and illness severity in manifest HD. Subtle abnormalities in UHDRS motor and cognitive domains may differentiate at-risk individuals who do or do not carry the HD gene.[20-23]

Total Functional Capacity (TFC) represents a standardized rating of functions and disability that is part of the UHDRS and has been used extensively in clinical research of manifest HD.[24] This scale ranges from a score of 13 (normal) to 0 (completely incapacitated), and assesses a patient's capacity in five functional domains of capacity: employability, financial abilities, domestic tasks, activities of daily living, and care provisions.[24] Longitudinal studies have shown an annual decline in TFC of approximately 0.8 to 1 unit per year.[25-27] This consistency across populations has made TFC a useful tool for the evaluation of potential therapeutic interventions. The TFC scale seems to be of limited value, however, in characterizing the subtle disability of emerging signs and symptoms in premanifest HD.[28]

HEREDITY AND RISK OF HUNTINGTON DISEASE

HD is an autosomal dominant, adult-onset neurodegenerative disorder whereby offspring of an affected parent carry a nominal 50:50 risk of having inherited (or not) the causally related mutant gene. Without knowledge of the extent of CAGn expansion of the affected parent, the risk of having inherited the HD gene depends more precisely on the age of the offspring, and the sex and age at onset of the affected parent. Because the peak age at clinical onset of HD is about 40 years and the average age at death is about 60 years,[11] the actuarial risk of an unaffected adult at risk for HD begins to diminish by age 55 to 60 years.[8] If the affected parent is the father, clinical onset of HD is on average slightly earlier than if the affected parent is the mother. Unaffected offspring of an affected father tend to reduce their actuarial risk slightly earlier than unaffected offspring of an affected mother.

GENOTYPE AND RISK OF HUNTINGTON DISEASE

The foregoing estimates were based on the information that had accrued from studying hereditary patterns and age at clinical onset in families and populations affected by HD. In the 1980s, advances in molecular genetics led to identification of the gene causing HD and transformed how and to what extent at-risk individuals are able to learn of their gene-carrier status. Largely through the study of extended families in the Lake Maracaibo region of Venezuela and the application of molecular genetic techniques, the single gene mutation responsible for HD was identified in 1993.[3] Much has been learned about the pathogenesis of HD from this seminal genetic discovery, including how the mutant *huntingtin* protein leads to the pathological hallmarks of disease. These discoveries are addressed Chapter 24 dealing with the etiology, pathology, and pathogenesis of HD. Much has also been learned about the relationship of expanded CAGn with the clinical manifestations of HD and the premanifest period when clinical changes can first be discerned.

Clinical Diagnosis

The signs and symptoms of HD vary depending on age at clinical onset, clinical stage of illness, and extent of clinical scrutiny. The clinical characteristics of HD have traditionally been categorized as motor, cognitive, and behavioral, but these domains are highly inter-related and stem from a common process of selective neuronal degeneration and resulting gliosis and atrophy. The first signs of HD detected by a clinician or family member are often not reflected by expressed symptoms or complaints. Individuals with emerging signs of HD tend not to complain of cognitive or motor impairments, perhaps partly as a result of denial or impaired insight. In retrospect, seemingly subtle changes in behavior and especially in personality, mood, and temperament often herald the onset of disease.

Motor and cognitive impairments develop in all HD patients, but the resulting disability and handicap depend on many psychosocial and other modifying factors. Identification of the gene and the resulting ability to detect gene-carrier status has had a major impact on how and when HD is diagnosed. Individuals at risk for HD are under great scrutiny by themselves, family members, and others for emerging clinical features. Many symptoms and concerns may not be specific to HD, rather reflecting the general background of health and illness. Although the clinical recognition of manifest HD is seemingly straightforward, the diagnosis is typically confirmed only months or years after the insidious emergence of signs and symptoms referable to motor, cognitive, behavioral, and functional impairments.[15,25-27,29-32] Even demonstrable motor and cognitive abnormalities may be fleeting and unrelated to HD, perhaps resulting from medications, pregnancy, infections, immunological disorders, depression, or stress.[33] In contrast to these identifiable disorders, the cognitive and motor signs of HD tend to progress over months and years until disability becomes evident.

In an adult known to be at risk for HD, the emergence of an otherwise unexplained, sustained or progressive extrapyramidal movement disorder, especially associated with oculomotor impairment or cognitive decline, may be viewed as strong presumptive evidence of manifest disease.[3,34] This constellation of clinical findings is accurate and usually sufficient for making the diagnosis of HD,[35] especially in the setting of a positive family history. Evidence of striatal atrophy by magnetic resonance imaging (MRI) is usually, but not always, an accompaniment of early HD.

When clinical features resemble HD, but the family history is absent or sketchy, DNA testing for the HD gene can be informative. The inaugural diagnosis of HD in a family carries major implications and confers new risks on the siblings and offspring of the individual who has been diagnosed. DNA testing for the HD gene, including the number of CAGn, is reserved primarily for informed, consenting, and counseled adults, whether to help confirm the diagnosis of manifest HD or for unaffected individuals at risk for HD who wish to learn if they have inherited the HD gene. The complex decision to be tested, the currently irreversible consequences of learning of one's HD gene-carrier status, and the research implications for premanifest HD are discussed later.

MOTOR PHENOTYPE

Chorea is the most characteristic and conspicuous movement disorder of HD, occurring in nearly all affected adults. A wide range of other motor abnormalities may occur early, however, and antedate the onset of chorea, including impaired ocular motility, rapid alternating movements, and impaired fine motor coordination.[15,25,36-45] Chorea represents fast, arrhythmic, semipurposeful and involuntary movements; HD patients seem to have an uncanny ability to blend chorea into voluntary movements, often in the forms of crossing and uncrossing of the legs, smoothing of the hair, or rubbing of the chin or brow (parakinesias). Patterns of choreic movements may appear stereotyped in an individual patient, but vary considerably from patient to patient. What may begin as subtle, fleeting movement of the fingers and toes typically evolves into slower writhing movements in association with axial posturing or dystonia of the arms, legs, or torso (choreoathetosis). Motor impersistence may develop whereby individuals are unable to maintain tongue protrusion or eye closure.

Impairment in oculomotor function may be evidenced by increased latency of response, insuppressible eye blinks or head movements associated with saccade initiation, and slowing of saccade velocity.[25,36,43,44,46-48] The slower and more sustained abnormal postures of dystonia may be seen early, especially in individuals with younger onset, who on average have more expanded CAGn than individuals with older onset. Dystonia may also develop and predominate as typical adult-onset HD advances, a phenomenon that may be exacerbated by neuroleptic drugs that block dopamine receptors.[15,26,40] Other movement disorders commonly develop with progression of disease, including bradykinesia, rigidity, myoclonus, tics, bruxism, and ataxia.[37,38,42,49-51] Hypertonicity, representing pyramidal (spasticity) and extrapyramidal (rigidity) tone abnormalities, may be seen, even in the same patient. Other signs of pyramidal tract dysfunction are also seen, including, hyperreflexia, clonus, and extensor plantar responses.[51]

Dysarthria can occur at any stage of the illness and may progress to make speech unintelligible. In contrast to Alzheimer's disease, central (cortical) language is largely unaffected in HD. Dysphagia tends to be most prominent in the terminal stages of the disease, and aspiration is a common cause of death.[39,52] Gait, station, and balance become increasingly impaired in HD. Superimposed chorea may give the gait a dancelike or lurching appearance. Patients have a remarkable ability to maintain their balance and move in a zigzag pattern despite appearing to be thrown off balance by sudden involuntary movements. Station is typically broad-based, and postural reflexes are eventually lost, leading to falls and injury.

Generally, clinical onset of HD before age 30 and particularly in adolescence or childhood is more likely to show motor features characterized by dystonia, oculomotor impairment, incoordination, and bradykinesia compared with the more chorea-predominant and hyperkinetic features associated with clinical onset after age 30.[53]

COGNITIVE PHENOTYPE

Intellectual impairment, similar to motor impairment, is a cardinal clinical feature of HD that occurs early and is a major source of progressive disability. The profile of cognitive impairment is characterized by selective deficits in psychomotor, executive, and visuospatial abilities.[14,54-57] Memory, the ability to shift cognitive sets, visuospatial processing, cognitive speed, sensorimotor function, concentration, and the acquisition and encoding of sensory stimuli are typically impaired.[54,55,58-60] Some individuals with HD are prone to cognitive inflexibility whereby they may perseverate incessantly about specific and seemingly unimportant issues. Such cognitive inflexibility, which may be extremely distressing to caregivers, is thought to result from dysfunction of frontostriatal loops.[54,61,62] Higher cortical language and gnostic operations that are typically impaired in Alzheimer's disease are generally spared in HD, where insight is relatively preserved. Frank dementia, defined by global intellectual performance 2 standard deviations below the mean for healthy controls, is a common but not inevitable consequence of advanced illness.[14,59]

Measurable cognitive impairments may precede the early motor manifestations of HD. Studies evaluating cognitive measures in seemingly unaffected individuals who have inherited the gene show early impairment in psychomotor tasks, memory, and frontal executive function, frequently antedating motor symptoms.[12,15,30,31,46,63-68] Other studies have failed to show early cognitive impairment in asymptomatic individuals.[69-73]

Two large prospective studies involving individuals at risk for HD who have chosen not to undergo predictive DNA testing (Prospective Huntington At Risk Observational Study [PHAROS]) and individuals who have been tested (Neurobiological Predictors of HD [PREDICT-HD]) are under way to help clarify the specificity, pattern, and temporal sequence of the earliest cognitive and motor abnormalities among HD gene carriers.[74,75] Initial data from PHAROS and PREDICT-HD indicate that psychometric impairment was detected very early, perhaps months to years before extrapyramidal motor abnormalities appeared.[28] It remains to be clarified to what extent these early detectable abnormalities are a source of disability or predictive of future disability.

BEHAVIORAL PHENOTYPE

Psychiatric illness and the "tendency to insanity and suicide," were recognized by Huntington as an important feature of hereditary chorea.[1] A wide array of psychiatric and behavioral disturbances, including mood disorders, psychosis, anxiety, obsessions, compulsions, aggression, irritability, and apathy, are now recognized as common and disabling features of HD.[76] In contrast to the motor and cognitive impairments, the behavioral disorders of HD are more varied and may be florid in some patients, but minimal or absent in other patients.

Affective disorders are an important and a potentially treatable manifestation of HD. Depression may occur in 50% of HD patients,[6,76] and manic features develop in about 10% of patients.[6,77] Affective disorders may be related to the disruption of specific frontal-subcortical neural pathways regulating mood.[78] Apathy, characterized by a loss of emotion resulting in an internal feeling of disinterest or a behavioral state of inaction,[79] is a problem commonly mentioned by caregivers of patients with HD, and may occur independent of depression.[80]

The suicide rate in HD patients is five times more frequent than in the general population and may account for 2% of HD mortality.[81] Suicidal behavior and completed suicides are not always linked to depression and other mood disorders. Impulsivity, access to firearms and medications, and life events such as loss of employment or a driver's license seem to be predisposing and potentially treatable suicidal factors.

Psychosis is also more common in HD than in the general population, occurring in 15% of HD patients,[76,77] and may be more common in young-onset cases.[6] Frank auditory or visual hallucinations are rare,[82] but paranoia is a common psychotic manifestation. Psychotic features usually emerge in an insidious fashion; the acute onset of hallucinations should alert the clinician to other causes of psychiatric disturbance, such as drug intoxication.

Anxiety disorders, consisting of generalized anxiety, panic attacks, and obsessive and compulsive symptoms, are common[82]; nearly two thirds of HD patients showed increased indices of aggression using a standardized rating scale.[79] Aggressive behavior may vary in severity from short-temperedness and overreaction to relatively trivial issues to overt violence. Irritability, reflecting an inability to control temper or a reduced threshold for the development of anger, may be linked to aggressive behavior and not be recognized by patients themselves. If left untreated, irritability may lead to aggressive behaviors and psychiatric hospitalization.[83] Aggressive behavior may also reflect other underlying psychopathology, such as paranoia, depression, or anxiety.

Psychiatric disturbances may be early manifestations of HD and seemingly predate motor and cognitive abnormalities. It has been suggested that psychiatric disturbances are more common in at-risk individuals who have inherited the HD gene compared with their counterparts who have not inherited the gene,[30,84] but such differences have not been uniformly observed.[64,67] Although features may develop very early, the HD specificity of subtle psychiatric symptoms before clinical diagnosis has not yet been established.[85]

Search for a Systemic Phenotype

Individuals who have inherited the HD gene have expanded CAGn and mutant *huntingtin* in all their cells; neural tissues bear the pathological brunt of selective degeneration. Nonetheless, it is surprising that more systemic and widespread metabolic abnormalities do not become manifest in HD patients. Difficulty maintaining body weight in the face of seemingly adequate caloric intake has been long recognized as a clinically relevant problem that often heralds or accompanies functional decline. Cellular metabolic inefficiencies involving mitochondrial electron transport and glucose metabolism may represent systemic abnormalities that contribute to the progressive clinical decline of HD.[86]

Difficulty in maintaining body weight is a phenomenon that occurs in premanifest and very early and more advanced manifest HD.[87] In manifest HD, weight loss usually occurs in a setting of a healthy-appearing appetite and high caloric intake that cannot keep pace with the steady loss of body mass. HD patients have lower body mass index (weight/height) than age-matched controls,[87-91] and these differences are more apparent with advancing disease.[88-90] Indirect calorimetry shows about 11% to 14% higher 24-hour energy expenditure in HD patients compared with normal controls, which has been attributable largely to voluntary and involuntary movements.[92,93] If provided with sufficient caloric intake, some of these individuals were capable of a positive energy balance and maintaining their weight.[93] Weight loss in manifest HD seems to be multifactorial, partly related to a relative reduction in caloric intake and increased energy expenditure owing to physical activity.[92,93]

In the PHAROS cohort of unaffected adults at risk for HD, individuals who have inherited the HD gene have a lower body mass index compared with their counterparts who do not carry the gene.[94] The lower body mass index of premanifest HD is also associated with increased energy expenditure, caused by either physical activity that is clinically unrecognized or alterations in energy efficiency. In premanifest HD, the apparently normal physical activity suggests systemic metabolic abnormalities, possibly leading to a hypermetabolic state.[95,96] It is unclear to what extent weight loss reflects early neuronal vulnerability and brain pathology[96] or the ubiquitous HD gene that may be expressed subtly in peripheral somatic cells.

In the context of low body mass index and weight loss in HD, it is surprising that glucose intolerance and non–insulin-dependent diabetes mellitus occur in HD.[97-99] A carefully conducted study has shown reduced insulin secretion in 29 normoglycemic HD patients compared with 22 control participants who were administered intravenous glucose tolerance tests. This initially sluggish insulin response was associated with reduced insulin sensitivity and increased insulin resistance.[100] Hypothalamic dysfunction, perhaps involving altered growth hormone secretion, may be a contributing factor.[101] Of investigative interest, transgenic HD mice commonly develop diabetes as a terminal consequence of progressive disease.[102] Altered insulin secretion; insulin resistance; and subtle pathology in pancreas, liver, and skeletal muscle[103,104] require more systematic examination as factors leading to the peculiar bioenergetic features of HD. Further metabolic research in unaffected HD gene carriers and in patients with manifest disease should help elucidate bioenergetic mechanisms, which would inform about therapeutic strategies aimed at maintaining body mass and slowing the progression of disease.

Juvenile-onset Huntington Disease

Young-onset HD accounts for about 10% to 15% of affected individuals. Clinical onset in childhood shows a unique clinical phenotype that is often associated with 50 or more expanded CAGn. The juvenile variant of HD, where age of onset occurs before 20, is typically manifested by an akinetic-rigid phenotype, which often emerges as rigidity, dystonia, and bradykinesia.[13,25,105-117] Juvenile-onset of HD may not always fit this stereotype, however. Cognitive and behavioral changes in the young, relatively immature brain may antedate the onset of motor abnormalities. Paternal inheritance of the HD gene is the rule for onset before age 10 years and still predominates (~3:1 paternal:maternal) for onset between ages 10 and 20.[13,105]

Care of the Huntington Disease Patient and Family

Because of the profound hereditary nature of HD, care of the patient is also care of the family. This expansion of care is unavoidable and preferable in providing the necessary information, counseling, and treatment that have implications beyond the traditional one-on-one patient-clinician relationship. Generally, the family approach to care is becoming increasingly applicable in the age of molecular genetics, and DNA predictive testing remains challenging because of often complicated and unique family dynamics and interactions. Topics for ongoing discussion with the patient and family include the boundaries of sharing genetic and hereditary information, the implications for family members who are unaware of HD and its hereditary features, and the precautions and safeguards required to protect individual privacy and confidentiality. The increasing amount of new knowledge about the mutant gene, the virtual inevitability of manifest illness in gene carriers, the strong relationship of clinical onset to CAGn, and the current lack of disease-modifying treatments have added to the burdens and uncertainties confronted by HD patients and families, particularly those who learn of the at-risk status and choose to undergo DNA testing.

PREDICTIVE DNA TESTING

Since DNA testing for the HD gene became available in about 1993, less than 10% of individuals who are at immediate risk (50:50) for HD have chosen to be tested, and only about 500 predictive DNA tests are performed in the United States annually[118]; rates of testing seem to be slightly higher in Canada and Europe.[112] There are myriad reasons for deciding not to be tested, including an increased risk to offspring if the test were positive, lack of effective treatment, potential loss of health and life insurance,[119] costs of testing, and inability to "undo" the test results.[120] The impact of the results may affect entire families and reach far beyond the individual tested.[121]

Fears about testing are understandable and should be respected rather than challenged. Individuals who choose to remain at risk for HD rather than learn definitively of their HD gene carrier status often cite their comfort level in living with ambiguity and uncertainty.[122] The relief from a negative result is offset by the grim reality of a positive one. In evaluating the impact of HD DNA testing, some investigators have not found a negative psychological impact of predictive testing,[123,124] but others have reported adverse psychosocial effects in individuals who received nonexpanded (negative) CAGn results and individuals who have received expanded (positive) CAGn test results.[125]

Studies also indicate that some individuals who undergo DNA testing may fear or experience discrimination, especially if they are refused employment or insurance based on genetic risk.[126-129] The enactment in the United States of the Genetic Information Nondiscrimination Act (GINA), taking effect in 2009, is intended to protect individuals from discrimination by employers and health insurers on the basis of genetic or hereditary information that may have been learned through participation in DNA testing or clinical research.[130,131] It remains to be determined how GINA and similar legislation will influence the participation of HD family members in DNA testing and clinical research involving genetic information.

PRENATAL TESTING

Direct prenatal DNA testing, involving detection of the actual CAG expansion in fetal cells, is accurate, but also reveals the HD gene-carrier status of the at-risk parent. Exclusion testing using linkage analysis can exclude the allele of the at-risk grandparent while the at-risk parent remains nominally at 50% risk and unaware of individual gene status. In either approach to prenatal testing, the implication is that a pregnancy would be aborted if the fetus is found to be at high risk for HD. Experiences with prenatal testing vary, and prenatal testing is a highly personal decision.[132] In a European study where 305 individuals underwent prenatal testing between 1993-1998, 131 (43%) tests were high risk for HD, and 8 of these pregnancies continued.[133] There is controversy about prenatal screening for HD where gene carriers may remain healthy for 30 to 50 years before the onset of illness.[133-135]

For a potential parent who is at risk for or known to carry the HD gene, preimplantation genetic diagnosis of HD is an alternative to prenatal testing that may not carry the same ethical dilemmas.[136] This scenario involves in vitro fertilization to prompt ovulation and the development of multiple fertilized eggs, which are retrieved, fertilized, and screened for the HD gene. Embryos not containing the HD gene are returned to the mother to complete pregnancy.[137,138] This highly technical and expensive approach is not without its own ethical dilemmas and societal implications.[139]

GENETIC TESTING AND COUNSELING

The decision facing HD family members to undergo predictive or prenatal DNA testing is personal, complex, and life-changing. Individuals at risk for HD may choose the irreversible decision to learn of their HD gene-carrier status. A potential parent at risk for or known to carry the HD gene may choose prenatal testing and the potential consequences and dilemmas that arise from such reproductive planning options. Considerable effort and time must be devoted to the education, counseling, and ongoing care of individuals at risk for HD and individuals known to carry the HD gene. Skilled and experienced genetic and psychological counseling is essential before and after the administration of the predictive or prenatal test.[140,141] These choices are best assessed within the context of the family care paradigm because of the far-reaching implications of test results.

Medical Care and Treatment of Manifest Huntington Disease

General medical care of the HD patient is similar to the care of an otherwise healthy child or adult who manifests the motor, cognitive, and behavioral features of HD. With the exception of the tendency for glucose intolerance and progressive weight loss associated with HD, there are no systemic medical problems that require clinical attention. The clinician should remain mindful, however, of the potential for impaired compensation in the setting of organ dysfunction or comorbid disease because the HD gene is present in all somatic cells, including skeletal muscle wherein dysfunction have been shown in HD transgenic mice.[103]

Reasonably effective pharmacotherapy has been developed for temporary treatment of the motor, cognitive, and behavioral symptoms of HD notwithstanding the progressive underlying neurodegeneration. Most symptomatic therapies used in HD have not been rigorously evaluated. The reader is referred to a more recent evidence-based review by Bonelli and Wenning[142] of symptomatic and disease-modifying pharmacological treatments for HD. This comprehensive review is also a useful guide and helpful starting point for clinicians and clinical investigators by which to measure success in addressing the many unmet needs of HD. Most therapies have focused on ameliorating chorea, and there have been few controlled studies of treatments for the cognitive, affective, or behavioral disorders of HD.

TREATMENT OF MOVEMENT DISORDER

Treatment of chorea has been a major focus of therapeutic development because of the relative ease and potency by which dopamine-blocking agents (neuroleptics) and dopamine-depleting agents ameliorate the involuntary movements of HD. Not all chorea requires treatment, however, and the drawbacks of antichoreic therapy should be carefully considered and reconsidered. Antichoreic treatments should be reserved for patients who have prominent chorea interfering with gait, balance, activities of daily living, or self-care functions. Many treated patients show functional benefits, but antichorea therapy is also attended by risks of worsening the same functional impairments that are the target of treatment. The natural pattern of HD progression is also characterized by diminishing intensity of chorea and increasing dystonic posturing.[25] These observations support the need for periodic assessment of HD patients treated with antichoreic therapies. Physical and occupational therapies are sensible, but there are no controlled studies of benefit.

Agents that block postsynaptic dopamine receptors (e.g., fluphenazine,[143] haloperidol[144]) are generally effective in suppressing chorea, but treatment is often associated with nagging long-term risks of promoting superimposed tardive dyskinesia and the more immediate adverse effects of dysphoria, apathy, and bradykinesia. The so-called atypical antipsychotic drugs might be expected to lessen chorea; however, only clozapine has been subjected to short-term rigorous assessment and with weak results.[145]

Tetrabenazine, which selectively depletes presynaptic vesicular-stored dopamine, was evaluated in a randomized placebo-controlled trial in 84 patients for 12 weeks and showed clear antichoreic effects associated with improvement in the (blinded) investigators' judgment of overall change.[146] Tetrabenazine treatment predisposed to parkinsonian features (bradykinesia, dysphagia) and depression, which could be remedied by reduction in dosage or discontinuation of tetrabenazine. Although tetrabenazine treatment is without risk of tardive dyskinesia, the potency and narrow therapeutic window of this catecholamine-depleting drug require careful dosage adjustment and periodic clinical re-evaluation.

Amantadine, an antiviral and anti-Parkinson agent that exerts partial N-methyl-D-aspartate (NMDA) antagonist effects, has shown conflicting results in treating chorea in randomized controlled trials.[147,148] Riluzole, which retards presynaptic glutamate release and is used in amyotrophic lateral sclerosis, shows mild beneficial effect on chorea at doses of 200 mg/day; however, its cost and the need to monitor liver function tests are drawbacks.[149] The fatty acid ethyl-EPA has been tested in randomized placebo-controlled studies of ambulatory HD patients who were treated for up to 12 months. No major adverse effects were encountered, but the antichoreic effects were modest and of unclear clinical relevance.[53]

There are no controlled trials evaluating dopaminergic treatment of the akinetic-rigid features of HD, but judicious use of levodopa or dopamine agonists seems helpful when parkinsonian features predominate and are disabling. Drugs that increase dopaminergic neurotransmission may increase the severity of chorea, dystonia, and other hyperkinetic movements. There is no systematic research examining whether physical or occupational therapy improves the movement disorder of HD, or whether speech therapy improves dysarthria, intelligibility, or dysphagia.

TREATMENT OF COGNITIVE IMPAIRMENT

Although cognitive impairment is a major source of disability, there is meager evidence of benefit from medications used to improve cognition temporarily in other neurological disorders. Acetylcholinesterase inhibitors show modest and so far unimpressive results. No benefit was found in HD patients who were randomly assigned to donepezil 10 mg/day or placebo and followed for 12 weeks.[150] In an open-label study of rivastigmine,[151,152] there was a suggestion of benefit. Dimebolin hydrochloride (Dimebon), a novel antihistamine that has enhanced cognition in experimental models of Alzheimer's disease[153] and in a small controlled study of Alzheimer's patients (www.medivation.com), is currently being evaluated in HD to treat cognitive impairment (ClinicalTrials.gov Identifier NCT00497159).

TREATMENT OF MOOD AND BEHAVIORAL DISORDERS

Antidepressants have not been systematically evaluated in depressed HD patients, but traditional tricyclic and selective serotonin reuptake inhibitor antidepressants are widely considered to benefit HD.[142] The extent and duration of benefit have not been examined. Generally, a carefully monitored trial of selective serotonin reuptake inhibitor or tricyclic antidepressants should be considered for HD patients who are depressed or suspected to have a unipolar mood disorder. Suicidal behavior and completed suicide are common outcomes in HD. Depression is likely a predisposing factor, but impulsivity, alcohol and substance abuse, and access to harmful or lethal agents contribute to the increased suicidal risks of HD.

There are no controlled studies of treatments comparing antidepressant, mood-stabilizing, or antipsychotic treatments in HD. A randomized placebo-controlled trial of fluoxetine in 30 nondepressed HD patients who were followed for 4 months did not show any benefit on functional, neurological, or cognitive batteries, but did show slight improvement in agitation.[154] Clozapine may improve chorea and psychosis,[155,156] but requires monitoring for the rare occurrence of leukopenia. Although obsessive-compulsive symptoms, apathy, irritability, and aggressive behavior may accompany HD, treatments for these distressing and disabling disorders have not been systematically examined.

EXPERIMENTAL TREATMENTS FOR HUNTINGTON DISEASE

The major difference between so-called symptomatic and neuroprotective treatments for neurodegenerative disorders rests in the duration of the therapeutic effect. Symptomatic therapies improve the signs and symptoms of illness without affecting underlying disease progression; benefits are only temporary in the setting of progressive neurodegeneration. Neuroprotection refers to interventions aimed at producing enduring benefits by favorably influencing underlying etiology or pathogenesis.[157] Although it is desirable to mount biological evidence of neuroprotection, enduring benefit of relevant clinical outcomes over months and years is tantamount to disease modification for disorders such as HD wherein steady and relatively rapid functional decline parallels progressive neurodegeneration.

Restorative therapies promote regrowth or repair of areas of neuronal injury or cell loss. Neuroprotective and restorative treatments exert disease-modifying effects, which could be measured by slowing clinical decline in manifest HD or forestalling onset of illness in premanifest HD ("secondary prevention"). In their evidence-based review, Bonelli and Wenning[142] summarized the outcomes of disease-modifying clinical trials for HD. The scientific rationale for these trials is addressed in Chapter 24.

To date, no studies have decisively shown a slowing of clinical progression in manifest HD. The randomized controlled trial in ambulatory HD patients of coenzyme Q10, an antioxidant and cofactor involved in mitochondrial electron transfer, and remacemide, a noncompetitive NMDA receptor antagonist, illustrates a multicenter effort to ameliorate distal pathogenetic mechanisms in HD.[158] Employing a double-blind, placebo-controlled, parallel group, 2×2 factorial design, 347 patients with early HD were evaluated for a minimum of 30 months by HSG investigators at 23 sites in the United States and Canada. Research participants were randomly assigned to one of four treatment groups: coenzyme Q10 600 mg daily, remacemide 600 mg daily, the combination of coenzyme Q10 and remacemide, or placebo. Remacemide exerted a modest antichoreic effect, but did not slow functional capacity, which was the prespecified primary outcome. In contrast, individuals treated with coenzyme Q10 showed about a 13% slowing in functional decline ($P = .15$) and a benefit on cognitive measures compared with individuals not receiving coenzyme Q10. (Fig. 25–2).[159] These encouraging findings using relatively low-dose coenzyme Q10 and studies of coenzyme Q10 showing good tolerability at doses of 2400 mg/day (K. Kieburtz, personal communication) have prompted a 5-year placebo-controlled study (2-CARE) of coenzyme Q10 2400 mg/day in early HD patients (clintrials.gov registration # NCT00608881).

Creatine increases cytoplasmic brain phosphocreatine to maintain cellular adenosine triphosphate levels and buffer energy metabolism.[160] Similar to coenzyme Q10, creatine is a nutritional supplement that exerts antioxidative effects and neuroprotective effects in HD animal models.[161,162] Creatine, 8 g/day, was safe and well tolerated, and reduced blood indices of oxidative DNA injury in 64 HD patients.[163] Creatine, 10 g/day, in 13 HD patients for 2 years was safe and well tolerated, and associated with weight stabilization.[164] The disease-modifying rationale and dose-ranging and safety studies in HD have prompted the development of a multicenter, placebo-controlled, randomized controlled trial of high-dosage creatine (CREST-E), which is being conducted by HSG and enrolling research participants (CREST-E clintrials.gov registration# pending).

Minocycline is a caspase inhibitor and second-generation tetracycline that exerts various antiapoptotic, antioxidant, and antiexcitotoxic effects of potential neuroprotective benefit in HD.[165,166] Minocycline is safe and well tolerated in doses of 200 mg/day in HD,[167] but a subsequent study showed no persuasive evidence of benefit.[168] (ClinicalTrials.gov Identifier NCT00277355).

Inhibition of histone deacetylase is a treatment strategy for some types of cancer[169,170] and favorably affects transcriptional dysregulation that is observed in HD models.[171] A more recently completed study of phenylbutyrate, a histone deacetylase inhibitor, has shown sufficient safety and tolerability to consider further trials of this compound.[172]

The failure of disease-modifying interventions in HD so far may be related to many factors, including selection of drug and dosage, penetration into the brain, duration of exposure and follow-up, and sensitivity of clinical outcome measures. A lingering concern is that irreversible pathogenic processes have already developed in early HD patients, reducing the likelihood of neuroprotective action and outcomes. If so, potential disease-modifying treatments might best be initiated before the onset of HD when pathogenic mechanisms are potentially more reversible.[173] To address this concern, a randomized, controlled study (PREQUEL) has been designed to examine the safety, tolerability, and dosage of coenzyme Q10 in unaffected (premanifest) individuals who through predictive DNA testing are known to carry the HD gene (clintrials.gov registration# NCT00920699). This study will soon be under way as a prelude to more definitive studies aimed at forestalling the clinical onset and attendant disability of HD.

To inform better about research methodology and potential biomarkers in premanifest HD, two large prospective observational studies are under way to inform about the feasibility of conducting clinical trials in this population and to identify the sensitive and specific early precursors of HD onset and correlative biomarkers of premanifest disease. PHAROS enrolled 1001 clinically unaffected adults at risk for HD who chose not to undergo predictive DNA testing.[74]

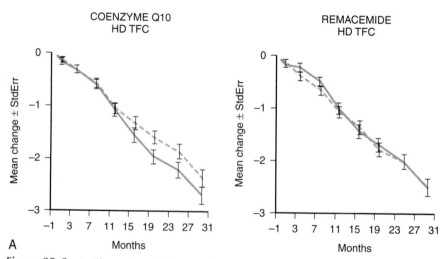

Figure 25–2 A, Change in total functional capacity (TFC) from randomization (*baseline*) to 30 months of prospective follow-up for coenzyme Q10, 600 mg/day (*solid line*), versus no coenzyme Q10 (*dashed line*) on the left and remacemide, 600 mg/day (*solid line*), versus no remacemide (*dashed line*) on the right.

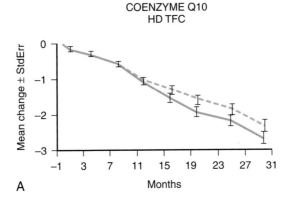

A

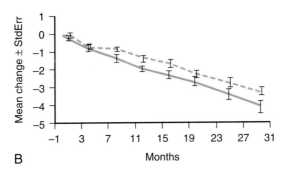

B

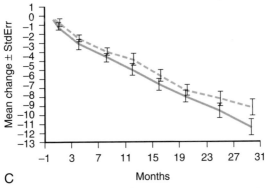

C

Figure 25–2, cont'd B, Treatment effects of coenzyme Q10, 600 mg (*solid line*), versus no coenzyme Q10 (*dashed line*) comparing functional outcomes measures of TFC (*top*), the HD Functional Assessment checklist (*middle*) and the HD Independence Scale (*bottom*). HD, Huntington's disease. (From Huntington Study Group: A randomized, placebo-controlled trial on coenzyme Q10 and remacemide in Huntington's disease. *Neurology*. 2001;57:397-404.)

Beginning in 1999 and using procedures to deidentify data and protect the confidentiality of genetic status, 1001 PHAROS research participants consented to be followed in a multiyear, double-blinded longitudinal study to examine the precursors of clinical onset and the specificity of emerging phenotype to CAGn length. PREDICT-HD is a similarly large prospectively observational study that largely involves unaffected adults who have chosen to undergo predictive DNA testing and have been informed that they have inherited the HD gene. PREDICT-HD research participants have also consented to be followed prospectively and undergo extensive cognitive assessments and standardized MRI to assess the predictive value of quantitative clinical assessments and emerging biomarkers relative to the clinical onset of HD.[75] The clinical and biological markers corresponding to clinical onset from these and other longitudinal studies are expected to provide useful clinical end points, needed experience, and potential biomarkers for clinical trials aimed at postponing the onset and corresponding disability of HD.

RESTORATIVE STRATEGIES

Prompted by animal models studies in which transplanted striatal cells have been shown to survive, differentiate, grow, and reverse some motor and behavioral abnormalities,[174-176] restorative approaches using transplantation of fetal tissue have been undertaken in HD patients. In preliminary, small, uncontrolled trials in HD patients,[177-180] implantation of striatal fetal tissue has been considered safe. Functional neuroimaging studies have shown increased metabolic activity in some patients treated with fetal tissue allografts and prolonged survival of these grafts; however, these biomarker changes have not been accompanied by sustained clinical benefit.[178,179,181-183] Motor deterioration and mood changes have also developed in some patients.[177,179] Clinical research guidelines for tissue transplantation in HD have been developed,[184] but the investigative experience is limited to small numbers of patients without blinded assessments or controlled interventions.

Ciliary neurotrophic factor has been shown to protect striatal neurons in HD animal models,[185] and has been administered intraventricularly in HD patients.[186] An innovative approach to restorative therapy has emerged from knowledge about how growth factors such as brain-derived neurotrophic factor can coax periventricular stem cells to become neurons. By overexpressing the Noggin gene that promotes neuronal differentiation and using intraventricular administration of adenovirus vectors to overexpress brain-derived neurotrophic factor and Noggin, investigators have been successful in inducing neurogenesis of medium-sized spiny neurons, which have enhanced performance and survival in HD transgenec (R6/2) mice.[187] Clinical translation of this animal research to HD depends on replication in other animal experiments and the development of safe and effective methods of vector administration in humans.

Participation in Huntington Disease Clinical Research

Identification of the HD gene and advances in drug discovery have improved prospects for the development of treatments that slow the progression of manifest HD and delay the clinical onset of premanifest HD. Experimental therapeutics has become the focus of scientific inquiry in HD, largely as a result of the concerted efforts of the HD community and scientists, and substantive research sponsorship from nonprofit HD-focused organizations, government, and industry. Still, it is expected that it will take many years and sustained participation in clinical research before the ultimate therapeutic objectives are realized.

Research participation by HD family members, including individuals with manifest and premanifest HD, is key for advancing scientific knowledge and facilitating the development of safe and effective treatments. In addition to aforementioned therapeutic trials in manifest HD and planned trials in premanifest HD, HSG (www.huntington-study-group.org), through the sponsorship of the nonprofit foundation CHDI Inc, New York, NY (www.CHDI-inc.org), is enrolling HD patients and their family members in the North American COHORT observational study (www.huntingtonproject.org and www.clinicaltrials.gov), to develop biological markers of HD gene expression and disease progression, improve understanding of genotype-phenotype relationships, and identify genetic factors that may modify the onset and course of HD. Eligible COHORT research participants include individuals with manifest HD, individuals at nominal 50:50 risk to have HD who have chosen not to be tested, individuals who have chosen to undergo predictive DNA testing and been found to carry the HD gene (premanifest HD) or not carry the gene (controls), and spouse controls of individuals with manifest or premanifest HD.

A parallel observational and biomarker study in Europe called REGISTRY, conducted by the European HD Network (EHDN) (www.euro-hd.net) and sponsored by CHDI Inc, is enrolling similar HD family research participants. COHORT and REGISTRY include annual clinical assessments, the provision of samples for biomarker research, and information about HD clinical research. Neither study precludes participation in experimental interventional studies. For current information on HD clinical trials, the reader is referred to www.clinicaltrials.gov and www.HDtrials.org.

Conclusions

Identification of the HD gene, the rapid pace of scientific discovery, and expanding knowledge about the clinical and biological features of premanifest and manifest HD hold great promise for substantive therapeutic advances. The therapeutic gains are expected to be incremental over the coming years, and require the commitment and patience of HD patients and the clinicians who care for them. In the meantime, there are manifold unmet clinical needs to address. The option to learn of one's gene carrier status, the expanding group of individuals who learn they have premanifest HD, technological advances such as preimplantation genetic diagnosis, and incremental gains in developing disease-modifying therapies carry potential drawbacks as well as benefit. There remains an unmet need for improved treatments to lessen the disability associated with the signs and symptoms of manifest illness and the emerging predictors of disability associated with premanifest HD. The challenges remain, but there is a rational and evidence-based pathway forward to lessen the burden and improve the quality of life for patients and families affected by HD.

REFERENCES

1. Huntington G: On chorea. Medical and Surgical Reporter 1872;26:317-321.
2. Giron L Jr, Koller W: A critical survey and update on the epidemiology of Huntington's disease. In Gorelick P, Alter M, eds: Handbook of Neuroepidemiology. New York: Marcel Dekker 1994, pp 181-292.
3. A novel gene containing a trinucleotide repeat that is expanded and unstable on Huntington's disease chromosomes. The Huntington's Disease Collaborative Research Group. Cell 1993;72: 971-983.
4. Harper PS: The epidemiology of Huntington's disease. Hum Genet 1992;89:365-376.
5. Hayden MR, MacGregor JM, Beighton PH: The prevalence of Huntington's chorea in South Africa. South Afr Med J 1980;58:193-196.
6. Folstein SE, Chase GA, Wahl WE, et al: Huntington disease in Maryland: clinical aspects of racial variation. Am J Hum Genet 1987;41:168-179.
7. Kokmen E, Ozekmekci FS, Beard CM, et al: Incidence and prevalence of Huntington's disease in Olmsted County, Minnesota (1950 through 1989). Arch Neurol 1994;51:696-698.
8. Conneally PM: Huntington disease: genetics and epidemiology. Am J Hum Genet 1984;36: 506-526.
9. Tanner CM, Goldman SM: Epidemiology of movement disorders. Curr Opin Neurol 1994;7: 340-345.
10. Farrer LA, Conneally PM: A genetic model for age at onset in Huntington disease. Am J Hum Genet 1985;37:350-357.
11. Lanska DJ, Lavine L, Lanska MJ, Schoenberg BS: Huntington's disease mortality in the United States. Neurology 1988;38:769-772.
12. Foroud T, Gray J, Ivashina J, Conneally PM: Differences in duration of Huntington's disease based on age at onset. J Neurol Neurosurg Psychiatry 1999;66:52-56.
13. van Dijk JG, van der Velde EA, Roos RA, Bruyn GW: Juvenile Huntington disease. Hum Genet 1986;73:235-239.
14. Josiassen RC, Curry LM, Mancall EL: Development of neuropsychological deficits in Huntington's disease. Arch Neurol 1983;40:791-796.
15. Penney JB Jr, Young AB, Shoulson I, et al: Huntington's disease in Venezuela: 7 years of follow-up on symptomatic and asymptomatic individuals. Mov Disord 1990;5:93-99.
16. Ravina B, Romer M, Constantinescu R, et al: The relationship between CAG repeat length and clinical progression in Huntington's disease. Mov Disord 2008;23(9):1223-1227.
17. The Huntington Study Group; Kieburtz K: The Unified Huntington's Disease Rating Scale: reliability and consistency. Mov Disord 1996;11:136-142.
18. Hogarth P, Kayson E, Kieburtz K, et al: Interrater agreement in the assessment of motor manifestations of Huntington's disease. Mov Disord 2005;20:293-297.
19. Siesling S, van Vugt JP, Zwinderman KA, et al: Unified Huntington's Disease Rating Scale: a follow up. Mov Disord 1998;13:915-919.
20. Saft C, Andrich J, Meisel NM, et al: Assessment of simple movements reflects impairment in Huntington's disease. Mov Disord 2006;21:1208-1212.
21. Kipps CM, Duggins AJ, Mahant N, et al: Progression of structural neuropathology in preclinical Huntington's disease: a tensor based morphometry study. J Neurol Neurosurg Psychiatry 2005;76:650-655.
22. Snowden JS, Craufurd D, Thompson J, Neary D: Psychomotor, executive, and memory function in preclinical Huntington's disease. J Clin Exp Neuropsychol 2002;24:133-145.
23. Langbehn DR, Paulsen JS: Predictors of diagnosis in Huntington disease. Neurology 2007;68: 1710-1717.
24. Shoulson I, Kurlan R, Rubin A: Assessment of functional capacity in neurodegenerative movement disorders: Huntington's disease as a prototype. In Munsat TL, ed: Quantification of Neurologic Deficit. Boston: Butterworths, 1989, pp 285-306.
25. Young AB, Shoulson I, Penney JB, et al: Huntington's disease in Venezuela: neurologic features and functional decline. Neurology 1986;36:244-249.
26. Feigin A, Kieburtz K, Bordwell K, et al: Functional decline in Huntington's disease. Mov Disord 1995;10:211-214.
27. Shoulson I, Odoroff C, Oakes D, et al: A controlled clinical trial of baclofen as protective therapy in early Huntington's disease. Ann Neurol 1989;25:252-259.
28. Biglan KM, Zhao H, Oakes D, et al: HSG PHAROS Investigators. Longitudinal analysis of the UHDRS in individuals at-risk for Huntington's disease [Abstract]. Ann Neurol 2008;64(12):S51.

29. Greenamyre J, Shoulson I: Huntington's disease. In Calne D, ed: Neurodegenerative Diseases. Philadelphia: Saunders 1986, pp 685–704.
30. McCusker E, Richards F, Sillence D, et al: Huntington's disease: neurological assessment of potential gene carriers presenting for predictive DNA testing. J Clin Neurosci 2000;7:38-41.
31. Hahn-Barma V, Deweer B, Durr A, et al: Are cognitive changes the first symptoms of Huntington's disease? A study of gene carriers. J Neurol Neurosurg Psychiatry 1998;64:172-177.
32. Baxter LR Jr, Mazziotta JC, Pahl JJ, et al: Psychiatric, genetic, and positron emission tomographic evaluation of persons at risk for Huntington's disease. Arch Gen Psychiatry 1992;49:148-154.
33. Shoulson I: On chorea. Clin Neuropharmacol 1986;9(Suppl 2):S85-S99.
34. Folstein SE, Leigh RJ, Parhad IM, Folstein MF: The diagnosis of Huntington's disease. Neurology 1986;36:1279-1283.
35. Bateman D, Boughey AM, Scaravilli F, et al: A follow-up study of isolated cases of suspected Huntington's disease. Ann Neurol 1992;31:293-298.
36. Tian JR, Zee DS, Lasker AG, Folstein SE: Saccades in Huntington's disease: Predictive tracking and interaction between release of fixation and initiation of saccades. Neurology 1991;41:875-881.
37. Carella F, Scaioli V, Ciano C, et al: Adult onset myoclonic Huntington's disease. Mov Disord 1993;8:201-205.
38. Jankovic J, Ashizawa T: Tourettism associated with Huntington's disease. Mov Disord 1995;10:103-105.
39. Leopold NA, Kagel MC: Dysphagia in Huntington's disease. Arch Neurol 1985;42:57-60.
40. Louis ED, Lee P, Quinn L, Marder K: Dystonia in Huntington's disease: prevalence and clinical characteristics. Mov Disord 1999;14:95-101.
41. van Vugt JP, van Hilten BJ, Roos RA: Hypokinesia in Huntington's disease. Mov Disord 1996;11:384-388.
42. Racette BA, Perlmutter JS: Levodopa responsive parkinsonism in an adult with Huntington's disease. J Neurol Neurosurg Psychiatry 1998;65:577-579.
43. Beenen N, Buttner U, Lange HW: The diagnostic value of eye movement recordings in patients with Huntington's disease and their offspring. Electroencephalogr Clin Neurophysiol 1986;63:119-127.
44. Collewijn H, Went LN, Tamminga EP: Vegter-Van der Vlis M. Oculomotor defects in patients with Huntington's disease and their offspring. J Neurol Sci 1988;86(2-3):307-320.
45. Siemers E, Foroud T, Bill DJ, et al: Motor changes in presymptomatic Huntington disease gene carriers. Arch Neurol 1996;53:487-492.
46. Kirkwood SC, Siemers E, Bond C, et al: Confirmation of subtle motor changes among presymptomatic carriers of the Huntington disease gene. Arch Neurol 2000;57:1040-1044.
47. Oepen G, Clarenbach P, Thoden U: Disturbance of eye movements in Huntington's chorea. Arch Psychiatr Nervenkrank 1981;229:205-213.
48. Blekher T, Johnson SA, Marshall J, et al: Saccades in presymptomatic and early stages of Huntington disease. Neurology 2006;67:394-399.
49. Reuter I, Hu MT, Andrews TC, et al: Late onset levodopa responsive Huntington's disease with minimal chorea masquerading as Parkinson plus syndrome. J Neurol Neurosurg Psychiatry 2000;68:238-241.
50. Tan EK, Jankovic J, Ondo W: Bruxism in Huntington's disease. Mov Disord 2000;15:171-173.
51. Paulson GW: Diagnosis of Huntington's disease. In Chase TN, Wexler NS, Barbeau A, eds: Huntington's Disease. New York: Raven Press 1979, pp 177-184.
52. Edmonds C: Huntington's chorea, dysphagia and death. Med J Aust 1966;2:273-274.
53. Dorsey ER: Huntington Study Group TREND-HD Investigators. Randomized, controlled trial of ethyl eicosapentaenoic acid in Huntington disease: the TREND study. Arch Neurol 2008;65(12):1582-1589.
54. Bamford KA, Caine ED, Kido DK, et al: Clinical-pathologic correlation in Huntington's disease: a neuropsychological and computed tomography study. Neurology 1989;39:796-801.
55. Lawrence AD, Sahakian BJ, Hodges JR, et al: Executive and mnemonic functions in early Huntington's disease. Brain 1996;119(Pt 5):1633-1645.
56. Wilson RS, Garron DC: Cognitive and affective aspects of Huntington's disease. In Chase TN, Wexler NS, Barbeau A, eds: Huntington's Disease. New York: Raven Press, 1979, pp 193-201.
57. Shelton PA, Knopman DS: Ideomotor apraxia in Huntington's disease. Arch Neurol 1991;48: 35-41.
58. Morris M: Dementia and cognitive changes in Huntington's disease. In Weiner WJ, Lang A, eds: Behavioral Neurology of Movement Disorders. New York: Raven Press 1995, pp 187-200.

59. Pillon B, Dubois B, Ploska A, Agid Y: Severity and specificity of cognitive impairment in Alzheimer's, Huntington's, and Parkinson's diseases and progressive supranuclear palsy. Neurology 1991;41:634-643.
60. Huber SJ, Paulson GW: Memory impairment associated with progression of Huntington's disease. Cortex 1987;23:275-283.
61. Watkins LH, Rogers RD, Lawrence AD, et al: Impaired planning but intact decision making in early Huntington's disease: implications for specific fronto-striatal pathology. Neuropsychologia 2000;38:1112-1125.
62. Lawrence AD, Weeks RA, Brooks DJ, et al: The relationship between striatal dopamine receptor binding and cognitive performance in Huntington's disease. Brain 1998;121(Pt 7):1343-1355.
63. Paulsen JS, Zhao H, Stout JC, et al: Clinical markers of early disease in persons near onset of Huntington's disease. Neurology 2001;57:658-662.
64. Strauss ME, Brandt J: Are there neuropsychologic manifestations of the gene for Huntington's disease in asymptomatic, at-risk individuals? Arch Neurol 1990;47:905-908.
65. Diamond R, White RF, Myers RH, et al: Evidence of presymptomatic cognitive decline in Huntington's disease. J Clin Exp Neuropsychol 1992;14:961-975.
66. Jason GW, Pajurkova EM, Suchowersky O, et al: Presymptomatic neuropsychological impairment in Huntington's disease. Arch Neurol 1988;45:769-773.
67. Rosenberg NK, Sorensen SA, Christensen AL: Neuropsychological characteristics of Huntington's disease carriers: a double blind study. J Med Genet 1995;32:600-604.
68. Lawrence AD, Hodges JR, Rosser AE, et al: Evidence for specific cognitive deficits in preclinical Huntington's disease. Brain 1998;121(Pt 7):1329-1341.
69. Giordani B, Berent S, Boivin MJ, et al: Longitudinal neuropsychological and genetic linkage analysis of persons at risk for Huntington's disease. Arch Neurol 1995;52:59-64.
70. de Boo GM, Tibben A, Lanser JB, et al: Early cognitive and motor symptoms in identified carriers of the gene for Huntington disease. Arch Neurol 1997;54:1353-1357.
71. Blackmore L, Simpson SA, Crawford JR: Cognitive performance in UK sample of presymptomatic people carrying the gene for Huntington's disease. J Med Genet 1995;32:358-362.
72. Rothlind JC, Brandt J, Zee D, et al: Unimpaired verbal memory and oculomotor control in asymptomatic adults with the genetic marker for Huntington's disease. Arch Neurol 1993;50:799-802.
73. Wexler NS: Perceptual-motor, cognitive, and emotional characteristics of persons at risk for Huntington's disease. In Chase TN, Wexler NS, Barbeau A, eds: Huntington's Disease. New York: Raven Press, 1979, pp 257-271.
74. Huntington Study Group PHAROS Investigators: At risk for Huntington disease: The PHAROS (Prospective Huntington At Risk Observational Study) cohort enrolled. Arch Neurol 2006;63:991-996.
75. Paulsen JS, Hayden M, Stout JC, et al: Preparing for preventive clinical trials: the Predict-HD study. Arch Neurol 2006;63:883-890.
76. Caine ED, Shoulson I: Psychiatric syndromes in Huntington's disease. Am J Psychiatry 1983;140:728-733.
77. Mendez MF: Huntington's disease: update and review of neuropsychiatric aspects. Int J Psychiatry Med 1994;24:189-208.
78. Mayberg HS, Starkstein SE, Peyser CE, et al: Paralimbic frontal lobe hypometabolism in depression associated with Huntington's disease. Neurology 1992;42:1791-1797.
79. Burns A, Folstein S, Brandt J, Folstein M: Clinical assessment of irritability, aggression, and apathy in Huntington and Alzheimer disease. J Nerv Mental Dis 1990;178:20-26.
80. Levy ML, Cummings JL, Fairbanks LA, et al: Apathy is not depression. J Neuropsychiatry Clinical Neurosci 1998;10:314-319.
81. Schoenfeld M, Myers RH, Cupples LA, et al: Increased rate of suicide among patients with Huntington's disease. J Neurol Neurosurg Psychiatry 1984;47:1283-1287.
82. Guttman M, Alpay M, Chouinard S: Clinical management of psychosis and mood disorders in Huntington's disease. In Bedard MA, Agid Y, Chouinard G et al, eds: Mental and Behavioral Dysfunction in Movement Disorders. Totowa, NJ: Humana Press, 2002.
83. Dewhurst K, Oliver JE, McKnight AL: Socio-psychiatric consequences of Huntington's disease. Br J Psychiatry 1970;116:255-258.
84. Shiwach RS, Norbury CG: A controlled psychiatric study of individuals at risk for Huntington's disease. Br J Psychiatry 1994;165:500-505.
85. Duff K, Paulsen JS, Beglinger LJ, et al. Psychiatric symptoms in Huntington's disease before diagnosis. Biol Psychiatry 2007;62(12):1341-1346.

86. Schapira AH: Mitochondrial function in Huntington's disease: clues for pathogenesis and prospects for treatment. Ann Neurol 1997;41:141-142.
87. Djousse L, Knowlton B, Cupples LA, et al: Weight loss in early stage of Huntington's disease. Neurology 2002;59:1325-1330.
88. Morales LM, Estevez J, Suarez H, et al: Nutritional evaluation of Huntington disease patients. Am J Clin Nutr 1989;50:145-150.
89. Hamilton JM, Wolfson T, Peavy GM, et al: Rate and correlates of weight change in Huntington's disease. J Neurol Neurosurg Psychiatry 2004;75:209-212.
90. Robbins AO, Ho AK, Barker RA: Weight changes in Huntington's disease. Eur J Neurol 2006; 13:e7.
91. Trejo A, Tarrats RM, Alonso ME, et al: Assessment of the nutrition status of patients with Huntington's disease. Nutrition 2004;20:192-196.
92. Pratley RE, Salbe AD, Ravussin E, Caviness JN: Higher sedentary energy expenditure in patients with Huntington's disease. Ann Neurol 2000;47:64-70.
93. Gaba AM, Zhang K, Marder K, et al: Energy balance in early-stage Huntington disease. Am J Clin Nutr 2005;81:1335-1341.
94. Marder K, Zhao H, Eberly S, et al: On behalf of the Huntington Study Group. Dietary intake in adults at risk for Huntington disease: Analysis of PHAROS research participants. Neurology 2009;68:A230.
95. Mochel F, Charles P, Seguin F, et al: Early energy deficit in Huntington disease: identification of a plasma biomarker traceable during disease progression. PLoS ONE 2007;2:e647.
96. Petersen A, Bjorkqvist M: Hypothalamic-endocrine aspects in Huntington's disease. Eur J Neurosci 2006;24:961-967.
97. Podolsky S, Leopold NA, Sax DS: Increased frequency of diabetes mellitus in patients with Huntington's chorea. Lancet 1972;1:1356-1358.
98. Podolsky S, Leopold NA: Abnormal glucose tolerance and arginine tolerance tests in Huntington's disease. Gerontology 1977;23:55-63.
99. Farrer LA: Diabetes mellitus in Huntington disease. Clin Genet 1985;27:62-67.
100. Lalic NM, Maric J, Svetel M, et al: Glucose homeostasis in Huntington disease: abnormalities in insulin sensitivity and early-phase insulin secretion. Arch Neurol 2008;65:476-480.
101. Leopold NA, Podolsky S: Exaggerated growth hormone response to arginine infusion in Huntington's disease. J Clin Endocrinol Metab 1975;41:160-163.
102. Hurlbert MS, Zhou W, Wasmeier C, et al: Mice transgenic for an expanded CAG repeat in the Huntington's disease gene develop diabetes. Diabetes 1999;48:649-651.
103. Strand AD, Aragaki AK, Shaw D, et al: Gene expression in Huntington's disease skeletal muscle: a potential biomarker. Hum Mol Genet 2005;14:1863-1876.
104. Turner C, Cooper JM, Schapira AH: Clinical correlates of mitochondrial function in Huntington's disease muscle. Mov Disord 2007;22:1715-1721.
105. Rasmussen A, Macias R, Yescas P, et al: Huntington disease in children: genotype-phenotype correlation. Neuropediatrics 2000;31:190-194.
106. Siesling S: Vegter-van der Vlis M, Roos RA. Juvenile Huntington disease in the Netherlands. Pediatr Neurol 1997;17:37-43.
107. Gomez-Tortosa E, del Barrio A, Garcia Ruiz PJ, et al: Severity of cognitive impairment in juvenile and late-onset Huntington disease. Arch Neurol 1998;55:835-843.
108. Roos RA, Vegter-van der Vlis M, Hermans J, et al: Age at onset in Huntington's disease: effect of line of inheritance and patient's sex. J Med Genet 1991;28:515-519.
109. Cannella M, Gellera C, Maglione V, et al: The gender effect in juvenile Huntington disease patients of Italian origin. Am J Med Genet B Neuropsychiatr Genet 2004;125B:92-98.
110. Nance MA: Genetic testing of children at risk for Huntington's disease. US Huntington Disease Genetic Testing Group. Neurology 1997;49:1048-1053.
111. Oliva D, Carella F, Savoiardo M, et al: Clinical and magnetic resonance features of the classic and akinetic-rigid variants of Huntington's disease. Arch Neurol 1993;50:17-19.
112. Laccone F, Engel U, Holinski-Feder E, et al: DNA analysis of Huntington's disease: five years of experience in Germany, Austria, and Switzerland. Neurology 1999;53:801-806.
113. Squitieri F, Berardelli A, Nargi E, et al: Atypical movement disorders in the early stages of Huntington's disease: clinical and genetic analysis. Clin Genet 2000;58:50-56.
114. Wexler NS, Lorimer J, Porter J, et al: Venezuelan kindreds reveal that genetic and environmental factors modulate Huntington's disease age of onset. Proc Natl Acad Sci U S A 2004;101:3498-3503.
115. Duesterhus P, Schimmelmann BG, Wittkugel O, Schulte-Markwort M: Huntington disease: a case study of early onset presenting as depression. J Am Acad Child Adolesc Psychiatry 2004;43: 1293-1297.

116. Squitieri F, Pustorino G, Cannella M, et al: Highly disabling cerebellar presentation in Huntington disease. Eur J Neurol 2003;10:443-444.
117. Ribai P, Nguyen K, Hahn-Barma V, et al: Psychiatric and cognitive difficulties as indicators of juvenile Huntington disease onset in 29 patients. Arch Neurol 2007;64:813-819.
118. Nance M, Myers RH: Trends in predictive and prenatal testing for Huntington's disease 1993-1999. The US Huntington Disease Genetic Testing Group. Am J Hum Genet 1999;65:A406.
119. Oster E, Dorsey ER, Bausch J, et al: Huntington Study Group PHAROS Investigators. Fear of health insurance among individuals at risk for Huntington disease. Am J Med Genet Part A 2008;146A:2070-2077.
120. Quaid KA, Morris M: Reluctance to undergo predictive testing: the case of Huntington disease. Am J Med Genet 1993;45:41-45.
121. Hayes CV: Genetic testing for Huntington's disease—a family issue. N Engl J Med 1992;327:1449-1451.
122. Quaid KA, Sims SL, Swenson MM, et al: Living at risk: concealing risk and preserving hope in Huntington disease. J Genet Couns 2008;17:117-128.
123. Wiggins S, Whyte P, Huggins M, et al: The psychological consequences of predictive testing for Huntington's disease. Canadian Collaborative Study of Predictive Testing. N Engl J Med 1992;327:1401-1405.
124. Duncan RE, Gillam L, Savulescu J, et al: "Holding your breath": interviews with young people who have undergone predictive genetic testing for Huntington disease. Am J Med Genet A 2007;143:1984-1989.
125. Tibben A, Frets PG, van de Kamp JJ, et al: On attitudes and appreciation 6 months after predictive DNA testing for Huntington disease in the Dutch program. Am J Med Genet 1993;48:103-111.
126. Alper JS, Geller LN, Barash CI, et al: Genetic discrimination and screening for hemochromatosis. J Public Health Policy 1994;15:345-358.
127. Low L, King S, Wilkie T: Genetic discrimination in life insurance: empirical evidence from a cross sectional survey of genetic support groups in the United Kingdom. BMJ (Clin Res Ed) 1998;317:1632-1635.
128. Billings PR, Kohn MA, de Cuevas M, et al: Discrimination as a consequence of genetic testing. Am J Hum Genet 1992;50:476-482.
129. Lapham EV, Kozma C, Weiss JO: Genetic discrimination: perspectives of consumers. Science (New York) 1996;274:621-624.
130. Slaughter LM: Genetic testing and discrimination: how private is your information? Stanford Law Policy Rev 2006;17:67-81.
131. Slaughter LM: Your genes and privacy. Science (New York) 2007;316:797.
132. Post SG: Huntington's disease: prenatal screening for late onset disease. J Med Ethics 1992;18:75-78.
133. Simpson SA, Zoeteweij MW, Nys K, et al: Prenatal testing for Huntington's disease: a European collaborative study. Eur J Hum Genet 2002;10:689-693.
134. Creighton S, Almqvist EW, MacGregor D, et al: Predictive, pre-natal and diagnostic genetic testing for Huntington's disease: the experience in Canada from 1987 to 2000. Clin Genet 2003;63:462-475.
135. Tassicker RJ, Marshall PK, Liebeck TA, et al: Predictive and pre-natal testing for Huntington disease in Australia: results and challenges encountered during a 10-year period (1994-2003). Clin Genet 2006;70:480-489.
136. Braude PR, De Wert GM, Evers-Kiebooms G, et al: Non-disclosure preimplantation genetic diagnosis for Huntington's disease: practical and ethical dilemmas. Prenat Diag 1998;18:1422-1426.
137. Sermon K, De Rijcke M, Lissens W, et al: Preimplantation genetic diagnosis for Huntington's disease with exclusion testing. Eur J Hum Genet 2002;10:591-598.
138. Stern HJ, Harton GL, Sisson ME, et al: Non-disclosing preimplantation genetic diagnosis for Huntington disease. Prenat Diag 2002;22:503-507.
139. De Wert GM: Ethical aspects of prenatal testing and preimplantation genetic diagnosis for late-onset neurogenetic disease: the case of Huntington disease. In Evers-Kiebooms G, Harper P, Zoeteweij MW, eds: Prenatal Testing for Late-onset Neurogenetic Diseases. Routeledge, UK 2002, pp 129–158.
140. Tibben A, Duivenvoorden HJ, Vegter-van der Vlis M, et al: Presymptomatic DNA testing for Huntington disease: identifying the need for psychological intervention. Am J Med Genet 1993;48:137-144.
141. Quaid KA, Brandt J, Faden RR, Folstein SE: Knowledge, attitude, and the decision to be tested for Huntington's disease. Clin Genet 1989;36:431-438.

142. Bonelli RM, Wenning GK: Pharmacological management of Huntington's disease: an evidence-based review. Curr Pharmaceut Design 2006;12:2701-2720.
143. Fahn S: Perphenazine in Huntington's chorea. In Barbeau A, Chase TN, Paulson GW, eds: Advances in Neurology, Vol. 1: Huntington's Chorea, 1872-1972. New York: Raven Press, 1973.
144. Leonard DP, Kidson MA, Shannon PJ, Brown J: Double-blind trial of lithium carbonate and haloperidol in Huntington's chorea [Letter]. Lancet 1974;2:1208-1209.
145. van Vugt JP, Siesling S, Vergeer M, et al: Clozapine versus placebo in Huntington's disease: a double blind randomised comparative study. J Neurol Neurosurg Psychiatry 1997;63:35-39.
146. Huntington Study Group: Tetrabenazine as antichorea therapy in Huntington disease: a randomized controlled trial. Neurology 2006;66:366-372.
147. Verhagen Metman L, Morris MJ, Farmer C, et al: Huntington's disease: a randomized, controlled trial using the NMDA-antagonist amantadine. Neurology 2002;59:694-699.
148. O'Suilleabhain P, Dewey RB Jr: A randomized trial of amantadine in Huntington disease. Arch Neurol 2003;60:996-998.
149. Huntington Study Group: Dosage effects of riluzole in Huntington's disease: a multicenter placebo-controlled study. Neurology 2003;61:1551-1556.
150. Cubo E, Shannon KM, Tracy D, et al: Effect of donepezil on motot and cognitive function in Huntington disease. Neurology 2006;67:1268-1271.
151. de Tommaso M, Specchio N, Sciruicchio V, et al: Effects of rivastigmio on motor and cognitive impairment in Huntington's disease. Mov Disord 2004;19:1516-1518.
152. de Tommaso M, Difruscolo O, Sciruicchio V, et al: Two years' follow-up of rivastigmine treatment in Huntington disease. Clin Neuropharmacol 2007;30:43-46.
153. Lermontova NN, Lukoyanov NV, Serkova TP, et al: Dimebon improves learning in animals with experimental Alzheimer's disease. Bull Exp Biol Med 2000;129:544-546.
154. Como PG, Rubin AJ, O'Brien CF, et al: A controlled trial of fluoxetine in nondepressed patients with Huntington's disease. Mov Disord 1997;12:397-401.
155. Bonuccelli U, Ceravolo R, Maremmani C, et al: Clozapine in Huntington's chorea. Neurology 1994;44:821-823.
156. Sajatovic M, Verbanac P, Ramirez LF, Meltzer HY: Clozapine treatment of psychiatric symptoms resistant to neuroleptic treatment in patients with Huntington's chorea. Neurology 1991;41:156.
157. Shoulson I: DATATOP: a decade of neuroprotective inquiry. Parkinson Study Group. Deprenyl And Tocopherol Antioxidative Therapy Of Parkinsonism. Ann Neurol 1998;44(3 Suppl. 1): S160-S166.
158. Huntington Study Group: A randomized, placebo-controlled trial of coenzyme Q10 and remacemide in Huntington's disease. Neurology 2001;57:397-404.
159. Shults CW, Oakes D, Kieburtz K, et al: Effects of coenzyme Q10 in early Parkinson disease: evidence of slowing of the functional decline. Arch Neurol 2002;59:1541-1550.
160. Hemmer W, Wallimann T: Functional aspects of creatine kinase in brain. Dev Neurosci 1993;15 (3-5):249-260.
161. Ferrante RJ, Andreassen OA, Jenkins BG, et al: Neuroprotective effects of creatine in a transgenic mouse model of Huntington's disease. J Neurosci 2000;20:4389-4397.
162. Matthews RT, Yang L, Jenkins BG, et al: Neuroprotective effects of creatine and cyclocreatine in animal models of Huntington's disease. J Neurosci 1998;18:156-163.
163. Hersch SM, Gevorkian S, Marder K, et al: Creatine in Huntington disease is safe, tolerable, bioavailable in brain and reduces serum 8OH2'dG. Neurology 2006;66:250-252.
164. Tabrizi SJ, Blamire AM, Manners DN, et al: High-dose creatine therapy for Huntington disease: a 2-year clinical and MRS study. Neurology 2005;64:1655-1656.
165. Chen M, Ona VO, Li M, et al: Minocycline inhibits caspase-1 and caspase-3 expression and delays mortality in a transgenic mouse model of Huntington disease. Nat Med 2000;6:797-801.
166. Yrjanheikki J, Tikka T, Keinanen R, et al: A tetracycline derivative, minocycline, reduces inflammation and protects against focal cerebral ischemia with a wide therapeutic window. Proc Natl Acad ci U S A 1999;96:13496-13500.
167. Huntington Study Group: Minocycline safety and tolerability in Huntington disease. Neurology 2004;63:547-549.
168. Cudkowicz ME, McDermott M, Doolan R, et al: A phase 2 trial of minocycline in Huntington's disease. Mov Disord 2009;24(suppl 1),pS164.
169. Butler LM, Agus DB, Scher HI, et al: Suberoylanilide hydroxamic acid, an inhibitor of histone deacetylase, suppresses the growth of prostate cancer cells in vitro and in vivo. Cancer Res 2000;60:5165-5170.

170. Warrell RP Jr, He LZ, Richon V, et al: Therapeutic targeting of transcription in acute promyelocytic leukemia by use of an inhibitor of histone deacetylase. J Natl Cancer Inst 1998;90:1621-1625.

171. Steffan JS, Bodai L, Pallos J, et al: Histone deacetylase inhibitors arrest polyglutamine-dependent neurodegeneration in Drosophila. Nature 2001;413:739-743.

172. Hersch S: PHEND- HD: A safety, tolerability, and biomarker study of phenylbutyrate in symptomatic HD [Abstract]. Neurotherapeutics 2008;5:363.

173. Gomez-Tortosa E, MacDonald ME, Friend JC, et al: Quantitative neuropathological changes in presymptomatic Huntington's disease. Ann Neurol 2001;49:29-34.

174. Armstrong RJ, Watts C, Svendsen CN, et al: Survival, neuronal differentiation, and fiber outgrowth of propagated human neural precursor grafts in an animal model of Huntington's disease. Cell Transplant 2000;9:55-64.

175. Nakao N, Itakura T: Fetal tissue transplants in animal models of Huntington's disease: the effects on damaged neuronal circuitry and behavioral deficits. Progr Neurobiol 2000;61:313-338.

176. Borlongan CV, Koutouzis TK, Poulos SG, et al: Bilateral fetal striatal grafts in the 3-nitropropionic acid-induced hypoactive model of Huntington's disease. Cell Transplant 1998;7:131-135.

177. Bachoud-Levi A, Bourdet C, Brugieres P, et al: Safety and tolerability assessment of intrastriatal neural allografts in five patients with Huntington's disease. Exp Neurol 2000;161:194-202.

178. Philpott LM, Kopyov OV, Lee AJ, et al: Neuropsychological functioning following fetal striatal transplantation in Huntington's chorea: three case presentations. Cell Transplant 1997;6:203-212.

179. Hauser RA, Furtado S, Cimino CR, et al: Bilateral human fetal striatal transplantation in Huntington's disease. Neurology 2002;58:687-695.

180. Rosser AE, Barker RA, Harrower T, et al: Unilateral transplantation of human primary fetal tissue in four patients with Huntington's disease: NEST-UK safety report ISRCTN no. 36485475. J Neurol Neurosurg Psychiatry 2002;73:678-685.

181. Bachoud-Levi AC, Remy P, Nguyen JP, et al: Motor and cognitive improvements in patients with Huntington's disease after neural transplantation. Lancet 2000;356:1975-1979.

182. Bachoud-Levi AC, Gaura V, Brugieres P, et al: Effect of fetal neural transplants in patients with Huntington's disease 6 years after surgery: a long-term follow-up study. Lancet Neurol 2006;5:303-309.

183. Keene CD, Sonnen JA, Swanson PD, et al: Neural transplantation in Huntington disease: long-term grafts in two patients. Neurology 2007;68:2093-2098.

184. Quinn N, Brown R, Craufurd D, et al: Core Assessment Program for Intracerebral Transplantation in Huntington's Disease (CAPIT-HD). Mov Disord 1996;11:143-150.

185. Emerich DF, Winn SR: Neuroprotective effects of encapsulated CNTF-producing cells in a rodent model of Huntington's disease are dependent on the proximity of the implant to the lesioned striatum. Cell Transplant 2004;13:253-259.

186. Bloch J, Bachoud-Levi AC, Deglon N, et al: Neuroprotective gene therapy for Huntington's disease, using polymer-encapsulated cells engineered to secrete human ciliary neurotrophic factor: results of a phase I study. Hum Gene Ther 2004;15:968-975.

187. Cho SR, Benraiss A, Chmielnicki E, et al: Induction of neostriatal neurogenesis slows disease progression in a transgenic murine model of Huntington disease. J Clin Invest 2007;117:2889-2902.

26 | The Genetics and Pathogenesis of Dystonia

THOMAS T. WARNER

Introduction

The dystonias are an unusual group of hyperkinetic movement disorders whose main feature is involuntary muscle contraction or spasm.[1] The term *dystonia* was originally introduced by Oppenheim in 1911 to describe altering muscle tone and postural abnormalities that are seen in this condition. The concept of dystonia can be confusing because the term has been used to describe a symptom (e.g., a dystonic arm posture), a disease (primary torsion dystonia), and a syndrome. Overall, dystonias represent a common group of movement disorders that encompass a wide range of conditions—from those in which the only manifestation is dystonic muscle spasms to those in which dystonia is one part of a more severe neurological condition.[2]

This chapter explores more recent advances in understanding of the etiology of dystonia. We start with the role of genetic factors and molecular pathogenesis and then consider the abnormalities seen at the level of neural networks. First, a brief description of the etiological classification of dystonia is required. Dystonia can be divided into primary and secondary (or symptomatic) dystonia.[3] Primary torsion dystonia (PTD) comprises a group of dystonias that are unaccompanied by other neurological abnormalities except for tremor (arms or head and neck) and have no known cause apart from genetic causes that have been identified in some cases.[3,4] There is no evidence of neurodegeneration in PTD; it represents a disorder of abnormal function of the sensorimotor pathways.

Primary generalized dystonia is a progressive, disabling disorder that usually begins in childhood and is linked to several genetic loci.[4] Later onset primary focal dystonias are more common (~10 times as common as generalized PTD); nearly always occur in adults; and are focal, involving muscles of the neck, face, or arms, with leg involvement rare. Other inherited causes include the dystonia-plus syndromes, which are characterized by the presence of dystonia plus selected other neurological features (see later) and have a genetic basis without evidence of neurodegeneration.[5]

Secondary dystonias comprise syndromes in which dystonic symptoms arise from other disease states or brain injury.[3,6] They represent a large and diverse group of disorders with many causes, which can be divided into inherited, complex, and acquired causes. Dystonia can also be part of a more widespread neurological disorder in which there is underlying neurodegeneration (e.g., Wilson's disease); these are referred to as heredodegenerative causes.[6]

This chapter focuses on PTD and dystonia plus syndromes. The first section deals with genetic etiology, with particular emphasis on *DYT1* dystonia and dystonia-plus syndromes, where there have been the greatest advances in understanding of genetic features in the last 5 years. These forms of dystonia are described briefly (clinical features and treatment are discussed in Chapter 27), and our knowledge of genetic and molecular pathogenesis is explored. The second section describes findings from neurophysiological and imaging studies that have shaped current views on the pathogenesis of PTD.

Molecular Genetics of Primary Torsion Dystonia

Most forms of early-onset PTD are genetic in origin; Table 26–1 lists the genetic forms that have been identified to date. Most are autosomal dominant with reduced penetrance. This low penetrance suggests that a "second hit," such as inheritance of other genetic traits or environmental insults, may be required to trigger the onset of dystonia. The first gene to be identified was the *DYT1* gene, and most is known regarding its molecular pathogenesis.

EARLY-ONSET *DYT1* PRIMARY TORSION DYSTONIA (DYSTONIA MUSCULORUM DEFORMANS, OPPENHEIM'S DYSTONIA)

The most common cause of early-onset PTD (~80%) is a mutation in the *DYT1* gene on chromosome 9q34, which is inherited as an autosomal dominant trait with reduced penetrance of approximately 30% to 40%.[7] All cases of typical *DYT1* dystonia are caused by an in-frame GAG deletion (ΔGAG302/303; ΔE) in the

TABLE 26–1	**Genetics of Primary Torsion Dystonia**			
Type	Clinical Features	Frequency	Age of Onset	Inheritance/ Locus/Gene
DYT1	Limb onset; generalizes; can present as focal	50% cases early onset in non-Jews, 90% in Ashkenazi Jews	Childhood, most present by 26 yr	AD, *TOR1A*, protein torsinA
DYT2	Focal and generalized	Spanish gypsy families and single Iranian	Childhood to adult	AR, locus unknown
DYT4	Laryngeal and cervical; some generalize	Single Australian family	13-37 yr	AD, locus unknown
DYT6	Focal or generalized; cranial, cervical, or limb	Two Mennonite Amish families	Mean age of onset 19 yr	AD, *DYT6* chromosome 8p21-q22
DYT7	Focal dystonia; cervical and laryngeal	Single German family	28-70 yr	AD, *DYT7* chromosome 18p
DYT13	Cranial or cervical; some generalize	Single Italian family	Childhood to adult	AD, *DYT13* chromosome 1p36

AD, autosomal dominant; AR, autosomal recessive.

DYT1 gene, resulting in the loss of a glutamic acid in the C-terminal region of the encoded protein, torsinA.[8]

DYT1 dystonia typically manifests in childhood or adolescence (mean age of onset 12 years), during a distinct developmental window that overlaps with a period of high motor learning.[9] Onset of dystonia is often with posturing of a foot, leg, or arm. Dystonia is usually first apparent with specific actions (e.g., writing or walking), but becomes evident with less specific actions with time and spreads to other body regions. No other neurological abnormalities are present apart from postural arm tremor. Disease severity varies considerably even within the same family, and isolated writer's cramp may be the only sign. Approximately 60% to 70% of individuals have progression to generalized or multifocal dystonia involving at least a leg and an arm, and often axial muscles. Ten percent develop segmental dystonia (involving two contiguous body regions), and in only 25% does dystonia remain focal. The cranial muscles are involved in about 10% of individuals.[10]

There is a higher prevalence of *DYT1* PTD in the Ashkenazi Jewish population, where it accounts for 80% of early-onset cases starting in a limb and is believed to be the result of a founder mutation that appeared about 250 years ago during a population bottleneck.[11] In non-Jewish populations, 16% to 53% of cases of generalized early-onset PTD have been shown to be due to the *DYT1* gene.[9]

To gain insight into genetic factors that may influence penetrance, a more recent study analyzed three *DYT1* single nucleotide polymorphisms.[12] This included

D216H, a coding sequence variation that moderates the effects of the GAG deletion in cellular models.[13] The frequency of the 216H allele was increased in *DYT1*-deletion carriers without dystonia and decreased in carriers with dystonia compared with control individuals. Haplotype analysis showed a highly protective effect of the H allele in *trans* with the GAG deletion. There was also some evidence to support that the D216 allele in *cis* is required for the disease to be penetrant. This finding was relevant for genetic counseling because further analysis showed that the penetrance associated with carrying the D216 allele in *trans* was approximately 35%, and for the 216H allele was approximately 3%. Although the protective effect of the 216H allele is potent, it explains only a small proportion of the reduced penetrance associated with carrying the *DYT1* GAG-deletion mutation because it is an uncommon allele in the population.[12]

TorsinA is a member of the AAA ATPase superfamily of chaperone-like proteins.[14] In mammalian neuronal cells, torsinA is found throughout the cytoplasm, neurite processes, and growth cones.[15,16] TorsinA also has been found in the lumen of endoplasmic reticulum and in the space between the inner and the outer membrane of the nuclear envelope.[17-20] In contrast, in cells overexpressing the mutant (ΔE-torsinA), the protein was redistributed from endoplasmic reticulum to nuclear envelope, and accumulated in large perinuclear membranous inclusions, which arise from the nuclear envelope.[16,21-23] TorsinA-positive inclusions have been found in specific midbrain regions (pedunculopontine nucleus, periaqueductal gray) of four *DYT1* patients, suggesting they are relevant to the pathogenesis of *DYT1* dystonia.[24] In cell systems, the presence of the H216 variant of torsinA led to development of inclusions similar to the inclusions associated with ΔGAG-torsinA, but when H216 was introduced into ΔGAG-torsinA, there was a reduced tendency to form inclusions, suggesting the two changes offset each other.[13]

The finding of perinuclear inclusions has also been replicated in animal models, in transgenic mice overexpressing mutant ΔE torsinA[25,26] and in male *DYT1* ΔGAG knockin mice.[27] These mouse models did not have overt dystonia, but had motor deficits including hyperactivity, circling activity, and impaired beam walking. They also had reduced levels of striatal dopamine and dopamine metabolites. Transgenic mice expressing human mutant torsinA also have motor learning deficits without apparent changes in the level of dopamine receptors, transporters, or metabolites.[23,24] In addition, abnormalities in cholinergic interneuron physiology have been found in striatal slices.[28]

The redistribution of mutant ΔE-torsinA to the nuclear envelope has also been shown in torsinA null and homozygous mutant knockin mice that develop abnormalities of the nuclear envelope in postmigratory neurons.[29] These mice die at birth, which indicates that mutant torsinA leads to a loss of function.

Biochemical studies have identified numerous binding partners for torsinA, including the nuclear envelope protein LAP1 and the related endoplasmic reticulum protein LULL1/NET9[30] and kinesin light chain 1.[31] These interactions also point to roles for torsinA in regulating some aspect of nuclear envelope organization or in regulating microtubule-based movement of membrane compartments within cells, or both.

The lack of neuronal cell death in *DYT1* dystonia has led to the hypothesis that this condition is due to neuronal dysfunction or a neurochemical disturbance. Cell bodies of dopaminergic neurons seem to be enlarged in brains from dystonia patients.[32] Consistent with these observations, torsinA is highly expressed in dopaminergic neurons of the substantia nigra in human and rat brain.[33,34] Other evidence to support a neurochemical basis comes from a study in SH-SY5Y neuroblastoma cells, where the ΔE-enriched inclusions contain the vesicular monoamine transporter 2 (VMAT2), a membrane-associated protein involved in loading dopamine vesicles.[23]

Indirect evidence for abnormal dopaminergic function in *DYT1* dystonia comes from cell models showing that torsinA affects the membrane distribution of the dopamine transporter and influences the activation of dopaminergic D2 receptors in a transgenic mouse model.[28,35] More recent work in brain slices from a transgenic mouse model overexpressing ΔE-torsinA has suggested that mutant torsinA may interfere with the transport or release of dopamine, but does not alter presynaptic transporters or postsynaptic dopamine receptors.[36] Finally, a recent study has shown that in a cell system, torsinA interacts with the SNARE protein snapin to regulate synaptic vesicle turnover, and that ΔE-torsinA exerts its pathological effects through a loss of function mechanism.[37] Mutant ΔE-torsinA may lead to abnormal neurotransmission and disrupt the highly organized neuronal firing that occurs in the motor pathways involving the cortex and basal ganglia, leading to dystonic movements.

MIXED PRIMARY TORSION DYSTONIA

Clinical and genetic analysis has been performed on two Mennonite families with idiopathic torsion dystonia showing an autosomal dominant inheritance pattern with incomplete penetrance.[38] Linkage analysis mapped the gene in both families to chromosome 8p21-8q22 (*DYT6*). Some affected individuals had a phenotype indistinguishable from that found with the *DYT1* mutation. The site of onset was cranial or cervical in about half of the patients, however, and individuals who presented with limb symptoms later developed cranial or cervical symptoms. The age of onset was also later (average 18.9 years in *DYT6* dystonia versus 13.6 years in *DYT1* dystonia). In two of the cases with *DYT6* dystonia, the symptoms remained focal. Recently, mutations in the THAP1 gene have been shown to cause DYT6 dystonia in Mennonite and German families.[39] A subsequent study detected mutations in this gene in European patients with laryngeal/oromandicular dystonia that became generalized.[40]

An Italian family has also been reported in which there is focal or segmental dystonia, usually of adult onset and affecting the craniocervical region.[41] In this respect, the clinical features resemble the features of idiopathic late-onset focal dystonia. Some patients had early-onset dystonia (age 5 years), however, and a few developed generalized dystonia, suggesting that the dystonia in this family should be classified as the mixed type. Inheritance was autosomal dominant with incomplete penetrance, estimated to be less than 60%. The chromosomal locus in this family, *DYT13,* has been localized to a 22-cM interval on 1p36.13-36.32.[41]

ADULT-ONSET FOCAL PRIMARY TORSION DYSTONIA

Most cases of focal adult-onset PTD seem to be sporadic. Numerous families have been described with late-onset dystonia, however, some of which have affected individuals with the same type of dystonia (e.g., cervical dystonia, focal hand dystonia, or blepharospasm).[42] In these families, dystonia is inherited as an autosomal dominant trait with reduced penetrance. Linkage analysis performed in one such family, identified the *DYT1* gene in a kindred with focal hand dystonia.[43] Linkage to *DYT6* and *DYT13* has never been described in families with pure late-onset dystonia.[44]

In a large German family with cervical and laryngeal dystonia, a genetic locus mapped (*DYT7*) to the short arm of chromosome 18.[45] Subsequently, a small Bulgarian family with writer's cramp was reported in which analysis was compatible (although not definitively proven) with linkage to the *DYT7* locus.[46] Analysis of other patients with adult-onset focal dystonia from northwestern Germany and Central Europe revealed similar haplotypes to the original *DYT7* family, suggesting a founder effect,[47] but these data have not been confirmed.[48]

Many clinical series have been reported in which relatives of an index case of focal PTD have been examined. In most cases, no more than one affected first-degree relative could be found. These studies indicate, however, that in 27% of cases, additional individuals with dystonia can be identified, suggesting the presence of an autosomal dominant gene or genes with reduced penetrance.[49,50] A meta-analysis of four of these studies found that there was more likely to be phenotypic concordance in proband-relative pairs if the proband had either cervical dystonia or focal hand dystonia.[40] In these case series, the data suggest that inheritance does not seem to be mendelian. This implies that the adult-onset focal primary dystonias are a multifactorial condition, in which several genes, along with environmental factors, combine to reach the threshold of dystonia. This implication has led to a search for potential susceptibility genes in population studies.

More recently, numerous studies have suggested an association between common *DYT1* haplotypes and adult focal PTD.[51-53] The picture is unclear, however, because two other studies did not find an association.[54,55] The D216H single nucleotide polymorphism was specifically examined in two of these studies, and in both cases, no association was found,[51,52] suggesting that other single nucleotide polymorphisms in the *DYT1* gene may play a role in focal dystonia.

Another potential susceptibility locus for development of focal dystonia was identified by studying polymorphisms in the dopamine receptor genes. An association with a multiallelic polymorphism of the D5 receptor gene and cervical dystonia was found.[56] Subsequent studies have found an association between this polymorphism and blepharospasm and cervical dystonia,[57,58] although lack of association has also been reported.[54]

Genetics of Dystonia-plus Syndromes

Dystonia-plus syndromes describe a group of conditions that can be distinguished from PTD based on clinical characteristics found in addition to dystonia, or specific pharmacological responses. They usually have a genetic etiology, but do not have underlying neurodegeneration. The group comprises three distinct conditions: dopa-responsive dystonia (DRD), myoclonus-dystonia syndrome (MDS), and rapid-onset dystonia parkinsonism.

DOPA-RESPONSIVE DYSTONIA

DRD was first described in Japan by Segawa and colleagues.[59] Patients typically present in childhood with gait disturbance owing to foot dystonia. The dystonia frequently worsens as the day goes on (diurnal variation) and is relieved by rest or sleep. Progression varies; some patients develop severe generalized dystonia, whereas others develop features suggestive of lower limb spasticity. Parkinsonian features such as bradykinesia and rigidity can develop in later life in some individuals, but also can be the presenting feature in adult life in a few cases. Occasionally, patients with DRD can present with adult-onset limb dystonia (e.g., writer's cramp), cranial or cervical dystonia, or signs resembling spastic paraplegia. In most cases, DRD is inherited as an autosomal dominant trait with reduced penetrance.

The key feature is that DRD shows a dramatic and sustained response to small doses of levodopa, sometimes 50 to 200 mg. Benefit is usually apparent within days to weeks, and the motor complications of levodopa treatment seen with Parkinson's disease rarely develop, even with long-term treatment.[60]

The gene for autosomal dominant DRD has been mapped to chromosome 14 (*DYT5*), and mutations within the gene for GTP cyclohydrolase 1 have been identified.[61] More than 60 mutations have been identified in all five exons, including point mutations and deletions. The gene is necessary for the production of tetrahydrobiopterin, a key cofactor required for dopamine synthesis, and in vitro studies have shown that patients have reduced GTP cyclohydrolase 1 activity leading to low levels of pterins and monoamines.[62] Most of the missense mutations seem to lie within the core of the protein and impair its tertiary structure or stability or both.[63] Other, extremely rare forms of DRD have been reported, including an autosomal recessive form with genetic deficiency of tyrosine hydroxylase, and defects in other enzymes involved in pterin synthesis.[64] These forms usually have additional features, such as parkinsonism, cognitive impairment, hypotonia, and seizures.

The importance of recognizing DRD is that it is treatable and responds extremely well to levodopa. DRD also highlights the potential role for abnormal dopaminergic neurotransmission in the pathogenesis of dystonia. A GCH1-deficient mouse model of *DYT5* shows metabolic parameters that are similar to those in humans with low levels of tetrahydrobiopterin, catecholamines, serotonin, and their metabolites, but not apparent motor phenotype.[65]

MYOCLONUS-DYSTONIA SYNDROME

MDS is characterized by the presence of dystonia in combination with brief lightning-like myoclonic jerks.[66] MDS usually has onset in childhood or early adolescence, with myoclonic jerks affecting the upper limbs and axial muscles (trunk and neck). The myoclonus can occur on rest and can be precipitated by action. Dystonia occurs in about two thirds of patients, with cervical dystonia and writer's cramp the most common forms. Occasionally, dystonia affects the legs. Several reports have identified psychiatric features associated with MDS, including obsessive-compulsive disorder, panic attacks, and anxiety.[67] Most patients note significant relief of symptoms with alcohol or benzodiazepines, and can have marked rebound of symptoms after administration of these.

MDS is frequently inherited as an autosomal dominant trait, caused by a heterozygous mutation in the gene for ε-sarcoglycan (*DYT11*) on chromosome 7q21.3, although sporadic cases also occur.[68] Numerous point mutations and small deletions have been reported. Maternal imprinting of the ε-sarcoglycan gene has been found to explain the highly reduced penetrance after maternal transmission of mutations.[69]

The sarcoglycans are a family of single pass transmembrane proteins that are part of the dystrophin-associated glycoprotein complex that links the actin cytoskeleton to the extracellular matrix in cardiac and skeletal muscle.[70] In contrast to α-δ sarcoglycans, which can cause autosomal recessive limb-girdle muscular dystrophies, ε-sarcoglycan is expressed in a wide variety of tissues. In the brain, it is highly expressed during development and is found in midbrain monaminergic neurons, cerebellar Purkinje cells, and other regions including the hippocampus and cortex.[71] It is located at the plasma membrane in neurons, muscle, and transfected cells. A study of the effect of missense mutations on ε-sarcoglycan in cultured cells showed that the mutant proteins had impaired trafficking to the plasma membrane and were retained intracellularly where they became polyubiquitinated and degraded by the proteasome.[72] TorsinA was shown to bind and promote degradation of ε-sarcoglycan mutants when they were coexpressed. The effect of this dysfunctional trafficking of ε-sarcoglycan on cell function and the nature of the torsinA interaction remains uncertain. A further autosomal dominant locus (DYT15) has been mapped to chromosome 18p11, but the causative gene has not been identified to date.[73]

RAPID-ONSET DYSTONIA PARKINSONISM

Rapid-onset dystonia parkinsonism is a rare autosomal dominant movement disorder with reduced penetrance. It is characterized by abrupt or subacute onset of dystonia and parkinsonism with prominent bulbar involvement.[74] Symptoms develop over hours to days with dystonic posturing of the limbs, bradykinesia, dysarthria, dysphagia, and postural instability, followed by little or no progression. Onset is usually in adolescence or young adulthood, and the subacute extrapyramidal storm can be preceded by stable mild limb dystonia for many years. Potential triggers in some families include emotional trauma, extreme heat, or physical exertion.

Investigations with magnetic resonance imaging, computed tomography, and positron emission tomography of the presynaptic dopamine uptake sites have been normal. In some patients, reduced levels of cerebrospinal fluid dopamine metabolites have been detected, but there is no clinical response to dopaminergic medication. The current assumption is that rapid-onset dystonia parkinsonism is due to neuronal dysfunction, rather than neurodegeneration, although no postmortem evaluations have been reported to date.

The condition is rare, and only a few families have been described with evidence for autosomal dominant inheritance with reduced penetrance. The gene was mapped to chromosome 19q13.2 (DYT12), and mutations in the gene for the Na+,K+-ATPase α3 subunit (ATP1A3) have been identified.[75] This finding implicates the Na+,K+-ATPase pump, which is crucial for maintaining the electrochemical gradient across the cell membrane, in dystonia and parkinsonism. A structural model of the α3 subunit showed that two of the identified mutations seem to reduce Na+ affinity and decrease pump activity.[76]

A new young-onset dystonia parkinsonism disorder has been described in two Brazilian families with autosomal recessive inheritance.[77] The patients have progressive, early-onset dystonia with axial muscle involvement, oromandibular and laryngeal dystonia, and, in some cases, parkinsonian features. The condition has been found to be due to mutations in the gene protein kinase, interferon-inducible, double-stranded RNA–dependent activator (DYT16), although the role of this gene in causing dystonia is unclear.

Pathophysiology of Dystonia

NEUROPHYSIOLOGICAL STUDIES

Numerous neurophysiological abnormalities have been identified at various levels of the motor and sensory system in patients with dystonia.[78] The hallmark of dystonia is involuntary sustained muscle contractions, which are characterized by an abnormal pattern of electromyogram (EMG) activity with excessive cocontraction of antagonist muscles during an action and overflow into extraneous muscles. Other findings include prolongation of EMG bursts. These findings were originally described in patients with primary focal hand dystonia, and it was noted that there was loss of selectivity to perform independent finger movements, occasional failure of willed activity, and tremor. These features emphasize that in dystonia there is excessiveness of movements and lack of fine control.[79]

Loss of Inhibition

The problem of excessive cocontraction of agonist and antagonist muscles seems to be due partly to loss of reciprocal inhibition, a mechanism present at many levels in the central nervous system. Reciprocal inhibition can be evaluated in humans by the stimulation of the radial nerve at various times before producing an H-reflex with median nerve stimulation. The radial nerve afferents come from muscles that are antagonist to median nerve muscles. Via various pathways, the radial afferent traffic can inhibit motor neuron pools of median nerve muscles. Reciprocal inhibition is impaired in generalized dystonia, writer's cramp, spasmodic torticollis, and blepharospasm.

Valls-Sole and Hallett[80] evaluated the effects of radial nerve stimulation on the EMG activity of the wrist flexor muscles during a sustained contraction, and showed that the first inhibitory period was reduced in patients with writer's cramp consistent with reduced reciprocal inhibition during movement. This deficit is not limited to the symptomatic body part. The soleus H-reflex of the lower limb is also abnormal in patients with cervical dystonia. Additionally, the H-reflex recovery curve showed greater disinhibition in subjects with generalized dystonia compared with subjects with cervical dystonia and normal subjects during the early inhibition phase. The late facilitation phase of the recovery curve showed higher facilitation in generalized and cervical dystonia compared with normal controls.[81] Study of other spinal and brainstem inhibitory reflexes (e.g., blink and perioral reflexes) has also confirmed that a common theme in various forms of primary dystonia is the reduction in inhibitory processes within the motor system.[78]

Abnormalities of Sensory Input

It has become clear in recent years that dystonia is not a pure motor disorder, and that individuals with dystonia have sensory abnormalities that play an important role in causing motor dysfunction. The importance of the sensory system in dystonia is also evident from study of sensory tricks (*gestes antagoniste*), which are various maneuvers used by patients with focal dystonia to relieve temporarily the dystonic spasms: a finger placed on the face of an individual with cervical dystonia can eliminate neck muscle spasm. There is also evidence to suggest that abnormal sensory input can trigger dystonia, such as trauma to a body part preceding the dystonia.

Studies have shown evidence of abnormal somatosensory spatial discrimination, and temporal discrimination (the shortest time two successive stimuli are perceived as separate). The degree of temporal discrimination impairment is positively correlated with the severity of dystonia.[82-85] Another line of evidence comes from study of processing of muscle spindle input. In patients with hand cramps, vibration can induce dystonia, and cutaneous input similar to that which produces the sensory trick can reverse this vibration-induced dystonia.[86]

Abnormal Motor and Sensory Cortex Excitability

Studies of intracortical inhibition using transcranial magnetic stimulation (TMS) paradigms have shown that motor cortex hyperexcitability is present in dystonia. With the paired pulse method of TMS, an initial conditioning subthreshold stimulus activates cortical neurons and, at intervals of less than 5 ms, inhibits the size of a second subthreshold test stimulus.[87] This inhibition is largely a GABA-A effect. Intracortical inhibition is reduced in patients with focal hand dystonia on the affected and the unaffected hand,[88,89] and decreased intracortical inhibition related to hand muscles has been reported in patients who have blepharospasm without hand dystonia.[90] The decreased intracortical inhibition suggests increased excitability of the cortical motor area. One consequence of decreased inhibition is a loss of "surround inhibition," which could explain the phenomenon of overflow of dystonia that is seen in patients.[91]

The cortical silent period is another marker of cortical motor excitability that can be studied by TMS. It is a pause in the ongoing voluntary EMG activity elicited by a single magnetic stimulus and is mediated by GABA-B receptors.[92] The duration of the cortical silent period is reduced in the affected muscles of patients with cranial, cervical, and hand dystonia.[93,94] These findings of reduced intracortical inhibition, shorter silent period, and abnormal spinal reciprocal inhibition have also been shown in manifesting and nonmanifesting carriers of the abnormal DYT1 gene, although nonmanifesting carriers had normal reciprocal inhibition as assessed by the H-reflex.[95]

It is believed that the excessive muscle contractions that occur in dystonia are generated by loss of inhibition, in particular, loss of surround inhibition—the suppression of unwanted movements when performing a specific motor task. Surround inhibition is believed to be essential for the production of precise, functional movement, just as surround inhibition in the visual system leads to more precise perceptions. In one study in focal hand dystonia, task-dependent modulation of inhibition was studied; it was shown that during the selected task, conditioned motor evoked potentials of synergistic and agonist muscles increased in dystonia patients, showing a disturbed surround inhibition in dystonia.[96] Likewise, Sohn and Hallett[91] were able to show an inhibition of the adductor digiti minimi (an uninvolved muscle in the "surround") when the flexor digitorum superficialis of the second digit was activated. This effect was less in patients with focal hand dystonia.

Studies of sensory function have also suggested that the inhibitory integration of afferent inputs, mainly proprioceptive, coming from adjacent body parts is abnormal in dystonia. It was believed that this inefficient integration was likely to be due to altered surround inhibition, and could give rise to abnormal motor output and contribute to the genesis of dystonic movements.[97] It seems that deficient intracortical inhibition leads to hyperexcitability of the motor cortex, which could lead to the excessive movement seen in dystonia.

NEURAL NETWORKS IN DYSTONIA

Most of the clinical evidence points to the basal ganglia as the site of the pathology in dystonia. There is experimental evidence that the basal ganglia output can influence cortical inhibition, and that the basal ganglia are anatomically organized to work in a center-surround mechanism, which would allow surround inhibition.[98] The direct pathway of the corticobasal ganglia circuits is a net excitatory pathway (with two inhibitory synapses), and the indirect pathway (with three inhibitory synapses) is a net inhibitory pathway. It is believed that the direct pathway represents the center, and the indirect pathway represents the surround, of a center-surround mechanism.

Studies of PET and neurophysiology in *DYT1* and other genetic forms of dystonia have identified a potential endophenotype in asymptomatic carriers of the mutated genes. Abnormal neural networks have been identified in *DYT1* gene carriers.[99,100] Manifesting and nonmanifesting carriers of the *DYT1* mutation exhibited increased resting metabolic activity in the lentiform nuclei, cerebellum, and supplementary motor area. This suggests that in dystonia, there is a substrate of an abnormal motor system that may develop into clinical dystonia in certain circumstances. One example is that of repetitive activity; in a primate model, repetitive activity of the hand induced a motor disorder akin to dystonia associated with enlargement of somatosensory receptive fields of neurons in primary sensory cortex.[101] These findings have been reflected in functional magnetic resonance imaging studies in humans, which have shown that, in the absence of a specific dystonia-inducing task, patients with blepharospasm and focal hand dystonia have overactivity of the primary sensorimotor cortex and caudal part of the supplementary motor area.[102-104]

BRAIN PLASTICITY AND MOTOR LEARNING

The concept that repetitive activity or excessive sensory stimulation can lead to dystonia is supported by more recent studies showing that plasticity is abnormal. Using a technique of paired associative stimulation that can produce motor learning similar to long-term potentiation, Quatarone and colleagues[105] showed abnormal motor cortex plasticity in patients with focal hand dystonia. In the dystonic patients, paired associative stimulation produced a larger increase in the motor evoked potential than that seen in controls. Subsequent studies confirmed these findings in patients with writer's cramp.[106] A similar increase in plasticity has been shown in patients with blepharospasm, where there is an exaggerated R2 phase of the blink reflex when paired with high-frequency stimulation of the supraorbital nerve.[107] A TMS study in patients with limb dystonia also found evidence to implicate short-term cortical plasticity and long-term potentiation.[108] Finally, a study of manifesting and nonmanifesting *DYT1* mutation carriers revealed abnormal motor cortex plasticity in the manifesting carriers only, suggesting that in genetically susceptible individuals this may be an important mechanism in the pathogenesis of dystonic movements.[109]

STRUCTURAL IMAGING STUDIES IN DYSTONIA

Studies using various imaging techniques have identified abnormalities in focal and generalized PTD. Volumetric imaging of the basal ganglia has shown significantly larger putamina in patients with cranial and focal hand dystonia than in healthy controls.[110] More recent voxel-based morphometry studies have shown changes in gray matter density in several areas of the brain in patients with blepharospasm, cervical dystonia, and focal hand dystonia.[111-113] Typically, there was a bilateral increase in gray matter density in primary somatosensory and motor cortex, whereas basal ganglia changes were seen in blepharospasm and cervical dystonia. A study using voxel-based morphometry included patients with generalized primary dystonia and cervical and focal hand dystonia.[114] A common pattern of gray matter changes was found compared with controls with increased volume in the globus pallidus internus, nucleus accumbens, and prefrontal cortex, and unilaterally in the left inferior parietal lobe.

Using diffusion tensor imaging, subtle morphological and microstructural abnormalities in sensorimotor circuitry have also been shown. Studies in *DYT1* dystonia patients have shown that there were abnormalities (reduced fractional anisotropy) in subgyral white matter in manifesting and nonmanifesting carriers of the mutant gene.[115] This was more pronounced in the manifesting carriers. Abnormal fractional anisotropy has also been seen in the lentiform nucleus and surrounding white matter in patients with focal hand dystonia and cervical dystonia.[116-118] These changes reversed after treatment with botulinum toxin, suggesting that the microstructural changes seen may be secondary to metabolic or structural alterations in fibers as a result of dystonic symptoms.[118]

Overview of Pathogenesis and Treatment Targets

The available evidence suggests that dystonia is a disorder of central nervous system inhibition that affects motor and sensory function. Abnormal surround inhibition could lead to the generation of uncontrolled excessive movements that arise from the basal ganglia failing to focus the movement command. Study of secondary dystonias points to the basal ganglia as a pivotal brain region in the development of dystonia. The sensorimotor circuits apparently are impaired in dystonia, and can be disrupted by many causes at numerous levels resulting in a susceptibility state that may allow secondary insults (e.g., physiological stress, environmental insults, increased sensory input, repetitive activity) to push these pathways into a "dystonic state." The studies described in this chapter suggest that this state begins with reduced inhibition and abnormal plasticity in these regions, which lead to overrepresentation of body parts in the sensorimotor cortex. This creates a situation in which this imbalance in circuitry becomes perpetuated by feedback reinforcement. In some ways, the dystonia is abnormally learned.

Studies of genes and their cell biology, animal models, and patient imaging studies have identified factors that lead to dynamic changes in the neural networks that occur in dystonia. These include disruption of neurotransmitter communication involving dopaminergic and cholinergic systems and an overall loss of GABAergic inhibition, possibly by abnormal secretory vesicle dynamics. Subtle abnormalities of brain microstructure and development have been identified, as have defective channels and transporters that result in abnormal responses to stress and toxins. There may be multiple ways in which the vulnerable circuitry can be altered to unbalance sensorimotor pathways and lead to the abnormal motor learning that is dystonia.

The vast increase in understanding of the abnormal cellular, circuitry, and neural networks in dystonia is expected to lead to new areas to target therapy. If dystonia is due to an abnormal motor learning, can it be "unlearned"? This may be the process that is seen in patients with generalized dystonia in whom globus pallidus internus deep brain stimulation is successful, or in patients with task-specific focal dystonia who benefit from constraint-induced therapy. At a more fundamental level, understanding of the genetic and cellular pathogenesis may lead to specific therapies at a protein or enzymatic level. Gene therapy may also have a role to switch off abnormal genes, or introduce wild-type versions in cases such as DRD and GTP cyclohydrolase I, in which the mutant form leads to reduced level or function of the protein. Just as there may be multiple ways in which the sensorimotor control of voluntary movements can be altered in dystonia, there may also be many ways that these can be specifically targeted as therapy.

REFERENCES

1. Fahn S: Concept and classification of dystonia. Adv Neurol 1988;50:1-8.
2. Tarsy D, Simon DK: Dystonia. N Engl J Med 2006;355:818-829.
3. Geyer H, Bressman SB: The diagnosis of dystonia. Lancet Neurol 2006;5:780-790.
4. Warner TT, Bressmann SB: Overview of the genetic forms of dystonia. In Warner TT, Bressman SB, eds: Clinical Diagnosis and Management of Dystonia. London: Informa Healthcare, 2007, pp 27-34.
5. Albanese A, Barnes MP, Bhatia KP, et al: A systematic review on the diagnosis and treatment of primary (idiopathic) dystonia and dystonia plus syndromes: report of an EFNS/MDS-ES Task Force. Eur J Neurol 2006;13:433-444.
6. Bordelon Y, Frucht S: Secondary and heredodegenerative dystonia. In Warner TT, Bressman SB, eds: Clinical Diagnosis and Management of Dystonia. London: Informa Healthcare, 2007: 131-148.
7. Ozelius L, Bressman SB: DYT1 dystonia. In Warner TT, Bressmann SB, eds: Clinical Diagnosis and Management of Dystonia. London: Informa Healthcare, 2007, pp 53-64.
8. Ozelius L, Kramer P, Page CE, et al: The early-onset torsion dystonia gene (DYT1) encodes an ATP-binding protein. Nat Genet 1997;17:40-48.
9. Bressman SB, Sabati C, Raymond D, et al: The DYT1 phenotype and guidelines for diagnostic testing. Neurology 2000;54:1746-1752.
10. Bressman SB, Raymond D, Wendt K, et al: Diagnostic criteria for dystonia in DYT1 families. Neurology 2002;59:1780-1782.
11. Risch N, de Leon D, Ozelius L, et al: Genetic analysis of idiopathic torsion dystonia in Ashkenazi Jews and their recent descent from a small founder population. Nat Genet 1995;9:152-159.
12. Risch N, Bressman SB, Senthil G, Ozelius L: Intragenic cis and trans modification of genetic susceptibility in DYT1 dystonia. Am J Hum Genet 2007;80:1188-1193.
13. Kock N, Naismith T, Boston H, et al: Effects of genetic variations in the dystonia protein torsinA: identification of polymorphism at residue 216 as protein modifier. Hum Mol Genet 2006;15:1355-1364.
14. Neuwald AF, Aravind L, Spouge JL, Koonin E: AAA+: A class of chaperone-like ATPases associated with the assembly, operation and disassembly of protein complexes. Genomic Res 1999;9:27-43.
15. Kamm C, Boston H, Hewett J, et al: The early onset dystonia protein torsinA interacts with kinesin light chain 1. J Biol Chem 2004;279:19882-19892.

16. Hewett J, Gonzalez-Agosti C, Slater D, et al: Mutant torsinA, responsible for early onset torsion dystonia, forms membrane inclusions in cultured neural cells. Hum Mol Genet 2000;22:1403-1413.

17. Hewett J, Ziefer P, Bergeron D, et al: TorsinA in PC12 cells: localization in the endoplasmic reticulum and response to stress. J Neurosci Res 2003;72:158-168.

18. Liu Z, Zolkiewska A, Zolkiewska M: Characterization of human torsinA and its dystonia-associated mutant form. Biochem J 2003;374:117-122.

19. Callan AC, Bunning S, Jones OT, et al: Biosynthesis of the dystonia-associated AAA + ATPase torsinA at the endoplasmic reticulum. Biochem J 2007;401:607-612.

20. Kustedjo K, Bracey MH, Cravatt BF: Torsin A and its torsion dystonia-associated mutant forms are lumenal glycoproteins that exhibit distinct subcellular localizations. J Biol Chem 2000;275:27933-27939.

21. Goodchild R, Dauer WT: Mislocalisation of the nuclear envelope: an effect of the dystonia causing torsinA mutation. Proc Natl Acad Sci U S A 2004;1001:847-852.

22. Naismith TV, Heuser JE, Breakefield XO, Hanson PI: TorsinA in the nuclear envelope. Proc Natl Acad Sci U S A 2004;101:7612-7617.

23. Misbahuddin A, Placzek MR, Taanman JW, et al: Mutant torsinA, which causes early-onset primary torsion dystonia, is redistributed to membranous structures enriched in vesicular monoamine transporter in cultured human SH-SY5Y cells. Mov Disord 2005;20:432-440.

24. McNaught KS, Kapustin A, Jackson T, et al: Brainstem pathology in DYT1 primary torsion dystonia. Ann Neurol 2004;56:540-547.

25. Shashidharan P, Sandu D, Potla U, et al: Transgenic mouse model of early-onset DYT1 dystonia. Hum Mol Genet 2005;14:125-133.

26. Grundmann K, Reischmann B, Vanhoutte G, et al: Overexpression of human wildtype torsinA and human deltaGAG torsinA in a transgenic mouse model causes phenotypic abnormalities. Neurobiol Dis 2007;27:190-206.

27. Dang MT, Yokoi F, McNaught K, et al: Generation and characterisation of DYT1 delta GAG knock-in mouse as a model for early onset dystonia. Exp Neurol 2005;196:452-463.

28. Pisani A, Martella G, Tscherter A, et al: Altered response to dopaminergic D2 receptor activation and N-type calcium currents in striatal cholinergic interneurons in a mouse model of DYT1 dystonia. Neurobiol Dis 2006;24:318-325.

29. Goodchild RE, Kim CE, Dauer WT: Loss of the dystonia-associated protein torsinA selectively disrupts the neuronal nuclear envelope. Neuron 2005;48:923-932.

30. Goodchild RE, Dauer WT: The AAA+ protein torsinA interacts with a conserved domain present in LAP1 and a novel ER protein. Cell Biol 2005;168:855-862.

31. Kamm C, Boston H, Hewett J, et al: The early onset dystonia protein torsinA interacts with kinesin light chain 1. J Biol Chem 2004;279:19882-19992.

32. Rostasy K, Augood SJ, Hewett JW, et al: TorsinA protein and neuropathology in early onset generalized dystonia with GAG deletion. Neurobiol Dis 2003;12:11-24.

33. Augood SJ, Martin DM, Ozelius LJ, et al: Distribution of the mRNAs encoding torsinA and torsinB in the adult human brain. Ann Neurol 1999;46:761-769.

34. Shashidharan P, Kramer C, Walker R, et al: Immunohistochemical localization and distribution of torsinA in normal human and rat brain. Brain Res 2000;853:197-206.

35. Torres GE, Sweeney AL, Beaulieu JM, et al: Effect of torsinA on membrane proteins reveals a loss of function and a dominant negative phenotype of the dystonia-associated ΔE-torsinA mutant. Proc Natl Acad Sci U S A 2004;101:15650-15655.

36. Balcioglu A, Kim M, Sharma N, et al: Dopamine release is impaired in a mouse model of DYT1 dystonia. J Neurochem 2007;102:783-788.

37. Granata A, Watson R, Collinson L, et al: The dystonia-associated protein torsinA modulates synaptic vesicle recycling. J Biol Chem 2008;283:7568-7579.

38. Almasy L, Bressman SB, Kramer PL, et al: Idiopathic torsion dystonia linked to chromosome 8 in two Mennonite families. Ann Neurol 1997;42:670-673.

39. Fuchs T, Gavarini S, Saunders-Pullma R, et al: Mutations in the THAP1 gene are responsible for DYT6 primary torsion dystonia. Nature Genet 2009;41:286-288.

40. Djarmati A, Schneider J, Lohmann K, et al: Mutations in THAP1 gene (DYT6) are associated with generalised dystonia with prominent spasmodic dysphonia: a genetic screening study. Lancet Neurol 2009;8:441-446.

41. Valente EM, Bentivoglio AR, Cassetta E, et al: DYT13, a novel primary torsion dystonia locus, maps to chromosome 1p36.13-36.32 in an Italian family with cranial-cervical or upper limb onset. Ann Neurol 2001;49:363-364.

42. Defazio G, Berardelli A, Hallett M: Do primary adult-onset focal dystonias share aetiological factors? Brain 2007;130:1183-1193.
43. Gasser T, Windgassen K, Bereznai B, et al: Phenotypic expression of the DYT1 mutation: a family with writer's cramp of juvenile onset. Ann Neurol 1998;44:126-128.
44. Defazio G, Brancati F, Valente EM, et al: Familial blepharospasm is inherited as an autosomal dominant trait and relates to a novel unassigned gene. Mov Disord 2003;18:207-212.
45. Leube B, Doda R, Ratzlaff T, et al: Idiopathic torsion dystonia: assignment of a gene to chromosome 18p in a German family with adult onset, autosomal inheritance and purely focal distribution. Hum Mol Genet 1996;5:1673-1677.
46. Bhidayasiri R, Jen JC, Baloh RW: Three brothers with a very late onset writer's cramp. Mov Disord 2005;10:819-824.
47. Leube B, Kessler KR, Goecke T, et al: Frequency of familial inheritance among 488 index patients with idiopathic torsion focal dystonia and clinical variability in a large family. Mov Disord 1997;12:1000-1006.
48. Klein C, Ozelius L, Hagenah J, et al: Search for a founder mutation in idiopathic focal dystonia from Northern Germany. Am J Hum Genet 1998;63:1777-1782.
49. Waddy HM, Fletcher NA, Harding AE, Marsden CD: A genetic study of idiopathic focal dystonias. Ann Neurol 1991;29:320-324.
50. Martino D, Aniello MS, Masi G, et al: Validity of family history data on primary adult-onset dystonia. Arch Neurol 2004;61:1569-1573.
51. Clarimon J, Asgeirsson H, Singleton A, et al: Torsin A haplotype predisposes to idiopathic dystonia. Ann Neurol 2005;57:765-767.
52. Clarimon J, Brancati F, Peckham E, et al: Assessing the role of DRD5 and DYT1 in tow different case-control series with primary blepharospasm. Mov Disord 2007;22:162-166.
53. Kamm C, Asmus F, Mueller J, et al: Strong genetic evidence for association of TOR1A-TOR1B with idiopathic dystonia. Neurology 2006;67:1857-1859.
54. Sibbing D, Asmus F, Konig IR, et al: Candidate gene studies in focal dystonia. Neurology 2003;61:1097-1101.
55. Hague S, Klaffke S, Clarimon J, et al: Lack of association with TorsinA haplotype in German patients with sporadic dystonia. Neurology 2006;66:951-952.
56. Placzek MR, Misbahuddin A, Chaudhuri KR, et al: Cervical dystonia is associated with a polymorphism in the dopamine (D5) receptor gene. J Neurol Neurosurg Psychiatry 2001;71:262-264.
57. Misbahuddin A, Placzec MR, Chaudhuri KR, et al: A polymorphism in the dopamine receptor DRD5 is associated with blepharospasm. Neurology 2002;58:124-126.
58. Brancati F, Valente EM, Castori M, et al: Role of the dopamine D5 receptor (DRD5) as a susceptibility gene for cervical dystonia. J Neurol Neurosurg Psychiatry 2003;74:665-666.
59. Segawa M, Hosaka A, Miyagawa F, et al: Hereditary progressive dystonia with marked diurnal fluctuation. Adv Neurol 1976;14:215-233.
60. Nygaard TG, Marsden CD, Fahn S: Dopa-responsive dystonia: long-term treatment response and prognosis. Neurology 1991;41:174-181.
61. chinose H, Ohye T, Takahiashi E, et al: Hereditary progressive dystonia with marked diurnal fluctuation caused by mutations in the GTP cyclohydrolase I gene. Nat Genet 1994;8:236-242.
62. Furukawa Y, Nygaard TG, Gutlich M, et al: Striatal biopterin and tyrosine hydroxylase protein reduction in dopa-responsive dystonia. Neurology 1999;53:1032-1041.
63. Maita N, Hatakeyama K, Okada K, Hakoshima T: Structural basis of biopterin induced inhibition of GTP cyclohydrolase 1 by GFRP, its feedback regulatory protein. J Biol Chem 2004;279:51524-51540.
64. Ludecke B, Knappskog PM, Clayton PT, et al: Recessively inherited L-DOPA-responsive parkinsonism in infancy caused by a point mutation (L205P) in the tyrosine hydroxylase gene. Hum Mol Genet 1996;5:1023-1028.
65. Hyland K, Gunasekara R, Munk-Martin T, et al: The hph-1 mouse: a model for dominantly inherited GTP-cyclohydrolase deficiency. Ann Neurol 2003;6:S46-S48.
66. Gasser T: Inherited myoclonus-dystonia syndrome. Adv Neurol 1998;78:325-334.
67. Hess CW, Raymond D, Aguiar Pde C, et al: Myoclonus-dystonia, obsessive compulsive disorder, and alcohol dependence in SGCE mutation carriers. Neurology 2007;68:522-524.
68. Zimprich A, Grabowski M, Asmus F, et al: Mutations in the gene encoding epsilon-sarcoglycan cause myoclonus-dystonia syndrome. Nat Genet 2001;29:66-69.
69. Muller B, Hedrich K, Kock N, et al: Evidence that paternal expression of the epsilon-sarcoglycan gene accounts for reduced penetrance in myoclonus-dystonia. Am J Hum Genet 2002;71:1303-1311.

70. Blake DJ, Weir A, Newey SE, Davies KE: Function and genetics of dystrophin and dystrophin-related proteins in muscle. Physiol Rev 2002;82:291-329.

71. Chan P, Gonzalez-Maeso J, Ruff F, et al: Epsilon-sarcoglycan immunoreactivity and mRNA expression in mouse brain. J Comp Neurol 2005;482:50-73.

72. Esapa C, Waite A, Lock M, et al: SGCE mutations that cause myoclonus dystonia syndrome impair epsilon sarcoglycan trafficking to the plasma membrane: modulation by ubiquitination and torsinA. Hum Mol Genet 2007;16:327-342.

73. Han F, Racacho L, Lang AE, et al: Refinement of the DYT15 locus in myoclonus dystonia. Mov Disord 2007;22:888-892.

74. Brashear A, Dobyns W, de Carvalho Aguiar P, et al: The phenotypic spectrum of rapid-onset dystonia-parkinsonism (RDP) and mutations in the ATP1A3 gene. Brain 2007;130:828-835.

75. de Carvalho Aguiar P, Sweadner KJ, Penniston JT, et al: Mutations in the Na+/K+-ATPase alpha3 gene ATP1A3 are associated with rapid-onset dystonia parkinsonism. Neuron 2004;43:169-175.

76. Rodacker V, Toustrup-Jensen M, Vilsen B: Mutations Phe785Leu and Thr618Met in the Na+, K+ ATPase, associated with familial rapid onset dystonia-parkinsonism, interfere with Na+ interaction by distinct mechanisms. J Biol Chem 2006;281:18539-18548.

77. Camargos S, Scholz S, Simon-Sanchez J, et al: DYT16, a novel young onset dystonia-parkinsonism disorder: identification of a segregating mutation in the stress response protein prka. Lancet Neurol 2008;7:215-222.

78. Kanchana S, Hallett M: Pathophysiology of dystonia. In Warner TT, Bressman SB, eds: Clinical Diagnosis and Management of Dystonia. London: Informa Healthcare, 2007, pp 35-43.

79. Hallett M: Dystonia: abnormal movements result from loss of inhibition. Adv Neurol 2004;94:1-9.

80. Valls-Sole J, Hallett M: Modulation of electromyographic activity of wrist flexor and extensor muscles in patients with writer's cramp. Mov Disord 1995;10:741-748.

81. Sabbahi M, Etnyre B, Al-Jawayad I, Jankovic J: Soleus H-reflex measures in patients with focal and generalized dystonia. Clin Neurophysiol 2003;114:288-294.

82. Bara-Jimenez W, Shelton P, Hallett M: Spatial discrimination is abnormal in focal hand dystonia. Neurology 2000;55:1869-1873.

83. Molloy F, Carr T, Zeuner K, et al: Abnormalities of spatial discrimination in focal and generalized dystonia. Brain 2003;126:2175-2182.

84. Fiorio M, Tinazzi M: Bertolasi, Aglioti S. Temporal processing of visuotactile and tactile stimuli in writer's cramp. Ann Neurol 2003;53:630-635.

85. Tinazzi M, Fiorio M, Bertolasi L, Aglioti S: Timing of tactile and visuotactile events is impaired in patients with cervical dystonia. J Neurol 2004;251:85-90.

86. Kaji R, Rothwell J, Katayama M, et al: Tonic vibration reflex and muscle afferent block in writer's cramp: implications for a new therapeutic approach. Ann Neurol 1995;38:155-162.

87. Curra A, Modugna N, Inghilleri M, et al: Transcranial magnetic stimulation techniques in clinical investigation. Neurology 2002;59:1851-1859.

88. Ridding M, Sheean G, Rothwell J, et al: Changes in the balance between motor cortical excitation and inhibition in focal task specific dystonia. J Neurol Neurosurg Psychiatry 1995;59:493-498.

89. Gilio F, Curra A, Lorenzano C, et al: Effects of Botulinum toxin type A on intracortical inhibition in patients with dystonia. Ann Neurol 2000;48:20-26.

90. Sommer M, Ruge D, Tergau F, et al: Intracortical excitability in the hand motor representation in hand dystonia and blepharospasm. Mov Disord 2002;17:1017-1025.

91. Sohn Y, Hallett M: Disturbed surround inhibition in focal hand dystonia. Ann Neurol 2004;56:595-599.

92. Werhahn K, Kunesch E, Noachtar S, et al: Differential effects on motor cortical inhibition by blockade of GABA uptake in humans. J Physiol 1999;591-597.

93. Rona S, Berardelli A, Vacca L, et al: Alterations of motor cortical inhibition in patients with dystonic movement disorders. Mov Disord 1998;13:118-124.

94. Curra A, Romaniello A, Berardelli A, et al: Shortened cortical silent period in facial muscles of patients with cranial dystonia. Neurology 2000;54:130-135.

95. Edwards MJ, Huang YZ, Wood NW, et al: Different patterns of electrophysiological deficits in manifesting and non-manifesting carriers of the DYT1 gene mutation. Brain 2003;126:2074-2080.

96. Butefisch C, Boroojerdi B, Chen R, et al: Task-dependent intracortical inhibition in impaired in focal hand dystonia. Mov Disord 2005;20:545-551.

97. Tinazzi M, Priori A, Bertolasi L, et al: Abnormal central integration of a dual somatosensory input in dystonia: evidence for sensory overflow. Brain 2000;123:42-50.

98. Mink J: The basal ganglia: focused selection and inhibition of competing motor programs. Prog Neurobiol 1996;50:381-425.
99. Eidelberg D, Moeller J, Antonini A, et al: Functional networks in DYT1 dystonia. Ann Neurol 1998;44:303-312.
100. Carbon M, Ghilardi M, Dhawan V, et al: Abnormal brain networks in primary torsion dystonia. Adv Neurol 2004;94:155-161.
101. Byl N, Merzenich M, Jenkins W: A primate genesis model of focal dystonia and repetitive strain injury: learning-induced de-differentiation of the representation of the hand in the primary somatosensory cortex in adult monkeys. Neurology 1996;47:508-520.
102. Oga T, Honda M, Toma K, et al: Abnormal cortical mechanisms of voluntary muscle relaxation in patients with writer's cramp. Brain 2002;125:895-903.
103. Baker R, Andersen A, Morecraft R, Smith C: A functional magnetic resonance imaging study in patients with benign essential blepharospasm. J Neuro-ophthalmol 2003;23:11-15.
104. Dresel G, Haslinger B, Castrop F, et al: Silent event-related fMRI reveals deficient motor and enhanced somatosensory activation in orofacial dystonia. Brain 2006;129:36-46.
105. Quatarone A, Bagnato S, Rizzo V, et al: Abnormal associative plasticity of the human motor cortex in writer's cramp. Brain 2003;126:2586-2596.
106. Weise D, Schram A, Stefan K, et al: The two sides of associative plasticity in writer's cramp. Brain 2006;129:2709-2721.
107. Quatarone A, Sant'Angelo A, Battaglia F, et al: Enhanced long-term potentiation-like plasticity of the trigeminal blink reflex circuit in blepharospasm. J Neurosci 2006;26:716-721.
108. Gilio F, Suppa A, Bologna M, et al: Short term cortical plasticity with dystonia: a study with repetitive transcranial magnetic stimulation. Mov Disord 2007;22:1436-1443.
109. Edwards M, Huang Y-Z, Mir P, et al: Abnormalities in motor cortical plasticity differentiate manifesting from nonmanifesting DYT1 carriers. Mov Disord 2006;21:2181-2186.
110. Black J, Ongur D, Perlmutter J: Putamen volume in idiopathic focal dystonia. Neurology 1998;51:819-824.
111. Draganski B, Thun-Hohenstein C, Bogdahn U, et al: Motor circuit gray matter changes in idiopathic cervical dystonia. Neurology 2003;13:1017-1020.
112. Garraux G, Bauer A, Hanakawa T, et al: Changes in the brain anatomy in focal hand dystonia. Ann Neurol 2004;55:736-739.
113. Delmaire C, Vidailhet M, Elbaz A, et al: Structural abnormalities in the cerebellum and sensorimotor circuit in writer's cramp. Neurology 2007;69:376-380.
114. Egger K, Mueller J, Schocke M, et al: Voxel based morphometry reveals specific gray matter changes in primary dystonia. Mov Disord 2007;22:1538-1542.
115. Carbon M, Kingsley P, Su S, et al: Microstructural white matter changes in carriers of the DYT1 gene mutation. Ann Neurol 2004;56:283-286.
116. Blood A, Tuch D, Makris N, et al: White matter abnormalities in dystonia normalise after Botulinum toxin. Neuroreport 2006;17:1251-1255.
117. Colosimo C, Pantono P, Calistri V, et al: Diffusion tensor imaging in primary cervical dystonia. J Neurol Neurosurg Psychiatry 2005;76:1591-1593.
118. Bonhila L, de Vries P, Vincent D, et al: Structural white matter abnormalities in patients with idiopathic dystonia. Mov Disord 2007;22:1110-1116.

27 Management

ELENA MORO • MARIE VIDAILHET

Introduction

With the introduction of deep brain stimulation (DBS) surgery into clinical practice, the symptomatic treatment of dystonias has seen remarkable advances.[1] To some extent, the practice of DBS surgery in dystonia has brought the same revolutionary effect that botulinum toxin (BTX) had in the 1980s.[2] The surgical approach is indicated when dystonia is disabling and refractory to trials with several drugs. Medical therapy should be always the first line of treatment.

Medical treatment can be very specific for particular types of dystonias, such as levodopa for dopa-responsive dystonia[3] and decoppering therapy including chelators for dystonia secondary to Wilson's disease,[4] or broad spectrum for treating dystonia/hyperkinetic movements in primary and secondary dystonias.[5] Dystonic storm or status dystonicus also requires prompt and specific treatment.[6]

The choice of which antidystonia medication should be tried first is related to the type of dystonia, severity of the dystonic movements, age of patients, concomitant drugs, medical conditions, and potential risk of adverse effects. Because of the extreme variability in etiology and type of dystonias, it is not surprising that there is no evidence of effectiveness for most of the currently used medications.[7] Only BTX in cervical dystonias and high-dose trihexyphenidyl in generalized and segmental dystonias have reached level A evidence of efficacy.[7-9]

Overall, the choice of therapy is often guided by personal experience or the results of open-label trials. Focal and segmental dystonias are more likely to be treated with local therapies (BTX injections, physiotherapy), whereas more severe or generalized dystonias are more likely to receive oral treatments (before any possibility of surgery) (Table 27–1 and Fig. 27–1).

The assessment of therapeutic effects should be performed using the clinical global impression of the patient and the semiquantitative evaluations of standardized rating scales, such as the Toronto Western Spasmodic Torticollis Rating Scale

TABLE 27–1	Therapies for Dystonia		
	Medical Treatments	**Surgical Treatments**	**Other Treatments**
Focal dystonias	Botulinum toxin injections (A, B)*	DBS: thalamus, GPi, STN	Occupational therapy
	Benzodiazepines	Motor cortex stimulation	Physiotherapy
	Trihexyphenidyl	Lesions†	Supportive therapy
	Benztropine	Peripheral (posterior ramisection, myotomy, and myectomy)	Immobilization, constraint therapies
	Tetrabenazine	Central (thalamotomy, pallidotomy)	
	Oral baclofen Antiepileptic drugs		
Segmental/ generalized dystonias	Levodopa	DBS: thalamus, GPi, STN	Occupational therapy
	Trihexyphenidyl	Motor cortex stimulation	Physiotherapy
	Benztropine	Intrathecal baclofen pump	Supportive therapy
	Botulinum toxin injections (A, B)*	Lesions†	Immobilization, constraint therapies
	Clozapine	Peripheral (posterior ramisection, myotomy, and myectomy)	
	Tetrabenazine	Central (thalamotomy, pallidotomy)	
	Oral baclofen Antiepileptic drugs		

*Most commonly used types of botulinum toxin.
†Lesions have progressively been abandoned in favor of neurostimulation (i.e., better benefit/risk ratio).
DBS, deep brain stimulation; GPi, globus pallidus internus; STN, subthalamic nucleus.

(TWSTRS)[10-11] and the Tsui scale[12] for cervical dystonia, or the Global Dystonia Scale (GDS)[13] and the Burke Fahn Marsden Dystonia Scale (BFMDS)[14] for segmental/generalized dystonia. In some cases, such as upper limb dystonias, the assessment of the beneficial effect of treatment is more problematic because various types of scales have been developed, but each is focused on different items. Assessment of the quality of life using generic scales or more specific evaluation of the burden of dystonia (i.e., in cervical dystonia, the Cervical Dystonia Impact Profile Scale [CDIP-58][15] and the craniocervical dystonia questionnaire [CDQ-24][16]) should be also done, although these are mainly performed as part of clinical trials, and not as part of routine assessment.

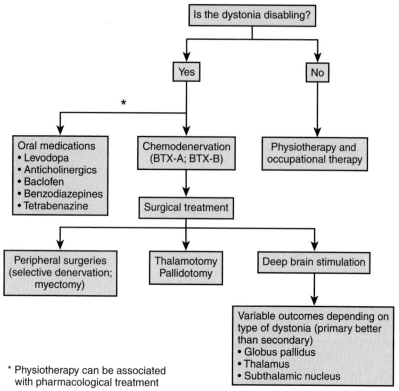

Figure 27–1   Flow chart for the treatment of dystonia. BTX-A, botulinum toxin type A; BTX-B, botulinum toxin type B.

Medical Treatment

FOCAL AND SEGMENTAL DYSTONIAS

BTX injections directly into affected muscles represent the first-line treatment of focal dystonias.[5,17] Results from more than 10 years of follow-up in various types of dystonias and movement disorders have been reported.[18] An evidence-based review of BTX treatment of movement disorders has also been published more recently.[19]

BTX type A (Botox, Dysport, Xeomin)[2] is the most widely used, but BTX type B (Myobloc/Neurobloc)[12] may be used in cases of secondary resistance to toxin A with similar effects. BTX type F has little clinical application because of its short-lasting effect (1 month). To date, there is no clear consensus on the conversion factor between the two main commercial formulations of BTX-A (Botox and Dysport); reports vary from 1:2 to 1:6, but most frequently it is 1:4 (Botox versus Dysport), depending on the studies, the dilution, and the muscles.[18,20-23] A new formulation of BTX-A, NT 201 (Xeomin) has shown a 1:1 dose ratio compared with Botox.[24] Overall, equivalent results were reported in large series with mild differences in the duration of effects and adverse event rates, suggesting that use of the different preparations should be based on the experience of the movement disorders neurologist more than on safety profile differences.[25,26]

Cervical Dystonia

In a meta-analysis of 13 studies comparing BTX with placebo, the Cochrane group found that both BTX formulations (Botox and Dysport) were equally used to treat cervical dystonias.[27] Significant clinical motor improvement on objective rating scales (Tsui scale, TWSTRS)[28] and significant pain relief using subjective scales was obtained for 75% or more of patients. There was a clear dose-response relationship for subjective and objective benefit, and for frequency and severity of adverse events (neck weakness, dysphagia, sore throat, voice change, local pain). Safety data were similar for both formulations.[27]

Only a few long-term studies of BTX treatment in cervical dystonia have been published. Several groups have reported that about two thirds of the patients had sustained benefit after 10 years of follow-up.[29-31] Incomplete long-term beneficial effect may be related to modification or worsening of the pattern of dystonia or secondary resistance to BTX-A.

Overall, the most frequent clinical practice involves BTX injections every 3 to 4 months. The muscles most frequently injected are the sternocleidomastoid and the contralateral splenius capitis, plus additional injections in the trapezius, levator scapulae, semispinalis, and sometimes scalene muscle, depending on the dystonic posture. Some studies have suggested that electromyogram (EMG) guidance improves clinical outcome.[32] EMG guidance should be used in patients with very complex postures and especially in patients with poor outcomes from earlier treatment before considering them a treatment failure.[33]

In long-term published series, 5% to 10% of patients became resistant to BTX-A and received BTX-B as alternative and efficacious treatment.[34] In a double-blind controlled trial[35] of 122 patients treated with BTX-B, about 77% were found to be improved at 1 month, and this beneficial effect was confirmed in other studies.[36,37] The adverse effects observed with BTX-B and BTX-A were very similar, although dry mouth was more frequently reported in patients treated with BTX-B.[34-37]

Blepharospasm

The effectiveness of BTX in blepharospasm was first shown in a double-blind placebo-controlled study in 1987.[38] Since then, most studies have confirmed that significant improvement is obtained in more than 90% of patients, with a long-term beneficial effect (≤10 years) in 80% to 90% of the subjects.[29,39,40]

The clinical benefit starts on average 4 days after injection and can last 3 to 4 months. The orbicularis oculi is injected in the orbital or pretarsal portions, or both, the number of sites depending on severity, dosage, and injector experience.[41] In Meige's syndrome, other muscles, such as frontalis, corrugator, masseter, and platysma, may be injected, depending on their involvement in the dystonia. The most frequent adverse effects of treatment are ptosis, tearing, blurry vision, diplopia, and local hematomas.[38-41] Special attention should be given to eyelid-opening apraxia, which may need pretarsal injections.[41]

Upper Limb Dystonia and Writer's Cramp

Several open and double-blind controlled trials have concluded that BTX injections in carefully selected muscles of the hand and forearm provide beneficial effect in upper limb dystonia, with special attention to task-specific dystonias (e.g., writer's cramps).[42-44] EMG-guided injections seem to be more effective because this approach precisely targets the specific muscles.[45] Voluntary activity of the hand immediately after BTX injection, and performed for 30 minutes, may enhance the weakness—hence the beneficial effect—produced by the injection.[46] Despite the relative difficulty managing writer's cramps, in a placebo-controlled study, about 50% of patients were still under treatment after 1 year.[47] One more recent study attempted to determine the "best candidates" for BTX injections in writer's cramp; patients with flexion/pronation of the wrist were found to have a significantly better prognosis, whereas patients with pure writing tremor had minimal or no effect.[48]

In cervical and upper limb dystonia, physiotherapy can be combined with BTX injections.[49,50] Although there is no standard program, some guidelines can be used when approaching different clinical forms (e.g., in tonic forms, emphasis is placed on reinforcing corrector muscles). Physiotherapy and BTX can mutually interact in reducing symptoms.

SEGMENTAL AND GENERALIZED DYSTONIA

In addition to BTX injections, which can be used focally in segmental and generalized dystonias, several medications have been used over the years to treat segmental and generalized dystonias. The effectiveness of most medications has not been supported, however, by rigorous double-blind controlled trials. Besides the use of evidence-based reviews[5,9] and expert's opinion,[5] the treatment options are based on personal experience and careful balance between benefits and risks of the treatment.

Dopaminergic Drugs

Without clinical evidence, a diagnostic levodopa trial is warranted in patients with early-onset dystonia without an alternative diagnosis. Dopa-responsive dystonia[3] can be misdiagnosed because it has a multifaceted clinical presentation as cerebral palsy, spastic diplegia, paroxysmal dystonia or adult-onset dystonia, and adult-onset levodopa-responsive parkinsonism.[51] Despite the fact that dopa-responsive dystonia accounts for only 5% of childhood dystonia, the substantial and sustained improvement or even the complete resolution of dystonia with low doses of levodopa support the systematic prescription of levodopa for at least 3 months (upto 200 mg three times a day).[52]

Although levodopa (and sometimes anticholinergic drugs or dopaminergic agonists) is markedly effective in dopa-responsive dystonia, little or no effect is obtained in primary dystonias.[53] In some cases, mild improvement of 20% may be obtained.[17,54] A placebo effect cannot be excluded in these cases, however, because 3 days' withdrawal of levodopa in patients with primary generalized dystonia did not reveal any significant change.[55] Some clinical improvement with levodopa doses in the range of antiparkinsonian treatment has been observed occasionally in dystonia as part of heredodegenerative diseases (spinocerebellar ataxia type 2 and spinocerebellar ataxia type 3), young-onset parkinsonism with dystonia (e.g., with *parkin* mutations; here the response can be profound), secondary dystonias such as tardive dystonia (although improvement is only modest in tardive dystonia),[5] but not in other forms of secondary dystonia, such as rapid-onset dystonia parkinsonism or manganese-induced parkinsonism with dystonia.

Antidopaminergic Drugs

Although antidopaminergic therapy (mainly using "typical" neuroleptics, sometimes combined with tetrabenazine and high-dose anticholinergic treatment) was recommended in the past[54] and produced some beneficial effects, most clinical trials have produced mixed and generally disappointing results. "Typical" neuroleptics have progressively been abandoned, in part because of the risk of parkinsonism, worsening of dystonia, tardive dystonia, or sedation.[5]

Atypical neuroleptics (clozapine, olanzapine, quetiapine, risperidone) have been reported to be useful. In a small open-label trial with clozapine, a mild improvement was reported in patients with segmental and generalized dystonia, but the use was limited by potential side effects and the need for frequent blood cell counts.[56] Rarely, clozapine may improve tardive dystonia.[57]

Tetrabenazine, an inhibitor of the vesicular monoamine transporter, does not cause tardive dyskinesia, in contrast to other antidopaminergic drugs. Transient acute dyskinesia can be observed, but does not preclude long-term use of tetrabenazine. Some benefit can be obtained in primary and especially tardive dystonia; the initial dose can be aimed at 75 mg daily (upto 200 mg/day) with long-term beneficial effect and tolerance.[58] No specific trial has been designed for dystonia, but a few double-blind crossover studies have been published in various hyperkinetic movement disorders[59] and, more recently, in chorea. In addition, numerous open-label studies with a long-term follow-up provide support for trying tetrabenazine in some dystonic patients, although drowsiness, anxiety, depression, restlessness, and parkinsonism may limit the use of the drug.[7,9,58] Tetrabenazine has also been used in childhood dystonia with good tolerance, but with only mild to moderate efficacy.

Anticholinergic Drugs

Anticholinergic drugs are the only substance class for which controlled studies (using 30 to 60 mg of trihexyphenidyl and benzhexol) are available.[7,9,60] Dosages should be increased very slowly to prevent side effects such as cognitive and memory deficits, which are often dose-limiting. Nevertheless, young patients, especially children, can tolerate much higher doses than adults, and a substantial clinical improvement (≤50%) may be observed in some patients with generalized dystonia.[54,61] In adults, anticholinergics may be useful as add-on therapy in segmental and focal dystonia (especially cervical dystonia) in addition to botulinum toxin injections.[7,9]

Other Drugs

A wide range of drugs have been proposed on the basis of single reports or small series, with variable results.

Benzodiazepines

Many patients with dystonia require a combination of several treatments. Benzodiazepines (clonazepam, lorazepam, diazepam) may provide additional benefit to dystonia and accompanying tremor or myoclonus.[5]

Muscle Relaxants

Several muscle relaxants have been explored, including agents approved for the treatment of spasticity (e.g., tizanidine, although it is still unclear whether this drug is actually useful in dystonia). Oral baclofen has been proposed in oromandibular dystonia in adults or generalized dystonia in children at a mean dose of 90 mg/day (range 40 to 180 mg), with variable results.[62] Intrathecal baclofen infusion has been proposed since the early 1990s, with some relief reported in patients with dystonia associated with spasticity (e.g., cerebral palsy), but with limited effect on functional capacity.[63] Nevertheless, the beneficial effects are variable with a relatively high rate of adverse events (≤38%), mainly related to dysfunction of the implanted device (e.g., catheter disconnections, infections).[64-66]

Antiepileptic Drugs

Leviracetam has been proposed for treating dystonia,[67] but dystonia may also occur as an adverse event of antiepileptic drugs.[68]

Morphine and Opioids

Opioids have been shown to improve levodopa-induced dyskinesia in Parkinson's disease. By analogy, they have been proposed in a few cases of primary dystonia and tardive dystonia. Open-label studies on a small number of patients (<10) have shown some improvement in tardive dystonia and rarely in primary dystonia with 20 to 60 mg/day of morphine sulfate in a controlled release preparation.[69]

Cannabinoid agonists

The effects of cannabinoids in dystonia are still under investigation.[70]

Physiotherapy

Physiotherapy and the use of various types of devices date to the time of Duchenne de Boulogne or before. Since then, various approaches have been proposed, including immobilization (4 to 5 weeks) by splints in writer's cramp[71] and immobilization of one or more digits (the so-called constraint-induced movement therapy,[72] by analogy with stroke rehabilitation programs). Although these treatments provide some relief, at the cost of mild loss of dexterity at the time of the splint removal, it is unclear whether a sustained and prolonged benefit can be obtained. To date, the effects of these treatments have not been precisely evaluated in dystonia. Another simple treatment that is effective in selected patients with writer's cramp is the use of a writing device that supports the pen and allows the patient to relax the fingers and forearm with the more proximal muscles directing the writing task (akin to writing with large strokes on a blackboard).[73]

Sensory training to restore sensory representations of the hand has also been proposed, with some improvement in focal hand dystonia after training to read

Braille for 30 to 60 minutes daily for 8 weeks,[74] or after sensory discrimination training.[75] More recently, tailored physiotherapy, based on the analysis of the characteristics of dystonia, has been proposed.[76] This rehabilitation approach is designed as a relearning process. The first step is to use relaxing techniques until the patient can actively relax the muscles responsible for the dystonic posture. The second step is to perform exercises to improve independence and precision of fingers and wrist movements. Next, the muscles involved in the correction of dystonic postures are trained by drawing of loops, curves, and arabesques related to the clinical forms of writer's cramp. Graphic exercises are made increasingly complex and fast. The aim of this rehabilitation is not to enable patients to write as they used to, but to help their dysgraphia evolve toward a more relaxed, more flexible, and better controlled writing gesture.[76]

Relaxation is frequently added for patients who have excessive anxiety because of their handwriting difficulties. Jacobson's progressive relaxation leads to a passive progressive muscular relaxation (sensation of "dead arm"). Shultz-type autogenic training allows an active state of muscular relaxation (sensation of "heavy arm").[77] This sensation of "heavy arm" should be present during the rehabilitation sessions while relaxing, performing graphomotor exercises, and performing writing activity. The long-term effects of these physiotherapy techniques require careful evaluation before they can be routinely recommended.

Surgical Treatment

LESIONS

With the increasing use of DBS surgery for dystonic patients, ablative surgeries are not currently commonly performed.[1] Several brain targets have been lesioned in the past, particularly the lateral thalamus and the globus pallidus internus (GPi).[78] Reported clinical outcomes have been quite variable, mostly because of differences in inclusion criteria and lack of standardized scales to measure outcome and neuroimaging to review location and size of the lesions.[78]

Thalamotomy

Overall, moderate to marked clinical benefit in patients with generalized and focal dystonia has been reported after thalamotomy, together with a relatively high incidence of dysarthria/dysphonia with bilateral lesions.[79,80] Remarkable benefit has been reported with thalamotomy in patients with writer's cramp and musician's dystonias.[81,82]

Pallidotomy

Renaissance of pallidal lesions for generalized dystonia occurred in the early 1990s encouraged by the benefits observed in parkinsonian patients after pallidotomy.[83] Remarkable improvement has been reported by different centers after unilateral or bilateral pallidotomy,[84,85] together with the observation of some loss of benefit over time.[86]

Peripheral Surgery

Selective denervation procedures are considered efficacious and safe in cervical dystonia.[7,87,88] The clinical improvement with posterior ramisectomy, the most currently used procedure, has been reported to be approximately 70%. More recently, the trend is to offer DBS surgery for cervical dystonia.[89-91]

DEEP BRAIN STIMULATION

There is growing evidence from long-term follow-up that DBS for dystonia is safe and effective.[92-96] The U.S. Food and Drug Administration has approved pallidal and subthalamic DBS for primary generalized and segmental dystonia under the Humanitarian Device Exemption provision.

Thalamic Stimulation

The ventralis oralis anterior and ventralis oralis posterior nuclei of the thalamus can be targeted by DBS in patients with secondary dystonia, in patients with dystonic tremor, or in the case of pallidal stimulation failure.[97] Thalamic stimulation overall seems to be less effective than pallidal stimulation,[97,98] but some successful cases have been reported.[99,100]

Pallidal Stimulation

The GPi is presently considered the target of choice for DBS treatment in generalized and segmental dystonia, and well-designed clinical trials provide considerable evidence that bilateral GPi DBS is effective in treating primary dystonia.[92-96,101-111] The clinical improvement, measured using the BFMRS, has been reported to be 40% to 70% in generalized and segmental primary dystonias, including Meige's syndrome.[92,93,101,104,107-109]

In the short-term[92] and long-term[94] follow-up of a French study involving 22 patients with primary generalized dystonia, bilateral GPi DBS was reported to improve dystonic features significantly. The patients were assessed and video-taped on alternate days with stimulation "on" or "off" in double-blind fashion. At 1-year follow-up, the motor part of the BFMRS improved by 55% and the disability BFMRS score improved by 44% compared with before surgery.[92] At 3-year follow-up, the motor BFMRS scores and the disability BFMRS scores were improved by 58% and 46% compared with baseline.[94]

A class I study examined the effects of bilateral GPi DBS in 40 patients with primary segmental or generalized dystonia.[93] Patients were randomly assigned to receive GPi stimulation or sham treatment for 3 months (sham-treated patients had electrodes implanted, but received stimulation at 0 V). All patients then entered an open-label phase of the trial and were assessed at 6 months. At the double-blind assessment performed at 3 months, the motor BFMRS scores were improved significantly by 40% in the group of patients with active stimulation, but only by 5% in the group with sham stimulation. Similarly, the disability BFMRS scores improved significantly by 38% in the patients with stimulation and by only 11% in the patients without stimulation. In the open phase at 6 months, there was 45% improvement in the motor BFMRS and 41% improvement in the disability BFMRS scores compared with baseline.[93] Quality of life (measured with the SF-36) was also significantly improved at 6 months in the same group of patients compared with baseline.[96]

Although initially the impression was that patients with *DYT1* dystonia improved to a greater extent than non-*DYT1* patients with GPi DBS,[101-103] more recent studies have reported similar benefit.[92-94,104] Phasic movements show a better and more rapid response to stimulation than tonic and fixed postures.[92]

In cervical dystonias, clinical improvement with bilateral GPi DBS has been reported to be about 50% to 70%.[90,91,95,109,110] Similar to patients with generalized dystonias, patients with cervical dystonia show faster improvement of phasic movements and pain relief with DBS.[91] The clinical improvement also seems to be stable in the long-term.[91] A Canadian multicenter, prospective, single-blind study with double-blinded assessment involving 10 cervical dystonia patients has also confirmed significant benefit from bilateral GPi DBS.[95]

More variable results from DBS have been reported in patients with secondary dystonias, heredodegenerative dystonias, and dystonia-plus.[111] Similar to the outcome observed in primary dystonias, patients with tardive dystonia have shown a clinical improvement of about 50% to 70% with GPi DBS.[112-114] These results have been confirmed by a more recent prospective, multicenter, phase II double-blind study in 10 patients with tardive dystonia 6 months after surgery.[115] GPi DBS has also been used in post-traumatic,[116] postanoxic, postencephalitic, perinatal, or poststroke dystonia with very unpredictable outcomes.[99,103,111] An improvement of 50% to 80% at 2-year follow-up has also been reported in patients with pantothenate kinase–associated neurodegeneration,[117] although the benefit has been reported to decline markedly in patients at longer term follow-up (3 to 5 years).[118] Pallidal stimulation has also been reported to be effective in patients with myoclonic dystonia[119,120] and "Lubag."[121] Cognitive changes have not been reported after GPi DBS to date,[122] although at least two suicides have occurred after surgery.[123]

Subthalamic Stimulation

The subthalamic nucleus has been reported more recently to be another effective target in improving generalized, segmental, and focal dystonia.[124-127] Overall, despite clinical evidence of effectiveness, various issues still need to be clarified in DBS for dystonia, including the mechanism of action of DBS[128] and preoperative predictive signs of surgical outcome.

MOTOR CORTEX STIMULATION

Although motor cortex stimulation has been reported to improve dystonia,[129] safety and efficacy need to be clarified in well-designed studies.[130]

REFERENCES

1. Hamani C, Moro E: Surgery for other movement disorders—dystonia, tics. Curr Opin Neurol 2007;20:470-476.
2. Jankovic J, Brin MF: Therapeutic uses of botulinum toxin. N Engl J Med 1991;324:1186-1194.
3. Ichinose H, Ohye T, Takashi E, et al: Hereditary progressive dystonia with marked diurnal fluctuation caused by mutations in the GTP cyclohydrolase I gene. Nat Genet 1994;8:236-242.

4. Svetel M, Kozic D, Stefanoval E, et al: Dystonia in Wilson's disease. Mov Disord 2001;16: 719-723.
5. Jankovic J: Treatment of dystonia. Lancet Neurol 2006;5:864-872.
6. Mariotti P, Fasano A, Contarino MF, et al: Management of status dystonicus: our experience and review of the literature. Mov Disord 2007;22:963-968.
7. Balash Y, Giladi N: Efficacy of pharmacological treatment of dystonia: evidence-based review including meta-analysis of the effect of botulinum toxin and other cure options. Eur J Neurol 2004;11:361-370.
8. Jankovic J, Esquenazi A, Fehling D, et al: Evidence-based review of patient reported outcomes with botulinum toxin type A. Clin Neuropharmacol 2004;27:234-244.
9. Albanese A, Barnes MP, Bhatia KP, et al: A systematic review on the diagnosis and treatment of primary (idiopathic) dystonia and dystonia plus syndromes: report of an EFNS/MDS-ES Task Force. Eur J Neurol 2006;13:433-444.
10. Consky ES, Lang AE: Clinical assessments of patients with cervical dystonia. In Jankovic J, Hallet M (eds): Therapy with Botulinum Toxin. New York: Marcel Dekker, 1994, pp 211-237.
11. Comella CL, Stebbins GT, Goetz CG, et al: Teaching tape for the motor section of the Toronto Western Spasmodic Torticollis Scale. Mov Disord 1997;12:570-575.
12. Tsui JK, Hayward M, Mak EK, Schulzer M: Botulinum toxin type B in the treatment of cervical dystonia: a pilot study. Neurology 1995;45:2109-2110.
13. Comella CL, Leurgans S, Wuu J, et al: Dystonia study group. Rating scales for dystonia: a multi-center assessment. Mov Disord 2003;18:303-312.
14. Burke RE, Fahn S, Marsden CD, et al: Validity and reliability of a rating scale for the primary torsion dystonia. Neurology 1985;35:73-77.
15. Cano SJ, Warner TT, Linacre JM, et al: Capturing the true burden of dystonia on patients: the Cervical Dystonia Impact Profile (CID-58). Neurology 2004;63:1629-1633.
16. Muller J, Wissel J, Kemmler G, et al: Craniocervical dystonia questionnaire (CDQ-24): development and validation of a disease-specific quality of life instrument. J Neurol Neurosurg Psychiatry 2004;75:749-753.
17. Jankovic J: Dystonia: medical therapy and botulinum toxin. Adv Neurol 2004;94:275-286.
18. Mejia NI, Vuong KD, Jankovic J: Long-term botulinum toxin efficacy, safety and immunogenicity. Mov Disord 2005;20:592-597.
19. Simpson DM, Blitzer A, Brashear A, et al: Assessment: botulinum neurotoxin for the treatment of movement disorders (an evidence-based review): report of the Therapeutics and Technology Assessment Subcommittee of the American Academy of Neurology. Neurology 2008;70:1699-1706.
20. Odergren T, Hjaltason H, Kaakkola S, et al: A double blind, randomised, parallel group study to investigate the dose equivalence of Dysport and Botox in the treatment of cervical dystonia. J Neurol Neurosurg Psychiatry 1998;64:6-12.
21. Ranoux D, Gury C, Fondarai J, et al: Respective potencies of Botox and Dysport: a double blind, randomised, crossover study in cervical dystonia. J Neurol Neurosurg Psychiatry 2002;72: 459-462.
22. Bihari K: Safety, effectiveness, and duration of effect of BOTOX after switching from Dysport for blepharospasm, cervical dystonia, and hemifacial spasm dystonia, and hemifacial spasm. Curr Med Res Opin 2005;21:433-438.
23. Marchetti A, Magar R, Findley L, et al: Retrospective evaluation of the dose of Dysport and BOTOX in the management of cervical dystonia and blepharospasm: the REAL DOSE study. Mov Disord 2005;20:937-944.
24. Jost WH, Blümel J, Grafe S: Botulinum neurotoxin type A free of complexing proteins (XEOMIN) in focal dystonia. Drugs 2007;67:669-683.
25. Truong D, Duane DD, Jankovic J, et al: Efficacy and safety of botulinum type A toxin (Dysport) in cervical dystonia: results of the first US randomized, double-blind, placebo-controlled study. Mov Disord 2005;20:783-791.
26. Chapman MA, Barron R, Tanis DC, et al: Comparison of botulinum neurotoxin preparations for the treatment of cervical dystonia. Clin Ther 2007;29:1325-1537.
27. Costa J, Espírito-Santo C, Borges A, et al: Botulinum toxin type A therapy for cervical dystonia. Cochrane Database Syst Rev 2005;1:CD003633.
28. Tarsy D: Comparison of clinical rating scales in treatment of cervical dystonia with botulinum toxin. Mov Disord 1997;12:100-102.
29. Hsiung GY, Das SK, Ranawaya R, et al: Long-term efficacy of botulinum toxin A in treatment of various movement disorders over a 10-year period. Mov Disord 2002;17:1288-1293.

30. Haussermann P, Marczoch S, Klinger C, et al: Long-term follow-up of cervical dystonia patients treated with botulinum toxin A. Mov Disord 2004;19:303-308.
31. Skogseid IM, Kerty E: The course of cervical dystonia and patient satisfaction with long-term botulinum toxin A treatment. Eur J Neurol 2005;12:163-170.
32. Comella CL, Buchman AS, Tanner CM, et al: Botulinum toxin injection for spasmodic torticollis: increased magnitude of benefit with electromyographic assistance. Neurology 1992;42:878-882.
33. Jankovic J: Needle EMG guidance is rarely required. Muscle Nerve 2001;24:1568-1570.
34. Brin MF, Lew MF, Adler CH, et al: Safety and efficacy of NeuroBloc (botulinum toxin type B) in type-A resistant cervical dystonia. Neurology 1999;53:1431-1438.
35. Lew MF, Adornato BT, Duane DD, et al: Botulinum toxin type B: a double-blind, placebo-controlled, safety and efficacy study in cervical dystonia. Neurology 1997;49:701-707.
36. Brashear A, Lew MF, Dykstra DD, et al: Safety and efficacy of Neurobloc (botulinum toxin type B) in type A responsive cervical dystonia. Neurology 1999;53:1439-1446.
37. Costa J, Espírito-Santo C, Borges A, et al: Botulinum toxin type B for cervical dystonia. Cochrane Database Syst Rev 2005;1:CD004315.
38. Jankovic J, Orman J: Botulinum A toxin for cranial-cervical dystonia: a double-blind, placebo-controlled study. Neurology 1987;37:616-623.
39. Calace P, Cortese G, Piscopo R, et al: Treatment of blepharospasm with botulinum neurotoxin type A: long-term results. Eur J Ophthalmol 2003;13:331-336.
40. Costa J, Espírito-Santo C, Borges A, et al: Botulinum toxin type A therapy for blepharospasm. Cochrane Database Syst Rev 2005;1:CD004900.
41. Jankovic J: Pretarsal injection of botulinum toxin for blepharospasm and apraxia of eyelid opening. J Neurol Neurosurg Psychiatry 1996;60:704.
42. Quirk JA, Sheean GL, Marsden CD, Lees AJ: Treatment of nonoccupational limb and trunk dystonia with botulinum toxin. Mov Disord 1996;11:377-383.
43. Wissel J, Kabus C, Wenzel R: Botulinum toxin in writer's cramp: objective response evaluation in 31 patients. J Neurol Neurosurg Psychiatry 1996;61:172-175.
44. Cole R, Hallet M, Cohen LG: Double-blind trial of botulinum toxin for treatment of focal hand dystonia. Mov Disord 1995;10:466-471.
45. Molloy FM, Shill HA, Kaelin-Lang A, Karp BI: Accuracy of muscle localization without EMG: implications for treatment of limb dystonia. Neurology 2002;58:805-807.
46. Chen R, Karp BI, Goldstein SR, et al: Effect of muscle activity immediately after botulinum toxin injection for writer's cramp. Mov Disord 1999;14:307-312.
47. Kruisdijk JJ, Koelman JH, Ongerboer de Visser BW, et al: Botulinum toxin for writer's cramp: a randomised, placebo-controlled trial and 1-year follow-up. J Neurol Neurosurg Psychiatry 2007;78:264-270.
48. Djebbari R, du Montcel ST, Sangla S, et al: Factors predicting improvement in motor disability in writer's cramp treated with botulinum toxin. J Neurol Neurosurg Psychiatry 2004;75:1688-1691.
49. Tassorelli C, Mancini F, Balloni L, et al: Botulinum toxin and neuromotor rehabilitation: an integrated approach to idiopathic cervical dystonia. Mov Disord 2006;21:2240-2243.
50. Sheean G: Restoring balance in focal limb dystonia with botulinum toxin. Disabil Rehabil 2007;29:1778-1788.
51. Harwood G, Hierons R, Fletcher NA, Mardsen CD: Lessons from a remarkable family with dopa-responsive dystonia. J Neurol Neurosurg Psychiatry 1994;57:460-463.
52. Nygaard TG, Marsedn CD, Duvoisin RC: Dopa-responsive dystonia. Adv Neurol 1988;50:377-384.
53. Lang AE: Dopamine agonists and antagonists in the treatment of idiopathic dystonia. Adv Neurol 1988;50:561-570.
54. Marsden CD, Marion MH, Quinn N: The treatment of severe dystonia in children and adults. J Neurol Neurosurg Psychiatry 1984;47:1166-1173.
55. Dewey RB Jr, Muenter MD, Kishore A, Snow BJ: Long-term follow-up of levodopa responsiveness in generalized dystonia. Arch Neurol 1998;55:1320-1323.
56. Karp BI, Goldstein SR, Chen R, et al: An open trial of clozapine for dystonia. Mov Disord 1999;14:652-657.
57. Trugman JM, Leadbetter R, Zalis ME, et al: Treatment of severe axial tardive dystonia with clozapine: case report and hypothesis. Mov Disord 1994;9:441-446.
58. Kenney C, Hunter C, Jankovic J: Long-term tolerability of tetrabenazine in the treatment of hyperkinetic movement disorders. Mov Disord 2007;22:193-197.

59. Jankovic J: Treatment of hyperkinetic movement disorders with tetrabenazine: a double-blind crossover study. Ann Neurol 1982;11:41-47.
60. Burke RE, Fahn S, Marsden CD: Torsion dystonia: a double-blind, prospective trial of high-dosage trihexyphenidyl. Neurology 1986;36:160-164.
61. Hoon AH Jr, Freese PO, Reinhardt EM, et al: Age-dependent effects of trihexyphenidyl in extrapyramidal cerebral palsy. Pediatr Neurol 2001;25:55-58.
62. Anca MH, Falic Zaccai T, Badarna S, et al: Natural history of Oppenheim's dystonia (DYT-1) in Israel. J Child Neurol 2003;18:325-330.
63. Ford B: Intrathecal baclofen in the treatment of dystonia. Adv Neurol 1998;78:199-210.
64. Albright AL, Barry MJ, Shafton DH, Ferson SS: Intrathecal baclofen for generalized dystonia. Dev Med Child Neurol 2001;43:652-657.
65. Richard I, Menei P: Intrathecal baclofen in the treatment of spasticity, dystonia and vegetative disorders. Acta Neurochir Suppl 2007;97:213-218.
66. Motta F, Buonaguro V, Stignani C: The use of intrathecal baclofen pump implants in children and adolescents: safety and complications in 200 consecutive cases. J Neurosurg 2007;107; (Suppl 1):32-35.
67. Hering S, Wenning GK, Seppi K, et al: An open trial of levetiracetam for segmental and general-ized dystonia. Mov Disord 2007;22:1649-1651.
68. Pina MA, Modrego PJ: Dystonia induced by gabapentin. Ann Pharmacother 2005;39:380-382.
69. Berg D, Becker G, Naumann M, Reiners K: Morphine in tardive and idiopathic dystonia (short communication). J Neural Transm 2001;108:1035-1041.
70. Fox SH, Kellet M, Moore AP, et al: Randomised, double-blind, placebo-controlled trial to assess the potential of cannabinoid receptor stimulation in the treatment of dystonia. Mov Disord 2002;17:145-149.
71. Priori A, Pesenti A, Cappellari A, et al: Limb immobilization for the treatment of focal occupa-tional dystonia. Neurology 2001;57:405-409.
72. Candia V, Elbert T, Altenmüller E, et al: Constraint-induced movement therapy for focal hand dystonia in musicians. Lancet 1999;53:42.
73. Ranawaya R, Lang AE: Usefulness of a writing device in writer's cramp. Neurology 1991;41: 1136-1138.
74. Zeuner KE, Bara-Jimenez W, Noguchi PS, et al: Sensory training for patients with focal hand dystonia. Ann Neurol 2002;51:593-598.
75. Byl NN, Nagajaran S, McKenzie AL: Effect of sensory discrimination training on structure and function in patients with focal hand dystonia: a case series. Arch Phys Med Rehabil 2003;84: 1505-1514.
76. Bleton JP: Role of the physiotherapist. In Werner TT, Bressman SB (eds): Clinical Diagnosis and Management of Dystonia. London: Informa Healthcare, 2007, pp 223-233.
77. de Ajuriaguerra J, Garcia Badaracco J, Trillat E, Soubiran G: Traitement de la crampe des écri-vains par la relaxation: le processus de guérison à partir de l'expérience tonique. L'Encéphale 1956;45:141-171.
78. Lang AE: Surgical treatment of dystonia. Adv Neurol 1998;78:185-198.
79. Tasker RR, Doorly T, Yamashiro K: Thalamotomy in generalized dystonia. Adv Neurol 1988;50:615-631.
80. Loher TJ, Pohle T, Krauss JK: Functional stereotactic surgery for treatment of cervical dystonia: review of the experience from the lesional era. Stereotact Funct Neurosurg 2004;82:1-13.
81. Taira T, Ochiai T, Goto S, et al: Multimodal neurosurgical strategies for the management of dystonias. Acta Neurochir Suppl 2006;99:29-31.
82. Shibata T, Hirashima Y, Ikeda H, et al: Stereotactic Voa-Vop complex thalamotomy for writer's cramp. Eur Neurol 2005;53:38-39.
83. Laitinen LV, Bergenheim AT, Hariz MI: Leksell's posteroventral pallidotomy in the treatment of Parkinson's disease. J Neurosurg 1992;76:53-61.
84. Lozano AM, Kumar R, Gross RE, et al: Globus pallidus internus pallidotomy for generalized dystonia. Mov Disord 1997;12:865-870.
85. Yoshor D, Hamilton WJ, Ondo W, et al: Comparison of thalamotomy and pallidotomy for the treatment of dystonia. Neurosurgery 2001;48:818-824.
86. Ford B: Pallidotomy for generalized dystonia. Adv Neurol 2004;94:287-299.
87. Cohen-Gadol AA, Ahlskog JE, Matsumoto JY, et al: Selective peripheral denervation for the treatment of intractable spasmodic torticollis: experience with 168 patients at the Mayo Clinic. J Neurosurg 2003;98:1247-1254.

88. Bertrand CM, Molina-Negro P: Selective peripheral denervation in 111 cases of spasmodic torticollis: rationale and results. Adv Neurol 1988;50:637-643.
89. Krauss JK, Loher TJ, Pohle T, et al: Pallidal deep brain stimulation in patients with cervical dystonia and severe cervical dyskinesias with cervical myelopathy. J Neurol Neurosurg Psychiatry 2002;72:249-256.
90. Bittar RG, Yianni J, Wang S, et al: Deep brain stimulation for generalised dystonia and spasmodic torticollis. J Clin Neurosci 2005;12:12-16.
91. Hung SW, Hamani C, Lozano AM, et al: Long-term outcome of bilateral pallidal deep brain stimulation for primary cervical dystonia. Neurology 2007;68:457-459.
92. Vidailhet M, Vercueil L, Houeto JL, et al: Bilateral deep-brain stimulation of the globus pallidus in primary generalized dystonia. N Engl J Med 2005;352:459-467.
93. Kupsch A, Benecke R, Muller J, et al: Pallidal deep-brain stimulation in primary generalized or segmental dystonia. N Engl J Med 2006;355:1978-1990.
94. Vidailhet M, Vercueil L, Houeto JL, et al: Bilateral, pallidal, deep-brain stimulation in primary generalized dystonia: a prospective 3 year follow-up study. Lancet Neurol 2007;6:223-229.
95. Kiss ZH, Doig-Beyaert K, Eliasziw M, et al: The Canadian multicenter trial of deep brain stimulation for cervical dystonia. Brain 2007;130:2879-2886.
96. Mueller J, Skogseid JM, Benecke R, et al: Pallidal deep brain stimulation improves quality of life in segmental and generalized dystonia: results from a prospective, randomized sham-controlled trial. Mov Disord 2008;23:131-134.
97. Vercueil L, Pollak P, Fraix V, et al: Deep brain stimulation in the treatment of severe dystonia. J Neurol 2001;248:695-700.
98. Holloway KL, Baron MS, Brown R, et al: Deep brain stimulation for dystonia: a meta-analysis. Neuromodulation 2006;9:253-261.
99. Ghika J, Villemure JG, Miklossy J, et al: Postanoxic generalized dystonia improved by bilateral Voa thalamic deep brain stimulation. Neurology 2002;58:311-313.
100. Fukaya C, Katayama Y, Kano T, et al: Thalamic deep brain stimulation for writer's cramp. J Neurosurg 2007;107:977-982.
101. Krauss JK, Loher TJ, Weigel R, et al: Chronic stimulation of the globus pallidus internus for treatment of non-DYT1 generalized dystonia and choreoathetosis: 2-year follow up. J Neurosurg 2003;98:785-792.
102. Katayama Y, Fukaya C, Kobayashi K, et al: Chronic stimulation of the globus pallidus internus for control of primary generalized dystonia. Acta Neurochir Suppl 2003;87:125-128.
103. Krause M, Fogel W, Kloss M, et al: Pallidal stimulation for dystonia. Neurosurgery 2004;55:1361-1368.
104. Coubes P, Cif L, El Fertit H, et al: Electrical stimulation of the globus pallidus internus in patients with primary generalized dystonia: long-term results. J Neurosurg 2004;101:189-194.
105. Diamond A, Shahed J, Azher S, et al: Globus pallidus deep brain stimulation in dystonia. Mov Disord 2006;21:692-695.
106. Goto S, Yamada K, Shimazu H, et al: Impact of bilateral pallidal stimulation on DYT1-generalized dystonia in Japanese patients. Mov Disord 2006;21:1785-1787.
107. Foote KD, Sanchez JC, Okun MS: Staged deep brain stimulation for refractory craniofacial dystonia with blepharospasm: case report and physiology. Neurosurgery 2005;56:E415.
108. Houser M, Waltz T: Meige syndrome and pallidal deep brain stimulation. Mov Disord 2005;20:1203-1205.
109. Ostrem JL, Marks WJ, Volz MM, et al: Pallidal deep brain stimulation in patients with cranial-cervical dystonia (Meige syndrome). Mov Disord 2007;22:1885-1891.
110. Krauss JK, Loher TJ, Pohle T, et al: Pallidal deep brain stimulation in patients with cervical dystonia and severe cervical dyskinesias with cervical myelopathy. J Neurol Neurosurg Psychiatry 2002;72:249-256.
111. Eltahawy HA, Saint-Cyr J, Giladi N, et al: Primary dystonia is more responsive than secondary dystonia to pallidal interventions: outcome after pallidotomy or pallidal deep brain stimulation. Neurosurgery 2004;54:613-619.
112. Eltahawy HA, Feinstein A, Khan F, et al: Bilateral globus pallidus internus deep brain stimulation in tardive dyskinesia: a case report. Mov Disord 2004;19:969-972.
113. Trottenberg T, Volkmann J, Deuschl G, et al: Treatment of severe tardive dystonia with pallidal deep brain stimulation. Neurology 2005;64:344-346.
114. Franzini A, Marras C, Ferroli P, et al: Long-term high-frequency bilateral pallidal stimulation for neuroleptic-induced tardive dystonia: report of two cases. J Neurosurg 2005;102:721-725.

115. Damier P, Thobois S, Witjas T, et al: Bilateral deep brain stimulation of the globus pallidus to treat tardive dyskinesia. Arch Gen Psychiatry 2007;64:170-176.
116. Capelle HH, Grips E, Weigel R, et al: Posttraumatic peripherally-induced dystonia and multifocal deep brain stimulation: case report. Neurosurgery 2006;59:E702.
117. Castelnau P, Cif L, Valente EM, et al: Pallidal stimulation improves pantothenate kinase-associated neurodegeneration. Ann Neurol 2005;57:738-741.
118. Krause M, Fogel W, Tronnier V, et al: Long-term benefit to pallidal deep brain stimulation in a case of dystonia secondary to pantothenate kinase-associated neurodegeneration. Mov Disord 2006;21:2255-2257.
119. Cif L, Valente EM, Hemm S, et al: Deep brain stimulation in myoclonus-dystonia syndrome. Mov Disord 2004;19:724-727.
120. Magarinos-Ascone CM, Regidor I, Martinez-Castrillo JC, et al: Pallidal stimulation relieves myoclonus-dystonia syndrome. J Neurol Neurosurg Psychiatry 2005;76:989-991.
121. Evidente VG, Lyons MK, Wheeler M, et al: First case of X-linked dystonia-parkinsonism ("Lubag") to demonstrate a response to bilateral pallidal stimulation. Mov Disord 2007;22: 170-179.
122. Pillon B, Ardouin C, Dujardin K, et al: Preservation of cognitive function in dystonia treated by pallidal stimulation. Neurology 2006;66:1556-1558.
123. Foncke EM, Schuurman PR, Speelman JD: Suicide after deep brain stimulation of the internal globus pallidus for dystonia. Neurology 2006;6:142-143.
124. Pastor-Gomez J, Hernando-Requejo V, Luengo-Dos Santos A, et al: Treatment of a case of generalized dystonia using subthalamic stimulation. Rev Neurol 2003;37:529-531.
125. Chou KL, Hurtig HI, Jaggi JL, et al: Bilateral subthalamic nucleus deep brain stimulation in a patient with cervical dystonia and essential tremor. Mov Disord 2005;20:377-380.
126. Sun B, Chen S, Zhan S, et al: Subthalamic nucleus stimulation for primary dystonia and tardive dystonia. Acta Neurochir Suppl 2007;97:207-214.
127. Kleiner-Fisman G, Liang GS, Moberg PJ, et al: Subthalamic nucleus deep brain stimulation for severe idiopathic dystonia: impact on severity, neuropsychological status, and quality of life. J Neurosurg 2007;107:29-36.
128. Tish S, Rothwell JC, Limousin P, et al: The physiological effects of pallidal deep brain stimulation in dystonia. IEEE Trans Neural Syst Rehabil Eng 2007;15:166-172.
129. Romito LM, Franzini A, Perani D, et al: Fixed dystonia unresponsive to pallidal stimulation improved by motor cortex stimulation. Neurology 2007;68:875-876.
130. Espay AJ, Chen R, Moro E, Lang AE: Fixed dystonia unresponsive to pallidal stimulation improved by motor cortex stimulation [Reply]. Neurology 2007;69:1062-1063.

28 Paroxysmal Dyskinesias

KAILASH P. BHATIA • SUSANNE A. SCHNEIDER

Introduction

Paroxysmal movement disorders are a heterogeneous group of disorders characterized by episodes of abnormal involuntary movements without change in consciousness. Phenomenologically, the episodic involuntary movements may be dystonic, choreiform, ballistic, or a complex combination of these—referred to as paroxysmal dyskinesias (PxD).[1] Although their exact prevalence is uncertain, PxD are rare. In one study by Blakeley and Jankovic,[2] only 92 cases with PxD were

TABLE 28–1	Secondary Causes of Paroxysmal Kinesigenic Dyskinesia, Paroxysmal Nonkinesigenic Dyskinesia, Paroxysmal Exercise-Induced Dyskinesia, and Paroxysmal Hypnogenic Dyskinesia

Demyelination, such as multiple sclerosis
Vasculopathy, such as ischemia, hemorrhage, moyamoya disease
Infectious disease (encephalitis, HIV, CMV, after streptococcal pharyngitis)
Cerebral and peripheral trauma
Migraine
Hormonal and metabolic dysfunction (diabetes mellitus, hyperthyroidism, hypopara-
thyroidism, Albright pseudohypoparathyroidism, antiphospholipid syndrome,
kernicterus)
Neurodegenerative disease (Huntington's disease)
Neoplasm (parasagittal meningioma)
Chiari malformation, cervical syringomyelia
Cerebral palsy after perinatal hypoxia
Drug-induced (methylphenidate therapy)

CMV, cytomegalovirus; HIV, human immunodeficiency virus.

reported out of 12,063 movement disorder patients (0.76%) seen over 19 years. Because of the fact that PxD episodes are typically of short duration and often remain unwitnessed, and because neurological examination is typically normal between attacks, these conditions may be underdiagnosed.

With regard to etiology, PxD may be a primary disorder (often familial or sporadic) or due to an acquired (secondary) cause. There are many secondary etiological causes (Table 28–1) over a wide range of onset age. An identifiable cause, suggesting secondary paroxysmal kinesigenic dyskinesia (PKD), could be identified in 7 (28%) of 25 patients.[3] All secondary causes should be considered and ruled out as deemed appropriate before making the diagnosis of primary PxD.

Over the years, various classifications for these disorders have been proposed, mainly according to attack duration (brief, intermediate, and prolonged), etiology (primary/idiopathic versus secondary/acquired), and triggering factors. The classification by Demirkiran and Jankovic,[4] based on triggering factors (i.e., whether attacks are induced by sudden movement, as in PKD, or other triggers, as in the nonkinesigenic form paroxysmal nonkinesigenic dyskinesia [PNKD]), is most widely accepted. Apart from PKD and PNKD, two further forms, paroxysmal exercise-induced dyskinesia (PED) and nocturnal hypnogenic dyskinesia (PHD), can be distinguished. Not all patients fall easily into either group, however, and some forms of PxD are unclassifiable as per the current accepted definition,[5,6] and some of these have a mixed phenotype, particularly in secondary PxD. In one study of 17 cases of secondary dystonia (identified among 76 PxD cases), 2 patients (12%) who had multiple short episodes of less than 5 minutes duration per day were classified as "pure PKD"; 9 cases (52%) of cases were diagnosed as "pure PNKD"; another 5 cases (29%) had mixed symptoms with features of both PKD and PNKD.[2]

There have been recent advances regarding the genetic underpinnings underlying some of these disorders, such as identification of the *MR1* gene causing PNKD, and historically described cases could be genetically confirmed in hindsight.

Clinical data of genetically proven cases have been published. We review here main forms of PxD, including PKD, PNKD, PED, and nocturnal PxD/PHD, and the episodic ataxias and some rare variants of PxD.

Paroxysmal Kinesigenic Dyskinesia

PKD episodes are by definition triggered by sudden movement; the attacks are typically brief lasting seconds. Some families with this condition have been linked to chromosome 16, but so far no gene have been identified (see later for more details).

HISTORICAL BACKGROUND

In 1901, Gowers[7] first described attacks of an "unusual character" that occurred after sudden movement. He noted that in contrast to epileptic seizures, consciousness was not lost, and movements were tonic without a clonic component. Despite this observation, Gowers[7] classified them as epileptic, and following this terms including "extrapyramidal epilepsy," "striatal epilepsy," "tonic seizures," "tonic motor attacks," and "reflex epilepsy" were coined. Other links to epilepsy were the observations of a good treatment response to antiepileptics[8] or surgical excision of a cortical scar.[9] The first detailed description of clinical features was presented by Kertesz[10] in a seminal review including 31 cases from the literature and 10 new cases, including 1 autopsied. Brain pathology was found to be normal except for slight loss of neurons of the nucleus caeruleus.[10]

CLINICAL PRESENTATION

In addition to single case reports, two studies review clinical features in larger cohorts, including the study by Houser and colleagues[11] on 26 patients with PKD and the more recent study by Bruno and colleagues,[12] who reviewed features of 121 affected individuals with a presumptive diagnosis of idiopathic PKD and referred for genetic studies. On this basis, the latter authors also proposed new diagnostic criteria (Table 28–2).

Age of onset in PKD ranges from 6 months to 33 years, but onset is usually between 7 and 15 years. There seems to be a higher prevalence in males (4:1 to 8:1) in the sporadic form, but not in familial cases.

Typically, an attack is induced by a sudden movement, such as getting up quickly to answer the doorbell or the telephone. Even a sudden increase in speed, amplitude, or force strength or sudden additions of new actions during ongoing steady movements may induce an attack.[13] An example may be sudden acceleration from a walk to a run (trying to catch a bus) or a change in direction. Startle, sound and photo stimulation, vestibular stimulation, hyperventilation, or stress may also trigger attacks. Many patients report an abnormal sensation before the movement, such as numbness or "pins and needles" in the affected limb or the epigastric region.[14] Such an "aura" preceding the attack was reported by almost 70% to 80% of patients.[11,12] Some patients learn to use the aura positively as a warning sign and to prevent subsequent attacks by slowing down or "holding tight" of the affected limb.

TABLE 28–2	Suggested Clinical Criteria for Paroxysmal Kinesigenic Dyskinesia* and for Paroxysmal Nonkinesigenic Dyskinesia[†]

Paroxysmal Kinesigenic Dyskinesia:
  Identified Kinesigenic Trigger for the Attacks
  Short duration of attacks (<1 min)
  No loss of consciousness
  Onset age 1-20 yr, if no family history
  Control of attacks with phenytoin or carbamazepine
  Normal neurological examination; exclusion of other causes
Paroxysmal Nonkinesigenic Dyskinesia:
  Onset of Attacks in Infancy or Early Childhood
  Precipitation by caffeine and alcohol consumption
  Attack duration 10 min–1 hr (≤4 hr)
  Normal neurological examination between attacks; exclusion of other causes
  Family history of movement disorders meeting these criteria

*Based on clinical evaluation of 121 patients.[12]
†Based on genetic testing.[35]

The clinical manifestation may exhibit dystonia, chorea, ballismus, or a combination of these. Among these, dystonia is most common.[2] Typically, attacks affect limbs on one side, although generalized attacks also occur. About 30% of patients experience speech disturbance (dysarthria or anarthria), which may be due to facial involvement.[11] In case of multiple attacks, there may be a refractory period of about 20 minutes during which no further attacks can be induced.[15] Most attacks (88% to 100%) are very brief, lasting only seconds.[11,12] In the series by Houser and colleagues,[11] attacks lasted less than 2 minutes in 88% and 30 to 60 seconds in two thirds of patients. Similarly, Bruno and colleagues[12] reported that attacks were shorter than 1 minute in 95% of patients. Long PKD-like attacks should thus make the clinician suspicious of a secondary cause, including the possibility of psychogenic PxD. There is usually no loss of consciousness (in 98%), and no "postictal" confusion or drowsiness.[11,12]

PKD attacks are frequent. Most patients have 1 to 20 attacks per day; some patients may have more than 20 attacks per day.[12] The frequency of PKD episodes usually peaks in puberty with 30 to 100 attacks,[13] and becomes less after age 20. Attacks may even remit completely after age 30.

PATHOPHYSIOLOGICAL MECHANISMS

Over the years, there has been debate whether PxD are an epileptic or nonepileptic disorder. The brief, stereotyped nature and the dramatic response to anticonvulsant agents argue for an epileptic origin. Electroencephalogram (EEG) studies and sleep EEGs fail to show typical ictal or interictal changes,[16] however, with few exceptions.[17-19] A subcortical origin of the epileptogenic source located in the basal ganglia has been speculated.

Other neurophysiological findings share features seen in basal ganglia disorders (e.g., dystonia), such as abnormal H-reflexes and contingent negative variation. Two studies[20,21] investigated patients with idiopathic PKD using transcranial magnetic stimulation; in one of the studies, a proportion of patients was assessed on and off treatment. Mir and coworkers[21] found reduced short intracortical inhibition, a reduced early phase of transcallosal inhibition, and a reduced first phase of spinal reciprocal inhibition. The cortical silent period, the startle response, and the second and third phases of reciprocal inhibition were normal. The abnormalities in transcallosal inhibition could be normalized by carbamazepine, whereas the other parameters did not change with treatment. The authors concluded that the abnormalities in cortical and spinal inhibitory circuits may be useful to differentiate PKD from primary dystonia and epilepsy. Kang and associates[20] reported normal measures for thresholds, intracortical facilitation, and silent period. In contrast to Mir and coworkers,[21] they found normal short intracortical inhibition. Functional imaging studies such as single photon emission computed tomography (SPECT) scans showing altered perfusion of the basal ganglia contralaterally to the affected side or bilaterally support the basal ganglia theory.[22,23]

GENETICS

Among the primary forms, 65% to 72% of PKD patients had a family history of a similar disorder, and autosomal dominant inheritance was noted. Penetrance was complete in more than half of the cases.[24] A genetic breakthrough of this disorder came about with the recognition of similarities between PKD and paroxysmal movements noted in the context of the syndrome labeled "ICCA" because of presence of infantile convulsions and paroxysmal choreoathetosis. The ICCA syndrome had been mapped to a 10-cM interval of the pericentromere region on chromosome 16. Subsequently, numerous families with pure PKD were also linked to the same area.

Since then, idiopathic PKD cases have also been linked to the pericentromeric region of chromosome 16 (spanning a 24-cM segment between D16S3131 and D16S408), and this was designated the DYT10 locus.[25,26] Despite various attempts and detailed analysis of 157 genes in this area, no mutations could be identified yet that were shared by unrelated families.[26] More recently, two nonsynonymous substitutions affecting the *SCNN1G* and *ITGAL* genes, which were segregated with disease in two families, have been proposed to play a role.[26] There is also evidence of genetic heterogeneity with two independent loci identified in some patients—one on chromosome 16[27] (recently designed the DYT19 locus) and a third locus elsewhere[28] after linkage to chromosome 16 was excluded.

An overlap with the syndrome of rolandic epilepsy, paroxysmal exercise-induced dyskinesia and writer's cramp (RE-PED-WC) was also noted.[29] In RE-PED-WC syndrome, there was a strong relationship between symptom expression and age; seizures and paroxysmal dystonia peaked in childhood. Onset of writer's cramp also was in childhood, but did not cease with age. In contrast to typical PKD (as well as *GLUT1*-associated PED (see below)), inheritance was autosomal recessive. Genome-wide linkage analysis identified a critical region spanning 6 cM on chromosome 16. ICCA syndrome entirely included these 6 cM of the RE-PED-WC critical region. It is unclear, however, whether these conditions are caused by mutations of the same gene or two different genes.

TREATMENT AND PROGNOSIS

PKD attacks usually respond well to anticonvulsants, and carbamazepine is the drug of choice. In the study by Bruno and colleagues,[12] 86% of patients responded well to either carbamazepine or phenytoin. The phenytoin dose required for

PKD control in children is comparable to the dose used for epileptic seizures. In adults, a lower dose is sufficient. Houser and colleagues[11] suggested doses of 5 mg/kg/day of phenytoin for adults and 7 to 15 mg/kg/day of carbamazepine. Acetazolamide is also a useful alternative or adjunct to carbamazepine in the treatment of PKD, especially when due to demyelinating lesions. Other options may include hydantoin, topiramate, or barbiturates. Benzodiazepines were reported to be beneficial in patients with human immunodeficiency virus–associated PKD.

The prognosis is overall good because attack frequency decreases with age,[13] and patients have a normal life expectancy. If undiagnosed, this disorder can have a great impact on the quality of life, however, and in rare instances there have been reports of suicide of patients with PxD.[10] During pregnancy, 50% of affected women may note improvement.[12]

Paroxysmal Nonkinesigenic Dyskinesia (Paroxysmal Dystonic Choreoathetosis)

PNKD has a longer duration compared with PKD and is not induced by sudden movement, but by alcohol, coffee, or strong emotion. More recently, associations with the *MR1* gene were identified, and since this identification, clinical data of genetically proven cases have become available (see later). These cases mostly confirm previous historical reports based on clinical criteria.

HISTORICAL ASPECTS

The first distinct clinical description of "familial paroxysmal choreoathetosis" was by Mount and Reback,[30] who reported a large family with 28 affected members in five generations. Precipitating factors were alcohol, coffee, and fatigue, and improvement was noted after rest and sleep. Symptoms were relieved by scopolamine hydrobromide. Descriptions of similar families followed.[31] Lance[32] presented a review of 100 cases and one new family, and established a classification of PxD syndromes dividing them into three groups according to the duration of episodes (brief, intermediate, and prolonged attacks). More cases were described,[33,34] and the terms "familial paroxysmal dystonia" and "paroxysmal dystonic choreoathetosis" were coined, which were later adopted by Lance and are still frequently used.

CLINICAL ASPECTS

Attacks occur spontaneously at rest or after provocation by alcohol or coffee (reported by almost 100% of gene-positive cases; see later).[35] Other triggering factors include coke, tobacco, emotional excitement, hunger, concentration, or fatigue.[30] Female patients may experience attacks more frequently during menstruation or ovulation periods. Similar to PKD, attacks may begin with premonitory symptoms (41% of genetically proven cases), such as a sensation of tightness (80% of the genetically proven cases) in one limb or involuntary movements of the mouth or anxiety.[35] Movements usually begin on one side and tend to spread or even generalize.[32] Of genetically proven cases, 80% were found to have a combination of dystonia and chorea; 12% had dystonia only.[35] During severe episodes, patients may develop dysarthria or anarthria, with full awareness (reported by 45% of genetically proven cases).[30,35]

In contrast to PKD, in which attacks occur daily, PNKD attacks occur only a few times per year (up to several times per week) and last longer (10 minutes to 12 hours, although usually not longer than 1 hour).[35,36] There is no consistent correlation between duration and frequency.[2] Data about male-to-female ratios are inconsistent and vary between 2:1 for sporadic cases and 1:1 for genetically proven cases. Onset of primary PNKD is in early childhood (mean age 8 years).[30] Onset of symptoms of secondary paroxysms has a wider range (2.5 to 79 years) with a peak in the 20s when caused by trauma and a mean age of 60 years when caused by vascular events.[2] A similar but distinct syndrome co-occurring with spastic paraparesis has been reported, called "choreoathetosis/spasticity" by Auburger and coworkers.[37] (designated the DYT9 locus); however, this may in fact etiologically be more closely linked to PED (see below).

PATHOPHYSIOLOGICAL MECHANISMS

EEGs are generally normal. An invasive videoelectroencephalographic study by Lombroso and Fischman[38] showed discharge from the caudate nuclei, whereas cortical recordings were normal.

SPECT scans revealed hyperperfusion of the right caudate and thalamus.[39] Reduced density of presynaptic dopa decarboxylase activity in the striatum and increased density of postsynaptic dopamine D2 receptors could be shown by fluorodopa F 18 (^{18}F-dopa) and C 11 raclopride PET,[38] thought to reflect chronic upregulation of postsynaptic dopa receptors. Fludeoxyglucose F 18 (^{18}FDG) and [^{11}C]dihydrotetrabenazine (DTBZ) PET did not show any metabolic abnormalities or abnormal binding.[40] It has been suggested that dopaminergic abnormalities, if present, may be due to altered regulation of dopamine release or to postsynaptic mechanisms, rather than to an altered density of nigrostriatal innervation.

GENETIC INSIGHTS

The mode of inheritance in PNKD was recognized as autosomal dominant with a high but incomplete penetrance of approximately 80%.[41] A causative gene was identified by Rainier and coworkers,[42] who detected a missense mutation in the myofibrillogenesis regulator 1 (*MR1*) gene (DYT8), and findings were confirmed by others.[43,44] Substitution of valine for alanine at amino positions 7 and 9 resulted in alteration of the amino-terminal α helix in the two unrelated kindreds.[42] Functional studies by Lee and associates[45] revealed that of the two existing MR isoforms, MR-1L and MR-1S, the former is exclusively expressed in the cell membrane of the brain, whereas the latter is ubiquitously expressed and shows diffuse cytoplasmic and nuclear localization. Functionally, there may be involvement in a stress-related pathway. The homologue, the hydroxyacylglutathione hydrolase (HAGH), plays a role in a pathway to detoxify methylglyoxal, a compound present in coffee and alcoholic beverages and produced as a by-product of oxidative stress, suggesting a possible mechanism whereby alcohol, coffee, and stress precipitate attacks in PNKD (Fig. 28–1). There is genetic heterogeneity with a locus on chromosome 2q31, termed PNKD2, described by Spacey and colleagues.[46]

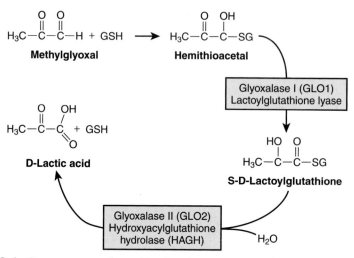

Figure 28–1 Stress response pathway. The glyoxalase system comprises two enzymes, glyoxalase I (GLOI, lactoylglutathione lyase) and glyoxalase II (GLOII, hydroxyacylglutathione hydrolase [HAGH]). Methylglyoxal and glutathione nonenzymatically form a hemithioacetal intermediate and then GLOI catalyzes formation of S-D-lactoylglutathione. HAGH catalyzes the hydrolysis of S-D-lactoylglutathione to D-lactate and reduced glutathione (GSH). (From Lee HY, Xu Y, Huang Y, et al. The gene for paroxysmal non-kinesigenic dyskinesia encodes an enzyme in a stress response pathway. *Hum Mol Genet.* 2004;13:3161-3170.)

The condition of "paroxysmal choreoathetosis/spasticity" (DYT9), a combination of PNKD and spasticity, has been mapped to a region of 2 cM between D1S443 and D1S197 on chromosome 1p coding for a cluster of related potassium channel genes, but the gene is unknown.[37] In view of the proximity to the localisation of the *GLUT1* gene associated with PED (see below), we wonder whether this condition may aslo be associated with *GLUT1* gene mutation confirmation is awaited.

TREATMENT AND PROGNOSIS

First, triggering factors such as caffeine, alcohol, or stress should be clarified and avoided or reduced. Clonazepam is the drug of first choice. In a study of 49 genetically proven *MR1* gene mutation carriers, 97% of subjects who had tried benzodiazepines had a favorable response.[35] The response to antiepileptic treatment is limited; there may be an initial response, which is lost over the years.[35] Haloperidol, gabapentin, acetazolamide, and levodopa may be mildly beneficial. Botulinum toxin can improve PNKD symptoms secondary to stroke.[2] Overall prognosis is good, and attack frequency tends to decrease with age.[35]

Paroxysmal Exercise-Induced Dyskinesia

HISTORICAL ASPECTS

In 1977, Lance[32] recognized the group of "intermediate-type" PxD. In the family described, attacks lasted 5 to 30 minutes, longer than the typically very brief PKD attacks (<5 minutes, normally only seconds). Attacks were not brought on by sudden movement, but by physical exhaustion after continuous exertion. In 1984, Plant and colleagues[47] described a second family with a mother and daughter being affected. Both families suggested an autosomal dominant inheritance. Sporadic cases have also been reported.[48]

CLINICAL ASPECTS

PED is a rare form of paroxysmal movement disorder with a male-to-female ratio of 2:3.[4] Mean onset age is in childhood (5 years), and ranges from 2 to 30 years. By definition, episodes are typically precipitated by prolonged or sustained exercise. In some cases, muscle vibration, passive movements, electrical nerve stimulation, and exposure to cold can trigger attacks.[49]

Although the episodes can vary, the most common presentation is dystonia. In one report of eight cases, hemidystonic distribution was the most common distribution (50% of cases).[48] Generalization was unusual. In a review of 19 patients (including the 8 mentioned), feet were most commonly (79%) affected, and hemidystonia was the next most common presentation.[50]

Attacks last 2 to 5 minutes on average (≤2 hours), and cease within about 10 minutes after discontinuation of the exercise. Frequency of attacks varies and depends on the amount of physical exercise. Episodes occurred once or twice a month in a young girl described by Nardocci and associates.[51]

PED may be accompanied by migraine without aura[52] or a combination of alternating hemiplegia, epilepsy, and ataxia.[53] A combination with rolandic epilepsy and writer's cramp (RE-PED-WC) has also been reported.[29] In some patients, PED may be the presenting sign of young-onset idiopathic Parkinson's disease[54] (e.g., caused by the *parkin* gene).

PATHOPHYSIOLOGICAL MECHANISMS

EEG recordings are typically normal. Other neurophysiological studies, including somatosensory evoked potentials by stimulation of the median nerve, somatosensory evoked potentials by posterior tibial nerve stimulation, brainstem auditory evoked potentials, visual evoked potentials, motor evoked potentials, and electromyography, are suggestive of hyperexcitability at the muscular and brain membrane levels.[55]

Outside the attacks, cortical excitability and inhibitory neuronal mechanisms (response threshold and amplitudes, duration of the silent period ipsilaterally and contralaterally, corticocortical inhibition and facilitation) have been found normal,[56] in contrast to focal task–related dystonia where abnormal motor cortex inhibition is also present during isometric muscle contraction.[57] SPECT studies during motor attacks[58] revealed reduced perfusion of the frontal cortex and basal ganglia, and increased perfusion of the cerebellum, a SPECT pattern compatible with other forms of idiopathic and symptomatic forms of dystonia.[58]

A twofold increase of homovanillic acid and 5-hydroxyindoleacetic acid was measured in cerebrospinal fluid after motor attacks compared with baseline,[50] supporting the hypothesis of dopamine involvement in the pathophysiology of PED. More recently, in some families PED has been recognized to be due to mutations in the glucose transporter 1 gene (see following section on genetics).[42] In affected members from these *GLUT1* families, investigations of cerebrospinal fluid may show glucose levels at or below the lower limit of the normal range.

GENETICS

Mutations in the *GLUT1* gene on chromosome 1p35-p31.3 (designated the DYT18 locus) have been identified in a three-generation family with PED.[59] Findings were confirmed by studying two independent families in which two additional mutations were detected. The gene encodes the transporter of glucose into erythrocytes and across the blood-brain barrier. This explains why glucose levels in the cerebrospinal fluid have been found at or below the lower limit of the normal range.[59] Sporadic cases gene-proven for *GLUT1* gene mutations have also been described.[60] PED is likely to be genetically heterogeneous, however, and *GLUT1* gene mutations may explain only some of the families with PED or sporadic cases. There has also been linkage to 6 cM on chromosome 16 in the same site as PKD in one family with autosomal recessive writer's cramp, PED, and rolandic epilepsy (see also earlier).[61]

TREATMENT

Based on the molecular findings in *GLUT1*-related cases, a ketogenic diet has been recommended.[59] Pharmacologically, anticonvulsants are not useful in patients with PED except for gabapentin, which may reduce frequency and severity of attacks. Levodopa had beneficial effects in one of five patients in whom it was tried.[4] Trihexiphenidyl and acetazolamide showed some benefit in one case each.[50] In another patient reported, acetazolamide dramatically worsened the condition, however.[62] One case responded to pallidotomy.[63]

Paroxysmal Hypnogenic Dyskinesia (Nocturnal Paroxysmal Dyskinesia)

The syndrome of PHD is defined as intermittent (sometimes complex) motor events such as dystonic, choreoathetoid, and ballistic movements arising from non–rapid eye movement (REM) sleep, in particular sleep stages 2 and 3.[64] PHD is newly recognized, however, as a form of nocturnal frontal lobe epilepsy (NFLE), a distinct sleep-related syndrome characterized by nocturnal paroxysmal dyskinesias, very brief paroxysmal arousals, and prolonged somnambulism behavior (also known as episodic nocturnal wanderings).[64] Symptoms often coexist.

CLINICAL ASPECTS

Attacks may occur several times per night over years. Tonic movements affect the trunk and limbs. Automatisms, affective mimicry, vocalization causing subsequent sleep fragmentation, and insomnia are also characteristic.[65] Clusters of 20 attacks lasting about 30 to 60 seconds each are typical,[66] whereas long-lasting variants are rare. NFLE is more common in men (male-to-female ratio 7:3), and onset of symptoms is usually during adolescence. Some patients may be affected by additional epileptic attacks during the day. Marked intrafamilial and interfamilial variability is common.

PATHOPHYSIOLOGY

Classic sleep parameters are normal; however, sleep instability and arousal fluctuations can be measured by microstructure analysis.[67] A polysomnographic study of 40 patients showed ictal epileptiform abnormalities over frontal areas in 32% of cases.[68] Interictal EEG is normal in half of NFLE cases; in other cases, there may be discharge patterns with resemblance to frontal lobe seizures arising mesially or in depth.[64] SPECT studies showed hyperperfusion of the anterior cingulate gyrus.[69]

GENETIC ASPECTS

About 40% of NFLE patients have a family history of nocturnal paroxysmal episodes.[64] Provini and colleagues[64] reported autosomal dominant inheritance in 6% of documented cases. Penetrance is reduced to 80%.[68] The eponym ADNFLE (autosomal dominant nocturnal frontal lobe epilepsy) refers to this autosomal dominant variant,[66,70] and mutations of nicotinic acetylcholine receptors *CHRNA4* and *CHRNB2*, precisely in the α4 and α2 subunits, on chromosomes 15q24 and 20q13.2-13.3 could be identified.[70] Since then, further reports of missense mutations[71] leading to the replacement of serine 248 by phenylalanine in the second transmembrane segment and a three–base pair insertion in the *CHRNA4* gene have been reported.[72]

TREATMENT AND PROGNOSIS

Generally, short-lasting nocturnal dyskinesias respond well to low doses of carbamazepine. Phenytoin and acetazolamide may also alleviate symptoms. Only a few data are published on prognosis; however, it seems that NFLE does not show a tendency to spontaneous remission.

Miscellaneous Movement Disorders Occurring in Bursts or as Paroxysmal Attacks

Other, intermittently occurring disorders that do not easily fit into any of the four described subtypes have been described in the literature, some of which are briefly discussed. Major symptoms include dystonia, ataxia, and tremor.

PAROXYSMS WITH DYSTONIA AS MAJOR SYMPTOM

Orthostatic Paroxysmal Dystonia

"Orthostatic paroxysmal dystonia" refers to attacks provoked by assuming an upright position after sitting or lying.[73] Vascular changes were present on magnetic resonance imaging in the case described. Ictal PET showed reduced perfusion in the contralateral frontoparietal cortex.

Transient Paroxysmal Dystonia or Torticollis in Infancy

Toddlers with intermittent head rotation or tilting, usually alternating from side to side, which may in some cases be associated with irritability, vomiting, pallor, agitation, abnormal truncal posture, and gait disturbance, may have transient paroxysmal dystonia/torticollis in infancy.[74] Rarely, there may be additional infantile migraine or seizures. Episodes usually last 2 to 3 days and range from 10 minutes to 14 days. The disorder is of benign character and self-limiting, and disappears by age 2 years, so treatment is not needed. However, secondary conditions, such as posterior fossa tumor, cervical dislocation, ocular palsy, dystonia owing to side effects of drugs, and Sandifer's syndrome (prolonged head-tilting in children after eating because of hiatal hernia and gastroesophageal reflux),[75] should be excluded.[76] In Sandifer's syndrome, children or infants present with vomiting and feeding difficulties and occasionally with an iron-deficiency anemia. A characteristic feature of Sandifer's syndrome is the bizarre posturing that occurs immediately after feeding and subsides with fasting. More recent genetic studies suggest involvement of calcium channels.[77]

PAROXYSMS WITH ATAXIA AS MAJOR SYMPTOM

Paroxysmal Ataxias

Episodic ataxia (EA) is a rare, familial disorder characterized by brief attacks of generalized ataxia with normal or near-normal neurological function between attacks. Intermittent attacks of ataxia may occur in isolation (EA-2) or in association with interictal myokymia (rippling of muscles, also referred to as neuromyotonia) (EA-1). Inheritance is autosomal dominant. Duration is seconds to minutes in EA-1 and longer (hours to days) in EA-2. Physical and emotional stress and startle or sudden movements may bring on the events. Dysarthria, tremor, or visual disturbances may be present in some cases during episodes.[78] Vertigo is more frequent in EA-2.[79] The presence of interictal myokymia is a sign of EA-1. Drug treatment includes acetazolamide (EA-2) and the potassium channel blocker 4-aminopyridine.[80] EA-1 and EA-2 have been identified as channelopathies. EA-1 was linked to missense mutations on chromosome 12p13 in the gene encoding for the voltage-gated K^+ channel, *KCNA1*. EA-2 typically results from nonsense mutations in the *CACNA1A* gene located on chromosome 19p13.2, which encodes the α1A subunit of the P/Q-type calcium channel.

More recently, other forms of EA have been described, enumerated as EA-3 through EA-6 in the Online Mendelian Inheritance of Man (OMIM).[81] EA-3[82] refers to a Canadian kindred of Mennonite heritage that presented with autosomal dominant EA responsive to acetazolamide. Associated features were vestibular ataxia and tinnitus, which are not seen in EA-1 or EA-2, and presence of interictal myokymia. Age of onset varied. The family was later linked to a 4-cM region on chromosome 1q42; however, three affected individuals did not have the putative disease haplotype, and four unaffected individuals carried the disease haplotype.[83]

EA-4, also known as periodic vestibulocerebellar ataxia, refers to two unrelated North Carolina families described by Farmer and Mustian[84] and Vance and colleagues.[85] Affected individuals had recurrent attacks of ataxia, vertigo, and diplopia with onset in early adulthood. In some, the cerebellar ataxia was slowly progressive. Inheritance was autosomal dominant. Linkage to EA-1, EA-2, and spinocerebellar ataxia types 1 through 5 was excluded.[86]

Escayg and associates[87] studied the role of the calcium channel β4-subunit gene *CACNB4* on chromosome 2q22-23, and detected mutations in this gene in a French-Canadian family with clinical similarities to EA-2 but that was negative for *CACNA1A* gene mutations. This condition is referred to as EA-5. The same mutation was also detected in a German family, however, with generalized epilepsy and praxis-induced seizures (but no ataxia), and functional studies showed only subtle changes in calcium channel function.[87]

A heterozygous mutation in *SLC1A3*, which encodes the glutamate transporter excitatory amino acid transporter (EAAT) 1 was detected in a patient with episodic ataxia, seizures, migraine, and alternating hemiplegia without mutations in either *CACNA1A* or *ATP1A2*.[88] The condition has been referred to as EA-6.

Finally, Kerber and colleagues[89] reported a family with attacks of EA (which they suggested to be called EA-7) lasting hours to days, triggered by exercise and excitement. Associated symptoms included weakness and dysarthria. Some individuals also had associated vertigo. Interictal neurological examination was normal except for some who had a history of migraine. Linkage to chromosome 19q13 was reported and mutations in the *KCNC3* and *SLC17A7* genes and linkage to the EA-3 locus on 1q42 were excluded.

This demonstrated that episodic ataxias are genetically and phenotypically heterogeneous. From the clinician's point of view, EA-1 and EA-2 remain the most common forms.

PAROXYSMS OF THE FACE AND EYES

Paroxysms with Tonic Conjugate Deviation of the Eyes

Clinically, there is sudden sustained upward deviation of the eyes in early childhood (onset age ~9 months). This condition may be associated with mild ataxia with down beating nystagmus on attempted downgaze and apparently preserved horizontal eye movements.[90,91] Symptoms can be exacerbated by fatigue, illness, or vaccination, and are relieved by sleep. A nocturnal polysomnographic study revealed focal or generalized paroxysmal discharges during non-REM sleep in the form of polyspike waves and spike waves[92] and shortened REM sleep latency. The prognosis is usually good with spontaneous disappearance of symptoms around age 2.5 years. A long-term follow-up of 10 years supported the good prognosis of this disorder whether or not treated with antiepileptic medication.[93] Another study reported developmental delay, however, in almost 70%. Tics are an important differential diagnosis because the association of involuntary gaze deviation and tics is common.[94]

Paroxysmal Superior Oblique Myokymia

Orbicularis myokymia (manifesting as eyelid flickering) is common in young, otherwise healthy individuals.[4] The intermittent muscle fasciculations are transient, generally disappear with time, and do not require treatment.[95] Muscle relaxants or botulinum toxin may be considered in severe cases.

Paroxysms of the Tongue

Paroxysms of the tongue are characterized by a delayed onset of episodic, rhythmic, involuntary movements of the tongue after head or neck trauma.[96] Focal tongue contractions are usually slow (three per second), and episodes last approximately 10 seconds, persisting for 2 to 4 months. A similar disorder occurring mainly in sleep has also been described.[97]

REFERENCES

1. Lotze T, Jankovic J: Paroxysmal kinesigenic dyskinesias. Semin Pediatr Neurol 2003;10:68-79.
2. Blakeley J, Jankovic J: Secondary paroxysmal dyskinesias. Mov Disord 2002;17:726-734.
3. Bressman SB, Fahn S, Burke RE: Paroxysmal non-kinesigenic dystonia. Adv Neurol 1988;50: 403-413.
4. Demirkiran M, Jankovic J: Paroxysmal dyskinesias: clinical features and classification. Ann Neurol 1995;38:571-579.
5. De Grandis E, Mir P, Edwards MJ, et al: Paroxysmal dyskinesia with interictal myoclonus and dystonia: a report of two cases. Parkinsonism Relat Disord 2008;14(3):250-25.
6. Pourfar MH, Guerrini R, Parain D, Frucht SJ: Classification conundrums in paroxysmal dyskinesias: a new subtype or variations on classic themes? Mov Disord 2005;20:1047-1051.
7. Gowers WR: Epilepsy and other chronic convulsive diseases: their causes, symptoms and treatment. In Gowers WR, ed: London: J & A Churchill, 1901, p 109.
8. Smith LA, Heersema PH: Periodic dystonia. Proc Mayo Clin 1941;16:842-846.
9. Falconer M, Driver M, Serafetinides E: Seizures induced by movement: report of a case relieved by operation. J Neurol Neurosurg Psychiatry 1963;26:300-307.
10. Kertesz A: Paroxysmal kinesigenic choreoathetosis: an entity within the paroxysmal choreoathetosis syndrome: description of 10 cases, including 1 autopsied. Neurology 1967;17:680-690.
11. Houser MK, Soland VL, Bhatia KP, et al: Paroxysmal kinesigenic choreoathetosis: a report of 26 patients. J Neurol 1999;246:120-126.
12. Bruno MK, Hallett M, Gwinn-Hardy K, et al: Clinical evaluation of idiopathic paroxysmal kinesigenic dyskinesia: new diagnostic criteria. Neurology 2004;63:2280-2287.
13. Fahn S: The paroxysmal dyskinesias. In Marsden CD, Fahn S, eds: Movement Disorders. Oxford: Butterworth Heinmann, 1994, pp 310-345.
14. Jung SS, Chen KM, Brody JA: Paroxysmal choreoathetosis: report of Chinese cases. Neurology 1973;23:749-755.
15. Lishman WA, Symonds CP, Whitty CW, Willison RG: Seizures induced by movement. Brain 1962 Mar;85:93-108.
16. Sadamatsu M, Masui A, Sakai T, et al: Familial paroxysmal kinesigenic choreoathetosis: an electrophysiologic and genotypic analysis. Epilepsia 1999;40:942-949.
17. Hirata K, Katayama S, Saito T, et al: Paroxysmal kinesigenic choreoathetosis with abnormal electroencephalogram during attacks. Epilepsia 1991;32:492-494.
18. Lombroso CT: Paroxysmal choreoathetosis: an epileptic or non-epileptic disorder? Ital J Neurol Sci 1995;16:271-277.
19. Ohmori I, Ohtsuka Y, Ogino T, et al: The relationship between paroxysmal kinesigenic choreoathetosis and epilepsy. Neuropediatrics 2002;33:15-20.
20. Kang SY, Sohn YH, Kim HS, et al: Corticospinal disinhibition in paroxysmal kinesigenic dyskinesia. Clin Neurophysiol 2006;117:57-60.
21. Mir P, Huang YZ, Gilio F, et al: Abnormal cortical and spinal inhibition in paroxysmal kinesigenic dyskinesia. Brain 2005;128(Pt 2):291-299.
22. Ko CH, Kong CK, Ngai WT, Ma KM: Ictal (99m)Tc ECD SPECT in paroxysmal kinesigenic choreoathetosis. Pediatr Neurol 2001;24:225-227.
23. Joo EY, Hong SB, Tae WS, et al: Perfusion abnormality of the caudate nucleus in patients with paroxysmal kinesigenic choreoathetosis. Eur J Nucl Med Mol Imaging 2005;32:1205-1209.
24. Nagamitsu S, Matsuishi T, Hashimoto K, et al: Multicenter study of paroxysmal dyskinesias in Japan—clinical and pedigree analysis. Mov Disord 1999;14:658-663.
25. Swoboda KJ, Soong B, McKenna C, et al: Paroxysmal kinesigenic dyskinesia and infantile convulsions: clinical and linkage studies. Neurology 2000;55:224-230.
26. Kikuchi T, Nomura M, Tomita H, et al: Paroxysmal kinesigenic choreoathetosis (PKC): confirmation of linkage to 16p11-q21, but unsuccessful detection of mutations among 157 genes at the PKC-critical region in seven PKC families. J Hum Genet 2007;52:334-341.
27. Valente EM, Spacey SD, Wali GM, et al: A second paroxysmal kinesigenic choreoathetosis locus (EKD2) mapping on 16q13-q22.1 indicates a family of genes which give rise to paroxysmal disorders on human chromosome 16. Brain 2000;123(Pt 10):2040-2045.
28. Spacey SD, Valente EM, Wali GM, et al: Genetic and clinical heterogeneity in paroxysmal kinesigenic dyskinesia: evidence for a third EKD gene. Mov Disord 2002;17:717-725.
29. Guerrini R, Bonanni P, Nardocci N, et al: Autosomal recessive rolandic epilepsy with paroxysmal exercise-induced dystonia and writer's cramp: delineation of the syndrome and gene mapping to chromosome 16p12-11.2. Ann Neurol 1999;45:344-352.

30. Mount LA, Reback S: Familial paroxysmal choreoathetosis. Arch Neurol Psychiatry 1940;44: 841-847.
31. Lance JW: Sporadic and familial varieties of tonic seizures. J Neurol Neurosurg Psychiatry 1963;26:51-59.
32. Lance JW: Familial paroxysmal dystonic choreoathetosis and its differentiation from related syndromes. Ann Neurol 1977;2:285-293.
33. Forsman H: Hereditary disorder characterized by attacks of muscular contractions, induced by alcohol amongst other factors. Acta Med Scand 1961;170:517-533.
34. Richards RN, Barnett HJ: Paroxysmal dystonic choreoathetosis: a family study and review of the literature. Neurology 1968;18:461-469.
35. Bruno MK, Lee HY, Auburger GW, et al: Genotype-phenotype correlation of paroxysmal nonkinesigenic dyskinesia. Neurology 2007;68:1782-1789.
36. Fink JK, Rainer S, Wilkowski J, et al: Paroxysmal dystonic choreoathetosis: tight linkage to chromosome 2q. Am J Hum Genet 1996;59:140-145.
37. Auburger G, Ratzlaff T, Lunkes A, et al: A gene for autosomal dominant paroxysmal choreoathetosis/spasticity (CSE) maps to the vicinity of a potassium channel gene cluster on chromosome 1p, probably within 2 cM between D1S443 and D1S197. Genomics 1996;31:90-94.
38. Lombroso CT, Fischman A: Paroxysmal non-kinesigenic dyskinesia: pathophysiological investigations. Epileptic Disord 1999;1:187-193.
39. del Carmen Garcia M, Intruvini S, Vazquez S, et al: Ictal SPECT in paroxysmal non-kinesigenic dyskinesia: case report and review of the literature. Parkinsonism Relat Disord 2000;6:119-121.
40. Bohnen NI, Albin RL, Frey KA, et al: (+)-alpha-[11C]Dihydrotetrabenazine PET imaging in familial paroxysmal dystonic choreoathetosis. Neurology 1999;52:1067-1069.
41. Zorzi G, Conti C, Erba A, et al: Paroxysmal dyskinesias in childhood. Pediatr Neurol 2003;28: 168-172.
42. Rainier S, Thomas D, Tokarz D, et al: Myofibrillogenesis regulator 1 gene mutations cause paroxysmal dystonic choreoathetosis. Arch Neurol 2004;61:1025-1029.
43. Hempelmann A, Kumar S, Muralitharan S, Sander T: Myofibrillogenesis regulator 1 gene (MR-1) mutation in an Omani family with paroxysmal nonkinesigenic dyskinesia. Neurosci Lett 2006;402(1-2):118-120.
44. Stefanova E, Djarmati A, Momcilovic D, et al: Clinical characteristics of paroxysmal nonkinesigenic dyskinesia in Serbian family with myofibrillogenesis regulator 1 gene mutation. Mov Disord 2006;21:2010-2015.
45. Lee HY, Xu Y, Huang Y, et al: The gene for paroxysmal non-kinesigenic dyskinesia encodes an enzyme in a stress response pathway. Hum Mol Genet 2004;13:3161-3170.
46. Spacey SD, Adams PJ, Lan PJ et al: Genetic heterogeneity in paroxysmal nonkinesigenic dyskinesia. Neurology 2006;66:1588-1590.
47. Plant GT, Williams AC, Earl CJ, Marsden CD: Familial paroxysmal dystonia induced by exercise. J Neurol Neurosurg Psychiatry 1984;47:275-279.
48. Bhatia KP, Soland VL, Bhatt MH, et al: Paroxysmal exercise-induced dystonia: eight new sporadic cases and a review of the literature. Mov Disord 1997;12:1007-1012.
49. Wali GM: Paroxysmal hemidystonia induced by prolonged exercise and cold. J Neurol Neurosurg Psychiatry 1992;55:236-237.
50. Bhatia KP: The paroxysmal dyskinesias. J Neurol 1999;246:149-155.
51. Nardocci N, Lamperti E, Rumi V, et al: Typical and atypical forms of paroxysmal choreoathetosis. Dev Med Child Neurol 1989;31:670-674.
52. Munchau A, Valente EM, Shahidi GA, et al: A new family with paroxysmal exercise induced dystonia and migraine: a clinical and genetic study. J Neurol Neurosurg Psychiatry 2000;68:609-614.
53. Neville BG, Besag FM, Marsden CD: Exercise induced steroid dependent dystonia, ataxia, and alternating hemiplegia associated with epilepsy. J Neurol Neurosurg Psychiatry 1998;65:241-244.
54. Bozi M, Bhatia KP: Paroxysmal exercise-induced dystonia as a presenting feature of young-onset Parkinson's disease. Mov Disord 2003;18:1545-1547.
55. Margari L, Perniola T, Illiceto G, et al: Familial paroxysmal exercise-induced dyskinesia and benign epilepsy: a clinical and neurophysiological study of an uncommon disorder. Neurol Sci 2000;21:165-172.
56. Meyer BU, Irlbacher K, Meierkord H: Analysis of stimuli triggering attacks of paroxysmal dystonia induced by exertion. J Neurol Neurosurg Psychiatry 2001;70:247-251.
57. Rona S, Berardelli A, Vacca L: Alteration of motor cortical inhibition in patients with dystonia. Mov Disord 1998;13:118-124.

58. Kluge A, Kettner B, Zschenderlein R, et al: Changes in perfusion pattern using ECD-SPECT indicate frontal lobe and cerebellar involvement in exercise-induced paroxysmal dystonia. Mov Disord 1998;13:125-134.

59. Weber YG, Storch A, Wuttke TV, et al: GLUT1 mutations are a cause of paroxysmal exertion-induced dyskinesias and induce hemolytic anemia by a cation leak. J clin Invest. 2008 Jun;118(6):2157-2168.

60. Schneider SA, Paisan-Ruiz C, Garcia-Gorostiaga I, et al: GLUT 1 gene mutations cause sporadic paroxysmal exercise induced dyskinesias. Mov Disord (in press).

61. Guerrini R, Parmeggiani L, Bonanni P, et al: Locus for paroxysmal kinesigenic dyskinesia maps to human chromosome 16. Neurology 2000;55:738-739.

62. Guimaraes J, Vale-Santos JE: Paroxysmal dystonia induced by exercise and acetazolamide. Eur J Neurol 2000;7:237-240.

63. Bhatia KP, Marsden CD, Thomas D: Posteroventral pallidotomy can ameliorate attacks of paroxysmal dystonia induced by exercise. J Neurol Neurosurg Psychiatry 1998;65:604-605.

64. Provini F, Plazzi G, Montagna P, Lugaresi E: The wide clinical spectrum of nocturnal frontal lobe epilepsy. Sleep Med Rev 2000;4:375-386.

65. Hirsch E, Sellal F, Maton B, et al: Nocturnal paroxysmal dystonia: a clinical form of focal epilepsy. Neurophysiol Clin 1994;24:207-217.

66. Scheffer IE, Bhatia KP, Lopes-Cendes I, et al: Autosomal dominant nocturnal frontal lobe epilepsy: a distinctive clinical disorder. Brain 1995;118(Pt 1):61-73.

67. Zucconi M, Ferini-Strambi L: NREM parasomnias: arousal disorders and differentiation from nocturnal frontal lobe epilepsy. Clin Neurophysiol 2000;111(Suppl 2):S129-S135.

68. Oldani A, Zucconi M, Asselta R, et al: Autosomal dominant nocturnal frontal lobe epilepsy: a video-polysomnographic and genetic appraisal of 40 patients and delineation of the epileptic syndrome. Brain 1998;121:205-223.

69. Schindler K, Gast H, Bassetti C, et al: Hyperperfusion of anterior cingulate gyrus in a case of paroxysmal nocturnal dystonia. Neurology 2001;57:917-920.

70. Bhatia KP: Familial (idiopathic) paroxysmal dyskinesias: an update. Semin Neurol 2001;21:69-74.

71. Weiland S, Witzemann V, Villarroel A, et al: An amino acid exchange in the second transmembrane segment of a neuronal nicotinic receptor causes partial epilepsy by altering its desensitization kinetics. FEBS Lett 1996;398:91-96.

72. Steinlein OK, Mulley JC, Propping P, et al: A missense mutation in the neuronal nicotinic acetylcholine receptor alpha 4 subunit is associated with autosomal dominant nocturnal frontal lobe epilepsy. Nat Genet 1995;11:201-203.

73. Sethi K, Lee KH, Deuskar V, et al: Orthostatic paroxysmal dystonia. Mov Disord 2002;17:841-845.

74. shida T, Hattori S, Ueda T, et al: Benign paroxysmal torticollis in infancy: case report. No To Hattatsu 1990;22:274-278.

75. Menkes JH, Ament ME: Neurologic disorders of gastroesophageal function. Adv Neurol 1988;49:409-416.

76. Guerrero VJ, de Paz AP, Luengo Casasola JL, et al: [Benign infantile paroxysmal torticollis: apropos of 3 cases]. An Esp Pediatr 1988;29:149-152.

77. Giffin NJ, Benton S, Goadsby PJ: Benign paroxysmal torticollis of infancy: four new cases and linkage to CACNA1A mutation. Dev Med Child Neurol 2002;44:490-493.

78. Klein A, Boltshauser E, Jen J, Baloh RW: Episodic ataxia type 1 with distal weakness: a novel manifestation of a potassium channelopathy. Neuropediatrics 2004;35:147-149.

79. Brandt T, Strupp M: Episodic ataxia type 1 and 2 (familial periodic ataxia/vertigo). Audiol Neurootol 1997;2:373-383.

80. Strupp M, Kalla R, Dichgans M, et al: Treatment of episodic ataxia type 2 with the potassium channel blocker 4-aminopyridine. Neurology 2004;62:1623-1625.

81. Jen JC, Graves TD, Hess EJ, et al: Primary episodic ataxias: diagnosis, pathogenesis and treatment. Brain 2007 Oct;130(Pt 10):2484-2493.

82. Steckley JL, Ebers GC, Cader MZ, McLachlan RS: An autosomal dominant disorder with episodic ataxia, vertigo, and tinnitus. Neurology 2001;57:1499-1502.

83. Cader MZ, Steckley JL, Dyment DA, et al: A genome-wide screen and linkage mapping for a large pedigree with episodic ataxia. Neurology 2005;65:156-158.

84. Farmer T, Mustian VM: Vestibulo-cerebellar ataxia: a newly defined hereditary syndrome with periodic manifestations [Abstract]. Arch Neurol 1963;8:471-480.

85. Vance J, Pericak-Vance M, Payne CS, et al: Linkage and genetic analysis in adult onset periodic vestibulo-cerebellar ataxia: report of a new family [Abstract]. Am J Hum Genet 1984;36:78S.
86. Damji KF, Allingham RR, Pollock SC, et al: Periodic vestibulocerebellar ataxia, an autosomal dominant ataxia with defective smooth pursuit, is genetically distinct from other autosomal dominant ataxias. Arch Neurol 1996;53:338-344.
87. Escayg A, De Waard M, Lee DD, et al: Coding and noncoding variation of the human calcium-channel beta4-subunit gene CACNB4 in patients with idiopathic generalized epilepsy and episodic ataxia. Am J Hum Genet 2000;66:1531-1539.
88. Jen JC, Wan J, Palos TP, et al: Mutation in the glutamate transporter EAAT1 causes episodic ataxia, hemiplegia, and seizures. Neurology 2005;65:529-534.
89. Kerber KA, Jen JC, Lee H, et al: A new episodic ataxia syndrome with linkage to chromosome 19q13. Arch Neurol 2007;64:749-752.
90. Lispi ML, Vigevano F: Benign paroxysmal tonic upgaze of childhood with ataxia. Epileptic Disord 2001;3:203-206.
91. Ouvrier RA, Billson F: Benign paroxysmal tonic upgaze of childhood. J Child Neurol 1988;3: 177-180.
92. Merino-Andreu M, Arcas J, al Linares E, et al: [Is benign childhood paroxysmal eye deviation a non-epileptic disorder?]. Rev Neurol 2004;39:129-132.
93. Verrotti A, Trotta D, Blasetti A, et al: Paroxysmal tonic upgaze of childhood: effect of age-of-onset on prognosis. Acta Paediatr 2001;90:1343-1345.
94. Frankel M, Cummings JL: Neuro-ophthalmic abnormalities in Tourette's syndrome: functional and anatomic implications. Neurology 1984;34:359-361.
95. Jordan DR, Anderson RL, Thiese SM: Intractable orbicularis myokymia: treatment alternatives. Ophthalmic Surg 1989;20:280-283.
96. Keane JR: Galloping tongue: post-traumatic, episodic, rhythmic movements. Neurology 1984;34:251-252.
97. Jabbari B, Coker SB: Paroxysmal, rhythmic lingual movements and chronic epilepsy. Neurology 1981;31:1364-1367.

29 Essential Tremor and Other Tremors

GÜNTHER DEUSCHL • ALFONSO FASANO

Introduction

Tremor is the most common movement disorder encountered in clinical neurology. Tremor denotes a rhythmic involuntary movement of one or several regions of the body.[1] Although most tremors are pathological, a low-amplitude physiological action tremor can be detected in healthy subjects, and may be of functional relevance for normal motor control. Pathological tremor is visible to the naked eye and mostly interferes with normal motor function. The disabilities caused by these tremors are as diverse as their clinical appearance, pathophysiology, and etiologies. Although there are numerous medical treatment options, their efficacy is limited, and refined stereotactic surgical approaches have become increasingly important for the most severe cases.

Clinical Definitions

The clinical examination of tremor patients should focus on certain aspects of the tremor that are the basis for the differential diagnosis and should always be documented (Table 29–1), as follows:

Topography: Tremors can occur in any joint or muscle that is free to oscillate. The patient should be examined carefully under different conditions (see later) to be able to detect all the affected body parts. The most common locations are the arms and hands, but these can be spared, and arm and hand tremors are typically combined with tremor in other regions. Symmetry on the two sides can be important.

Condition of activation: Tremor is also described depending on the activation condition leading to appearance or a marked increase of tremor severity. *Resting tremor* occurs when the muscles of the affected body part are not voluntarily activated. Rest tremor must cease or be suppressed when a voluntary movement is initiated or performed. *Action tremor* is any tremor that is produced by voluntary contraction of muscles, and covers postural and kinetic tremor. *Postural tremor* is present while voluntarily maintaining a position; *kinetic tremor* occurs during voluntary movement. *Simple kinetic tremor* is seen during purposeless voluntary movements. *Goal-directed tremor* (most commonly labeled as intention tremor) occurs when a target is reached. Rarer forms of action tremor occur only during certain positions or tasks (*task-specific* or *position-specific tremor* or *isometric tremor*).

Frequency: For exact frequency measurement, a signal analysis of accelerometric or electromyography (EMG) recordings is necessary. With some experience, the three main frequency ranges can be separated on inspection: high (>7 Hz), medium (4 to 7 Hz) and low (<4 Hz).

Additional symptoms: Additional signs and symptoms are equally important as the tremor characteristics. A parkinsonian syndrome, cerebellar ataxia, and dystonia are important diagnostic and etiologic hints (see later).

TABLE 29–1 **Clinical and Instrumental Features of the Tremor Syndromes***

Diagnosis	Definition	Symmetry	Activation R	P	GD	TP	Frequency (Hz)	Additional Symptoms	Course	Family History	Specific Drug Response	DaTSCAN/ ^{18}F-dopa PET	Brain MRI	Notes
Enhanced physiological tremor	Increase of amplitude of normal physiological tremor. Other neurological symptoms or diseases that could cause tremor must be excluded	+		+		+	6-13	–	Reversible	–	Propranolol	–	–	Tremor is typically short-lived and reversible when cause is removed
Essential tremor	Bilateral tremor of hands or forearms with predominant kinetic tremor and resting tremor only in advanced stages; or isolated head tremor without evidence of abnormal posture, *and* absence of other neurological signs except for cogwheel phenomenon and slight gait disturbances	+	±	+		+	4-11	Cogwheel phenomenon (no rigidity); mild ataxia when advanced (typically abnormal tandem gait)	Slowly progressive	++/–	Alcohol, propranolol	–	–	Rarely tremor may occur in isolation also in voice or chin. Experts believe that duration >3 yr, alcohol responsiveness, and family history support diagnosis, although prospective studies on their diagnostic value are not yet available

Parkinsonian tremors

Type	Description				Frequency (Hz)	Other features		Drug			Typical examples
Type I	Unilateral (or asymmetrical) resting tremor that increases in amplitude under mental stress, and is suppressed during initiation of movement and often during course of movement. "Re-emergent" tremor is same tremor occurring after some latency under postural and action conditions	−	++	±	±	4–7	Other parkinsonian features (rigidity, bradykinesia)	Variable	±	Levodopa	+	−	Typical examples: pill-rolling tremor of hand seen during walking or when sitting; unilateral leg tremor. Pseudo-orthostatic tremor is resting tremor affecting trunk
Type II	Tremor coexisting with type I (frequency should be at least 1.5 Hz higher than type I); bilateral (usually asymmetrical) postural/kinetic tremor of hands	±	+	+		6–13	Other parkinsonian features (rigidity, bradykinesia)	Variable	±	Propranolol	+	−	
Type III	Postural/kinetic tremor of hands without resting component	±	+	+		6–13	Other parkinsonian features (rigidity, bradykinesia)	Variable	±	Propranolol	+	−	

Table continued on following page

TABLE 29–1   Clinical and Instrumental Features of the Tremor Syndromes* (Continued)

Diagnosis	Definition	Symmetry	R	P	GD	TP	Frequency (Hz)	Additional Symptoms	Course	Family History	Specific Drug Response	DaTSCAN/ 18F-dopa PET	Brain MRI	Notes
Orthostatic tremors														
Primary orthostatic tremor	High-frequency trunk tremor present only during standing. None of the patients have problems when sitting and lying. Tremor may also involve upper limbs	+	±	±		+	13-18	–	Stable	±	(Gabapentin)	±	–	Patients have subjective feeling of unsteadiness during stance (in severe cases during gait). Some patients have sudden falls
Orthostatic tremor–plus	Association of orthostatic tremor and other primary neurological disorders	+	±	±		+	13-18	Depending on associated condition	Stable	–	?	±	–	Patients have subjective feeling of unsteadiness during stance (in severe cases during gait). Some patients have sudden falls
Symptomatic orthostatic tremor	Association of orthostatic tremor and structural acquired lesion of brain	+	±	±		+	13-18	Depending on associated condition	Stable	–	?	–	+	Patients have subjective feeling of unsteadiness during stance (in severe cases during gait). Some patients have sudden falls

Dystonic tremors

Dystonic tremor	Postural/kinetic tremor, rarely at rest, occurring in body region affected by dystonia. Usually, focal with irregular amplitudes and frequencies; antagonistic gestures lead to reduction of tremor amplitude	−	±	+	+	±	5-10	Slowly progressive	±	(Anticholinergics, botulinum toxin)	−	±	Typical examples: head tremor in torticollis, hand tremor in writer's cramp, jaw tremor in orofacial dystonias. Some patients exhibit focal tremors even without overt signs of dystonia (e.g., SWEDDs) or very mild posturing. Thalamic tremor is dystonic tremor secondary to thalamic lesions
Tremor associated with dystonia	Postural/kinetic tremor in body region not affected by dystonia, but dystonia is present elsewhere. Usually it affects hands (e.g., in patients with spasmodic torticollis ["essential tremor–like tremor"])	+	+	+			6-12	Slowly progressive/ stable	±	(Propranolol)	−	−	Isolated jaw tremor in patients affected by dystonia not involving facial muscles has been included in this type of tremor

Table continued on following page

TABLE 29-1   Clinical and Instrumental Features of the Tremor Syndromes* (Continued)

Diagnosis	Definition	Symmetry	Activation R	Activation P	Activation GD	Activation TP	Frequency (Hz)	Additional Symptoms	Course	Family History	Specific Drug Response	DaTSCAN/ ^{18}F-dopa PET	Brain MRI	Notes
Dystonia gene–associated tremor	Postural/kinetic tremor usually affecting hands ("essential tremor–like tremor"). No signs of dystonia, but dystonia is present in relatives	+		+	+		6-12	–	Slowly progressive/stable	+	(Propranolol)	–	–	Endophenotype of dystonia causing genes
Task- and position-specific tremor	Focal and irregular task-specific tremor. Tremor predominantly or only occurs during specific motor task (type A) or positions (type B)	–		±	±	+	5-10	–	Stable	–	Anticholinergics	–	–	Typical examples: primary writing tremor; jaw tremor induced by drinking, lip tremor induced by smiling
Cerebellar tremor	Pure or dominant intention tremor; postural tremor (>5 Hz) resembling essential tremor may be present. Titubation is slow-frequency tremor involving axial body parts (head or trunk)	±		+	+	++	<5	Other cerebellar signs (gait ataxia, dysmetria, hypotonia)	Progressive	±	–	–	+	Lesions of archicerebellum usually result in titubation, whereas lesions of neocerebellum produce intention tremor of limbs

Tremor	Description					Frequency (Hz)	Clinical features		Levodopa			Comments
Holmes' tremor (myorhythmia, Benedikt's syndrome, rubral, midbrain, or mixed extrapyramidal tremor)	Slow-frequency and irregular resting tremor that seems to spill into voluntary movements, giving rise to intention tremor of same frequency as resting component	−	+	+	+	3-6	Parkinsonian and cerebellar features	Progressive	−	+	+	Symptomatic tremor that manifests within variable time after lesion within Guillaret-Mollaret triangle (described after hemorrhage, ischemia, vascular malformations, trauma, demyelinating plaques, and neoplasm) Alternatively, it may occur in patients with cerebellar disorder and subsequent Parkinson's disease tremor
Neuropathic tremor	Postural/kinetic variable tremor affecting limbs; frequency can be higher in proximal arm muscles. Two criteria should be fulfilled: confirmed diagnosis of neuropathy (abnormal position sense need not be present) and exclusion of other neurological diseases associated with tremor	+	+			5-10	Peripheral sensory loss (and peripheral weakness)	Variable	− (+ in hereditary sensorimotor neuropathy)	−	−	Usually late manifestation of demyelinating neuropathies

Table continued on following page

Diagnosis	Definition	Symmetry	Activation R	P	GD	TP	Frequency (Hz)	Additional Symptoms	Course	Family History	Specific Drug Response	DaTSCAN/ ^{18}F-dopa PET	Brain MRI	Notes
Palatal tremors														
Essential palatal tremor	Rhythmic movement of roof of soft palate owing to contractions of tensor veli palatine muscle (CNV)	+	+				2-5	Ear click	Stable	−	−	?	−	Inferior olivary pseudohypertrophy is typical feature. Oculopalatal tremor is characterized by eye muscle involvement producing oscillopsia; progressive ataxia and palatal tremor has been reported in sporadic (sometimes compatible with diagnosis of "olivopontocerebellar atrophy") and familial forms, occasionally owing to adult-onset Alexander's syndrome
Symptomatic palatal tremor	Rhythmic movement of edge of soft palate owing to contractions of levator veli palatine muscle (CN IX and X). Other muscles innervated by cranial nerves may be involved (e.g., eye, eyelid, chin, tongue, pharynx). More rarely patients have synchronous diaphragmatic tremor or postural/kinetic tremor of arms	±	+	±	±		1-7	Cerebellar and brainstem signs	Stable (remission in selected cases)	±	−	±	+	

| Psycho-genic tremor | Irregular tremor with variable frequency and amplitude. Decrease of tremor amplitude during distraction or positive "coactivation sign" (see text for details) | – | ± | + | + | 4-9 | Somatizations or other psychiatric disorders | Highly variable | – | – | – | – | Often sudden onset or spontaneous remissions |

*For toxic and drug-induced tremors, see Table 29–6.

GD, goal-directed; P, posture; R, rest; TP, task- or position-specific.

Drugs into brackets are probably but not unequivocally effective.

Physiological and Enhanced Physiological Tremor

DEFINITION AND DIFFERENTIAL DIAGNOSIS

Normal physiological tremor is an action tremor and usually is not visible. It can be measured only with sensitive accelerometers. An increase of the amplitude leads to the visible enhanced physiological tremor (see Table 29–1). The pathological tremor amplitudes are typically short-lived and reversible when the cause is removed. Other neurological symptoms or diseases that could cause tremor must be excluded.[1]

Enhanced physiological tremor and early essential tremor (ET) sometimes can be difficult to distinguish. The positive family history in ET, its chronic course, and the lack of an overt cause for the tremor are important hints. Enhanced physiological tremor is usually bilateral, and any tremor presenting unilaterally even with a high frequency and a pure postural component must be suspected to be a symptomatic tremor. Electrophysiology (spectral analysis of accelerometry and EMG) can be helpful in cases in which enhanced physiological tremor emerges from a reflex enhancement of physiological tremor because ET is a centrally driven tremor.[2,3] EMG bursts less than 8 Hz seem to be in favor of ET rather than enhanced physiological tremor.[4]

EPIDEMIOLOGY

A cross-sectional population-based study found the prevalence of enhanced physiological tremor to be 9.5% in subjects older than 50 years. Enhanced physiological tremor was much more common than ET (3.06%), parkinsonian tremor (2.05%), or Parkinson's disease (PD) (4.49%).[5] No studies are available on the natural cause of the condition. Because most of the causes of enhanced physiological tremor are treatable or reversible, it is believed that it can be corrected for many causes.

PATHOPHYSIOLOGY

Enhanced physiological tremor relies on the same physiological mechanism as normal physiological tremor, and the physiology of normal tremor has been intensively studied.[67]

ETIOLOGY

Most causes of enhanced physiological tremor are related to drugs or toxins that can enhance the peripheral or central component of physiological tremor (Table 29–2). The most important problem is to uncover the cause of enhanced physiological tremor.

TREATMENT

Depending on the etiology, causative treatment is always the first step. Short-lived emotional trembling in certain situations requires treatment only rarely. A single dose of a β-blocking agent (e.g., propranolol 30 to 100 mg) just before a stressful

TABLE 29–2	Causes of Enhanced Physiological Tremor

Drugs
  Neuroleptics, metoclopramide, antidepressants (tricyclics), lithium, cocaine, alcohol, sympathomimetics, steroids, valproate, antiarrhythmics (amiodarone), thyroid hormones, cytostatics, immunodepressants
Toxins
  Mercury, lead, manganese, alcohol, DDT, lindane
Metabolic disturbances
  Hyperthyroidism, hyperparathyroidism, hypoglycemia, hepatic encephalopathy, magnesium deficiency, hypocalcemia, hyponatremia
Others
  Anxiety, fatigue, sympathetic reflex dystrophy, withdrawal of alcohol or drugs

situation can usually help to suppress this transient tremor that may interfere with important (e.g., professional) functions. Other β-blockers (atenolol <200 mg daily), metoprolol (<200 mg), acebutolol (<400 mg), oxprenolol (<160 mg), and nadolol (<80 mg) have a similar effect. Propranolol improves the tremor of ophthalmic surgeons when given before surgery.[8] Treatment of thyrotoxic tremor is recommended with propranolol (<160 mg).

Essential Tremor

DEFINITION AND DIFFERENTIAL DIAGNOSIS

ET is a slowly progressive tremor disorder that sometimes causes severe disability, but is not life-limiting. The traditional view of ET as a monosymptomatic disorder has been revised because this disorder is more complex and heterogeneous. A physiological or laboratory test for the validation of the diagnosis is still lacking because many other conditions may manifest with a slowly progressive action tremor. The heterogeneity may partly be due to diagnostic uncertainty, with different sets of diagnostic criteria all using only medical history and clinical findings (Table 29–3). Some criteria involve the severity of the tremor,[9] which is inadequate when applied to a slowly developing condition, but may be adequate for research purposes.

CLINICAL FEATURES

See Table 29–1.

Motor Features

The topographic distribution shows hand tremor in 94%, head tremor in 33%, voice tremor in 16%, jaw tremor in 8%, facial tremor in 3%, leg tremor in 12%, and tremor of the trunk in 3% of patients.[11,12] In some topographic regions (e.g., head, voice, and chin), tremor may occur in isolation.[10] Fifty percent to 90% of patients improve with ingestion of alcohol, which can be an important feature of the medical history.

TABLE 29–3	**Diagnostic Criteria for Essential Tremor**

Core Criteria

Bilateral tremor of hands or forearms with predominant kinetic tremor *or*
Isolated head tremor without evidence of abnormal posture *and*
Absence of other neurological diagnosis with except for cogwheel phenomenon and
  slight gait disturbances

Supporting Criteria

Family history of uncomplicated tremor
Alcohol sensitivity of trembling
Long duration

"Red Flags" for Diagnosis of Essential Tremor

Isolated tremor in voice, tongue, chin, or legs
Unilateral tremor or leg tremor
Presence of known causes of enhanced physiological tremor (e.g., drugs, anxiety,
  depression, hyperthyroidism)
History of recent trauma preceding the onset of tremor
History or presence of psychogenic tremor
Sudden onset or stepwise progression
Isolated head tremor with abnormal postures (e.g., dystonia)
Drugs
Other systemic disorders (e.g. endocrine, renal)
Primary orthostatic tremor
Isolated position-specific or task-specific tremors, including occupational tremors and
  primary writing tremor

Adapted from references 1 and 10.

ET starts with a postural tremor, which can still be suppressed during goal-directed movements. In advanced stages, an intention tremor can develop, and is accompanied by signs of cerebellar dysfunction of hand movements, such as movement overshoot and slowness of movements.[13] Also, a mild gait disorder prominent during tandem gait is frequently found.[14] In more advanced stages, a tremor at rest can develop.[15] The features of this tremor at rest need to be evaluated in more detail. Subtle signs of cerebellar dysfunction are important for the pathophysiology of the condition, and have been shown for hand and elbow movements,[13,16] gait,[14] subclinical eye movements,[17] cerebellar rhythm generation,[18] and motor learning deficits during an eye blink conditioning protocol.[19]

Nonmotor Features

Several more recent studies have described clinically subtle attentional and executive dysfunction accompanying ET, such as deficits on tests of verbal fluency, naming, mental set-shifting, verbal and working memory, complex auditory attention, visual attention, and response inhibition.[20-24] A deficit of hearing[25] and olfaction was found independent of disease duration and severity,[26] albeit the report of mild olfactory impairment has been subsequently questioned.[27,28]

A distinct personality profile has been found in ET with lower psychoticism scores on the Eysenck personality questionnaire, suggesting that patients are more tender minded and less aggressive than the normal population, with a trend toward social introversion[29] matching with higher scores in the harm avoidance scale of the tridimensional personality questionnaire in another study.[30] Behavioral symptoms that are found to be associated with ET include anxiety, phobic anxiety, and psychoticism.[31-33] The mild frontal dysexecutive syndrome and the slight personality changes have been interpreted to reflect a relative dysfunction of frontal areas resulting from a remote effect within the cerebellothalamocortical circuits as a consequence of cerebellar dysfunction[34] or as an independent frontal dysfunction.[32]

One prevalence study described an association of elderly-onset ET with dementia.[24] The same cohort of patients was prospectively studied, and ET cases with tremor onset after age 65 years were twice as likely to develop incident dementia than were controls; most (71.4%) of the patients had probable Alzheimer's disease.[35] The significance of these results is unclear because of limitations of the study, such as uncertainty about the diagnosis of dementia in this group; a different group size of older and younger onset ET cases; and the fact that the older onset ET patients were twice as likely to be illiterate and almost twice as likely to be depressed, both of which are recognized risk factors for Alzheimer's disease.[36] Because of the high prevalence of enhanced physiological tremor in the elderly population,[5] diagnostic difficulties are a specific concern for an age-related effect such as the incidence of dementia. Further studies on independent cohorts are mandatory.

CLINICAL COURSE

The condition may begin in childhood, but the incidence increases after 40 years, with a mean onset of 35 to 45 years in different studies and an almost complete penetrance at age 60.[12,37] Rarely, older age of onset is found.[38] So far, only a few data are available on the progression of the condition and have shown a decrease of tremor frequency and a tendency to develop larger amplitudes.[39] Intention tremor develops at various intervals between 3 and 30 years after the onset of postural tremor.[40] The disease-related disability varies significantly and depends on the severity of intention tremor.[41] On a generic quality-of-life questionnaire, ET patients scored worse in all eight domains of the SF-36. Tremor severity correlated with some of the physical domains and with social function of the mental domains.[29] An ET-specific quality-of-life questionnaire has been validated more recently.[42] Twenty-five percent of patients seeking medical attention must change jobs or retire from work.[43,44]

EPIDEMIOLOGY

ET is the most common adult movement disorder, although its epidemiology is still unclear. As a result of application of imprecise and variable diagnostic criteria, prevalence estimates range from 0.008% to 22%, with an increase with age. Even in more recent studies using similar criteria, there are 10-fold differences between studies (0.4% to 3.9%).[45] More recently, three large population-based surveys with narrow diagnostic criteria found prevalence data of 4%, 4.8% and 3.06%.[5,46,47] In a retrospective 45-year study performed in Rochester, New York, the age-adjusted incidence was estimated to be 17.5/100,000/year[48]; a large population-based study in Spain reported an incidence rate of 616/100,000/year in a population older than 65 years.[49]

Patients with ET were assumed to have mortality rates similar to the general population.[48] In retrospective studies, patients with ET were found to live longer, however, than individuals without ET,[50] whereas in a longitudinal prospective population-based study the risk of mortality was slightly increased.[51] Other studies failed to find any difference. These controversial results suggest only a minor effect of the disease on mortality, but additional studies are needed.

ETIOLOGY AND GENETICS

Most cases are hereditary. The families that have been described have shown an autosomal dominant inheritance with an almost complete penetrance at age 60 to 70 years. Twin studies allow an estimation of the heritability; in a small study, the pairwise concordance was found to be 0.60 and 0.27 in monozygotic and dizygotic twins,[52] but it was found to be 0.93 and 0.29 in a larger study of twins older than 70 years.[38] In familial ET, the heritability seems to be extremely high, and the role of environmental factors is probably limited.

Twenty percent to 40% of patients are sporadic cases. Possible causes for phenomenologically identical sporadic ET include reduced or age-dependent penetrance of autosomal dominant mutations, new mutations, and phenocopies. Alternative explanations include a polygenic or mitochondrial origin,[53] or autosomal recessive and X-linked patterns of inheritance.[54] A nonmendelian preferential transmission of the affected allele in several families with multiple affected members and apparent autosomal dominant inheritance was found.[55] Because of the questionable diagnostic criteria, a misdiagnosis cannot be excluded, particularly misinterpretation as enhanced physiological tremor. A hitherto unknown nongenetic cause also cannot be excluded.

Linkage mapping studies have found at least three loci for familial ET. On chromosome 3q13 (*ETM1*, OMIM190300),[56] a Ser9Gly variant in the *DRD3* gene, located in the *ETM1* locus, was found to be associated with risk and age at onset of ET.[57] The *DRD3* gene encodes the dopamine D3 receptor, expressed in Purkinje cells. In vitro studies have shown that the functional Gly9 variant represents a gain-of-function mutation because it increases dopamine affinity four to five times, mediates cyclic adenosine monophosphate response, and prolongs the mitogen-associated protein kinase signal compared with the Ser9 variant.[57] It is unclear whether the Ser9Gly variant has been shown to cosegregate with the disease in the original 16 Icelandic families linked to *ETM1*,[56] and no significant association of the Ser9Gly variant with ET has been found in an Asian population.[58]

The second locus is on chromosome 2p24.1 (*ETM2*, OMIM 602134),[59,60] for which a rare variant of the gene encoding the hematopoietic lineage cell-specific protein 1–binding protein 3 (HS1-BP3) has been described[61] that binds to motor neurons and Purkinje cells and regulates the Ca^{2+}/calmodulin-dependent protein kinase activation of tyrosine and tryptophan hydroxylase. The association with the *HS1-BP3* gene was not confirmed by other extended studies.[62,63]

Genetic heterogeneity in ET has been proved by studies in several families in which the *ETM1* and *ETM2* loci have been excluded. More recently, genome-wide nonparametric and parametric linkage analyses were conducted in seven multigenerational North American families totaling 65 patients. In two families, the third ET susceptibility locus (*ETM3*, OMIM 611456)[64] was revealed on chromosome 6p23. Fifteen genes were selected as plausible candidates, and none of them was found to bear pathogenic mutations.[64]

The gene for the α1 subunit of the γ-aminobutyric acid (GABA) receptors (*GABA-A1* gene) has been proposed as a candidate gene because the knock-out mouse model exhibits a postural and kinetic, propranolol-responsive and alcohol-responsive tremor.[65] One pilot study in ET patients could not show novel mutations in the coding region of the *GABA-A1* gene, however.[66]

The environmental factors that may cause tremor are understudied and only more recently investigated. β-carboline alkaloids (including harmine and harmane) are known to cause tremor in animals and humans, and were found to be elevated in the blood of patients with ET.[67] Other studies describe an association between ET and blood lead concentration, and a possible interaction with allele status for the *d*-aminolevulinic acid dehydratase, a principal enzyme involved in lead kinetics.[68]

PATHOLOGY AND PATHOPHYSIOLOGY

ET is likely to be enhanced by peripheral reflex mechanisms, but its main origin must be within the central nervous system for several reasons; either a preformed mechanism in the brain that is producing rhythmic movements is overactive, or pathology has induced a system, which is usually stable, to oscillate. Several lines of evidence suggest that the oscillator is located within the Guillain-Mollaret triangle (rubral nucleus, olivary nucleus, and cerebellum), assuming that the tremor may result from abnormal intrinsic oscillations originating in the inferior olive and spreading throughout the olivocerebellar network.[7,40,69] Hypotheses on the pathophysiology of ET are based on the above-cited studies on environmental and genetic factors and on other evidence.

Neuropathology

No consistent pathology has been described in more than 30 cases reported between 1903-2005. Since then, a further 33 patients and 21 controls have been reported[70] proposing two different patterns of pathology: 24.2% of the cases had Lewy bodies in the brainstem, mainly in the locus caeruleus, whereas 75.8% had changes in the cerebellum characterized by a nonsignificant reduction of the number of Purkinje cells and cell torpedoes in the survivor neurons. ET cases with Lewy bodies were older, had shorter disease duration, and had lower occurrence of gait difficulty and family history than ET cases without Lewy bodies. After more than 100 years of negative pathology for ET, these findings seem promising, but their relevance remains uncertain. For the Lewy body variant, preclinical PD cannot be excluded, although according to the Braak staging system, the occurrence of Lewy bodies in the locus caeruleus should be preceded by involvement of the dorsal vagal nucleus.[71]

Imaging

Previous positron emission tomography (PET) studies have provided evidence for bilateral overactivity of cerebellar connections in ET.[72-75] More recent magnetic resonance spectroscopy studies reported a reduced N-acetyl aspartate-to-creatine ratio in ET, possibly indicating neuronal damage or loss in ET, which raised the question of neurodegeneration in ET.[76,77] One study using voxel-based morphometry[78] and a controlled diffusion-weighted magnetic resonance imaging (MRI) study[79] could not show any structural abnormalities in ET patients as an argument against a progressive neurodegenerative process in ET. Ultrasound in patients with ET revealed a hyperechogenicity of the substantia nigra in 16%. Nine percent of normal individuals and 90% of patients with PD have this feature.[80] The significance of this result remains unclear.

Neurophysiology

Rhythmic discharges are likely mediated through the brainstem to the motor neurons or through the thalamus to the premotor and motor cortex projecting down to the motor neurons. At the cortical level, tremor-related activity can be detected with electrophysiological techniques. Electroencephalography and magnetoencephalography have been used to analyze the relationship between activity of the motor cortex and the muscles[81] or between different muscles. A high coherence has been shown between the muscles of one limb, but not between different limbs, indicating separate central oscillators for the different extremities.[82,83] Coherence tests have shown coherence between activity in the motor cortex and the contralateral hand tremor,[84,85] indicating a transcortical pathway of these tremor-related signals. Even the premotor cortex is intermittently involved in the generation or transmission of these rhythmic signals to the spinal cord.[86] The findings have been interpreted to represent a spatio-temporal pattern of intermittent synchronization within a complex cortical network that is responsible for tremor.[83] Evidence for a particular dysfunction of the generator of the N30 within the prefrontal cortex has been provided with a somatosensory evoked potentials study.[87]

Animal Models

Harmaline, which induces synchronized rhythmic activity of inferior olive neurons by increasing their electrotonic coupling, induces a postural/kinetic tremor in laboratory animals that is similar to ET in humans.[88] The above-mentioned GABA-A1 knockout mouse represents a novel model.[65]

TREATMENT

Medical Therapy

Presently, the medical treatment of ET involves numerous drugs, but only some of them have been studied within randomized double-blind studies. Table 29–4 summarizes dosages, side effects, and contraindications. An evidence-based review of treatments for ET confirmed the first-line pharmacological agents are propranolol, primidone, gabapentin, and topiramate, although the last-mentioned is less well established. Second-line drugs that are probably effective include alprazolam, atenolol, clonazepam, and sotalol. Third-line drugs with only a possible effect include clozapine, nadolol, and nimodipine, and botulinum toxin, type A, injections for hand, head, and voice tremor in ET patients.[89]

Propranolol and primidone are the drugs of first choice for treatment of ET, and both have been carefully studied.[90] Propranolol, a β_1 and β_2 blocker, was introduced in 1971[91] as a treatment for ET. Only 25% of patients maintain their initial good response for 2 years. Patients who need only intermittent tremor reduction (e.g., for attendance at a social event) might benefit from taking oral propranolol,

10 to 40 mg, about 30 minutes before the event. Ingesting small amounts of alcohol is similarly beneficial in this setting, and the risk of secondary alcoholism has been considered low in these patients.[92] The anticonvulsant primidone has shown efficacy in placebo-controlled trials at doses of 750 mg/day,[93] but tachyphylaxis may occur. In addition, primidone can result in multiple side effects, especially during the titration phase, even when a very low initial dose and a graduated titration schedule is used.[94] The combination of propranolol and primidone is recommended whenever one of the drugs is insufficient.

Second-line treatments include gabapentin and topiramate. Gabapentin was effective in two double-blind studies,[95] but another double-blind study showed no convincing effect.[96] Likewise, topiramate was shown to be effective in two double-blind studies,[97,98] whereas another study failed to prove benefit.[99]

Alprazolam is helpful especially when anxiety causes transient worsening of the tremor.[100] Clonazepam is recommended for patients with predominant action and intention tremor in ET,[101] but is ineffective in uncomplicated ET.[102]

Other β-adrenergic receptor antagonists, such as atenolol and sotalol, might reduce tremor.[103] Arotinolol has been tested in a crossover study and found to have a similar effect as propranolol.[104] Generally, drugs with predominant β_1 effects have been shown to be less effective than drugs acting on the β_2-receptor, and none has proved superior to propranolol. One double-blind[105] and one open study[106] showed no effect of levetiracetam, whereas a positive effect was found in a double-blind acute challenge with 1000 mg.[107] The anticonvulsant pregabalin has been reported to be effective in an open study[108] and a double-blind study.[109] Zonisamide, another antiepileptic agent, was tested in a small double-blind, placebo-controlled trial including 20 ET patients, but did not provide significant improvements in clinical rating scales, and was only modestly well tolerated.[110] An open-label trial with sodium oxybate, which is the sodium salt form of γ-hydroxybutyric acid, showed improvements in postural and kinetic tremor.[111,112] The barbiturate T2000 was tested in a phase II study of 34 ET patients; a significant improvement and adverse events including rashes and pruritus occurred in 2 patients.[113]

Pharmacological treatment of head and voice tremor is less efficient than treatment of hand tremor. Propranolol and primidone, each alone or both combined, have been recommended[114,115] for essential head tremor. Clonazepam is often recommended for this indication, but careful studies are unavailable. Botulinum toxin, type A, injection has been proposed because of the efficacy reported in vocal cords and head tremors in the context of spasmodic dysphonia and cervical dystonia.

Botulinum Toxin

Botulinum toxin, type A, has been proposed as a treatment for ET because it may reduce tremor by weakening the muscles or by blocking gamma motor efferents and muscle spindle afferents. Objective acoustic measures have shown the efficacy of botulinum toxin for voice tremor in only a few treated patients.[116] Subjective evaluations reported benefit in most patients.[117-120] If oral treatment does not work, botulinum toxin should be considered as an option. Head tremor can also be significantly improved.[89] Botulinum toxin also was used for hand tremor in a carefully controlled study, but showed only limited effect.[121]

TABLE 29–4	Pharmacological Management of Tremors					
Drug	Daily Dosage (mg)	Daily Doses	Specific Effect	Contraindications/ Side Effects	Indication	Note
Propranolol	30–320	2–3 standard 1–2 long-acting	Postural/action tremor Hand tremor +++ Head tremor +	Bradycardia, congestive heart failure, atrioventricular block, hypotension, depression fatigue, bronchospasm, male impotence	ET (level of evidence: 1A) PD: double-blind study Cerebellar tremor: single cases Neuropathic tremor: single cases	First choice in ET patients
Primidone	62.5–500	1 in the evening	Postural/action tremor Hand tremor +++ Head tremor +	Ataxia, vertigo, diplopia, somnolence, megaloblastic anemia, osteoporosis	ET (level of evidence: 1A) Neuropathic tremor: single cases	First choice in ET, preferentially for patients >60 yr old
Combination: Propranolol/ primidone	Maximum dosage for each	see above	Postural/action tremor Hand tremor +++ Head tremor +	Ataxia, vertigo, diplopia, somnolence, megaloblastic anemia, osteoporosis	ET (level of evidence: IIB)	First choice in ET; try always before using second and third choice drugs
Gabapentin	1800–2400	3	Action tremor	Dizziness, somnolence, peripheral edema	ET: conflicting results of three double-blind-studies: one without, two with benefit (level of evidence: IIB) Neuropathic tremor: single cases Primary orthostatic tremor: double-blind study	Second choice in ET

Topiramate	<400	2-3	Action tremor	Paresthesias, weight decrease, somnolence, anorexia, dizziness, amnesia, depression, insomnia, acute or chronic metabolic acidosis, nephrolithiasis, elevated intraocular pressure	ET: conflicting results of three double-blind studies: one without, two with benefit (II) Cerebellar tremor: open study	Second choice in ET
Clonazepam	0.75-6	2-3	For predominant kinetic tremor	Confusion, depression, amnesia, paradoxical reactions (agitation, nervousness), respiratory depression	ET (level of evidence: IIB) Cerebellar tremor (single cases) Dystonic tremor (single cases)	Second choice in ET
Alcohol	Small amounts	Intermittent treatment before meals or social events	Postural/action tremor Hand tremor +++ Head tremor +	CNS depression (interaction with sedating drugs)	ET (level of evidence: IIB)	Second choice in ET; can be used judiciously
Alprazolam	0.75-4	Intermittent treatment	Postural/action tremor Hand tremor ++	Confusion, depression, amnesia, paradoxical reactions (agitation, nervousness), respiratory depression	ET (level of evidence: IIB)	Second choice in ET (for mild cases)
Botulinum toxin	Botox doses: vocal muscle: 1.25-3.75 U; cervical muscles: 40-400 U; forearm muscles: 50-100 U; tensor veli palatine: 4-10 U	Every 3rd month	Postural/action tremor Voice tremor +++ Head tremor ++ Ear click ++ Hand tremor +	Muscular weakness	ET (level of evidence: IIB) Dystonic tremor (double-blind studies) Essential palatal tremor: single cases	Second choice in ET. Injections are made under EMG guidance. Dysport U doses are 3- to 5-fold higher than Botox

Table continued on following page

TABLE 29–4	Pharmacological Management of Tremors (Continued)				
Drug	Daily Dosage (mg)	Daily Doses	Specific Effect	Contraindications/ Side Effects	Indication	Note
Clozapine	12.5 (test) 25-100	1 in the evening (+ 1-2 additional doses during the morning)	Resting tremor	Agranulocytosis, seizures, myocarditis, orthostatic hypotension	ET (level of evidence: IIIC) PD: several small open and double-blind studies Holmes' tremor: single cases	Third choice in ET. Less well documented effect than for PD (indicate if concomitant psychosis). Effectiveness of clozapine in particular patient can be predicted after single dose of 12.5 mg of clozapine
Flunarizine	10	1 in the evening	Postural/action tremor	Confusion, depression, parkinsonism	ET: one study for, one against mild therapeutic effect (level of evidence: IID)	Third choice in ET
Tryptophan	<1000	3	Intention tremor	Nausea	Cerebellar tremor: open studies	
Carbamazepine	400-600	3 standard 2 long-acting	For predominant kinetic tremor	Aplastic anemia, agranulocytosis, ataxia, vertigo, diplopia, nystagmus	Cerebellar tremor: small controlled studies	

Levodopa	<1200	4 standard 3 long-acting	Resting tremor	Orthostatic hypotension, psychosis, nausea and vomiting, somnolence	PD: ample documented evidence Holmes' tremor: single cases	
Dopamine agonist	Medium to high	3 standard 1-2 long-acting 1 transdermal patch (rotigotine)	Resting tremor	Orthostatic hypotension, psychosis, nausea and vomiting, somnolence	PD: double-blind studies Holmes' tremor: single cases	Daily doses: bromocriptine: 5-20 mg; lisuride: 0.1-1.2 mg; pergolide: 0.15-3 mg; pramipexole: 1.5-4.5 mg; ropinirole: 3-24 mg; cabergoline: 1-6 mg; rotigotine: 2-6 mg
Anticholinergics	Bornaprine: 3-12 mg Trihexyphenidyl: 1-10 mg Biperiden: 1-12 mg Metixene: 7.5-60 mg	3	Resting tremor Postural/action tremor	Especially in elderly subjects. Dryness of mouth, blurred vision, dizziness, nausea, paralytic ileus, psychosis, amnesia, urinary hesitancy or retention, tachycardia, increased intraocular pressure	PD: Poorly documented Holmes' tremor: Single cases Bornaprine: two double blind-studies in PD Trihexyphenidyl: open and controlled studies in PD	Slow titration is strictly recommended. Sudden discontinuation may induce severe rebound effect

Table continued on following page

TABLE 29–4	Pharmacological Management of Tremors (Continued)				
Drug	Daily Dosage (mg)	Daily Doses	Specific Effect	Contraindications/ Side Effects	Indication	Note
Levetiracetam	1000-3000	2-3	For predominant kinetic tremor	Dizziness, somnolence, confusion	ET: 1 double-blind study and open trials showing no effect; positive effect in 1 double-blind acute study Cerebellar tremor: open study with benefit Holmes' tremor: single case	
Pregabalin	150-600	2	Postural > action tremor	Ataxia, confusion, asthenia	ET: single cases and 1 double-blind study	Third choice in ET

CNS, central nervous system; ET, essential tremor; PD, Parkinson's disease.

Surgical Therapy

Surgery is the accepted treatment for patients with severe disability and resistance to medical treatment. Multicenter studies have shown that deep brain stimulation (DBS) of the thalamus is effective,[122-125] and one study showed that ventral intermediate nucleus (Vim) DBS has a better effect than Vim thermocoagulation and, more importantly, fewer side effects.[126]

DBS reduces tremor severity by about 60% (functionally relevant) in 80% of ET cases. The standard stereotactic coordinates for thalamic DBS cover a region including the ventral border of the Vim and the adjacent subthalamic white matter (zona incerta, prelemniscal radiation).[127] Standard treatment improved tremor in all locations, a small case series reported that stimulation within the posterior subthalamic area may have a better impact on proximal arm muscles, trunk, or legs.[128] In patients with limb tremor, unilateral stimulation sometimes may be sufficient to reduce the disability. In the case of disabling bilateral limb tremor, or head, voice, and trunk tremor, a bilateral procedure is necessary. Because bilateral thalamotomies carry a high risk of dysarthria,[129,130] mostly Vim stimulation is applied.[124,131] Gamma Knife surgery for the treatment of tremors is proposed in some centers,[132] but cases with slowly growing lesions over months (running lesions) and subsequent worsening of tremor have been published.[133]

Parkinsonian Tremors

Parkinsonian tremor has been defined as tremor that occurs in PD.[1] The most common forms are types I, II, and III (see Table 29–1).

Classic parkinsonian tremor (type I) is the typical resting tremor. It may be seen in the hands during walking or when sitting as the characteristic pill-rolling tremor of the hand. Tremor frequency is 4 to 7 Hz, and can be 6 Hz especially in early PD. The postural/kinetic tremor seems to be a continuation of the resting tremor occurring after some latency under postural and action conditions. This "re-emergent tremor" has clinical characteristics similar to a resting tremor, including having the same frequency, asymmetry, and response to levodopa, and is thought to have the same pathophysiological mechanism as resting tremor.[134] Unilateral tremor and leg tremor are often seen and are typical for type I tremor.

A clinically important specific variant of PD is the so-called monosymptomatic tremor at rest or benign tremulous parkinsonism. This is defined as a classic PD type I tremor with no other symptoms sufficient to diagnose PD.[1]

In some patients, a second form of postural and action tremor with a different frequency from resting tremor (>1.5 Hz) may occur, which is labeled *type II tremor*. This postural/action tremor can be extremely disabling. Some patients have a predominant postural tremor in addition to the resting tremor. The postural/action tremor has a higher and non–harmonically related frequency to the resting tremor. This form is rare (<15% of patients with PD) and has often been described as a combination of an ET with PD.[135] Some of these patients had their postural tremor long before the onset of other symptoms of PD. A high-frequency action tremor also described as "rippling" is often found in PD and has been described as *type III tremor* in PD.[1]

EPIDEMIOLOGY

Tremor at rest is common in PD. It is estimated that 90% of all patients with PD have a classic rest tremor at any time of their disease, and 75% of all parkinsonian syndromes are idiopathic. The occurrence of the classic tremor at rest in a patient with parkinsonism has a likelihood of greater than 95% to reflect idiopathic PD.

ETIOLOGY AND PATHOPHYSIOLOGY

It is one of the mysteries of PD that the typical type I tremor is a symptom with such a high specificity for PD, but the symptom of tremor does not correlate with disease progression or with the amount of dopaminergic degeneration measured with PET or single photon emission computed tomography (SPECT).[136,137] Pathology suggests that in patients with predominant tremor, the retrorubral A8 part of the substantia nigra is specifically degenerating,[138-140] but there are no clear-cut differences of the PET imaging of the presynaptic or postsynaptic dopaminergic terminals in patients with monosymptomatic tremor at rest compared with patients with classic PD.[141,142] Reduction in 5-HT1A binding in the midbrain raphe region correlates with tremor severity, but not with rigidity or bradykinesia.[143] Degeneration of transmitter systems other than dopamine may be responsible for the erratic behavior of tremor as a symptom in PD. Nevertheless, levodopa and dopamine agonists are potent drugs to treat PD tremor.

Beyond all these unsolved problems, animal experiments and human data converge to suggest that parkinsonian tremor is generated within the basal ganglia.[144] In the 1-methyl-4-phenyl-1,2,3,6-tetrahydropyridine (MPTP) model of PD, it has been shown that the cells within the basal ganglia loop are topographically organized through the whole loop and well segregated for the different muscle groups and functional regions. In MPTP animals, these cells get abnormally synchronized, and this may be the reason for synchronized activity leading to peripheral tremor.[145] Recordings in humans are compatible with this view.[83]

TREATMENT

Medical Therapy

Drug treatments differ for the different forms of tremor in PD (for drug dosages, see Table 29–4). Levodopa is the most effective treatment for most symptoms in PD. Among the tremors in PD, mainly the resting tremor is improved, but other forms may also respond. Generally, the effect on tremor is highly variable, and the tremor may worsen, especially for the action tremor with frequencies different from the resting tremor frequency. Available double-blind studies of different dopamine agonists failed to give a hint at a superior effect of one or the other agonist on tremor.[146] In a small study, 0.5 mg of either pramipexole or pergolide acutely administered reduced PD resting tremor scores to a similar degree, significantly better than placebo.[147]

There are only a few small double-blind studies on the effect of anticholinergics. Bornaprine was found to be effective in two studies.[148,149] Trihexyphenidyl has been tested alone and compared with amantadine and levodopa.[150] The drugs are not recommended in elderly patients or patients with multiple morbidities because of possible confusional states, which are reversible after cessation of the drug. More importantly, a more recent study has provided ample evidence that patients treated with anticholinergics may have a higher incidence of Alzheimer's-type pathology.[151] Discontinuation may induce a severe rebound effect. Other possible side effects are dry mouth, visual disturbances, constipation, glaucoma, disturbance of micturition, and memory deficits.

The favorable effect of clozapine on resting tremor has been confirmed in several studies,[152,153] which have shown a good effect even when other drugs failed.[154] No tolerance has been observed over the course of 6 months. Sedation is a major side effect; leukopenia, as a serious, possibly lethal complication, is the main limitation for its use.

Although some studies support the use of propranolol,[155] a Cochrane Review found the results to be inconclusive.[156] Jaw tremor in PD sometimes does not respond well to oral medication. It has been reported that botulinum toxin injections into masseter muscles may improve jaw tremor without relevant side effects.[157]

Surgical Therapy

Sometimes, parkinsonian tremor can be very difficult to treat. Functional neurosurgery is a useful treatment for some patients who cannot be treated otherwise. Thalamic thermocoagulation and Vim DBS improve resting, postural, and kinetic tremors, but do not improve akinesia. Lesional surgery cannot be applied bilaterally because of speech disturbances (but DBS can) and is no longer recommended.[126] Pallidotomy and stimulation of the globus pallidus internus also improve tremor. Stimulation of the subthalamic nucleus (STN) successfully improves tremor,[158,159] and akinesia and rigidity, and is presently preferred.[160] Vim DBS can be considered for tremor-dominant elderly patients with a slow disease progression in whom other features of PD are not a source of disability because the Vim DBS operation is a shorter operative procedure, requires less postoperative adaptation of medication, and can be performed unilaterally. Sometimes tremor suppression requires high doses of levodopa with a higher risk of psychosis. STN DBS can be a therapeutic option for such patients[161] because this allows reduction of levodopa dosage by 50% on average.

Pragmatic Treatment

Treatment needs to be individualized. When a patient is seen for the first time, akinesia and rigidity as the target symptoms are addressed initially. After these symptoms are managed, we treat the patient according to Table 29–5 depending on the remaining tremor symptoms. Some treatment failures occur with PD tremors. The most common reason for failure is that the dosage of dopaminergics is too low. Also, the tremor can get worse initially when treatment with antirigidity agents is initiated. Waiting often helps. Sometimes the action tremor can also increase with increasing dosages preferentially in type II tremors. In this case, additional treatment with propranolol or primidone is worth trying. If all these procedures fail, a patient may be a candidate for DBS surgery only because of the tremor.

TABLE 29–5	Suggestions for Treatment of Tremors in Parkinson's Disease			
Tremor Type	Step 1	Step 2	Step 3	Step 4
Classic parkinsonian tremor or monosymptomatic rest tremor	Treat bradykinesia and rigidity (levodopa, dopamine agonists)	Levodopa, dopamine agonists (add on or increase), anticholinergics	Amantadine, propranolol, clozapine	STN stimulation
Rest and postural tremor with different frequencies		Propranolol, primidone	Dopamine, dopamine agonists, anticholinergics, clozapine	STN stimulation
Isolated action tremor		Propranolol, anticholinergics	Amantadine	

STN, subthalamic nucleus.

Orthostatic Tremor

Orthostatic tremor (OT) is a unique tremor syndrome[162,163] characterized by a subjective feeling of unsteadiness during stance, but only in severe cases during gait. Some patients experience sudden falls. None of the patients have problems when sitting and lying. OT is the only tremor with a pathognomonic frequency: surface EMG (e.g., from the quadriceps femoris muscle) while standing shows the typical 13- to 18-Hz burst pattern.[164] Arm tremor may occur in approximately half of the patients and is usually more evident during stance.[165,166]

The tremor cannot be seen with the naked eye, and sometimes the only clinical finding is the palpable fine-amplitude rippling of leg muscles. The diagnosis is suspected mainly based on the complaints of the patient rather than clinical findings. Besides asterixis, OT is the only tremulous condition for which EMG is mandatory for the diagnosis. Auscultation with the stethoscope over the muscles of the thigh and calf reveals a repetitive thumping sound, similar to the noise of a distant helicopter, and this sound has been proposed as a new clinical sign supporting diagnosis.[167]

The differential diagnosis is broad because other idiopathic tremors, such as ET, cerebellar tremor, and PD tremor, can manifest with similar complaints. Orthostatic myoclonus is a rare condition to consider in the differential diagnosis. The most important test to separate these entities is EMG.

EPIDEMIOLOGY AND ETIOLOGY

OT is rare, and epidemiologic data are lacking. The largest case series contains less than 50 patients. The condition occurs only in patients older than 40 years; the mean age at onset was younger for women (50 years) compared with men

(60 years) in one study.[168] It is not considered a hereditary disease, albeit familial cases have been described.[168,169]

OT may be classified according to the associated conditions (see Table 29–1). *Primary OT* is considered an idiopathic condition and may be divided further into two subgroups: patients with additional postural arm tremor and patients without postural arm tremor.[168] There has been debate whether OT is a separate entity or a variant of ET because it may be associated with this upper limb postural tremor.[170] In a relatively large series, OT patients with hand tremor had benefit from alcohol and frequent family history of tremor; however, electrophysiological assessments of postural arm tremors were not performed, and the authors did not report on the frequency of the tremor.[168]

Whether upper limb postural tremor represents ET or another form of tremor, perhaps even part of the syndrome of OT, has long been a matter of debate.[168] A different series reported that only 9 of 30 patients had a postural arm tremor on routine clinical examination; a 13- to 18-Hz arm tremor was present in 27 of the patients when the arms were involved in weight-bearing tasks, suggesting a common pathophysiology with OT, different from ET.[164] In contrast to ET, OT shows a high degree of synchrony between different muscles, and rarely responds to therapeutic agents such as propranolol and alcohol.[171] In addition, it was suggested that the 6- to 8-Hz postural arm tremor might be a subharmonic of the high-frequency OT tremor spreading throughout the body.[166]

OT-plus is defined when other primary neurological disorders occur together with OT[168]; so far, OT has been found in association with restless legs syndrome, orobuccal dyskinesias,[168] cerebellar ataxia,[172] progressive supranuclear palsy,[173] and PD.[174] Two types of tremor have been reported in PD patients: slow (sometimes asymmetrical) OT (range 4 to 6 Hz), improved by levodopa,[175] and fast (symmetrical) OT, mimicking primary OT (range 13 to 18 Hz).[176,174] The first is a different expression of the classic resting PD tremor, and it has been called "pseudo-OT."[177] *Symptomatic OT* has been described in nontumoral aqueduct stenosis, after head trauma,[178] in vascular lesions, or and in abscesses.[179]

PATHOPHYSIOLOGY

The high-frequency EMG pattern is coherent in all the muscles of the body,[171] leading to the hypothesis that a bilaterally descending system must underlie OT. It is unknown where in the nervous system the oscillator is located. Numerous reports have suggested possible sites as the origin of this activity, including the spinal cord,[180] the pons and cerebellum,[179,181] and the motor cortex.[182] Although to date no single site has emerged as the origin of this tremor, the generator for this tremor is assumed to be located within the brainstem or cerebellum.[181] Dopaminergic terminals in the striatum are significantly reduced in this condition,[183] however clinical trials with levodopa and dopamine agonists are usually unsuccessful.

TREATMENT

OT has been documented to be responsive to clonazepam and primidone.[184] Valproate and propranolol were applied in single cases with variable success. Levodopa has not consistently shown efficacy.[183,185] According to small double-blind studies,[186,187] gabapentin seems to have an excellent and consistent beneficial effect.[188] We use it as the first-choice drug for OT (1800 to 2400 mg daily). The second-choice drug is clonazepam.

Dystonic Tremor

Different forms of tremor can be associated with dystonia (see Table 29–1). Typical dystonic tremor (DT) occurs in the body region affected by dystonia; typical examples are head tremor in torticollis, hand tremor in writer's cramp, and jaw tremor in orofacial dystonias.[189] DT is defined as a postural/kinetic tremor usually not seen during complete rest.[190] Usually, these are focal tremors with irregular amplitudes and variable frequencies (mostly <7 Hz). Some patients exhibit focal tremors even without overt signs of dystonia.[191]

In many patients with DT, antagonistic gestures lead to a reduction of the tremor amplitude. This is well known for dystonic head tremor in the setting of spasmodic torticollis. A reduction in tremor is seen when the patient touches the head or lifts the arm.[192] Because this sign is absent in essential head tremor, it can be a differential diagnostic hint in unclear head tremors in which the dystonic posture is not obvious. The effect of these maneuvers can sometimes be difficult to observe clinically, and it can be helpful to record surface EMG from the affected muscles and look for EMG suppression.[192] Other important, but less specific differential diagnostic clues are the focal nature and low frequency of DT. Patients with DT may have a resting tremor mimicking PD tremor, especially in cases in which dystonic posturing is not well evident (sometimes only a dystonic thumb extension). Dystonic patients sometimes have jaw tremor, facial hypomimia,[193] loss of arm swing on the affected side, increased limb tone,[194] and clumsiness often misdiagnosed as bradykinesia. It has been proposed that some "PD patients" with scans without evidence of dopaminergic deficit (SWEDDs) actually are patients affected by focal adult-onset DT.[195]

Tremor associated with dystonia is a more generalized form of tremor in extremities that are not affected by the dystonia. This is a relatively symmetrical, postural, and kinetic tremor usually showing higher frequencies than actual DT, often seen in the upper limbs in patients with spasmodic torticollis.[196] More recently, isolated jaw tremor in patients affected by dystonia not involving facial muscles has been included in this type of tremor.[189] The tremor associated with dystonia is more difficult to separate from ET, especially when the accompanying dystonia has not evolved completely. Some neurophysiological techniques might be useful in the differential diagnosis.[196]

EPIDEMIOLOGY

The prevalence of DT is unknown. In one Brazilian cross-sectional study, it has been estimated that approximately 20% of patients with dystonia present with postural tremor.[197] This proportion does not differ between primary and secondary dystonia, but seems to be more common in cervical dystonia than other locations.[198] In a large survey among patients from an Indian movement disorder center, DT accounted for about 20% of all patients presenting with nonparkinsonian and noncerebellar tremor (ET accounted for 60%).[199]

PATHOPHYSIOLOGY AND ETIOLOGY

DT is still debated as a separate entity, and different definitions have been proposed by clinicians.[200-202] Virtually every dystonic syndrome may manifest with DT. Among secondary dystonias, a specific tremor syndrome associated with thalamic lesions has been labeled "thalamic tremor."[203] This tremor is part of a specific dystonia-athetosis-chorea-action tremor following lateral-posterior thalamic strokes.[204,205] In the setting of a well-recovered severe hemiparesis, the combination of tremor with an intentional component, dystonia, and a severe sensory loss seems to be the important clue for the diagnosis. Proximal segments are often involved. This tremor syndrome also may develop with a certain delay after the initial insult.

The pathophysiology of DT is largely unknown, but is likely related to the central nervous system (especially basal ganglia) abnormality postulated for dystonia itself.[190] Tremor associated with dystonia may be a forme fruste of ET.[201] It is unclear, however, if they share common genes (the *DYT1* locus is already excluded), and the pathophysiological mechanisms seem to be different in some patients.[196] During ballistic wrist flexion movements, the latency of the second agonist EMG burst was later in ET patients than in patients with tremor associated with cervical dystonia.[196] In addition, when assessing the reciprocal inhibition between forearm muscles, two different patterns have been described: patients with normal levels of presynaptic inhibition are affected by an ET-like tremor starting simultaneously with torticollis; in patients with reduced or absent presynaptic inhibition, arm tremor preceded onset of torticollis by a longer interval.[196]

TREATMENT

There is a paucity of information about the treatment of the DT syndromes. Several drugs (including anticholinergics, tetrabenazine, benzodiazepines) have been tried with inconsistent results (for drug dosages, see Table 29–4). Propranolol was found to be effective for dystonic head tremor. Levodopa sometimes can worsen the tremor.[195,206] The efficacy of botulinum toxin for dystonic head tremor[207] and tremulous spasmodic dysphonia is well documented. Tremor associated with dystonia often responds to the medication for classic ET.

Severe cases in the setting of a generalized dystonia have been successfully treated with DBS of the globus pallidus internus.[208] Stimulation of the thalamic Vim can also drastically alleviate the tremor, but can occasionally lead to worsening of the dystonia itself. Considering the potential worsening of other dystonic features, the suggested target is the globus pallidus internus.

Bilateral STN DBS has been reported to improve cervical dystonia, dystonic head tremor, and ET-like tremor of the hands in one patient.[209] Others reported that DBS of the subthalamic white matter, including the zona incerta, remarkably improved proximal DT that had been refractory to Vim thalamotomy.[210]

Ⅰ Primary Writing Tremor

Primary writing tremor is a condition in which tremor, usually characterized by prominent pronation/supination wrist movements, occurs predominantly or only during writing.[211] No other neurological signs are evident except for a slight postural and terminal intention tremor. Primary writing tremor can be task-induced (type A) or position-sensitive (type B). The epidemiology and the natural course of primary writing tremor are not well known. Age at onset varies; cases manifesting during childhood have been reported. The disorder begins slowly, progresses for years, and becomes stabilized. Familial history is generally negative.[212]

PATHOPHYSIOLOGY AND ETIOLOGY

Primary writing tremor is considered to be a focal task-specific tremor, which has been classified as among the ET syndromes, a form of focal dystonia, both, or neither.[213,214] In the first reported cases, the writing disorder and tremor were temporarily abolished by partial motor point anesthesia of the pronator teres, suggesting that the tremor was caused by an abnormal central response to muscle spindle discharges that originated in the pronator teres.[211] Although it resembles ET (where tremor is present on action, and on maintenance of a posture, and may affect hand writing), its focal task-specific nature, the lack of response to propranolol, and a well documented effect of central cholinergic drugs[212] have suggested that primary writing tremor may be more closely related to focal dystonia than ET.[213,214] The abnormal coactivation of antagonist muscles on EMG recording has been used to support this claim. Primary writing tremor is distinguished, however, from focal task-specific dystonia (writer's cramp) by the lack of excessive overflow of EMG activity into the proximal musculature, and the absence of reciprocal inhibition of the median nerve H-reflex on radial nerve stimulation.[215,216]

TREATMENT

No double-blind studies of primary writing tremor are available. Propranolol, primidone, levodopa, and neuroleptics were ineffective. Anticholinergics, when tolerated, may have a role.[212] Studies are available on the use of botulinum toxin, which was reported to be successful.[217] Nevertheless, treatment of primary writing tremor is often ineffective. The disability caused by this condition can vary from mild to considerable, depending on the profession of the patient. The handicap that it produces in Western cultures is not considered sufficient to merit the risks involved in stereotactic surgery. In Japan, where calligraphy is an important occupation, thalamotomy has been successfully performed for primary writing tremor because it can threaten the professional career of the patient.[218] Successful Vim DBS procedures have been reported.[219,220] A significant improvement with a simple hand orthotic device has been shown.[221]

Cerebellar Tremor Syndromes

Classic cerebellar tremor is an intention tremor that may occur unilaterally or bilaterally depending on the underlying cerebellar abnormality. The tremor frequency is almost always less than 5 Hz. Simple kinetic and postural tremor may also be present. Some patients with a mild cerebellar ataxia present with an isolated postural and simple kinetic tremor greater than 5 Hz resembling ET. *Titubation* is another tremor manifestation of cerebellar disease and is a low-frequency oscillation (~3 Hz) of the head and trunk depending on postural innervation. If the low-frequency action tremor is severe, it may sometimes be seen in a seemingly resting position because the patient is unable to relax completely.

Intention tremor is a unique form of tremor that usually can be separated from other tremor forms clinically. The fact that intention tremor can also occur in advanced ET can make the separation difficult sometimes. The most important clinical clue in this situation is the degree to which ataxia is present, and the absence of clinically detectable oculomotor abnormalities in ET. Although in ET only a mild dysmetria and tandem gait disturbance have been described, these are dominating the cerebellar syndrome. Oculomotor disturbance and lesions or atrophy often seen in brain imaging studies are additional distinctive features.

EPIDEMIOLOGY AND ETIOLOGY

Because cerebellar tremor can be caused by insults of various etiology and degenerations, no epidemiologic data are available. Demyelinating lesions in multiple sclerosis are one of the most common causes of cerebellar tremor; it is observed in 75% of cases and constitutes the predominant source of disability.[222] Cerebellar tremor may be the consequence of head trauma, cerebellar strokes (especially when the brainstem is involved[223]), or degenerations of cerebellar neurons of various etiologies. Although the hereditary ataxias are rare syndromes, toxic cerebellar degeneration secondary to alcohol abuse predominantly of the anterior lobe is common, and often manifests with low-frequency (2 to 3 Hz) stance tremor in the anteroposterior direction.[224]

PATHOPHYSIOLOGY

The pathophysiology of classic cerebellar intention tremor seems to be distinct from the mechanisms underlying most of the other central tremors in that it most likely does not emerge from oscillating groups or loops of neurons, but is due to altered characteristics of feedforward or feedback loops. It is well established in animals and humans[225-227] that a striking abnormality in cerebellar dysfunction is a delay of the second and third phase of the triphasic EMG pattern in ballistic movements,[228] or a delay of the reflexes regulating stance control.[229] During goal-directed movements or sway during stance, this delay causes the breaking movement to occur late and produce an overshoot, producing a quasirhythmic movement that is compatible with intention tremor during goal-directed movements or the low-frequency body tremor during stance. The higher frequency postural and action tremors in some patients with cerebellar disease more likely reflect the existence of a separate central oscillator.

TREATMENT

Cerebellar tremors are difficult to treat, and good results are rare. Double-blind studies are lacking for most commonly used drugs. Studies with cholinergic substances (e.g., physostigmine, lecithin, which is a precursor of choline) have shown improvement in some patients, but have failed in most. Isoniazid failed to show significant results.[230] 5-Hydroxy-L-tryptophan has been found to be effective in some patients.[231,232] More recently, administration of amantadine has been proposed. Open studies and single case observations have shown favorable results with propranolol (320 mg/day), clonazepam, carbamazepine, tetrahydrocannabinol, and trihexyphenidyl. Limited improvements have been observed after loading of the shaking extremity, but most clinicians do not use it because the patients adapt rapidly to the new weight. In a double-blind trial, cannabis was ineffective.[233]

Probably the best symptomatic improvement can be obtained in selected patients with Vim DBS or thalamotomy.[126,234,235] Functional outcome after surgery varies greatly, however. In one study,[234] patients with multiple sclerosis–related tremor with a frequency greater than 3 Hz and significant tremor-related disabilities were found to respond favorably. Post-hoc secondary analysis indicated that patients who have no superimposed ataxia, weakness, or sensory loss in the tremulous limb, and with shorter disease duration, younger age, more education, and purely distal preoperative tremor benefited more from thalamic DBS. Accelerometric tremor recordings and frequency and rhythmicity analysis may help to distinguish patients with predominant multiple sclerosis tremor from patients with tremor and ataxia. It has been proposed that a favorable response to propranolol may indicate that a major component of the patient's upper limb movement disorder is tremor. The long-term follow-up in a larger cohort has not yet been assessed. Generally, the response of titubation to DBS is poor.

Gamma Knife thalamotomy, although effective, may cause side effects. It has been proposed that Gamma Knife procedures should be offered to patients unable to tolerate or unwilling to undergo DBS.[236]

Holmes' Tremor

Holmes' tremor is a rare symptomatic tremor caused by a lesion in the region of the midbrain. It has been called different names in the past (rubral tremor, midbrain tremor, myorhythmia, mixed extrapyramidal tremor, Benedikt's syndrome); Holmes' tremor is the name suggested by the Movement Disorder Society.[1] Clinically, Holmes' tremor is the combination of a parkinsonian rest tremor and a cerebellar tremor: it is the only tremor with resting, postural, and intentional components (see Table 29–1). It typically has low (<4.5 Hz) and often irregular frequencies, not rhythmic frequencies similar to other tremors. If the date of the lesion is known (e.g., in the case of a cerebrovascular accident), a variable delay between the lesion and the first occurrence of the tremor is typical (mostly 2 weeks to 2 years).

Holmes' tremor is one of the most disabling forms of tremor because it disturbs rest and all kinds of voluntary and involuntary movements. It mainly affects the hands and proximal arm, and is mostly unilateral. Some DTs (e.g., "thalamic tremor") and cerebellar tremor can be difficult to differentiate from Holmes' tremor, especially when tremor continues under seemingly resting conditions because of a lack of relaxation. Clinical features (i.e., irregularity, lower frequency, and an accompanying parkinsonian syndrome) and imaging studies (DaTSCAN) can help in recognizing Holmes' tremor in these situations.

PATHOPHYSIOLOGY AND ETIOLOGY

It is generally accepted that this unique tremor form is caused by lesions that seem to be centered in the brainstem/cerebellum and the thalamus. The pathophysiological basis of Holmes' tremor is a combined lesion of the cerebellothalamic and nigrostriatal systems as suggested by autopsy data,[237] PET data,[238] and clinical observations.[239,240] Any lesion (hemorrhage, ischemia, vascular malformations, trauma, demyelinating plaques, and neoplasm) involving fiber tracts from both systems can produce this tremor. Also, metabolic disorders (e.g., nonketotic hyperglycemia) can induce "reversible Holmes' tremor."[241] The exact location of the lesions seen in these patients may vary. Because of these lesions, the tremors can be accompanied by a cerebellar and parkinsonian syndrome. Central oscillators cause this tremor. It seems likely that the rhythm of resting tremor is usually blocked during voluntary movements by the cerebellum. If this cerebellar compensation is absent, the rhythm of rest tremor spills into movements,[239] producing the low-frequency intention (action) tremor.

TREATMENT

No generally accepted therapy is available. Nevertheless, treatment is successful in a higher percentage of patients with Holmes' tremor than patients with cerebellar tremor. Some patients respond to levodopa, dopamine agonists, anticholinergics, or clonazepam (for drug dosages, see Table 29–4). The effect of functional neurosurgery for this tremor syndrome is poorly documented. Patients have been operated on, but their tremors have been diagnosed as post-traumatic tremors or poststroke tremors, and the clinical features have not been described in detail. Several patients underwent thalamic surgery (lesion or DBS[242-244]) with some improvement. Vim DBS is considered the target of choice. Based on the hypothesis that Holmes' tremor is caused by the combined imbalance of different cerebral circuits, different double approaches have been used in single cases: (1) Vim and STN DBS,[245] (2) ventralis oralis posterior/ventralis oralis anterior and Vim DBS,[246] (3) Vim DBS and pallidotomy,[247] and (4) Vim/ventralis oralis anterior border and globus pallidus internus DBS.[248]

▌ Tremor Syndromes in Peripheral Neuropathy

Several peripheral neuropathies regularly manifest with tremors (see Table 29–1). Usually it is a mild postural tremor; however, some cases involve very disabling action and intention tremor.

EPIDEMIOLOGY

Dysgammaglobulinemic neuropathies and chronic inflammatory demyelinating polyradiculopathy are acquired neuropathies manifesting most frequently with tremor. In a series of 62 patients with dysgammaglobulinemic polyneuropathy, postural and action tremor of the hands was present in 70% to 80% of cases.[249] Tremor only rarely represents the dominant source of disability in these patients, however.[250] A similar type of tremor can be observed in approximately 40% of patients with hereditary sensorimotor neuropathy. Many of these patients have a family history of tremor.[251]

PATHOPHYSIOLOGY AND ETIOLOGY

The tremor in dysimmune neuropathies seems to be related to the severity of the peripheral neuronal damage,[252] and it has been postulated that an abnormal peripheral feedback to central tremor-generating structures could be the basis for the tremor enhancement in this situation.[253] The tremor in hereditary sensorimotor neuropathy seems to be largely unrelated to the severity of neuropathic syndromes, and it may occur in family members without a neuropathy. It has been suggested that it is pathogenetically related to ET.[251] There is an ongoing debate as to whether the combination of a hereditary neuropathy with postural tremor (Roussy-Lévy syndrome) actually constitutes a distinct disease entity.[254]

Kinematic profiles of simple voluntary wrist movements (with duration of the bursts prolonged and the onset of the second agonist delayed at triphasic EMG patterns in agonist-antagonist-agonist muscles) and PET findings (abnormal activation of the cerebellum) have been found to be similar to ET.[253] The central pathways are considered normal in these patients, however, and the major pathological state seems to be the peripheral slowing and possibly distortion of afferent signals. In contrast to cerebellar disease, it may be hypothesized that not the feedforward control of movement, but the feedback control is the cause of the rhythmic disturbance in these patients.

TREATMENT

No convincing therapies are reported for this type of tremor. Successful treatment of the underlying neuropathy can improve the tremor in some patients.[252] Even when the neuropathy is improved, however, the tremor may not respond or may worsen. In our hands, propranolol, primidone, and clonazepam have been helpful for some patients at dosages similar to those for ET. One patient was successfully implanted with DBS electrodes in the Vim.[255] The rationale for performing stereotactic procedures would be to alter central processing.

Palatal Tremor Syndromes

Palatal tremors are rare tremor syndromes that were earlier classified among the myoclonias (palatal myoclonus).[256] Palatal tremor can be separated into at least two forms (see Table 29–1).[257,258] *Symptomatic palatal tremor (SPT)* is characterized by rhythmic movements of the soft palate (levator veli palatini). This tremor is clinically visible as a rhythmic movement of the edge of the palate. Other brainstem-innervated (leading to oscillopsia in case of eye muscle involvement) or extremity muscles can also be involved.[237] SPT typically follows a brainstem/cerebellar lesion with a variable delay,[259] and is often associated with a cerebellar syndrome.[260] SPT with a degeneration of the brainstem and cerebellum has been described as progressive ataxia with palatal tremor.[259] *Essential palatal tremor* occurs without any overt central nervous system pathology, and is characterized by rhythmic movements of the soft palate (tensor veli palatini), usually with an ear click. The tensor contraction is visible as a movement of the roof of the palate. Extremity or eye muscles are not involved, but more extensive involvement of pharyngeal and laryngeal muscles does occur.[261]

PATHOLOGY AND ETIOLOGY

The pathophysiology of essential palatal tremor is unknown, and it occurs without known pathology. In contrast, many aspects of SPT have been studied. After the cerebellar/brainstem lesion, an inferior olivary pseudohypertrophy, which can be shown by MRI, develops most likely as a consequence of an interruption of inhibitory GABAergic fibers terminating in the inferior olive.[258] Inferior olivary neurons are prone to oscillate spontaneously and can be synchronized through gap junctions.[262] The disinhibition and hypertrophy lead to enhanced synchronized oscillations and build the basis for the rhythmic movement disorder. This rhythm is also reflected in rhythmic EMG inhibition in extremity muscles sometimes leading to a mild postural tremor.[258,263] So far it is unknown why later hypertrophy turns into atrophy, although for most cases SPT continues. It has been postulated that the inferior olive (and the olivocerebellar system) may be a key structure in producing postural tremors.[7]

TREATMENT

The disability of patients with SPT is mostly due to other clinical symptoms of the underlying cerebellar lesion. The rhythmic palatal movement in SPT does not cause discomfort or disability for patients except when the eyes display oscillopsia, or when there is an extremity tremor. Oscillopsia is difficult to treat. Use of oral drugs clonazepam, trihexyphenidyl, and valproate has been described. Botulinum toxin can be injected into the retrobulbar fat tissue, or specific muscles can be targeted.[264,265] So far, controlled studies are unavailable. For the treatment of extremity tremors, case reports have described a response to clonazepam[266] or trihexiphenidyl.[267]

The only complaint of patients with essential palatal tremor is the ear click. Many medications have been reported to be successful, including valproate, trihexyphenidyl, flunarizine, and sumatriptan. The most frequently reported therapy is the treatment of the click by injection of botulinum toxin into the tensor veli palatini. Low doses (e.g., Botox 4 to 10 U) are injected under EMG guidance. Endoscopy and EMG through an EMG injection needle is recommended. Spread of botulinum toxin in the soft palate or too-large doses can cause severe side effects, and specific experience is necessary.

❚ Drug-induced and Toxic Tremors

Drug-induced tremors can manifest with the whole range of clinical features of tremors (rest and action tremors) depending on the drug and probably a further individual predisposition of the patient (e.g., older age, genetic predisposition, central nervous system structural lesions). Several drugs may induce tremors (Table 29–6). Different mechanisms are responsible for enhanced physiological tremor (after sympathomimetics or antidepressants) and resting parkinsonian

TABLE 29–6	Toxic and Drug-induced Tremors		
	Action or Postural Tremor	**Intention Tremor**	**Resting Tremor**
Antiarrhythmics	Amiodarone, mexiletine, procainamide		
Antibiotics, antivirals, and antimycotics		Vidarabine	Co-trimoxazole, amphotericin B
Antidepressants and mood stabilizers	Amitriptyline, lithium, SSRIs	Lithium	SSRIs, lithium
Antiepileptics	Valproic acid		Valproic acid
Bronchodilators	Salbutamol, salmeterol	Salbutamol, salmeterol	
Chemotherapeutics	Tamoxifen, cytarabine, ifosfamide	Cytarabine, ifosfamide	Thalidomide
Drugs of misuse	Cocaine, ethanol, MDMA, nicotine	Ethanol	Cocaine, ethanol, MDMA, MPTP
Gastrointestinal drugs	Metoclopramide, cimetidine		Metoclopramide
Hormones	Thyroxine, calcitonin, medroxyprogesterone	Epinephrine	Medroxyproges-terone
Immunosuppressants	Tacrolimus, cyclosporine, interferon alfa	Tacrolimus, cyclosporine	
Methylxanthines	Theophylline, caffeine		
Neuroleptics and dopamine depleters	Haloperidol, thioridazine, cinnarizine, reserpine, tetrabenazine		Haloperidol, thioridazine, cinnarizine, reserpine, tetrabenazine

MDMA, 3,4-methylenedioxymethamphetamine (ecstasy); MPTP, 1-methyl-4-phenyl-1,2,5,6-tetrahydropyridine; SSRIs, selective serotonin reuptake inhibitors.

From Morgan JC, Sethi KD. Drug-induced tremors. *Lancet Neurol.* 2005;4:866-876.

tremor (after antidopaminergic drugs, such as dopamine receptor blockers and dopamine-depleting drugs). Intention tremor may occur after lithium intoxication and some other substances. The withdrawal tremor from alcohol or other drugs has been characterized as enhanced physiological tremor with tremor frequencies mostly greater 6 Hz. This tremor has to be separated from the intention tremor of chronic alcoholism, however, which is most likely related to cerebellar damage after alcohol ingestion and is combined with a 3-Hz anteroposterior stance tremor in advanced cases.

Drug-induced tremor is symmetrical for most drugs, but in the setting of drug-induced parkinsonism, patients commonly develop unilateral resting tremor.[268] A specific variant is *tardive tremor* associated with long-term neuroleptic treatment.[269] The risk factors to develop this tremor are not well known, but many clinicians believe that patients with ET, older individuals, and women have a higher risk to develop this tremor. Its frequency range is 3 to 5 Hz; it is most prominent during posture, but it is also present at rest and during goal-directed movements.

The tremor in *Wilson's disease* can also be regarded as a toxic tremor because it results from copper toxicity. All kinds of movement disorders, including cerebellar syndromes, can be observed. Tremor is one of the most common neurological manifestations and occurs in approximately 30% to 50% of patients. Resting, postural, and kinetic tremors all have been described.

TREATMENT

After the diagnosis has been made, if the tremor does not affect social functioning or occupation, it is acceptable simply to monitor the patient. If the causative drug provides significant benefit for the patient, the morbidity of the tremor has to be weighed against the benefit of the drug. If the tremor becomes bothersome to the patient in social or occupational functioning, it is prudent to try to reduce the dosage or stop the drug. Switching to an effective, less tremorigenic drug is a good therapeutic choice for many patients (e.g., patients with tardive tremor should be switched to a more atypical neuroleptic).[268] If it is impossible to stop or change the medication, propranolol may be tried in action tremors if it does not have negative interactions with the causative drug. Propranolol has been shown to be effective in a small open series of valproate-induced tremors.[270] Treatment attempts for tardive tremor have included amantadine, trihexyphenidyl, clozapine, and tetrabenazine.[269]

The treatment of Wilson's disease with zinc and copper chelators also improves the tremor and other neurological manifestations.[271,272] In cases of severely disabling neurological symptoms (tremor), a liver transplantation may be considered even with normal liver function.[273]

Psychogenic Tremor

Psychogenic tremor is discussed in detail in Chapter 33 and is described only briefly here. Psychogenic movement disorders are seen in 3% to 5% of all cases of most movement disorder clinics and roughly half of the patients present with tremors.[274]

Most of psychogenic tremors are action tremors, but many show unusual combinations of tremors[275] often characterized by atypical features (see Table 29–1).[276] Two pathogenetic mechanisms seem to play a role in psychogenic tremor. (1) A voluntary-like rhythmic movement can be detected by coherent tremor oscillations in different limbs. In organic tremor, the oscillations are typically independent between different limbs.[82] Normal subjects mostly cannot maintain voluntarily rhythmic movements in different limbs at two completely independent rhythms.[277,278] Many patients with psychogenic tremor have a similar coupling that can be tested with the entrainment maneuver. (2) Rarely, independent rhythms can also be found in patients with psychogenic tremor.[279] They also represent physiological but involuntary oscillations on the basis of clonus-like mechanisms, which are enhanced by the ongoing cocontraction of antagonistic muscles. This mechanism can be detected with the coactivation sign (voluntary-like cocontraction can be felt in both movement directions when passive limb movements are imposed[276]). These findings may explain the motor control mechanisms underlying these tremors, but they do not allow conclusions on the underlying psychological mechanisms.

Therapies for psychogenic tremor are not established. One small study in psychogenic movement disorders including psychogenic tremor has shown some improvement with antidepressants.[280] Psychotherapy is helpful only in a few patients. We recommend physiotherapy aiming at decontraction of the muscles during voluntary movements. We also administer propranolol at medium or high dosages to desensitize the muscle spindles that are necessary to maintain the clonus mechanism in these patients. Conclusive data on the prognosis and long-term outcome in these patients are lacking, but the prognosis is generally believed to be poor.[281]

Rare (or Undetermined) Tremor Syndromes

The following tremors are not yet clearly classified and are reported here as undetermined tremors.

HEREDITARY CHIN TREMOR

Hereditary chin tremor ("hereditary quivering of the chin," "familial geniospasm," "hereditary essential chin myoclonus") is a rare condition characterized by episodes of involuntary oscillatory rhythmic movements of the chin muscles (mainly the mentalis muscle).[282] This tremor usually starts early in life and is not associated with tremor elsewhere. Symptoms peak in early adulthood and gradually improve or even disappear by the fifth decade.[283] The episodes last seconds to hours, and may be triggered by emotion or anxiety. The amplitude varies, and the tremor frequency ranges from 2 to 11 Hz.[284] Associated conditions have been described, including tongue biting, myoclonus, nystagmus, nocturnal bruxism, rapid eye movements, sleep behavioral disorder, otosclerosis, hereditary sensorimotor neuropathy, and PD.[282,285] Hereditary chin tremor must be separated from other rhythmical involuntary movements involving the lower face, such as PD tremor, ET, facial myoclonus and myokymia, and orofacial tardive dyskinesias.[282,286] Hereditary chin tremor is an autosomal dominant condition with high penetrance, and has been linked to chromosome 9q13-q21 in one kindred.[287] The condition has genetic heterogeneity.[288]

Benzodiazepine, phenytoin, haloperidol, and other sedatives have been reported to alleviate hereditary chin tremor. Botulinum toxin injections into the mentalis muscles seem to be the most effective treatment, however.[283,284,286]

FRAGILE X–ASSOCIATED TREMOR/ATAXIA SYNDROME

Fragile X–associated tremor/ataxia syndrome (FXTAS) is a recently recognized progressive disorder associated with the *FRM1* gene premutation.[289] FXTAS encompasses two main clinical features, cerebellar ataxia or intention tremor or both, and is more frequent and severe in men. The phenotype manifests typically with onset in the sixth decade and includes additional executive cognitive deficits, variable degrees of peripheral neuropathy, and occasionally mild parkinsonism.[289] Penetrance is close to 50% at age 60 and 100% for individuals older than 80. Occasional patients with FXTAS manifesting as an ET-like picture have been reported.[290] FXTAS is associated with a hyperdensity on T2-weighted MR images of the middle cerebellar peduncle.[291] It has been suggested that *FMR1* DNA testing should be performed in men older than 50 years with unexplained cerebellar ataxia, and in men older than 50 with action tremor, parkinsonism, or dementia who also have a family history of developmental delay, autism, or mental retardation.

BILATERAL HIGH-FREQUENCY SYNCHRONOUS DISCHARGES

A new form of tremor has been described in a patient affected by a hemorrhagic lesion of the midbrain and in two patients with sporadic olivopontocerebellar atrophy.[292,293] The tremor was characterized by a low-frequency postural tremor in the upper limbs with episodes of highly coherent tremor at a frequency of 14 Hz induced by maintaining the upper limbs outstretched. Because of the high frequency, patients complain of episodes of involuntary vibrations or contraction in the upper limb. In one of the cases, squared coherence and cospectral density was strong between agonist and antagonist muscles in the left and right upper limbs and across limbs for the high-frequency discharges.[293] Electrical stimulation over the posterior fossa reset the explosive high-frequency bursts.[293] These findings and the position-specific onset suggest that this disorder shares a common pathophysiology with OT.

MICROSACCADIC OSCILLATIONS AND LIMB TREMOR

A novel disorder of saccadic oscillations and fine hand tremor has been described in a mother and her daughter.[294] The patients complained since childhood of occasional brief episodes of blurring of vision and hand tremor, accentuated during periods of stress or anxiety. During attempted steady fixation, there were nearly continuous, small-amplitude, high-frequency saccadic oscillations (18 Hz) around all three axes of rotation (horizontal, vertical, and torsional). They showed a small-amplitude, high-frequency (12-Hz) postural and kinetic tremor of the upper limbs.[294]

ISOLATED TONGUE TREMOR

Tongue tremor is sometimes observed in patients with ET, parkinsonism, or SPT. Isolated tongue tremor is a very rare condition, however. Although this tremor can be recognized as a predominant or initial feature in ET[295] or Wilson's disease,[296] most cases are due to secondary lesions of the Guillain-Mollaret triangle, sharing a common pathophysiology with SPT. Isolated tongue tremor has been described after trauma, brainstem or cerebellar astrocytoma, electrical injury, or Gamma Knife radiosurgery.[297,298] Tremor usually affects the posterior part of the tongue with rhythmic alternating protrusion-retrogression movements at a frequency of 3 to 5 Hz. Tremor may be observed when the tongue is protruded, is at rest, or during both conditions. Isolated tongue tremor has been reported to follow a self-limiting course with duration of about 6 months. Regarding the response to treatment, scanty data are available for non-ET cases; in two cases, a favorable outcome was achieved using anticholinergics.[297,298]

TREMOR INDUCED BY PERIPHERAL NERVE INJURY

There is some evidence that peripheral trauma can cause tremor,[299-301] often associated with complex regional pain syndrome, paresthesia, or hyperpathia in the affected region.[302] Generally, trauma-induced tremor occurs in the hands after limb or cervical injury, although it can spread to other body regions. Usually, it is an asymmetrical, postural-kinetic tremor with a moderate frequency (5 to 7 Hz). Other movement disorders, such as dystonia or myoclonic-like jerking, may be occasionally associated.[299-301]

The pathophysiology is still debated. A possible predisposing factor is present in 65% of these cases, including family history of ET or dystonia, previous use of neuroleptics or stimulants, human immunodeficiency virus infection, coexisting tremor, seizure disorder, and mental retardation.[300] Central reorganization in response to peripheral injury may give rise to a motor disturbance, including tremor.[299,300] Modulation induced by the increased load applied or the persistence during sleep[299] suggest the contribution of a mechanical reflex mechanism (analogous to enhanced physiological tremor or a peripheral generator). Tremor generally starts within weeks after trauma, it worsens over the first year, then becomes less pronounced, but rarely recovers.[302] Some patients experienced improvement on propranolol or clonazepam.[299,301] A relationship with the dystonia-causalgia syndrome may be possible.[303]

RHYTHMIC MYOCLONUS

Rhythmic myoclonias may be misinterpreted as tremors. They are mentioned here as important differential diagnoses.

Rhythmic myoclonus is not well defined, but has been described as low-frequency (usually <5 Hz) muscle jerks topographically limited to segmental levels.

Orthostatic myoclonus is a rare condition to consider in the differential diagnosis of trunk tremors.[174]

Cortical tremor is considered a specific form of rhythmic myoclonus manifesting with high-frequency, irregular tremor-like postural and action myoclonus. This form is mostly hereditary, but has also been described in corticobasal degeneration[304,305] and after focal lesions[306] or celiac disease.[307] There is an overlap between these cortical myoclonias and epileptic phenomena being most obvious in *epilepsia partialis continua*, a focal epilepsy producing (mostly low-frequency) rhythmic jerks of an extremity. Resting and rarely postural/intention tremors (e.g., Holmes' tremor) can be mimicked by epilepsia partialis continua.

Asterixis occurs when an ongoing contraction is repetitively interrupted by inhibitions of different duration ("negative myoclonus"). It can manifest as a bilateral "flapping tremor," and typically results from endocrine dysfunction, intoxication, and liver disease.

Clonus is a rhythmic movement mostly around one joint elicited through the stretch reflex loop and increasing in strength (or amplitude) by maneuvers affecting the stretch reflex. Passive stretching of the muscles increases the force of clonus and serves as a diagnostic criterion.

REFERENCES

1. Deuschl G, Bain P, Brin M: Adhoc-Scientific-Committee. Consensus statement of the Movement Disorder Society on Tremor. Mov Disord 1998;13(Suppl 3):2-23.
2. Deuschl G, Krack P, Lauk M, Timmer J: Clinical neurophysiology of tremor. J Clin Neurophysiol 1996;13:110-121.
3. Raethjen J, Lindemann M, Morsnowski A, et al: Is the rhythm of physiological tremor involved in cortico-cortical interactions? Mov Disord 2004;19:458-465.
4. Elble RJ, Higgins C, Elble S: Electrophysiologic transition from physiologic tremor to essential tremor. Mov Disord 2005;20:1038-1042.
5. Wenning GK, Kiechl S, Seppi K, et al: Prevalence of movement disorders in men and women aged 50-89 years (Bruneck Study cohort): a population-based study. Lancet Neurol 2005;4:815-820.
6. Elble RJ: Central mechanisms of tremor. J Clin Neurophysiol 1996;13:133-144.
7. Deuschl G, Raethjen J, Lindemann M, Krack P: The pathophysiology of tremor. Muscle Nerve 2001;24:716-735.
8. Elman MJ, Sugar J, Fiscella R, et al: The effect of propranolol versus placebo on resident surgical performance. Trans Am Ophthalmol Soc 1998;96:283-291.
9. Louis ED, Ford B, Lee H, et al: Diagnostic criteria for essential tremor: a population perspective. Arch Neurol 1998;55:823-828.
10. Bain P, Brin M, Deuschl G, et al: Criteria for the diagnosis of essential tremor. *Neurology* 2000;54(11 Suppl. 4):S7.
11. Koller WC, Busenbark K, Miner K: The relationship of essential tremor to other movement disorders: report on 678 patients. Essential Tremor Study Group. Ann Neurol 1994;35:717-723.
12. Lou JS, Jankovic J: Essential tremor: clinical correlates in 350 patients. Neurology 1991;41(2 Pt 1):234-238.
13. Deuschl G, Wenzelburger R, Loffler K, et al: Essential tremor and cerebellar dysfunction clinical and kinematic analysis of intention tremor. Brain 2000;123(Pt 8):1568-1580.
14. Stolze H, Petersen G, Raethjen J, et al: The gait disorder of advanced essential tremor. Brain 2001;124(Pt 11):2278-2286.
15. Cohen O, Pullman S, Jurewicz E, et al: Rest tremor in patients with essential tremor: prevalence, clinical correlates, and electrophysiologic characteristics. Arch Neurol 2003;60:405-410.
16. Koster B, Deuschl G, Lauk M, et al: Essential tremor and cerebellar dysfunction: abnormal ballistic movements. J Neurol Neurosurg Psychiatry 2002;73:400-405.
17. Helmchen C, Hagenow A, Miesner J, et al: Eye movement abnormalities in essential tremor may indicate cerebellar dysfunction. Brain 2003;126(Pt 6):1319-1332.
18. Farkas Z, Szirmai I, Kamondi A: Impaired rhythm generation in essential tremor. Mov Disord 2006;21:1196-1199.
19. Kronenbuerger M, Gerwig M, Brol B, et al: Eyeblink conditioning is impaired in subjects with essential tremor. Brain 2007;130(Pt 6):1538-1551.
20. Gasparini M, Bonifati V, Fabrizio E, et al: Frontal lobe dysfunction in essential tremor: a preliminary study. J Neurol 2001;248:399-402.
21. Lombardi WJ, Woolston DJ, Roberts JW, Gross RE: Cognitive deficits in patients with essential tremor. Neurology 2001;57:785-790.
22. Lacritz LH, Dewey R Jr, Giller C, Cullum CM: Cognitive functioning in individuals with "benign" essential tremor. J Int Neuropsychol Soc 2002;8:125-129.
23. Troster AI, Woods SP, Fields JA, et al: Neuropsychological deficits in essential tremor: an expression of cerebello-thalamo-cortical pathophysiology? Eur J Neurol 2002;9:143-151.
24. Benito-Leon J, Louis ED, Bermejo-Pareja F: Elderly-onset essential tremor is associated with dementia. Neurology 2006;66:1500-1505.
25. Ondo WG, Sutton L, Dat Vuong K, et al: Hearing impairment in essential tremor. Neurology 2003;61:1093-1097.
26. Louis ED, Bromley SM, Jurewicz EC, Watner D: Olfactory dysfunction in essential tremor: a deficit unrelated to disease duration or severity. Neurology 2002;59:1631-1633.
27. Applegate LM, Louis ED: Essential tremor: mild olfactory dysfunction in a cerebellar disorder. Parkinsonism Relat Disord 2005;11:399-402.
28. Hawkes C, Shah M, Findley L: Olfactory function in essential tremor: a deficit unrelated to disease duration or severity. Neurology 2003;61:871-872.
29. Lorenz D, Schwieger D, Moises H, Deuschl G: Quality of life and personality in essential tremor patients. Mov Disord 2006;21:1114-1118.

30. Chatterjee A, Jurewicz EC, Applegate LM, Louis ED: Personality in essential tremor: further evidence of non-motor manifestations of the disease. J Neurol Neurosurg Psychiatry 2004;75:958-961.
31. Schneier FR, Barnes LF, Albert SM, Louis ED: Characteristics of social phobia among persons with essential tremor. J Clin Psychiatry 2001;62:367-372.
32. Louis ED: Behavioral symptoms associated with essential tremor. Adv Neurol 2005;96:284-290.
33. Tan EK, Fook-Chong S, Lum SY, et al: Non-motor manifestations in essential tremor: use of a validated instrument to evaluate a wide spectrum of symptoms. Parkinsonism Relat Disord 2005;11:375-380.
34. Schmahmann JD, Sherman JC: The cerebellar cognitive affective syndrome. Brain 1998;121(Pt 4):561-579.
35. Bermejo-Pareja F, Louis ED, Benito-Leon J: Risk of incident dementia in essential tremor: a population-based study. Mov Disord 2007;22:1573-1580.
36. Elble RJ, Dubinsky RM, Ala T: Alzheimer's disease and essential tremor finally meet. Mov Disord 2007;22:1525-1527.
37. Bain PG, Findley LJ, Thompson PD, et al: A study of hereditary essential tremor. Brain 1994;117 (Pt 4):805-824.
38. Lorenz D, Frederiksen H, Moises H, et al: High concordance for essential tremor in monozygotic twins of old age. Neurology 2004;62:208-211.
39. Elble RJ: Essential tremor frequency decreases with time. Neurology 2000;55:1547-1551.
40. Deuschl G, Elble RJ: The pathophysiology of essential tremor. Neurology 2000;54:S14-S20.
41. Louis ED, Ford B, Wendt KJ, Cameron G: Clinical characteristics of essential tremor: data from a community-based study. Mov Disord 1998;13:803-808.
42. Troster AI, Pahwa R, Fields JA, et al: Quality of life in Essential Tremor Questionnaire (QUEST): development and initial validation. Parkinsonism Relat Disord 2005;11:367-373.
43. Busenbark KL, Nash J, Nash S, et al: Is essential tremor benign? Neurology 1991;41:1982-1983.
44. Louis ED, Barnes L, Albert SM, et al: Correlates of functional disability in essential tremor. Mov Disord 2001;16:914-920.
45. Louis ED, Ottman R, Hauser WA: How common is the most common adult movement disorder? Estimates of the prevalence of essential tremor throughout the world. Mov Disord 1998;13:5-10.
46. Benito-Leon J, Bermejo-Pareja F, Morales JM, et al: Prevalence of essential tremor in three elderly populations of central Spain. Mov Disord 2003;18:389-394.
47. Dogu O, Louis ED, Sevim S, et al: Clinical characteristics of essential tremor in Mersin, Turkey—a population-based door-to-door study. J Neurol 2005;252:570-574.
48. Rajput AH, Offord KP, Beard CM, Kurland LT: Essential tremor in Rochester, Minnesota: a 45-year study. J Neurol Neurosurg Psychiatry 1984;47:466-470.
49. Benito-Leon J, Bermejo-Pareja F, Louis ED: Incidence of essential tremor in three elderly populations of central Spain. Neurology 2005;64:1721-1725.
50. Jankovic J, Beach J, Schwartz K, Contant C: Tremor and longevity in relatives of patients with Parkinson's disease, essential tremor, and control subjects. Neurology 1995;45:645-648.
51. Louis ED, Benito-Leon J, Ottman R, Bermejo-Pareja F: A population-based study of mortality in essential tremor. Neurology 2007;69:1982-1989.
52. Tanner CM, Goldman SM, Lyons KE, et al: Essential tremor in twins: an assessment of genetic vs environmental determinants of etiology. Neurology 2001;57:1389-1391.
53. Louis ED: Etiology of essential tremor: should we be searching for environmental causes? Mov Disord 2001;16:822-829.
54. Baughman FA Jr, Higgins JV, Mann JD: Sex chromosome anomalies and essential tremor. Neurology 1973;23:623-625.
55. Ma S, Davis TL, Blair MA, et al: Familial essential tremor with apparent autosomal dominant inheritance: should we also consider other inheritance modes? Mov Disord 2006;21:1368-1374.
56. Gulcher JR, Jonsson P, Kong A, et al: Mapping of a familial essential tremor gene, FET1, to chromosome 3q13. Nat Genet 1997;17:84-87.
57. Jeanneteau F, Funalot B, Jankovic J, et al: A functional variant of the dopamine D3 receptor is associated with risk and age-at-onset of essential tremor. Proc Natl Acad Sci U S A 2006;103:10753-10758.
58. Tan EK, Prakash KM, Fook-Chong S, et al: DRD3 variant and risk of essential tremor. Neurology 2007;68:790-791.
59. Higgins JJ, Loveless JM, Jankovic J, Patel PI: Evidence that a gene for essential tremor maps to chromosome 2p in four families. Mov Disord 1998;13:972-977.

60. Higgins JJ, Jankovic J, Lombardi RQ, et al: Haplotype analysis of the ETM2 locus in familial essential tremor. Neurogenetics 2003;4:185-189.
61. Higgins JJ, Lombardi RQ, Pucilowska J, et al: A variant in the HS1-BP3 gene is associated with familial essential tremor. Neurology 2005;64:417-421.
62. Deng H, Le WD, Guo Y, et al: Extended study of A265G variant of HS1BP3 in essential tremor and Parkinson disease. Neurology 2005;65:651-652.
63. Shatunov A, Jankovic J, Elble R, et al: A variant in the HS1-BP3 gene is associated with familial essential tremor. Neurology 2005;65:1995. author reply 1995.
64. Shatunov A, Sambuughin N, Jankovic J, et al: Genomewide scans in North American families reveal genetic linkage of essential tremor to a region on chromosome 6p23. Brain 2006;129(Pt 9):2318-2331.
65. Kralic JE, Criswell HE, Osterman JL, et al: Genetic essential tremor in gamma-aminobutyric acidA receptor alpha1 subunit knockout mice. J Clin Invest 2005;115:774-779.
66. Deng H, Xie WJ, Le WD, et al: Genetic analysis of the GABRA1 gene in patients with essential tremor. Neurosci Lett 2006;401(1-2):16-19.
67. Louis ED, Zheng W, Mao X, Shungu DC: Blood harmane is correlated with cerebellar metabolism in essential tremor: a pilot study. Neurology 2007;69:515-520.
68. Louis ED, Applegate L, Graziano JH, et al: Interaction between blood lead concentration and delta-amino-levulinic acid dehydratase gene polymorphisms increases the odds of essential tremor. Mov Disord 2005;20:1170-1177.
69. Pinto AD, Lang AE, Chen R: The cerebellothalamocortical pathway in essential tremor. Neurology 2003;60:1985-1987.
70. Louis ED, Faust PL, Vonsattel JP, et al: Neuropathological changes in essential tremor: 33 cases compared with 21 controls. Brain 2007;130(Pt 12):3297-3307.
71. Braak H, Bohl JR, Muller CM, et al: Stanley Fahn Lecture 2005: the staging procedure for the inclusion body pathology associated with sporadic Parkinson's disease reconsidered. Mov Disord 2006;21:2042-2051.
72. Jenkins IH, Bain PG, Colebatch JG, et al: A positron emission tomography study of essential tremor: evidence for overactivity of cerebellar connections. Ann Neurol 1993;34:82-90.
73. Wills AJ, Jenkins IH, Thompson PD, et al: Red nuclear and cerebellar but no olivary activation associated with essential tremor: a positron emission tomographic study. Ann Neurol 1994;36:636-642.
74. Wills AJ, Jenkins IH, Thompson PD, et al: A positron emission tomography study of cerebral activation associated with essential and writing tremor. Arch Neurol 1995;52:299-305.
75. Boecker H, Wills AJ, Ceballos-Baumann A, et al: The effect of ethanol on alcohol-responsive essential tremor: a positron emission tomography study. Ann Neurol 1996;39:650-658.
76. Louis ED, Shungu DC, Chan S, et al: Metabolic abnormality in the cerebellum in patients with essential tremor: a proton magnetic resonance spectroscopic imaging study. Neurosci Lett. 2002;333:17-20.
77. Pagan FL, Butman JA, Dambrosia JM, Hallett M: Evaluation of essential tremor with multi-voxel magnetic resonance spectroscopy. Neurology 2003;60:1344-1347.
78. Daniels C, Peller M, Wolff S, et al: Voxel-based morphometry shows no decreases in cerebellar gray matter volume in essential tremor. Neurology 2006;67:1452-1456.
79. Martinelli P, Rizzo G, Manners D, et al: Diffusion-weighted imaging study of patients with essential tremor. Mov Disord 2007;22:1182-1185.
80. Stockner H, Sojer M, Seppi K, et al: Midbrain sonography in patients with essential tremor. Mov Disord 2007;22:414-417.
81. Salenius S, Hari R: Synchronous cortical oscillatory activity during motor action. Curr Opin Neurobiol 2003;13:678-684.
82. Raethjen J, Lindemann M, Schmaljohann H, et al: Multiple oscillators are causing parkinsonian and essential tremor. Mov Disord 2000;15:84-94.
83. Hurtado JM, Rubchinsky LL, Sigvardt KA, et al: Temporal evolution of oscillations and synchrony in GPi/muscle pairs in Parkinson's disease. J Neurophysiol 2005;93:1569-1584.
84. Halliday DM, Conway BA, Farmer SF, et al: Coherence between low-frequency activation of the motor cortex and tremor in patients with essential tremor. Lancet 2000;355:1149-1153.
85. Hellwig B, Haussler S, Schelter B, et al: Tremor-correlated cortical activity in essential tremor. Lancet 2001;357:519-523.
86. Raethjen J, Govindan RB, Kopper F, et al: Cortical involvement in the generation of essential tremor. J Neurophysiol 2007;97:3219-3228.

87. Restuccia D, Valeriani M, Barba C, et al: Abnormal gating of somatosensory inputs in essential tremor. Clin Neurophysiol 2003;114:120-129.
88. Wilms H, Sievers J, Deuschl G: Animal models of tremor. Mov Disord 1999;14:557-571.
89. Zesiewicz TA, Elble R, Louis ED, et al: Practice parameter: therapies for essential tremor: report of the Quality Standards Subcommittee of the American Academy of Neurology. Neurology 2005;64:2008-2020.
90. Findley LJ: The pharmacological management of essential tremor. Clin Neuropharmacol 1986;9(Suppl 2):S61-S75.
91. Winkler GF, Young RR: The control of essential tremor by propranolol. Trans Am Neurol Assoc. 1971;96:66-68.
92. Koller WC: Alcoholism in essential tremor. Neurology 1983;33:1074-1076.
93. Findley LJ, Cleeves L, Calzetti S: Primidone in essential tremor of the hands and head: a double blind controlled clinical study. J Neurol Neurosurg Psychiatry 1985;48:911-915.
94. O'Suilleabhain P, Dewey RB Jr.: Randomized trial comparing primidone initiation schedules for treating essential tremor. Mov Disord 2002;17:382-386.
95. Gironell A, Kulisevsky J, Barbanoj M, et al: A randomized placebo-controlled comparative trial of gabapentin and propranolol in essential tremor. Arch Neurol 1999;56:475-480.
96. Pahwa R, Lyons K, Hubble JP, et al: Double-blind controlled trial of gabapentin in essential tremor. Mov Disord 1998;13:465-467.
97. Connor GS: A double-blind placebo-controlled trial of topiramate treatment for essential tremor. Neurology 2002;59:132-134.
98. Ondo WG, Jankovic J, Connor GS, et al: Topiramate in essential tremor: a double-blind, placebo-controlled trial. Neurology 2006;66:672-677.
99. Frima N, Grunewald RA: A double-blind, placebo-controlled, crossover trial of topiramate in essential tremor. Clin Neuropharmacol 2006;29:94-96.
100. Huber SJ, Paulson GW: Efficacy of alprazolam for essential tremor. Neurology 1988;38:241-243.
101. Biary N, Koller W: Kinetic predominant essential tremor: successful treatment with clonazepam. Neurology 1987;37:471-474.
102. Thompson C, Lang A, Parkes JD, Marsden CD: A double-blind trial of clonazepam in benign essential tremor. Clin Neuropharmacol 1984;7:83-88.
103. Leigh PN, Jefferson D, Twomey A, Marsden CD: Beta-adrenoreceptor mechanisms in essential tremor: a double-blind placebo controlled trial of metoprolol, sotalol and atenolol. J Neurol Neurosurg Psychiatry 1983;46:710-715.
104. Lee KS, Kim JS, Kim JW, et al: A multicenter randomized crossover multiple-dose comparison study of arotinolol and propranolol in essential tremor. Parkinsonism Relat Disord 2003;9:341-347.
105. Handforth A, Martin FC: Pilot efficacy and tolerability: a randomized, placebo-controlled trial of levetiracetam for essential tremor. Mov Disord 2004;19:1215-1221.
106. Ondo WG, Jimenez JE, Vuong KD, Jankovic J: An open-label pilot study of levetiracetam for essential tremor. Clin Neuropharmacol 2004;27:274-277.
107. Bushara KO, Malik T, Exconde RE: The effect of levetiracetam on essential tremor. Neurology 2005;64:1078-1080.
108. Zesiewicz TA, Ward CL, Hauser RA, et al: Pregabalin (Lyrica) in the treatment of essential tremor. Mov Disord 2007;22:139-141.
109. Zesiewicz TA, Ward CL, Hauser RA, et al: A pilot, double-blind, placebo-controlled trial of pregabalin (Lyrica) in the treatment of essential tremor. Mov Disord 2007;22:1660-1663.
110. Zesiewicz TA, Ward CL, Hauser RA, et al: A double-blind placebo-controlled trial of zonisamide (zonegran) in the treatment of essential tremor. Mov Disord 2007;22:279-282.
111. Frucht SJ, Bordelon Y, Houghton WH, Reardan D: A pilot tolerability and efficacy trial of sodium oxybate in ethanol-responsive movement disorders. Mov Disord 2005;20:1330-1337.
112. Frucht SJ, Houghton WC, Bordelon Y, et al: A single-blind, open-label trial of sodium oxybate for myoclonus and essential tremor. Neurology 2005;65:1967-1969.
113. Melmed C, Moros D, Rutman H: Treatment of essential tremor with the barbiturate T2000 (1,3-dimethoxymethyl-5,5-diphenyl-barbituric acid). Mov Disord 2007;22:723-727.
114. Calzetti S, Sasso E, Negrotti A, et al: Effect of propranolol in head tremor: quantitative study following single-dose and sustained drug administration. Clin Neuropharmacol 1992;15:470-476.
115. Massey EW, Paulson GW: Essential vocal tremor: clinical characteristics and response to therapy. South Med J 1985;78:316-317.

116. Warrick P, Dromey C, Irish JC, et al: Botulinum toxin for essential tremor of the voice with multiple anatomical sites of tremor: a crossover design study of unilateral versus bilateral injection. Laryngoscope 2000;110:1366-1374.

117. Hertegard S, Granqvist S, Lindestad PA: Botulinum toxin injections for essential voice tremor. Ann Otol Rhinol Laryngol 2000;109:204-209.

118. Adler CH, Bansberg SF, Hentz JG, et al: Botulinum toxin type A for treating voice tremor. Arch Neurol 2004;61:1416-1420.

119. Ludlow CL: Treatment of speech and voice disorders with botulinum toxin. JAMA 1990;264: 2671-2675.

120. Blitzer A, Brin MF, Fahn S, Lovelace RE: Localized injections of botulinum toxin for the treatment of focal laryngeal dystonia (spastic dysphonia). Laryngoscope 1988;98:193-197.

121. Brin MF, Lyons KE, Doucette J, et al: A randomized, double masked, controlled trial of botulinum toxin type A in essential hand tremor. Neurology 2001;56:1523-1528.

122. Kolek M, Mrozek V, Schenk P: [Cardiac manifestations of Friedreich's ataxia]. Cas Lek Cesk 2004;143:48-51.

123. Koller W, Pahwa R, Busenbark K, et al: High-frequency unilateral thalamic stimulation in the treatment of essential and parkinsonian tremor. Ann Neurol 1997;42:292-299.

124. Limousin P, Speelman JD, Gielen F, Janssens M: Multicentre European study of thalamic stimulation in parkinsonian and essential tremor. J Neurol Neurosurg Psychiatry 1999;66:289-296.

125. Pahwa R, Lyons KL, Wilkinson SB, et al: Bilateral thalamic stimulation for the treatment of essential tremor. Neurology 1999;53:1447-1450.

126. Schuurman PR, Bosch DA, Bossuyt PM, et al: A comparison of continuous thalamic stimulation and thalamotomy for suppression of severe tremor. N Engl J Med 2000;342:461-468.

127. Herzog J, Hamel W, Wenzelburger R, et al: Kinematic analysis of thalamic versus subthalamic neurostimulation in postural and intention tremor. Brain 2007;130(Pt 6):1608-1625.

128. Plaha P, Patel NK, Gill SS: Stimulation of the subthalamic region for essential tremor. J Neurosurg 2004;101:48-54.

129. Koller WC, Lyons KE, Wilkinson SB, Pahwa R: Efficacy of unilateral deep brain stimulation of the VIM nucleus of the thalamus for essential head tremor. Mov Disord 1999;14:847-850.

130. Ondo W, Almaguer M, Jankovic J, Simpson RK: Thalamic deep brain stimulation: comparison between unilateral and bilateral placement. Arch Neurol 2001;58:218-222.

131. Pollak P, Benabid AL, Gervason CL, et al: Long-term effects of chronic stimulation of the ventral intermediate thalamic nucleus in different types of tremor. Adv Neurol 1993;60:408-413.

132. Ohye C, Shibazaki T, Sato S: Gamma knife thalamotomy for movement disorders: evaluation of the thalamic lesion and clinical results. J Neurosurg 2005;102(Suppl):234-240.

133. Siderowf A, Gollump SM, Stern MB, et al: Emergence of complex, involuntary movements after gamma knife radiosurgery for essential tremor. Mov Disord 2001;16:965-967.

134. Jankovic J, Schwartz KS, Ondo W: Re-emergent tremor of Parkinson's disease. J Neurol Neurosurg Psychiatry 1999;67:646-650.

135. Koller WC, Vetere-Overfield B, Barter R: Tremors in early Parkinson's disease. Clin Neuropharmacol 1989;12:293-297.

136. Leenders KL, Oertel WH: Parkinson's disease: clinical signs and symptoms, neural mechanisms, positron emission tomography, and therapeutic interventions. Neural Plast 2001;8(1-2): 99-110.

137. Tissingh G, Bergmans P, Booij J, et al: Drug-naive patients with Parkinson's disease in Hoehn and Yahr stages I and II show a bilateral decrease in striatal dopamine transporters as revealed by [123I]beta-CIT SPECT. J Neurol 1998;245:14-20.

138. Hirsch EC, Mouatt A, Faucheux B, et al: Dopamine, tremor, and Parkinson's disease. Lancet 1992;340:125-126.

139. Jellinger KA: Post mortem studies in Parkinson's disease—is it possible to detect brain areas for specific symptoms? J Neural Transm Suppl 1999;56:1-29.

140. Paulus W, Jellinger K: The neuropathologic basis of different clinical subgroups of Parkinson's disease. J Neuropathol Exp Neurol 1991;50:743-755.

141. Brooks DJ, Playford ED, Ibanez V, et al: Isolated tremor and disruption of the nigrostriatal dopaminergic system: an 18F-dopa PET study. Neurology 1992;42:1554-1560.

142. Ghaemi M, Raethjen J, Hilker R, et al: Monosymptomatic resting tremor and Parkinson's disease: a multitracer positron emission tomographic study. Mov Disord 2002;17:782-788.

143. Doder M, Rabiner EA, Turjanski N, et al: Tremor in Parkinson's disease and serotonergic dysfunction: an 11C-WAY 100635 PET study. Neurology 2003;60:601-605.

144. Bergman H, Deuschl G: Pathophysiology of Parkinson's disease: from clinical neurology to basic neuroscience and back. Mov Disord 2002;17(Suppl 3):S28-S40.
145. Bergman H, Raz A, Feingold A, et al: Physiology of MPTP tremor. Mov Disord 1998;13(Suppl 3):29-34.
146. Pogarell O, Gasser T, van Hilten JJ, et al: Pramipexole in patients with Parkinson's disease and marked drug resistant tremor: a randomised, double blind, placebo controlled multicentre study. J Neurol Neurosurg Psychiatry 2002;72:713-720.
147. Navan P, Findley LJ, Jeffs JA, et al: Double-blind, single-dose, cross-over study of the effects of pramipexole, pergolide, and placebo on rest tremor and UPDRS part III in Parkinson's disease. Mov Disord 2003;18:176-180.
148. Cantello R, Riccio A, Gilli M, et al: Bornaprine vs placebo in Parkinson disease: double-blind controlled cross-over trial in 30 patients. Ital J Neurol Sci 1986;7:139-143.
149. Piccirilli M, D'Alessandro P, Testa A, et al: [Bornaprine in the treatment of parkinsonian tremor]. Riv Neurol 1985;55:38-45.
150. Koller WC: Pharmacologic treatment of parkinsonian tremor. Arch Neurol 1986;43:126-127.
151. Perry EK, Kilford L, Lees AJ, et al: Increased Alzheimer pathology in Parkinson's disease related to antimuscarinic drugs. Ann Neurol 2003;54:235-238.
152. Fischer PA, Baas H, Hefner R: Treatment of parkinsonian tremor with clozapine. J Neural Transm Park Dis Dement Sect 1990;2:233-238.
153. Pakkenberg H, Pakkenberg B: Clozapine in the treatment of tremor. Acta Neurol Scand 1986;73:295-297.
154. Jansen EN: Clozapine in the treatment of tremor in Parkinson's disease. Acta Neurol Scand 1994;89:262-265.
155. Koller WC, Herbster G: Adjuvant therapy of parkinsonian tremor. Arch Neurol 1987;44:921-923.
156. Crosby NJ, Deane KH, Clarke CE: Beta-blocker therapy for tremor in Parkinson's disease. Cochrane Database Syst Rev 2003(1):CD003361.
157. Schneider SA, Edwards MJ, Cordivari C, et al: Botulinum toxin A may be efficacious as treatment for jaw tremor in Parkinson's disease. Mov Disord 2006;21:1722-1724.
158. Krack P, Benazzouz A, Pollak P, et al: Treatment of tremor in Parkinson's disease by subthalamic nucleus stimulation. Mov Disord 1998;13:907-914.
159. Sturman MM, Vaillancourt DE, Metman LV, et al: Effects of subthalamic nucleus stimulation and medication on resting and postural tremor in Parkinson's disease. Brain 2004;127(Pt 9):2131-2143.
160. Deuschl G, Schade-Brittinger C, Krack P, et al: A randomized trial of deep-brain stimulation for Parkinson's disease. N Engl J Med 2006;355:896-908.
161. Katayama Y, Kasai M, Oshima H, et al: Subthalamic nucleus stimulation for Parkinson disease: benefits observed in levodopa-intolerant patients. J Neurosurg 2001;95:213-221.
162. Heilman KM: Orthostatic tremor. Arch Neurol 1984;41:880-881.
163. Pazzaglia P, Sabattini L, Lugaresi E: [On an unusual disorder of erect standing position (observation of 3 cases)]. Riv Sper Freniatr Med Leg Alien Ment 1970;94:450-457.
164. McManis PG, Sharbrough FW: Orthostatic tremor: clinical and electrophysiologic characteristics. Muscle Nerve 1993;16:1254-1260.
165. Boroojerdi B, Ferbert A, Foltys H, et al: Evidence for a non-orthostatic origin of orthostatic tremor. J Neurol Neurosurg Psychiatry 1999;66:284-288.
166. McAuley JH, Britton TC, Rothwell JC, et al: The timing of primary orthostatic tremor bursts has a task-specific plasticity. Brain 2000;123(Pt 2):254-266.
167. Brown P: New clinical sign for orthostatic tremor. Lancet 1995;346:306-307.
168. Gerschlager W, Munchau A, Katzenschlager R, et al: Natural history and syndromic associations of orthostatic tremor: a review of 41 patients. Mov Disord 2004;19:788-795.
169. Contarino MF, Welter ML, Agid Y, Hartmann A: Orthostatic tremor in monozygotic twins. Neurology 2006;66:1600-1601.
170. Wee AS, Subramony SH, Currier RD: "Orthostatic tremor" in familial-essential tremor. Neurology 1986;36:1241-1245.
171. Britton TC, Thompson PD: Primary orthostatic tremor. BMJ 1995;310:143-144.
172. Setta F, Jacquy J, Hildebrand J, Manto MU: Orthostatic tremor associated with cerebellar ataxia. J Neurol 1998;245:299-302.
173. de Bie RM, Chen R, Lang AE: Orthostatic tremor in progressive supranuclear palsy. Mov Disord 2007;22:1192-1194.

174. Leu-Semenescu S, Roze E, Vidailhet M, et al: Myoclonus or tremor in orthostatism: an under-recognized cause of unsteadiness in Parkinson's disease. Mov Disord 2007;22:2063-2069.
175. Kim JS, Lee MC: Leg tremor mimicking orthostatic tremor as an initial manifestation of Parkinson's disease. Mov Disord 1993;8:397-398.
176. Apartis E, Tison F, Arne P, et al: Fast orthostatic tremor in Parkinson's disease mimicking primary orthostatic tremor. Mov Disord 2001;16:1133-1136.
177. Thomas A, Bonanni L, Antonini A, et al: Dopa-responsive pseudo-orthostatic tremor in parkinsonism. Mov Disord 2007;22:1652-1656.
178. Sanitate SS, Meerschaert JR: Orthostatic tremor: delayed onset following head trauma. Arch Phys Med Rehabil 1993;74:886-889.
179. Benito-Leon J, Rodriguez J, Orti-Pareja M, et al: Symptomatic orthostatic tremor in pontine lesions. Neurology 1997;49:1439-1441.
180. Norton JA, Wood DE, Day BL: Is the spinal cord the generator of 16-Hz orthostatic tremor? Neurology 2004;62:632-634.
181. Wu YR, Ashby P, Lang AE: Orthostatic tremor arises from an oscillator in the posterior fossa. Mov Disord 2001;16:272-279.
182. Tsai CH, Semmler JG, Kimber TE, et al: Modulation of primary orthostatic tremor by magnetic stimulation over the motor cortex. J Neurol Neurosurg Psychiatry 1998;64:33-36.
183. Katzenschlager R, Costa D, Gerschlager W, et al: [123I]-FP-CIT-SPECT demonstrates dopaminergic deficit in orthostatic tremor. Ann Neurol 2003;53:489-496.
184. Poersch M: Orthostatic tremor: combined treatment with primidone and clonazepam. Mov Disord 1994;9:467.
185. Wills AJ, Brusa L, Wang HC, et al: Levodopa may improve orthostatic tremor: case report and trial of treatment. J Neurol Neurosurg Psychiatry 1999;66:681-684.
186. Evidente VG, Adler CH, Caviness JN, Gwinn KA: Effective treatment of orthostatic tremor with gabapentin. Mov Disord 1998;13:829-831.
187. Onofrj M, Thomas A, Paci C, D'Andreamatteo G: Gabapentin in orthostatic tremor: results of a double-blind crossover with placebo in four patients. Neurology 1998;51:880-882.
188. Rodrigues JP, Edwards DJ, Walters SE, et al: Gabapentin can improve postural stability and quality of life in primary orthostatic tremor. Mov Disord 2005;20:865-870.
189. Schneider SA, Bhatia KP: The entity of jaw tremor and dystonia. Mov Disord 2007;22:1491-1495.
190. Deuschl G: Dystonic tremor. Rev Neurol (Paris) 2003;159(10 Pt 1):900-905.
191. Rivest J, Marsden CD: Trunk and head tremor as isolated manifestations of dystonia. Mov Disord 1990;5:60-65.
192. Masuhr F, Wissel J, Muller J, et al: Quantification of sensory trick impact on tremor amplitude and frequency in 60 patients with head tremor. Mov Disord 2000;15:960-964.
193. Micheli S, Fernandez-Pardal M, Quesada P, et al: Variable onset of adult inherited focal dystonia: a problem for genetic studies. Mov Disord 1994;9:64-68.
194. Sheehy MP, Marsden CD: Writers' cramp—a focal dystonia. Brain 1982;105(Pt 3):461-480.
195. Schneider SA, Edwards MJ, Mir P, et al: Patients with adult-onset dystonic tremor resembling parkinsonian tremor have scans without evidence of dopaminergic deficit (SWEDDs). Mov Disord 2007;22:2210-2215.
196. Munchau A, Schrag A, Chuang C, et al: Arm tremor in cervical dystonia differs from essential tremor and can be classified by onset age and spread of symptoms. Brain 2001;124(Pt 9):1765-1776.
197. Ferraz HB, De Andrade LA, Silva SM, et al: [Postural tremor and dystonia. Clinical aspects and physiopathological considerations]. Arq Neuropsiquiatr 1994;52:466-470.
198. Bartolome FM, Fanjul S, Cantarero S, et al: [Primary focal dystonia: descriptive study of 205 patients]. Neurologia 2003;18:59-65.
199. Shukla G, Behari M: A clinical study of non-parkinsonian and non-cerebellar tremor at a specialty movement disorders clinic. Neurol India 2004;52:200-202.
200. Jedynak CP, Bonnet AM, Agid Y: Tremor and idiopathic dystonia. Mov Disord 1991;6:230-236.
201. Marsden CD: Dystonia: the spectrum of the disease. Res Publ Assoc Res Nerv Ment Dis 1976;55:351-367.
202. Vidailhet M, Jedynak CP, Pollak P, Agid Y: Pathology of symptomatic tremors. Mov Disord 1998;13(Suppl 3):49-54.
203. Miwa H, Hatori K, Kondo T, et al: Thalamic tremor: case reports and implications of the tremor-generating mechanism. Neurology 1996;46:75-79.

204. Kim JS: Delayed onset mixed involuntary movements after thalamic stroke: clinical, radiological and pathophysiological findings. Brain 2001;124(Pt 2):299-309.
205. Lehericy S, Grand S, Pollak P, et al: Clinical characteristics and topography of lesions in movement disorders due to thalamic lesions. Neurology 2001;57:1055-1066.
206. Hensman DJ, Bain PG: Levodopa can worsen tremor associated with dystonia. Mov Disord 2006;21:1778-1780.
207. Jankovic J, Schwartz K: Botulinum toxin treatment of tremors. Neurology 1991;41:1185-1188.
208. Coubes P, Roubertie A, Vayssiere N, et al: Treatment of DYT1-generalised dystonia by stimulation of the internal globus pallidus. Lancet 2000;355:2220-2221.
209. Chou KL, Hurtig HI, Jaggi JL, Baltuch GH: Bilateral subthalamic nucleus deep brain stimulation in a patient with cervical dystonia and essential tremor. Mov Disord 2005;20:377-380.
210. Plaha P, Khan S, Gill SS: Bilateral stimulation of the caudal zona incerta nucleus for tremor control. J Neurol Neurosurg Psychiatry 2008;79:504-513.
211. Rothwell JC, Traub MM, Marsden CD: Primary writing tremor. J Neurol Neurosurg Psychiatry 1979;42:1106-1114.
212. Klawans HL, Glantz R, Tanner CM, Goetz CG: Primary writing tremor: a selective action tremor. Neurology 1982;32:203-206.
213. Elble RJ, Moody C, Higgins C: Primary writing tremor: a form of focal dystonia? Mov Disord 1990;5:118-126.
214. Soland VL, Bhatia KP, Volonte MA, Marsden CD: Focal task-specific tremors. Mov Disord 1996;11:665-670.
215. Bain PG, Findley LJ, Britton TC, et al: Primary writing tremor. Brain 1995;118(Pt 6):1461-1472.
216. Modugno N, Nakamura Y, Bestmann S, et al: Neurophysiological investigations in patients with primary writing tremor. Mov Disord 2002;17:1336-1340.
217. Papapetropoulos S, Singer C: Treatment of primary writing tremor with botulinum toxin type a injections: report of a case series. Clin Neuropharmacol 2006;29:364-367.
218. Ohye C, Miyazaki M, Hirai T, et al: Primary writing tremor treated by stereotactic selective thalamotomy. J Neurol Neurosurg Psychiatry 1982;45:988-997.
219. Minguez-Castellanos A, Carnero-Pardo C, Gomez-Camello A, et al: Primary writing tremor treated by chronic thalamic stimulation. Mov Disord 1999;14:1030-1033.
220. Racette BA, Dowling J, Randle J, Mink JW: Thalamic stimulation for primary writing tremor. J Neurol 2001;248:380-382.
221. Espay AJ, Hung SW, Sanger TD, et al: A writing device improves writing in primary writing tremor. Neurology 2005;64:1648-1650.
222. Alusi SH, Worthington J, Glickman S, Bain PG: A study of tremor in multiple sclerosis. Brain 2001;124(Pt 4):720-730.
223. Louis ED, Lynch T, Ford B, et al: Delayed-onset cerebellar syndrome. Arch Neurol 1996;53:450-454.
224. Neiman J, Lang AE, Fornazzari L, Carlen PL: Movement disorders in alcoholism: a review. Neurology 1990;40:741-746.
225. Flament D, Hore J: Movement and electromyographic disorders associated with cerebellar dysmetria. J Neurophysiol 1986;55:1221-1233.
226. Flament D, Hore J: Comparison of cerebellar intention tremor under isotonic and isometric conditions. Brain Res. 1988;439(1-2):179-186.
227. Hore J, Flament D: Evidence that a disordered servo-like mechanism contributes to tremor in movements during cerebellar dysfunction. J Neurophysiol 1986;56:123-136.
228. Hallett M, Shahani BT, Young RR: EMG analysis of patients with cerebellar deficits. J Neurol Neurosurg Psychiatry 1975;38:1163-1169.
229. Mauritz KH, Schmitt C, Dichgans J: Delayed and enhanced long latency reflexes as the possible cause of postural tremor in late cerebellar atrophy. Brain 1981;104(Pt 1):97-116.
230. Hallett M, Ravits J, Dubinsky RM, et al: A double-blind trial of isoniazid for essential tremor and other action tremors. Mov Disord 1991;6:253-256.
231. Rascol A, Clanet M, Montastruc JL, et al: L5H tryptophan in the cerebellar syndrome treatment. Biomedicine 1981;35:112-113.
232. Trouillas P, Xie J, Getenet JC, et al: [Effect of buspirone, a serotonergic 5-HT-1A agonist in cerebellar ataxia: a pilot study: preliminary communication]. Rev Neurol (Paris) 1995;151:708-713.
233. Fox P, Bain PG, Glickman S, et al: The effect of cannabis on tremor in patients with multiple sclerosis. Neurology 2004;62:1105-1109.

234. Alusi SH, Aziz TZ, Glickman S, et al: Stereotactic lesional surgery for the treatment of tremor in multiple sclerosis: a prospective case-controlled study. Brain 2001;124(Pt 8):1576-1589.
235. Lozano AM: Vim thalamic stimulation for tremor. Arch Med Res. 2000;31:266-269.
236. Mathieu D, Kondziolka D, Niranjan A, et al: Gamma knife thalamotomy for multiple sclerosis tremor. Surg Neurol 2007;68:394-399.
237. Masucci EF, Kurtzke JF, Saini N: Myorhythmia: a widespread movement disorder: clinicopathological correlations. Brain 1984;107:53-79.
238. Remy P, de Recondo A, Defer G, et al: Peduncular 'rubral' tremor and dopaminergic denervation: a PET study. Neurology 1995;45(3 Pt 1):472-477.
239. Deuschl G, Wilms H, Krack P, et al: Function of the cerebellum in Parkinsonian rest tremor and Holmes' tremor. Ann Neurol 1999;46:126-128.
240. Krack P, Deuschl G, Kaps M, et al: Delayed onset of "rubral tremor" 23 years after brainstem trauma. Mov Disord 1994;9:240-242.
241. Tan JH, Chan BP, Wilder-Smith EP, Ong BK: A unique case of reversible hyperglycemic Holmes' tremor. Mov Disord 2006;21:707-709.
242. Kim MC, Son BC, Miyagi Y, Kang JK: Vim thalamotomy for Holmes' tremor secondary to midbrain tumour. J Neurol Neurosurg Psychiatry 2002;73:453-455.
243. Kudo M, Goto S, Nishikawa S, et al: Bilateral thalamic stimulation for Holmes' tremor caused by unilateral brainstem lesion. Mov Disord 2001;16:170-174.
244. Nikkhah G, Prokop T, Hellwig B, et al: Deep brain stimulation of the nucleus ventralis intermedius for Holmes (rubral) tremor and associated dystonia caused by upper brainstem lesions: report of two cases. J Neurosurg 2004;100:1079-1083.
245. Romanelli P, Bronte-Stewart H, Courtney T, Heit G: Possible necessity for deep brain stimulation of both the ventralis intermedius and subthalamic nuclei to resolve Holmes tremor: case report. J Neurosurg 2003;99:566-571.
246. Foote KD, Okun MS: Ventralis intermedius plus ventralis oralis anterior and posterior deep brain stimulation for posttraumatic Holmes tremor: two leads may be better than one: technical note. Neurosurgery 2005;56(2 Suppl). E445.
247. Goto S, Yamada K: Combination of thalamic Vim stimulation and GPi pallidotomy synergistically abolishes Holmes' tremor. J Neurol Neurosurg Psychiatry 2004;75:1203-1204.
248. Lim DA, Khandhar SM, Heath S, et al: Multiple target deep brain stimulation for multiple sclerosis related and poststroke Holmes' tremor. Stereotact Funct Neurosurg 2007;85:144-149.
249. Yeung KB, Thomas PK, King RH, et al: The clinical spectrum of peripheral neuropathies associated with benign monoclonal IgM, IgG and IgA paraproteinaemia: comparative clinical, immunological and nerve biopsy findings. J Neurol 1991;238:383-391.
250. Busby M, Donaghy M: Chronic dysimmune neuropathy: a subclassification based upon the clinical features of 102 patients. J Neurol 2003;250:714-724.
251. Cardoso F, Jankovic J: Movement disorders. Neurol Clin 1993;11:625-638.
252. Dalakas MC, Teravainen H, Engel WK: Tremor as a feature of chronic relapsing and dysgammaglobulinemic polyneuropathies: incidence and management. Arch Neurol 1984;41:711-714.
253. Bain PG, Britton TC, Jenkins IH, et al: Tremor associated with benign IgM paraproteinaemic neuropathy. Brain 1996;119(Pt 3):789-799.
254. Plante-Bordeneuve V, Guiochon-Mantel A, Lacroix C, et al: The Roussy-Levy family: from the original description to the gene. Ann Neurol 1999;46:770-773.
255. Ruzicka E, Jech R, Zarubova K, et al: VIM thalamic stimulation for tremor in a patient with IgM paraproteinaemic demyelinating neuropathy. Mov Disord 2003;18:1192-1195.
256. Lapresle J: Palatal myoclonus. Adv Neurol 1986;43:265-273.
257. Deuschl G, Mischke G, Schenck E, et al: Symptomatic and essential rhythmic palatal myoclonus. Brain 1990;113(Pt 6):1645-1672.
258. Deuschl G, Toro C, Valls SJ, et al: Symptomatic and essential palatal tremor, 1: clinical, physiological and MRI analysis. Brain 1994;117:775-788.
259. Samuel M, Torun N, Tuite PJ, et al: Progressive ataxia and palatal tremor (PAPT): clinical and MRI assessment with review of palatal tremors. Brain 2004;127(Pt 6):1252-1268.
260. Deuschl G, Jost S, Schumacher M: Symptomatic palatal tremor is associated with signs of cerebellar dysfunction. J Neurol 1996;243:553-556.
261. Deuschl G, Toro C, Hallett M: Symptomatic and essential palatal tremor, 2: differences of palatal movements. Mov Disord 1994;9:676-678.
262. Llinas R, Volkind RA: The olivo-cerebellar system: functional properties as revealed by harmaline-induced tremor. Exp Brain Res 1973;18:69-87.

263. Elble RJ: Inhibition of forearm EMG by palatal myoclonus. Mov Disord 1991;6:324-329.
264. Leigh RJ, Averbuch HL, Tomsak RL, et al: Treatment of abnormal eye movements that impair vision: strategies based on current concepts of physiology and pharmacology. Ann Neurol 1994;36:129-141.
265. Repka MX, Savino PJ, Reinecke RD: Treatment of acquired nystagmus with botulinum neurotoxin A. Arch Ophthalmol 1994;112:1320-1324.
266. Bakheit AM, Behan PO: Palatal myoclonus successfully treated with clonazepam [Letter]. J Neurol Neurosurg Psychiatry 1990;53:806.
267. Jabbari B, Scherokman B, Gunderson CH, et al: Treatment of movement disorders with trihexyphenidyl. Mov Disord 1989;4:202-212.
268. Morgan JC, Sethi KD: Drug-induced tremors. Lancet Neurol 2005;4:866-876.
269. Stacy M, Jankovic J: Tardive tremor. Mov Disord 1992;7:53-57.
270. Karas BJ, Wilder BJ, Hammond EJ, Bauman AW: Treatment of valproate tremors. Neurology 1983;33:1380-1382.
271. Starosta-Rubinstein S, Young AB, Kluin K, et al: Clinical assessment of 31 patients with Wilson's disease: correlations with structural changes on magnetic resonance imaging. Arch Neurol 1987;44:365-370.
272. Takahashi W, Yoshii F, Shinohara Y: Reversible magnetic resonance imaging lesions in Wilson's disease: clinical-anatomical correlation. J Neuroimaging 1996;6:246-248.
273. Schumacher G, Platz KP, Mueller AR, et al: Liver transplantation: treatment of choice for hepatic and neurological manifestation of Wilson's disease. Clin Transplant 1997;11:217-224.
274. Factor SA, Podskalny GD, Molho ES: Psychogenic movement disorders: Frequency, clinical profile, and characteristics. J Neurol Neurosurg Psychiatry 1995;59:406-412.
275. Kim YJ, Pakiam AS, Lang AE: Historical and clinical features of psychogenic tremor: a review of 70 cases. Can J Neurol Sci 1999;26:190-195.
276. Deuschl G, Koster B, Lucking CH, Scheidt C: Diagnostic and pathophysiological aspects of psychogenic tremors. Mov Disord 1998;13:294-302.
277. Brown P, Thompson PD: Electrophysiological aids to the diagnosis of psychogenic jerks, spasms, and tremor. Mov Disord 2001;16:595-599.
278. McAuley JH, Rothwell JC, Marsden CD, Findley LJ: Electrophysiological aids in distinguishing organic from psychogenic tremor. Neurology 1998;50:1882-1884.
279. Raethjen J, Kopper F, Govindan RB, et al: Two different pathogenetic mechanisms in psychogenic tremor. Neurology 2004;63:812-815.
280. Voon V, Lang AE: Antidepressant treatment outcomes of psychogenic movement disorder. J Clin Psychiatry 2005;66:1529-1534.
281. Feinstein A, Stergiopoulos V, Fine J, Lang AE: Psychiatric outcome in patients with a psychogenic movement disorder: a prospective study. Neuropsychiatry Neuropsychol Behav Neurol 2001;14:169-176.
282. Danek A: Geniospasm: hereditary chin trembling. Mov Disord 1993;8:335-338.
283. Soland VL, Bhatia KP, Sheean GL, Marsden CD: Hereditary geniospasm: two new families. Mov Disord 1996;11:744-746.
284. Bakar M, Zarifoglu M, Bora I, et al: Treatment of hereditary trembling chin with botulinum toxin. Mov Disord 1998;13:845-846.
285. Erer S, Jankovic J: Hereditary chin tremor in Parkinson's disease. Clin Neurol Neurosurg 2007;109:784-785.
286. Destee A, Cassim F, Defebvre L, Guieu JD: Hereditary chin trembling or hereditary chin myoclonus? J Neurol Neurosurg Psychiatry 1997;63:804-807.
287. Jarman PR, Wood NW, Davis MT, et al: Hereditary geniospasm: linkage to chromosome 9q13-q21 and evidence for genetic heterogeneity. Am J Hum Genet. 1997;61:928-933.
288. Devetag Chalaupka F, Bartholini F, Mandich G, Turro M: Two new families with hereditary essential chin myoclonus: clinical features, neurophysiological findings and treatment. Neurol Sci. 2006;27:97-103.
289. Hagerman PJ, Hagerman RJ: Fragile X-associated tremor/ataxia syndrome (FXTAS). Ment Retard Dev Disabil Res Rev 2004;10:25-30.
290. Hall DA, Hagerman RJ, Hagerman PJ, et al: Prevalence of FMR1 repeat expansions in movement disorders: a systematic review. Neuroepidemiology 2006;26:151-155.
291. Berry-Kravis E, Abrams L, Coffey SM, et al: Fragile X-associated tremor/ataxia syndrome: clinical features, genetics, and testing guidelines. Mov Disord 2007;22:2018-2030.

292. Vengud E, Jacquy J, Vanderkelen B, Manto MU: [High-frequency synchronous bursts firing associated with asynchronous midbrain tremor]. Rev Neurol (Paris) 2001;157(6-7):682-687.
293. Manto MU, Pandolfo M, Moore J: Bilateral high-frequency synchronous discharges: a new form of tremor in humans. Arch Neurol 2003;60:416-422.
294. Shaikh AG, Miura K, Optican LM, et al: A new familial disease of saccadic oscillations and limb tremor provides clues to mechanisms of common tremor disorders. Brain 2007;130(Pt 11): 3020-3031.
295. Biary N, Koller WC: Essential tongue tremor. Mov Disord 1987;2:25-29.
296. Topaloglu H, Gucuyener K, Orkun C, Renda Y: Tremor of tongue and dysarthria as the sole manifestation of Wilson's disease. Clin Neurol Neurosurg 1990;92:295-296.
297. Chung SJ, Im JH, Lee JH, et al: Isolated tongue tremor after gamma knife radiosurgery for acoustic schwannoma. Mov Disord 2005;20:108-111.
298. Kim SJ, Lee WY, Kim BJ, et al: Isolated tongue tremor after removal of cerebellar pilocytic astrocytoma: functional analysis with SPECT study. Mov Disord 2007;22:1825-1828.
299. Costa J, Henriques R, Barroso C, et al: Upper limb tremor induced by peripheral nerve injury. Neurology 2006;67:1884-1886.
300. Jankovic J, Van der Linden C: Dystonia and tremor induced by peripheral trauma: predisposing factors. J Neurol Neurosurg Psychiatry 1988;51:1512-1519.
301. Koller WC, Wong GF, Lang A: Posttraumatic movement disorders: a review. Mov Disord 1989;4:20-36.
302. Ellis SJ: Tremor and other movement disorders after whiplash type injuries. J Neurol Neurosurg Psychiatry 1997;63:110-112.
303. Bhatia KP, Bhatt MH, Marsden CD: The causalgia-dystonia syndrome. Brain 1993;116(Pt 4):843-851.
304. Chen R, Ashby P, Lang AE: Stimulus-sensitive myoclonus in akinetic-rigid syndromes. Brain 1992;115:1875-1888.
305. Thompson PD, Day BL, Rothwell JC, et al: The myoclonus in corticobasal degeneration: evidence for two forms of cortical reflex myoclonus. Brain 1994;44:578-591.
306. Wang HC, Hsu WC, Brown P: Cortical tremor secondary to a frontal cortical lesion. Mov Disord 1999;14:370-374.
307. Fung VS, Duggins A, Morris JG, Lorentz IT: Progressive myoclonic ataxia associated with celiac disease presenting as unilateral cortical tremor and dystonia. Mov Disord 2000;15:732-734.

30 Other Choreas

RUTH H. WALKER

Introduction

The term *chorea* refers to involuntary movements of the limbs, trunk, neck, or face that rapidly flit from region to region in an irregular pattern. This movement disorder may be due to numerous neurological disorders, and the specific diagnosis may be suggested by features of the patient's history and examination (Table 30–1). The work-up of a patient with chorea can be extensive (Table 30–2). The development of genetic tests has resulted in the molecular identification of many hereditary causes of chorea, and in many cases has expanded the phenotype of genetically defined disorders. There are many well-characterized genetic disorders that typically cause chorea, and others in which it may occur less often, for example as part of a phenotype of a mixed movement disorder (Tables 30–3 and 30–4). Chorea may also be a feature of metabolic disturbances that affect neuronal function in a manner apparently identical to that seen in neurodegenerative diseases. Similarly, structural lesions can physically disrupt neuronal pathways with the same phenotypic result.

TABLE 30–1	History and Clinical Features in the Evaluation of a Patient with Chorea
Key Element	**Possible Diagnosis**
Onset: acute versus chronic	Stroke, metabolic disorder (e.g., hyperglycemia) versus neurodegenerative disease
Medication	Medication effect or tardive syndrome
Systemic illness	Metabolic effect (e.g., thyroid disease, diabetes); CNS involvement (e.g., autoimmune disease, metastatic disease, paraneoplastic syndrome)
Family history	AD, AR, X-linked, mitochondrial disease
Psychiatric features, cognitive impairment	Frontotemporal cortical involvement; subcortical dementia
Localizing neurological features	Structural lesion; multifocal disease

AD, autosomal dominant; AR, autosomal recessive; CNS, central nervous system.

Pathophysiology of Chorea

The model developed by Albin and colleagues,[1] despite criticisms of its limitations,[2-4] can still be used to understand many of the pathophysiological aspects of movement disorders. It is postulated that the direct pathway is responsible for activation of a motor program after an input from the motor cortex, and that the indirect pathway focuses and selects the movements (Fig. 30–1A).[5] This process most likely happens at several levels of the basal ganglia, including the caudate/putamen, subthalamic nucleus (STN), and globus pallidus internus (GPi) because disruption of the pathway at different sites may result in similar movements. Signal selection is likely controlled by temporally and spatially distributed mechanisms.

According to the classic model,[1,6] chorea may be attributed to a decrease in activity of the indirect pathway from the caudate/putamen to the globus pallidus externus (see Fig. 30–1). This results in overactivity of this nucleus, and increased inhibition and decreased activity of its projection targets, the STN, the GPi, and the substantia nigra pars reticularis. This model correlates with the fact that lesions of the STN are also well known to cause chorea (hemiballismus) (see Fig. 30–1B). According to the model, this hyperkinetic movement disorder is due to a decrease in the afferents from the STN to the GPi (indirect pathway) (see Fig. 30–1C), resulting in a loss of selection of motor signals that have arrived from the striatum via the direct pathway.[5] The motor thalamus is disinhibited, and an increased signal is conveyed to the motor cortex, resulting in the production of involuntary movements.

At present, this explanation of chorea remains a model, and the pathophysiology of chorea in vivo is not well understood. Apart from involvement of the caudate/putamen, neuropathological studies have not been informative in understanding the mechanisms of production of chorea. In early Huntington's disease (HD), the biological data support the model, in that the enkephalinergic neurons of the indirect pathway typically degenerate first.[7] In other circumstances, the

TABLE 30–2	**Laboratory Evaluation of the Patient with Chorea**
Test	**Possible Diagnosis**
Blood chemistry	Hyper-/hypoglycemia; hyper-/hyponatremia; hypomagnesemia; hyper-/hypocalcemia; Lesch-Nyhan syndrome
CBC with smear	Neuroacanthocytosis syndrome (chorea-acanthocytosis, McLeod syndrome, HDL2, PKAN)
Liver function tests	Wilson's disease; choreoacanthocytosis; McLeod syndrome
Thyroid function tests	Hypo-/hyperthyroidism
Parathyroid levels	Hypo-/hyperparathyroidism
Pregnancy test	Chorea gravidarum
Creatine phosphokinase	Choreoacanthocytosis; McLeod syndrome
Ceruloplasmin	Wilson's disease; aceruloplasminemia
Ferritin	Neuroferritinopathy
Erythrocyte sedimentation rate, antinuclear antibodies	Autoimmune disease
Lupus anticoagulant	Systemic lupus erythematosus
Antiphospholipid antibodies	Antiphospholipid syndrome
ASO titers	Sydenham's chorea
HIV test	HIV/AIDS-related infection
Antigliadin antibodies	Celiac disease
Antineuronal antibodies (anti-CRMP-5, anti-Hu, anti-Yo)	Paraneoplastic syndromes
RBC Kell and Kx antigens	McLeod syndrome
Genetic testing	See Table 30-3
MRI/CT with contrast enhancement	Structural lesions; iron deposition; calcification
EEG	Seizure-related syndrome; Creutzfeldt-Jakob disease
CSF (14-3-3 protein; cell count, chemistry, microbiology)	Creutzfeldt-Jakob disease; chronic infection
Urinary and serum organic and amino acids	Organic/amino acidopathies

CBC, complete blood count; CSF, cerebrospinal fluid; EEG, electroencephalography; HDL2, Huntington's disease–like 2; HIV, human immunodeficiency virus; PKAN, pantothenate kinase–associated neurodegeneration; RBC, red blood cell.

model does not fit the experimental data so well, however, and these data are discussed in detail elsewhere.[2-4] Most other neurodegenerative choreas are rare, and come to postmortem examination only at advanced stages of disease when there is typically marked and nonspecific atrophy of the caudate/putamen. Decreased numbers of several classes of interneurons, including large cholinergic and various GABAergic subtypes, in a single case of benign hereditary chorea type 1[8] suggest that the loss of inhibition of projection neurons of the indirect pathway by these interneurons[9] may be a potential mechanism for the generation of chorea.

Functional imaging studies have similarly been uninformative in shedding light on the pathophysiology of chorea. Metabolic activity may be decreased in the putamen in neurodegenerative,[10-12] structural,[13] metabolic,[14] and benign[15] choreas, but normal[16,17] or increased in metabolic or benign choreas.[18-21]

Metabolic Causes

A common cause of reversible chorea in adults is nonketotic hyperglycemia in diabetics, which may manifest acutely with hemichorea. Neuroimaging in these cases shows hyperintensity of the contralateral putamen on T1-weighted and T2-weighted magnetic resonance imaging (MRI).[22,23] These studies suggest that this hyperintensity may be due to breakdown of the blood-brain barrier as a result of inflammation and edema,[24] or possibly hyperviscosity.[25] The movement disorder usually reverses with correction of the metabolic abnormality, but may persist for months after resolution of hyperglycemia.[26] It is unknown why this syndrome is typically unilateral.

Autoimmune Disorders

An autoimmune mechanism may be the etiology of movement disorders in systemic lupus erythematosus,[27,28] Sjögren's syndrome,[29] and other autoimmune disorders in light of reports of antibodies against components of basal ganglia neurons. The association of chorea with antiphospholipid antibodies (including anticardiolipin antibodies and lupus anticoagulant), as part of an antiphospholipid antibody syndrome is reported in the literature,[30] but more recently has been subject to debate.[31-33] Anti–basal ganglia antibodies have been reported in patients with various movement disorders,[34,35] including estrogen/progesterone-related chorea.[36]

Paraneoplastic chorea may occur occasionally,[37-42] and has been reported in renal carcinoma, small cell lung carcinoma, breast cancer, Hodgkin's lymphoma, and non-Hodgkin's lymphoma. This chorea seems to be due to anti-CRMP-5[41,43,44] or, less commonly, anti-Hu[42] neuronal autoantibodies. A case of chorea in a patient with anti-Yo antibodies and the more typical cerebellar degeneration has been reported.[45]

Polycythemia rubra vera may manifest with chorea.[46,47] It is unclear whether this chorea is due to the presence of autoantibodies or to hyperviscosity resulting in basal ganglia ischemia.

Celiac disease has been associated with numerous neurological complications. Chorea may occasionally be seen, which responds to a gluten-free diet.[48]

Drug-induced Choreas

Drug-induced choreas usually are not considered as choreiform disorders because the diagnosis is self-evident. Chorea induced by levodopa in Parkinson's disease is the most commonly seen drug-induced chorea in neurological practice. Despite extensive study of humans and animal models with levodopa-induced dyskinesias, and some significant progress,[49,50] the underlying mechanisms remain obscure.[51,52]

TABLE 30-3   Molecular Features of Genetic Choreiform Disorders

Diagnosis	Mode of Inheritance	Gene	Location	Protein Product	Mutation
HD	AD	HD	4p15	Huntingtin	Expanded CAG repeats
HDL1	AD	PRNP	20p12	Prion protein	192 nucleotide insertion
HDL2	AD	JPH	16q24.3	Junctophilin-3	Expanded CAG/CTG repeats
Spinocerebellar ataxia 1	AD	SC1	6p23	Ataxin-1	Expanded CAG repeats
Spinocerebellar ataxia 2	AD	SCA2	12q24	Ataxin-2	Expanded CAG repeats
Spinocerebellar ataxia 3	AD	MJD1	14q32.1	Ataxin-3	Expanded CAG repeats
Spinocerebellar ataxia 17	AD	TBP	6q.27	TATA-binding protein	Expanded CAA/CAG repeats
DRPLA	AD	DRPLA	12p13.31	Atrophin-1	Expanded CAG repeats
Benign hereditary chorea	AD	TITF-1 (NKX2.1); other	14q13.1	Thyroid transcription factor 1; other	Transversions, deletions, substitutions
Neuroferritinopathy	AD	FTL	19q13.3	Ferritin light chain	Adenine insertion
Paroxysmal kinesigenic dyskinesia	AD	EKD1; EKD2; EKD3	16p11-q12; 16q13-22.1; other	—	—
Paroxysmal nonkinesigenic dyskinesia	AD	MR-1	2q33	Myofibrillogenesis regulator	Missense
Paroxysmal exertional dyskinesia	AD	GLUT1/ SLC2A1	1p34.2	Glucose transporter	Frameshift, missense, deletions
Paroxysmal choreoathetosis/ episodic ataxia	AD	KCNA1	12p13; other	Potassium channel	Point mutation
Paroxysmal choreoathetosis/ spasticity	AD	—	1p.21	Potassium channels (?)	—

Disease	Inheritance	Gene	Locus	Protein	Mutation
Choreoacanthocytosis	AR	VPS13	9q21	Chorein	Many
PKAN	AR	PANK2	20p.13	Pantothenate kinase 2	Deletions, missense mutations
Karak syndrome	AR	PLA2G6	22q12-q13	Phospholipase A	Many
Aceruloplasminemia	AR	CP	3q23	Ceruloplasmin	Nonsense
Wilson's disease	AR	ATP7B	13q14.3	Copper-transporting ATPase 2	Many
HDL3	AR	NK	4p15.3	NK	NK
Infantile bilateral striatal necrosis	AR, Mitochondrial	NK	19q13.32-13.41, mitochondrial	—	—
Ataxia-telangiectasia	AR	ATM	11q22.3	Serine-protein kinase ATM	Many
Ataxia with oculomotor apraxia 1	AR	APTX	9p13.3	Aprataxin	Many
Ataxia with oculomotor apraxia 2	AR	SETX	9q34	senataxin	Truncation
Friedreich's ataxia	AR	frataxin	9p13	Frataxin	Trinucleotide expansion, deletion
McLeod syndrome	X-linked recessive	XK	Xp21	XK	Deletions, missense, insertions
Lubag	X-linked recessive	DYT3	Xq13.1	Multiple transcript system	Missense, deletions
Lesch-Nyhan syndrome	X-linked recessive	HPRT	Xq26-27	Hypoxanthine phosphoribosyltransferase	Many
Leigh syndrome	Mitochondrial	Many	Many	Many	Many

AD, autosomal dominant; AR, autosomal recessive; DPRLA, dentatorubropallidoluysian atrophy; HD, Huntington's disease; HDL2, Huntington's disease–like 2; NK, not known; PKAN, pantothenate kinase–associated neurodegeneration.

TABLE 30–4   Clinical Features of Genetic Choreiform Disorders

Diagnosis	Useful Blood Tests	Movement Disorder	Dementia	Other Neurological Features	Usual Age of Onset	Ethnic Predominance
HD	—	Chorea, dystonia, parkinsonism	+++	Ataxia, seizures (juvenile onset)	Inversely related to repeats	—
HDL1		Chorea, rigidity	+++	Seizures (variable)	20-40 yr	Swedish
HDL2	Acanthocytosis ±	Chorea, dystonia parkinsonism	+++	Hyperreflexia	Inversely related to repeats	African
Spinocerebellar ataxia 1	—	Chorea, dystonia	+	Ataxia, supranuclear ophthalmoplegia	Inversely related to repeats	—
Spinocerebellar ataxia 2	—	Chorea, dystonia, parkinsonism, tremor	++	Ataxia, supranuclear ophthalmoplegia	Inversely related to repeats	—
Spinocerebellar ataxia 3	—	Chorea, dystonia parkinsonism	+	Ataxia	Inversely related to repeats	—
Spinocerebellar ataxia 17	—	Chorea, dystonia parkinsonism	+++	Ataxia, hyperreflexia	Inversely related to repeats	—
DRPLA	—	Chorea, myoclonus	+++	Ataxia, seizures	Inversely related to repeats	Japanese
Benign hereditary chorea	—	Chorea	–	Mild ataxia	Childhood	—
Neuroferritinopathy	Reduced serum ferritin	Chorea, dystonia, parkinsonism	–	Spasticity, rigidity	40-55 yr	Northern English, French
Paroxysmal kinesigenic dyskinesia	—	Chorea, dystonia	–	(Seizures in ICCA)	Childhood	—
Paroxysmal nonkinesigenic dyskinesia	—	Chorea, dystonia	–	—	Childhood	—

	Lab findings	Movement disorder		Other features	Age of onset	Ethnicity
Paroxysmal exertional dyskinesia	—	Chorea, dystonia	-	—	Childhood	—
Paroxysmal choreoathetosis/episodic ataxia	—	Chorea, dystonia	-	Ataxia, myokymia, dysarthria	Childhood	—
Paroxysmal choreoathetosis/spasticity	—	Chorea, dystonia	+	Spasticity, dysarthria	Childhood	—
Chorea-acanthocytosis	Acanthocytosis; elevated CK, LFTs	Chorea, dystonia, parkinsonism	++	Seizures, orofacial self-mutilation, peripheral neuropathy	20-50 yr	Japanese
PKAN	Acanthocytosis ±	Chorea, dystonia	++	Spasticity, rigidity, retinal degeneration	Childhood (occasionally older)	—
Karak syndrome	—	Chorea, dystonia	++	Ataxia	Childhood	Arab
Aceruloplasminemia	Ceruloplasmin, glucose	Chorea, dystonia	++	Ataxia, retinal degeneration	30-50 yr	Japanese
Wilson's disease	Ceruloplasmin	Coarse tremor, parkinsonism	++	Psychiatric disease	6-55 yr	—
HDL3	—	Chorea, dystonia	+++	Seizures, spasticity, ataxia	Childhood	Arab
Infantile bilateral striatal necrosis	—	Chorea	+++	Pendular nystagmus, dysarthria, optic atrophy	Infancy	Israeli bedouin
Ataxia-telangiectasia	Elevated α-fetoprotein	Chorea	-	Ataxia, oculomotor apraxia, dysarthria	Early childhood	—
Ataxia with oculomotor apraxia I	Hypoalbuminemia, high cholesterol	Chorea, dystonia	++	Ataxia, oculomotor apraxia, peripheral neuropathy	Childhood	—

Table continued on following page

TABLE 30–4	Clinical Features of Genetic Choreiform Disorders (Continued)				
Ataxia with oculomotor apraxia 2	Elevated α-fetoprotein, high cholesterol	Chorea, dystonia	–	Ataxia, oculomotor apraxia, peripheral neuropathy	Childhood	—
Friedreich's ataxia	—	Dystonia, chorea	–	Ataxia, spasticity, myoclonus	Childhood	—
McLeod syndrome	Acanthocytosis; negative Kx antigen, decreased Kell antigens; increased CK, LFTs	Chorea, dystonia, parkinsonism, orofacial dyskinesias	++	Seizures, peripheral neuropathy, myopathy	40-70 yr	—
Lubag	—	Dystonia, chorea parkinsonism, tremor, myoclonus	–	—	10-40 yr	Filipino
Lesch-Nyhan syndrome	Hyperuricemia	Chorea, dystonia	+++	Spasticity, self-mutilation	Infancy	—
Leigh syndrome	Elevated lactate/pyruvate	Chorea, dystonia	+++	Hypotonia, cranial neuropathy, ataxia, seizures	Infancy	—

CK, creatine kinase; DRPLA, dentatorubropallidoluysian atrophy; HD, Huntington's disease; HDL1, HDL2, HDL3, Huntington's disease–like 1, 2, 3; ICCA, benign infantile convulsions and paroxysmal choreoathetosis; LFTs, liver function tests; PKAN, pantothenate kinase–associated neurodegeneration.

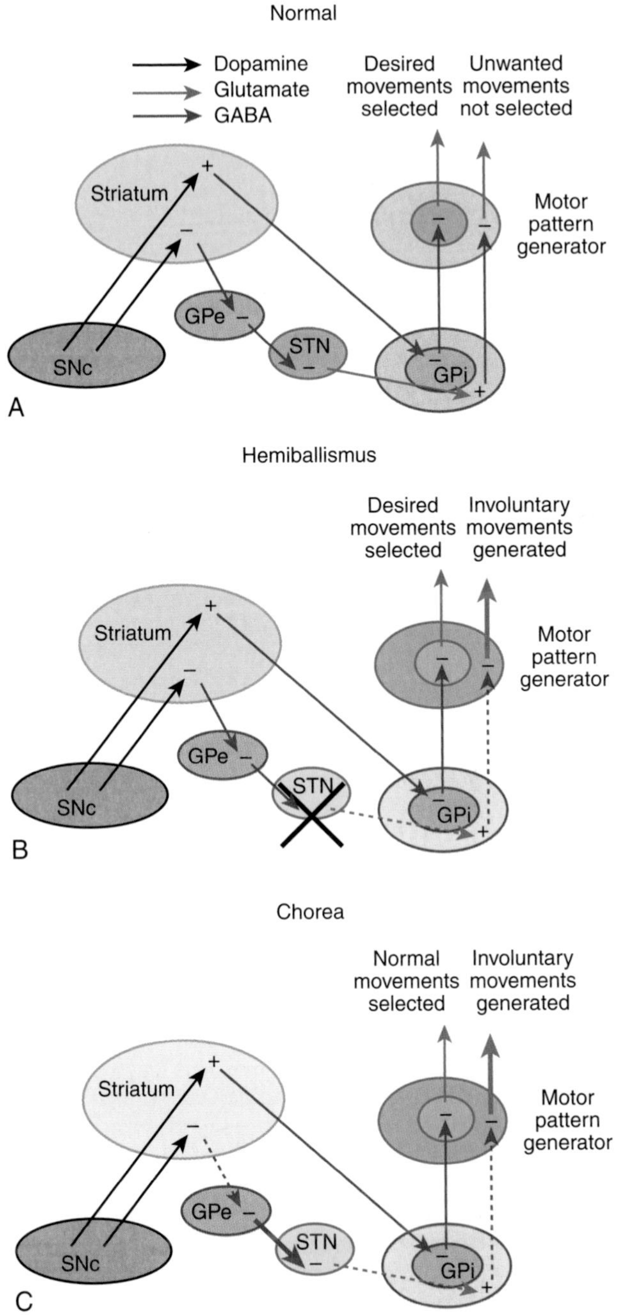

Figure 30–1 Classic model of basal ganglia circuitry. **A,** In normal conditions. **B,** Lesion of the subthalamic nucleus. **C,** Striatal pathology with decreased activity of the indirect pathway resulting in chorea. GABA, γ-aminobutyric acid; GPe, globus pallidus externus; GPi, globus pallidus internus; SNc, substantia nigra pars compacta; STN, subthalamic nucleus.

The pathophysiology of chorea in levodopa-induced dyskinesias may be shared by other conditions, however, and treatment may likewise be derived from insights gained from studies of animal models of this hyperkinetic disorder.

Tardive dyskinesia appears after the initiation of a dopamine-blocking medication, typically the classic neuroleptics, or other dopaminergic antagonists, such as prochlorperazine and metoclopramide. Of the second-generation antipsychotics, occasional cases of tardive dyskinesia have been reported with most agents, including risperidone,[53] olanzapine,[54,55] quetiapine,[56] ziprasidone,[56] clozapine, and aripiprazole. Use of these medications to treat tardive dyskinesia induced by other antipsychotics may also reduce symptom severity. The lesser risk of developing tardive dyskinesia with these medications should be balanced against other factors, such as the increased risk of metabolic syndrome and lengthening of the Q–T interval. The timing of the emergence of the symptoms, and the fact that tardive dyskinesia often does not resolve (and may even worsen) with discontinuation of the medication, makes it hard to confirm or refute the association of other medications with this disorder, but selective serotonin reuptake inhibitors (SSRIs), lithium, and anticonvulsant medications have also been implicated.

The use of estrogens in the contraceptive pill and as hormone replacement therapy[57] may result in chorea, presumably by the same mechanism that causes chorea gravidarum in pregnancy. Other medications, including anticonvulsants, acetylcholinesterase inhibitors,[58] and lithium,[59] may cause chorea. Stimulants, including those used therapeutically[60] and drugs used recreationally, such as amphetamine, cocaine, and specifically "crack" cocaine, may result in chorea ("crack-dancing"). The neuropharmacology of these agents, specifically the release of catecholamines, is the likely explanation for the appearance of the movement disorder. Usually the timing and the resolution of the movements with discontinuation of the offending agent makes the diagnosis and treatment straightforward.

Infectious and Postinfectious Causes

Sydenham's chorea is a common cause of reversible chorea in childhood, seen after a streptococcal throat infection. The recognition of tubulin[61] in basal ganglia neurons by antistreptococcal antibodies[62] seems to be the cause, although the pathophysiology of chorea remains obscure. Similarly, poststreptococcal anti–basal ganglia antibodies have been reported in patients with various other movement disorders, and it has been postulated that this might be a more common cause of movement disorders than was previously recognized.[34,35]

Various movement disorders have been associated with human immunodeficiency virus (HIV) infection.[63] Sometimes these are due to a mass lesion, such as lymphoma or abscess, whereas in other cases they may be a direct effect of HIV encephalopathy.[64,65] Creutzfeldt-Jakob disease, particularly new variant, related to bovine spongiform encephalopathy, should be considered,[66,67] especially if the course is of subacute deterioration over months.

In children, striatal necrosis may occur as a complication of measles encephalitis[68] or after undefined febrile illness.[69] A similar picture can be seen after *Mycoplasma pneumoniae* infection,[70] with a mixture of chorea and dystonia, hyperreflexia, and encephalopathy. Chorea has also been reported in the setting of encephalopathy secondary to parvovirus infection.[71]

Genetic Causes of Chorea

See Tables 30–3 and 30–4 for summaries of the genetic causes of chorea.

AUTOSOMAL DOMINANT CHOREAS

New genetic causes of chorea are being rapidly identified. HD remains the prototype of the autosomal dominantly–inherited choreiform disorder, but a few families with a Huntington's disease–like (HDL) phenotype lack the CAG repeat expansion in the huntingtin (*htt*) gene. In other families, the inheritance pattern of the neurological disorder seems to be autosomal recessive, X-linked, or pseudo-dominant. In addition to differences in inheritance, phenotypic presentation may help distinguish these disorders from HD.

Huntington's Disease–like 1

HDL1 is a rare inherited disorder resulting from mutations of the prion protein located at 20p12.[72,73] Patients develop personality change in early to middle adulthood, followed by chorea, rigidity, dysarthria, myoclonus, ataxia, and occasional seizures. Neuropathology of one patient showed generalized neuronal loss and gliosis.

Huntington's Disease–like 2

HDL2 is an autosomal dominantly–inherited disorder manifesting in the third or fourth decade with various movement disorders, including chorea, dystonia, or parkinsonism,[74] which may change with evolution of the disease and progressive cognitive and neuropsychiatric deficits.[75] Acanthocytosis can sometimes be seen, confusing the diagnosis with that of other neuroacanthocytosis syndromes.[76]

HDL2 is due to an uninterrupted CTG/CAG trinucleotide repeat expansion located within a variably spliced exon (labeled 2A) between exon 1 and exon 2B of junctophilin-3 (*JPH3*) on chromosome 16q24.3.[77] The repeat size is polymorphic, ranging from 6 to 28 CTG/CAG triplets in the normal population, whereas affected individuals have repeat expansions of 40 to 59 triplets; 29 to 39 repeats seems to be unstable with inheritance. Anticipation seems to be likely with longer repeat expansions correlating with a younger age of onset,[78] although it is unclear that expansion size affects clinical phenotype.

Junctophilin-3 seems to be involved in junctional membrane structures, and may play a role in the regulation of intracellular calcium. Mice without junctophilin-3 show impaired motor coordination, but examination of neuropathology has been limited.[79]

Neuropathology of HDL2 is identical to that seen in HD with intranuclear inclusions immunoreactive for ubiquitin and expanded polyglutamine repeats[75,80,81]; however, the pathophysiology may also be related to intracytoplasmic mRNA inclusions.[82] These were reduced in cell culture by cotransfection with the protein muscleblind-like 1, similar to the RNA inclusions in myotonic dystrophy, another CTG repeat expansion disorder.[82]

Most HDL2 patients reported have been of African ancestry,[75,77,83] and very few patients of white or Asian ancestry have yet been found.[83-86] The implications of this finding await haplotype analysis and comparison of the range of normal alleles in various African and non-African populations, but suggest either a rare common ancestral mutation or a population skewed toward longer alleles prone to expansion. Preliminary evidence may suggest the latter.[87]

Spinocerebellar Ataxias and Dentatorubropallidoluysian Atrophy

The phenotypes of the spinocerebellar ataxias (SCAs) can involve various movement disorders attributable to basal ganglia dysfunction, in addition to cerebellar signs. Most of these neurodegenerative disorders are due to expanded trinucleotide repeats with various proteins, but the size of the expansions does not generally seem to correlate with the phenotype.

SCA 3 (Machado-Joseph disease) can manifest with parkinsonism, dystonia, and chorea, usually in association with the typical cerebellar signs and eye findings. SCA 1, along with the cerebellar findings, may rarely manifest with or develop chorea during the evolution of the disease.[88,89] Patients with SCA 2 may also develop chorea occasionally (personal observations). Various movement disorders may be seen in SCA 17, which has also been referred to as HDL4, including parkinsonism, dystonia, and chorea.[83,90-93] An HD-like presentation was reported in a patient who was homozygous for the TBP expansion.[94]

Dentatorubropallidoluysian atrophy, more often found in Japanese populations, but occasionally in white[95-97] or African-American[98] families, may manifest with movement disorders, including chorea and myoclonus. Usual features are ataxia and dementia. Seizures are common in patients with onset before age 20, but tend to decrease with time, and are rare in older onset patients.

Benign Hereditary Chorea

Benign hereditary chorea type 1 has been associated with mutations of the gene for thyroid transcription factor 1 (*TITF-1*),[99-101] also known as *NKX2.1*. The chorea may respond to levodopa,[102] and may occasionally be accompanied by other movements such as dystonia and myoclonus.[103] Neuropathological findings are subtle and reflect alterations in a subset of striatal interneurons,[8] which are likely to be due to aberrant neuronal migration.[101] Striatal hypermetabolism[21] and hypometabolism[156] have been reported. Chorea has also been reported as part of a multisystem disorder resulting from a mutation of the same gene, causing congenital hypothyroidism, hypotonia, and pulmonary problems.[104-106]

Mutations of *TITF-1* are not found in all families with this disorder, which seems to be genetically heterogeneous.[107] Linkage has been identified for a locus on chromosome 8q21.3-q23.3 for benign hereditary chorea type 2, in which chorea develops in middle age.[108]

Neuroferritinopathy

Neuroferritinopathy is a disorder that falls under the classification of neurodegeneration with brain iron accumulation (see later) as the mutation of ferritin light chain results in iron deposition in the basal ganglia.[109] In contrast to the other disorders, most of which are inherited in autosomal recessive fashion (described later), this disorder is inherited in an autosomal dominant manner. Various movement disorders, including chorea, dystonia, and parkinsonism,[110-112] result, with onset at 40 to 55 years. Cognitive impairment is only occasionally a feature.[113]

Fahr's Disease

Fahr's disease (idiopathic basal ganglia calcification) refers to a heterogeneous group of disorders in which there is deposition of calcium in the basal ganglia and other cerebral regions, particularly the deep cerebellar nuclei. The clinical picture may include dystonia, parkinsonism, chorea, ataxia, cognitive impairment, and behavioral changes. In one family, linkage was shown to 14q (IBC1),[114] although the gene has not yet been identified. In several other families with autosomal dominant inheritance, linkage to this locus was excluded.[115-117] In other families, the pattern of inheritance and additional clinical features suggest mitochondrial inheritance.[118,119]

AUTOSOMAL RECESSIVE CHOREAS

Choreoacanthocytosis

The molecular diagnosis has never been confirmed of the original families reported with the disorder termed *Levine-Critchley syndrome,* or neuroacanthocytosis. Now that the various neuroacanthocytosis syndromes have been molecularly defined, the term *choreoacanthocytosis* is preferred for the autosomal recessive form, as confirmed by molecular or protein findings. The classic neuroacanthocytosis series by Hardie and colleagues[120] was heterogeneous, consisting of cases of choreoacanthocytosis, McLeod syndrome, and probable pantothenate kinase–associated neurodegeneration (PKAN).[121]

The typical neurological presentation of choreoacanthocytosis is the development in early to middle adulthood of chorea with marked lingual-buccal-facial dyskinesia and self-mutilation.[122-124] Similar to many other basal ganglia neurodegenerative disorders, the motor presentation may be preceded by psychiatric disease, behavioral changes, or subtle cognitive dysfunction. The use of neuroleptics may mask the development of the movement disorder.

In addition to chorea, vocal and motor tics[125] and parkinsonism[122] can be seen. Seizures are found in 40% of patients, and are often of temporal lobe origin. Peripheral neuropathy with areflexia is typical. Weight loss and nutritional compromise are frequent problems because of severe feeding dystonia, in particular due to tongue protrusion,[126] and dysphagia. Tongue and lip biting and other forms of self-mutilation, such as chronic scratching or finger biting, may be severe, and may be related to behavioral compulsions.[124]

The head of caudate nucleus is most vulnerable as observed neuroradiologically[127] and neuropathologically.[120] There is severe neuronal loss and gliosis primarily of the head of the caudate nucleus, but to a lesser extent of the putamen, globus pallidus, and substantia nigra. There is no evidence of inclusion bodies or other protein aggregates. The cortex seems to be relatively spared.

Laboratory testing frequently reveals elevated creatine kinase and liver enzymes, although hepatosplenomegaly seems to be less common than in McLeod syndrome (see later).[122] The appearance of acanthocytosis can vary,[128] and its absence does not exclude this diagnosis. Examination of wet peripheral blood smears diluted 1:1 in normal saline and 10 U/mL heparin may increase the likelihood of acanthocyte detection.[129]

Causative mutations are found in VPS13A (initially called CHAC) localized to chromosome 9q21.[130,131] This gene encodes for chorein, which seems to participate in protein sorting, suggesting that its dysfunction may result in cell membrane disruption, possibly explaining the abnormality of erythrocyte shape.[130] Absence of chorein in RBCs on Western blot confirms the diagnosis.[132]

Occasional Japanese families have been reported in which apparent autosomal dominant choreoacanthocytosis has been reported with a mutation of chorein in one allele.[133,134] Some of these patients appear phenotypically identical to patients with autosomal recessive inheritance, although others may have a milder or transient phenotype. Other pedigrees have been described in which dominant inheritance seems to have occurred,[135] although pseudodominant inheritance owing to consanguinity is a likely explanation.

Neurodegeneration with Brain Iron Accumulation

Several disorders caused by various different genetic mutations result in abnormal brain iron accumulation. This term includes autosomal dominantly–inherited neuroferritinopathy (described previously) and autosomal recessive PKAN (described subsequently). This term is also used for cases phenotypically and neuroradiologically resembling PKAN, but in which there is no mutation of PANK2, also including aceruloplasminemia and neuroaxonal dystrophy (see later). The signature MRI finding in all these disorders, is to iron deposition in the basal ganglia. Some NBIA cases remain undiagnosed.

Pantothenate Kinase–Associated Neurodegeneration

The disorder now known as PKAN is due to mutations of pantothenate kinase 2 (PANK2) located on chromosome 20p13.[136] The course in typical cases is of disease onset by age of 10 years, with dystonia and a rapid progression over the next 10 years.[137] Orofacial and limb dystonia, choreoathetosis, and spasticity are characteristic early features. Approximately one third of typical cases developed cognitive impairment, and two thirds had retinopathy. Eight percent of these patients had acanthocytosis. The typical MRI "eye-of-the-tiger" pattern of iron deposition in the globus pallidus is seen in most, but not all, of these patients.[138] HARPP syndrome (hypoprebetalipoproteinemia, acanthocytosis, retinitis pigmentosa, and pallidal degeneration)[139,140] is allelic with PKAN.[141]

In atypical cases, disease onset is in adulthood, with dystonia, rigidity, and gait freezing, but with slower progression and no retinopathy. Early speech difficulty, with pallilalia or dysarthria, is common, as is cognitive decline and personality change. In one third of these, there is a mutation of PANK2 and the diagnostic MRI finding, whereas in two thirds, neither of these was found.[137]

Most clinically typical cases are due to mutations of PANK2 causing protein truncation. Pantothenate kinase catalyzes the rate-limiting step in the synthesis of coenzyme A from vitamin B_5 (pantothenate). The amount of active enzyme correlates with the disease phenotype because typical patients have no active enzyme, but atypical patients, in whom there is a missense mutation of *PANK2*, may have some function.[137,138] The distribution of the neurological lesions is thought to relate to the accumulation of iron and other neurotoxic substances, and to local tissue demand for coenzyme A.[136] Impaired lipid synthesis may account for erythrocyte membrane abnormalities and acanthocytosis.

Neuroaxonal Syndrome

Karak syndrome, a rare syndrome of neurodegeneration with brain iron accumulation, reported to date in a single family,[142] is caused by mutation of *PLA2G6*, which codes for phospholipase A.[143] Mutation of the same gene also result in infantile neuroaxonal dystrophy, with movement disorders occurring in a typical forms of this syndrome. The cause of the phenotypic variation is unclear.

Aceruloplasminemia

Autosomal recessive inheritance of mutations of the gene for ceruloplasmin results in iron deposition in the cerebellum and basal ganglia.[144,145] Ceruloplasmin functions as a ferroxidase—iron oxidation from Fe^{2+} to Fe^{3+} is impaired, and neurons are more vulnerable to oxidative stress. The typical presentation is of retinal degeneration and diabetes mellitus in the 20s. In the 40s and 50s, neurological signs appear, usually ataxia, and subsequently dystonia (especially orofacial), parkinsonism, and chorea may develop. Dementia may manifest in later years. Symptomatic heteroplasmic carriers have also been reported. All cases to date have been Japanese apart from a single white American case, which was atypical in that iron was not seen on brain MRI.[146] Neuropathologically, astrocytes and neurons laden with iron are found in the cerebellum, basal ganglia, and cortex.[144,145]

Wilson's Disease

Chorea may be seen,[147,148] but is rarely reported as a presenting symptom of Wilson's disease. This treatable disease should always be considered, however, especially if serum liver enzyme levels are elevated.

Huntington's Disease–like 3

HDL3 was described in several young children in a consanguineous family who developed chorea, dystonia, dysarthria, cognitive impairment, and seizures.[149] Cortical and caudate nucleus atrophy were seen on neuroimaging. The genetic locus for this disorder was localized to 4p15.3, and was distinct from the HD locus, but this finding has been challenged.[150]

Infantile Bilateral Striatal Necrosis

Infantile bilateral striatal necrosis, with onset in infancy of chorea or dystonia or both, may be inherited in an autosomal recessive manner,[151] but also seems to be due to mitochondrial mutations.[152] The diagnostic findings are of bilateral lesions in the striatum on neuroimaging.

Autosomal Recessive Ataxias

Similar to the autosomal dominant ataxias, the autosomal recessive ataxias may also present with chorea. Friedreich's ataxia is the most common inherited autosomal recessive ataxia in Western populations, and chorea may occasionally develop, or may even be a presenting symptom before the development of the other features.[153-155] Chorea may also be seen in ataxia-telangiectasia and ataxia with oculomotor apraxia type 1 and type 2.

X-LINKED CHOREAS

McLeod Syndrome

The X-linked McLeod neuroacanthocytosis syndrome[156,157] is similar to autosomal recessive choreoacanthocytosis in its neurological presentation, with additional involvement of other organs. The blood group phenotype is defined by absent Kx and reduced Kell antigen expression on red blood cells (RBCs).[158] Mutation of the *XK* gene results in absent or dysfunctional XK protein, and absent expression of the Kx protein on the RBC membrane. In the RBC membrane, the XK protein is linked to the Kell protein via a disulfide bond, so Kell antigen expression is also affected.[159] The diagnosis can usually be confirmed at regional blood banks, which have the requisite panel of anti-Kell and anti-Kx antibodies. XK is postulated to be a membrane transport protein,[160] and is found in muscle and brain in addition to RBCs.[161-164] Acanthocytosis is typical, but occasionally may be absent.[165]

McLeod syndrome typically develops in middle-aged men.[157,161] Patients are often identified before the appearance of neurological symptoms by blood antigen typing, as was the eponymous patient. Patients with the mutation, but without any neurological or other abnormalities, have been reported.[166,167] Occasionally, carrier females are symptomatic, presumably due to X-chromosome inactivation.[120,161,168] The lack of genotype-phenotype correlation is suggested by the variability within families.[169,170]

Patients may present initially with psychiatric disease or subtle neurobehavioral changes, and the movement disorder may be attributed to medications. In addition to chorea, dystonia and parkinsonism may be seen. Facial hyperkinesias with dysarthria and involuntary vocalizations are frequent, although the self-mutilating lip biting seen in autosomal recessive choreoacanthocytosis is not characteristic. Peripheral sensorimotor neuropathy and areflexia are typical. Seizures are seen in 50%, and usually can be controlled with standard anticonvulsant medications.

Cardiomyopathy is seen in approximately two thirds of patients, and cardiac arrhythmias may be a significant source of morbidity and mortality.[157] Myopathy is primarily secondary to neuropathy,[171] but may be severe.[157,172] Elevated creatine kinase (often >1000 U/L) is seen in most cases and may evolve to rhabdomyolysis.[173] Liver enzymes are elevated, and hepatosplenomegaly is present in one third of patients. Hepatic failure may occasionally be a cause of morbidity.[165]

Neuroimaging typically shows decreased basal ganglia volume,[157] although white matter changes have been reported.[174] Neuropathological findings appear nonspecific, with neuronal loss and reactive gliosis.[175]

Because the RBC phenotype is characterized by decreased Kell and Kx antigen expression, transfusion with heterologous blood may result in production of anti-Kell antibodies. The anti-Kell antibodies may cause massive hemolysis with any subsequent heterologous transfusions.

Lubag

Lubag is an X-linked disorder characterized by dystonia and parkinsonism, and is found solely among Filipinos from the province of Capiz on the island of Panay.[176] A range of movement disorders have been reported, including chorea, tremor, and myoclonus.[177] Although mostly males are affected, occasional affected carrier females have been reported, one of whom had chorea.[178,179] The gene has been identified as coding for a multiple transcript system whose function is not yet known.[180]

Lesch-Nyhan Syndrome

Lesch-Nyhan syndrome is an X-linked disorder that is due to mutation of hypoxanthine phosphoribosyl transferase; it manifests at 3 to 6 months with psychomotor retardation and hypotonia. Subsequently, spasticity, dystonia and choreoathetosis develop. A typical feature is self-mutilation with biting of the hands and lips, but this is not an invariable feature.[181] The enzyme deficiency results in the accumulation of uric acid, due to impaired phosphorylation of hypoxanthine and guanine.

▎ Other Pediatric Metabolic Causes of Chorea

LEIGH'S SYNDROME

Leigh's syndrome is due to numerous different mutations of mitochondrial DNA, and manifests in early childhood, although adult-onset presentation has been reported.[182] Characteristically, lesions in the thalamus or caudate/putamen are seen on neuroimaging. Various neurological signs may be present, including acute encephalopathy, psychomotor retardation, hypotonia, spasticity, myopathy, dysarthria, seizures, dystonia, and chorea. An overlap with MELAS (mitochondrial encephalomyopathy, lactic acidosis and stroke-like episodes) may occur.[183] Other mitochondrial disorders may also manifest with chorea.[184]

OTHER INHERITED METABOLIC DISORDERS

Various movement disorders may be present in numerous metabolic diseases. These are typically part of a constellation of neurological abnormalities, which may vary with the age of presentation. Dystonia seems to be more common than chorea, possibly because of the coexistence of rigidity or spasticity from pyramidal tract involvement. Autosomal recessive inheritance of mutations of crucial enzymes is the cause. These disorders are diagnosed by assaying blood and urine for amino acids, by enzyme assays in lymphocytes, or by genetic testing.

Glutaricaciduria typically manifests with generalized dystonia, although chorea is sometimes seen,[185,186] in addition to features of encephalopathy. Often the presentation is catastrophic in early infancy, but occasionally this disorder may manifest more insidiously in later childhood or even adulthood. On MRI, dilation of the sylvian fissures and lesions of the putamen can be seen. Chorea, typically mild, can be seen in propionicacidemia, due to propionic–CoA carboxylase deficiency.[187,188] Other aminoacidopathies in which chorea may occasionally be seen include 3-methylglutaconicaciduria[189] and succinate-semialdehyde dehydrogenase deficiency. Chorea may occur in Niemann-Pick disease type C,[190,191] chronic GM_2 and late-onset GM_1 gangliosidoses, neuronal intranuclear inclusion disease, and metachromatic leukodystrophy.

Treatment of Chorea

As long as there are no definitive therapies for the underlying causative disease, treatment of chorea is purely symptomatic. The paucity of understanding of the pathophysiology of chorea at the neuronal level has not been facilitated by the multiplicity of potential mechanisms. Presently, medical therapies aimed at decreasing dopaminergic function are the mainstay, with some evidence that drugs with other modes of action, such as N-methyl-D-aspartate receptor antagonism or membrane stabilization, may be useful. A few cases of patients who underwent surgical therapies, specifically deep brain stimulation or ablative procedures, have been reported, with mixed outcomes.

Reduction in chorea may not result in functional improvement, and should be employed only if the involuntary movements are disabling or distressing. Most experience has been obtained with HD, and this experience can be extrapolated to other choreiform conditions because of presumed similarity of pathophysiology.

Treatment of neuropsychiatric aspects of many of these disorders, specifically depression and psychosis, is important for maintaining quality of life, particularly because these conditions may be amenable to pharmacotherapy than the movement disorder. Selective serotonin reuptake inhibitors and tricyclic antidepressants may be useful, in addition to mood-stabilizing medications. The second-generation neuroleptics may improve psychosis and chorea with less risk of adverse effects than the classic neuroleptics.

DOPAMINE-BLOCKING AGENTS

Although so far there are few published data, clinical experience suggests that second-generation antipsychotic agents may reduce chorea with fewer concerns of causing parkinsonism or tardive dyskinesia, specifically quetiapine, olanzapine, and clozapine. Reports of the efficacy of clozapine for chorea in HD have been mixed.[192,193] Preliminary experience with aripiprazole (personal observations), ziprasidone,[194] and tiapride[24,195] suggests these agents may be promising.

Tetrabenazine depletes monoamines from presynaptic terminals[196] and blocks dopamine receptors, and may be useful in various hyperkinetic movement disorders,[197,198] including HD,[199-201] cerebral palsy, and others. The side effects of depression and parkinsonism may be limiting,[202] however, and this agent should be used with care. Reserpine may occasionally play a role in the treatment of tardive dyskinesia; its use carries the same caveats as tetrabenazine.[203,204]

ANTICONVULSANTS

Levetiracetam is reported to be beneficial in tardive dyskinesia,[205,206] in HD,[207] and in tics associated with choreoacanthocytosis,[208] although results vary. Other anticonvulsants have been used with some positive results, possibly related to a membrane-stabilizing effect. Sodium valproate and carbamazepine have been shown to be useful in Sydenham's chorea,[209,210] although in some cases it may worsen the movement disorder, as may lamotrigine in choreoacanthocytosis.[211]

OTHER AGENTS

In chorea secondary to cerebral palsy, intrathecal baclofen has proven useful.[212] Its efficacy may be due to an upper motor neuron component of the condition because intrathecal baclofen is not of clear benefit in hyperkinetic disorders of other etiologies.[213,214]

SURGICAL THERAPIES

Deep brain stimulation or lesioning of the STN or the GPi has been used to treat chorea of various etiologies in small numbers of cases.[21,215-218] Case reports of deep brain stimulation of the GPi in HD[215,219] and "senile" chorea[21] were promising, although in choreoacanthocytosis[220,221] and McLeod syndrome[222] results are mixed. In chorea secondary to cerebral palsy, results were mixed.[223] The motor thalamus has also been proposed as a potentially promising site for deep brain stimulation in benign "senile" chorea[21] and chorea from cerebral palsy,[216] and has been reported as being beneficial in a patient with choreoacanthocytosis.[220,222,224] The optimal site and frequency of stimulation for treatment of chorea remain to be identified.[222] Patients with Lesch-Nyhan syndrome may benefit from deep brain stimulation, in particular from lead placement in the ventral GPi resulting in behavioral improvements rather than a direct effect on involuntary movements.[225]

NONMEDICAL THERAPIES

In the absence of effective medical therapies to reverse or reduce the symptoms of neurodegenerative choreas, adjunctive nonmedical therapies are invaluable. A multidisciplinary team approach, involving the patient and family, may be valuable.[226]

The pharyngeal musculature is often affected by hyperkinetic movement disorders, and evaluation of swallowing is important to avoid aspiration and to maintain adequate oral intake. If the patient is at high risk for aspiration, placement of a feeding tube may be necessary. Weight loss is often a major feature of these disorders; careful monitoring of nutritional status and supplementation is vital.

Dysarthria may be significant, and patients may benefit from speech therapy and assistive devices. The use of computers, and specifically the Internet, has become an invaluable mechanism of communication for individuals with limited physical mobility and speech problems.

Physical therapy aimed at improving gait and balance may be useful to improve stability, but ultimately assistive devices for walking become essential for safety.

Although unwieldy, these devices may enable patients with moderately advanced disease to stay mobile.

Social and psychological supports are essential components of care for patients and families with these disorders. These supports can be facilitated by judicious use of the Internet. Genetic counseling requires accurate diagnosis and should be made available to the patient and family members.

❘ Conclusions

Chorea is a common movement disorder that may arise from multiple causes. Advances in molecular medicine have facilitated the diagnosis of many patients with inherited choreas. Details of the medical history and neurological examination may be informative, but numerous patients typically remain undiagnosed.

Approaches to understanding the underlying pathophysiology focus primarily on the caudate/putamen, but the precise mechanism for the generation of involuntary movements remains obscure. Treatment is often challenging and is essentially based on empirical observations; further developments in understanding of the etiology of this symptom are awaited.

REFERENCES

1. Albin RL, Young AB, Penney JB: The functional anatomy of basal ganglia disorders. Trends Neurosci 1989;12:366-375.
2. Marsden CD, Obeso JA: The functions of the basal ganglia and the paradox of stereotaxic surgery in Parkinson's disease. Brain 1994;117(Pt 4):877-897.
3. Chesselet MF, Delfs JM: Basal ganglia and movement disorders: an update. Trends Neurosci 1996;19:417-422.
4. Obeso JA, Rodriguez-Oroz MC, Lanciego JL, et al: Pathophysiology of the basal ganglia in Parkinson's disease. Trends Neurosci 2000;23(10 Suppl):S8-S19.
5. Mink JW: The basal ganglia and involuntary movements—impaired inhibition of competing motor patterns. Arch Neurol 2003;60:1365-1368.
6. Wichmann T, DeLong MR: Models of basal ganglia function and pathophysiology of movement disorders. Neurosurg Clin N Am 1998;9:223-236.
7. Albin RL, Reiner A, Anderson KD, et al: Preferential loss of striato-external pallidal projection neurons in presymptomatic Huntington's disease. Ann Neurol 1992;31:425-430.
8. Kleiner-Fisman G, Calingasan NY, Putt M, et al: Alterations of striatal neurons in benign hereditary chorea. Mov Disord 2005;20:1353-1357.
9. Tepper JM, Bolam JP: Functional diversity and specificity of neostriatal interneurons. Curr Opin Neurobiol 2004;14:685-692.
10. Sporer B, Linke R, Seelos K, et al: HIV-induced chorea: evidence for basal ganglia dysregulation by SPECT. J Neurol 2005;252:356-358.
11. Muller-Vahl KR, Berding G, Emrich HM, Peschel T: Chorea-acanthocytosis in monozygotic twins: clinical findings and neuropathological changes as detected by diffusion tensor imaging, FDG-PET and (123)I-beta-CIT-SPECT. J Neurol 2007;254:1081-1088.
12. Kuwert T, Lange HW, Langen KJ, et al: Cortical and subcortical glucose consumption measured by PET in patients with Huntington's disease. Brain 1990;113(Pt 5):1405-1423.
13. Morigaki R, Uno M, Suzue A, Nagahiro S: Hemichorea due to hemodynamic ischemia associated with extracranial carotid artery stenosis: report of two cases. J Neurosurg 2006;105:142-147.
14. Joo EY, Hong SB, Tae WS, et al: Perfusion abnormality of the caudate nucleus in patients with paroxysmal kinesigenic choreoathetosis. Eur J Nucl Med Mol Imaging 2005;32:1205-1209.
15. Mahajnah M, Inbar D, Steinmetz A, et al: Benign hereditary chorea: clinical, neuroimaging, and genetic findings. J Child Neurol 2007;22:1231-1234.

16. Suchowersky O, Muthipeedika J: A case of late-onset chorea. Nat Clin Pract Neurol 2005;1:113-116.
17. Kuwert T, Lange HW, Langen KJ, et al: Normal striatal glucose consumption in two patients with benign hereditary chorea as measured by positron emission tomography. J Neurol 1990;237:80-84.
18. Wu SW, Graham B, Gelfand MJ, et al: Clinical and positron emission tomography findings of chorea associated with primary antiphospholipid antibody syndrome. Mov Disord 2007;22:1813-1815.
19. Lee PH, Nam HS, Lee KY, et al: Serial brain SPECT images in a case of Sydenham chorea. Arch Neurol 1999;56:237-240.
20. Citak EC, Gucuyener K, Karabacak NI, et al: Functional brain imaging in Sydenham's chorea and streptococcal tic disorders. J Child Neurol 2004;19:387-390.
21. Yianni J, Nandi D, Bradley K, et al: Senile chorea treated by deep brain stimulation: a clinical, neurophysiological and functional imaging study. Mov Disord 2004;19:597-602.
22. Lee BC, Hwang SH, Chang GY: Hemiballismus-hemichorea in older diabetic women: a clinical syndrome with MRI correlation. Neurology 1999;52:646-648.
23. Lin JJ, Chang MK: Hemiballism-hemichorea and non-ketotic hyperglycaemia. J Neurol Neurosurg Psychiatry 1994;57:748-750.
24. Iwata A, Koike F, Arasaki K, Tamaki M: Blood brain barrier destruction in hyperglycemic chorea in a patient with poorly controlled diabetes. J Neurol Sci 1999;163:90-93.
25. Chu K, Kang DW, Kim DE, et al: Diffusion-weighted and gradient echo magnetic resonance findings of hemichorea-hemiballismus associated with diabetic hyperglycemia: a hyperviscosity syndrome? Arch Neurol 2002;59:448-452.
26. Ahlskog JE, Nishino H, Evidente VG, et al: Persistent chorea triggered by hyperglycemic crisis in diabetics. Mov Disord 2001;16:890-898.
27. Font J, Cervera R, Espinosa G, et al: Systemic lupus erythematosus (SLE) in childhood: analysis of clinical and immunological findings in 34 patients and comparison with SLE characteristics in adults. Ann Rheum Dis 1998;57:456-459.
28. Watanabe T, Onda H: Hemichorea with antiphospholipid antibodies in a patient with lupus nephritis. Pediatr Nephrol 2004;19:451-453.
29. Venegas FP, Sinning M, Miranda M: Primary Sjogren's syndrome presenting as a generalized chorea. Parkinsonism Relat Disord 2005;11:193-194.
30. Ciubotaru CR, Esfahani F, Benedict RH, et al: Chorea and rapidly progressive subcortical dementia in antiphospholipid syndrome. J Clin Rheumatol 2002;8:332-339.
31. Chapman J, Rand JH, Brey RL, et al: Non-stroke neurological syndromes associated with antiphospholipid antibodies: evaluation of clinical and experimental studies. Lupus 2003;12:514-517.
32. Kiechl-Kohlendorfer U, Ellemunter H, Kiechl S: Chorea as the presenting clinical feature of primary antiphospholipid syndrome in childhood. Neuropediatrics 1999;30:96-98.
33. Sanna G, Bertolaccini ML, Cuadrado MJ, et al: Neuropsychiatric manifestations in systemic lupus erythematosus: prevalence and association with antiphospholipid antibodies. J Rheumatol 2003;30:985-992.
34. Edwards MJ, Dale RC, Church AJ, et al: A dystonic syndrome associated with anti-basal ganglia antibodies. J Neurol Neurosurg Psychiatry 2004;75:914-916.
35. Martino D, Giovannoni G: Antibasal ganglia antibodies and their relevance to movement disorders. Curr Opin Neurol 2004;17:425-432.
36. Miranda M, Cardoso F, Giovannoni G, Church A: Oral contraceptive induced chorea: another condition associated with anti-basal ganglia antibodies. J Neurol Neurosurg Psychiatry 2004;75:327-328.
37. Kujawa KA, Niemi VR, Tomasi MA, et al: Ballistic-choreic movements as the presenting feature of renal cancer. Arch Neurol 2001;58:1133-1135.
38. Tani T, Piao Y, Mori S, et al: Chorea resulting from paraneoplastic striatal encephalitis. J Neurol Neurosurg Psychiatry 2000;69:512-515.
39. Batchelor TT, Platten M, Palmer-Toy DE, et al: Chorea as a paraneoplastic complication of Hodgkin's disease. J Neurooncol 1998;36:185-190.
40. Albin RL, Bromberg MB, Penney JB, Knapp R: Chorea and dystonia: a remote effect of carcinoma. Mov Disord 1988;3:162-169.
41. Vernino S, Tuite P, Adler CH, et al: Paraneoplastic chorea associated with CRMP-5 neuronal antibody and lung carcinoma. Ann Neurol 2002;51:625-630.
42. Dorban S, Gille M, Kessler R, et al: [Chorea-athetosis in the anti-Hu syndrome]. Rev Neurol (Paris) 2004;160:126-129.

43. Muehlschlegel S, Okun MS, Foote KD, et al: Paraneoplastic chorea with leukoencephalopathy presenting with obsessive-compulsive and behavioral disorder. Mov Disord 2005;20:1523-1527.
44. Kellinghaus C, Kraus J, Blaes F, et al: CRMP-5-autoantibodies in testicular cancer associated with limbic encephalitis and choreiform dyskinesias. Eur Neurol 2007;57:241-243.
45. Krolak-Salmon P, Androdias G, Meyronet D, et al: Slow evolution of cerebellar degeneration and chorea in a man with anti-Yo antibodies. Eur J Neurol 2006;13:307-308.
46. Nazabal ER, Lopez JM, Perez PA, Del Corral PR: Chorea disclosing deterioration of polycythaemia vera. Postgrad Med J 2000;76:658-659.
47. Cohen AM, Gelvan A, Yarmolovsky A, Djaldetti M: Chorea in polycythemia vera: a rare presentation of hyperviscosity. Blut 1989;58:47-48.
48. Pereira AC, Edwards MJ, Buttery PC, et al: Choreic syndrome and coeliac disease: a hitherto unrecognised association. Mov Disord 2004;19:478-482.
49. Picconi B, Centonze D, Hakansson K, et al: Loss of bidirectional striatal synaptic plasticity in L-DOPA-induced dyskinesia. Nat Neurosci 2003;6:501-506.
50. Carta M, Carlsson T, Kirik D, Bjorklund A: Dopamine released from 5-HT terminals is the cause of L-DOPA-induced dyskinesia in Parkinsonian rats. Brain 2007;130:1819-1833.
51. Brotchie JM, Lee J, Venderova K: Levodopa-induced dyskinesia in Parkinson's disease. J Neural Transm 2005;112:359-391.
52. Brotchie JM: Nondopaminergic mechanisms in levodopa-induced dyskinesia. Mov Disord 2005;20:919-931.
53. Harrison TS, Goa KL: Long-acting risperidone: a review of its use in schizophrenia. CNS Drugs 2004;18:113-132.
54. Bella VL, Piccoli F: Olanzepine-induced tardive dyskinesia. Br J Psychiatry 2003;182:81-82.
55. Bressan RA, Jones HM, Pilowsky LS: Atypical antipsychotic drugs and tardive dyskinesia: relevance of D2 receptor affinity. J Psychopharmacol 2004;18:124-127.
56. Ghaemi SN, Hsu DJ, Rosenquist KJ, et al: Extrapyramidal side effects with atypical neuroleptics in bipolar disorder. Prog Neuropsychopharmacol Biol Psychiatry 2006;30:209-213.
57. Suchowersky O, Muthipeedika J: A case of late-onset chorea. Nat Clin Pract Neurol 2005;1:113-116.
58. Nozaki I, Inao G, Yamada M: Donepezil-induced chorea in Alzheimer's disease. J Neurol 2007;254:1752-1753
59. Stemper B, Thurauf N, Neundorfer B, Heckmann JG: Choreoathetosis related to lithium intoxication. Eur J Neurol 2003;10:743-744.
60. Weiner WJ, Nausieda PA, Klawans HL: Methylphenidate-induced chorea: case report and pharmacologic implications. Neurology 1978;28:1041-1044.
61. Kirvan CA, Cox CJ, Swedo SE, Cunningham MW: Tubulin is a neuronal target of autoantibodies in Sydenham's chorea. J Immunol 2007;178:7412-7421.
62. Church AJ, Cardoso F, Dale RC, et al: Anti-basal ganglia antibodies in acute and persistent Sydenham's chorea. Neurology 2002;59:227-231.
63. Tse W, Cersosimo MG, Gracies JM, et al: Movement disorders and AIDS: a review. Parkinsonism Relat Disord 2004;10:323-334.
64. Passarin MG, Alessandrini F, Nicolini GG, et al: Reversible choreoathetosis as the early onset of HIV-encephalopathy. Neurol Sci 2005;26:55-56.
65. Sporer B, Linke R, Seelos K, et al: HIV-induced chorea: evidence for basal ganglia dysregulation by SPECT. J Neurol 2005;252:356-358.
66. Bowen J, Mitchell T, Pearce R, Quinn N: Chorea in new variant Creutzfeldt-Jacob disease. Mov Disord 2000;15:1284-1285.
67. McKee D, Talbot P: Chorea as a presenting feature of variant Creutzfeldt-Jakob disease. Mov Disord 2003;18:837-838.
68. Cambonie G, Houdon L, Rivier F, et al: Infantile bilateral striatal necrosis following measles. Brain Dev 2000;22:221-223.
69. Yamamoto K, Chiba HO, Ishitobi M, et al: Acute encephalopathy with bilateral striatal necrosis: favourable response to corticosteroid therapy. Eur J Paediatr Neurol 1997;1:41-45.
70. Zambrino CA, Zorzi G, Lanzi G, et al: Bilateral striatal necrosis associated with *Mycoplasma pneumoniae* infection in an adolescent: clinical and neuroradiologic follow up. Mov Disord 2000;15:1023-1026.
71. Fong CY, de Sousa C: Childhood chorea-encephalopathy associated with human parvovirus B19 infection. Dev Med Child Neurol 2006;48:526-528.
72. Moore RC, Xiang F, Monaghan J, et al: Huntington disease phenocopy is a familial prion disease. Am J Hum Genet 2001;69:1385-1388.

73. Lewis V, Collins S, Hill AF, et al: Novel prion protein insert mutation associated with prolonged neurodegenerative illness. Neurology 2003;60:1620-1624.
74. Walker RH, Jankovic J, O'Hearn E, Margolis RL: Phenotypic features of Huntington disease-like 2. Mov Disord 2003;18:1527-1530.
75. Margolis RL, O'Hearn E, Rosenblatt A, et al: A disorder similar to Huntington's disease is associated with a novel CAG repeat expansion. Ann Neurol 2001;50:373-380.
76. Walker RH, Rasmussen A, Rudnicki D, et al: Huntington's disease-like 2 can present as chorea-acanthocytosis. Neurology 2003;61:1002-1004.
77. Holmes SE, O'Hearn E, Rosenblatt A, et al: A repeat expansion in the gene encoding junctophilin-3 is associated with Huntington disease-like 2. Nat Genet 2001;29:377-378.
78. Margolis RL, Holmes SE, Rosenblatt A, et al: Huntington's disease-like 2 (HDL2) in North America and Japan. Ann Neurol 2004;56:670-674.
79. Nishi M, Hashimoto K, Kuriyama K, et al: Motor discoordination in mutant mice lacking junctophilin type 3. Biochem Biophys Res Commun 2002;292:318-324.
80. Walker RH, Morgello S, Davidoff-Feldman B, et al: Autosomal dominant chorea-acanthocytosis with polyglutamine-containing neuronal inclusions. Neurology 2002;58:1031-1037.
81. Greenstein PE, Vonsattel JP, Margolis RL, Joseph JT: Huntington's disease like-2 neuropathology. Mov Disord 2007;22:1416-1423.
82. Rudnicki DD, Holmes SE, Lin MW, et al: Huntington's disease-like 2 is associated with CUG repeat-containing RNA foci. Ann Neurol 2007;61:272-282.
83. Stevanin G, Fujigasaki H, Lebre AS, et al: Huntington's disease-like phenotype due to trinucleotide repeat expansions in the TBP and JPH3 genes. Brain 2003;126:1599-1603.
84. Andrew SE, Goldberg YP, Kremer B, et al: Huntington disease without cag expansion-phenocopies or errors in assignment. Am J Hum Genet 1994;54:852-863.
85. Stevanin G, Camuzat A, Holmes SE, et al: CAG/CTG repeat expansions at the Huntington's disease-like 2 locus are rare in Huntington's disease patients. Neurology 2002;58:965-967.
86. Bauer I, Gencik M, Laccone F, et al: Trinucleotide repeat expansions in the junctophilin-3 gene are not found in Caucasian patients with a Huntington's disease-like phenotype. Ann Neurol 2002;51:662.
87. Bardien S, Abrahams F, Soodyall H, et al: A South African mixed ancestry family with Huntington disease-like 2: Clinical and genetic features. Mov Disord 2007;22:2083-2089.
88. Namekawa M, Takiyama Y, Ando Y, et al: Choreiform movements in spinocerebellar ataxia type 1. J Neurol Sci 2001;187(1-2):103-106.
89. Geschwind DH, Perlman S, Figueroa CP, et al: The prevalence and wide clinical spectrum of the spinocerebellar ataxia type 2 trinucleotide repeat in patients with autosomal dominant cerebellar ataxia. Am J Hum Genet 1997;60:842-850.
90. Zuhlke C, Gehlken U, Hellenbroich Y, et al: Phenotypical variability of expanded alleles in the TATA-binding protein gene: reduced penetrance in SCA17? J Neurol 2003;250:161-163.
91. Schneider SA, van de Warrenburg BP, Hughes TD, et al: Phenotypic homogeneity of the Huntington disease-like presentation in a SCA17 family. Neurology 2006;67:1701-1703.
92. Richfield EK, Vonsattel JP, Macdonald ME, et al: Selective loss of striatal preprotachykinin neurons in a phenocopy of Huntington's disease. Mov Disord 2002;17:327-332.
93. Stevanin G, Brice A: Spinocerebellar ataxia 17 (SCA17) and Huntington's disease-like 4 (HDL4). Cerebellum 2007;6:1-9.
94. Toyoshima Y, Yamada M, Onodera O, et al: SCA17 homozygote showing Huntington's disease-like phenotype. Ann Neurol 2004;55:281-286.
95. Martins S, Matama T, Guimaraes L, et al: Portuguese families with dentatorubropallidoluysian atrophy (DRPLA) share a common haplotype of Asian origin. Eur J Hum Genet 2003;11:808-811.
96. Le Ber I, Camuzat A, Castelnovo G, et al: Prevalence of dentatorubral-pallidoluysian atrophy in a large series of white patients with cerebellar ataxia. Arch Neurol 2003;60:1097-1099.
97. Wardle M, Majounie E, Williams NM, et al: Dentatorubral pallidoluysian atrophy in South Wales. J Neurol Neurosurg Psychiatry 2008;79:804-807.
98. Burke JR, Wingfield MS, Lewis KE, et al: The Haw River syndrome: dentatorubropallidoluysian atrophy (DRPLA) in an African-American family. Nat Genet 1994;7:521-524.
99. Willemsen MA, Breedveld GJ, Wouda S, et al: Brain-thyroid-lung syndrome: a patient with a severe multi-system disorder due to a de novo mutation in the thyroid transcription factor 1 gene. Eur J Pediatr 2005;164:28-30.
100. Breedveld GJ, van Dongen JW, Danesino C, et al: Mutations in TITF-1 are associated with benign hereditary chorea. Hum Mol Genet 2002;11:971-979.

101. Kleiner-Fisman G, Lang AE. Benign hereditary chorea revisited: a journey to understanding. Mov Disord 2007;22:2297-2305.
102. Asmus F, Horber V, Pohlenz J, et al: A novel TITF-1 mutation causes benign hereditary chorea with response to levodopa. Neurology 2005;64:1952-1954.
103. Asmus F, Devlin A, Munz M, et al: Clinical differentiation of genetically proven benign hereditary chorea and myoclonus-dystonia. Mov Disord 2007;22:2104-2109.
104. Krude H, Schutz B, Biebermann H, et al: Choreoathetosis, hypothyroidism, and pulmonary alterations due to human NKX2-1 haploinsufficiency. J Clin Invest 2002;109:475-480.
105. Doyle DA, Gonzalez I, Thomas B, Scavina M: Autosomal dominant transmission of congenital hypothyroidism, neonatal respiratory distress, and ataxia caused by a mutation of NKX2-1. J Pediatr 2004;145:190-193.
106. Devos D, Vuillaume I, De Becdelievre A, et al: New syndromic form of benign hereditary chorea is associated with a deletion of TITF-1 and PAX-9 contiguous genes. Mov Disord 2006;21:2237-2240.
107. Bauer P, Kreuz FR, Burk K, et al: Mutations in TITF1 are not relevant to sporadic and familial chorea of unknown cause. Mov Disord 2006;21:1734-1737.
108. Shimohata T, Hara K, Sanpei K, et al: Novel locus for benign hereditary chorea with adult onset maps to chromosome 8q21.3 q23.3. Brain 2007;130(Pt 9):2302-2309.
109. Curtis AR, Fey C, Morris CM, et al: Mutation in the gene encoding ferritin light polypeptide causes dominant adult-onset basal ganglia disease. Nat Genet 2001;28:350-354.
110. Crompton DE, Chinnery PF, Bates D, et al: Spectrum of movement disorders in neuroferritinopathy. Mov Disord 2004;20:95-99.
111. Mir P, Edwards MJ, Curtis AR, et al: Adult-onset generalized dystonia due to a mutation in the neuroferritinopathy gene. Mov Disord 2004;20:243-245.
112. Chinnery PF, Crompton DE, Birchall D, et al: Clinical features and natural history of neuroferritinopathy caused by the FTL1 460InsA mutation. Brain 2007;130(Pt 1):110-119.
113. Wills AJ, Sawle GV, Guilbert PR, Curtis AR: Palatal tremor and cognitive decline in neuroferritinopathy. J Neurol Neurosurg Psychiatry 2002;73:91-92.
114. Geschwind DH, Loginov M, Stern JM: Identification of a locus on chromosome 14q for idiopathic basal ganglia calcification (Fahr disease). Am J Hum Genet 1999;65:764-772.
115. Brodaty H, Mitchell P, Luscombe G, et al: Familial idiopathic basal ganglia calcification (Fahr's disease) without neurological, cognitive and psychiatric symptoms is not linked to the IBGC1 locus on chromosome 14q. Hum Genet 2002;110:8-14.
116. Oliveira JR, Spiteri E, Sobrido MJ, et al: Genetic heterogeneity in familial idiopathic basal ganglia calcification (Fahr disease). Neurology 2004;63:2165-2167.
117. Wszolek ZK, Baba Y, Mackenzie IR, et al: Autosomal dominant dystonia-plus with cerebral calcifications. Neurology 2006;67:620-625.
118. Younes-Mhenni S, Thobois S, Streichenberger N, et al: [Mitochondrial encephalomyopathy, lactic acidosis and stroke-like episodes (MELAS) associated with a Fahr disease and cerebellar calcifications]. Rev Med Interne 2002;23:1027-1029.
119. Reske-Nielsen E, Jensen PK, Hein-Sorensen O, Abelskov K: Calcification of the central nervous system in a new hereditary neurological syndrome. Acta Neuropathol (Berl) 1988;75:590-596.
120. Hardie RJ, Pullon HW, Harding AE, et al: Neuroacanthocytosis: a clinical, haematological and pathological study of 19 cases. Brain 1991;114:13-49.
121. Gandhi S, Hardie RJ, Lees AJ: An update on the Hardie neuroacanthocytosis series. In Walker RH, Saiki S, Danek A (eds): Neuroacanthocytosis Syndromes II. Berlin: Springer-Verlag, 2008, pp 43-51.
122. Rampoldi L, Danek A, Monaco AP: Clinical features and molecular bases of neuroacanthocytosis. J Mol Med 2002;80:475-491.
123. Walker RH, Danek A, Dobson-Stone C, et al: Developments in neuroacanthocytosis: expanding the spectrum of choreatic syndromes. Mov Disord 2006;21:1794-1905.
124. Walker RH, Liu Q, Ichiba M, et al: Self-mutilation in chorea-acanthocytosis—manifestation of movement disorder or psychopathology? Mov Disord 2006;21:2268-2269.
125. Saiki S, Hirose G, Sakai K, et al: Chorea-acanthocytosis associated with Tourettism. Mov Disord 2004;19:833-836.
126. Schneider SA, Aggarwal A, Bhatt M, et al: Severe tongue protrusion dystonia: clinical syndromes and possible treatment. Neurology 2006;67:940-943.
127. Henkel K, Danek A, Grafman J, et al: Head of the caudate nucleus is most vulnerable in chorea-acanthocytosis: a voxel-based morphometry study. Mov Disord 2006;21:1728-1731.

128. Sorrentino G, De Renzo A, Miniello S, et al: Late appearance of acanthocytes during the course of chorea-acanthocytosis. J Neurol Sci 1999;163:175-178.
129. Storch A, Kornhass M, Schwarz J: Testing for acanthocytosis: a prospective reader-blinded study in movement disorder patients. J Neurol 2005;252:84-90.
130. Rampoldi L, Dobson-Stone C, Rubio JP, et al: A conserved sorting-associated protein is mutant in chorea-acanthocytosis. Nat Genet 2001;28:119-120.
131. Velayos-Baeza A, Vettori A, Copley RR, et al: Analysis of the human *VPS13* gene family. Genomics 2004;84:536-549.
132. Dobson-Stone C, Velayos-Baeza A, Filippone LA, et al: Chorein detection for the diagnosis of chorea-acanthocytosis. Ann Neurol 2004;56:299-302.
133. Saiki S, Sakai K, Kitagawa Y, et al: Mutation in the *CHAC* gene in a family of autosomal dominant chorea-acanthocytosis. Neurology 2003;61:1614-1616.
134. Ichiba M, Nakamura M, Kusumoto A, et al: Clinical and molecular genetic assessment of a chorea-acanthocytosis pedigree. J Neurol Sci 2007;263(1-2):124-132.
135. Andermann E, Badhwar A, Al-Asmi A, et al: Chorea-acanthocytosis in a large French-Canadian kindred with dominant or pseudo-dominant inheritance. Neurology 2004;60(Suppl 1). A248.
136. Zhou B, Westaway SK, Levinson B, et al: A novel pantothenate kinase gene (*PANK2*) is defective in Hallervorden-Spatz syndrome. Nat Genet 2001;28:345-349.
137. Hayflick SJ, Westaway SK, Levinson B, et al: Genetic, clinical, and radiographic delineation of Hallervorden-Spatz syndrome. N Engl J Med 2003;348:33-40.
138. Hartig MB, Hortnagel K, Garavaglia B, et al: Genotypic and phenotypic spectrum of PANK2 mutations in patients with neurodegeneration with brain iron accumulation. Ann Neurol 2006;59:248-256.
139. Malandrini A, Cesaretti S, Mulinari M, et al: Acanthocytosis, retinitis pigmentosa, pallidal degeneration: report of two cases without serum lipid abnormalities. J Neurol Sci 1996;140(1-2):129-131.
140. Orrell RW, Amrolia PJ, Heald A, et al: Acanthocytosis, retinitis pigmentosa, and pallidal degeneration: a report of three patients, including the second reported case with hypoprebetalipoproteinemia (HARP syndrome). Neurology 1995;45(3 Pt 1):487-492.
141. Ching KH, Westaway SK, Gitschier J, et al: HARP syndrome is allelic with pantothenate kinase-associated neurodegeneration. Neurology 2002;58:1673-1674.
142. Mubaidin A, Roberts E, Hampshire D, et al: Karak syndrome: a novel degenerative disorder of the basal ganglia and cerebellum. J Med Genet 2003;40:543-546.
143. Morgan NV, Westaway SK, Morton JE, et al: PLA2G6, encoding a phospholipase A2, is mutated in neurodegenerative disorders with high brain iron. Nat Genet 2006;38:752-754.
144. Xu X, Pin S, Gathinji M, et al: Aceruloplasminemia: an inherited neurodegenerative disease with impairment of iron homeostasis. Ann N Y Acad Sci 2004;1012:299-305.
145. Miyajima H: Aceruloplasminemia, an iron metabolic disorder. Neuropathology 2003;23:345-350.
146. Skidmore FM, Drago V, Foster P, et al: Aceruloplasminemia with progressive atrophy without brain iron overload: treatment with oral chelation. J Neurol Neurosurg Psychiatry 2008;79:467-470.
147. Machado A, Fen CH, Mitiko DM, et al: Neurological manifestations in Wilson's disease: report of 119 cases. Mov Disord 2006;21:2192-2196.
148. Taly AB, Meenakshi-Sundaram S, Sinha S, et al: Wilson disease: description of 282 patients evaluated over 3 decades. Medicine (Baltimore) 2007;86:112-121.
149. Kambouris M, Bohlega S, Al Tahan A, Meyer BF: Localization of the gene for a novel autosomal recessive neurodegenerative Huntington-like disorder to 4p15.3. Am J Hum Genet 2000;66:445-452.
150. Lesperance MM, Burmeister M: Interpretation of linkage data for a Huntington-like disorder mapping to 4p15.3. Am J Hum Genet 2000;67:262-263.
151. Basel-Vanagaite L, Straussberg R, Ovadia H, et al: Infantile bilateral striatal necrosis maps to chromosome 19q. Neurology 2004;62:87-90.
152. De Meirleir L, Seneca S, Lissens W, et al: Bilateral striatal necrosis with a novel point mutation in the mitochondrial ATPase 6 gene. Pediatr Neurol 1995;13:242-246.
153. Hanna MG, Davis MB, Sweeney MG, et al: Generalized chorea in two patients harboring the Friedreich's ataxia gene trinucleotide repeat expansion. Mov Disord 1998;13:339-340.
154. Zhu D, Burke C, Leslie A, Nicholson GA: Friedreich's ataxia with chorea and myoclonus caused by a compound heterozygosity for a novel deletion and the trinucleotide GAA expansion. Mov Disord 2002;17:585-589.

155. Spacey SD, Szczygielski BI, Young SP, et al: Malaysian siblings with Friedreich ataxia and chorea: a novel deletion in the frataxin gene. Can J Neurol Sci 2004;31:383-386.
156. Symmans WA, Shepherd CS, Marsh WL, et al: Hereditary acanthocytosis associated with the McLeod phenotype of the Kell blood group system. Br J Haematol 1979;42:575-583.
157. Danek A, Rubio JP, Rampoldi L, et al: McLeod neuroacanthocytosis: genotype and phenotype. Ann Neurol 2001;50:755-764.
158. Allen FH, Krabbe SM, Corcoran PA: A new phenotype (McLeod) in the Kell blood-group system. Vox Sang 1961;6:555-560.
159. Russo D, Redman C, Lee S: Association of XK and Kell blood group proteins. J Biol Chem 1998;273:13950-13956.
160. Ho M, Chelly J, Carter N, et al: Isolation of the gene for McLeod syndrome that encodes a novel membrane transport protein. Cell 1994;77:869-880.
161. Jung HH, Hergersberg M, Kneifel S, et al: McLeod syndrome: a novel mutation, predominant psychiatric manifestations, and distinct striatal imaging findings. Ann Neurol 2001;49:384-392.
162. Ho M, Chelly J, Carter N, et al: Isolation of the gene for McLeod syndrome that encodes a novel membrane transport protein. Cell 1994;77:869-880.
163. Russo D, Wu X, Redman CM, Lee S: Expression of Kell blood group protein in nonerythroid tissues. Blood 2000;96:340-346.
164. Jung HH, Russo D, Redman C, Brandner S: Kell and XK immunohistochemistry in McLeod myopathy. Muscle Nerve 2001;24:1346-1351.
165. Klempir J, Roth J, Zarubova K, et al: The McLeod syndrome without acanthocytes. Parkinsonism Relat Disord 2008;14:364-366.
166. Jung HH, Hergersberg M, Vogt M, et al: McLeod phenotype associated with a XK missense mutation without hematologic, neuromuscular, or cerebral involvement. Transfusion 2003;43:928-938.
167. Walker RH, Danek A, Uttner I, et al: McLeod phenotype without the McLeod syndrome. Transfusion 2006;47:299-305.
168. Ueyama H, Kumamoto T, Nagao S, et al: A novel mutation of the McLeod syndrome gene in a Japanese family. J Neurol Sci 2000;176:151-154.
169. Walker RH, Jung HH, Tison F, et al: Phenotypic variation among brothers with the McLeod neuroacanthocytosis syndrome. Mov Disord 2007;22:244-248.
170. Miranda M, Castiglioni C, Frey BM, et al: Phenotypic variability of a distinct deletion in McLeod syndrome. Mov Disord 2007;22:1358-1361.
171. Hewer E, Danek A, Schoser BG, et al: McLeod myopathy revisited—more neurogenic and less benign. Brain 2007;130:3285-3296.
172. Kawakami T, Takiyama Y, Sakoe K, et al: A case of McLeod syndrome with unusually severe myopathy. J Neurol Sci 1999;166:36-39.
173. Jung HH, Brandner S: Malignant McLeod myopathy. Muscle Nerve 2002;26:424-427.
174. Nicholl DJ, Sutton I, Dotti MT, et al: White matter abnormalities on MRI in neuroacanthocytosis. J Neurol Neurosurg Psychiatry 2004;75:1200-1201.
175. Brin MF, Hays A, Symmans WA, et al: Neuropathology of McLeod phenotype is like chorea-acanthocytosis (CA). Can J Neurol Sci 1993;20(Suppl 4):234.
176. Lee LV, Pascasio FM, Fuentes FD, Viterbo GH: Torsion dystonia in Panay, Philippines. Adv Neurol 1976;14:137-151.
177. Evidente VG, Advincula J, Esteban R, et al: Phenomenology of "Lubag" or X-linked dystonia-parkinsonism. Mov Disord 2002;17:1271-1277.
178. Waters CH, Takahashi H, Wilhelmsen KC, et al: Phenotypic expression of X-linked dystonia-parkinsonism (lubag) in two women. Neurology 1993;43:1555-1558.
179. Evidente VG, Nolte D, Niemann S, et al: Phenotypic and molecular analyses of X-linked dystonia-parkinsonism ("lubag") in women. Arch Neurol 2004;61:1956-1959.
180. Nolte D, Niemann S, Muller U: Specific sequence changes in multiple transcript system DYT3 are associated with X-linked dystonia parkinsonism. Proc Natl Acad Sci U S A 2003;100:10347-10352.
181. Chiong MA, Marinaki A, Duley J, et al: Lesch-Nyhan disease in a 20-year-old man incorrectly described as developing 'cerebral palsy' after general anaesthesia in infancy. J Inherit Metab Dis 2006;29:594.
182. Goldenberg PC, Steiner RD, Merkens LS, et al: Remarkable improvement in adult Leigh syndrome with partial cytochrome c oxidase deficiency. Neurology 2003;60:865-868.
183. Crimi M, Galbiati S, Moroni I, et al: A missense mutation in the mitochondrial ND5 gene associated with a Leigh-MELAS overlap syndrome. Neurology 2003;60:1857-1861.
184. Caer M, Viala K, Levy R, et al: Adult-onset chorea and mitochondrial cytopathy. Mov Disord 2005;20:490-492.

185. Ojwang PJ, Pegoraro RJ, Deppe WM, et al: Biochemical and molecular diagnosis of glutaric aciduria type 1 in a black South African male child: case report. East Afr Med J 2001;78:682-685.
186. Friedman JR, Thiele EA, Wang D, et al: Atypical GLUT1 deficiency with prominent movement disorder responsive to ketogenic diet. Mov Disord 2006;21:241-245.
187. Sethi KD, Ray R, Roesel RA, et al: Adult-onset chorea and dementia with propionic acidemia. Neurology 1989;39:1343-1345.
188. Surtees RA, Matthews EE, Leonard JV: Neurologic outcome of propionic acidemia. Pediatr Neurol 1992;8:333-337.
189. Gascon GG, Ozand PT, Brismar J: Movement disorders in childhood organic acidurias: clinical, neuroimaging, and biochemical correlations. Brain Dev 1994;16(Suppl):94-103.
190. Josephs KA, Van Gerpen MW, Van Gerpen JA: Adult onset Niemann-Pick disease type C presenting with psychosis. J Neurol Neurosurg Psychiatry 2003;74:528-529.
191. Shulman LM, Lang AE, Jankovic J, et al: Case 1 psychosis, dementia, chorea, ataxia, and supranuclear gaze dysfunction. Mov Disord 1995;1995(10):257-262.
192. van Vugt JP, Siesling S, Vergeer M, et al: Clozapine versus placebo in Huntington's disease: a double blind randomised comparative study. J Neurol Neurosurg Psychiatry 1997;63:35-39.
193. Bonuccelli U, Ceravolo R, Maremmani C, et al: Clozapine in Huntington's chorea. Neurology 1994;44:821-823.
194. Bonelli RM, Mayr BM, Niederwieser G, et al: Ziprasidone in Huntington's disease: the first case reports. J Psychopharmacol 2003;17:459-460.
195. Deroover J, Baro F, Bourguignon RP, Smets P: Tiapride versus placebo: a double-blind comparative study in the management of Huntington's chorea. Curr Med Res Opin 1984;9:329-338.
196. Pearson SJ, Reynolds GP: Depletion of monoamine transmitters by tetrabenazine in brain tissue in Huntington's disease. Neuropharmacology 1988;27:717-719.
197. Jankovic J, Orman J: Tetrabenazine therapy of dystonia, chorea, tics, and other dyskinesias. Neurology 1988;38:391-394.
198. Chatterjee A, Frucht SJ: Tetrabenazine in the treatment of severe pediatric chorea. Mov Disord 2003;18:703-706.
199. Ondo WG, Tintner R, Thomas M, Jankovic J: Tetrabenazine treatment for Huntington's disease-associated chorea. Clin Neuropharm 2002;25:300-302.
200. Kenney C, Hunter C, Davidson A, Jankovic J: Short-term effects of tetrabenazine on chorea associated with Huntington's disease. Mov Disord 2007;22:10-13.
201. Tetrabenazine as antichorea therapy in Huntington disease: a randomized controlled trial. Neurology 2006;66:366-372.
202. Moss JH, Stewart DE: Iatrogenic parkinsonism in Huntington's chorea. Can J Psychiatry 1986;31:865-866.
203. Markham CH, Clark WG, Winters WD: Effects of Alpha-methyl dopa and reserpine in Huntington's chorea, Parkinson's disease and other movement disorders. Life Sci (Oxford) 1963;9:697-705.
204. Fahn S: A therapeutic approach to tardive dyskinesia. J Clin Psychiatry 1985;46(4 Pt 2):19-24.
205. Meco G, Fabrizio E, Epifanio A, et al: Levetiracetam in tardive dyskinesia. Clin Neuropharm 2006;29:265-268.
206. Konitsiotis S, Pappa S, Mantas C, Mavreas V: Levetiracetam in tardive dyskinesia: an open label study. Mov Disord 2006;21:1219-1221.
207. Zesiewicz TA, Sullivan KL, Hauser RA, Sanchez-Ramos J: Open-label pilot study of levetiracetam (Keppra) for the treatment of chorea in Huntington's disease. Mov Disord 2006;21:1998-2001.
208. Lin FC, Wei LJ, Shih PY: Effect of levetiracetam on truncal tic in neuroacanthocytosis. Acta Neurol Taiwan 2006;15:38-42.
209. Genel F, Arslanoglu S, Uran N, Saylan B: Sydenham's chorea: clinical findings and comparison of the efficacies of sodium valproate and carbamazepine regimens. Brain Dev 2002;24:73-76.
210. Harel L, Zecharia A, Straussberg R, et al: Successful treatment of rheumatic chorea with carbamazepine. Pediatr Neurol 2000;23:147-151.
211. Al-Asmi A, Jansen AC, Badhwar A, et al: Familial temporal lobe epilepsy as a presenting feature of choreoacanthocytosis. Epilepsia 2005;46:1256-1263.
212. Albright AL: Intrathecal baclofen in cerebral palsy movement disorders. J Child Neurol 1996;11(Suppl 1):S29-S35.
213. Walker RH, Danisi FO, Swope DM, et al: Intrathecal baclofen for dystonia: benefits and complications during six years experience. Mov Disord 2000;15:1242-1247.
214. Ford B, Greene P, Louis ED, et al: Use of intrathecal baclofen in the treatment of patients with dystonia. Arch Neurol 1996;53:1241-1246.

215. Moro E, Lang AE, Strafella AP, et al: Bilateral globus pallidus stimulation for Huntington's disease. Ann Neurol 2004;56:290-294.
216. Thompson TP, Kondziolka D, Albright AL: Thalamic stimulation for choreiform movement disorders in children: report of two cases. J Neurosurg 2000;92:718-721.
217. Kyriagis M, Grattan-Smith P, Scheinberg A, et al: Status dystonicus and Hallervorden-Spatz disease: treatment with intrathecal baclofen and pallidotomy. J Paediatr Child Health 2004;40 (5-6):322-325.
218. Castelnau P, Cif L, Valente EM, et al: Pallidal stimulation improves pantothenate kinase-associated neurodegeneration. Ann Neurol 2005;57:738-741.
219. Hebb MO, Garcia R, Gaudet P, Mendez IM: Bilateral stimulation of the globus pallidus internus to treat choreathetosis in Huntington's disease: technical case report. Neurosurgery 2006;58:E383.
220. Burbaud P, Rougier A, Ferrer X, et al: Improvement of severe trunk spasms by bilateral high-frequency stimulation of the motor thalamus in a patient with chorea-acanthocytosis. Mov Disord 2002;17:204-207.
221. Wihl G, Volkmann J, Allert N, et al: Deep brain stimulation of the internal pallidum did not improve chorea in a patient with neuro-acanthocytosis. Mov Disord 2001;16:572-575.
222. Burbaud P: Deep brain stimulation in neuroacanthocytosis. Mov Disord 2005;20:1681-1682.
223. Krauss JK, Loher TJ, Weigel R, et al: Chronic stimulation of the globus pallidus internus for treatment of non-dYT1 generalized dystonia and choreoathetosis: 2-year follow up. J Neurosurg 2003;98:785-792.
224. Burbaud P, Vital A, Rougier A, et al: Minimal tissue damage after stimulation of the motor thalamus in a case of chorea-acanthocytosis. Neurology 2002;59:1982-1984.
225. Cif L, Biolsi B, Gavarini S, et al: Antero-ventral internal pallidum stimulation improves behavioral disorders in Lesch-Nyhan disease. Mov Disord 2007;22:2126-2129.
226. McIntosh J: Multidisciplinary neurorehabilitation in chorea-acanthocytosis: a case study. In Walker RH, Saiki S, Danek A, eds: Neuroacanthocytosis Syndromes II. Berlin: Springer, 2008, pp 271-284.

31 | Restless Legs Syndrome

WAYNE HENING[†] • CLAUDIA TRENKWALDER

Introduction

Restless legs syndrome (RLS) was a relatively unknown disorder until several years ago. Now that there is convincing evidence that RLS is a common disorder (at least in European populations[1,2]), that good therapeutic options for RLS exist,[3-5] and that there are established genetic variants conferring differential risk,[6] RLS has been clearly established as a significant and important element of clinical practice.[7] For this reason, RLS has become an important disorder in the field of movement disorders, within which it fits the category of hyperkinetic disorders, and the category of sleep disorders because RLS symptoms are circadian in nature and cause major problems to affected individuals in the evening and at night. Numerous reviews[8-10] are available, as are books for the lay public[11-13] and health care professionals. Because the field of RLS is developing so rapidly, published works become obsolete quickly.

[†]Deceased

Definition, Diagnosis, and Assessment of Restless Legs Syndrome

DEFINITION

RLS is a sensorimotor sleep/wake disorder in which the key symptom is an urge to move provoked by rest. As defined by the International Restless Legs Syndrome Study Group (IRLSSG),[14,15] there are four key diagnostic features of RLS (Table 31–1), which can be remembered by the acronym *URGE*, as follows:

Urge to move the legs, usually associated with unpleasant leg sensations
Rest induces symptoms
Getting active (physically and mentally) brings relief
Evening and night make symptoms worse

IRLSSG[15] delineated several supportive and associated features (see Table 31–1) that may also play a role in diagnosis.[16]

RLS patients fall into two major groups: idiopathic and secondary RLS. Idiopathic, usually familial, RLS has early onset and slow symptom progression. So-called secondary RLS is associated with various conditions including iron deficiency, kidney failure, and pregnancy, with a later onset and more rapid progression.[17]

DIAGNOSIS

RLS has been diagnosed primarily through clinical means, especially a good clinical interview with the patient and, if possible, the bed partner. RLS cannot be securely diagnosed without the patient's communication of at least the four diagnostic features. Other conditions may "mimic" RLS,[18,19] however, and diagnoses may require either a more detailed understanding of the four features or additional investigations related to the supportive and associated features (see Table 31–1).[16,19-21] A study at Johns Hopkins has found that the specificity of the four features is only 84%; another study by Benes and Kohnen[22] found, that using a diagnostic index specificity was higher in items related to supportive or associated diagnostic information (95.7%) than in those related to the essential diagnostic criteria (81.7%).

Four Key Diagnostic Features

Urge to Move the Legs, Usually Associated with Unpleasant Leg Sensations

RLS has been termed a *focal akathisia*,[19] emphasizing that the primary symptom is one of a need to move, and that the symptoms are specifically localized in the legs. Patients say, "I cannot keep still," or "I just need to move." They admit that they cannot resist moving when their symptoms occur, similar to the compelled movements of tic disorder (which may have some association with RLS).[23-25] Patients are particularly bothered by confined, restraining conditions, such as a prolonged airplane journey or lengthy theater event. They describe these conditions as intolerable, anxiety-provoking, or torture, and state that such conditions would cause them to "go crazy," and that, no matter what, they would move (one former U.S. marine mentioned that in Vietnam he had to move even when he was lying in ambush, whereas an older woman stated that she "walked all the way to China" when on a flight).

TABLE 31–1	Essential, Supportive, and Associated Features of Restless Legs Syndrome

Essential Diagnostic Criteria

1. Urge to move the legs, usually accompanied or caused by uncomfortable and unpleasant sensations in the legs (sometimes the urge to move is present without the uncomfortable sensations, and sometimes the arms or other body parts are involved in addition to the legs)
2. Urge to move or unpleasant sensations begin or worsen during periods of rest or inactivity such as lying or sitting
3. Urge to move or unpleasant sensations are partially or totally relieved by movement, such as walking or stretching, at least as long as the activity continues
4. Urge to move or unpleasant sensations are worse in the evening or at night than during the day or occur only in the evening or at night (when symptoms are very severe, the worsening at night may not be noticeable, but must have been previously present)

Supportive Clinical Features

Family history: Prevalence of RLS among first-degree relatives of individuals with RLS is 3-5 times greater than among individuals without RLS

Response to dopaminergic therapy: Nearly all individuals with RLS show at least an initial positive therapeutic response to either levodopa or a dopamine receptor agonist at doses considered to be very low in relation to the traditional doses of these medications used for the treatment of Parkinson's disease. This initial response is not universally maintained

Periodic limb movements (during wakefulness or sleep): PLMS occur in at least 85% of individuals with RLS; PLMS also commonly occur in other disorders and in elderly individuals. PLMS are much less common in children than in adults

Associated Features

Natural clinical course: Clinical course of the disorder varies considerably, but certain patterns have been identified that may be helpful to the experienced clinician. When the age of onset of RLS symptoms is <50 years, the onset is often more insidious; when the age of onset is >50 years, the symptoms often occur more abruptly and more severely. In some patients, RLS can be intermittent and may spontaneously remit for many years

Sleep disturbance: Disturbed sleep is a common major morbidity for RLS and warrants special consideration in planning treatment. Sleep disturbance is often the primary reason the patient seeks medical attention

Medical evaluation/physical examination: Physical examination is generally normal and does not contribute to the diagnosis except for conditions that may be comorbid or secondary causes of RLS. Iron status, in particular, should be evaluated because decreased iron stores are a significant potential risk factor that can be treated. The presence of peripheral neuropathy and radiculopathy should also be determined because these conditions have a possible, although uncertain, association and may require different treatment

PLMS, periodic limb movements in sleep; RLS, restless legs syndrome.
From Allen RP, Picchietti D, Hening WA, et al. Restless legs syndrome: diagnostic criteria, special considerations, and epidemiology. A report from the Restless Legs Syndrome Diagnosis and Epidemiology Workshop at the National Institutes of Health. *Sleep Med.* 2003;4:101-119.

TABLE 31–2	Descriptive Terms for Restless Legs Syndrome

Creepy-crawly
Ants crawling
Jittery
Pulling
Worms moving
Soda bubbling in the veins
Electric current
Shocklike feelings
Pain
The gotta moves
Burning
Jimmy legs
Heebie jeebies
Tearing
Throbbing
Tight feeling
Grabbing sensation
Elvis legs
Itching bones
Crazy legs
Fidgets

From Allen RP, Picchietti D, Hening WA, et al. Restless legs syndrome: diagnostic criteria, special considerations, and epidemiology. A report from the Restless Legs Syndrome Diagnosis and Epidemiology Workshop at the National Institutes of Health. *Sleep Med.* 2003;4:101-119.

The associated unpleasant feelings are diverse. They are generally felt deep in the legs, although either the upper or lower part of the leg may be selectively involved (and sometimes the foot or hip), or the entire leg may be involved. The most common area affected is that between the ankle and knee, typically in the region of the gastrocnemius. The feelings are usually bilateral, although they may alternate sides, be predominate on one side, or, in unusual cases (perhaps associated with some focal lesion), be strictly unilateral. Descriptions vary widely (Table 31–2) (see Buchfuhrer and colleagues[12] for 86 different terms that are not exhaustive). The classic descriptors include *creepy-crawly, shocklike, water moving,* or *ants crawling.* Some patients cannot describe their sensations at all, or mention only their need to move. These feelings can be considered spontaneous and can occur without any impinging sensory input; they are a central phenomenon, perhaps similar to neuropathic pain (and sharing some treatments).

Although patients may describe pain, mostly as an ache,[26] this is usually more common in patients with severe RLS.[27] Many patients may experience leg cramps and state that leg cramps are "really" painful, in contrast to RLS symptoms.

RLS is in some sense a misnomer because in severe cases the arms can also be involved.[26,28] This is also true of the associated involuntary movements, termed *periodic limb movements of sleep (PLMS).*[29] Almost always, leg involvement precedes arm involvement, although rare cases may manifest initially with arm symptoms alone.[30] Patients occasionally may have involvement of other body parts, including the pelvis, trunk, genitals, or even the face, but this is unusual, and if not associated with leg symptoms, this involvement may represent a different disorder, even if the character of the symptoms is otherwise typical of RLS. Such anomalous or incomplete presentations[31] may warrant a trial of a dopaminergic medication.

Rest Induces Symptoms

RLS is different from most hyperkinetic disorders (but similar to tics) in that symptoms emerge when the patient is mentally and physically relaxed. Rest can be in any position, but sitting and lying are most typical; rare patients report symptoms when standing quietly. Generally, the longer that the patient is at rest, the more severe the symptoms become.[32,33] In circumstances where the freedom to move is reduced, there is an increase not only in leg symptoms, but also in mental distress. RLS is not provoked only by specific postures, but some younger patients with mild RLS are able to lie down and fall asleep within such a short time that symptoms do not emerge, and consequently report symptoms when only sitting.

Getting Active (Physically and Mentally) Brings Relief

Patients with RLS invariably know that moving around, getting up, and walking bring at least temporary relief. Generally, the more severe the symptoms, the more activity is required to relieve them. All manner of motor activity can provide relief, and patients select the particular activities that are most effective or appropriate to a given situation. In most patients, relief begins as soon as activity starts, but in some cases it may take some minutes for relief to be experienced. For patients with severe RLS having an episode, relief is only temporary, and as soon as they resume sitting or lying, the symptoms recur, often very quickly. These patients may report that walking is not helpful, meaning that its benefits do not persist.

Mental activities can also reduce RLS symptoms, and patients may find that engrossing tasks—computer work, video games, exciting television programs, arguments—also reduce or mask RLS symptoms. Patients very rarely report that symptoms persist or begin during walking; this may occur, however, in severe and debilitated elderly patients who cannot achieve the intensity of walking needed for full relief.

Evening and Night Make Symptoms Worse

In the evening, individuals relax and prepare for sleep, so activity is less. It is now clear, however, that in addition to the provocation of rest, RLS symptoms have a circadian rhythm with symptoms maximal from late evening to early morning (~10 P.M. to 5 A.M.),[32,34-36] at least for patients with regular sleep-wake cycles. There is anecdotal evidence that symptoms show a phase lag when shifting time zones. The morning hours, especially from 9 A.M. to noon, provide a "protected" zone when symptoms are less pronounced.

The basis for this variation is uncertain, but dopamine and iron show circadian rhythms in humans. Cerebrospinal fluid studies show that dopamine and metabolites are higher in the morning,[37,38] whereas melatonin levels are highest synchronous with the peak of RLS symptoms.[36] RLS patients also show greater response to exogenous levodopa administered at night.[39] Dopamine pathways may be crucial in the generation of RLS, and one means for this influence to be exerted might be through an insufficiently damped circadian rhythm, with excess dopamine early in the day and too little dopamine at night.[40-42] One study investigated the relationship between cortisol levels and RLS severity by giving nighttime hydrocortisone in RLS patients, and concluded that low cortisol level may be related to RLS symptoms.[43]

In patients with very severe RLS, symptoms may be present throughout the day and may lose a distinct nocturnal accentuation; this happens in patients who experience severe augmentation. Circadian studies have also established that, with sufficient imposed rest, many patients have symptoms at all hours.[32,34,36] Patients whose nighttime symptoms are well treated may become more aware of symptoms earlier in the day.

Supportive Features

Periodic Limb Movements

As first noted by the Bologna group,[44] most patients with RLS have frequent, repetitive, periodic involuntary movements, periodic limb movements (PLM), at night (Fig. 31–1).[45] These movements vary in form,[46-48] but often take the form of flexion at the ankle, knee, and hip, resembling a flexion reflex.[49] These can occur awake (PLMW) and asleep (PLMS); they have been operationally defined (see Table 31–3).[50-52] The close link of these movements to RLS is supported by one associated gene variant that is closely tied to PLM in RLS.[53]

PLM can be measured during the night in a sleep study, or while the patient is awake with imposed immobility, the suggested immobilization test (SIT).[54,55] Electromyography, measuring muscle electrical activity, and actigraphy, usually measuring acceleration, can be used to detect these movements;[56] automatic programs can also enumerate them by using the operational definition: PLMS consist of movements lasting more than 0.5 second with an amplitude of at least 25% of the calibration amplitude and intermovement intervals of 4 to 90 seconds, and occurring in a series of at least four consecutive movements.[57] New criteria especially for research purposes have modified the definition and include a greater variability of the parameters.[52] Although a key observable feature of these movements is their regularity (see Fig. 31–1), the operational definition does not require strict periodicity. A measure of periodicity, the periodicity index, has been proposed and an increased trend of periodicity in PLM has been shown in RLS patients compared to narcolepsy patients;[58] a longer mean duration of PLM single movements and higher number of sequences were found in RLS compared to controls.[59] In the future, a stricter definition for PLM may be provided.

Because frequent PLM are associated with RLS, the measurement of PLM has been proposed as a diagnostic test. The Montreal group has taken the lead in validating such a test, finding that the number of PLMW during a sleep study best discriminates RLS patients from normals.[60] PLM can occur in many conditions other than RLS (especially narcolepsy and rapid eye movement [REM] sleep behavior disorder),[61] however, and in elderly individuals,[62,63] so the specificity of finding PLM is low. The possibility that testing for PLM may confirm diagnoses in unclear cases of RLS needs to be explored further.[20]

Response to Dopaminergic Medications

Dopaminergic drugs have been the most thoroughly tested in RLS, and are considered the first-line agents for RLS.[4,5] This supportive criterion is based on the expert clinical impression that RLS patients almost invariably respond to dopaminergics.

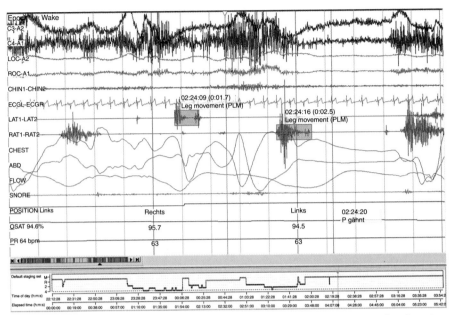

Figure 31–1 Periodic limb movements (PLM) during waking within polysomnography of a patient with restless legs syndrome without medication. There is alternating rhythm (right and left leg) within the periodicity. *Below,* Sleep profile (*blue,* wake; *red,* rapid eye movement sleep).

If a patient does not benefit, the diagnosis of RLS needs to be questioned. A specific test using levodopa and a visual analog scale to measure symptoms has been proven to identify most true RLS cases in a group with at least suggestive RLS, and excluded all subjects determined not to have RLS.[64] The high specificity of this test makes it quite useful for excluding cases with an ambiguous presentation, but not true RLS. The authors report that all patients who responded positively to the test—with at least 50% symptom reduction—subsequently benefited by dopaminergic therapy. Some patients with RLS did not respond positively, however, so a negative result may not be as conclusive.

Family History of Restless Legs Syndrome

RLS is a familial disorder: most patients are aware of affected family members. Finding an affected relative, especially a first-degree relative (biological parent, sibling, or child) raises the likelihood that a patient also has RLS. This may be especially important in diagnosing children, in whom a clear history of the four diagnostic features may be impossible.

Associated Features

Sleep Disruption

Sleep disruption is a primary morbidity of RLS,[45,65,66] and has been the usual chief complaint of RLS patients. Patients may have difficulty getting to sleep, have difficulty going back to sleep once wakened, and have sleep disrupted, often by PLMS;

overall total sleep is reduced, and the sleep period is highly fragmented.[17,45,65,67] Most patients who require medical management of RLS have some sleep complaint. RLS patients complain about sleep deprivation more than patients with any other sleep disorder or movement disorder because they may have been sleeping only 3 or 4 hours per night for years. Only a few patients describe fatigue or excessive daytime sleepiness, either because the situations that induce sleepiness also induce RLS symptoms, causing the patients to move, or because RLS patients have unusually enhanced alertness. If a patient presents with a chief complaint of severe excessive daytime sleepiness, additional causes of sleep disruption, such as sleep-related breathing disorders, need to be considered.

Physical Examination in Idiopathic Restless Legs Syndrome

Patients with idiopathic RLS generally do not have any abnormalities on physical examination. They only rarely display their restlessness when they are in the physician's office. Physical examination is undertaken mainly to ascertain the presence of disorders that might be confused with RLS, to determine comorbidities, or to support a diagnosis of potentially causative conditions (e.g., peripheral neuropathy).

Clinical Course

Patients generally present with a progressive, worsening condition, with patients with early-onset familial RLS having a slowly progressive disorder.[17] Older patients, perhaps with symptoms provoked by some underlying condition, may have a more rapidly progressive course. Generally, the course of the disease is variable, but RLS is a chronic condition. There may be remissions and a rare disappearance of symptoms, but unless there is a provocative condition, cures are not to be found. In the Hopkins family study, the average duration of symptoms in family members of patients and controls was nearly 20 years.[68] Less than 5% of subjects who ever reported symptoms lacked current symptoms, even though most of these individuals had not been diagnosed with RLS, were less severe on average than patients, and often had a stable or even improving course.

Diagnostic Instruments

Questionnaires

Questionnaires for RLS can be used to screen patients in clinical practice or to ascertain cases of RLS in epidemiological studies of large populations. A single question has proven highly sensitive in detecting RLS patients, and has reasonable specificity in many populations.[69] Available in several languages (for many European languages, see Ferri and colleagues[69]), the English version is as follows: When you try to relax in the evening or sleep at night, do you ever have unpleasant, restless feelings in your legs that can be relieved by walking or movement? A small pilot study suggests that the last part is unnecessary.

Several multiquestion instruments have been developed for epidemiological studies. Two have been validated. One 3-question instrument developed by Berger and endorsed at the National Institutes of Health diagnostic consensus conference[15] had an inter-rater κ of 0.67 between two experts, who, however, had access to the questionnaire results.[70] Another questionnaire developed at Johns Hopkins was validated by independent clinician interview and had a specificity of 80% in an American primary care practice.[71]

Structured Diagnostic Evaluations

Two different approaches have been taken to make more definitive diagnoses for clinical or research purposes. First is a telephone interview, the Hopkins Telephone Diagnostic Interview for RLS.[72] This interview includes not only questions that address the diagnostic features, but also questions to assist with differential diagnosis and uncover mimics. Finally, there are questions concerning key aspects of the disorder. Agreement with expert interviews was found to be 92%, approaching the inter-rater reliability of two expert face-to-face interviews of 96%.[72]

A second approach is a protocol that begins with questions about diagnostic features, but then includes tests related to the supportive and associated features (see Table 31–1). This diagnostic interview (RLS-DI) includes questions on sleep disorders, family history, a dopaminergic challenge test, and, in cases still diagnostically unclear, a sleep study to look for PLM and a neurological physical examination and a dopaminergic challenge test to exclude other causes for symptoms.[22] With the RLS-DI, persistent acute RLS and intermittent acute RLS can be diagnosed, but not sporadic RLS. Because it gives higher scores to patients with more frequent symptoms, the RLS-DI may not correctly identify patients with sporadic symptoms. Because it may require laboratory evaluation or a therapeutic trial, it is less useful for screening large populations. In essence, the RLS-DI makes a diagnosis of clinically significant RLS.

Diagnosis in Children and Elderly Individuals

Children

Because children have limited ability to communicate their symptoms, the diagnosis of RLS in children includes additional elements. As indicated in Table 31–3, diagnosis in children may depend more on supportive or associated features, such as family history, the presence of PLM, or sleep disturbance.[15] Additional categories of probable or possible RLS are also defined, primarily for research purposes.[15] A more recent study indicated, however, that many children who originally meet criteria only for possible or probable RLS go on to meet criteria for definite RLS.[73] Adolescents 12 years or older can generally communicate well enough to be diagnosed using adult standards.

Elderly and Cognitively Impaired Individuals

Elderly individuals may be able to describe their condition sufficiently to be diagnosed in the usual way. In the oldest (>85 years old) patients, a significant fraction fall into the groups with dementia, however. As in other individuals with cognitive impairment, it may be possible to determine the diagnostic criteria for their interview. In this situation, several strategies may lead to a necessarily tentative diagnosis of RLS: observation of motor restlessness in the evening and at night or of patients massaging their legs; history of RLS obtained earlier in life; reports from close relatives, bed partners, or co-residents; sleep disruption; numerous PLM (>25/hr at night); and response to dopaminergic medications.

TABLE 31–3	Criteria for the Diagnosis of Definite Restless Legs Syndrome in Children

1. The child meets all four essential adult criteria for RLS
and
2. The child relates a description in his or her own words that is consistent with leg discomfort. The child may use terms such as *oowies, tickle, spiders, boo-boos, want to run,* and *a lot of energy in my legs* to describe symptoms. Age-appropriate descriptors are encouraged
or
1. The child meets all four essential adult criteria for RLS
and
2. Two of three supportive criteria are present

Supportive Criteria for Diagnosis of Definite RLS in Children
Sleep disturbance for age
Biological parent or sibling has definite RLS
Child has polysomnographically documented periodic limb movement index of ≥5 per hour of sleep

RLS, restless legs syndrome.
From Allen RP, Picchietti D, Hening WA, et al. Restless legs syndrome: diagnostic criteria, special considerations, and epidemiology. A report from the Restless Legs Syndrome Diagnosis and Epidemiology Workshop at the National Institutes of Health. *Sleep Med.* 2003;4:101-119.

Differential Diagnosis

Two sets of conditions may produce symptoms that are similar to those of RLS: first, conditions of restlessness such as subtypes of major depression, anxiety disorder, akathisia, attention-deficit/hyperactivity disorder (ADHD), and drug-induced restlessness, and second, conditions of leg discomfort secondary to local pathology, such as peripheral neuropathy, myelopathy, and pain owing to venous congestion or disease, which may be more intense or appreciated at night. To discriminate between RLS and such "mimic" conditions, the key is to pay close attention to the four diagnostic features to ensure they are met. RLS can be differentiated from positional discomfort by the fact that although the latter is relieved by a change in position, in RLS the symptoms reoccur after movement is discontinued, which is covered by essential criterion number 2. The diagnosis tends to be more secure in more severe and frequent RLS.

INITIAL WORK-UP AND ASSESSMENT OF RESTLESS LEGS SYNDROME SEVERITY

Initial Work-up

When a diagnosis of RLS has been made, the work-up is quite abbreviated. Measurement of serum ferritin values, the basic measure of iron stores, is required, and percent saturation of transferrin is highly recommended. This requirement is due to the key role of iron deficiency as a precipitating cause of RLS, which can be treated with iron supplementation. Patients should be screened for diabetes and kidney failure, which can be done with a basic serum chemical screen. Other laboratory values are

TABLE 31–4	**Scales for Assessing Restless Legs Syndrome**

Severity Scales

IRLS (Severity Scale of the International RLS study group)[77]
RLS-6[80]
Johns Hopkins Severity Scale (JHSS)[78]

Quality of Life Scales

RLS QoL questionnaire (Kohnen)[275]
RLS QoL questionnaire (Allen)[276]
RLS-QLI instrument[277]
SF 36 (Short-Form 36 Health Survey)[278]

Other Scales for RLS

Clinical Global Impression (CGI), Patient Global Impression (PGI)[279]
RLS Diagnostic Index (RLS-DI)[22]
Augmentation Severity Rating Scale of the European RLS study group (ASRS)[280]
Structured Interview for Diagnosis of Augmentation (SIDA)[281]

From Hogl B, Gschliesser V. RLS assessment and sleep questionnaires in practice—lessons learned from Parkinson's disease. *Sleep Med.* 2007;8(Suppl 2):S7-S12.[76]

necessary only if there are further clinical indications; routine screening for rheumatologic abnormalities has not been found to be useful.[74] Many patients may have a thyroid disorder, although the role of thyroid metabolism in RLS is unclear.

Imaging, electromyography and nerve conduction studies, and sleep studies should be undertaken only when evidence of some comorbid or causative disorder is noted on evaluation. In the United States, it has been explicitly stated that a sleep study (polysomnography) is not indicated for the routine diagnosis of RLS.[75] It is, however, necessary when a sleep-related breathing disorder is suspected or when the diagnosis remains uncertain.

Subjective Assessment Measures

Because RLS is primarily a subjective disorder, the major assessments have relied on subjective instruments (Table 31–4).[76] The two most common instruments used in therapeutic trials are the IRLSSG rating scale (IRLS) and the Clinical Global Impression. The IRLS is a validated 10-item scale with five levels ranging from no symptoms (0) to very severe symptoms (4).[77] The summed score is generally used (0 to 40), with a score 1 to 10 labeled as mild RLS, 11 to 20 labeled as moderate RLS, 21 to 30 labeled as severe RLS, and 31 to 40 labeled as very severe RLS. The Johns Hopkins RLS Severity Scale is based on the usual time of day for onset of RLS symptoms. Severity is graded as "no symptoms at all," "bedtime-only symptoms," "evening symptoms," and "RLS symptoms during the day (before 6 P.M.)."[78]

Factor analysis has shown that it can also be broken down into two subscales: one on symptoms and the second on impact. The Clinical Global Impression is a collection of four generic scales that assess disease severity and response to treatment. The most used are two 7-point scales on current severity and on change since baseline.[79] An alternative rating scale is the RLS-6, which includes questions on symptom severity at different times of the day and daytime sleepiness.[80,81] The

Johns Hopkins RLS rating scale categorizes patients by the time of onset of symptoms; earlier onset indicates more severe disease (but mainly restricted to patients with daily symptoms).[78] Additional rating scales used frequently include general (SF-36) and specific quality-of-life scales, sleep assessments, and daytime somnolence questionnaires (for general review, see Kohnen and colleagues).[81] Sleep diaries have sometimes been used to assess RLS,[82] and in the future, perhaps in an electronic format, they may be more frequently used, as they currently are in Parkinson's disease.

Objective Assessment Measures

The primary objective measure of RLS severity has been measuring PLM during a sleep study, using either polysomnography[83-85] or activity recording. Frequency of PLM correlates with subjective severity measures in some studies,[78,86] but individual patients may show large discrepancies and therefore changes of PLM by medication correlated much better than baseline values.[87] Night-to-night variability, although stable for groups,[88] may be high for individuals.[89] Actigraphic assessment for 3 or more days may give a more accurate picture, especially in patients with fewer PLM (<25/hr). Because RLS is a subjective disorder, and some patients do not have numerous PLM, PLM indices remain an incomplete measure in RLS.

Assessing sleep studies according to standard measures, such as total sleep time, sleep efficiency (time asleep/time in bed), measures of deeper sleep stages (slow wave or REM sleep), wake during sleep, or the amount of sleep disruption (arousals, awakenings, or sleep stage changes), has not proven as useful as PLM measures in RLS. Although sleep disruption is a primary complaint in RLS and can be objectively established,[67] studies have often not found significant improvements in such sleep measures; this might be due to the contaminating sleep-disruptive effects of the measures themselves. In patients with severely compromised sleep because of RLS, successful treatment would include notable improvement in individual patient sleep measures.

A third approach to measure RLS severity objectively is the use of a provocative test, the SIT.[54,55,60,90] During the SIT, the patient remains seated and inactive in bed for 1 hour while PLM are measured and periodic ratings are made of subjective discomfort[91]; the SIT is most typically carried out in the evening, perhaps as a prelude to polysomnography. The current status of the SIT as a measure of severity remains experimental.[92] Similar to polysomnography PLM measures, there can be large individual day-to-day variation in measured PLMW.[93] Correlations between nighttime and SIT PLM measures and general and SIT subjective measures are often not robust. To date, no blood or cerebrospinal fluid values, no electromyography or nerve conduction velocity measures, and no imaging methods have developed that can be useful either for diagnosis or for assessment of RLS severity. One exception may be in patients with low serum ferritin levels (<45 µg/L); increasing the ferritin level may be distinctly associated with RLS improvement within weeks.

Pathophysiology of Restless Legs Syndrome

Pathophysiology of RLS is a complex topic because it is still unknown how RLS symptoms evolve. An overall pathophysiological concept cannot be given. We describe here current research approaches into different aspects of RLS pathophysiology. We present results derived from diverse studies using neurophysiological, neuropharmacological, neuroimaging, and neurogenetic approaches.

CORTICAL STRUCTURES

In contrast to positron emission tomography (PET) results and measurements of preparatory cortical activation,[94] no cortical activation was detected in functional magnetic resonance imaging (MRI) during PLMW[95] with a lack of the Bereitschaftspotential before PLM.[96] Increased cortical excitability has been described in RLS using paired pulse techniques with transcranial magnetic stimulation[97]; this excitability could be reversed by cabergoline.[98] These findings may be related to MRI-detected structural changes of decreased gray matter volume of the bihemispheric primary somatosensory cortex, the study reflecting[99] a primary structural change in association with RLS, and not a secondary correlate of neuroplasticity. Conflicting gray matter results are reported in two other studies, however.[100,101] A cognitive decline in RLS, presumably related to cortical dysfunction, was comparable to the cognitive decline caused by a loss of 1 night's sleep,[102] suggesting an acquired deficit, in contrast to another study, which found cognitive deficits in RLS patients relatively resistant to sleep deprivation.[103] One possible explanation for cortical changes might lie in the actions of RLS-predisposing genes during development (see section on genetic epidemiology of RLS).

BASAL GANGLIA

The basal ganglia have always been a location of major interest for RLS because dopaminergic treatment is so effective for RLS; the role of the nigrostriatal dopaminergic system has been explored in several studies. Conflicting data arise from PET and single photon emission computed tomography (SPECT) studies. Several studies showed slightly reduced dopamine receptor binding on the postsynaptic level, although methodological problems in these early studies may have influenced the outcome. These studies comprised RLS patients and patients with pure PLMS, including patients with and without dopaminergic pretreatment; most had severe RLS. Other studies observed normal presynaptic and postsynaptic bindings in RLS patients.[104,105] One PET study using presynaptic and postsynaptic receptor binding ligands in nontreated patients with mild RLS gives evidence for a generalized reduced level of endogenous dopamine or, alternatively, an increased dopamine D2 receptor availability.[106]

One study assessed opioid binding with diprenorphine C 11.[107] The study found that the endogenous opiate system may show redistributed binding, which could compensate for unpleasant RLS symptoms in proportion to RLS severity in a pattern of changes similar to that in chronic pain conditions.

Substantia nigra abnormalities have been found in RLS. Several studies show that iron stores are low, and that cells show signs of altered iron regulation pathology in female patients with early onset of RLS.[108,109] Several specialized MRI studies detected low brain iron in vivo,[110,111] a finding confirmed by transcranial ultrasound, which detected a hypoechogenic substantia nigra indicating low iron stores.[112,113] A more recent ultrasound publication compared RLS and Parkinson's disease patients and confirmed that RLS subjects had low brain iron, whereas Parkinson's disease subjects had high levels.[114]

One leading pathogenetic hypothesis is that RLS is due, at least in some cases, to deficient brain iron. This hypothesis has been supported not only by autopsy and imaging studies, but also by studies that show low cerebrospinal fluid ferritin, suggesting decreased iron stores.[115,116] A consequence of such depleted iron stores may be altered function of the dopamine system.[41] Support for such a link comes from studies that show a synaptic protein, Thy 1, necessary for dopamine synapses is deficient in RLS substantia nigra neurons.[117] In addition, RLS patients show aberrant circadian rhythm of dopamine metabolites in cerebrospinal fluid,[37] and iron-deprived animals show altered circadian dopamine rhythms.[118] Such animals can also show altered sleep-wake and activity patterns.[119,120]

BRAINSTEM AND SPINAL CORD

Beneath the basal ganglia, several studies have focused on the role of A11 cells, the only source of spinal dopaminergic innervation.[121,122] Proposed animal models for RLS involve lesioning of these A11 cells,[121,123,124] although it is hard to know how complete and selective the lesions might be because this is small, ill-defined nuclear group. In a more recent study, the relationship of the dopaminergic and iron systems was investigated. Increased animal motor activity was observed in 6-hydroxydopamine A11 lesioned rodents additionally subjected to iron deprivation, mimicking one feature of RLS (excessive motor activity).[120] This augmented activity was relieved with dopamine agonist treatment. It is still unclear whether degeneration of the A11 neurons plays an active role in RLS symptoms in elderly patients.[122,125]

Other brainstem nuclei, including the red nucleus, the inferior olive, and the cerebellar nuclei, form a network that is able to attenuate sensory information during movement.[126] They were found to be activated during PLMW in a functional MRI pilot study.[95] The increased incidence of RLS in spinocerebellar ataxias[127] may indicate involvement of further brainstem or cerebellar structures, however, with the inferior olive as the key site of abnormal activity.[126]

A hyperexcitability of the spinal motor system[49,128] and the spinal sensory system including pain tracts may be involved in RLS. A study with pin-prick stimuli showed that patients with RLS exhibit a profound static mechanical hyperalgesia, but no dynamic mechanical hyperalgesia, a characteristic sign of neuropathic pain.[129] Differential responses of early and late flexor reflexes to dopaminergic and opioid therapy in experimental studies may explain why a dopaminergic-induced hyperexcitability can occur in dopaminergic-induced augmentation, and may make opioids a good choice to treat augmentation.[130]

PERIPHERAL NERVOUS SYSTEM

The involvement of the peripheral nervous system in RLS pathology is still speculative, but many patients with neuropathy have disturbing RLS symptoms in addition to their neuropathic complaints and deficits. Several different types of neuropathy have reported to be associated with RLS, including amyloid neuropathy,[131] cryoglobulinemic neuropathy,[132] Charcot-Marie-Tooth disease type 2,[133] axonal neuropathy,[134] subclinical sensory neuropathy,[134-136] and diabetic neuropathy.[137] More recent investigations detected RLS symptoms in 30% of patients with small fiber–type sensory neuropathy.[138] Together with the study of Stiasny-Kolster and colleagues,[129] these findings indicate that deficits in temperature perception measured in idiopathic RLS are not due to peripheral small fiber damage, but rather indicate a functional impairment of central somatosensory processing.[125]

Epidemiology and Genetics of Restless Legs Syndrome

PREVALENCE OF RESTLESS LEGS SYNDROME

Although Ekbom[139] noted in 1945 that RLS could be diagnosed in 5% of clinic patients, the general impression for the succeeding decades was that RLS was uncommon. The first population-wide study to suggest that RLS was common in the general population was a Canadian study published in 1994, which found that 10% to 15% of adults reported symptoms of RLS.[140] After the consensus clinical definition of RLS was published in 1995,[14] single-question[141] and multiple-question[70] survey instruments were based on the four diagnostic criteria. In Western populations, these have led to an endorsement rate of 7% to 13% in adults.[2] These rates were not corrected, however, for the likely less than perfect specificity of these instruments or the need for treatment.

Major risk factors for RLS are increasing age (at least through the sixth decade) and gender. Increasing age likely reflects the chronic nature of RLS; as population groups age, ever larger numbers shift from the non-RLS to the RLS subgroups, whereas the reverse shift is unlikely. In children, RLS is less common. A large-scale population study found that approximately 2% of children 8 to 17 years old met criteria for definite RLS[142]; 0.25% of children 12 years old and younger and 0.5% of the older children met criteria for more severe RLS (two or more episodes of RLS per week and moderate or greater bothersomeness of symptoms). Female gender may reflect the greater iron stresses and lower iron stores in women. Two studies have now found that having been pregnant may account for much of the gender difference.[143] Consistent with this possibility is the finding that gender is not a risk factor in children.[142] Family history together with certain specific disorders and conditions also increase the likelihood of RLS.

In the general population, there is a wide spectrum of RLS severity. Several studies found that {1/5} to {1/6} of subjects who report RLS symptoms experience them on a daily basis, with relatively equal amounts of the rest of subjects (i.e., ~40%) having either weekly, but not daily, symptoms or less than weekly symptoms.[144,145] These figures reflect the expected decrease in severity measures compared with patient samples, in which most subjects may have daily symptoms.

Prevalence figures for non–European-derived populations vary widely.[1,2] Most studies have been undertaken in Asia and find prevalences that range from near zero[146] to about 1%[147] to several percent[148,149] to more than 10%[150]; a more recent study in Korea reported a prevalence of 7.5%.[151] These differences, sometimes seen in the same population, are likely due in part to different instruments, languages, and cultural attitudes toward responses. Although the discrepancies between studies make any definitive conclusion impossible, it does seem that Asians may have a lower biological tendency toward RLS than Europeans.

There are no studies to date in African populations. Only one study in a Native American population found an estimated prevalence of 2%.[152] In one study, similar frequencies of RLS in African-American (4.7%) adults were found compared with whites (3.8%).[153,154]

RLS is more common in clinical than general populations.[65] In one U.S. clinical practice, 24% of patients reported RLS symptoms; 15% had symptoms at least weekly.[71] A subsequent validation of the questionnaire indicated that approximately 60% of these individuals did have true RLS.[71] A similar high endorsement rate was found in another primary care study.[155]

It seems that RLS is a common disorder in most populations, and that any physician who sees patients with movement disorders would see patients with RLS. Despite increased awareness, only few patients with RLS received an accurate diagnosis or appropriate treatment for clinically significant symptoms.[65,66,145] The substantial increase in patient treatment with the approval of RLS medications in Europe and the United States is a testimony to the unmet clinical needs of these patients.

GENETICS OF RESTLESS LEGS SYNDROME

It was appreciated early on that RLS patients had a positive family history for the disorder.[139,156] Subsequently, several large case series found that more than 50% of RLS patients were aware of affected first-degree relatives.[45,157-159] Formal case-control family studies showed that the relative risk of RLS to first-degree relatives of RLS cases was approximately 3 to 7,[160] with greater relative risk for cases with early onset of RLS.

Consistent with the familial aggregation of RLS, large pedigrees were located with many affected members.[161] These pedigrees permitted the application of segregation analyses to see which possible model for inheritance (or environmental factors) could account for the observed family distribution of cases. Two analyses in different populations found that a dominant autosomal genetic model best fit the family patterns either in younger onset RLS cases[162] or in all primary cases.[163] Both analyses found a high frequency of phenocopies unrelated to the genetic factor. In the second analysis,[163] age of onset was found to be under multigenic and environmental control.

The large families with multiple affected members also led to numerous efforts to find linkage of RLS to specific chromosome loci.[164] Beginning in 2001, at least seven loci have now been reported in specific families or groups of families, and have been designated RLS1 through RLS7 (on 12q, 14q, 9p, 2q, and 20p, 4q and 17p);[165] despite much effort, no specific gene mutations have been found.[166] Another possible linkage has been reported on chromosome 19q.[164] Several loci have been replicated in different populations,[166] in families,[167,168] or by association studies.[169,170] In two of the linkages, affected family members were likely to have frequent PLM (12q, 14q).

More recently, genome-wide association studies have detected gene variants in four chromosomal regions that convey differential risk for RLS,[6,53,171] and have been calculated to make a substantial contribution to the presence of RLS in the population. As has happened in other genome-wide association studies, the genes involved have no clear relationship to RLS pathophysiological concepts; they are primarily active in embryonic development, and their adult function is not well established. It had been expected that genes in the iron, dopamine, or endogenous opiate pathways might be important for RLS because these pathways are important for pathogenesis or therapy, but studies of these candidate genes have been unavailing so far.

One associated gene, *BTBD9* on 6p, was found by two groups. In the Iceland/American study, it was more associated with PLM in the cases than subjective symptoms of RLS, and was associated with body iron stores.[53] This finding underscores further the important but little understood link between RLS and PLM: they share an array of risk factors and some common pathophysiology. In the German study, the clinical population consisted of severely affected RLS patients seeking treatment. The genetic variants of this study were within the *MEIS 1* gene, *BTBD9*, and another region in which the genes *MAP2K5* and *LBXCOR1* were annotated and were highly associated with RLS.

ASSOCIATED AND COMORBID DISORDERS AND SECONDARY RESTLESS LEGS SYNDROME

Associated Disorders

As mentioned previously, RLS with onset later in life tends to be less familial, and is often associated with a predisposing factor.[17,159] This finding led to the suggestion that one could differentiate primary, familial RLS from cases of secondary RLS in which the RLS was due to a specific cause, such as kidney failure.[160] The more recent genetic discoveries suggest a different picture, however, in which RLS is likely to arise from an interplay of predisposing genetic variants with environmental factors, including numerous disorders. Genetic factors are present at birth, but it may take time for them to become fully manifest. Acquired risk factors, such as diseases, tend to accumulate over time as well. Both trends may contribute to the growing frequency of RLS in older age groups. In one segregation analysis, it was shown that the likely determinants of RLS age of onset were multigenic and environmental.[166]

When two disorders are comorbid, either may be the cause of the other, or both may share a common cause. In the case of RLS, most linkages to other disorders or conditions can be considered associations with no clear indication of causality. These associations may be of lesser (e.g., small case series) or greater (e.g., case-control studies) evidentiary value. A few disorders or conditions have been studied in ways that provide some evidence of causality, however. Conditions that RLS may cause are considered elements of RLS morbidity. Most are speculative. When RLS arises in the context of a disorder that likely precedes RLS, or when treatment of the disorder alleviates RLS, there is evidence of a potential causative condition. One association that may involve a common cause is the link between RLS and ADHD. It has been found that childhood ADHD and RLS are associated.[172,173] There is also preliminary evidence that adults with RLS have an increased frequency of attention-deficit disorder.[174] A common link between RLS and ADHD may be iron deficiency[175,176]; it has been speculated that a third disorder that seems more prevalent in ADHD and RLS, Gilles de la Tourette syndrome, may also share an iron deficiency diathesis.[25]

Secondary Restless Legs Syndrome

Several conditions seem to have a causative influence on RLS, including anemia and iron deficiency, kidney failure, pregnancy, and certain medications, because treating them or removing their influence is likely to alleviate RLS symptoms. Iron deficiency is a common thread among many of these provocative factors; anemia, kidney failure, blood donation, and pregnancy all put stress on iron stores, or result from iron deficiency.[41]

There is evidence that RLS patients have an elevated frequency of iron deficiency, and that lower iron stores are related to more severe RLS.[178] There is some evidence, although it is a surprisingly modest amount, to support a higher frequency of RLS in iron-deficient individuals.[178] Broad population studies have not found iron stores to be strongly related to RLS frequency.[70] However, oral[179] and intravenous[180-182] iron have not or only partially relieved RLS in iron-deficient patients. Some female patients may benefit from intravenous iron sucrose, patients with normal iron stores may not receive similar benefits.[183] Iron deficiency induced by gastrointestinal bleeding may explain the association between use of nonsteroidal anti-inflammatory drugs and RLS,[184] and reports that RLS can be the presenting symptom of colon cancer.[185,186]

Elevated frequencies of RLS in kidney failure have been found in Europe and Asia, including in patients on dialysis[187-193] (ranging from 6.6% in India[189] to 70% in China).[188] Some of this association can be explained by uremia-induced iron deficiency, but not all of it. The character of RLS in uremia is quite similar to that of idiopathic RLS, although higher frequencies of PLMS have been observed.[194] RLS in dialysis patients is associated with greater sleep disturbance, poorer quality of life, and higher mortality.[187,195,196] Although dialysis seems to have little impact on RLS symptoms, kidney transplantation usually relieves RLS symptoms.[197] Recurring RLS is associated with declining renal function[197] and is a risk factor for mortality after transplant.[198] Better treatment of anemia and iron deficiency seems to be helpful in reducing RLS in these patients.

Another probable provocative factor for RLS is pregnancy; similar rates of 20% to 27% are seen around the world.[199-201] Approximately two thirds of RLS in pregnancy is due to initial manifestation of the disease; patients with preexisting RLS often find RLS worsening. Patients with initial symptoms of RLS usually find relief near the time of delivery.[202] Although pregnancy may be a risk factor for developing RLS later in life,[143] it has not yet been established that this is especially true for women who develop RLS during pregnancy.

Elevated frequencies of RLS have been reported in Parkinson's disease.[203-205] This finding is surprising because brain iron is low in RLS, but high in Parkinson's disease,[112] and most RLS patients do not show signs of Parkinson's disease. In one study,[203] it was found that most RLS in Parkinson's disease had a late onset, in most cases after the beginning of Parkinson's disease. This finding is typical of what has been considered secondary RLS. A possible intervening factor may be the administration of dopaminergic medications in Parkinson's disease. These medications have been implicated in causing augmentation in RLS, an iatrogenic worsening of RLS owing to treatment.[206]

Neuropathy has been frequently cited as a possible cause of RLS, but this has not been easy to establish. Some more recent studies have documented an elevated frequency of RLS in neuropathy, especially small-fiber neuropathy.[207] Because nerve pathology has been found in some RLS patients without neuropathic complaints,[134,136] it is also possible that RLS and small-fiber neuropathy share some common causality. If neuropathy is causative, it may be a cause for the high frequency of RLS reported in diabetic patients.[208]

Although the literature is sparse, any antidopaminergic may likely cause or aggravate RLS. This includes antiemetics and gastrointestinal medications, such as metoclopramide. Administration of metoclopramide to asymptomatic patients in the afternoon did not robustly induce symptoms, however.[209] Similarly, there are scattered reports of antidepressants aggravating or provoking RLS.

Morbidity Associated with Restless Legs Syndrome

RLS is associated with significant medical and psychiatric comorbidities. There are few studies, however, that go beyond association to support causation by RLS. Depression and anxiety have been associated with RLS,[210,211] with some suggestion that depression could be reactive to RLS symptoms.[210] Hypertension and cardiovascular disease have also been found to be associated with RLS symptoms in population studies.[212,213] RLS symptoms can acutely precipitate premature termination of dialysis, and compromise or cause abandonment of surgical procedures, and conditions of stress and unrelieved symptoms have been suggested to precipitate cardiovascular or cerebrovascular events.

A major morbidity of RLS is disruption of sleep. Disrupted sleep may be responsible for many of the daytime consequences of RLS, such as decreased alertness and emotional distress.[214] Generally, sleep deprivation and fragmentation are associated with various daytime consequences; reduced sleep (<6 hours a night) is a risk factor for mortality. There is even some support for the proposition that sleep deprivation can cause hypertension and impair insulin function. RLS patients often have sleep that is severely deprived, averaging fewer than 5 hours per night.[17,65] Sleep deprivation reduces vitality and concentration, and can aggravate a depressive mood. Another possible intermediary factor is the presence of PLMS, especially PLMS with arousal, which have been associated with autonomic arousal, including significant elevations of heart rate and blood pressure.[215-221]

If we become more certain that RLS has all these complications, or that PLMS alone may lead to poorer outcomes, the treatment of RLS would take on an even greater urgency. To support such an attitude, studies need to show that treating RLS can ameliorate the putative sequelae. The discovery that PLM may involve central nervous system arousals that are associated with sleep fragmentation raises the question of whether PLM should be treated, if severe, more for preventive reasons than merely to suppress the often asymptomatic movements.

Management of Restless Legs Syndrome

GENERAL CONSIDERATIONS

The high prevalence of RLS does not mean that all patients with RLS should be treated with pharmacological therapy. No data are available about mild or intermittent RLS and its need and response to common treatment concepts. Before starting a pharmacological treatment, however, sleep hygiene measures should be recommended, and all causes of secondary RLS should be considered. Patients with serum ferritin values even in the low to normal range may benefit from iron supplementation.[178] Such patients exhibit increased rates of augmentation on dopaminergic therapy.[222]

Based on clinical trials and expert experience, long-term therapy with one substance and stable dosages may cause increasing problems over time. The best strategy is to start pharmacological therapy cautiously and at the lowest recommended dosage. RLS and its chronic sleep disturbance may have a significant impact on sleep, social life, and working life,[7,223,224] and adequate treatment should not be withheld from patients in need.

Pharmacological intervention in RLS is symptomatic and can relieve subjective symptoms or improve the sleep disturbance or both. PLMS are closely related to RLS and are the target of therapy in polysomnographically controlled trials. PLMW and PLMS may reflect the amount of RLS motor symptoms. Neuroprotective treatment strategies for RLS and a cure for RLS are not yet known.

Nonpharmacological treatments such as exercise[225] have rarely been investigated. None such treatments are considered efficacious according to evidence-based medicine criteria. More recently, approaches for additional psychotherapeutic interventions have been described and are currently being investigated in clinical trials.[226]

AUGMENTATION AND REBOUND

Before discussing specific RLS medications and their benefits, it is important to introduce the concepts of rebound and augmentation, two phenomena that can limit therapeutic efficacy, especially for dopaminergic agents. The most important complication of dopaminergic therapy is augmentation, which was first described in 1996 by Allen and Earley[227] as a paradoxical worsening of RLS symptoms after an initially successful dopaminergic treatment.[15] Augmentation is characterized by the advance of RLS symptoms to earlier in the day, then, by a shorter latency at rest, increased intensity of symptoms, and a spreading of RLS symptoms to previously unaffected areas of the body. Onset of symptoms earlier in the day is the most common phenomenon.[50]

Augmentation is assumed to be a specific problem associated with dopaminergic medications, although two case reports are documented with possible augmentation under tramadol[228,229]; the mechanisms underlying the development of augmentation are still under debate.[52] A dopaminergic overstimulation of the striatal dopamine D1 receptors, such as occurs with levodopa, may play a key role in the development of augmentation.[130,230] Tolerance to treatment has been described in some cases of dopaminergic therapy[53] as the loss of therapeutic efficacy of an RLS treatment that had previously been efficacious.

Rebound should be distinguished from augmentation. Rebound is the appearance of RLS symptoms at a time that is compatible with the half-life of the drug, when the effects of the drug are wearing off, and is equivalent to withdrawal. Rebound was first noticed in the morning with increases of leg movements in about one fourth of RLS patients treated with levodopa.[231] It occurs after morning awakening and consists of more severe RLS symptoms in the morning than without treatment.

TREATMENT

Levodopa/Decarboxylase Inhibitor

Eight randomized controlled trials[54,232-238] showed the efficacy of levodopa/decarboxylase inhibitor in RLS therapy. Four of these trials were placebo-controlled mostly giving levodopa/decarboxylase inhibitor as a single bedtime dose for nocturnal RLS symptoms.[54,232,233,236] Two other trials, one of which was an open-label trial, investigated the sustained-release formulation of levodopa[233,235]; others investigated levodopa compared with other agents, such as pergolide,[234] valproic acid,[237] gabapentin,[239] and cabergoline.[238] The dosages ranged from 100 to 300 mg as a single dose per night, with a second dose 3 hours after bedtime or in combination with a sustained-release formulation.

Levodopa has been shown to control the motor and sensory disturbances of RLS as measured by subjective RLS rating scales and improves quality of life, RLS severity,[232] and polysomnographic parameters.[54,232,236] In comparative trials of dopamine agonists such as pergolide (mean dose 0.159 mg) or cabergoline (1 to 3 mg) compared with up to 300 mg levodopa, the dopamine agonists were shown to be superior to levodopa as far as efficacy measured and augmentation were concerned. Levodopa caused fewer side effects such as nausea and dizziness, however. In another comparative trial of valproate 600 mg versus controlled-release levodopa/benserazide 200/50 mg, both drugs significantly improved RLS, but only valproic acid decreased the intensity of RLS for more than the first 4 hours after intake.[237] In a comparison between gabapentin (100 to 200 mg) and levodopa/carbidopa (100/25 mg/day) both given as single dosages, sleep improved more with gabapentin than levodopa/carbidopa when measured in the sleep laboratory.[239]

Levodopa is a short-acting medication, and it seems to be appropriate for treating mild and intermittent RLS, although all treatment trials to date have been performed with moderate to severe RLS. Levodopa/benserazide is licensed for RLS therapy in some European countries and Brazil. The limitation of levodopa relates mainly to its lack of efficacy with the dosage used and its long-term side effect of augmentation (see previous definition).

Dopamine Agonists

Ergot-Dopamine Agonists

The ergot-DA, bromocriptine, pergolide, and cabergoline, have been investigated in RLS therapy, and all have proven effective according to evidence-based medicine level 1 studies.[230] Ergot-DA are no longer the first-choice treatment, however, in Parkinson's disease or in RLS because of the risk of developing fibrosis (i.e., valvulopathy), a class effect of ergot derivatives.

Bromocriptine was the first DA used in RLS therapy. Pergolide, in a double-blind controlled study with a long-term observation of 1 year, was shown to be efficacious. In a large multicenter (PEARLS) study with 100 patients, the IRLS score improved (IRLS score 12.2 for pergolide versus 1.8 for placebo); these effects were maintained for 12 months at a mean dosage of 0.52 to 0.72 mg/day. No significant improvements were seen in sleep efficiency (11.3% versus 6.1%; $P = .196$) or total sleep time ($P = .145$). The largest trial that has been carried out with cabergoline was a comparative trial with levodopa and cabergoline in 361 patients with severe RLS:[238] 2 to 3 mg of cabergoline ($n = 178$) and 200/50 to 300/75 mg of levodopa/benserazide ($n = 183$) (CALDIR study). Both treatments were efficient regarding improvement in subjective rating of the IRLS score. Augmentation has reliably been assessed by clinical interviews in several trials, revealing a lower incidence with cabergoline compared with levodopa. Special concerns about "sleep attacks" have not been raised.[240]

Because of the increasing knowledge about valvular fibrosis as a side effect of the ergot-DA, we focus on the currently used nonergot DA in this chapter. Lisuride, which behaves as a 5-HT_{2B} receptor antagonist and is a strong 5-HT_{1A} agonist, has been investigated as a transdermal patch (fixed dose 3 mg or 6 mg) in a small 1-week randomized, double-blind, parallel treatment with nine patients, and was found effective in patients with mild RLS in one small proof-of-principle study (1 patch, 3 mg—IRLS 23.3 ± 11.6; 2 patches, 6 mg—IRLS 22 ± 12.5).[241]

Nonergot Dopamine Agonists: Ropinirole, Pramipexole, and Rotigotine

Seven randomized, placebo-controlled trials[84,242-247] have been reported with ropinirole in the treatment of RLS, four of them large-scale clinical trials. In a sleep laboratory trial, there was a significant decrease in sleep laboratory parameters, including PLMS/hr and PLMW/hr; sleep efficiency was not different from placebo-treated patients.[84]

In two 12-week prospective, double-blind, placebo-controlled trials comprising more than 550 patients (18 to 79 years old) with RLS with an IRLS score of 15 or more, the patients were treated with 0.25 to 4 mg/day of ropinirole administered 1 to 3 hours before bedtime or placebo. Improvement in IRLS scores at week 12 was greater in the ropinirole group (mean [SD] dose 1.90 [1.13] mg/day) compared with placebo (mean [SE] –11.04 (0.719) versus –8.03 [0.738] points). All secondary end points also improved. Side effects included nausea, headache, and daytime somnolence. Bogan and coworkers[246] confirmed the results in a similar design. Daytime somnolence did not change ($P = .10$). Montplaisir and colleagues[248] investigated the long-term efficacy of ropinirole in treating idiopathic RLS patients who received open ropinirole for 24 weeks and were then randomly assigned to double-blind treatment with either ropinirole or placebo for a further 12 weeks in a withdrawal design study.[248] Significantly fewer patients relapsed on ropinirole than on placebo (32.6% versus 57.8%; $P = .0156$).

Currently, more than 1000 patients with idiopathic RLS have been included in controlled trials with ropinirole, and positive results have been shown; adverse reactions were similar to those reported for ropinirole in studies in Parkinson's disease patients, and included nausea, somnolence, and dizziness. No cases of dyskinesia or sleep attacks have been observed. Patients were usually followed for 12 weeks in sleep laboratory studies, but some were followed only for 4 weeks. The mean effective daily dose of ropinirole reported in clinical trials was about 2 mg, which is currently used in clinical practice as a single dose at night; the maximum licensed dose is 4 mg.

For pramipexole treatment in RLS, five randomized, placebo-controlled trials[85,249-252] have been published. The first small study using sleep laboratory outcome measures was in 1999 by Montplaisir and colleagues.[249] In a polysomnographic study, Partinen and associates[85] investigated 109 patients for 3 weeks in a double-blind, placebo-controlled, dose-finding study. Pramipexole significantly improved PLM-Index (number of PLM per hour) (PLMI) ($P < .0001$) and IRLS scores ($P = .0274$, 0.125 mg; $P < .0001$, all other doses).

Two randomized, placebo-controlled trials with a total of more than 600 patients (pramipexole 0.125 to 0.75 mg/day as either a flexible or a fixed dose) confirmed the efficacy shown in earlier trials with an improvement of the IRLS by –12.4 for pramipexole ($P < .0001$) in the 6-week study[252] and –12.8 (1.0) for 0.25 mg/day, −13.8 (1.0) for 0.50 mg/day, and −14 (1.0) for 0.75 mg/day (all $P < .01$) in the 12-week study.[250]

Using a controlled withdrawal design, 150 RLS patients who had responded to pramipexole (mean dose 0.50 mg) during a 6-month open run-in period were randomly assigned to receive placebo or to continue with pramipexole for 3 months. Significantly more patients on placebo experienced a worsening in symptoms compared with patients receiving pramipexole (85.5% versus 20.5%; $P < .0001$).[251]

More than 1000 patients with idiopathic RLS have been included in controlled trials that all were in favor of pramipexole; adverse reactions were similar to those reported for pramipexole in studies in Parkinson's disease patients and included nausea, somnolence, and dizziness. Sleep attacks were not observed within the clinical trials, which is different from trials in Parkinson's disease patients. In clinical trials pramipexole was used in dosages of 0.125 to 0.75 mg (0.088 to 0.54 mg, respectively), and this reflects the current clinical use of the drug in RLS. A more detailed prospective analysis of side effects, such as dopamine dysregulation syndrome, sleepiness, or sudden sleep onset, would be required in long-term studies, although one retrospective study did not show an increased risk of sleepiness with pramipexole therapy.[253]

Rotigotine, a D3/D2/D1 dopamine agonist developed as a matrix-type transdermal patch for once-daily dosing, has been studied for treating RLS. Three randomized controlled trials with more than 800 patients treated with dosages of 1 mg, 2 mg or 3 mg rotigotine/24 h showed a significant improvement on the IRLS score compared with placebo.[254-256] In a 6-month randomized, double-blind, placebo-controlled trial, 1 to 3 mg of rotigotine was effective in relieving the nighttime and the daytime symptoms of RLS.[255] Low doses of 1 mg and 2 mg were already effective; the 3-mg dose did not additionally improve RLS symptoms. In one study, 43% of patients had local site reactions,[255] although most of those were mild, and did not lead to study withdrawal.

Opiates

Opiates have been used for treating RLS since 1684, when Willis first described the therapy.[257] Despite this, data on opioidergic therapy in RLS are sparse, and not one large-scale trial has been conducted so far. Opioids are regarded as second-choice medications. In patients who cannot tolerate dopaminergic agents, they are also given as first-choice medications. Although only case reports are available, many patients with more severe forms of RLS have been efficiently treated with a combination of dopaminergic agents and an opioid. In an early double-blind randomized crossover trial, oxycodone at an average dose of 15.9 mg reduced sensory symptoms and motor restlessness at night and during the day.[258] A significant reduction in PLMS and PLMS arousal index was also found polysomnographically.[257] A second double-blind study of opiates in PLMS found a low dose of propoxyphene, which is a less potent opioid than oxycodone, to be effective—although less effective than levodopa—in the treatment of PLMS.[259] Long-term observations are available only as case series,[260] and show a minimal risk of dependency, but some worsening of sleep apnea on long-term opioids may occur.[260]

Gabapentin and Other Anticonvulsants

Gabapentin has been shown to be an effective treatment for RLS,[247,261,262] although as is the case with opioids, large-scale trials and long-term observations are lacking. To recommend anticonvulsants as first-line treatments of RLS therapy, head-to-head trials with dopaminergics and a better exploration of long-term side effects in RLS patients are necessary. In a controlled study with a mean dose of 1855 mg/day[261] the IRLS was significantly improved compared with placebo. In a further controlled comparative study gabapentin (mean dose of 800 mg) and ropinirole (mean dose of 0.78 mg), both provided a similarly well-tolerated and effective treatment of PLMS and sensorimotor symptoms in patients with RLS.[247] In hemodialysis patients, a reduced dose of 200 to 300 mg is recommended.[262] XP13512, a gabapentin-precursor to improve gabapentin resorption and plasma levels was taken once daily ata dosage of 1200 mg in a controlled trial and significantly improved RLS symptoms compared with placebo. Main side effects were somnolence and dizziness.[263]

Today, the use of carbamazepine and valproic acid in the treatment of RLS is limited because other drugs with a sufficient efficacy and a more appropriate side-effect profile are available. Early controlled studies with small patient sizes showed significant effects on treating RLS; the outcome measures are not comparable, however, to more recent trials with dopaminergic agents.[264,265] In a controlled trial of 600 mg of slow-release valproic acid compared with 200 mg of slow-release levodopa, there was no major difference in efficacy, whereas levodopa, but not valproic acid, significantly increased arousals not associated with PLMS.[237]

Benzodiazepines and Other Hypnosedatives

Only small trials are available for clonazepam, mostly with a population of RLS and PLMS patients.[266-269] In these trials, 0.5 mg of clonazepam was ineffective in improving either polysomnographic or subjective RLS parameters. Currently, there is no evidence of the efficacy of clonazepam in patients with RLS; this applies also for triazolam[270] in patients with pure PLMS and for zolpidem.[271] No recent trials using the current definition criteria and scales have been performed with clonazepam.

Oral and Intravenous Administration of Iron

To treat RLS patients with iron, patients have to be differentiated between patients with normal or low iron storage. Only small studies with different compounds are available, and data from different studies cannot be compared. In a randomized, double-blind, placebo-controlled trial with 28 RLS patients, iron sulfate was not shown to improve RLS symptoms, but in this study patients were not selected according to their serum ferritin levels.[183] In another study, high-dose iron dextran infusion was associated with a significant, but transient, reduction in symptoms of RLS in patients with end-stage renal disease.[181] In a single open study, in which 10 RLS patients received a single 1000-mg intravenous iron infusion, 7 subjects showed a substantial improvement in RLS symptoms 2 weeks later.[180]

In a small study with ferrous sulfate, 325 mg twice daily, or placebo for 12 weeks, clinical efficacy was not different in the two groups, but three patients in the iron group dropped out of the study because of adverse events.[183] In another study, 200 mg three times daily of oral ferrous sulfate for 8 to 20 weeks in 18 RLS patients was shown to be efficient in RLS patients with a serum ferritin less than 45 µg/L at baseline.[179] Two further studies investigating the effect of intravenous iron found that 1000 mg of iron dextran was clinically efficacious.[181,182]

One patient had a possible allergic reaction (shortness of breath) after 30 mg of iron had been infused and was excluded from the study.[182] Because of a possible iron overload especially in patients with hemochromatosis, iron status needs to be monitored before and periodically during treatment. The major adverse effects of oral iron involve gastrointestinal discomfort, including nausea, reflux, abdominal pain, and diarrhea, and especially constipation. In addition, with the dextran formulation, there is the risk of an anaphylactoid reaction, which is increased in patients with preexisting autoimmune or rheumatoid disorders.

Other Therapies

Clonidine,[271] amantadine,[273] and magnesium[274] have been tested in open trials or case series, but not been studied in any controlled or large-scale trial. Although a promising open study on magnesium was conducted, these results have not be confirmed in a double-blind trial. Other approaches using nonpharmacological therapy, such as exercise, have proven to be efficacious.

Pharmacological treatment in RLS should be individually tailored to the symptomatology and severity of the patient's symptoms. Dopaminergic agents should be considered first line treatment, but dosages need to be carefully adjusted and have to remain as low as possible to avoid the development of augmentation. Additional non-pharmacological strategies should be considered for long-term treatment.

REFERENCES

1. Garcia-Borreguero D, Egatz R, Winkelmann J, Berger K: Epidemiology of restless legs syndrome: the current status. Sleep Med Rev 2006;10:153-167.
2. Berger K, Kurth T: RLS epidemiology—frequencies, risk factors and methods in population studies. Mov Disord 2007;22(Suppl 18):S420-423.
3. Hening WA, Allen RP, Earley CJ, et al: An update on the dopaminergic treatment of restless legs syndrome and periodic limb movement disorder. Sleep 2004;27:560-583.
4. Trenkwalder C, Hening WA, Montagna P, et al: Treatment of restless legs syndrome: an evidence-based review and implications for clinical practice. Mov Disord 2008 Dec 15;23(16): 2267-2302.
5. Vignatelli L, Billiard M, Clarenbach P, et al: EFNS guidelines on management of restless legs syndrome and periodic limb movement disorder in sleep. Eur J Neurol 2006;13:1049-1065.
6. Winkelmann J, Schormair B, Lichtner P, et al: Genome-wide association study of restless legs syndrome identifies common variants in three genomic regions. Nat Genet 2007;39:1000-1006.
7. Hening WA, Allen RP, Chaudhuri KR, et al: The clinical significance of RLS. Mov Disord 2007;22(Suppl 18):S395-400.
8. Hogl B, Poewe W: Restless legs syndrome. Curr Opin Neurol 2005;18:405-410.
9. Gamaldo CE, Earley CJ: Restless legs syndrome: a clinical update. Chest 2006;130:1596-1604.
10. Kushida CA: Clinical presentation, diagnosis, and quality of life issues in restless legs syndrome. Am J Med 2007;120:S4-S12.
11. Wilson V: *Sleep Thief: Restless Legs Syndrome*. Orange Park, FL: Galaxy Books, 1996.
12. Buchfuhrer MJ, Hening WA, Kushida CA: *The Restless Legs Syndrome*. New York: Demos, 2006.
13. Yoakum R: *Nightwalkers: Sleepless Victims of a Hidden Epidemic*. New York: Simon & Schuster, 2006.

14. The International Restless Legs Syndrome Study Group: Towards a better definition of the restless legs syndrome. Mov Disord 1995;10:634-642.
15. Allen RP, Picchietti D, Hening WA, et al: Restless legs syndrome: diagnostic criteria, special considerations, and epidemiology. A report from the Restless Legs Syndrome Diagnosis and Epidemiology Workshop at the National Institutes of Health. Sleep Med 2003;4:101-119.
16. Hening WA: Subjective and objective criteria in the diagnosis of the restless legs syndrome. Sleep Med 2004;5:285-292.
17. Allen RP, Earley CJ: Defining the phenotype of the restless legs syndrome (RLS) using age-of-symptom-onset. Sleep Med 2000;1:11-19.
18. Hening WA, Allen RP, Washburn M, et al: The four diagnostic criteria for Restless Legs Syndrome are unable to exclude confounding conditions ("mimics"). Sleep Med 2009. [Epub ahead of print].
19. Benes H, Walters AS, Allen RP, et al: Definition of restless legs syndrome, how to diagnose it, and how to differentiate it from RLS mimics. Mov Disord 2007;22(Suppl 18):S401-408.
20. Allen RP: Improving RLS diagnosis and severity assessment: polysomnography, actigraphy and RLS-sleep log. Sleep Med 2007;8(Suppl 2):S13-18. Epub 2007 Jun 12.
21. Ferini-Strambi L: RLS-like symptoms: differential diagnosis by history and clinical assessment. Sleep Med 2007;8(Suppl 2):S3-6. Epub 2007 Jun 12.
22. Benes H, Kohnen R: Validation of an algorithm for the diagnosis of restless legs syndrome: The Restless Legs Syndrome-Diagnostic Index (RLS-DI). Sleep Med 2009;10(5):515-523. Epub 2008 Sep 26.
23. Lipinski JF, Sallee FR, Jackson C, Sethuraman G: Dopamine agonist treatment of Tourette disorder in children: results of an open-label trial of pergolide. Mov Disord 1997;12:402-407.
24. Lesperance P, Djerroud N, Diaz Anzaldua A, et al: Restless legs in Tourette syndrome. Mov Disord 2004;19:1084.
25. Cortese S, Lecendreux M, Bernardina BD, et al: Attention-deficit/hyperactivity disorder, Tourette's syndrome, and restless legs syndrome: The iron hypothesis. Med Hypotheses 2008;70(6):128-1132. Epub 2007 Dec 2.
26. Bassetti CL, Mauerhofer D, Gugger M, et al: Restless legs syndrome: a clinical study of 55 patients. Eur Neurol 2001;45:67-74.
27. Hening WA, Allen RP, Earley CJ: Pain in the restless legs syndrome is more common in patients with frequent RLS [Abstract]. Mov Disord 2007;22:S274.
28. Michaud M, Chabli A, Lavigne G, Montplaisir J: Arm restlessness in patients with restless legs syndrome. Mov Disord 2000;15:289-293.
29. Chabli A, Michaud M, Montplaisir J: Periodic arm movements in patients with the restless legs syndrome. Eur Neurol 2000;44:133-138.
30. Freedom T, Merchut MP: Arm restlessness as the initial symptom in restless legs syndrome. Arch Neurol 2003;60:1013-1015.
31. Bassetti CL, Kretzschmar U, Werth E, Baumann CR: Restless legs and restless legs-like syndrome. Sleep Med 2006;7:534.
32. Michaud M, Dumont M, Paquet J, et al: Circadian variation of the effects of immobility on symptoms of restless legs syndrome. Sleep 2005;28:843-846.
33. Birinyi PV, Allen RP, Lesage S, et al: Investigation into the correlation between sensation and leg movement in restless legs syndrome. Mov Disord 2005;20:1097-1103.
34. Hening WA, Walters AS, Wagner M, et al: Circadian rhythm of motor restlessness and sensory symptoms in the idiopathic restless legs syndrome. Sleep 1999;22:901-912.
35. Trenkwalder C, Hening WA, Walters AS, et al: Circadian rhythm of periodic limb movements and sensory symptoms of restless legs syndrome. Mov Disord 1999;14:102-110.
36. Michaud M, Dumont M, Selmaoui B, et al: Circadian rhythm of restless legs syndrome: relationship with biological markers. Ann Neurol 2004;55:372-380.
37. Earley CJ, Hyland K, Allen RP: Circadian changes in CSF dopaminergic measures in restless legs syndrome. Sleep Med 2006;7:263-268.
38. Poceta JS, Parsons L, Engelland S, Kripke DF: Circadian rhythm of CSF monoamines and hypocretin-1 in restless legs syndrome and Parkinson's disease. Sleep Med 2009;10(1):129-33. Epub 2008 Jan 22.
39. Garcia-Borreguero D, Larrosa O, Granizo JJ, et al: Circadian variation in neuroendocrine response to L-dopa in patients with restless legs syndrome. Sleep 2004;27:669-673.
40. Winkelman JW: Considering the causes of RLS. Eur J Neurol 2006;13(Suppl 2):8-14.
41. Allen RP, Earley CJ: The role of iron in restless legs syndrome. Mov Disord 2007;22 Suppl 18:S440-448.

42. Zucconi M, Manconi M, Ferini Strambi L: Aetiopathogenesis of restless legs syndrome. Neurol Sci 2007;28(Suppl 1):S47-S52.
43. Hornyak M, Rupp A, Riemann D, et al: Low-dose hydrocortisone in the evening modulates symptom severity in restless legs syndrome. Neurology 2008;70:1620-1622.
44. Lugaresi E, Coccagna G, Berti Ceroni G, Ambrosetto C: Restless legs syndrome and nocturnal myoclonus. In Gastaut H, Lugaresi E, Berti Ceroni G, Coccagna G, eds: The Abnormalities of Sleep in Man. Bologna: Aulo Gaggi Editore, 1968, pp 285-294.
45. Montplaisir J, Boucher S, Poirier G, et al: Clinical, polysomnographic, and genetic characteristics of restless legs syndrome: a study of 133 patients diagnosed with new standard criteria. Mov Disord 1997;12:61-65.
46. Trenkwalder C, Bucher SF, Oertel WH: Electrophysiological pattern of involuntary limb movements in the restless legs syndrome. Muscle Nerve 1996;19:155-162.
47. Provini F, Vetrugno R, Meletti S, et al: Motor pattern of periodic limb movements during sleep. Neurology 2001;57:300-304.
48. de Weerd AW, Rijsman RM, Brinkley A: Activity patterns of leg muscles in periodic limb movement disorder. J Neurol Neurosurg Psychiatry 2004;75:317-319.
49. Bara-Jimenez W, Aksu M, Graham B, et al: Periodic limb movements in sleep: state-dependent excitability of the spinal flexor reflex. Neurology 2000;54:1609-1616.
50. Diagnostic Classification Steering Committee of the American Sleep Disorders Association: *The International Classification of Sleep Disorders: Diagnostic and Coding Manual–Second Version.* Chicago: American Association of Sleep Medicine, 2005.
51. Walters AS, Lavigne G, Hening W, et al: The scoring of movements in sleep. J Clin Sleep Med 2007;3:155-167.
52. Zucconi M, Ferri R, Allen R, et al: The official World Association of Sleep Medicine (WASM) standards for recording and scoring periodic leg movements in sleep (PLMS) and wakefulness (PLMW) developed in collaboration with a task force from the International Restless Legs Syndrome Study Group (IRLSSG). Sleep Med 2006;7:175-183.
53. Stefansson H, Rye DB, Hicks A, et al: A genetic risk factor for periodic limb movements in sleep. N Engl J Med 2007;357:639-647.
54. Brodeur C, Montplaisir J, Godbout R, Marinier R: Treatment of restless legs syndrome and periodic movements during sleep with L-Dopa: a double-blind controlled study. Neurology 1988;38:1845-1848.
55. Michaud M, Lavigne G, Desautels A, et al: Effects of immobility on sensory and motor symptoms of restless legs syndrome. Mov Disord 2002;17:112-115.
56. Sforza E, Johannes M, Claudio B: The PAM-RL ambulatory device for detection of periodic leg movements: a validation study. Sleep Med 2005;6:407-413.
57. Coleman RM: Periodic movements in sleep (nocturnal myoclonus) and restless legs syndrome. In Guilleminault C (ed): Sleeping and Waking Disorders: Indications and Techniques. Menlo Park, CA: Addison-Wesley, Medical/Nursing Division, 1982, pp 265-295.
58. Ferri R, Zucconi M, Manconi M, et al: Different periodicity and time structure of leg movements during sleep in narcolepsy/cataplexy and restless legs syndrome. Sleep 2006;29:1587-1594.
59. Boehm G, Wetter TC, Trenkwalder C: Periodic leg movements in RLS patients as compared to controls: Are there differences beyond the PLM index? Sleep Med. 2009;10(5):566-71. Epub 2008 Aug 26.
60. Michaud M, Paquet J, Lavigne G, et al: Sleep laboratory diagnosis of restless legs syndrome. Eur Neurol 2002;48:108-113.
61. Hornyak M, Feige B, Riemann D, Voderholzer U: Periodic leg movements in sleep and periodic limb movement disorder: prevalence, clinical significance and treatment. Sleep Med Rev 2006;10:169-177.
62. Bliwise DL, Petta D, Seidel W, Dement W: Periodic leg movements during sleep in the elderly. Arch Gerontol Geriatr 1985;4:273-281.
63. Ancoli-Israel S, Kripke DF, Klauber MR, et al: Periodic limb movements in sleep in community-dwelling elderly. Sleep 1991;14:496-500.
64. Stiasny-Kolster K, Kohnen R, Moller JC, et al: Validation of the "L-DOPA test" for diagnosis of restless legs syndrome. Mov Disord 2006;21:1333-1339.
65. Hening W, Walters AS, Allen RP, et al: Impact, diagnosis and treatment of restless legs syndrome (RLS) in a primary care population: the REST (RLS epidemiology, symptoms, and treatment) primary care study. Sleep Med 2004;5:237-246.
66. Allen RP, Walters AS, Montplaisir J, et al: Restless legs syndrome prevalence and impact: REST general population study. Arch Intern Med 2005;165:1286-1292.

67. Hornyak M, Feige B, Voderholzer U, et al: Polysomnography findings in patients with restless legs syndrome and in healthy controls: a comparative observational study. Sleep 2007;30: 861-865.

68. Hening W, Washburn T, Allen R, Earley C: Characteristics of restless legs syndrome in affected individuals ascertained through a population study [Abstract]. Mov Disord 2002;17:1109.

69. Ferri R, Lanuzza B, Cosentino FI, et al: A single question for the rapid screening of restless legs syndrome in the neurological clinical practice. Eur J Neurol 2007;14:1016-1021.

70. Rothdach AJ, Trenkwalder C, Haberstock J, et al: Prevalence and risk factors of RLS in an elderly population: the MEMO study. Memory and Morbidity in Augsburg Elderly. Neurology 2000;54:1064-1068.

71. Nichols DA, Allen RP, Grauke JH, et al: Restless legs syndrome symptoms in primary care: a prevalence study. Arch Intern Med 2003;163:2323-2329.

72. Hening WA, Allen RP, Washburn M, et al: Validation of the Hopkins telephone diagnostic interview for restless legs syndrome. Sleep Med 2008;9(3):283-289. Epub 2007 Jul 17.

73. Picchietti DL, Stevens HE: Early manifestations of restless legs syndrome in childhood and adolescence. Sleep Med 2008;9(7):770-781. Epub 2007 Nov 19.

74. Ondo W, Tan EK, Mansoor J: Rheumatologic serologies in secondary restless legs syndrome. Mov Disord 2000;15:321-323.

75. Kushida CA, Littner MR, Morgenthaler T, et al: Practice parameters for the indications for polysomnography and related procedures: an update for 2005. Sleep 2005;28:499-521.

76. Hogl B, Gschliesser V: RLS assessment and sleep questionnaires in practice—lessons learned from Parkinson's disease. Sleep Med 2007;8(Suppl 2):S7-S12.

77. Walters AS, LeBrocq C, Dhar A, et al: Validation of the International Restless Legs Syndrome Study Group rating scale for restless legs syndrome. Sleep Med 2003;4:121-132.

78. Allen RP, Earley CJ: Validation of the Johns Hopkins restless legs severity scale. Sleep Med 2001;2:239-242.

79. National Institute of Mental Health: CGI. Clinical Global Impressions. In Guy W, ed: ECDEU Assessment Manual for Psychopharmacology. Rockville, MD: National Institute of Mental Health, 1976, pp 218-222.

80. Kohnen R, Oertel WH, Stiasny-Kolster K, et al: Severity rating of restless legs syndrome: review of ten years of experience with the RLS-6 scales in clinical trials [Abstract]. Sleep 2003;26. A342.

81. Kohnen R, Allen RP, Benes H, et al: Assessment of restless legs syndrome: methodological approaches for use in practice and clinical trials. Mov Disord 2007;22(Suppl 18):S485-494.

82. Earley CJ, Yaffee JB, Allen RP: Randomized, double-blind, placebo-controlled trial of pergolide in restless legs syndrome. Neurology 1998;51:1599-1602.

83. Trenkwalder C, Hundemer HP, Lledo A, et al: Efficacy of pergolide in treatment of restless legs syndrome: the PEARLS Study. Neurology 2004;62:1391-1397.

84. Allen R, Becker PM, Bogan R, et al: Ropinirole decreases periodic leg movements and improves sleep parameters in patients with restless legs syndrome. Sleep 2004;27:907-914.

85. Partinen M, Hirvonen K, Jama L, et al: Efficacy and safety of pramipexole in idiopathic restless legs syndrome: a polysomnographic dose-finding study—the PRELUDE study. Sleep Med 2006;7:407-417.

86. Garcia-Borreguero D, Larrosa O, de la Llave Y, et al: Correlation between rating scales and sleep laboratory measurements in restless legs syndrome. Sleep Med 2004;5:561-565.

87. Hornyak M, Hundemer HP, Quail D, et al: Relationship of periodic leg movements and severity of restless legs syndrome: a study in unmedicated and medicated patients. Clin Neurophysiol 2007;118:1532-1537.

88. Sforza E, Haba-Rubio J: Night-to-night variability in periodic leg movements in patients with restless legs syndrome. Sleep Med 2005;6:259-267.

89. Hornyak M, Kopasz M, Feige B, et al: Variability of periodic leg movements in various sleep disorders: implications for clinical and pathophysiologic studies. Sleep 2005;28:331-335.

90. Aksu M, Demirci S, Bara-Jimenez W: Correlation between putative indicators of primary restless legs syndrome severity. Sleep Med 2007;8(1):84-89. Epub 2006 Jun 5.

91. Allen RP, Dean T, Earley CJ: Effects of rest-duration, time-of-day and their interaction on periodic leg movements while awake in restless legs syndrome. Sleep Med 2005;6:429-434.

92. Michaud M: Is the suggested immobilization test the "gold standard" to assess restless legs syndrome? Sleep Med 2006;7:541-543.

93. Haba-Rubio J, Sforza E: Test-to-test variability in motor activity during the suggested immobilization test in restless legs patients. Sleep Med 2006;7:561-566.

94. Rau C, Hummel F, Gerloff C: Cortical involvement in the generation of "involuntary" movements in restless legs syndrome. Neurology 2004;62:998-1000.
95. Bucher SF, Seelos KC, Oertel WH, et al: Cerebral generators involved in the pathogenesis of the restless legs syndrome. Ann Neurol 1997;41:639-645.
96. Trenkwalder C, Bucher SF, Oertel WH, et al: Bereitschaftspotential in idiopathic and symptomatic restless legs syndrome. Electroencephalogr Clin Neurophysiol 1993;89:95-103.
97. Tergau F, Wischer S, Paulus W: Motor system excitability in patients with restless legs syndrome. Neurology 1999;52:1060-1063.
98. Nardone R, Ausserer H, Bratti A, et al: Cabergoline reverses cortical hyperexcitability in patients with restless legs syndrome. Acta Neurol Scand 2006;114:244-249.
99. Unrath A, Juengling FD, Schork M, Kassubek J: Cortical grey matter alterations in idiopathic restless legs syndrome: an optimized voxel-based morphometry study. Mov Disord 2007;22(12):1751-1756.
100. Etgen T, Draganski B, Ilg C, et al: Bilateral thalamic gray matter changes in patients with restless legs syndrome. Neuroimage 2005;24:1242-1247.
101. Hornyak M, Ahrendts JC, Spiegelhalder K, et al: Voxel-based morphometry in unmedicated patients with restless legs syndrome. Sleep Med 2007;9(1):22-26. Epub 2007 May 18.
102. Pearson VE, Allen RP, Dean T, et al: Cognitive deficits associated with restless legs syndrome (RLS). Sleep Med 2006;7:25-30.
103. Gamaldo CE, Benbrook AR, Allen RP, et al: A further evaluation of the cognitive deficits associated with restless legs syndrome (RLS). Sleep Med 2007;9(1):22-26. Epub 2007 May 18.
104. Tribl GG, Asenbaum S, Klosch G, et al: Normal IPT and IBZM SPECT in drug naive and levodopa-treated idiopathic restless legs syndrome. Neurology 2002;59:649-650.
105. Wetter TC, Eisensehr I, Trenkwalder C: Functional neuroimaging studies in restless legs syndrome. Sleep Med 2004;5:401-406.
106. Cervenka S, Palhagen SE, Comley RA, et al: Support for dopaminergic hypoactivity in restless legs syndrome: a PET study on D2-receptor binding. Brain 2006;129:2017-2028.
107. von Spiczak S, Whone AL, Hammers A, et al: The role of opioids in restless legs syndrome: an (11C)diprenorphine PET study. Brain 2005;128:906-917.
108. Connor JR, Boyer PJ, Menzies SL, et al: Neuropathological examination suggests impaired brain iron acquisition in restless legs syndrome. Neurology 2003;61:304-309.
109. Connor JR, Wang XS, Patton SM, et al: Decreased transferrin receptor expression by neuromelanin cells in restless legs syndrome. Neurology 2004;62:1563-1567.
110. Allen RP, Barker PB, Wehrl F, et al: MRI measurement of brain iron in patients with restless legs syndrome. Neurology 2001;56:263-265.
111. Earley CJ, Barker PB, Horska A, Allen RP: MRI-determined regional brain iron concentrations in early- and late-onset restless legs syndrome. Sleep Med 2006;7:458-461.
112. Schmidauer C, Sojer M, Seppi K, et al: Transcranial ultrasound shows nigral hypoechogenicity in restless legs syndrome. Ann Neurol 2005;58:630-634.
113. Godau J, Schweitzer KJ, Liepelt I, et al: Substantia nigra hypoechogenicity: definition and findings in restless legs syndrome. Mov Disord 2007;22:187-192.
114. Berg D: Disturbance of iron metabolism as a contributing factor to SN hyperechogenicity in Parkinson's disease: implications for idiopathic and monogenetic forms. Neurochem Res 2007;32:1646-1654.
115. Earley CJ, Connor JR, Beard JL, et al: Abnormalities in CSF concentrations of ferritin and transferrin in restless legs syndrome. Neurology 2000;54:1698-1700.
116. Clardy SL, Earley CJ, Allen RP, et al: Ferritin subunits in CSF are decreased in restless legs syndrome. J Lab Clin Med 2006;147:67-73.
117. Wang X, Wiesinger J, Beard J, et al: Thy1 expression in the brain is affected by iron and is decreased in restless legs syndrome. J Neurol Sci 2004;220:59-66.
118. Nelson C, Erikson K, Pinero DJ, Beard JL: In vivo dopamine metabolism is altered in iron-deficient anemic rats. J Nutr 1997;127:2282-2288.
119. Dean T Jr, Allen RP, O'Donnell CP, Earley CJ: The effects of dietary iron deprivation on murine circadian sleep architecture. Sleep Med 2006;7:634-640.
120. Qu S, Le W, Zhang X, et al: Locomotion is increased in A11-lesioned mice with iron deprivation: a possible animal model for restless legs syndrome. J Neuropathol Exp Neurol 2007;66:383-388.
121. Ondo WG, He Y, Rajasekaran S, Le WD: Clinical correlates of 6-hydroxydopamine injections into A11 dopaminergic neurons in rats: a possible model for restless legs syndrome. Mov Disord 2000;15:154-158.

122. Paulus W, Schomburg ED: Dopamine and the spinal cord in restless legs syndrome: does spinal cord physiology reveal a basis of augmentation? Sleep Med Rev 2006;10:185-196.

123. Zhao H, Zhu W, Pan T, et al: Spinal cord dopamine receptor expression and function in mice with 6-OHDA lesion of the A11 nucleus and dietary iron deprivation. J Neurosci Res 2007;85:1065-1076.

124. Qu S, Ondo WG, Zhang X, et al: Projections of diencephalic dopamine neurons into the spinal cord in mice. Exp Brain Res 2006;168:152-156.

125. Paulus W, Dowling P, Rijsman RM, et al: Update of the pathophysiology of the restless-legs-syndrome. Mov Disord 2007;22:S431-S439.

126. Trenkwalder C, Paulus W: Why do restless legs occur at rest? Pathophysiology of neuronal structures in RLS. Neurophysiology of RLS (part 2). Clin Neurophysiol 2004;115:1975-1988.

127. Schols L, Haan J, Riess O, et al: Sleep disturbance in spinocerebellar ataxias: is the SCA3 mutation a cause of restless legs syndrome? Neurology 1998;51:1603-1607.

128. Rijsman RM, Stam CJ, de Weerd AW: Abnormal H-reflexes in periodic limb movement disorder: impact on understanding the pathophysiology of the disorder. Clin Neurophysiol 2005;116:204-210.

129. Stiasny-Kolster K, Magerl W, Oertel WH, et al: Static mechanical hyperalgesia without dynamic tactile allodynia in patients with restless legs syndrome. Brain 2004;127:773-782.

130. Paulus W, Trenkwalder C: Less is more: pathophysiology of dopaminergic-therapy-related augmentation in restless legs syndrome. Lancet Neurol 2006;5:878-886.

131. Salvi F, Montagna P, Plasmati R, et al: Restless legs syndrome and nocturnal myoclonus: initial clinical manifestation of familial amyloid polyneuropathy. J Neurol Neurosurg Psychiatry 1990;53:522-525.

132. Gemignani F, Marbini A, Di Giovanni G, et al: Cryoglobulinaemic neuropathy manifesting with restless legs syndrome. J Neurol Sci 1997;152:218-223.

133. Gemignani F, Marbini A, Di Giovanni G, et al: Charcot-Marie-Tooth disease type 2 with restless legs syndrome. Neurology 1999;52:1064-1066.

134. Iannaccone S, Zucconi M, Marchettini P, et al: Evidence of peripheral axonal neuropathy in primary restless legs syndrome. Mov Disord 1995;10:2-9.

135. Happe S, Zeitlhofer J: Abnormal cutaneous thermal thresholds in patients with restless legs syndrome. J Neurol 2003;250:362-365.

136. Polydefkis M, Allen RP, Hauer P, et al: Subclinical sensory neuropathy in late-onset restless legs syndrome. Neurology 2000;55:1115-1121.

137. Gemignani F, Brindani F, Vitetta F, et al: Restless legs syndrome in diabetic neuropathy: a frequent manifestation of small fiber neuropathy. J Peripher Nerv Syst 2007;12:50-53.

138. Schattschneider J, Bode A, Wasner G, et al: Idiopathic restless legs syndrome: abnormalities in central somatosensory processing. J Neurol 2004;251:977-982.

139. Ekbom KA: Restless legs: a clinical study. Acta Med Scand Suppl 1945;158:1-122.

140. Lavigne GJ, Montplaisir JY: Restless legs syndrome and sleep bruxism: prevalence and association among Canadians. Sleep 1994;17:739-743.

141. Phillips B, Young T, Finn L, et al: Epidemiology of restless legs symptoms in adults. Arch Intern Med 2000;160:2137-2141.

142. Picchietti D, Allen RP, Walters AS, et al: Restless legs syndrome: prevalence and impact in children and adolescents—the Peds REST study. Pediatrics 2007;120:253-266.

143. Berger K, Luedemann J, Trenkwalder C, et al: Sex and the risk of restless legs syndrome in the general population. Arch Intern Med 2004;164:196-202.

144. Tison F, Crochard A, Leger D, et al: Epidemiology of restless legs syndrome in French adults: a nationwide survey. The INSTANT Study. Neurology 2005;65:239-246.

145. Hadjigeorgiou GM, Stefanidis I, Dardiotis E, et al: Low RLS prevalence and awareness in central Greece: an epidemiological survey. Eur J Neurol 2007;14:1275-1280.

146. Tan EK, Seah A, See SJ, et al: Restless legs syndrome in an Asian population: a study in Singapore. Mov Disord 2001;16:577-579.

147. Mizuno S, Miyaoka T, Inagaki T, Horiguchi J: Prevalence of restless legs syndrome in non-institutionalized Japanese elderly. Psychiatry Clin Neurosci 2005;59:461-465.

148. Sevim S, Dogu O, Camdeviren H, et al: Unexpectedly low prevalence and unusual characteristics of RLS in Mersin, Turkey. Neurology 2003;61:1562-1569.

149. Rangarajan S, Rangarajan S, D'Souza GA: Restless legs syndrome in an Indian urban population. Sleep Med 2007;9(1):88-93. Epub 2007 Sep 6.

150. Kim J, Choi C, Shin K, et al: Prevalence of restless legs syndrome and associated factors in the Korean adult population: The Korean Health and Genome Study. Psychiatry Clin Neurosci 2005;59:350-353.

151. Cho YW, Shin WC, Yun CH, et al: Epidemiology of restless legs syndrome in Korean adults. Sleep 2008;31:219-223.
152. Castillo PR, Kaplan J, Lin SC, et al: Prevalence of restless legs syndrome among native South Americans residing in coastal and mountainous areas. Mayo Clin Proc 2006;81:1345-1347.
153. Lee HB, Hening WA, Allen RP, et al: Race and restless legs syndrome symptoms in an adult community sample in east Baltimore. Sleep Med 2006;7(8):642-645. Epub 2006 Oct 4.
154. Berger K. A message of restless legs on ethnicity. Sleep Med 2006;7(8):597-598. Epub 2006 Nov 13.
155. Alattar M, Harrington JJ, Mitchell CM, Sloane P: Sleep problems in primary care. A North Carolina Family Practice Research Network (NC-FP-RN) study. J Am Board Fam Med 2007;20:365-374.
156. Oppenheim H: *Lehrbuch der Nervenkrankheiten.* Berlin: Karger, 1923.
157. Walters AS, Hickey K, Maltzman J, et al: A questionnaire study of 138 patients with restless legs syndrome: the 'Night-Walkers' survey. Neurology 1996;46:92-95.
158. Ondo W, Jankovic J: Restless legs syndrome: clinicoetiologic correlates. Neurology 1996;47:1435-1441.
159. Winkelmann J, Wetter TC, Collado-Seidel V, et al: Clinical characteristics and frequency of the hereditary restless legs syndrome in a population of 300 patients. Sleep 2000;23:597-602.
160. Allen RP, La Buda MC, Becker P, Earley CJ: Family history study of the restless legs syndrome. Sleep Med 2002;3(Suppl):S3-S7.
161. Montplaisir J, Boucher S, Poirier G, et al: Clinical, polysomnographic, and genetic characteristics of restless legs syndrome: a study of 133 patients diagnosed with new standard criteria. Mov Disord 1997;12(1):61-65.
162. Winkelmann J, Muller-Myhsok B, Wittchen HU, et al: Complex segregation analysis of restless legs syndrome provides evidence for an autosomal dominant mode of inheritance in early age at onset families. Ann Neurol 2002;52:297-302.
163. Mathias RA, Hening W, Washburn M, et al: Segregation analysis of restless legs syndrome: possible evidence for a major gene in a family study using blinded diagnoses. Hum Hered 2006;62:157-164.
164. Kemlink D, Plazzi G, Vetrugno R, et al: Suggestive evidence for linkage for restless legs syndrome on chromosome 19p13. Neurogenetics 2008;9(2):75-82. Epub 2008 Jan 10.
165. Trenkwalder C, Högl B, Winkelmann J. Recent advances in the diagnosis, genetics and treatment of restless legs syndrome. J Neurol. 2009;256(4):539-553. Epub 2009 Apr 27.
166. Winkelmann J, Muller-Myhsok B: Genetics of restless legs syndrome: a burning urge to move. Neurology 2008;70:664-665.
167. Lohmann-Hedrich K, Neumann A, Kleensang A, et al: Evidence for linkage of restless legs syndrome to chromosome 9p. Neurology 2008;70(9):686-694. Epub 2007 Nov 21.
168. Liebetanz KM, Winkelmann J, Trenkwalder C, et al: RLS3: fine-mapping of an autosomal dominant locus in a family with intrafamilial heterogeneity. Neurology 2006;67:320-321.
169. Kemlink D, Polo O, Montagna P, et al: Family-based association study of the restless legs syndrome loci 2 and 3 in a European population. Mov Disord 2007;22:207-212.
170. Kemlink D, Polo O, Frauscher B, et al: J Med Genet. 2009;46(5):315-318. Epub 2009 Mar 10.
171. Schormair B, Kemlink D, Roeske D, et al: PTPRD (protein tyrosine phosphatase receptor type delta) is associated with restless legs syndrome. Nat Genet 2008;40:946-948.
172. Picchietti DL, England SJ, Walters AS, et al: Periodic limb movement disorder and restless legs syndrome in children with attention-deficit hyperactivity disorder. J Child Neurol 1998;13:588-594.
173. Chervin RD, Archbold KH, Dillon JE, et al: Associations between symptoms of inattention, hyperactivity, restless legs, and periodic leg movements. Sleep 2002;25:213-218.
174. Wagner ML, Walters AS, Fisher BC: Symptoms of attention-deficit/hyperactivity disorder in adults with restless legs syndrome. Sleep 2004;27:1499-1504.
175. Konofal E, Cortese S, Marchand M, et al: Impact of restless legs syndrome and iron deficiency on attention-deficit/hyperactivity disorder in children. Sleep Med 2007.
176. Oner P, Dirik EB, Taner Y, et al: Association between low serum ferritin and restless legs syndrome in patients with attention deficit hyperactivity disorder. Tohoku J Exp Med 2007;213:269-276.
177. Sun ER, Chen CA, Ho G, et al: Iron and the restless legs syndrome. Sleep 1998;21:371-377.
178. Aspenstroem G: Pica and restless legs in iron deficiency. Sven Läkartidningen 1964;61:1174-1177.
179. Davis BJ, Rajput A, Rajput ML, et al: A randomized, double-blind placebo-controlled trial of iron in restless legs syndrome. Eur Neurol 2000;43:70-75.

180. Sloand JA, Shelly MA, Feigin A, et al: A double-blind, placebo-controlled trial of intravenous iron dextran therapy in patients with ESRD and restless legs syndrome. Am J Kidney Dis 2004;43: 663-670.
181. Earley CJ, Heckler D, Allen RP: Repeated IV doses of iron provides effective supplemental treatment of restless legs syndrome. Sleep Med 2005;6:301-305.
182. Earley CJ, Heckler D, Allen RP: The treatment of restless legs syndrome with intravenous iron dextran. Sleep Med 2004;5:231-235.
183. Grote L, Leissner L, Hedner J, et al: A randomized, double-blind, placebo controlled, multicenter study of intravenous iron sucrose and placebo in the treatment of restless legs syndrome. Mov Disord 2009;24(10):1445-1452.
184. Leutgeb U, Martus P: Regular intake of non-opioid analgesics is associated with an increased risk of restless legs syndrome in patients maintained on antidepressants. Eur J Med Res 2002;7: 368-378.
185. Ekbom KA: [Restless legs as an early symptom of cancer]. Sven Lakartidn 1955;52:1875-1883.
186. Morcos Z: Restless legs syndrome, iron deficiency and colon cancer. J Clin Sleep Med 2005;1:433.
187. Winkelman JW, Chertow GM, Lazarus JM: Restless legs syndrome in end-stage renal disease. Am J Kidney Dis 1996;28:372-378.
188. Hui D, Wong T, Li T, et al: Prevalence of sleep disturbances in Chinese patients with end stage renal failure on maintenance hemodialysis. Med Sci Monit 2002;8:CR331-CR336.
189. Bhowmik D, Bhatia M, Gupta S, et al: Restless legs syndrome in hemodialysis patients in India: a case controlled study. Sleep Med 2003;4:143-146.
190. Gigli GL, Adorati M, Dolso P, et al: Restless legs syndrome in end-stage renal disease. Sleep Med 2004;5:309-315.
191. Kavanagh D, Siddiqui S, Geddes CC: Restless legs syndrome in patients on dialysis. Am J Kidney Dis 2004;43:763-771.
192. Murtagh FE, Addington-Hall JM, Donohoe P, Higginson IJ: Symptom management in patients with established renal failure managed without dialysis. Edtna Erca J 2006;32:93-98.
193. Bastos JP, Sousa RB, Nepomuceno LA, et al: Sleep disturbances in patients on maintenance hemodialysis: role of dialysis shift. Rev Assoc Med Bras 2007;53:492-496.
194. Wetter TC, Stiasny K, Kohnen R, et al: Polysomnographic sleep measures in patients with uremic and idiopathic restless legs syndrome. Mov Disord 1998;13:820-824.
195. Unruh ML, Levey AS, D'Ambrosio C, et al: Restless legs symptoms among incident dialysis patients: association with lower quality of life and shorter survival. Am J Kidney Dis 2004;43: 900-909.
196. Kawauchi A, Inoue Y, Hashimoto T, et al: Restless legs syndrome in hemodialysis patients: health-related quality of life and laboratory data analysis. Clin Nephrol 2006;66:440-446.
197. Molnar MZ, Novak M, Ambrus C, et al: Restless legs syndrome in patients after renal transplantation. Am J Kidney Dis 2005;45:388-396.
198. Molnar MZ, Szentkiralyi A, Lindner A, et al: Restless legs syndrome and mortality in kidney transplant recipients. Am J Kidney Dis 2007;50:813-820.
199. Manconi M, Govoni V, De Vito A, et al: Pregnancy as a risk factor for restless legs syndrome. Sleep Med 2004;5:305-308.
200. Tunc T, Karadag YS, Dogulu F, Inan LE: Predisposing factors of restless legs syndrome in pregnancy. Mov Disord 2007;22:627-631.
201. Suzuki K, Ohida T, Sone T, et al: The prevalence of restless legs syndrome among pregnant women in Japan and the relationship between restless legs syndrome and sleep problems. Sleep 2003;26:673-677.
202. Manconi M, Govoni V, De Vito A, et al: Restless legs syndrome and pregnancy. Neurology 2004;63:1065-1069.
203. Ondo WG, Vuong KD, Jankovic J: Exploring the relationship between Parkinson disease and restless legs syndrome. Arch Neurol 2002;59:421-424.
204. Nomura T, Inoue Y, Miyake M, et al: Prevalence and clinical characteristics of restless legs syndrome in Japanese patients with Parkinson's disease. Mov Disord 2006;21:380-384.
205. Gomez-Esteban JC, Zarranz JJ, Tijero B, et al: Restless legs syndrome in Parkinson's disease. Mov Disord 2007.
206. Garcia-Borreguero D, Allen RP, Benes H, et al: Augmentation as a treatment complication of restless legs syndrome: concept and management. Mov Disord 2007.
207. Gemignani F, Brindani F, Negrotti A, et al: Restless legs syndrome and polyneuropathy. Mov Disord 2006;21:1254-1257.

208. Merlino G, Fratticci L, Valente M, et al: Association of restless legs syndrome in type 2 diabetes: a case-control study. Sleep 2007;30:866-871.
209. Winkelmann J, Schadrack J, Wetter TC, et al: Opioid and dopamine antagonist drug challenges in untreated restless legs syndrome patients. Sleep Med 2001;2:57-61.
210. Winkelmann J, Prager M, Lieb R, et al: Anxietas tibiarum" depression and anxiety disorders in patients with restless legs syndrome. J Neurol 2005;252:67-71.
211. Lee HB, Hening WA, Allen RP, et al: Restless legs syndrome is associated with DSM IV major depressive disorder and panic disorder in the community. J Neuropsychiatry Clin Neurosci 2008;20(1):101-105.
212. Winkelman JW, Finn L, Young T: Prevalence and correlates of restless legs syndrome symptoms in the Wisconsin Sleep Cohort. Sleep Med 2006;7(7):545-552. Epub 2006 Jun 5.
213. Winkelman JW, Shahar E, Sharief I, Gottlieb DJ: Association of restless legs syndrome and cardiovascular disease in the Sleep Heart Health Study. Neurology 2008;70:35-42.
214. Kushida CA, Allen RP, Atkinson MJ: Modeling the causal relationships between symptoms associated with restless legs syndrome and the patient-reported impact of RLS. Sleep Med 2004;5: 485-488.
215. Winkelman JW: The evoked heart rate response to periodic leg movements of sleep. Sleep 1999;22:575-580.
216. Ferrillo F, Beelke M, Canovaro P, et al: Changes in cerebral and autonomic activity heralding periodic limb movements in sleep. Sleep Med 2004;5:407-412.
217. Sforza E, Pichot V, Barthelemy JC, et al: Cardiovascular variability during periodic leg movements: a spectral analysis approach. Clin Neurophysiol 2005;116:1096-1104.
218. Ferri R, Zucconi M, Rundo F, et al: Heart rate and spectral EEG changes accompanying periodic and non-periodic leg movements during sleep. Clin Neurophysiol 2007;118(2):438-448. Epub 2006 Nov 30.
219. Sforza E, Pichot V, Cervena K, et al: Cardiac variability and heart-rate increment as a marker of sleep fragmentation in patients with a sleep disorder: a preliminary study. Sleep 2007;30: 43-51.
220. Siddiqui F, Strus J, Ming X, et al: Rise of blood pressure with periodic limb movements in sleep and wakefulness. Clin Neurophysiol 2007;118(9):1923-1930. Epub 2007 Jun 27.
221. Guggisberg AG, Hess CW, Mathis J: The significance of the sympathetic nervous system in the pathophysiology of periodic leg movements in sleep. Sleep 2007;30:755-766.
222. Trenkwalder C, Hogl B, Benes H, Kohnen R: Augmentation in restless legs syndrome is associated with low ferritin. Sleep Med 2008;9(5):572-574. Epub 2007 Oct 24.
223. Allen RP, Ritchie SY: Clinical efficacy of ropinirole for restless legs syndrome is not affected by age at symptom onset. Sleep Med 2008;9(8):899-902. Epub 2007 Nov 19.
224. Trenkwalder C: Restless legs syndrome: overdiagnosed or underdiagnosed? Nat Clin Pract Neurol 2007;3(9):474-475. Epub 2007 Jun 26.
225. Aukerman MM, Aukerman D, Bayard M, et al: Exercise and restless legs syndrome: a randomized controlled trial. J Am Board Fam Med 2006;19:487-493.
226. Hornyak M, Grossmann C, Kohnen R, et al: Cognitive behavioral group therapy to improve patients scoping strategies with restless legs syndrome: a proof-of-concept trial. J Neurol Neurosurg Psychiatry 2008;79(7):823-825. Epub 2008 Feb 26.
227. Allen RP, Earley CJ: Augmentation of the restless legs syndrome with carbidopa/levodopa. Sleep 1996;19:205-213.
228. Earley CJ, Allen RP: Restless legs syndrome augmentation associated with tramadol. Sleep Med 2006;7:592-593.
229. Vetrugno R, La Morgia C, D'Angelo R, et al: Augmentation of restless legs syndrome with long-term tramadol treatment. Mov Disord 2007;22:424-427.
230. Trenkwalder C, Hening WA, Montagna P, et al: Treatment of restless legs syndrome: an evidence-based review and implications for clinical practice. Mov Disord 2008;23(16):2267-2302.
231. Guilleminault C, Cetel M, Philip P: Dopaminergic treatment of restless legs and rebound phenomenon. Neurology 1993;43:445.
232. Trenkwalder C, Stiasny K, Pollmacher T, et al: L-dopa therapy of uremic and idiopathic restless legs syndrome: a double-blind, crossover trial. Sleep 1995;18:681-688.
233. Walker SL, Fine A, Kryger MH: L-DOPA/carbidopa for nocturnal movement disorders in uremia. Sleep 1996;19:214-218.
234. Staedt J, Wassmuth F, Ziemann U, et al: Pergolide: treatment of choice in restless legs syndrome (RLS) and nocturnal myoclonus syndrome (NMS). A double-blind randomized crossover trial of pergolide versus L-Dopa. J Neural Transm 1997;104:461-468.

235. Collado-Seidel V, Kazenwadel J, Wetter TC, et al: A controlled study of additional sr-L-dopa in L-dopa-responsive restless legs syndrome with late-night symptoms. Neurology 1999;52: 285-290.

236. Benes H, Kurella B, Kummer J, et al: Rapid onset of action of levodopa in restless legs syndrome: a double-blind, randomized, multicenter, crossover trial. Sleep 1999;22:1073-1081.

237. Eisensehr I, Ehrenberg BL, Rogge Solti S, Noachtar S: Treatment of idiopathic restless legs syndrome (RLS) with slow-release valproic acid compared with slow-release levodopa/benserazid. J Neurol 2004;251:579-583.

238. Trenkwalder C, Benes H, Grote L, et al: Cabergoline compared to levodopa in the treatment of patients with severe restless legs syndrome: results from a multi-center, randomized, active controlled trial. Mov Disord 2007;22:696-703.

239. Micozkadioglu H, Ozdemir FN, Kut A, et al: Gabapentin versus levodopa for the treatment of restless legs syndrome in hemodialysis patients: an open-label study. Ren Fail 2004;26:393-397.

240. Walters AS, Hening WA, Kavey N, et al: A double-blind randomized crossover trial of bromocriptine and placebo in restless legs syndrome. Ann Neurol 1988;24:455-458.

241. Benes H: Transdermal lisuride: short-term efficacy and tolerability study in patients with severe restless legs syndrome. Sleep Med 2006;7:31-35.

242. Adler CH, Hauser RA, Sethi K, et al: Ropinirole for restless legs syndrome: a placebo-controlled crossover trial. Neurology 2004;62:1405-1407.

243. Trenkwalder C, Garcia-Borreguero D, Montagna P, et al: Ropinirole in the treatment of restless legs syndrome: results from a 12-week, randomised, placebo-controlled study in 10 European countries. J Neurol Neurosurg Psychiatry 2004;75:92-97.

244. Walters AS, Ondo WG, Dreykluft T, et al: Ropinirole is effective in the treatment of restless legs syndrome. TREAT RLS 2: a 12-week, double-blind, randomized, parallel-group, placebo-controlled study. Mov Disord 2004;19:1414-1423.

245. Bliwise DL, Freeman A, Ingram CD, et al: Randomized, double-blind, placebo-controlled, short-term trial of ropinirole in restless legs syndrome. Sleep Med 2005;6:141-147.

246. Bogan RK, Fry JM, Schmidt MH, et al: Ropinirole in the treatment of patients with restless legs syndrome: a US-based randomized, double-blind, placebo-controlled clinical trial. Mayo Clin Proc 2006;81:17-27.

247. Happe S, Sauter C, Klosch G, et al: Gabapentin versus ropinirole in the treatment of idiopathic restless legs syndrome. Neuropsychobiology 2003;48:82-86.

248. Montplaisir J, Karrasch J, Haan J, Volc D: Ropinirole is effective in the long-term management of restless legs syndrome: a randomized controlled trial. Mov Disord 2006;21:1627-1635.

249. Montplaisir J, Nicolas A, Denesle R, Gomez-Mancilla B: Restless legs syndrome improved by pramipexole: a double-blind randomized trial. Neurology 1999;52:938-943.

250. Winkelman JW, Sethi KD, Kushida CA, et al: Efficacy and safety of pramipexole in restless legs syndrome. Neurology 2006;67:1034-1039.

251. Trenkwalder C, Stiasny-Kolster K, Kupsch A, et al: Controlled withdrawal of pramipexole after 6 months of open-label treatment in patients with restless legs syndrome. Mov Disord 2006;21:1404-1410.

252. Oertel WH, Stiasny-Kolster K, Bergtholdt B, et al: Efficacy of pramipexole in restless legs syndrome: a six-week, multicenter, randomized, double-blind study (effect-RLS study). Mov Disord 2007;22:213-219.

253. Stiasny K, Moller JC, Oertel WH: Safety of pramipexole in patients with restless legs syndrome. Neurology 2000;55:1589-1590.

254. Stiasny-Kolster K, Kohnen R, Schollmayer E, et al: Patch application of the dopamine agonist rotigotine to patients with moderate to advanced stages of restless legs syndrome: a double-blind, placebo-controlled pilot study. Mov Disord 2004;19:1432-1438.

255. Trenkwalder C, Benes H, Poewe W, et al: Efficacy of rotigotine for treatment of moderate-to-severe restless legs syndrome: a randomised, double-blind, placebo-controlled trial. Lancet Neurol 2008;7:595-604.

256. Oertel WH, Benes H, Garcia-Borreguero D, et al: Efficacy of rotigotine transdermal system in severe restless legs syndrome: a randomized, double-blind, placebo-controlled, six-week dose-finding trial in Europe. Sleep Med 2008;9:228-239.

257. Willis T: *The London Practice of Physick*. London: Bassett & Croke, 1685.

258. Walters AS, Wagner ML, Hening WA, et al: Successful treatment of the idiopathic restless legs syndrome in a randomized double-blind trial of oxycodone versus placebo. Sleep 1993;16: 327-332.

259. Kaplan PW, Allen RP, Buchholz DW, Walters JK: A double-blind, placebo-controlled study of the treatment of periodic limb movements in sleep using carbidopa/levodopa and propoxyphene. Sleep 1993;16:717-723.
260. Walters AS, Winkelmann J, Trenkwalder C, et al: Long-term follow-up on restless legs syndrome patients treated with opioids. Mov Disord 2001;16:1105-1109.
261. Garcia-Borreguero D, Larrosa O, de la Llave Y, et al: Treatment of restless legs syndrome with gabapentin: a double-blind, cross-over study. Neurology 2002;59:1573-1579.
262. Thorp ML, Morris CD, Bagby SP: A crossover study of gabapentin in treatment of restless legs syndrome among hemodialysis patients. Am J Kidney Dis 2001;38:104-108.
263. Kushida CA, Becker PM, Ellenbogen AL et al: XP052 Study Group. Neurology 2009;72(5): 439-446.
264. Lundvall O, Abom PE, Holm R: Carbamazepine in restless legs: a controlled pilot study. Eur J Clin Pharmacol 1983;25:323-324.
265. Telstad W, Sorensen O, Larsen S, et al: Treatment of the restless legs syndrome with carbamazepine: a double blind study. BMJ (Clin Res Ed) 1984;288:444-446.
266. Montagna P, de Bianchi LS, Zucconi M, et al: Clonazepam and vibration in restless leg syndrome. Acta Neurol Scand 1984;69:428-430.
267. Saletu M, Anderer P, Saletu-Zyhlarz G, et al: Restless legs syndrome (RLS) and periodic limb movement disorder (PLMD): acute placebo-controlled sleep laboratory studies with clonazepam. Eur Neuropsychopharmacol 2001;11:153-161.
268. Peled R, Lavie P: Double-blind evaluation of clonazepam on periodic leg movements in sleep. J Neurol Neurosurg Psychiatry 1987;50:1679-1681.
269. Horiguchi J, Inami Y, Sasaki A, et al: Periodic leg movements in sleep with restless legs syndrome: effect of clonazepam treatment. Jpn J Psychiatry Neurol 1992;46:727-732.
270. Bonnet MH, Arand DL: The use of triazolam in older patients with periodic leg movements, fragmented sleep, and daytime sleepiness. J Gerontol 1990;45:M139-M144.
271. Bezerra ML, Martinez JV: Zolpidem in restless legs syndrome. Eur Neurol 2002;48:180-181.
272. Wagner ML, Walters AS, Coleman RG, et al: Randomized, double-blind, placebo-controlled study of clonidine in restless legs syndrome. Sleep 1996;19:52-58.
273. Evidente VG, Adler CH, Caviness JN, et al: Amantadine is beneficial in restless legs syndrome. Mov Disord 2000;15:324-327.
274. Hornyak M, Voderholzer U, Hohagen F, et al: Magnesium therapy for periodic leg movements-related insomnia and restless legs syndrome: an open pilot study. Sleep 1998;21:501-505.
275. Kohnen R, Benes H, Heinrich CR, Kurella B: Development of the disease-specific Restless Legs Syndrome Quality of Life (RLS-QoL) questionnaire. Mov Disord 2002;17. A232.
276. Abetz L, Arbuckle R, Allen RP, et al: The reliability, validity and responsiveness of the International Restless Legs Syndrome Study Group rating scale and subscales in a clinical-trial setting. Sleep Med 2006;7:340-349.
277. Atkinson MJ, Allen RP, DuChane J, et al: Validation of the Restless Legs Syndrome Quality of Life Instrument (RLS-QLI): findings of a consortium of national experts and the RLS. Foundation. Qual Life Res 2004;13:679-693.
278. Ware JE Jr, Sherbourne CD: The MOS 36-item short-form health survey (SF-36), I: conceptual framework and item selection. Med Care 1992;30:473-483.
279. Högl B, Leissner L, Poewe W: Clinical global impression-improvement (CGI-I) and patient global improvement (PGI) are equivalent and useful tools in measuring treatment effects in restless legs syndrome (RLS) patients. Eur J Neurol 2005;12:215.
280. Garcia-Borreguero D, Kohnen R, Hogl B, et al: Validation of the Augmentation Severity Rating Scale (ASRS): a multicentric, prospective study with levodopa on restless legs syndrome. Sleep Med 2007;8:455-463.
281. Högl B, Garcia-Borreguero D, Gschliesser V, et al: On the development of the "Structured Interview for Diagnosis of Augmentation during RLS treatment" (RLS-SIDA): first experiences. Sleep Med 2005;6:S158.

32 Startled People

PHILIP THOMPSON

Startle Response

Sudden unexpected visual, auditory, somatosensory, and vestibular stimuli elicit a startle response in normal subjects. It is augmented by fright or other emotional stimuli and habituates with repeated exposure to the same stimulus.[1] The response consists of a generalized myoclonic jerk affecting particularly the upper body, and has two components. The first component is a brief reflex at short latency. The second component follows at variable intervals encroaching on voluntary reaction time and is more prolonged. It is suggested that the clinical expression of an exaggerated startle response can be based on either component with different clinical implications in each case. Pathological enhancement of the initial short latency component is referred to as *hyperekplexia*.[2] Exaggeration of the later (secondary) component occurs in various neuropsychiatric and behavioral syndromes.[1,3]

The initial startle response consists of a blink, facial grimace, neck flexion, shoulder elevation, and bilateral flexion (less commonly extension) of the upper limbs and trunk. The sequence of muscle activation begins in the sternomastoid and upper trapezius at a latency of approximately 60 ms after auditory stimulation, and spreads rostrally to cranial muscles and caudally to the limbs and trunk over the following 100 ms or so.[1,2] This important physiological fact is easily measured, and provides a useful marker for identifying exaggeration of this component of the startle response and distinguishing it from events that occur beyond this time.[4,5] There is some variability in response latency, and responses habituate rapidly with repeated stimulation (within three to five trials) in normal individuals.[1,2]

The auditory startle response in orbicularis oculi follows and merges with the "tail" of the auditory blink reflex, the equivalent of the R2 component of the blink reflex that occurs at an earlier latency (30 to 40 ms) and does not habituate.[6] Facial muscle activation in the auditory startle reflex is most conveniently recorded from orbicularis oris or mentalis, rather than orbicularis oculi to avoid interference of the R2 component of the blink reflex.[6] Auditory startle responses in leg muscles are infrequent while sitting, but may be augmented by changing posture such as standing, with shortening of the response latency in tibialis anterior and soleus from 120 ms while sitting to 80 ms when standing.[7] This behavior may be explained by the preferential activation of one of the two or three successive bursts of muscle activity that characterize the typical startle response pattern. An unexplained finding is the disproportionately long latency of distal muscle contraction in the startle response.[6]

The following findings in humans are consistent with the startle reflex originating in the caudal pontine reticular formation with efferent projections in bilateral reticulospinal pathways as in experimental animal models:[8] (1) the response is bilateral[1,6]; (2) caudal propagation speed is roughly half that of conduction in corticospinal tracts[6]; (3) startle responses persist after corticospinal tract lesions causing hemiplegia[9]; and (4) lesions of the pontine reticular formation can result in symptomatic hyperekplexia,[10] or abolish the startle response as in Steele-Richardson-Olszewski syndrome (progressive supranuclear palsy).[11]

Descending cortical projections influence excitability of the startle circuit. The amygdala, frontostriatal and limbic structures have extensive reciprocal interconnections and mediate fear, anxiety and level of arousal. Amygdala projections to the pontine reticular formation influence the startle circuit in the rat.[12] Lesions of the amygdala abolish the fear-potentiated startle response, and electrical stimulation of the amygdala increases the startle response.[13] In humans, arousal potentiates the startle response, and amygdala lesions diminish both arousal and the startle response.[14] Ascending aminergic projections to amygdala and limbic regions from the brainstem link the pontine generators of the startle response with cortical control of emotional tone and arousal.

The second component of the startle response begins a variable interval after stimulation, usually 200 ms or more.[1,15] The duration is longer than the initial component, and may last several seconds. The latency and duration of the second component of the startle response fall within the range of voluntary reaction times. The pattern of response may be influenced by the nature of the startling stimulus, the situation in which it occurs,[1,15] and the general state of arousal and attention.[16] For these reasons, the clinical manifestations of this component of the startle response are complex, reflecting the prestimulus emotional state, incorporating emotional, behavioral, and voluntary responses to the startling stimulus. This component also has been considered an "orienting" response[15] as part of the behavioral reaction toward a stimulus.

The anatomical and physiological substrates of the second component are less well understood, but reciprocal connections between brainstem reticular networks and frontal and limbic regions, particularly the amygdala, seem likely to be important determinants of the "orienting" response. Connections of the amygdala with other cortical areas, hypothalamus, and brainstem autonomic centers provide an explanation for the brief sensation of arousal or anxiety and autonomic (piloerection) symptoms that may accompany the startle response in normal individuals.

Disorders of the First Component of the Startle Response

HYPEREKPLEXIA

Pathological exaggeration of the initial component of the startle reflex is the basis for startle disease, or hyperekplexia. This condition manifests in early infancy with stiffness, repetitive jerking, and hypertonia due to an exaggerated startle in response to various stimuli, such as noise, touch (when handling the infant), sudden perturbations, and tapping the mantle region, particularly the nose.[17-19] Hyperreflexia also is observed. Stiffness disappears during sleep. Abdominal hernias and hip dislocation may complicate persistent abdominal stiffness.[17,18] During childhood, sudden and unexpected noise, surprise, fright, and taps to the mantle continue to elicit dramatic startle responses.[17,18] The characteristic pattern of the exaggerated startle response ("jumps") involves facial muscle contraction, flexion or extension of the head and neck, shoulder elevation, and bilateral symmetrical flexion of the arms.[17] The myoclonic jerk may be followed by stiffness of the limbs and trunk leading to dramatic falls ("like a log") with head injury.[17,19]

During the period of stiffness, patients report they are suddenly unable to move and as a result cannot make any postural adjustments to restore balance or make protective limb movements to break the fall.[17] There is no disturbance of consciousness. Walking becomes slow, hesitant, and cautious on a wide base seeking support because of fear of falling during and after startles.

Familial hyperekplexia was originally divided into a major form, defined by severe exaggeration of the startle reflex and the presence hypertonia in infancy, hyperreflexia, falls, and an insecure gait, and a minor form comprising variable exaggeration of the startle reflex alone.[19] Subsequent genetic analysis has shown that only the major form is associated with genetic defects of the glycine receptor.[20] The latencies of cranial and proximal muscle responses during the exaggerated startle response were much shorter in the glycine receptor mutation (major) form than in the minor form, where latencies were similar to normal startle responses.[21]

Symptomatic hyperekplexia has been described after lesions affecting the brainstem reticular formation in the region of the nucleus pontis caudalis.[2,12,22] The clinical and electrophysiological features of the exaggerated startle response in symptomatic hyperekplexia are similar to hereditary hyperekplexia, including, in some cases, precipitous falls during episodes of generalized stiffness.[2]

Molecular Genetics of Hyperekplexia

The molecular genetic basis for sporadic and inherited hyperekplexia involves presynaptic and postsynaptic defects in glycinergic transmission. Postsynaptic causes include mutations in the alpha 1 subunit of the glycine receptor (*GLRA1*) inherited as autosomal recessive (including compound heterozygotes) and autosomal dominant traits leading to failure of the formation of adequate numbers of functional glycine receptors.[23]

The *GLAR1* mutation was the first identified in human hyperekplexia. Autosomal recessive mutations in beta subunit of the glycine receptor (GLRB) also have been identified.[24,25] Mutations in the *GLRA1* gene have been described in bovine myoclonus,[23] in autosomal recessive spasmodic[26] and oscillating mice,[27] and in the *GLRB* gene in spastic mice.[28] Phenotypic variation in the appearance of the mouse mutants is marked.[29] Other postsynaptic glycinergic defects (in humans and mice) are caused by mutations in gephyrin, which clusters glycine (and γ-aminobutyric acid [GABA]) receptors on the postsynaptic membrane,[30] and collybistin, which directs the location and fixes the position of gephyrin and therefore glycine receptor location.[31] Presynaptic defects in glycinergic transmission are caused by mutations in the gene coding for a glycine transporter (*GLYT2*), which controls the release and synaptic concentration of glycine in humans[32] and mice.[33]

Neurophysiology of Hyperekplexia

Tapping the forehead or nose produces a brisk reflex movement of the head with contraction of the trapezius and sternomastoid muscles at short latency (20 to 50 ms). This reflex has been referred to as a "head retraction reflex,"[17,34] and is the hallmark of myoclonus of brainstem origin.[2] The response then spreads to caudal muscles. In some cases of hyperekplexia, enhancement of long loop reflexes with enlarged cortical somatosensory responses and C reflexes (latency ~60 ms in intrinsic hand muscles after stimulation of the median nerve at the wrist) has been shown.[2,18]

STARTLE AND STIFF PERSON SYNDROME

Cases of stiff person syndrome in which myoclonus is prominent are referred to as the "jerking stiff man syndrome." The physiological basis for myoclonus in these cases includes enhanced exteroceptive reflexes[35] and brainstem myoclonus due to an exaggerated auditory startle response (latency of ~70 ms in neck muscles)[36] and the head retraction reflex.[34,36] A readily elicited head retraction reflex after taps to the nose and upper lip, and less commonly the glabella and chin was found in 61% of cases of stiff person syndrome and in 50% of cases of progressive encephalomyelitis with rigidity and myoclonus.[34] The response began in trapezius at short latency (12 to 20 ms) followed by a more variable, longer latency response (44 to 70 ms), then spread to sternomastoid and paraspinal muscles resulting in neck extension and retropulsion of the trunk.

The brisk head retraction reflex indicated involvement of brainstem circuits in stiff person syndrome even in the absence of continuous motor unit activity, spasm, or stiffness in craniocervical muscles.[36] This is consistent with previous suggestions that continuous motor unit activity and enhancement of exteroceptive reflexes is driven by abnormal descending inputs from brainstem to spinal motor neurons.[35] The similar reflex patterns in hyperekplexia and stiff person syndrome raise the possibility of common brainstem defects in glycine and GABA inhibitory transmission.[34] The significance of this concept is emphasized by one case of paraneoplastic stiff person syndrome with antibodies against gephyrin, a postsynaptic cytoplasmic protein that clusters glycine and GABA inhibitory receptors.[37] This patient exhibited prominent myoclonus due to an enhanced auditory startle response and a brisk head retraction reflex after stimulation of the face and jaw.[37] A recent report described a man with the clinical picture of progressive encephalomyelitis, rigidity and myoclonus (hyperekplexia) associated with a glycine receptor antibody.[38]

Disorders of the Second Component of the Auditory Startle Response

CULTURE BOUND STARTLE SYNDROMES

The *culture bound startle syndromes* have long attracted the attention of neurologists and psychiatrists. The best-known examples are latah, Jumping Frenchmen of Maine, and myriachit, but similar conditions have been described throughout the world.[3,39,40] These syndromes are characterized by "jumps" caused by exaggerated responses to unexpected stimuli, and are accompanied by numerous additional clinical features, including vocalizations, coprolalia, echolalia, echopraxia, and complex motor activities such as forced obedience, imitation behavior, and environmentally dependent behaviors. The behavioral manifestations can be prolonged, goal-directed, and potentially harmful.

Video recordings of startle-induced responses in latah and descendants of the Jumping Frenchmen show the onset of stimulus-induced behaviors beginning at intervals consistent with voluntary reaction times and continuing for long periods.[41-43] During this time, an "orienting response" directed toward the stimulus is frequently observed.[41-43] Whether these behaviors are an emotionally driven elaboration of the second component of the startle response or simply a voluntary reaction has not been established.

GILLES DE LA TOURETTE SYNDROME AND STARTLE

The aforementioned conundrum also applies to Gilles de la Tourette syndrome. Of patients with Gilles de la Tourette syndrome, 20% are reported to have an exaggerated startle response,[44] although studies of the startle response have confirmed an exaggerated response in some patients,[45] but not in others.[46] Reflex tics, vocalizations, coprolalia, and echolalia in Gilles de la Tourette syndrome may be triggered by ambient noises such as coughing, sniffing, or even particular words.[47] Similar stimulus-induced motor activities, obsessive-compulsive behaviors, rituals, touching, echopraxia, and echolalia occur in Gilles de la Tourette syndrome and the culture bound startle syndromes.[48]

A study of three cases with late-onset startle-induced tics revealed onset latencies (to various stimuli) 500 ms after stimulation, variable patterns of muscle activation, and motor behaviors lasting 2 minutes.[49] These features suggested a voluntary response, but a premovement cortical potential was not recorded, indicating the movements were not generated by voluntary motor pathways, findings similar to those described for simple motor tics.[50] The delayed onset of the motor responses and the associated neuropsychiatric and behavioral features (anxiety, panic attacks, screaming) suggest an interaction between the emotional state, level of arousal, and the second component of the startle response during which the complex responses occurred.

STARTLE IN PSYCHIATRIC CONDITIONS

The startle response is enhanced during states of high emotional tone, anxiety, and fear, and conversely is reduced during relaxed pleasurable states. This capacity for the startle response to mirror emotional tone has produced a growing body of work using excitability of the auditory startle response to explore modulation of emotional states, emotional tone, and arousal in affective disorders and generalized anxiety disorder. Studies in schizophrenia and drug withdrawal also are part of this expanding literature.[16] Abnormalities of the startle response in post-traumatic stress disorder, "war neurosis," "shell shock," or "startle neurosis"[51] are now an integral part of the diagnosis of post-traumatic stress disorder.[16] More recently, abnormal enhanced startle modulation was shown in patients with psychogenic movement disorders.[52]

The methodology in these studies involves recording and measuring the amplitude of rectified orbicularis oculi electromyographic activity for 250 ms after the acoustic stimulus.[14,16,52] These measures include electromyographic activity from the blink reflex and both components of the startle response. From a physiological point of view, as discussed previously, most of the affective modulation of the startle response should be reflected in the second component of the startle response that incorporates an "orienting" or behavioral response to the stimulus. Whether descending inputs from the amygdala and frontal regions influence the pontine reticular origin of all components of the startle response is unknown.

BEHAVIORAL PHENOMENA AND THE STARTLE RESPONSE

It is a common and normal experience that an unexpected startle may be accompanied by a transient sensation of fright, anxiety, or fear. The emotional arousal is accompanied by an orienting reaction that may include looking toward the stimulus; moving away from it; raising the hands in that direction; or vocalization, coprolalia, and dropping or throwing objects. The extent and nature of such responses are influenced by the emotional state, type of stimulus, and circumstances in which it occurs. When observing this response over the course of 1 or 2 seconds, it is difficult to distinguish what is reflex and when a voluntary elaboration of the response begins. Individuals in whom exaggerated responses are readily elicited can be found in most societies,[39,53] and some of these individuals also exhibit behavioral phenomena similar to those described in the culture bound startle syndromes and Gilles de la Tourette syndrome.

The additional elaborate and complex behavioral phenomena, such as environmental dependency, utilization behavior, imitation, echopraxia, and echolalia warrant further comment. Psychiatric explanations emphasize the role of fright and fear in shaping the responses to startle,[39,40] and construe such behaviors as a defense elaborated by local custom against such strong emotions.[40] From a neurological point of view, these can be interpreted as typical of a frontal lobe syndrome.[54,55] One postulate is that subtle disturbances of frontal lobe function influence the excitability of the startle response, and this modifies levels of arousal. The interaction between these influences determines the behavioral consequences of startle. Any behavioral manifestations may be magnified when there is a degree of disinhibition caused by diminished frontal lobe function.

REFERENCES

1. Wilkins D, Hallett M, Wess MM: Audiogenic startle reflex of man and its relationship to startle syndromes. Brain 1986;109:561-573.
2. Brown P, Rothwell JC, Thompson PD, et al: The hyperekplexias and their relationship to the normal startle reflex. Brain 1991;114:1903-1928.
3. Thompson PD: The phenomenology of startle, Latah and related conditions. In Hallett M, Fahn S, Jankovic J, et al (eds): Psychogenic Movement Disorders. Philadelphia: Lippincott Williams & Wilkins, 2006, pp 48-52.
4. Thompson PD, Colebatch JG, Brown P, et al: Voluntary stimulus sensitive jerks and jumps mimicking myoclonus or pathological startle syndromes. Mov Disord 1992;7:257-262.
5. Brown P, Thompson PD: Electrophysiological aids to the diagnosis of psychogenic jerks, spasms and tremor. Mov Disord 2001;16:595-599.
6. Brown P, Rothwell JC, Thompson PD, et al: New observations on the normal auditory startle reflex in man. Brain 1991;114:1891-1902.
7. Brown P, Day BL, Rothwell JC, et al: The effect of posture on the normal and pathological auditory startle reflex. J Neurol Neurosurg Psychiatry 1991;54:892-897.
8. Davis M, Gendelman DS, Tischler MD, Gendelman PM: Primary acoustic startle circuit: lesion and stimulation studies. J Neurosci 1982;2:791-805.
9. Jankelowitz SK, Colebatch JG: The acoustic startle reflex in ischaemic stroke. Neurology 2004;62:114-115.
10. Kimber TE, Thompson PD: Symptomatic hyperekplexia occurring as a result of pontine infarction. Mov Disord 1997;12:814-816.
11. Vidailhet M, Rothwell JC, Thompson PD, et al: The auditory startle response in the Steele-Richardson-Olszewski syndrome and Parkinson's disease. Brain 1992;115:1181-1192.
12. Hitchcock JM, Davis M: Efferent pathway of the amygdala involved in conditioned fear as measured with the fear-potentiated startle paradigm. Behav Neurosci 2001;105:826-842.
13. Rosen JB, Hitchcock JM, Sananes CB, et al: A direct projection from the central nucleus of the amygdala to the acoustic startle pathway: antegrade and retrograde tracing studies. Behav Neurosci 1991;105:817-825.
14. Angrilli A, Mauri A, Palomba D, et al: Startle reflex and emotion modulation impairment after a right amygdala lesion. Brain 1996;119:1991-2000.
15. Gogan P: The startle and orienting reactions in man: a study of their characteristics and habituation. Brain Res 1970;18:117-135.
16. Grillon C, Baas J: A review of the modulation of the startle reflex by affective states and its application in psychiatry. Clin Neurophysiol 2003;114:1557-1579.
17. Suhren O, Bruyn GW, Tuynman JA: Hyperexplexia: a hereditary startle pattern. J Neurol Sci 1966;3:577-605.
18. Markand ON, Garg BP, Weaver DD: Familial startle disease (hyperekplexia). Arch Neurol 1984;41:71-74.
19. Andermann F, Andermann E: Excessive startle syndromes: startle disease, jumping and startle epilepsy. Adv Neurol 1986;43:321-338.
20. Tijssen MAJ, Shiang R, van Deutekom J, et al: Molecular genetic reevaluation of the Dutch hyperekplexia family. Arch Neurol 1995;52:578-582.
21. Tjissen MAJ, Padberg GW, van Dijk JG: The startle pattern in the minor form of hyperekplexia. Arch Neurol 1996;53:608-613.
22. Watson SR, Colebatch JG: Focal pathological startle following pontine infarction. Mov Disord 2002;17:212-218.
23. Healy PJ, Pierce KD, Dennis JA, et al: Bovine myoclonus: model of human hyperekplexia. Mov Disord 2002;17:743-747.
24. Rees MI, Lewis TM, Vafa F, et al: Compound heterozygosity and nonsense mutations in the alpha (1) subunit of the inhibitory glycine receptor in hyperekplexia. Hum Genet 2001;109:267-270.
25. Rees MI, Lewis TM, Kwok JB, et al: Hyperekplexia associated with compound heterozygote mutations in the beta subunit of the human inhibitory glycine receptor (GLRB). Hum Mol Genet 2002;11:853-860.
26. Ryan SG, Buckwater MS, Lynch JW, et al: A missense mutation in the gene encoding the alpha 1 subunit of the inhibitory glycine receptor in the spasmodic mouse. Nat Genet 1994;7:131-135.
27. Kling C, Koch M, Saul B, Becker CM: The frameshift mutation oscillator (Glra1(spd-ot)) produces a complete loss glycine receptor alpha 1-polypeptide in mouse central nervous system. Neuroscience 1997;78:411-447.

28. Kingsmore SF, Giros B, Suh D, et al: Glycine receptor beta subunit gene mutation in spastic mouse associated with LINE-1 element insertion. Nat Genet 1994;7:136-141.
29. Simon ES: Phenotypic heterogeneity and disease course in three murine strains with mutations in genes encoding for alpha 1 and beta glycine subunits. Mov Disord 1997;12:221-228.
30. Rees MI, Harvey K, Ward H, et al: Isoform heterogeneity of the human gephyrin gene (GPHN) binding domains to the glycine receptor and mutation analysis in hyperekplexia. J Biol Chem 2003;278:853-860.
31. Harvey K, Duguid I, Alldred M, et al: The GDP-GTP exchange factor collybistin: an essential determinant of neuronal gephyrin clustering. J Neurosci 2004;24:24688-24696.
32. Rees MI, Harvey K, Pearce BR, et al: Mutations in the gene encoding GlyT2 (SLC6A5) define a presynaptic component of human startle disease. Nat Genet 2006;38:801-806.
33. Gomeza J, Ohno K, Hulsmann S, et al: Deletion of the mouse glycine transporter 2 results in a hyperekplexia phenotype and postnatal lethality. Neuron 2003;40:785-796.
34. Khasani S, Becker K, Meinck H-M: Hyperekplexia and stiff man syndrome: abnormal brainstem reflexes suggest a physiological relationship. J Neurol Neurosurg Psychiatry 2004;75:1265-1269.
35. Meinck H-M, Thompson PD: The stiff man syndrome and related disorders. Mov Disord 2002;17:853-866.
36. Berger C, Meinck H-M: Head retraction reflex in stiff man syndrome and related disorders. Mov Disord 2003;18:906-911.
37. Butler HM, Hatashi A, Ohkoshi N, et al: Autoimmunity to gephyrin in stiff-man syndrome. Neuron 2000;26:307-312.
38. Hutchinson M, Waters P, McHugh J, et al: Progressive encephalomyelitis, rigidity and myoclonus: a novel glycine receptor antibody. Neurology 2008;71:1291-1292.
39. Simons RC: The resolution of the Latah paradox. J Nerv Ment Dis 1980;168:195-206.
40. Howard R, Ford R: From the jumping Frenchmen of Maine to post-traumatic stress disorder: the startle response in neuropsychiatry. Psychol Med 1992;22:695-707.
41. Tanner CM, Chamberland J: Latah in Jakarta, Indonesia. Mov Disord 2001;16:526-529.
42. Saint-Hilaire M-H, Saint-Hilaire J-M: Jumping Frenchmen of Maine. Mov Disord 2001;16:530.
43. McFarling DA: The "Ragin' Cajuns" of Louisiana. Mov Disord 2001;16:531-532.
44. Lees AJ, Robertson M, Trimble MR, et al: A clinical study of Gilles de la Tourette syndrome in the United Kingdom. J Neurol Neurosurg Psychiatry 1984;47:1-8.
45. Stell R, Thickbroom GW, Mastaglia FL: The audiogenic startle response in Tourette's syndrome. Mov Disord 1995;10:723-730.
46. Sachdev P, Chee KY, Aniss AM: The audiogenic startle reflex in Tourette's syndrome. Biol Psychiatry 1997;41. 796–403.
47. Commander M, Corbett J, Prendergast M, Ridley C: Reflex tics in two patients with Gilles de la Tourette syndrome. Br J Psychiatry 1991;159:877-879.
48. Eapen V, Moriarty J, Robertson MM: Stimulus induced behaviours in Tourette's syndrome. J Neurol Neurosurg Psychiatry 1994;57:853-855.
49. Tijssen MAJ, Brown P, Morris HR, Lees A: Late onset startle induced tics. J Neurol Neurosurg Psychiatry 1999;67:782-784.
50. Obeso JA, Rothwell JC, Marsden CD: Simple tics in Gilles de la Tourette's syndrome are not prefaced by a normal premovement potential. J Neurol Neurosurg Psychiatry 1981;44:735-738.
51. Thorne FC: Startle neurosis. Am J Psychiatry 1944;101:105-109.
52. Seignourel PJ, Miller K, Kellison I, et al: Abnormal affective startle modulation in individuals with psychogenical movement disorders. Mov Disord 2007;22:1265-1271.
53. Hardison J: Are the jumping Frenchmen of Maine goosey? JAMA 1980;244:70.
54. Lhermitte F, Pillon B, Serdaru M: Autonomy and the frontal lobes, part I: imitation and utilization behaviour: a neuropsychological study of 75 patients. Ann Neurol 1986;19:326-334.
55. Lhermitte F: Human autonomy and the frontal lobes, part II: patient behaviour in complex and social situations: the "environmental dependency syndrome." Ann Neurol 1986;19:335-343.

33 Psychogenic Movement Disorders

MADHAVI THOMAS • JOSEPH JANKOVIC

Introduction

Psychogenic disorders have been increasingly recognized as a specific diagnostic group with unclear etiology, contributing to significant disability and socioeconomic burden. In classic descriptions of these disorders by Charcot, Gowers, and other traditional neurologists, terms such as *hysteria, nonorganic,* and *functional* disorders were used for this group of disorders, which overlapped in clinical manifestations between psychiatry, neurology, and other fields of medicine. Sommer first introduced the word *psychogenic* into psychiatric literature in 1894 referring to "disorders originating in mind or mental or emotional processes, having psychological rather than a physiologic origin."[1] Marsden[2] proposed six rules of hysteria, stating that patients who have hysterical disorders usually (1) do not have histrionic personalities, (2) are unlikely to conform to Briquet's syndrome (somatization disorder), (3) may have underlying recognized physical or psychiatric illness, (4) could have unrecognized physical or psychiatric illness, (5) require further neurological or psychiatric exploration, and (6) may exhibit abnormal illness behavior (assuming the sick role). These rules seem to hold true in patients diagnosed with psychogenic movement disorders (PMD).

PMD are best defined as conditions manifesting either as hyperkinetic or hypokinetic movement disorders, or a combination thereof, not fully explained by organic disease (as determined by clinical examination and full investigation), and occurring in association with underlying psychiatric or psychological factors. Patients with PMD seem to follow a pattern of illness that ranges in its spectrum from being unclassifiable into psychiatric illness to being associated with severe underlying psychiatric disorders, including Munchausen's syndrome or Munchausen's syndrome by proxy.[3,4]

Epidemiology and Risk Factors

The estimated prevalence of psychogenic disorders is 1% to 9% of the general population.[3] This variable range is partly attributed to differences in diagnostic criteria for PMD, assessment methods, and case ascertainment. Based on our own experience and other published studies, PMD has been estimated to account for 3.3% to 3.6% of all patients seen in a movement disorders clinic.[3,5,6] Of 25,063 patients seen at the Parkinson's Disease Center and Movement Disorders Clinic, Baylor College of Medicine since 1977, 911 (3.6%) patients were diagnosed with PMD. In a previously published series of PMD from our center, movement disorders were encountered in the following order of frequency: dystonia, 40.6%; tremor, 39.8%; myoclonus, 17%; tics, 4.3%; parkinsonism, 3.2%; dyskinesia, 1.5%; and chorea, 0.6%.[3] Organic disorders have been reported to coexist with PMD in about 10% to 15% of PMD patients,[7] similar to the frequency of PMD encountered in our series (16.7%).[5] Based on various studies of patients with PMD, the mean age at onset is 38.5 years (range 4 to 73 years) with a 61% to 87% female preponderance.[2,3,5-8]

Because there is limited information about the occurrence of PMD in children, a retrospective review of all medical records of children (≤17 years old) diagnosed at Baylor College of Medicine Movement Disorders Clinic with PMD between 1988–2007 was performed.[9] Of the 54 patients who satisfied the diagnostic criteria for probable PMD,[8] 40 (78%) were girls; the mean age at presentation was 14.2 years (range 7.6 to 17.7 years), and the mean duration of symptoms before evaluation was 12 ± 12 months (range 0.5 to 48 months). The onset of symptoms was abrupt in 46 (90%) patients and followed an identifiable trigger, often a minor injury, in 27 (53%). In 16 children, PMD had a single phenomenology, whereas the remaining 35 (69%) children exhibited multiple motor phenotypes. PMD was paroxysmal in 31 (61%) children; continuous in 14 (27%); and nearly continuous, but punctuated by unexplained remissions, in the remainder. The following phenomenologies were observed: tremor in 30 (59%); jerklike movements (often too slow to be termed myoclonus) in 20 (39%); dystonia in 19 (37%) (with fixed posturing in 6); unusual gait in 12 (24%); convergence spasm in 5 (10%); false weakness in 5 (10%); speech disturbance in 4 (8%); and severe bradykinesia, athetosis, and "apraxia of eyelid opening" in one child each. Symptoms were restricted to the nondominant side in only 2 (4%) children, whereas exclusively dominant limb involvement was noted in 16 (31%) patients. Of the 51 children with PMD, 12 (23.5%) had a total of 17 surgeries for symptoms related to PMD or for associated symptoms without an identifiable organic basis. Another study of PMD in children[10] reported 15 cases with average time from symptom onset to diagnosis at 9.4 months (sd 15.1). Psychiatric diagnoses showed conversion disorder in 12 and somatization disorder in 3 children, again highlighting the importance of psychiatric evaluation in patients with childhood onset PMD. All of their patients also had abrupt onset of disease, and most common phenotype was dystonia. Earlier diagnosis and improved education of health care providers about PMD may lessen the morbidity and avoid potentially risky procedures in this vulnerable population of patients.[9]

Diagnostic Criteria for Psychogenic Movement Disorders

Fahn and Williams proposed criteria for diagnosis of PMD based on the level of certainty of having a PMD (Table 33–1).[8,11-12] This classification into documented, clinically established, probable and possible PMD[8] has been used by many investigators in subsequent studies, and has proven to be very valuable in clinical practice. An essential element of the diagnosis of PMD is not only the exclusion of organic causes, but also the requirement for "positive" features, such as sudden onset, variable frequency, changing pattern and intensity of the movement, deliberate slowness of movement and speech, verbal gibberish, bizarre movement and gait, excessive startle, and movements that are incongruous with any recognized organic movement disorders.[3,6,8,13]

Shill and Gerber[14] have proposed new diagnostic classification of PMD using primary and secondary criteria. They define PMD as being "clinically proven" PMD (remits with psychotherapy, remits when patient is unobserved, or there is premovement Bereitschaftspotential on electroencephalography for myoclonus only). Primary criteria include inconsistent with organic disease, excessive pain or fatigue, previous exposure to a disease model, and potential for secondary gain. Secondary criteria include multiple somatizations and obvious psychiatric disturbance. The diagnosis of "clinically definite" PMD requires three primary and at least one secondary criteria, "clinically probable PMD" requires two primary and two secondary criteria, and "clinically possible PMD" requires one primary and two secondary or two primary and one secondary criteria. Although these criteria include motor phenomena and psychiatric diagnoses, the study by Shill and Gerber[14] is limited because it is based on a retrospective analysis with less emphasis on the nature of PMD itself. Gupta and Lang[15] recently proposed revised Fahn and Williams' criteria including clinically definite and laboratory supported definite criteria.

Most patients with PMD have a coexisting psychiatric illness. Although often told by psychiatrists and psychologists that they are "normal," approximately 20% of patients with PMD are considered to have histrionic personality.[2] Depression is seen in 38% to 71% of patients,[3,5,8,16-19] and "conversion disorder" has been diagnosed in 75% to 95.2% of patients.[8,16] The differentiation between "histrionic personality," somatoform disorder such as conversion or somatization (hysteria), factitious disorder, malingering, and other medically unexplained symptoms may not be always possible—hence the term *psychogenic*.

Evaluation of Patients with Psychogenic Movement Disorders

Because of poor insights into precipitating or contributing factors, frequent denial of any stress, and attribution of the symptoms by the patient to other causes, the clinician's interviewing skills are crucial for the diagnosis and for understanding

TABLE 33–1	Diagnostic Features of Psychogenic Movement Disorders
History before onset	Abrupt onset, trauma, surgery, major life event
Social factors	Work-related injuries, litigation, poor relationships, physical abuse, sexual abuse, substance abuse, secondary gain (financial or increased attention)
Multiple somatizations	Self-inflicted injuries, unwitnessed paroxysmal disorders such as spells of dizziness or loss of consciousness, gastrointestinal symptoms (irritable bowel syndrome), cardiopulmonary symptoms (chest pain, palpitations), reproductive symptoms (dyspareunia, menstrual irregularities), food allergies, chronic pain, chronic fatigue, sleep disorder
Psychiatric disorders	Depression, anxiety disorder, somatization disorder, malingering, factitious disorder
Physical findings	Incongruous movements, inconsistent movements, response to placebo or suggestion, selective disability, dramatic resolution, maximum early disability, deliberate slowing, rhythmic shaking
Other neurological findings	Transient weakness, sensory symptoms, seizures, convergence spasm, bursts of verbal gibberish, amnesia

of potential psychodynamic issues that may explain the reason for the observed behavior. A skillful and detailed interview often uncovers potential predisposing factors for PMD, such as physical trauma, sexual abuse or rape, adverse reaction to a prescribed drug, surgery, emotional stress, or a major life event.[2,5,8,10-19]

The average number of physicians seen by PMD patients before the correct diagnosis is established is 13, but many patients have seen 15 physicians or more.[18] Of the patients with PMD seen in the series by Factor and coworkers,[6] 54% had abrupt onset, 39% had selective disability, 36% had multiple somatizations, 61% had a precipitating event, and 64% had evidence of secondary gain.[6] In our series of patients with PMD,[5] most (82.7%) had abrupt onset of symptoms, and the most common precipitating event was personal life stress, noted by 33.5% patients. Coexistent neurological symptoms were seen in 30.7% of patients, higher than in other series,[20] and included sensory symptoms, weakness, seizures, diplopia, and other visual symptoms.[5] Organic movement disorders, along with PMD, were seen in 16.2% of our patients.[5]

Most patients with PMD have underlying psychiatric problems, such as depression, anxiety disorder, somatization disorder, psychological factors secondary to long-term physical illness, and malingering or factitious disorders (see Table 33–1).[21-25] These comorbid psychiatric disorders may be subtle, and it is not unusual for these patients to be told by psychiatrists or psychologists that they are "normal" and that "there is nothing psychologically wrong." Schrag and colleagues[26] reported a higher percentage of self-reported diagnoses, such as peptic ulcer disease, diverticulitis, angina, epilepsy, and other medical conditions in patients with neurologically unexplained disorders compared with controls, and a specific increase in functional symptoms, such as irritable bowel syndrome and noncardiac chest pain. Complex regional pain syndrome (CRPS), multiple somatizations, and other general medical complaints are also common in patients with PMD.[2,26-28]

Physical examination of PMD patients may reveal features that are incongruous with organic movement disorder. Other neurological findings include false weakness, midline sensory split, Hoover sign (hip extension while the patient's heel is pressing into examiner's hand is weak when tested directly, but normal when subject is asked to flex the contralateral hip), pseudoclonus (clonus with irregular, variable amplitude), and pseudo–waxy flexibility (maintenance of limb in a set position, and inability to change this position).[3,27,28] Pseudoptosis (excessive contraction of orbicularis, with apparent weakness of frontalis) and convergence spasm during near reflex with intermittent disconjugate gaze and miosis are typical eye findings in PMD. In our experience in a tertiary movement disorders clinic, convergence spasm is frequently associated with PMD.[29] Convergence spasm also may be seen as a sequela of brainstem injury or other head trauma, neoplasm, metabolic encephalopathies,[30] and other disorders, including attention-deficit disorders.[31]

All the aforementioned physical signs must be interpreted with caution because some of these may also be present in organic disease. The frequency of misdiagnoses and symptoms wrongly attributable to organic illness vary among reported studies, largely because of the retrospective nature of the studies, variable experience of the investigators, and differences in referral patterns among centers.[18,27,28]

Specific Psychogenic Movement Disorders

PMD can be classified based on the pattern of movement disorder. As discussed earlier, some patients may have an underlying organic movement disorder along with PMD. The following discussion should help the clinician identify the specific features indicative of different types of PMD.

PSYCHOGENIC TREMOR

Psychogenic tremor is the most common of all PMD, based on data from various studies.[5,32-36] Koller and associates[32] studied 24 patients with psychogenic tremor (9 men and 15 women 15 to 78 years old); 21 had abrupt onset of tremor, and 3 had undetermined onset. All patients had reduction of tremor with distraction, and 22 of 24 (91.6%) had a change in direction of tremor during the course of the examination.[32] Anatomically, psychogenic tremor was distributed as follows: hands (84%), legs (28%), and generalized tremor (20%), although stance tremor, an irregular up-and-down (bouncing). low-frequency leg and trunk movement is also typical of psychogenic tremor.

Some patients exhibit bizarre, dancelike movements, and complain of exhaustion because of shaking.[32-36] Most patients have combination, often difficult-to-classify tremors, but approximately 63% exhibit rest tremor, and 51% have postural or action tremor.[36] Variability of amplitude, frequency, and direction is seen in 88% of patients, and tremor starting in a focal area spreading to adjacent areas is seen in 70% patients. In our series of 127 patients with psychogenic tremor, 92 (72.4%) were female, the mean age at initial evaluation was 43.7 ± 14.1 years, and mean duration of symptoms was 4.6 ± 7.6 years. Characteristic features of psychogenic tremor were abrupt onset (78.7%), distractibility (72.4%), variable amplitude and frequency (62.2%), intermittent occurrence (35.4%), inconsistent movement (29.9%), and variable direction (17.3%).[34,35]

Among the distinguishing features, distractibility, coactivation sign, and entrainment are particularly characteristic of psychogenic tremor.[37] Distractibility is defined as a change (usually a suppression) of amplitude and frequency of the tremor while the patient is asked to perform rapid, sometimes complex, sequential movements with the less affected or unaffected limb, and when the patient performs some mental task, such as arithmetic problems or simply subtracting 7 from 100. Distractibility was shown in all patients in the study by Koller and associates,[32] whereas Deuschl and colleagues[33] in their study reported distractibility in 19 of 22 cases. Distractibility was noted in 92 of our 127 patients.[34,35]

Based on clinical observation, psychogenic tremor may be classified into three types: (1) long duration (either continuous or intermittent) tremor; (2) short-lived or paroxysmal tremors lasting less than 30 seconds; and (3) continuous tremor, with superimposed short paroxysmal episodes.[34] Testing muscle resistance for one or two limbs during slow arrhythmic passive movements would elicit the coactivation sign of psychogenic tremor. Active resistance against such passive movement and fluctuations in muscle tone are common features of psychogenic tremor. Increasing the range of passive movements usually eventually results in complete breakdown of enhanced muscle tone and resolution of tremor during this test. With appropriate challenge, the muscles can be completely relaxed. Coactivation may sometimes produce bizarre positioning in outstretched hands.[31] Entrainment is a change in the original tremor frequency to match the frequency of requested repetitive task in another limb (or with side-to-side tongue movement). When tremor continues, entrainment can be shown by a change in speed or rhythmicity of the other requested movement, which becomes irregular or incomplete.[3,33,37]

In a study at Baylor College of Medicine Movement Disorders Clinic,[37] distractibility and suggestibility scores were significantly higher in patients with psychogenic tremor compared with patients with essential tremor. Clinical features that quite reliably distinguished psychogenic tremor from essential tremor included sudden onset, spontaneous remission, distractibility, and suggestibility. Clinical differentiation based on comparative study between patients with essential tremor and patients with psychogenic tremor showed 72.7% sensitivity and 73.3% specificity for distraction and alternate finger tapping test.[37] This study used a video protocol to assess tremor, at rest tremor in wing-beating position, tremor during alternate finger tapping and other repetitive movements, and tremor with hyperventilation or a tuning fork along with a suggestion that this may either improve or worsen the tremor.

Investigations to determine the nature of tremor in difficult cases include electromyography (EMG), accelerometry, tremograms, and tremor frequency analysis. EMG recordings show that, in contrast to essential tremor of Parkinson's disease, psychogenic tremor is not maintained while tapping with the contralateral arm, and either dissipates or shifts to the frequency of external auditory input provided by a metronome.[38] Postural tremor in Parkinson's disease is often delayed before "re-emergent tremor" appears. Accelerometry in psychogenic tremor may show an increase in amplitude with increasing load, in contrast to reduced amplitude seen in organic tremor.[33] Koller and associates[32] found highly unusual tremograms with fluctuation in tremor amplitude, particularly a decrease in tremor with distraction. In Parkinson's disease and essential tremor, the amplitude changes are minimal during recording.

In one study, patients with psychogenic tremor, patients with essential tremor, Parkinson's disease patients, and normal volunteers were requested to perform a unilateral simple reaction time task (SRT) to a visual imperative signal at rest (rSRT) and during contralateral hand tremor (tSRT).[39] Reaction time was significantly longer in tSRT than in rSRT in patients with psychogenic tremor and in normal volunteers, but no significant differences were observed between Parkinson's disease patients and patients with essential tremor. This delay of unilateral tSRT with respect to rSRT suggests a dual-task interference in patients with psychogenic tremor.

Long-term prognosis of psychogenic tremor varies among studies, depending on ascertainment and other methodological issues.[32,34,40] McKeon et al[41] recently studied long term prognosis in patients with documented electrodiagnostic features of psychogenic tremor. All patients had tremor frequency fluctuations of greater than or equal to 1.5 Hz along with marked distractibility, and documented entrainment and cessation of tremor in opposite limb. Median change of tremor frequency was 5 Hz (range, 1.5-13 Hz). They report persistent disability in 21 of 33 patients after median follow up 3.2 years (range 2.8-4.8). In contrast to other studies, in which less than a third of the patients improved, in our long-term series, 56.6% of patients reported improvement in tremor. Factors that predicted a favorable outcome were elimination of stressors and patient's perception of effective treatment by the physician. Better prognosis in our series may be a result of more aggressive treatment and longer duration of follow-up.[34,35]

PSYCHOGENIC DYSTONIA

Psychogenic dystonia is a well-recognized disorder, but half of patients with psychogenic dystonia may also have organic dystonia.[42] Fahn and Williams[11] found that of 1186 patients with dystonia, 2.6% had psychogenic dystonia using documented and clinically definite criteria. When the probable and possible cases were included, the frequency was 4.6%.[12] In our series of 517 patients with PMD, 208 (40.2%) had dystonia.[5] In the long-term follow-up data on psychogenic dystonia patients out of 89 patients with psychogenic dystonia, 51 met "clinically established" criteria, 15 met criteria for "probable" psychogenic dystonia, 13 had "documented" psychogenic dystonia based on their response to placebo, and 10 had "possible" psychogenic dystonia based on Fahn and Williams criteria.[12] Average age at onset was 34.8 ± 13.8 years, average duration of illness was 3.9 ± 5.1 years, and average duration of follow-up was 3.6 ± 3.1 years. A comorbid psychiatric illness was identified in 62.9%, and clear precipitating factor (personal stress and trauma most common) was noted by 78.7%. The most common clinical features were distractibility (58.4%); intermittent, episodic symptoms (42.7%); inconsistent movements (21.3%); active resistance to passive movement (24.7%); and fixed posture (7.9%). Generalized dystonia was noted in 20% of patients, and 20.2% of patients had coexistent organic movement disorder. Associated psychogenic tremor was noted in 71.7% of patients.[43]

One of the most common sites for psychogenic dystonia is the foot, which is not usually involved in adult-onset primary dystonia, but may be the initial manifestation of Parkinson's disease.[12,42] In most patients with psychogenic dystonia, there is a spread to other areas, including the head, neck, and trunk.[12] Patients with psychogenic dystonia frequently have tenderness to touch, labored speech and strained voice, exaggeration of pain with passive movement of the dystonic limb, and active resistance against passive movement.[42,43]

Common clues to the diagnosis of psychogenic dystonia include bizarre movements; changing postures that are incongruous and inconsistent with typical dystonia; paroxysmal, intermittent, or resting dystonia; and fixed postures. Most patients report rapid progression to maximum disability early in the course, and selective disabilities or abilities are inconsistent with the muscle spasms. Attempted voluntary movement to command in the opposite direction of the dystonic posturing may activate antagonists with little apparent action in the agonists (limb or digit may do the opposite of what the examiner requests). Also important for diagnosis is the presence of other PMD, no family history, spontaneous and dramatic remissions, no improvement with sleep, the presence of a physical or psychological precipitant or a trigger, and a response to a suggestion (placebo). Patients with long-standing psychogenic dystonia sometimes develop contractures, which may need to be investigated under anesthesia.[12,42,43] Disappearance with placebo or by suggestion does not establish the diagnosis of psychogenic paroxysmal dystonia because the remission may be coincidental. If paroxysms are frequent, and the patient has prolonged attacks, repeated trials with placebo may be more informative.[16,44]

Abnormal movements and postures may follow brain, root, peripheral nerve, or soft tissue trauma. Although post-traumatic and peripherally induced dystonia is a well-accepted entity,[45] some of these patients exhibit features of psychogenic dystonia. Bhatia and coworkers[46] described causalgia-dystonia syndrome in 18 patients after often trivial peripheral injury. The patients were predominantly women, and mean age was 28.5 years, with initial onset in the leg being more frequent. The patients had causalgia, allodynia, and hyperpathia, and sudomotor, trophic, and vasomotor changes in the affected area. Fixed dystonia predominantly in the foot and hand appeared at the same time as the pain along with muscle spasms. The spread of the symptoms followed a hemiplegic, transverse, or triplegic distribution. The investigators found contractures often early in the course of the disease, but spontaneous recovery was seen in three patients.

Schrag and colleagues[47] examined 103 patients with fixed dystonia, of which 41 patients were prospectively studied. Prior injury was reported in 61% of patients; 56% had spread to other areas, with limb dystonia being most common. Of these patients, 20% had CRPS, and 37% had psychogenic dystonia. Dissociation and affective disorders were more common in the patients with fixed dystonia, possibly indicative of a specific subtype of patients with fixed dystonia and CRPS.[44] Van Hilten et al[48] reported association of CRPS with autonomic dysfunction and multifocal dystonia with HLA DR 13 in 26 patients. Subsequent studies by the same group[49] identified the presence of dystonia in 121 of 185 (91%) patients with CRPS. This subgroup of patients had younger age at onset and were at higher risk of developing dystonia in other extremities. Gieteling and coworkers[50] reported functional magnetic resonance imaging (MRI) findings in 8 patients with CRPS showing decreased activation in the ipsilateral premotor and adjacent prefrontal cortex, and in a cluster comprising the frontal operculum, anterior aspect of insular cortex, and superior temporal gyrus, and a decrease in activity in contralateral inferior parietal and primary sensory cortex during imaginary movement of the affected hand.

This association of dystonic posture with trophic changes and other obvious skin and other local changes highlights the difficulty in determining whether CRPS (previously termed *reflex sympathetic dystrophy*) associated with fixed deformities is mostly due to psychogenic causes, as some investigators have suggested,[44] or whether they represent a post-traumatic dystonia mediated by central disinhibition as a result of peripherally induced central reorganization.[45,48-51] Contralateral cortical silent period is short in patients with fixed dystonia and patients with organic dystonia, indicating a more complex cortical involvement in fixed dystonia.[52] Studies of central inhibition, resting short and long interval intracortical inhibition, and cortical silent period in patients with psychogenic dystonia have shown abnormalities similar to those observed in patients with organic dystonia, suggesting either common pathophysiological mechanisms or lack of specificity of the various neurophysiological tests.[52,53]

PSYCHOGENIC PAROXYSMAL DYSKINESIAS

Paroxysmal dyskinesias are often difficult to diagnose because of the intermittent, episodic nature of these disorders that may not be witnessed by the examiner. The clinician often has to rely on descriptions by relatives or friends, although rarely the episodes are documented by videos. We find the use of a tuning fork accompanied by a verbal suggestion that the vibration "often" induces abnormal movements to be a very effective and powerful way to trigger the dyskinesia in the clinic; this is particularly useful when captured on a video. There is usually no family history, and the nature of illness does not fit into any of the classic categories of paroxysmal kinesigenic or nonkinesigenic types of dyskinesias. Psychogenic paroxysmal dyskinesia is common, accounting for 21 of 76 (28%) patients in one series of patients with paroxysmal nonkinesigenic dystonia.[54]

In another series, 11 of 46 (24%) patients with paroxysmal dyskinesia were diagnosed with psychogenic paroxysmal dystonia.[51] Five patients had additional complex paroxysms of vocalizations, chest pounding, and running, and five patients had nonphysiological findings of fluctuation, give-way weakness, hemisensory loss, and bizarre gait. Benefit was noted with placebo, psychotherapy, and faith healing. Clinical clues to the diagnosis of paroxysmal dystonia were tonic-clonic movements, stiffening with violent tremor, arching of trunk or legs, tongue protrusion, oscillatory movement of trunk or limbs, lurching, running, posturing, and jaw deviations.[55]

Psychogenic paroxysmal dystonia can be superimposed on preexisting organic movement disorder.[7] In one series, the patients had spasmodic torticollis, writer's cramp, cranial dystonia, and essential tremor, but maximal disability was reported with a recent paroxysmal dystonia. The movements consisted of head, shoulder, and arm rocking; head shaking from side to side; and generalized or whole-body tremors. In addition, the patients had abnormal gait and hemisensory loss.[7] Psychogenic paroxysmal dyskinesia, similar to other PMD, may coexist with organic disorders, such as multiple sclerosis.[56]

PSYCHOGENIC SPASMODIC DYSPHONIA

Spasmodic psychogenic dysphonia sometimes can be difficult to distinguish from dystonic dysphonia. In psychogenic dysphonia, the patient may reveal a history of stress-related problems or evidence that stress was a precipitating factor. In contrast to typical organic spasmodic dysphonia, which is usually of the "adductor" type and manifested by strained voice interrupted by voiceless pauses, psychogenic dysphonia is often the "abductor" type, characterized by a whispering, breathy voice.

In one study, phonoscopic evaluation of the vocal cords of patients with psychogenic dysphonia showed no tremor, and hyperabduction was uniform across the tasks, there was no phonetic variability, and there was worsening at the end of the breath.[57] False fold constriction was constant across tasks (counting; production of certain voiced and voiceless utterances; counting; and utterances and sustained vowel sounds at low and high comfortable frequencies, and at soft, comfortable, and loud intensities), and relaxation was noted at high fundamental frequencies in patients with psychogenic dysphonia, whereas patients with organic spasmodic dysphonia had episodic false fold contraction across all tasks. Sphincteric constriction was consistent, and there were rare voice arrests in patients with psychogenic dysphonia. Hyperabduction was inappropriate during inspiration or expiration.[57] These findings may help in distinguishing psychogenic from organic spasmodic dysphonia.

In a study of 74 patients using the Giessen test and picture frustration test, patients with nonorganic voice disorders showed significant differences in conflict situations compared with patients with organic dysphonia, showing the psychosocial basis of the disease in this experimental paradigm.[58] In a more recent study using a structured clinical interview in patients with spasmodic dysphonia and patients with vocal fold paralysis, psychiatric comorbidity was twice as high in patients with spasmodic dysphonia, suggesting a correlation between somatic complaints and psychopathology in spasmodic dysphonia.[59]

PSYCHOGENIC MYOCLONUS

Myoclonus is defined as a sudden, shocklike brief involuntary movement caused by muscle contraction (positive myoclonus) or inhibitions (negative myoclonus). Depending on its origin, myoclonus may be generalized, segmental, focal, or multifocal. Psychogenic myoclonus is characterized by incongruous movements with a lack of consistency, continuously changing pattern with respect to amplitude, frequency, and anatomical distribution. In a study by Monday and Jankovic,[57] of 212 patients with myoclonus, 18 (8.5%) were psychogenic. There were 13 women and 5 men, and the age range was 22 to 75 years (mean age 49.5). Eleven patients had sudden or acute onset, and seven had gradual onset. Ten patients had segmental myoclonus, seven had generalized myoclonus, and one had focal myoclonus. Involved areas were limbs, head, and paraspinal regions, and one patient had scrotal and perianal involvement. Psychogenic myoclonus is characterized by inconsistent character of the movements (amplitude, frequency, and distribution), and other features incongruous with typical organic myoclonus; marked reduction of myoclonus with distraction; exacerbation and relief with placebo and suggestion; spontaneous periods of remission; acute onset and sudden resolution; and evidence of underlying psychopathology.[60]

EMG studies in patients with stimulus-sensitive jerks and jumps mimicking myoclonus or pathological startle syndromes showed that patients with stimulus-sensitive jerks had long latency and variability to onset of jerking after stimulation from trial to trial. The stimulus-induced responses also tended to habituate with repeated presentation of stimuli as in the normal startle response.[61] Jerks secondary to bursts of EMG activity with a mean duration of less than 70 ms are likely to be organic, particularly when there is cocontraction of agonist and antagonist muscle pairs. Jerks with longer EMG bursts, especially if there is a well organized triphasic pattern of activation of agonist and antagonist muscles, are likely to be psychogenic.

Using electroencephalography with back-averaging epochs preceding the EMG accompanying spontaneous jerks shows premovement or Bereitschaftspotential before any self-initiated voluntary movement.[61,62] This is a slow positive potential occurring about 1 second before the movement and maximal over the vertex. Similar potentials are found before psychogenic jerks. In contrast, preceding organic myoclonus, there is usually a brief cortical spike discharge or a sharp wave preceding the cortical myoclonus by an interval of 20 to 40 ms depending on whether the muscle under investigation is in the upper or lower limb. The technique of back-averaging has its limitations, including time constraints and difficulties capturing the epochs when the movement is infrequent.[61-63]

PSYCHOGENIC HEMIFACIAL SPASM

In the report by Tan and Jankovic,[64] the frequency of hemifacial spasm was 2.4% (5 patients out of 210). Patients exhibited at least four of the following features: acute onset of unilateral facial contractions; inconsistent features such as changes in side and pattern during examination; associated somatizations; reduction or abolishment of facial spasm with distraction; response to placebo, psychotherapy, or suggestion; lack of hemifacial spasm during sleep; spontaneous remissions; and normal brain MRI and MR angiography. Absence of worsening of spasms during voluntary facial muscle movement, lower face involvement at onset, bilateral facial spasms, and synchronous contractions may offer additional clues to the diagnosis.[64]

PSYCHOGENIC PARKINSONISM

The term *parkinsonism* includes tremor, rigidity, akinesia, and postural instability, with at least two features being present. Psychogenic parkinsonism is rare and is seen in a small percentage of patients with PMD. In our study of 228 patients with PMD, parkinsonism was the dominant feature in 6 (2.6%).[5] In another series of 14 patients with psychogenic parkinsonism, 10 had abrupt onset, 6 had unilateral limb symptoms, and 4 had bilateral asymmetrical limb symptoms with the dominant right side being more affected.[65]

Patients with psychogenic parkinsonism usually have rest and action tremor, often characterized by marked variation in frequency. Rigidity is uncommon, but a voluntary resistance is usually appreciated by the examiner, and some patients exhibit "waxy flexibility" as seen in catatonia. While performing synkinetic movements with opposite limbs, resistance to passive movements diminishes, in contrast to the cogwheeling seen in patients with Parkinson's disease. Patients with psychogenic parkinsonism typically have slowness of voluntary movement in the absence of classic decrementing amplitude on performance of repetitive or alternate movements.

Patients commonly exhibit an inordinate amount of difficulty in performing manual tasks, accompanied by sighing, seeming exhaustion, or whole-body movement in a forceful attempt to complete the movement. Slowness of movement varies with distraction. Patients may show inconsistent abilities while performing certain tasks when the rest of movements are slow. Patients often have stiff gait, with unusual positioning of the affected arm that may or may not persist while running. On postural stability testing, patients show an extreme response to even minor pull, sometimes flinging their arms and retropulsing and reeling backward without falling. The response to pull test may be inconsistent, for example, flinging both arms equally and symmetrically, whereas one arm is bradykinetic on the remainder of the examination.

Generally, patients have an abrupt onset, and a static course with early maximal disability; dominant side being most affected; and rest, postural, and action tremor, which reduces with distraction and concentration, and increases with attention. No true fatiguing is noted, but marked slowness, atypical positioning of the arm, extreme or bizarre response to posterior displacement, and other neurological and psychological features are usually seen.[65] Many of our patients with psychogenic parkinsonism respond just as well to carbidopa alone as to carbidopa/levodopa combination. The subsequent discussion, which includes disclosure of the use of carbidopa and our interpretation of the improvement as a "placebo response," focuses on gaining insights into the psychodynamic reasons for the symptoms and the response.[66]

PSYCHOGENIC GAIT DISORDERS

The spectrum of phenomenology associated with psychogenic gait disorders is broad, and there were several attempts in the past to classify these. Blocq introduced the term *astasia-abasia,* which means inability to stand and walk, and he included paralysis, jumping, fits, tremor, and bizarre behavior as part of this syndrome.[67] Paradoxical ability to use the legs normally except when standing (astasia) or walking (abasia) was described in 1860 by Jaccoud as *ataxia.* Other terms include *akinesia algera* (paralysis resulting from excruciating pain precipitated by the slightest movement), *stasobasophobia* (fear of walking), *saltatory reflex spasm* (patients with normal strength and control of the legs in bed who begin to jump, hop, run, and dance as soon as their feet touch the floor), and *aposexie* (robotic gait accompanied by birdlike head movements). Roussy and Lhermitte classified hysterical gait into "astasia-abasia," "pseudotabetic," "pseudopolyneuritic," "tightrope walker," "robot," "habit limping," "choreic," "knock-kneed," "as on a sticky surface," and "as through water."[3] Despite all these previous descriptions, it is difficult to categorize psychogenic gait strictly into one pattern or the other.

In a study of 60 patients with hysterical gait disorders, hemiparesis was the most common paralytic gait variant, and the patients showed foot movement varying from dragging to hopping with the hemiparetic leg, while the arm was functioning normally during walking or was held in rigid flexion or extension. In this study, ataxic gaits were common, and patients showed moderately exaggerated swaying without falling, staggering long distances to obtain support from opposite walls, classic tightrope balancing, and an aggressive variant where the person assisting was forcefully grabbed and every effort was made to drag him or her to the floor. Ataxic gaits can sometimes blend into trembling, but tremblers usually have tremor in other locations. Sometimes patients show dystonic and truncal myoclonus.[68]

Lempert and colleagues,[69] in their video survey of 37 patients with psychogenic disorders of stance and gait, attempted to classify gait into slow gait, astasia, pseudoataxia, and buckling. Characteristic features noted on gait examination were fluctuation of impairment, excessive slowness of movements, hesitation, "psychogenic Romberg test," "walking on ice" gait pattern, uneconomic postures with waste of muscle energy such as camptocormia, sudden buckling with and without falls, astasia, and vertical shaking or bouncing tremor.

"Psychogenic Romberg test" was a specific response noted in these patients while performing the Romberg test; this included a response with constant falls toward or away from the observer regardless of his or her position or clutching the physician to avoid a fall. There was large-amplitude body sway, building up after silent latency of a few seconds, and an improvement of postural stability when distracted. "Walking on ice" consists of cautious, usually broad-based steps with decreased stride length and height, stiffening of knees and ankles, some degree of antagonist innervation, and shuffling of feet. Other features suggestive of psychogenic gait include sudden side steps; flailing of the arms; dragging of the leg; continuous flexion of the knees; extension of toes; bizarre tremors; and expressive behavior with grasping of the leg, mannered postures of the hands, suffering or strained facial expression, moaning, and hyperventilation during walking.[64-66]

Gait abnormalities may show improvement after distraction or with suggestion.[68-70] Baik and Lang[71] identified two patterns of gait dysfunction in a study of gait abnormalities in PMD. Slowness of gait was common in patients with PMD plus gait disorder, whereas buckling of knees and astasia-abasia were more common in patients with pure psychogenic gait disorder. Occasionally, patients treated for various psychiatric disorders with neuroleptics develop peculiar, "ducklike" or other bizarre gaits, sometimes wrongly attributed to their underlying psychiatric disorder, but the possibility of one should also considered.[72]

Investigations in Psychogenic Movement Disorders

Diagnosis of PMD has been largely based on clinical examination; electrophysiological testing may be useful for conditions such as tremor and myoclonus. Growing interest in single photon emission computed tomography (SPECT) and functional MRI may improve understanding of these disorders. Benaderette and coworkers[73] studied patients with psychogenic parkinsonism using ioflupane 123I-ioflupane (FP-2-β-carbomethoxy-3-β (4-iodophenyl)-tropane [CIT]) SPECT, and found that patients with Parkinson's disease had decreased uptake showing dopaminergic denervation, which was not seen in patients with psychogenic parkinsonism. Gaig and associates[74] investigated nine patients with suspected psychogenic parkinsonism; one patient had decreased striatal uptake of ^{123}I-FP, but the uptake was normal in the rest of the patients. Based on this testing, an underlying neurodegenerative process can be identified even in patients with a diagnosis of psychogenic disorder. Reversible hypoactivity owing to decline in regional cerebral blood flow in the contralateral thalamus and basal ganglia after recovery is seen in hysterical sensory loss based on technetium 99mTc-ethylcysteinate dimer (99mTc-ECD) SPECT.[75] Hysterical conversion disorders may involve functional disorders in striatothalamocortical circuits controlling sensorimotor function and voluntary motor behavior.

Functional imaging has been used as an investigative tool in various neurological disorders. A study by Stone and colleagues[76] showed activation of putamen, lingual gyri, left inferior frontal gyrus, left insula, and deactivation in right middle frontal and orbitofrontal cortices in patients with unilateral ankle weakness owing to conversion disorder, but patients with simulated unilateral weakness had activation of the contralateral supplementary motor area. In patients with unilateral psychogenic sensory loss, there was normal activation of somatosensory areas.[77]

Mailis-Gagnon and associates[78] used functional MRI studies of brush-evoked and noxious stimulation–evoked brain responses in four patients with chronic pain, and nondermatomal somatosensory deficits revealed altered somatosensory-evoked responses in specific forebrain areas. Unperceived stimuli failed to activate areas such as thalamus, posterior region of the anterior cingulate cortex, and Brodmann area 44/45 that were activated with perceived touch and pain. Unperceived stimuli were associated with deactivations in primary and secondary somatosensory cortex (S1, S2), posterior parietal cortex, and prefrontal cortex. Finally, unperceived (but not perceived) stimuli activated the rostral anterior cingulate cortex. Diminished perception of innocuous and noxious stimuli is associated with altered activity in many parts of the somatosensory pathway or other supraspinal areas.

Treatment of Psychogenic Movement Disorders

Longitudinal data are needed to identify predictors of favorable outcomes so that they can be considered in planning a therapeutic strategy. Such a treatment plan must be individualized and tailored to the patient's specific diagnosis, degree of disability, prior treatments, and associated psychological comorbidities. In our study on long-term prognosis of PMD, 69 (56.6%) of 122 patients who completed the survey reported improvement, 27 (22.1%) reported worsening, and 26 (21.3%) reported no change in clinical status.[5] Based on logistic regression analysis, poor prognostic indicators are presence of inconsistent movements, dissatisfaction with physician, positive history of smoking, and long duration of illness. Favorable prognosis was associated with patient's perception of receiving effective treatment by physician, attribution of improvement to a specific medication, good physical health, positive social life perception, higher score on McMaster Health Index, elimination of stressor, and comorbid anxiety disorder.[5]

Factor and colleagues[6] reported resolution of symptoms in 35% of their patients over a 6-year period. Williams and associates[8] reported a permanent meaningful benefit in 52% of patients, with complete, considerable, and moderate relief in 25%, 21%, and 8%. Among patients who were previously employed, 25% were able to resume full-time work, 10% resumed part-time work, and 15% were functioning at home. Williams and associates[8] used psychotherapy in all patients, along with supplemental approaches including family sessions (58%), hypnosis (42%), and placebo therapy (13%). Antidepressants were used in 71% of their patients, and 8% underwent electroconvulsive therapy. One fourth of their patients needed extended psychiatric hospitalization because of poor response or suicidality.[8] Routine use of placebo therapy for PMD is usually ineffective and should be discouraged.[79-81] Placebo has a role in diagnosis, but if the patient discovers that a placebo was used without a full disclosure, it would lead to mistrust toward the physician.

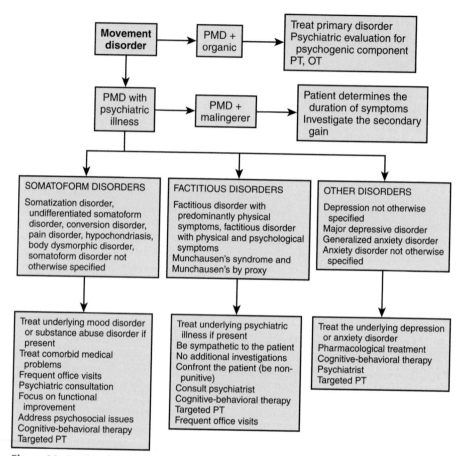

Figure 33–1   Flowchart for management of psychogenic movement disorders. OT, occupational therapy; PMD, psychogenic movement disorder; PT, physical therapy.

Only a few other studies have addressed the natural history and predictors of outcome in patients with PMD. In a 3.2-year study of outcome in 88 patients with PMD, the abnormal movements persisted during the follow-up in 90% with 52.5% of "survivors" interviewed.[16] Of these, 95% had active or remote primary psychiatric illness (major depression or anxiety or both); nearly half had personality disorders. The PMD remitted in only 10%, but half of these patients had new psychogenic symptoms. Patients with PMD did not acknowledge the psychiatric origin of their PMD.

Treatment of PMD is challenging even after establishing the diagnosis and often requires patience and a multidisciplinary approach to management (Fig. 33–1).[3,66] For therapeutic purposes, patients may be categorized into patients with preexisting organic illness with superimposed PMD, patients with underlying psychiatric disorders in addition to PMD, and malingerers presenting with a PMD. In patients with a primary organic movement disorder and coexisting PMD, the therapeutic intervention aimed at the primary organic illness along with supportive therapy for the underlying psychological factors would be beneficial to the patient.

PMD patients have been shown to be equally disabled compared with patients with Parkinson's disease, and they have higher scores on the depression and somatization subscales.[79] It is important to be aggressive in management of PMD to improve outcomes. Management starts with the initial encounter of the patient, who must believe that his or her symptoms are taken seriously by the physician and the management team. Unless requested otherwise, we usually prefer that the diagnosis is discussed in the presence of the patient's partner or caregiver because this individual is usually involved in the prescribed treatment and needs to understand the reasons for the diagnosis.

We use the terms *stress-induced* and *psychogenic* interchangeably. We emphasize that stress, whether specifically identified and recognized by the patient or not, can often cause various well-established symptoms, such as irritable colon, high blood pressure, and tremor, and it can cause other movement disorders. The word *psychosomatic* conveys a meaning that the symptoms are made up or imaginary, and this perception among patients negatively affects their outcome.[80] Sympathetic communication is vital to explore the psychodynamic issues adequately and fully, and to understand the underlying psychopathology. A collaborative team approach by the patient, family members, caregivers, neurologists, psychiatrists, psychologists, and primary care physicians is essential for improving patient outcomes.

In patients with PMD and psychiatric problems, the underlying psychiatric issue needs to be addressed. Common psychiatric diagnoses as discussed earlier include depression, anxiety, somatoform disorders, and factitious disorders. Voon and Lang[78] showed that treatment with antidepressants may be helpful in patients with chronic PMD with mixed etiology of somatization disorder, or conversion disorders in association with anxiety and depression. If PMD is better accounted for by underlying depression or anxiety disorder, pharmacological therapy and psychiatric consultation would be appropriate.

The approach to patients with underlying mood disorders includes cognitive-behavioral therapy (CBT) and pharmacological therapy. Pharmacological therapy for underlying anxiety and depression includes medications such as selective serotonin reuptake inhibitors and tricyclic antidepressants. Benzodiazepines such as alprazolam and clonazepam are useful for panic attacks. Therapy with antidepressants is indicated in the presence of moderate to severe major depression.[78] Patients must be informed that a resolution of the depressive symptoms with any individual agent may take about 4 months. Because of the numerous antidepressants available, it is important to follow certain guidelines. Antidepressant therapy should be continued for at least 6 months at a therapeutic dosage to decrease the chances of a recurrence. Anxiety disorders usually coexist with depression and respond to an anxiolytic combined with an antidepressant.[81-83]

After confirming the diagnosis of PMD, the physician must develop a planned treatment protocol.[66] If there is an underlying organic illness, treatment of the primary disorder in addition to supportive psychotherapy would help. If there are underlying psychiatric conditions such as depression or anxiety disorder or substance abuse or dependence, appropriate treatments must be initiated with the help of a psychiatrist. When a pure somatization disorder is diagnosed, the most important task of the physician is to understand the suffering of the patient and to develop a concerned attitude. Mistrust is common in patients with history of abuse. It is important to enlist the trust of the patient by being sympathetic.

Brief but regularly scheduled office visits every 3 to 4 weeks go a long way in avoiding unnecessary hospital visits and phone calls. During each visit, the physician must re-explore the psychosocial problems and help the patient understand the stressful situations responsible for precipitation of physical symptoms. Useful interventions include antidepressant medications, stress management, CBT, lifestyle changes, and harmless medical treatments (e.g., vitamins, heating pads). Conducting expensive and unnecessary investigations should be avoided. Patients with associated depression respond well to treatments. The physician needs to understand that a reasonable end point in treatment of the patient is to help the patient cope with the physical symptoms because the symptoms are unlikely to resolve, and it is important to stop unnecessary emergency department visits. Particular attention needs to paid to the fact that hypochondriacal patients, who may not agree or comply with psychiatric treatment.[84,85]

Treatment of factitious disorders including Munchausen's syndrome has not received enough attention, and there have been no published studies. Ethical and legal issues make the management of this disorder even more complicated.[4,81,82] The first goal of treatment in these cases should be reduction of expensive investigations or procedures. A definite therapeutic approach should be developed. Confrontation of the patient must be nonpunitive and nonadversarial. A sympathetic approach leads to a trusting patient-physician relationship. Involvement of a psychiatrist, psychotherapist, and other support staff is very helpful in management. It is important to schedule frequent visits even if the patient is seeing a psychiatrist because new episodes of illness or suicidal ideation may occur during therapy. Any comorbid psychiatric diagnoses must be evaluated and treated aggressively.[81-85] Factitious disorders have a better outlook than Munchausen's syndrome, although patients continue to deny their role in creation of symptoms and refuse to see or continue to see a psychiatrist. Malingerers generally have a secondary gain, such as worker's compensation, litigation, or sympathy from a spouse. Symptom resolution usually depends on the patient's insight and will to change.

Hinson and colleagues[86] conducted a single-blind study using psychotherapy in 10 patients using the Psychogenic Movement Disorders Rating Scale (PMDRS)[87] as one of the outcome measures. The PMDRS rates 10 different movement disorders categories in 14 body regions and two functions (gait and speech) with high inter-rater reliability and sensitivity to changes in response to treatment and validity compared with the Clinical Global Impression Scale (80A). In addition to the PMDRS, the investigators used the Hamilton Depression and Beck Anxiety scales, Minnesota Multiphasic Personality Inventory, and Global Assessment of Function, and showed significant benefits of psychotherapeutic intervention. Another study involving 91 patients with psychogenic neurological disorders showed that tailored psychotherapy is cost-effective and may achieve excellent success based on a quality-of-life questionnaire survey and patient outcomes research.[88] In addition to psychotherapy, inclusion of exercise and pharmacological therapy as a planned treatment approach seems to benefit patients with functional somatic syndromes, but abnormal illness behavior needs expert psychiatric input and treatment.[89]

Supportive therapies useful in PMD include CBT, biofeedback, and targeted physical therapy that can be tailored to the individual patient and his or her needs.

CBT also has been found to help patients develop insight into the beliefs and assumptions about their symptoms, and to modify factors that are responsible for behavior that facilitates secondary gain. Cognitive strategies include biofeedback, relaxation therapy, strategic family therapy, and relapse prevention, among other strategies, which can be individually tailored. In a large study of 48 patients with hypochondriasis, there was notable improvement with CBT.[90]

CBT was shown to be efficacious in a meta-analysis of various studies on CBT for somatization syndromes; 71% showed a definite or possible treatment effect.[86] Benefits of CBT on improvement of functional status were not as impressive with definite benefit in 46% studies and 26% studies showing possible benefit among 17 studies with functional benefit as their end point. Biofeedback is helpful in treatment of various PMD. A more recent PET study in eight healthy male volunteers showed changes in the anterior cingulate and cerebellar vermis during biofeedback relaxation, whereas relaxation alone was associated with increased activity in left anterior cingulate and globus pallidus, showing the involvement of cingulate cortex in biofeedback relaxation.[91] Allen and associates[92] also showed definitive improvement of physical symptoms after using CBT, particularly in somatization disorders.

Individualized therapy using psychotherapy, hypnosis, pharmacotherapy, and physical therapy is helpful in improving outcome of these patients.[90] Physical therapy targeted toward relaxing the agonist muscles may help prevent contractures in some patients with psychogenic dystonia. More recently, we have initiated a controlled trial of transcutaneous electrical nerve stimulation in patients with PMD at Baylor College of Medicine. The rationale for this study is based on the findings of studies evaluating the effectiveness of transcutaneous electrical nerve stimulation in dystonia showing sustained benefit possibly associated with a remodulating process of motor cortex.[94,95] Also, it is essential to prevent patients with psychogenic dystonia or tremor from undergoing procedures such as deep brain stimulation because the results of such therapy may not be favorable.[96] Overall, a combined multidisciplinary approach to PMD seems to yield the best therapeutic results. Further prospective studies are needed to evaluate the therapeutic options in these patients.

REFERENCES

1. Lewis A: "Psychogenic": a word and its mutations. Psychol Med 1972;2:209-215.
2. Marsden CD: Hysteria—a neurologist's view. Psychol Med 1986;16:277-288.
3. Thomas M, Jankovic J: Psychogenic movement disorders: diagnosis and management. CNS Drugs 2004;18:437-452.
4. Turner J, Reid S: Munchausen's syndrome. Lancet 2002;359:346-349.
5. Thomas M, Dat Vuong K, Jankovic J: Long-term prognosis of patients with psychogenic movement disorders. Parkinsonism Related Disord 2006;12:382-387.
6. Factor SA, Podskalny GD, Molho ES: Psychogenic movement disorders: frequency, clinical profile and characteristics. J Neurol Neurosurg Psychiatry 1995;59:409-412.
7. Ranawaya R, Riley D, Lang AE: Psychogenic dyskinesias in patients with organic movement disorders. Mov Disord 1990;5:127-133.
8. Williams DT, Ford B, Fahn S: Phenomenology and psychopathology related to psychogenic movement disorders. Adv Neurol 1995;65:231-257.
9. Ferrara J, Jankovic J: Psychogenic movement disorders in children. Mov Disord 2008;23:1875-1881.
10. Schwingenschuh P, Pont-Sunyer C, Surtees R: Psychogenic Movement Disorders in Children. A report of 15 cases and a Review of Literature. Mov Disord 2008;23:1882-1888.

11. Marjama J, Troster AI, Koller WC: Psychogenic movement disorders. Neurol Clin 1995;13:283-297.
12. Fahn S, Williams DT: Psychogenic dystonia. Adv Neurol 1988;50:431-455.
13. Hinson VK, Haren WB: Psychogenic movement disorders. Lancet Neurol 2006;5:695-700.
14. Shill H, Gerber P: Evaluation of clinical diagnostic criteria for psychogenic movement disorders. Mov Disord 2006;21:1163-1168.
15. Gupta A, Lang AE: Psychogenic Movement Disorders. Curr Opin Neurol 2009;22:430-436.
16. Feinstein A, Stergiopoulos V, Lang AE: Psychiatric outcome in patients with a psychogenic movement disorder: a prospective study. Neuropsychiatry Neuropsychol Behav Neurol 2001;14:169-176.
17. Vuilleumier P, Chicherio C, Assal F, et al: Functional neuroanatomical correlates of hysterical sensorimotor loss. Brain 2001;124:1077-1090.
18. Zeigler FJ, Imboden JB, Meyer E: Contemporary conversion reactions: a clinical study. Am J Psychiatry 1960;116:901-910.
19. Ron M: Explaining the unexplained: understanding hysteria. Brain 2001;124:1065-1066.
20. Schrag A, Lang AE: Psychogenic movement disorders. Curr Opin Neurol 2005;18:399-404.
21. Servan-Schreiber D, Kolb R, Tabas G: Mental health: the somatizing patient. Prim Care 1999;26:226-242.
22. Dimsdale JE, Dantzer R: A biological substrate for somatoform disorders: importance of pathophysiology. Psychosom Med 2007;69:850-854.
23. Stone J, Smyth R, Carson A, et al: La belle indifference in conversion symptoms and hysteria: systematic review. Br J Psychiatry 2006;188:204-209.
24. Cloninger CR: The origins of DSM and ICD criteria for conversion and somatization disorders. In Halligan PW, Bass C, Marshall JC (eds): Contemporary Approaches to the Study of Hysteria. Oxford: Oxford University Press, 2001, pp 49-62.
25. Wise MG, Ford CV: Factitious disorders. Prim Care 1999;26:315-326.
26. Schrag A, Brown RJ, Trimble MR: Reliability of self-reported diagnoses in patients with neurologically unexplained symptoms. J Neurol Neurosurg Psychiatry 2004;75:608-611.
27. Stone J, Zeman A, Sharpe M: Functional weakness and sensory disturbance. J Neurol Neurosurg Psychiatry 2002;73:241-245.
28. Carson AJ, Ringbauer B, Stone J, et al: Do medically unexplained symptoms matter? A study of 300 new referrals to neurology outpatient clinics. J Neurol Neurosurg Psychiatry 2000;68:207-210.
29. Mejia NI, Jankovic J: Convergence spasm and other psychogenic eye movement disorders. Neurology 2005(Suppl 1):A76.
30. Monteiro ML, Curi AL, Pereira A, et al: Persistent accommodative spasm after severe head trauma. Br J Ophthalmol 2003;87:243-244.
31. Gronlund MA, Aring E, Landgren M, Hellstrom A: Visual function and ocular features in children and adolescents with attention deficit hyperactivity disorder, with and without treatment with stimulants. Eye 2007;21:494-502.
32. Koller WC, Lang AE, Vetere-Overfield B, et al: Psychogenic tremors. Neurology 1989;39:1094-1099.
33. Deuschl G, Koster B, Lucking C, Scheidt C: Diagnostic and pathophysiological aspects of psychogenic tremors. Mov Disord 1998;13:294-302.
34. Jankovic J, Vuong KD, Thomas M: Psychogenic tremor: Long-term outcome. CNS Spectr 2006;11:501-508.
35. Jankovic J, Thomas M: Psychogenic tremor and shaking. In Hallett M, Fahn S, Jankovic J, eds: Psychogenic Movement Disorders: Neurology and Neuropsychiatry. Philadelphia: Lippincott Williams & Wilkins, 2006, pp 42-47.
36. Kim YJ, Anthony S, Pakiam I, Lang AE: Historical and clinical features of psychogenic tremor: a review of 70 cases. Can J Neurol Sci 1999;26:190-195.
37. Kenney C, Diamond A, Mejia N, et al: Distinguishing psychogenic and essential tremor. J Neurol Sci 2007;263:94-99.
38. O'Sulleabhain PE, Matsumoto J: Time-frequency analysis of tremors. Brain 1998;121:2127-2134.
39. Kumru H, Begeman M, Tolosa E, Valls-Sole J: Dual task interference in psychogenic tremor. Mov Disord 2007;22:2077-2082.
40. Bhatia KP, Schneider SA: Psychogenic tremor and related disorders. J Neurol 2007;254:569-574.
41. McKeon A, Ahlskog JE, Bower J, et al: Psychogenic tremor: Long term prognosis in patients with Electrophysiologically confirmed disease. Mov Disord 2009;24:72-76.
42. Lang AE: Psychogenic dystonia: a review of 18 cases. Can J Neurol Sci 1995;22:136-143.

43. Thomas M, Vuong KD, Jankovic J: Psychogenic dystonia: clinical characteristics and long-term progression. Mov Disord 2004;19(Suppl 9): S111.
44. Blakeley J, Jankovic J: Secondary causes of paroxysmal dyskinesia. Adv Neurol 2002;89:401-420.
45. Jankovic J: Can peripheral trauma induce dystonia and other movement disorders? Yes! Mov Disord 2001;16:7-12.
46. Bhatia KP, Bhatt MH, Marsden CD: The causalgia-dystonia syndrome. Brain 1993;116:843-851.
47. Schrag A, Trimble M, Quinn N, Bhatia K: The syndrome of fixed dystonia: an evaluation of 103 patients. Brain 2004;127:2360-2372.
48. van Hilten JJ, van de Beek WJ, Roep BO: Multifocal or generalized tonic dystonia of complex regional pain syndrome: a distinct clinical entity associated with HLA-DR13. Ann Neurol 2000;48:113-116.
49. van Rijn MA, Marinus J, Putter H, van Hilten JJ: Onset and progression of dystonia in complex regional pain syndrome. Pain 2007;130:287-293.
50. Gieteling EW, van Rijn MA, de Jong BM, et al: Cerebral activation during motor imagery in complex regional pain syndrome type 1 with dystonia. Pain 2008;134:302-309.
51. Navarro X, Vivó M, Valero-Cabré A: Neural plasticity after peripheral nerve injury and regeneration. Prog Neurobiol 2007;82:163-201.
52. Avanzino L, Martino D, van de Warrenburg BP, et al: Cortical excitability is abnormal in patients with the "fixed dystonia" syndrome. Mov Disord 2008;23:646-652.
53. Espay AJ, Morgante F, Purzner J, et al: Cortical and spinal abnormalities in psychogenic dystonia. Ann Neurol 2006;59:825-834.
54. Blakeley J, Jankovic J: Secondary paroxysmal dyskinesias. Mov Disord 2002;17:726-734.
55. Bressman SB, Fahn S, Burke RE: Paroxysmal non-kinesigenic dystonia. Adv Neurol 1988;50:403-413.
56. Morgan JC, Hughes M, Figueroa RE, Sethi KD: Psychogenic paroxysmal dyskinesia following paroxysmal hemidystonia in multiple sclerosis. Neurology 2005;65. E12.
57. Leonard R, Kendall K: Differentiation of spasmodic and psychogenic dysphonias with phonoscopic evaluation. Laryngoscope 1999;109:295-300.
58. Seifert E, Kollbrunner J: An update in thinking about nonorganic voice disorders. Arch Otolaryngol Head Neck Surg 2006;132:1128-1132.
59. Gündel H, Busch R, Ceballos-Baumann A, Seifert E: Psychiatric comorbidity in patients with spasmodic dysphonia: a controlled study. J Neurol Neurosurg Psychiatry 2007;78:1398-1400.
60. Monday K, Jankovic J: Psychogenic myoclonus. Neurology 1993;43:349-352.
61. Thompson PD, Colebatch JG, Brown P, et al: Voluntary stimulus-sensitive jerks and jumps mimicking myoclonus or pathological startle syndromes. Mov Disord 1992;7:257-262.
62. Terada K, Ikeda A, Van Ness PC, et al: Presence of Bereitschaftspotential preceding psychogenic myoclonus: clinical application of jerk-locked back averaging. J Neurol Neurosurg Psychiatry 1995;58:745-747.
63. Brown P, Thompson PD: Electrophysiological aids to jerks, spasms and tremor. Mov Disord 2001;16:595-599.
64. Tan EK, Jankovic J: Psychogenic hemifacial spasm. J Neuropsychiatry Clin Neurosci 2001;13:380-384.
65. Lang AE, Koller WC, Fahn S: Psychogenic parkinsonism. Arch Neurol 1995;52:802-810.
66. Jankovic J, Cloninger CR, Fahn S, et al: Therapeutic approaches to psychogenic movement disorders. In Hallett M, Fahn S, Jankovic J, eds: Psychogenic Movement Disorders: Neurology and Neuropsychiatry. Philadelphia: Lippincott Williams & Wilkins, 2006, pp 323-328.
67. Okun MS, Koehler PJ: Paul Blocq and (psychogenic) astasia abasia. Mov Disord 2007;22:1373-1378.
68. Keane JR: Hysterical gait disorders: 60 cases. Neurology 1989;39:586-589.
69. Lempert T, Brandt T, Dietrich M, Huppert D: How to identify psychogenic disorders of stance and gait: a video study in 37 patients. J Neurol 1991;238:140-146.
70. Hayes MW, Graham S, Heldorf P, et al: A video review of the diagnosis of psychogenic gait: appendix and commentary. Mov Disord 1999;14:914-921.
71. Baik JS, Lang AE: Gait abnormalities in psychogenic movement disorders. Mov Disord 2007;22:395-399.
72. Kuo SH, Jankovic J: Tardive gait. Clin Neurol Neurosurg 2008;110:198-201.
73. Benaderette S, Zanotti FP, et al: Psychogenic parkinsonism: a combination of clinical, electrophysiological, and ((123)I)-FP-CIT SPECT scan explorations improves diagnostic accuracy. Mov Disord 2006;21:310-317.

74. Gaig C, Martí MJ, Tolosa E, et al: 123I-Ioflupane SPECT in the diagnosis of suspected psychogenic Parkinsonism. Mov Disord 2006;21:1994-1998.
75. Vuilleumier P, Chicherio C, Assal F, et al: Functional neuroanatomical correlates of hysterical sensorimotor loss. Brain 2001;124:1065-1066.
76. Stone J, Zeman A, Simonotto E, et al: FMRI in patients with motor conversion symptoms and controls with simulated weakness. Psychosom Med 2007;69:961-969.
77. Hoechstetter K, Meinck HM, Henningsen P, et al: Psychogenic sensory loss: magnetic source imaging reveals normal tactile evoked activity of the human primary and secondary somatosensory cortex. Neurosci Lett 2002;323:137-140.
78. Mailis-Gagnon A, Giannoylis I, Downar J, et al: Altered central somatosensory processing in chronic pain patients with "hysterical" anesthesia. Neurology 2003;60:1501-1507.
79. Anderson KE, Gruber-Baldini AL, Vaughan CG, et al: Impact of psychogenic movement disorders versus Parkinson's on disability, quality of life, and psychopathology. Mov Disord 2007;22:2204-2209.
80. Stone J, Colyer M, Feltbower S, et al: "Psychosomatic": a systematic review of its meaning in newspaper articles. Psychosomatics 2004;45:287-290.
81. Voon V, Lang AE: Antidepressant treatment outcomes of psychogenic movement disorder. J Clin Psychiatry 2005;66:1529-1534.
82. Remick RA: Diagnosis and management of depression in primary care: a clinical update and review. Can Med Assoc J 2002;167:1253-1260.
83. Brawman-Mintzer O: Pharmacologic treatment of generalized anxiety disorder. Psychiatr Clin North Am 2001;24:119-137.
84. Barsky AJ: The patient with hypochondriasis. N Engl J Med 2001;345:1395-1399.
85. Wise MG, Ford CV: Factitious disorders. Prim Care 1999;26:315-326.
86. Hinson VK, Weinstein S, Bernard B, et al: Single-blind clinical trial of psychotherapy for treatment of psychogenic movement disorders. Parkinsonism Relat Disord 2006;12:177-180.
87. Hinson VK, Cubo E, Comella CL, et al: Rating scale for psychogenic movement disorders: scale development and clinimetric testing. Mov Disord 2005;20:1592-1597.
88. Reuber M, Burness C, Howlett S, et al: Tailored psychotherapy for patients with functional neurological symptoms: a pilot study. J Psychosom Res 2007;63:625-632.
89. Henningsen P, Zipfel S, Herzog W: Management of functional somatic syndromes. Lancet 2007;369:946-955.
90. Kroenke K, Swindle R: Cognitive behavioral therapy for somatization and symptom syndromes: a critical review of controlled clinical trials. Psychother Psychosom 2000;69:205-215.
91. Critchley HD, Melmed RN, Featherstone E, et al: Brain activity during biofeedback relaxation: a functional neuroimaging investigation. Brain 2001;124:1003-1012.
92. Allen LA, Woolfolk RL, Escobar JI, et al: Cognitive-behavioral therapy for somatization disorder: a randomized controlled trial. Arch Intern Med 2006;166:1512-1518.
93. Williams DT, Ford B, Fahn S: Treatment issues in psychogenic-neuropsychiatric movement disorders. Adv Neurol 2005;96:350-363.
94. Tinazzi M, Farina S, Bhatia K, et al: TENS for the treatment of writer's cramp dystonia: a randomized, placebo-controlled study. Neurology 2005;64:1946-1948.
95. Tinazzi M, Zarattini S, Massimiliano MV, et al: Effects of transcutaneous electrical nerve stimulation on motor cortex excitability in writer's cramp: neurophysiological and clinical correlations. Mov Disord 2006;21:1908-1913.
96. Bramstedt KA, Ford PJ: Protecting human subjects in neurosurgical trials: the challenge of psychogenic dystonia. Contemp Clin Trials 2006;27:161-164.

34 Tics and Gilles de la Tourette Syndrome

HARVEY S. SINGER

Introduction

This chapter provides a practical approach for understanding, evaluating, and treating tic disorders. Historically, these movement abnormalities have a long and storied past. Tic disorders are paroxysmal movement abnormalities that begin in childhood, are frequently associated with various comorbid problems, are capable of causing psychosocial difficulties, and may persist into adulthood. The specific etiologies and neuroanatomical localizations remain under investigation. Behavioral and pharmacological symptomatic treatments are available.

Historical Aspects

Several notable historical figures have been reported to have Gilles de la Tourette syndrome (TS), including the Roman Emperor Claudius, the musician Wolfgang Amadeus Mozart, and Dr. Samuel Johnson, the prominent 18th century literary scholar. The disorder itself is named after the French physician Georges Gilles de la Tourette, who in 1885 reported nine patients with chronic disorders characterized by the presence of involuntary motor and phonic tics.[1] In recent years, many diagnostic features have been redefined, coexisting problems have been clarified, prevalence figures have been established, neuroanatomic pathways have been suggested, and epigenetic etiologies have been proposed.

Tic Phenomenology

The diagnosis of a tic disorder is based on historical features and a clinical examination confirming their presence. Formal descriptions of tics include involuntary, sudden, rapid, abrupt, repetitive, nonrhythmic, simple, or complex motor movements or vocalizations (phonic productions). Nevertheless, observation either directly in the office or via homemade video is worth a thousand words. Brief rapid movements that involve only a single muscle or localized group are considered "simple" (eye blink, head jerk, shoulder shrug), whereas complex tics involve either a cluster of simple actions or a more coordinated sequence of movements. Complex motor tics can be nonpurposeful (facial or body contortions), appear purposeful but actually serve no purpose (touching, hitting, smelling, jumping, echopraxia), or have a dystonic character.

Simple phonations include various sounds and noises (grunts, barks, sniffs, and throat clearing), whereas complex vocalizations involve the repetition of words, syllables, or phrases; echolalia (repeating other people's words); palilalia (repeating one's own words); or coprolalia (repeating obscene words). Nontic movements that need to be distinguished include movements that are drug-induced (akathisia, dystonia, chorea, parkinsonism) or associated with common comorbidities, such as obsessive-compulsive disorder (OCD), attention-deficit/hyperactivity disorder (ADHD), and antisocial behaviors.[2]

Tics have several defining characteristics that are useful in confirming their presence. In individuals with a chronic course, a waxing and waning pattern of symptoms is to be expected. Brief exacerbations are often provoked by stress, anxiety, excitement, anger, fatigue, or infections, although the mechanism for prolonged tic exacerbations, whether environmental or biological, remains to be determined. Tic reduction often occurs when the affected individual is concentrating, focused, or emotionally pleased, or during sleep. The absence of tics during sleep is commonly reported by observers or parents; however, polysomnograms of TS subjects show tics in all phases of sleep.[3] About 90% of adults[4] and 37% of children[5] report a premonitory urge/sensation just before a motor or phonic tic, variously described as an impulse, tension, pressure, itch, or feeling. Lastly, attempts to suppress tics voluntarily often trigger an exacerbation of premonitory sensations or a sense of increased internal tension. Both of these conditions resolve when the tic is permitted to occur.

TABLE 34–1	Diagnostic Criteria for Gilles de la Tourette Syndrome

Onset by age 21
Multiple motor tics
At least one vocal tic
Gradual course with addition and subtraction of new and old tics
Duration of >1 yr
Tics not associated with the use of tic-provoking substances (e.g., stimulants)
Not associated with other medical conditions (e.g., Huntington's chorea, post–viral
　encephalitis, toxins, stroke, head trauma, or surgery)
Tics must be observed by a knowledgeable individual

From The Tourette Syndrome Classification Study Group. Definitions and classification of tic disorders. *Arch Neurol.* 1993;50:1013-1016.

Tic Disorders

TS actually represents only one entity in a spectrum of disorders that have tics as their cardinal feature, ranging from a mild transient form to TS.[6] Tic disorders are divided into two major categories based on their duration: transient (present for <12 months) and chronic (present for >12 months). *Tic disorder–diagnosis deferred* is a term used by the author to designate an individual with ongoing fluctuating tics that have been present for less than 1 year. This term is preferred because it is impossible to predict whether an individual's tics will persist for the requisite time interval required for a "chronic" designation. *Transient tic disorder,* the mildest and most common tic disorder, requires that tics resolve before 1 year, typically after several months' duration. *Chronic (motor or phonic) tic disorder* requires that tics be present for more than 1 year, and individuals have either entirely motor or, less commonly, solely vocal tics.

Criteria for *TS*[6] and *Tourette disorder*[7] are similar, but have minor differences. The formal criteria provided by the Tourette Syndrome Classification Study Group are shown in Table 34–1. Adult-onset tic disorders have been reported and are often associated with potential environmental triggers, severe symptoms, greater social morbidity, and a poorer response to medications.[8] *Tourettism, Tourette-like,* and *secondary disorder* are terms used for tic syndromes that do not meet the criteria for TS, such as those associated with another medical condition, including infection,[9,10] drugs,[11,12] toxins,[13] stroke,[14] head trauma,[15,16] and surgery,[17,18] or found in association with various sporadic, genetic, and neurodegenerative disorders.[19,20] *Tardive Tourette* is the term for individuals who develop tics after the use of neuroleptics.[21]

Outcome

Tics have a waxing and waning course, with many individuals having a maximum severity of tics between the ages of 8 and 12 years. Long-term, most studies support a decline in symptoms during the teenage to early adulthood years.[22,23]

I present the "rule of thirds": one third disappear, one third are better, and about one third continue.[24] Although tic resolution is reported by many adults, whether they fully resolve has been questioned, based on review of videotape assessments.[25] Proposed predictors of severity and longevity include tic severity, fine motor control, and volumetric size of caudate and subgenual volumes,[26,27] but all are controversial.[28] The presence of coexisting neuropsychiatric issues has a significant effect on impairment; individuals solely with chronic tics are less impaired than individuals with OCD, ADHD, or mood disorders.[29,30]

Epidemiology

The current prevalence figure (number of cases in a population at a given time) for tics in childhood is about 6% to 12% (range 4% to 24%).[31,32] The precise prevalence of chronic motor and vocal tics (TS) is unknown, with numbers varying widely in published reports. An estimated plausible prevalence of moderately severe cases is 1 to 10/1000 children and adolescents,[31,33,34] with an additional 10 to 30/1000 children and adolescents having mild unidentified "true" cases.[31,33,34] TS occurs worldwide with increasing evidence of common features in all cultures and races. TS is common in children with autism, Asperger's syndrome, and other autistic spectrum disorders, but its presence is unrelated to the severity of autistic symptoms.[35] Tics and related behaviors have not been found to be overrepresented among adult inpatients with psychiatric illnesses.[36]

Associated Problems

Numerous associated problems have been reported in individuals with tic disorders, although in most cases their link to tics remains undetermined.

ATTENTION-DEFICIT/HYPERACTIVITY DISORDER

ADHD is characterized by impulsivity, hyperactivity, and a decreased ability to maintain attention. Symptoms usually precede the onset of tics by 2 to 3 years. A genetic linkage has not been established except in cases in which each begins simultaneously. ADHD is reported to affect about 50% (range 21% to 90%) of referred cases with TS.[37] In patients with tics, the addition of ADHD symptoms correlates with increased psychosocial difficulties, disruptive behavior, functional impairment, and school problems.[30,38,39]

OBSESSIVE-COMPULSIVE BEHAVIORS

Obsessive-compulsive behaviors occur in 20% to 89% of patients with TS.[40] OCD, characterized by recurrent thoughts or repetitive behaviors or both that cause marked distress and interfere with normal functioning, is less common. Obsessive-compulsive behaviors generally emerge several years after the onset of tics, usually during early adolescence. Two subtypes of OCD based on differences in prevalence in age groups and implied etiological relationships have been proposed: a juvenile subtype and one related to tics.[41] Although sometimes differentiating obsessive-compulsive behaviors from tics may be difficult, clues favoring obsessive-compulsive behaviors include a cognitive-based drive and need to perform the action in a particular fashion (i.e., a certain number of times, until it feels "just right," or on both sides of the body).

ANXIETY AND DEPRESSION

An increased incidence of depression and anxiety in patients with TS has been reported in several studies.[30,42,43]

EPISODIC OUTBURSTS (RAGE) AND SELF-INJURIOUS BEHAVIOR

Episodic outbursts (rage) and self-injurious behavior have also been described in patients with TS.[44,45] Whether these behaviors are due to the presence of other disruptive psychopathology, such as obsessions, compulsions, ADHD-related impulsivity, risk-taking, rage, or affective disorders, is unclear.

ACADEMIC DIFFICULTIES

Poor school performance in children with tics can be secondary to several factors, including severe tics, psychosocial problems, ADHD, OCD, learning disabilities, or medications.[46] Individuals with TS typically have normal intellectual functioning, although there may be concurrent executive dysfunction, discrepancies between performance and verbal IQ testing, impairment of visual perceptual achievement, and decrease in visual-motor skills.[29,47-50]

SLEEP DISORDERS

Problems associated with sleep have been reported in about 20% to 50% of children and young adults with TS. Common symptoms include difficulties falling asleep, difficulties staying asleep, and parasomnias.[3,51] Sleep deficits may be associated with the presence of other comorbidities such as ADHD, anxiety, mood disorders, and OCD.[52]

Etiology

Strong support for a genetic disorder is provided by studies of monozygotic twins, which show an 86% concordance rate with chronic tic disorder compared with 20% in dizygotic twins.[53,54] A complex genetic etiology is also supported by a study of at-risk children free of tics at baseline who subsequently developed a tic disorder.[55] Several approaches have been used to identify the genetic site, including genetic linkage, cytogenetics, candidate gene studies, and molecular genetic studies.[56] Linkage analyses have suggested numerous chromosomal locations, but without a clear reproducible locus or convergence of findings.

One analysis performed in 238 affected sib pair families and 18 multigenerational families identified significant evidence for linkage to a marker on chromosome 2p32.2,[57] but studies remain inconsistent. Investigations after identification of a de novo chromosomal inversion at 13q31.1 in a child with TS have led to suggestions of an association with *SLITRK1*.[58] Results have not been confirmed in additional TS populations, however.[59] The possible effects of genomic imprinting, bilineal transmission,[60-62] and gene–environment interactions further complicate the understanding of TS genetics. Potential epigenetic risk factors that have been examined include timing of perinatal care, severity of mother's nausea and vomiting during the pregnancy, low proband birth weight, the Apgar score at 5 minutes, use of thimerosal,[63] and nonspecific maternal emotional stress.[64] Further replication of these latter studies is necessary before any significance can be truly assessed.

Several investigators have proposed that, in a subset of children, tic symptoms are caused by a preceding β-hemolytic streptococcal infection.[65,66] Labeled as pediatric autoimmune neuropsychiatric disorder associated with streptococcal infection (PANDAS), proposed criteria include a prepubertal abrupt onset and exacerbation of tics that occur in temporal association with a streptococcal infection. On the basis of a model proposed for Sydenham's chorea, it has been hypothesized that the underlying pathology in PANDAS involves an immune-mediated mechanism with molecular mimicry.[65] The PANDAS hypothesis remains controversial on clinical criteria grounds and measurement of antineuronal antibodies.[67-71] A longitudinal study in children with PANDAS showed little association between β-hemolytic streptococcal infection and symptom exacerbation,[72] and no correlation between exacerbation of symptoms and changes in antineuronal antibodies, anti-lysoganglioside GM$_1$ antibodies, or cytokines.[71]

Neurobiology

Convincing direct and indirect evidence indicates that corticostriatothalamocortical pathways are involved in the expression of TS and its accompanying neuropsychiatric problems.[73-75] Although there is general consensus of a corticostriatothalamocortical circuit abnormality, the precise pathophysiological location remains speculative. The presence of dopaminergic, glutamatergic, GABAergic, serotoninergic, cholinergic, noradrenergic, and opioid systems within corticostriatothalamocortical circuits raises the possibility that various transmitters may be involved in the pathobiology of TS.

A dopaminergic abnormality continues to receive strong support because of therapeutic response to neuroleptics, results from various nuclear imaging protocols,[76-80] cerebrospinal fluid analyses,[81] and postmortem studies.[82-85] Increased dopamine release, measured by positron emission tomography (PET), has been confirmed in two separate studies,[76,86] and a prefrontal dopaminergic abnormality has been proposed.[83,85] The finding that some individuals also had a combination of diminished serotonin transporter and elevated serotonin 2A receptor binding has suggested a possible serotoninergic modulatory effect.[86] PET of tryptophan metabolism has shown abnormalities in cortical and subcortical regions.[87]

Treatment

Recognizing that individuals not only have tics, but also various comorbid problems, the first step in treatment is a careful evaluation of all potential issues and determination of resulting impairment. In conjunction with the patient, family members, and school personnel, it is essential to determine whether tics or associated problems (e.g., ADHD, OCD, school problems, or behavioral disorders) represent the greatest handicap. Discussing and treating comorbid symptoms as separate entities from tics usually enables families and health care specialists to focus on the patient's needs more effectively. Therapeutically, just because a symptom exists, tics or otherwise, is not in and of itself an adequate reason to initiate pharmacotherapy. Medications should be targeted and reserved for only the problems that are functionally disabling and not remediable by nondrug interventions.

Physicians considering pharmacological treatment to suppress tics should be aware of their natural waxing and waning course and the influence of psychopathologies on outcome. Specific criteria for initiating tic-suppressing medication include the presence of psychosocial or physical difficulties, or both. There is no cure for tics, and all pharmacotherapy is symptomatic. The goal of treatment is not complete suppression of tics, but rather reduction to a level where they no longer cause significant psychosocial or physical disturbances.

NONPHARMACOLOGICAL BEHAVIORAL TREATMENTS

Nonpharmacological behavioral treatments include conditioning techniques, massed negative practice, awareness training, habit reversal, relaxation training, biofeedback, and hypnosis.[88-90] Few of these approaches have been adequately evaluated. Habit reversal training significantly improved tics compared with a supportive therapy group, and the beneficial effect persisted to a 10-month follow-up evaluation.[89,90]

PHARMACOTHERAPY

If medication is selected, a two-tiered approach is recommended: (1) nonneuroleptic (*tier 1*) drugs for milder tics, and (2) typical/atypical neuroleptics (*tier 2*) for more severe tics (Fig. 34–1). Only two medications have U.S. Food and Drug Administration approval: pimozide and haloperidol. The extent of supporting evidence for each medication is reviewed by Scahill and colleagues.[91]

Tier 1

Tier 1 medications include clonidine,[92] guanfacine,[93] baclofen,[94] and clonazepam.[95] Several anticonvulsant medications, such as topiramate[96] and levetiracetam,[97] have been used, although data are either limited or controversial.[91,98]

Tier 2

Tier 2 medications, including classic neuroleptics and D2 dopamine receptor antagonists, are effective tic-suppressing agents, but side effects may limit their usefulness. My order of preference is provided in Figure 34–1. Pimozide or fluphenazine is preferred to haloperidol because the observed frequency of side effects is reduced. Sulpiride and tiapride, substituted benzamides, have been

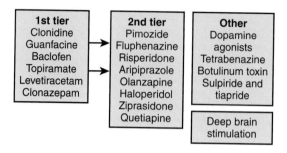

Figure 34–1 Pharmacotherapy for the treatment of tics.

beneficial in Europe, but neither is available in the United States. Newer a typical neuroleptics (risperidone, olanzapine, ziprasidone, and quetiapine) are characterized by a relatively greater affinity for 5-hydroxytryptamine receptors than for D2 receptors and a reduced potential for extrapyramidal side effects.

In this group, risperidone has been studied most extensively. In two randomized double-blind placebo-controlled trials, risperidone in a mean/median daily dose of 2.5 mg/day produced a significant reduction of tics compared with controls.[99,100] Several small studies have confirmed clinical effectiveness of olanzapine,[101,102] ziprasidone,[103,104] quetiapine,[105,106] and aripiprazole[107] Tetrabenazine, a benzoquinolizine derivative that depletes the presynaptic stores of catecholamines and blocks postsynaptic dopamine receptors, may also be effective.[108]

OTHER MEDICATIONS AND APPROACHES

Other medications and approaches include the dopamine agonists pergolide and ropinirole prescribed at lower doses than used in treating Parkinson's disease[109,110]; Δ-9-tetrahydrocannabinol, the major psychoactive ingredient of marijuana[111,112]; and botulinum toxin.[113,114] Preliminary studies using repetitive transcranial magnetic stimulation have been variable, in part based on stimulation site and parameters. Repetitive transcranial magnetic stimulation has been shown to be beneficial when targeting the supplemental motor area,[115] but of little success stimulating motor or premotor regions.[116,117] Deep brain stimulation, a stereotactic treatment proposed for use in other movement disorders, has had preliminary success in treating tics.[118,119] Other neurosurgical approaches, with target sites including the frontal lobe (bimedial frontal leucotomy and prefrontal lobotomy), limbic system (anterior cingulotomy and limbic leucotomy), cerebellum, and thalamus, have been tried in attempts to reduce severe tics.[120]

Conclusions

Although the diagnosis and treatment of tic disorders are often straightforward, many patients present with multiple complex issues. My recommended approach includes the following steps: evaluation and identification of all individual problems, determination of the degree of impairment and need for treatment for each concern, education of the patient and family about tic disorders (e.g., outcome, comorbidities, etiology, pathophysiology, treatment), selection of an appropriate treatment program, and establishment of a comprehensive multidisciplinary treatment approach.

REFERENCES

1. de la Tourette G: Étude sur une affection nerveuse caractérisée par l'incoordination motrice accompagnée d'écholalie et de copralalie. Arch Neurol 1885;19-42:158-200.
2. Kompoliti K, Goetz CG: Hyperkinetic movement disorders misdiagnosed as tics in Gilles de la Tourette syndrome. Mov Disord 1998;13:477-480.
3. Cohrs S, Rasch T, Altmeyer S, et al: Decreased sleep quality and increased sleep related movements in patients with Tourette's syndrome. J Neurol Neurosurg Psychiatry 2001;70:192-197.
4. Kwak C, Dat Vuong K, Jankovic J: Premonitory sensory phenomenon in Tourette's syndrome. Mov Disord 2003;18:1530-1533.
5. Banaschewski T, Woerner W, Rothenberger A: Premonitory sensory phenomena and suppressibility of tics in Tourette syndrome: developmental aspects in children and adolescents. Dev Med Child Neurol 2003;45:700-703.
6. The Tourette Syndrome Classification Study Group: Definitions and classification of tic disorders. Arch Neurol 1993;50:1013-1016.
7. American Psychiatric Association: *Diagnostic and Statistical Manual of Mental Disorders*, ed 4 (text revision) (DSM-IV-TR). Washington, DC: American Psychiatric Association, 2000.
8. Eapen V, Lees A, Lakke J, et al: Adult-onset tic disorders. Mov Disord 2002;17:735-740.
9. Northam RS, Singer HS: Postencephalitic acquired Tourette-like syndrome in a child. Neurology 1991;41:592-593.
10. Riedel M, Straube A, Schwarz MJ, et al: Lyme disease presenting as Tourette's syndrome. Lancet 1998;351:418-419.
11. Klawans HL, Falk DK, Nausieda PA, Weiner WJ: Gilles de la Tourette syndrome after long-term chlorpromazine therapy. Neurology 1978;28:1064-1066.
12. Luo F, Leckman JF, Katsovich L, et al: Prospective longitudinal study of children with tic disorders and/or obsessive-compulsive disorder: relationship of symptom exacerbations to newly acquired streptococcal infections. Pediatrics 2004;113:e578-e585.
13. Ko S, Ahn T, Kim J, et al: A case of adult onset tic disorder following carbon monoxide intoxication. Can J Neurol Sci 2004;31:268-270.
14. Kwak CH, Jankovic J: Tourettism and dystonia after subcortical stroke. Mov Disord 2002;17:821-825.
15. Majumdar A, Appleton RE: Delayed and severe but transient Tourette syndrome after head injury. Pediatr Neurol 2002;27:314-317.
16. Krauss J, Jankovic J: Tics secondary to craniocerebral trauma. Mov Disord 1997;12:776-782.
17. Singer HS, Dela Cruz PS, Abrams MT, et al: A Tourette-like syndrome following cardiopulmonary bypass and hypothermia: MRI volumetric measurements. Mov Disord 1997;12:588-592.
18. Chemali Z, Bromfield E: Tourette's syndrome following temporal lobectomy for seizure control. Epilepsy Behav 2003;4:564-566.
19. Jankovic J, Ashizawa T: Tourettism associated with Huntington's disease. Mov Disord 1995;10:103-105.
20. Scarano V, Pellecchia M, Filla A, Barone P: Hallervorden-Spatz syndrome resembling a typical Tourette syndrome. Mov Disord 2002;17:618-620.
21. Singer WD: Transient Gilles de la Tourette syndrome after chronic neuroleptic withdrawal. Dev Med Child Neurol 1981;23:518-521.
22. Leckman JF, Zhang H, Vitale A, et al: Course of tic severity in Tourette syndrome: the first two decades. Pediatrics 1998;102(1 Pt 1):14-19.
23. Bloch MH, Peterson BS, Scahill L, et al: Adulthood outcome of tic and obsessive-compulsive symptom severity in children with Tourette syndrome. Arch Pediatr Adolesc Med 2006;160:65-69.
24. Erenberg G, Cruse RP, Rothner AD: The natural history of Tourette syndrome: a follow-up study. Ann Neurol 1987;22:383-385.
25. Pappert EJ, Goetz CG, Louis ED, et al: Objective assessments of longitudinal outcome in Gilles de la Tourette's syndrome. Neurology 2003;61:936-940.
26. Bloch MH, Leckman JF, Zhu H, Peterson BS: Caudate volumes in childhood predict symptom severity in adults with Tourette syndrome. Neurology 2005;65:1253-1258.

27. Bloch MH, Sukhodolsky DG, Leckman JF, Schultz RT: Fine-motor skill deficits in childhood predict adulthood tic severity and global psychosocial functioning in Tourette's syndrome. J Child Psychol Psychiatry 2006;47:551-559.
28. Singer HS: Discussing outcome in Tourette syndrome. Arch Pediatr Adolesc Med 2006;160:103-105.
29. Channon S, Pratt P, Robertson MM: Executive function, memory, and learning in Tourette's syndrome. Neuropsychology 2003;17:247-254.
30. Sukhodolsky DG, Scahill L, Zhang H, et al: Disruptive behavior in children with Tourette's syndrome: association with ADHD comorbidity, tic severity, and functional impairment. J Am Acad Child Adolesc Psychiatry 2003;42:98-105.
31. Kurlan R, McDermott MP, Deeley C, et al: Prevalence of tics in schoolchildren and association with placement in special education. Neurology 2001;57:1383-1388.
32. Gadow K, Nolan E, Sprafkin J, Schwartz J: Tics and psychiatric comorbidity in children and adolescents. Dev Med Child Neurol 2002;44:330-338.
33. Robertson MM: Diagnosing Tourette syndrome: is it a common disorder? J Psychosom Res 2003;55:3-6.
34. Khalifa N, von Knorring AL: Prevalence of tic disorders and Tourette syndrome in a Swedish school population. Dev Med Child Neurol 2003;45:315-319.
35. Baron-Cohen S, Mortimore C, Moriarty J, et al: The prevalence of Gilles de la Tourette's syndrome in children and adolescents with autism. J Child Psychol Psychiatry 1999;40:213-218.
36. Eapen V, Laker M, Anfield A, et al: Prevalence of tics and Tourette syndrome in an inpatient adult psychiatry setting. J Psychiatry Neurosci 2001;26:417-420.
37. Comings DE, Comings BG: A controlled study of Tourette syndrome, I: attention-deficit disorder, learning disorders, and school problems. Am J Hum Genet 1987;41:701-741.
38. Hoekstra PJ, Steenhuis MP, Troost PW, et al: Relative contribution of attention-deficit hyperactivity disorder, obsessive-compulsive disorder, and tic severity to social and behavioral problems in tic disorders. J Dev Behav Pediatr 2004;25:272-279.
39. Spencer TJ, Biederman J, Faraone S, et al: Impact of tic disorders on ADHD outcome across the life cycle: findings from a large group of adults with and without ADHD. Am J Psychiatry 2001;158:611-617.
40. Robertson MM, Trimble MR, Lees AJ: The psychopathology of the Gilles de la Tourette syndrome: a phenomenological analysis. Br J Psychiatry 1988;152:383-390.
41. Scahill L, Kano Y, King RA, et al: Influence of age and tic disorders on obsessive-compulsive disorder in a pediatric sample. J Child Adolesc Psychopharmacol 2003;13(Suppl 1):S7-S17.
42. Rickards H, Robertson M: A controlled study of psychopathology and associated symptoms in Tourette syndrome. World J Biol Psychiatry 2003;4:64-68.
43. Coffey BJ, Park KS: Behavioral and emotional aspects of Tourette syndrome. Neurol Clin 1997;15:277-289.
44. Budman CL, Rockmore L, Stokes J, Sossin M: Clinical phenomenology of episodic rage in children with Tourette syndrome. J Psychosom Res 2003;55:59-65.
45. Mathews CA, Waller J, Glidden D, et al: Self injurious behaviour in Tourette syndrome: correlates with impulsivity and impulse control. J Neurol Neurosurg Psychiatry 2004;75:1149-1155.
46. Singer HS, Schuerholz LJ, Denckla MB: Learning difficulties in children with Tourette syndrome. J Child Neurol 1995;10(Suppl 1):S58-S61.
47. Brand N, Geenen R, Oudenhoven M, et al: Brief report: cognitive functioning in children with Tourette's syndrome with and without comorbid ADHD. J Pediatr Psychol 2002;27:203-208.
48. Schuerholz LJ, Singer HS, Denckla MB: Gender study of neuropsychological and neuromotor function in children with Tourette syndrome with and without attention-deficit hyperactivity disorder. J Child Neurol 1998;13:277-282.
49. Harris EL, Schuerholz LJ, Singer HS, et al: Executive function in children with Tourette syndrome and/or attention deficit hyperactivity disorder. J Int Neuropsychol Soc 1995;1:511-516.
50. Schuerholz LJ, Baumgardner TL, Singer HS, et al: Neuropsychological status of children with Tourette's syndrome with and without attention deficit hyperactivity disorder. Neurology 1996;46:958-965.
51. Kostanecka-Endress T, Banaschewski T, Kinkelbur J, et al: Disturbed sleep in children with Tourette syndrome: a polysomnographic study. J Psychosom Res 2003;55:23-29.
52. Allen RP, Singer HS, Brown JE, Salam MM: Sleep disorders in Tourette syndrome: a primary or unrelated problem? Pediatr Neurol 1992;8:275-280.
53. Price RA, Kidd KK, Cohen DJ, et al: A twin study of Tourette syndrome. Arch Gen Psychiatry 1985;42:815-820.

54. Hyde TM, Aaronson BA, Randolph C, et al: Relationship of birth weight to the phenotypic expression of Gilles de la Tourette's syndrome in monozygotic twins. Neurology 1992;42(3 Pt 1):652-658.
55. McMahon W, Carter AS, Fredine N, Pauls DL: Children at familial risk for Tourette's disorder: child and parent diagnoses. Am J Med Genet 2003;121B:105-111.
56. Cerullo J, Reimschisel T, Singer H: Genetic and neurobiological basis for Tourette syndrome. In Woods DW, Piacentini JC, Walkup JT (eds): Treating Tourette Syndrome and Tic Disorders: A Guide for Practitioners. New York: Guilford Press, 2007.
57. Pauls DL. Genome scan for Tourette's disorder in affected sib-pair and multigenerational families. The Tourette Syndrome Association International Consortium for Genetics, 2006.
58. Abelson JF, Kwan KY, O'Roak BJ, et al: Sequence variants in SLITRK1 are associated with Tourette's syndrome. Science 2005;310:317-320.
59. Deng H, Le WD, Xie WJ, Jankovic J: Examination of the SLITRK1 gene in Caucasian patients with Tourette Syndrome. Acta Neurol Scand 2006;114:400-402.
60. Eapen V, O'Neill J, Gurling HM, Robertson MM: Sex of parent transmission effect in Tourette's syndrome: evidence for earlier age at onset in maternally transmitted cases suggests a genomic imprinting effect. Neurology 1997;48:934-937.
61. Lichter DG, Dmochowski J, Jackson LA, Trinidad KS: Influence of family history on clinical expression of Tourette's syndrome. Neurology 1999;52:308-316.
62. Hanna PA, Janjua FN, Contant CF, Jankovic J: Bilineal transmission in Tourette syndrome. Neurology 1999;53:813-818.
63. Thompson WW, Price C, Goodson B, et al: Early thimerosal exposure and neuropsychological outcomes at 7 to 10 years. N Engl J Med 2007;357:1281-1292.
64. Burd L, Severud R, Klug MG, Kerbeshian J: Prenatal and perinatal risk factors for Tourette disorder. J Perinat Med 1999;27:295-302.
65. Swedo SE, Leonard HL, Garvey M, et al: Pediatric autoimmune neuropsychiatric disorders associated with streptococcal infections: clinical description of the first 50 cases. Am J Psychiatry 1998;155:264-271.
66. Snider LA, Swedo SE: Post-streptococcal autoimmune disorders of the central nervous system. Curr Opin Neurol 2003;16:359-365.
67. Kurlan R: Tourette's syndrome and 'PANDAS': will the relation bear out? Pediatric autoimmune neuropsychiatric disorders associated with streptococcal infection. Neurology 1998;50:1530-1534.
68. Kurlan R, Kaplan EL: The pediatric autoimmune neuropsychiatric disorders associated with streptococcal infection (PANDAS) etiology for tics and obsessive-compulsive symptoms: hypothesis or entity? Practical considerations for the clinician. Pediatrics 2004;113:883-886.
69. Kurlan R: The PANDAS hypothesis: losing its bite? Mov Disord 2004;19:371-374.
70. Singer HS, Loiselle CPANDAS: a commentary. J Psychosom Res 2003;55:31-39.
71. Singer H, Gause C, Morris C, Lopez P: Serial immune markers do not correlate with clinical exacerbations in PANDAS. Pediatrics 2008;121:1198-1205.
72. The Tourette's Syndrome Study Group, Johnson D, Kaplan EL: Streptococcal infection and exacerbation of childhood tics and obsessive-compulsive symptoms: a prospective blinded cohort study. Pediatrics 2008;121:1188-1197.
73. Singer HS, Harris K: Circuits to synapses: the pathophysiology of tourette syndrome. In Gilman S (ed): Neurobiology of Disease. Burlington, MA: Academic Press, 2006.
74. Berardelli A, Curra A, Fabbrini G, et al: Pathophysiology of tics and Tourette syndrome. J Neurol 2003;250:781-787.
75. Hoekstra PJ, Anderson GM, Limburg PC, et al: Neurobiology and neuroimmunology of Tourette's syndrome: an update. Cell Mol Life Sci 2004;61(7-8):886-898.
76. Singer HS, Szymanski S, Giuliano J, et al: Elevated intrasynaptic dopamine release in Tourette's syndrome measured by PET. Am J Psychiatry 2002;159:1329-1336.
77. Wong DF, Singer HS, Brandt J, et al: D2-like dopamine receptor density in Tourette syndrome measured by PET. J Nucl Med 1997;38:1243-1247.
78. Serra-Mestres J, Ring HA, Costa DC, et al: Dopamine transporter binding in Gilles de la Tourette syndrome: a [123I]FP-CIT/SPECT study. Acta Psychiatr Scand 2004;109:140-146.
79. Wolf SS, Jones DW, Knable MB, et al: Tourette syndrome: prediction of phenotypic variation in monozygotic twins by caudate nucleus D2 receptor binding. Science 1996;273:1225-1227.
80. Albin RL, Koeppe RA, Bohnen NI, et al: Increased ventral striatal monoaminergic innervation in Tourette syndrome. Neurology 2003;61:310-315.

81. Singer HS, Butler IJ, Tune LE, et al: Dopaminergic dysfunction in Tourette syndrome. Ann Neurol 1982;12:361-366.
82. Singer HS, Hahn IH, Moran TH: Abnormal dopamine uptake sites in postmortem striatum from patients with Tourette's syndrome. Ann Neurol 1991;30:558-562.
83. Minzer K, Lee O, Hong JJ, Singer HS: Increased prefrontal D2 protein in Tourette syndrome: a postmortem analysis of frontal cortex and striatum. J Neurol Sci 2004;219(1-2):55-61.
84. Anderson GM, Pollak ES, Chatterjee D, et al: Postmortem analysis of subcortical monoamines and amino acids in Tourette syndrome. Adv Neurol 1992;58:123-133.
85. Yoon DY, Gause CD, Leckman JF, Singer HS: Frontal dopaminergic abnormality in Tourette syndrome: a postmortem analysis. J Neurol Sci 2007;255(1-2):50-56.
86. Wong DF, Brasic JR, Singer HS, et al: Mechanisms of dopaminergic and serotonergic neurotransmission in Tourette syndrome: clues from an in vivo neurochemistry study with PET. Neuropsychopharmacology 2008;33:1239-1251.
87. Behen M, Chugani HT, Juhasz C, et al: Abnormal brain tryptophan metabolism and clinical correlates in Tourette syndrome. Mov Disord 2007;22:2256-2262.
88. Bergin A, Waranch HR, Brown J, et al: Relaxation therapy in Tourette syndrome: a pilot study. Pediatr Neurol 1998;18:136-142.
89. Wilhelm S, Deckersbach T, Coffey BJ, et al: Habit reversal versus supportive psychotherapy for Tourette's disorder: a randomized controlled trial. Am J Psychiatry 2003;160:1175-1177.
90. Woods DW, Twohig MP, Flessner CA, Roloff TJ: Treatment of vocal tics in children with Tourette syndrome: investigating the efficacy of habit reversal. J Appl Behav Anal 2003;36:109-112.
91. Scahill L, Erenberg G, Berlin CM Jr., et al: Contemporary assessment and pharmacotherapy of Tourette syndrome. NeuroRx 2006;3:192-206.
92. Gaffney GR, Perry PJ, Lund BC, et al: Risperidone versus clonidine in the treatment of children and adolescents with Tourette's syndrome. J Am Acad Child Adolesc Psychiatry 2002;41:330-336.
93. Scahill L, Chappell PB, Kim YS, et al: A placebo-controlled study of guanfacine in the treatment of children with tic disorders and attention deficit hyperactivity disorder. Am J Psychiatry 2001;158:1067-1074.
94. Singer HS, Wendlandt J, Krieger M, Giuliano J: Baclofen treatment in Tourette syndrome: a double-blind, placebo-controlled, crossover trial. Neurology 2001;56:599-604.
95. Gonce M, Barbeau A: Seven cases of Gilles de la Tourette's syndrome: partial relief with clonazepam: a pilot study. Can J Neurol Sci 1977;4:279-283.
96. Abuzzahab FS, Brown VL: Control of Tourette's syndrome with topiramate. Am J Psychiatry 2001;158:968.
97. Awaad Y, Michon AM, Minarik S: Use of levetiracetam to treat tics in children and adolescents with Tourette syndrome. Mov Disord 2005;20:714-718.
98. Smith-Hicks CL, Bridges DD, Paynter NP, Singer HS: A double blind randomized placebo control trial of levetiracetam in tourette syndrome. Mov Disord 2007;22:1764-1770.
99. Scahill L, Leckman JF, Schultz RT, et al: A placebo-controlled trial of risperidone in Tourette syndrome. Neurology 2003;60:1130-1135.
100. Dion Y, Annable L, Sandor P, Chouinard G: Risperidone in the treatment of tourette syndrome: a double-blind, placebo-controlled trial. J Clin Psychopharmacol 2002;22:31-39.
101. Stephens RJ, Bassel C, Sandor P: Olanzapine in the treatment of aggression and tics in children with Tourette's syndrome—a pilot study. J Child Adolesc Psychopharmacol 2004;14:255-266.
102. Budman CL, Gayer A, Lesser M, et al: An open-label study of the treatment efficacy of olanzapine for Tourette's disorder. J Clin Psychiatry 2001;62:290-294.
103. Sallee FR, Kurlan R, Goetz CG, et al: Ziprasidone treatment of children and adolescents with Tourette's syndrome: a pilot study. J Am Acad Child Adolesc Psychiatry 2000;39:292-299.
104. Sallee FR, Gilbert DL, Vinks AA, et al: Pharmacodynamics of ziprasidone in children and adolescents: impact on dopamine transmission. J Am Acad Child Adolesc Psychiatry 2003;42:902-907.
105. Mukaddes NM, Abali O: Quetiapine treatment of children and adolescents with Tourette's disorder. J Child Adolesc Psychopharmacol 2003;13:295-299.
106. Schaller JL, Behar D: Quetiapine treatment of adolescent and child tic disorders: two case reports. Eur Child Adolesc Psychiatry 2002;11:196-197.
107. Davies L, Stern JS, Agrawal N, Robertson MM: A case series of patients with Tourette's syndrome in the United Kingdom treated with aripiprazole. Hum Psychopharmacol 2006;21:447-453.
108. Jankovic J, Orman J: Tetrabenazine therapy of dystonia, chorea, tics, and other dyskinesias. Neurology 1988;38:391-394.

109. Gilbert DL, Dure L, Sethuraman G, et al: Tic reduction with pergolide in a randomized controlled trial in children. Neurology 2003;60:606-611.
110. Anca MH, Giladi N, Korczyn AD: Ropinirole in Gilles de la Tourette syndrome. Neurology 2004;62:1626-1627.
111. Muller-Vahl KR, Schneider U, Prevedel H, et al: Delta 9-tetrahydrocannabinol (THC) is effective in the treatment of tics in Tourette syndrome: a 6-week randomized trial. J Clin Psychiatry 2003;64:459-465.
112. Muller-Vahl KR, Schneider U, Koblenz A, et al: Treatment of Tourette's syndrome with Delta 9-tetrahydrocannabinol (THC): a randomized crossover trial. Pharmacopsychiatry 2002;35:57-61.
113. Awaad Y: Tics in Tourette syndrome: new treatment options. J Child Neurol 1999;14:316-319.
114. Trimble MR, Whurr R, Brookes G, Robertson MM: Vocal tics in Gilles de la Tourette syndrome treated with botulinum toxin injections. Mov Disord 1998;13:617-619.
115. Mantovani A, Leckman JF, Grantz H, et al: Repetitive transcranial magnetic stimulation of the supplementary motor area in the treatment of Tourette syndrome: report of two cases. Clin Neurophysiol 2007;118:2314-2315.
116. Munchau A, Bloem BR, Thilo KV, et al: Repetitive transcranial magnetic stimulation for Tourette syndrome. Neurology 2002;59:1789-1791.
117. Orth M, Kirby R, Richardson MP, et al: Subthreshold rTMS over pre-motor cortex has no effect on tics in patients with Gilles de la Tourette syndrome. Clin Neurophysiol 2005;116:764-768.
118. Vandewalle V, van der Linden C, Groenewegen HJ, Caemaert J: Stereotactic treatment of Gilles de la Tourette syndrome by high frequency stimulation of thalamus. Lancet 1999;353:724.
119. Hassler R, Dieckmann G: Stereotaxic treatment of tics and inarticulate cries or coprolalia considered as motor obsessional phenomena in Gilles de la Tourette's disease. Rev Neurol (Paris) 1970;123:89-100.
120. Temel Y, Visser-Vandewalle V: Surgery in Tourette syndrome. Mov Disord 2004;19:3-14.

INDEX

Pages followed by *f*, indicate figures; *t*, tables.